deWit's

Fundamental Concepts and Skills for Nursing

deWit's Fundamental Concepts and Skills for Nursing

5 EDITION

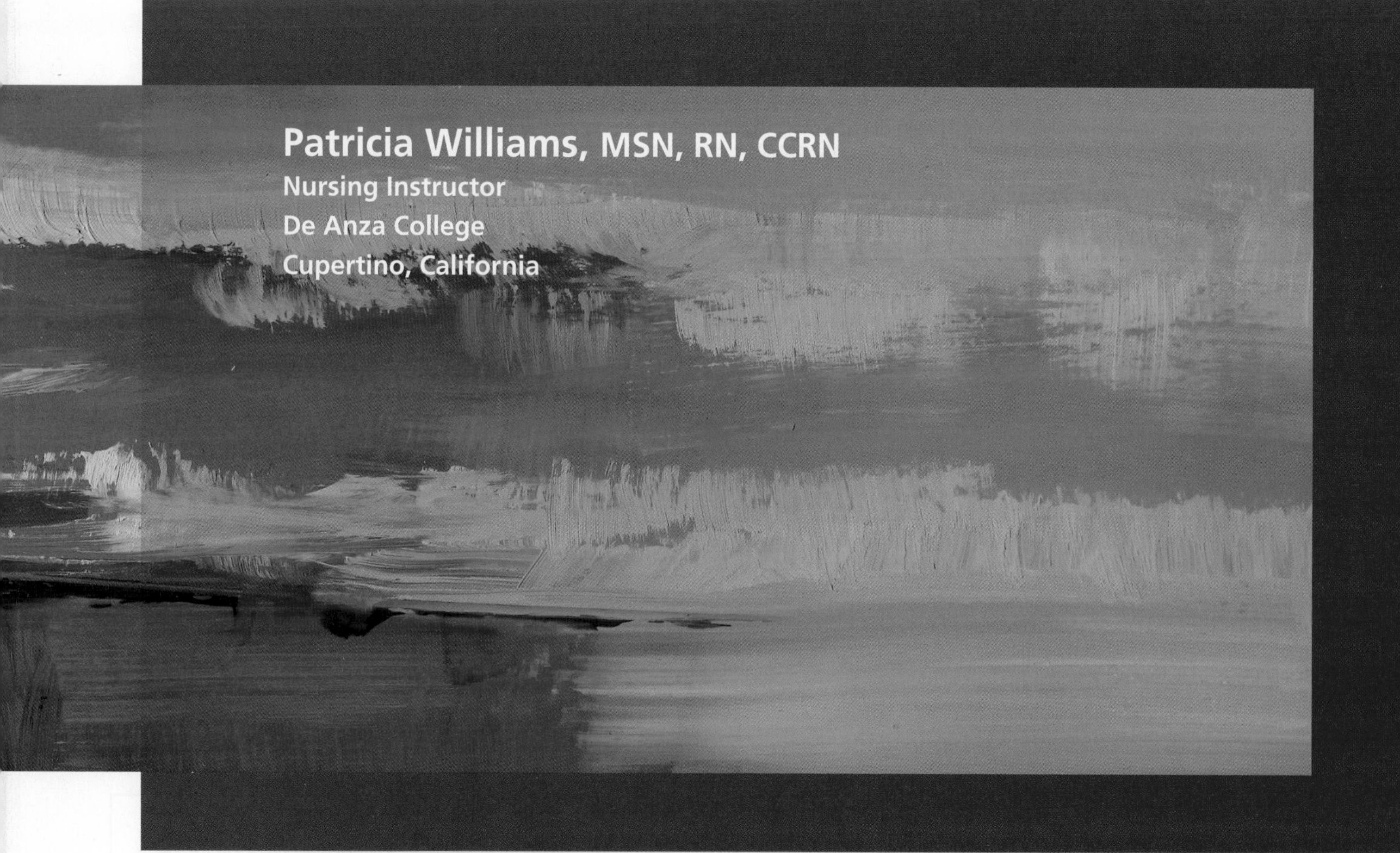

Patricia Williams, MSN, RN, CCRN
Nursing Instructor
De Anza College
Cupertino, California

ELSEVIER

ELSEVIER

3251 Riverport Lane
St. Louis, Missouri 63043

DEWIT'S FUNDAMENTAL CONCEPTS AND SKILLS FOR NURSING,
FIFTH EDITION
ISBN: 978-0-323-39621-9

International Standard Book Number: 978-0-323-39621-9

Content Strategist: Nancy O'Brien
Content Development Manager: Ellen Wurm-Cutter
Senior Content Development Specialist: Rebecca Leenhouts
Publishing Services Manager: Jeff Patterson
Book Production Specialist: Bill Drone
Design Direction: Renee Duenow

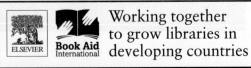

Printed in China

Last digit is the print number: 9 8 7 6 5 4 3 2 1

I dedicate this edition to my sister, Mary,
devoted wife and mom, proud new grandma, nurse,
and my best friend.
I love you.

Patricia Williams

Contributors and Reviewers

CONTRIBUTORS

Karen V. Anderson, MSN, RN
Associate Dean of Nursing
Nursing Department
Kaplan College, San Diego
San Diego, California

8 *Communication and the Nurse-Patient Relationship*
17 *Infection Prevention and Control in the Hospital and Home*
34 *Administering Oral, Topical, and Inhalant Medications*
36 *Administering Intravenous Solutions and Medications*
39 *Promoting Musculoskeletal Function*

Shelley Eckvahl, BSN, MSN
Professor
Nursing
Chaffey Community College
Rancho Cucamonga, California

3 *Legal and Ethical Aspects of Nursing*
5 *Assessment, Nursing Diagnosis, and Planning*
9 *Patient Education and Health Promotion*
16 *Infection Prevention and Control: Protective Mechanisms and Asepsis*

Louise S. Frantz, MHA, Ed, BSN, RN
Practical Nursing Program Coordinator
Continuing Education
Penn State Berks
Reading, Pennsylvania

26 *Concepts of Basic Nutrition and Cultural Considerations*
27 *Nutritional Therapy and Assisted Feeding*

Garry Johnson, DHSc, RN, CCRN, CMSRN
Nursing Professor
Evergreen Valley College
San Jose, California
Adjunct Nursing Professor
Samuel Merritt University
San Mateo, California
Mission College
Santa Clara, California

18 *Safely Lifting, Moving, and Positioning Patients*

Predrag Miskin, DrHS, MScN, RN, PHN, DMSRN
Nursing Faculty
Biological and Health Sciences
De Anza College
Cupertino, California
Adjunct Assistant Professor
School of Nursing
Samuel Merritt University
Oakland, California

14 *Cultural and Spiritual Aspects of Patient Care*
15 *Loss, Grief, and End-of-Life Care*

Susan M. Schmitz, RN, BSN, PHN
Associate Faculty
Health Occupations Department
Mission College
Santa Clara, California
Part-Time Faculty
Health Technology Department
De Anza College
Cupertino, California
American Heart Association ACLS, BLS, and First Aid Instructor
Nurse Education Workshops Inc
San Jose, California

19 *Assisting With Hygiene, Personal Care, Skin Care, and the Prevention of Pressure Injuries*
20 *Patient Environment and Safety*
22 *Assessing Health Status*
23 *Admitting, Transferring, and Discharging Patients*
28 *Assisting with Respiration and Oxygen Delivery*
29 *Promoting Urinary Elimination*
30 *Promoting Bowel Elimination*
31 *Pain, Comfort, and Sleep*
32 *Complementary and Alternative Therapies*
37 *Care of the Surgical Patient*

Gerald "Jerry" Thompson, MSN, RN, CNE
Assistant Professor
Undergraduate Nursing
Samuel Merritt University
Oakland, California

7 *Documentation of Nursing Care*
21 *Measuring Vital Signs*

REVIEWERS

Sherri L. Andrews, RN, MSN
Faculty
Bedford County Public Schools
Bedford County School of Practical Nurses
Bedford Science and Technology Center
Bedford, Virginia

Sharyn Boyle, MSN, RN-BC
LPN Instructor
Passaic County Technical Institute
LPN Program
Wayne, New Jersey

Fleurdeliz Cuyco, BS
Compliance Director/Instructor
Preferred College of Nursing
Los Angeles, California

Natalie O. DeLeonardis, MSN, RN
Coordinator, North Campus Outreach Practical Nursing Program
Pennsylvania College of Technology
Williamsport, Pennsylvania

Louise S. Frantz, MHA, Ed, BSN, RN
Coordinator Practical Nursing Program
Penn State University—Berks Campus
Continuing Education
Reading, Pennsylvania

Chasity Girvin, BSN, MSN, RN
Nursing Faculty/Sim Lab Coordinator
Fayette County Career & Technical Institute
LPN Program
Uniontown, Pennsylvania

Joanne Heck, RN, MSN
LPN Instructor
Parkland College
Health Professions
Champaign, Illinois

Kathleen Garrubba Hopkins, PhD, MSIE, RN
NINR/NIH Fellow
University of Pittsburgh
School of Nursing
Pittsburgh, Pennsylvania

Dawn Johnson, MSN, RN, Ed
Director of Practical Nursing Program
Great Lakes Institute of Technology
Nursing
Erie, Pennsylvania

Russlyn A. St. John, RN, MSN
Professor Emeritus
St. Charles Community College
Nursing & Allied Health
Cottleville, Missouri

Kelly Stone, RN, BSN
Coordinator
Practical Nursing Program
University of Arkansas Community College Batesville
Batesville, Arkansas

Judith M. Thompson, RN, MN, CMSRN
Nursing Faculty
Richmond Community College
Hamlet, North Carolina

LPN Advisory Board

Tawne D. Blackful, RN, MSN, MEd
Supervisor of Health Services and School Nurse
Lawrence Hall Youth Services
Chicago, Illinois

Barbara Carrig, BSN, MSN, APN
LPN Nurse Program Coordinator
Academic/Clinical Instructor, Passaic County Technical Institute
Wayne, New Jersey

Dolores Cotton, MSN, RN
Practical Nursing Coordinator
Meridian Technology Center
Stillwater, Oklahoma

Laurie F. Fontenot, BSN, RN
Department Head, Health Services Division
Acadiana Technical College—C.B. Coreil Campus
Ville Platte, Louisiana

Shelly R. Hovis, RN, MS
Director, Practical Nursing
Kiamichi Technology Centers
Antlers, Oklahoma

Patty Knecht, MSN, RN
Director of Practical Nursing
Center for Arts and Technology—Brandywine Campus
Coatesville, Pennsylvania

Hana Malik, MSN, FNP-BC
Family Nurse Practitioner
Take Care Health Systems
Villa Park, Illinois

Barb McFall-Ratliff, MSN, RN
Director of Nursing, Program of Practical Nurse Education
Butler Technology and Career Development Schools
Hamilton, Ohio

Toni L.E. Pritchard, BSN, MSN, EdD
Allied Health Professor, Practical Nursing Program
Central Louisiana Technical College—Lamar Salter Campus
Leesville, Louisiana

Pamela Reyes, RN, BSN, MSN
Assistant Director
Nursing, Porter and Chester Institute
Rocky Hill, Connecticut

Barbra Robins, BSN, MSN
Program Director
Leads School of Technology
New Castle, Delaware

Faye Silverman, RN, MSN/Ed, PHN, WOCN
Director of Nursing
Kaplan College
North Hollywood, California

Russlyn A. St. John, RN, MSN
Professor and Coordinator, Practical Nursing
Practical Nursing Department, St. Charles Community College
Cottleville, Missouri

Fleur de Liza S. Tobias-Cuyco, BSc, CPhT
Dean, Director of Student Affairs, and Instructor
Preferred College of Nursing
Los Angeles, California

To the Instructor

DeWit's Fundamental Concepts and Skills for Nursing, fifth edition, written especially for licensed practical nurse/licensed vocational nurse (LPN/LVN) students, incorporates aspects of nursing in all of the major settings in which LPN/LVNs are employed: hospitals, long-term care facilities, clinics, medical offices, home care agencies, and surgery centers. This edition further emphasizes the importance of evidence-based practice and the use of best practices.

This text teaches all the basic concepts and fundamental skills that an LPN/LVN needs in current practice. The material is presented from simple to complex, with clarity and conciseness of language, making the fundamental concepts and skills content readily comprehended by beginning nursing students. Because there are so many students with English as their second language entering nursing, this book has been reviewed and edited by an English-as-a-second-language specialist to make the language as clear as possible.

As the role of the LPN/LVN expands, there is an even greater need for a thorough knowledge of the nursing process and problem solving. The **nursing process** is the underlying theme of the text and is interwoven with these six threads: (1) focus on the patient as a consumer of health care with psychosocial as well as physical needs; (2) critical thinking as a tool for learning, problem solving, and developing clinical judgment; (3) communication as an essential tool for the art and practice of nursing; (4) collaboration with other health care workers and the use of management and supervision to provide coordinated, cost-effective patient care; (5) patient education for the maintenance of wellness and promotion of self-care; and (6) integration of cultural sensitivity and cultural competence into patient care.

Because of the difference in state laws, LPN/LVNs in some states may be certified to perform a variety of tasks related to intravenous (IV) fluid therapy, but in other states IV therapy is not within the scope of practice. We do include IV therapy because so many schools teach a separate short course on it for IV certification for their students. Consult your state nurse practice act for more information.

ORGANIZATION OF THE TEXT

CONTENT

The text is divided into the following nine units: *I,* Introduction to Nursing and the Health Care System; *II,* The Nursing Process; *III,* Communication in Nursing; *IV,* Developmental, Psychosocial, and Cultural Considerations; *V,* Basic Nursing Skills; *VI,* Meeting Basic Physiologic Needs; *VII,* Medication Administration; *VIII,* Care of the Surgical and Immobile Patient; *IX,* Caring for the Elderly.

In this fifth edition, we are pleased to include the following new content:

- Updated 2016 NPUAP Pressure Injury Stages
- Greater emphasis on QSEN (Quality and Safety Education for Nurses) with numerous boxed features throughout the text
- List of Giddens' Concepts presented at the beginning of each chapter
- The most current CPR guidelines from the American Heart Association
- The 2015 United States Department of Agriculture dietary guidelines
- Updated Joint Commission Pain Standards
- Greater emphasis on electronic MAR (eMAR), computerized order entry (CPOE), and computer documentation of medication administration
- Updated American Heart Association diet and lifestyle recommendations

The text emphasizes the following key content areas and major concepts:

- Evidence-based nursing and best practices
- Updated isolation information from the Centers for Disease Control and Prevention (CDC)
- Current immunization guidelines
- Ethnopharmacy
- Health care delivery, collaborative care, and changing and expanding role of the LPN/LVN
- Concepts of the nursing process and their application to clinical situations
- Nurse–patient and family communication
- Professional communication
- Management, supervision, and delegation
- Health promotion and patient education
- *Healthy People 2020* Objectives and National Patient Safety Goals
- Growth and development from infancy through adulthood, with special attention to the older adult
- Cultural sensitivity in nursing care
- Full chapter on loss, grief, end-of-life care, and palliative care
- Basic nursing skills, including current information about infection control in the health care setting and home, dangers of drug-resistant infections,

prevention of pressure injuries, patient safety, and assessment of health status
- Concepts and skills needed to meet basic physiologic needs
- Complete unit on medication knowledge and administration, with a section on blood product administration
- A chapter on the administration of intravenous fluids and medications
- Care of surgical patients; care of immobile patients, including those needing care of wounds and pressure injuries; promotion of musculoskeletal function
- Physiologic and psychosocial care of the older adult

SPECIAL FEATURES

The following pedagogic features help students to understand and apply the chapter content:
- **Overview of Structure and Function:** In chapters in which an understanding of anatomy and physiology is necessary to comprehend the chapter content, a brief **review of the body system** directly precedes the main text of the chapter.
- **Application of the Nursing Process:** After the basic concepts of nursing and the nursing process are introduced in Unit Two, the **nursing process** is integrated in succeeding chapters.
- Special features within the text, including **Clinical Cues, Complementary & Alternative Therapies, Cultural Considerations, Life-Span Considerations, Focused Assessment, Health Promotion, Home Care Considerations, Legal and Ethical Considerations, Patient Education, QSEN Considerations, Safety Alert, and Think Critically** boxes, enhance student learning and retention. More information on each of these boxes is provided on pp. xii-xiii.
- **Concept Maps** are visualizations of processes that help students to make sense of information that is typically more difficult to learn, and they are plentiful throughout the text.
- **NCLEX-PN Examination–Style Review Questions** at the end of each chapter include multiple-choice and alternate-format questions to help students to familiarize themselves with the format and prepare for the examination.
- **Nursing Care Plans:** These illustrate each step of the nursing process. Each nursing diagnosis is supported by the accompanying assessment data, and Critical Thinking Questions are provided at the end of each care plan. The nursing care plan has been chosen as the focus for care planning because it is such an integral part of teaching **the nursing process.** *Answers to Critical Thinking Questions in the Nursing Care Plans are provided on the Evolve website.*
- **Skills:** Seventy-five of the major skills that require mastery in most LPN/LVN programs are presented with full-color photographs in a step-by-step format that emphasizes use of the nursing process and includes rationales for each step, as well as Critical Thinking Questions at the end of each skill. Performance Checklists for all skills are located in the Student Learning Guide. *Answers to Critical Thinking Questions in these Skills are provided in the Instructor Resources on the Evolve website.*
- **Steps:** Steps are shorter versions of skills. These 37 other procedures that nurses are expected to perform are presented step by step with rationales. *Performance Checklists for all steps are found on the Evolve website.*
- **Appendixes:** *Appendix A* contains the Standard Steps protocol for the performance of each Skill and Step. *Appendix B* presents the NFLPN Nursing Practice Standards for the Licensed Practical/Vocational Nurse. *Appendix C* provides the ANA Code of Ethics. *Appendix D* contains the CDC Standard Precautions for the care of all patients. *Appendix E* contains a table of the basic common laboratory test values. *Appendix F* contains a listing of the NANDA definitions used in this text.
- **Bolded text** throughout the narrative emphasizes key concepts and practice.

LPN THREADS

The fifth edition of *deWit's Fundamental Concepts and Skills for Nursing* shares some feature and design elements with other Elsevier LPN/LVN textbooks. The purpose of these *LPN Threads* is to make it easier for students and instructors to use the variety of books required by the relatively brief and demanding LPN/LVN curriculum. The following features are included in the *LPN Threads*:
- A **reading level evaluation** is performed on every manuscript chapter during the book's development to increase the consistency among chapters and ensure the text is easy to understand.
- The **full-color design, cover, photos,** and **illustrations** are visually appealing and pedagogically useful.
- **Objectives** (numbered) begin each chapter and provide a framework for content and are especially important in providing the structure for the TEACH Lesson Plans for the textbook.
- **Key Terms** with phonetic pronunciations and page number references are listed at the beginning of each chapter. Key terms appear in color in the chapter and are defined briefly, with full definitions in the **Glossary.** The goal is to help the student reader with limited proficiency in English to develop a greater command of the pronunciation of scientific and nonscientific English terminology.
- A wide variety of **special features** relate to critical thinking, clinical practice, health promotion, safety, patient education, complementary and alternative therapies, communication, home health care, delegation and assignment, and more. Refer to the To the Student section of this introduction on pp. xii-xiii for descriptions.

- **Critical Thinking Questions** presented at the ends of chapters and with Nursing Care Plans give students opportunities to practice critical thinking and clinical decision-making skills with realistic patient scenarios. *Answers are provided on the Evolve website.*
- **Key Points** at the end of each chapter correlate to the objectives and serve as a useful chapter review.
- A full suite of **Instructor Resources** is available, including TEACH Lesson Plans and PowerPoint Slides, Test Bank, Image Collection, Open-Book Quizzes, and Answer Keys.
- In addition to consistent content, design, and support resources, these textbooks benefit from the advice and input of the **Elsevier LPN/LVN Advisory Board** (see p. viii).

TEACHING AND LEARNING PACKAGE

We provide a rich, abundant collection of supplemental resources for both instructors and students.

FOR THE INSTRUCTOR

- **ExamView Test Bank** contains more than 1300 NCLEX-PN Examination–Style Questions, including both multiple-choice and alternate-format questions.
- **TEACH Lesson Plans**, based on textbook chapter learning objectives, provide a roadmap to link and integrate all parts of the educational package. These concise and straightforward lesson plans can be modified or combined to meet scheduling and teaching needs.
- **PowerPoint Presentation** provides more than 1500 slides including text and images.
- **Open-Book Quizzes** for each chapter in the textbook vary instructor testing options.
- **Image Collection** includes illustrations and photographs from the book.
- **Answer Keys** to the Open Book Quizzes and to the Study Guide activities and exercises are included.

FOR THE STUDENT

- **Study Guide** contains various types of questions and activities, including *Terminology; Short Answer; Completion; Multiple Choice NCLEX-PN Examination Review Questions; Application of the Nursing Process; Priority Setting; Identification; Review of Structure and Function; Critical Thinking Activities; Clinical Activities;* and *Steps Toward Better Communication Activities.* The activities are designed to (1) reinforce material in the text chapter; (2) provide practice in priority setting; (3) guide practice in application of the nursing process; and (4) stimulate synthesis, analysis, and application necessary for the development of critical thinking skills and clinical judgment.
- **Performance Checklists** for Skills are included for each chapter, beginning with Chapter 15.
- **Application of the Nursing Process** helps students to make the connection between the conceptual nursing process, often very difficult to comprehend, and real-life patient care.
- The special section, **Steps Toward Better Communication,** is written by an English-as-a-second-language specialist to assist students with limited proficiency in English to gain a greater command of English pronunciation and medical language, while reinforcing chapter content. This section is subdivided into Vocabulary Building Glossary, Completion Exercise, Vocabulary Exercise, Word Attack Skills, Communication Exercise, and Cultural Points. There are examples and practice in appropriate dialogue needed for patient interaction and delegation of tasks.
- **Evolve Learning System Student Resources** include the Anatomy and Physiology Body Spectrum Coloring Book, a mathematics review, suggestions for further reading, and other bonus content. NCLEX-PN Examination–Style Interactive Review Questions test your students' knowledge and help in preparation for licensure.
- **Virtual Clinical Excursion (VCE)** is an interactive workbook CD-ROM that guides the student through a multifloor virtual hospital in a hands-on clinical experience. With limited clinical space for LPN/LVN students, the VCE is an excellent opportunity for "hands-on" practice.

Teaching nursing is one of the most exciting and gratifying experiences. I hope this textbook and its ancillaries make your job as an instructor easier and class preparation more time-efficient. May your students find excitement and joy in learning and applying the information you impart in the clinical setting.

Patricia Williams, MSN, RN, CCRN

To the Student

READING AND REVIEW TOOLS

- **Objectives** introduce the chapter topics.
- **Key Terms** are listed with page number references, and difficult medical, nursing, or scientific terms are accompanied by simple phonetic pronunciations. Key terms are considered essential to understanding chapter content and are defined within the chapter. Key terms are in color the first time they appear in the narrative and are briefly defined in the text, with complete definitions in the Glossary.
- Each chapter ends with a ***Get Ready for the NCLEX Examination!*** section that includes (1) **Key Points** that reiterate the chapter objectives and serve as a useful review of concepts; (2) a list of **Additional Resources**, including the Study Guide, Evolve Resources, and Online Resources; (3) an extensive set of **Review Questions for the NCLEX Examination;** and (4) **Critical Thinking Questions.**
- **Reader References** located in the back of the text cite evidence-based information and provide resources for enhancing knowledge.

CHAPTER FEATURES

Skills are presented in a logical format with defined *purpose,* relevant *illustrations,* and clearly defined and numbered nursing *steps.* Each Skill includes icons that serve as a reminder to perform the basic steps applicable to *all* nursing interventions:

- Check orders.
- Gather necessary equipment and supplies.
- Introduce yourself.
- Check patient's identification.
- Provide privacy.
- Explain the procedure or intervention.
- Perform hand hygiene.
- Don gloves (if applicable).

Steps are short, nonillustrated skills with Actions and Rationales.

Assignment Considerations address situations in which the registered nurse (RN) delegates tasks to the LPN/LVN or when the LPN/LVN assigns tasks to nurse assistants per the individual state nurse practice act.

Think Critically boxes encourage students to synthesize information and apply concepts beyond the scope of the chapter.

Home Care Considerations boxes focus on post-discharge adaptations of medical-surgical nursing care to the home environment.

Life-Span Considerations boxes highlight points of care for the older adult population and appear throughout the chapters to emphasize the changes that occur with age and the adjustments needed for delivery of nursing care to older adults.

Focused Assessment boxes are located in each body system overview chapter and include history taking and psychosocial assessment, physical assessment, and guidance on how to collect data/information for specific disorders.

Clinical Cues provide guidance and advice related to the application of nursing care.

Nursing Care Plans, developed around specific case studies, include nursing diagnoses with an emphasis on patient goals and outcomes and questions to promote critical thinking.

Safety Alerts emphasize the importance of maintaining safety in patient care to protect patients, family, health care providers, and the public from accidents, spread of disease, and medication-related issues.

Health Promotion boxes emphasize healthy lifestyle choices, preventive behaviors, and screening tests.

Cultural Considerations boxes explore select specific cultural preferences and how to address the needs of culturally diverse patients and families.

Patient Education boxes include step-by-step instructions and self-care guidelines.

Legal and Ethical Considerations boxes present pertinent information about the legal issues and ethical dilemmas that may face the practicing nurse.

Complementary and Alternative Therapies boxes contain information on how nontraditional treatments for medical-surgical conditions may be used to complement traditional treatment.

Materials available on **Evolve** are referenced with icons in the margins where related text appears.

Video clips portraying patient assessment available on Evolve are referenced with icons in the margins where applicable.

Evidence-Based Practice icons highlight current references to research in nursing and medical practice.

Acknowledgments

DeWit's Fundamental Concepts and Skills for Nursing is the result of the creative efforts of many people. First of all, I owe a deep debt of gratitude to Susan de Wit for being a wonderful mentor and passing along such a fine textbook and entrusting me with its future. You set the bar very high and have taught me so very much over the past several years.

I am especially grateful to the contributors, consultants, and reviewers for their expertise, suggestions, and finished work. Their perspectives from the various geographic areas of the United States and Canada have lent a broader viewpoint of current nursing practice.

The dedicated staff at Elsevier has provided tireless support and expertise from the initial concept of the book to the cohesive finished product. I am very grateful to Nancy O'Brien, Senior Content Strategist, who helped guide this project from start to finish and was never too busy to answer any question no matter how small. Bill Drone, Production Manager, made certain that problems were solved and skillfully attended to all aspects of production and printing of the text. Becky Leenhouts, Senior Content Development Specialist, was simply amazing with her creativity, diligence, and attention to detail. Brittany Clements, Marketing Manager, applied her creative ideas to promote the book and announce its presence to students and instructors. The design of the book, following the Threads design of other Elsevier LPN/LVN texts, was provided by Renee Duenow. Thanks for all the efforts of these diligent, creative, professional people.

The artistry, many hours, and creative eye of Jack Sanders, our photographer, lent the visual appeal and clinical detail needed to illustrate the concepts and skills of much of this edition, as well as the previous editions. Ginger Navarro, RN, did a wonderful job coordinating the photography shoots, facilities, and models at PeaceHealth for the past three editions of the book.

Many thanks also to PeaceHealth Southwest Washington Medical Center, the De Anza College Nursing Skills and Simulation Lab, and Bay Area Surgical Specialists Surgery Center for the opportunity to photograph within the facilities. Thanks to the many employees and nursing students who contributed their time and talents to the fifth edition as models. Much appreciation to all my nursing colleagues who comprise my e-mail network across the country and who contributed expertise and encouragement throughout the project.

Patricia Williams, MSN, RN, CCRN

Contents

chapter 1

Nursing and the Health Care System

http://evolve.elsevier.com/Williams/fundamental

Objectives

Upon completing this chapter, you should be able to do the following:

Theory

1. Describe Florence Nightingale's influence on nurses' training.
2. Explain why nursing is both an art and a science.
3. Define evidence-based practice and explain why it is important in nursing.
4. Trace the growth of nursing in the United States from the Civil War to the present.
5. Discuss the ways in which the desirable attributes of the nurse might be demonstrated.
6. Identify the educational ladder that is available to nurses.
7. Describe educational pathways open to the LPN/LVN upon graduation.
8. Compare methods of delivery of nursing care.
9. List four practice settings in which LPNs/LVNs may find employment.
10. Discuss today's health care system, its components, and changes proposed.
11. Explain how an HMO and a PPO differ.
12. Relate how the recent health care legislation has affected your own health care.

Clinical Practice

1. Write your own definition of *nursing.*
2. Discuss how the standards of practice for the LPN/LVN are applied in the clinical setting.
3. List the practice areas in the community in which you could be employed as a vocational nurse.

Key Terms

apprenticeship (ă-PRĔN-tĭ-shĭp, p. 2)
aseptically (ā-SĔP-tĭk-ăl-lē, p. 4)
capitated cost (p. 11)
clinical practice guidelines (p. 5)
diagnosis-related groups (DRGs) (dī-ăg-NŌS-ĭs, p. 9)
evidence-based nursing (p. 4)
health maintenance organizations (HMOs) (p. 10)
implement (ĬM-plĕ-mĕnt, p. 6)
interventions (p. 3)
invasive procedures (ĭn-VĀ-sĭv, p. 3)
nursing process (p. 6)
nursing theory (p. 4)
practice acts (p. 6)
preferred provider organizations (PPOs) (p. 10)
transition to practice (p. 6)

 **Concepts Covered in This Chapter**

- Care coordination
- Collaboration
- Communication
- Evidence
- Health care organizations
- Health policy
- Health care law
- Patient education
- Professionalism

HISTORICAL OVERVIEW

The art of nursing arose in primitive times, when one person simply cared for another who was sick. As family groups banded together into communities, certain individuals extended themselves to care for the ill, the helpless, and older adults. During this period, nursing consisted of comforting, caring for basic needs, and using herbal remedies.

NURSING IN ENGLAND AND EUROPE

As civilizations appeared, nurses were under the direction of the priest-physicians because illness was often believed to be caused by sin or the gods' displeasure. With the growth of Christianity, caring for the sick became a function of religious orders. The Christian St. Paul introduced a deaconess named Phoebe, a practical nurse, to Rome. She was the first visiting nurse. Both men and women tended the sick during this period. Nursing became a recognized vocation during the Crusades (AD 1100–1200) as hospitals were built to care for the large number of pilgrims needing health care.

The service provided by the religious orders in England changed with the break between King Henry VIII of England and the Catholic Church in the 1500s. The nuns and priests were sent out of the country. The patients in their hospitals were abandoned; the hospitals became the responsibility of the government. Criminals, widows, and orphans were recruited, and in exchange for housing and food, they tended the sick. The drunken nurse-midwives Sairey Gamp and Betsy Prig, as portrayed in Charles Dickens' 1849 novel *Martin Chuzzlewit,* were typical of hospital nurses at the time. Health care conditions became very bad.

Florence Nightingale

In the mid-1800s Florence Nightingale, an Englishwoman, felt a calling by God to become a nurse. Nightingale studied in Germany with a Protestant order of women who cared for the sick. She went on to reform and manage a charity hospital for ill governesses. During the Crimean War, Florence Nightingale asked the Secretary of War to allow her to train women to care for the sick and wounded. By cleaning up the wards and improving ventilation, sanitation, and nutrition, her group of 38 nurses lowered the death rate from 60% to 1%. The Nightingale nurses made their rounds after dark with the aid of a lighted oil lamp. The lamp became the official symbol of nursing. Florence Nightingale kept records and statistics that reinforced her theories of care, many of which are still valid today.

Funds were given out of gratitude by the service members and their families. These funds were used to begin the first Nightingale training school for nurses, located in England at St. Thomas Hospital, which operates to this day. Nightingale based her curriculum on the following beliefs:

- Nutrition is an important part of nursing care.
- Fresh, clean air is beneficial to the sick.
- Sick people need occupational and recreational therapy.
- Nurses should help identify and meet patients' personal needs, including providing emotional support.
- Nursing should be directed toward two conditions: health and illness.
- Nursing is distinct and separate from the practice of medicine and should be taught by nurses.
- Continuing education is needed for nurses.

These beliefs are still the foundation of nursing today.

? Think Critically

How is the tradition of combining religion and medical care still evident today?

NURSING IN NORTH AMERICA

Nursing care was sadly lacking during the Civil War in America. The Union government finally appointed Dorothea Dix, a social worker, to organize women volunteers to provide nursing care for the soldiers. These workers were similar to the nursing assistants of today. Clara Barton took volunteers into the field hospitals to care for soldiers of both armies. She later founded the American Red Cross. Lillian Wald took nursing out into the community, and in 1893, she and Mary Brewster established the Henry Street Settlement Service in New York City, which focused on the health needs of poor people who lived in tenements. In the period following the Civil War, nurses' training was essentially an **apprenticeship** (learning by doing). Over time, the schooling became more formal and the hospital-based training period lengthened from 6 months to 3 years. Graduates of the training program received a diploma. **In an era when women were expected to remain at home and be subservient to men, nurses' training became a way to obtain further education and employment that could provide independence for women.**

The training in the Nightingale schools varied considerably from that of the US nursing schools. The Nightingale program was well organized, with classes held separately from practical experience on the wards. The core curriculum was the same in all schools. Instruction was provided by a trained nurse and was focused on nursing care.

In the United States, the students staffed the hospital and worked without pay. There were no formal classes; education was achieved through work. There was no set curriculum, and content varied depending on the type of cases present in the hospital. Instruction was done at the bedside by the physician and, therefore, came from a medical viewpoint. In 1892, the New York Young Women's Christian Association (YWCA) started the first official school for practical nursing, the Ballard School, which offered a 3-month course. Students were trained to care for infants, children, and older adults in the home. The National League of Nursing Education issued formal standards for practical nursing education. In 1918, a group of women opened the Household Nursing School in Boston to train nurses to care for the sick at home. Later this school was called the Shepard-Gill School of Practical Nursing. During World War I, the Army School of Nursing was opened to train more practical nurses.

In the 20th century, nurses moved out into the community. They worked with the poor in the cities; provided midwifery services; and taught prenatal, obstetric, and child care (Fig. 1.1). The first African American nurses to serve in the US Army during World War I paved the way for others to follow (Fig. 1.2). World War II created a great demand for nurses in military hospitals, and training programs had to be increased (Fig. 1.3). Nurses served on many fronts and on hospital ships (Fig. 1.4). Congress passed a bill to draft nurses, but the declaration of peace occurred before it was

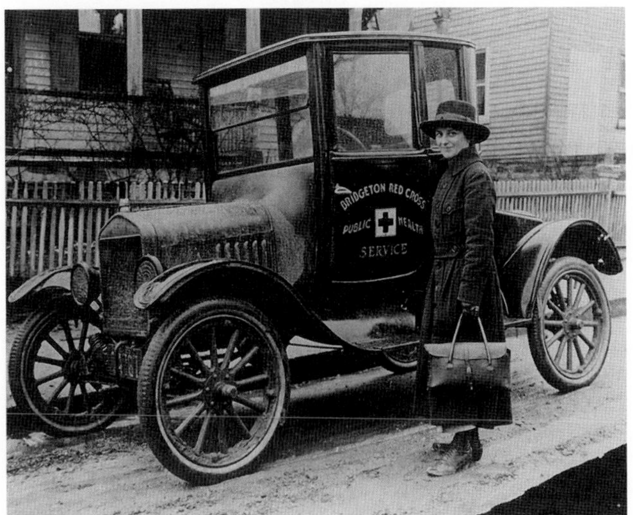

FIGURE 1.1 A Red Cross public health nurse poses with her Model T Ford before setting out on her rounds. (Photo courtesy American National Red Cross.)

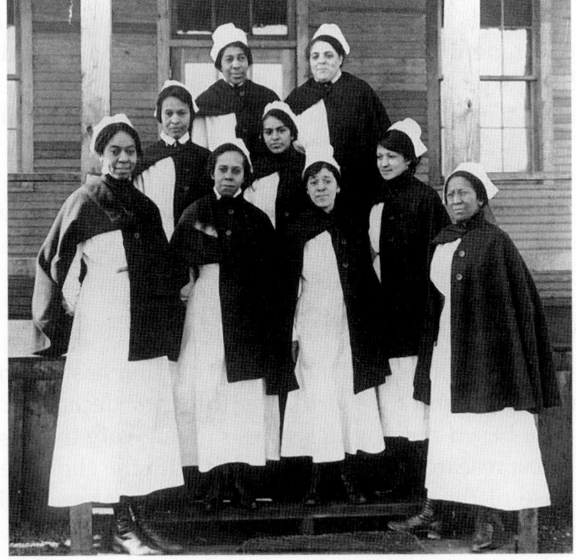

FIGURE 1.2 Some of the first African American nurses to serve with the US Army standing outside their quarters at Camp Sherman in Chillicothe, Ohio. (Photo courtesy American National Red Cross.)

enacted. Nurses continue to serve in times of military crisis, as in Iraq and Afghanistan, and American military nurses currently provide essential care to service members and local civilians whenever and wherever our armed services are deployed (Fig. 1.5).

THE ART AND SCIENCE OF NURSING

There are many definitions of *nursing*, and as you progress through your nursing career, ideas about what nursing is will grow and change. Among the various definitions, the following four common goals appear:

- To promote wellness
- To prevent illness
- To facilitate coping
- To restore health

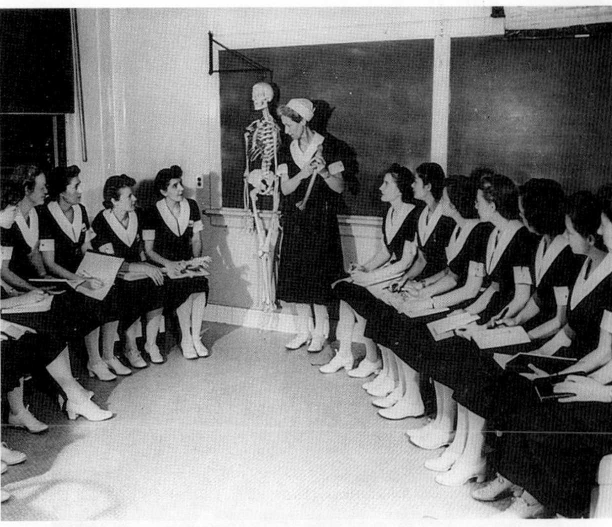

FIGURE 1.3 A group of nursing students during the 1930s or 1940s in an anatomy class at Walter Reed General Hospital, Washington, DC. (Photo courtesy of The US National Library of Medicine.)

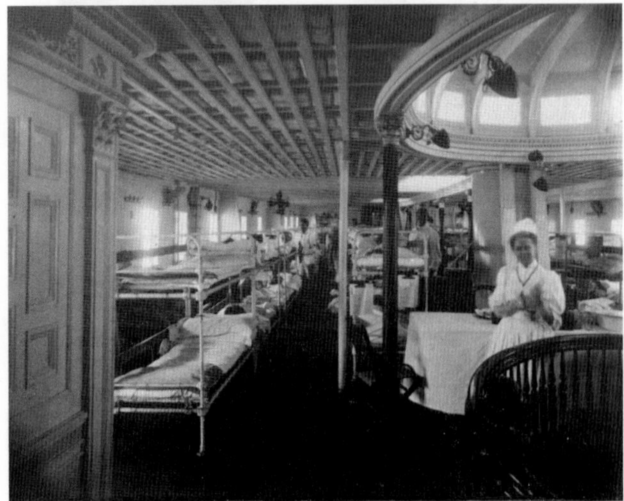

FIGURE 1.4 Nurses caring for patients on a hospital ship. (Photo courtesy of The US National Library of Medicine.)

To accomplish these goals, the practical nurse takes on the role of caregiver, educator, collaborator, advocate, and manager.

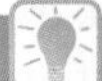 QSEN Considerations: Teamwork and Collaboration

Roles of the Practical Nurse

Collaboration with the health care team is an important role of the practical nurse.

Caregiving skills are interventions aimed at restoring and maintaining a person's health. **Interventions** are actions taken to improve, maintain, or restore health or prevent illness. An example would be assisting a patient with hygiene tasks such as bathing and brushing the teeth. Today, caregiving skills extend to using highly technical equipment for medical therapies and protecting the safety of the patient undergoing **invasive procedures** (procedures that require entry

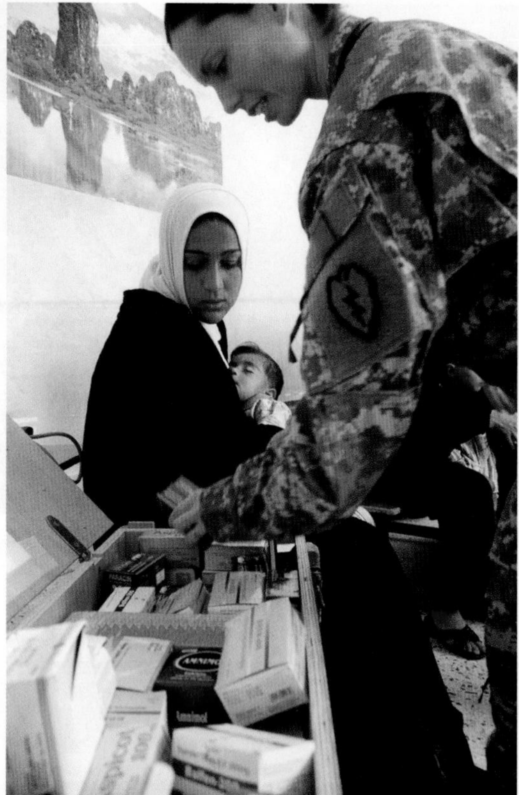

FIGURE 1.5 A nurse dispensing medication to a civilian patient in Iraq. (Courtesy of Sargent First Class Christina Bhatti.)

into the body). Nurses provide both physical and emotional care to patients. By performing various tasks and working closely with the patient, nurses develop a concern for the patient's well-being.

 QSEN Considerations: Patient-Centered Care

Growth Toward Wellness

The nurse's goal is to encourage growth toward wellness so that the patient can once again be self-reliant.

Patient education and health counseling are functions of the practical nurse and are directed toward promoting wellness and preventing illness. Teaching about medications and how to **aseptically** (without introducing infectious material) change dressings are examples of this role. Emotional support and comfort are incorporated in care, and the nurse is an advocate for the patient during times of health-related stress.

The licensed practical nurse (LPN), called a licensed vocational nurse (LVN) in California and Texas, collaborates with the registered nurse (RN) and other members of the health care team to provide continuity of care and care coordination.

 QSEN Considerations: Teamwork and Collaboration

Care Planning for the Patient

Care for the patient is planned jointly by all health care team members.

Minor tasks such as taking vital signs or giving a bed bath may be assigned to the nursing assistant or other ancillary personnel.

Therapeutic communication techniques facilitate a patient's ability to cope. Active listening is a therapeutic technique that helps the patient to consider possible solutions when a problem occurs. Establishing a good nurse-patient relationship is necessary to gain the patient's trust so that patient education and other communications are well received.

Initially nursing was an art: it consisted of performing certain acts of care skillfully, with intuition and creativity. Over time, a scientific base was combined with the art of nursing. From this body of knowledge, the nurse can choose interventions that are most likely to produce desired outcomes for the patient.

As this scientific base for nursing has developed, various scholars have proposed theories concerning the process of nursing. A **nursing theory** is a statement about relationships among concepts or facts, based on existing information. Nursing theorists generally base their beliefs on the relationships among humans, the environment, health, and nursing. Table 1.1 provides a brief explanation of some of the major nursing theories. A particular theory may be the basis of a nursing school's curriculum structure and part of its philosophy of how nursing care is delivered. Nursing strives to maintain recognition as a profession. For this reason, ongoing research is essential to add to the scientific knowledge base.

EVIDENCE-BASED PRACTICE

The promotion of **evidence-based nursing** has become stronger around the world over the last 2 decades. Evidence-based nursing describes nursing care that uses the best research evidence coupled with the clinical expertise of the clinician, considering the values of the patient (Stevens, 2013).

 QSEN Considerations: Quality Improvement

Interpreting Research

Learning the skills to discriminate between high-quality and flawed research and to interpret study results is important in becoming a practical nurse.

Nurses are being strongly encouraged to seek evidence for their practice throughout their careers. Evidence-based practice involves using the best scientific evidence from research to guide nursing care and improve patient outcomes (Academy of Medical-Surgical Nurses, 2014).

 QSEN Considerations: Evidence-Based Practice

About Evidence-Based Practice

Hypoglycemia is *always* a potential adverse effect of insulin therapy. Evidence-based practice consists of using your expertise, patient preferences and values, and a problem-solving approach to clinical practice to make decisions about

Table 1.1 Selected Nursing Theories

THEORIST	GOAL OF NURSING	PRACTICE FRAMEWORK
Virginia Henderson (1955)	To help patients gain independence in meeting their needs as quickly as possible	Fourteen fundamental needs
Dorothy Johnson (1968)	To reduce stress, allowing the patient to recover as quickly as possible	Seven behavioral subsystems in an adaptation model
Martha Rogers (1970)	To achieve maximum level of wellness	Concept of "unitary man" evolving along the life process
Dorothea Orem (1971)	To care for and help patients with various needs attain self-care	Self-care deficits
Betty Neumann (1972)	To help individuals, families, and groups attain and maintain maximum levels of total wellness through purposeful interventions	Systems model with stress reduction as its goal; nursing care occurs on various levels: primary prevention, secondary prevention, or tertiary prevention
Sister Callista Roy (1976)	To identify types of demands placed on the patient and the patient's adaptation to them	Four adaptive modes: physiologic, psychological, sociological, and independence
Jean Watson (1979)	To promote health, restore patients to health, and prevent illness	"Carative" factors, with caring as an interpersonal process used to meet human needs
Rosemarie Parse (1987)	To assist the patient in interaction with the environment and in co-creating health. To sustain a safe and protective environment	Human becoming: patients are open, mutual, and constantly interacting with the environment. Health is constantly changing
Patricia Benner and Judith Wrubel (1989)	To care about the patient as an individual	Primacy of caring: caring is central and allows for the giving and receiving of help. Caring extends to all aspects of care of the patient

patient care. Question the way things are done for patient care, and ask what does not make sense or what needs clarification. Ask yourself, Is there a better way to perform this procedure? An example of such a question would be, Is this the best solution to use for mouth care for this patient undergoing chemotherapy? Research the question topic and gather the best evidence available for an answer to the question. Critically look at the research for signs of validity of the data. Integrate the best evidence with your clinical expertise. Consider the patient's preferences and values when deciding on a course of action. Evaluate the outcome of the new action(s). Resources for research and guidelines for evidence-based practice include evidence-based journals, systematic reviews of studies, centers for evidence-based nursing, and evidence-based practice guidelines. A list of resources for evidence-based nursing is available from Virginia Commonwealth University at http://guides.library.vcu.edu/ebpsteps. A tutorial on understanding evidence-based practice is available at that website.

Evidence-based nursing is used to help determine "best practices." "Best practice means the use of care concepts, interventions, and techniques that are grounded in research and known to promote higher quality of care and living" (University of Iowa College of Nursing, 2015a, 2015b). Clinical field experience and evidence-based research are used to establish the best practices for patient care. Best practices are often provided in the form of clinical practice guidelines.

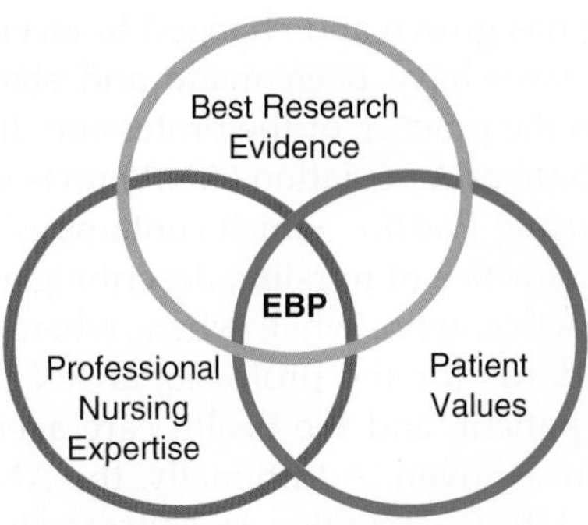

FIGURE 1.6 Evidence-based nursing.

Clinical practice guidelines are the product of evidence-based research, and they serve as a way for nurses to implement the evidence-based practices. For example, instead of performing catheter care a certain way "because we've always done it this way," the nursing staff adheres to a specific guideline that is evidence-based—has been shown with scientific evidence—to be safer and more effective. To sum up, evidence-based nursing is where the best research evidence, patient values and preferences, and professional nursing expertise come together (Fig. 1.6).

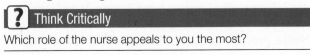

Think Critically

Which role of the nurse appeals to you the most?

Box 1.1 Standards of Practice for the Licensed Practical/Vocational Nurse

Practice

The licensed practical/vocational nurse:

1. Shall accept assigned responsibilities as an accountable member of the health care team.
2. Shall function within the limits of educational preparation and experience as related to the assigned duties.
3. Shall function with other members of the health care team in promoting and maintaining health, preventing disease and disability, caring for and rehabilitating individuals who are experiencing an altered health state, and contributing to the ultimate quality of life until death.
4. Shall know and utilize the nursing process in planning, implementing, and evaluating health services and nursing care for the individual patient or group.
   a. Planning: the planning of nursing includes:
      1) assessment/data collection of health status of the individual patient, the family, and community groups
      2) reporting information gained from assessment/data collection
      3) the identification of health goals
   b. Implementation: The plan for nursing care is put into practice to achieve the stated goals and includes:
      1) observing, recording, and reporting significant changes, which require intervention or different goals
      2) applying nursing knowledge and skills to promote and maintain health, to prevent disease and disability, and to optimize functional capabilities of an individual patient
      3) assisting the patient and family with activities of daily living and encouraging self-care as appropriate
      4) carrying out therapeutic regimens and protocols prescribed by personnel pursuant to authorized state law
   c. Evaluations: The plan for nursing care and its implementations are evaluated to measure the progress toward the stated goals and will include appropriate persons and/or groups to determine:
      1) the relevancy of current goals in relation to the progress of the individual patient
      2) the involvement of the recipients of care in the evaluation process
      3) the quality of the nursing action in the implementation of the plan
      4) a re-ordering of priorities or new goal setting in the care plan
5. Shall participate in peer review and other evaluation processes.
6. Shall participate in the development of policies concerning the health and nursing needs of society and in the roles and functions of the LP/VN.

CURRENT NURSING PRACTICE

As nursing has grown and changed to meet the needs of society, laws have been made and standards set that govern the practice of the profession. In 2015, the American Nurses Association (ANA) revised the *Standards of Nursing Practice,* which contains 17 standards of national practice of nursing, describing all facets of nursing practice: who, what, when, where, and how. These standards for the professional RN protect the nurse, the patient, and the health care agency where nursing care is given. Additionally, the ANA revised and updated the *Code of Ethics for Nurses with Interpretive Statements,* including areas addressing social media, the importance of intra-professional collaboration, and consideration of social justice (Epstein & Turner, 2015). The National League for Nursing published a vision statement describing the practical nurse's role in advancing the nation's health, emphasizing the importance of the practical nurse's contribution as professional partners in the health care team (National League for Nursing, 2014). The practical nurse follows standards written by the National Federation of Licensed Practical Nurses to deliver safe, knowledgeable nursing care (Box 1.1, Appendix B). The National Association for Practical Nurse Education and Service (NAPNES) has formulated an additional set of standards for practical nurses (see Chapter 3). In Canada, a set of similar standards guides the practice of nursing. Nurse practice acts have been established in each of the US states and in the provinces of Canada to regulate the practice of nursing. Each state has a regulatory body that makes and enforces rules and regulations for the nursing profession. The **practice acts** generally define activities in which nurses may engage, state the legal requirements and titles for nursing licensure, and establish the education needed for licensure. **The practice acts are designed to protect the public, and they define the legal scope of practice.** Policy and procedure books are established by each facility that hires nurses. These books define which procedures each professional can perform in that facility and specify step-by-step guidelines for the way that facility wants a procedure performed.

The National Council of State Boards of Nursing (NCSBN) has a proposal to enact rules for **transition to practice** for all newly licensed nurses. All newly licensed nurses will be required to complete a transition to practice program that meets the board criteria if the rule becomes a criterion for license renewal. The program would involve a minimum 6-month preceptorship with ongoing support through the first year of practice.

The **nursing process** emerged during the 1970s and 1980s as an organized, deliberate, systematic way to deliver nursing care. The nursing process provides a way to **implement** (to put into action) caregiving, and it combines the science and the art of nursing. The nurse focuses on the patient as an individual, identifies

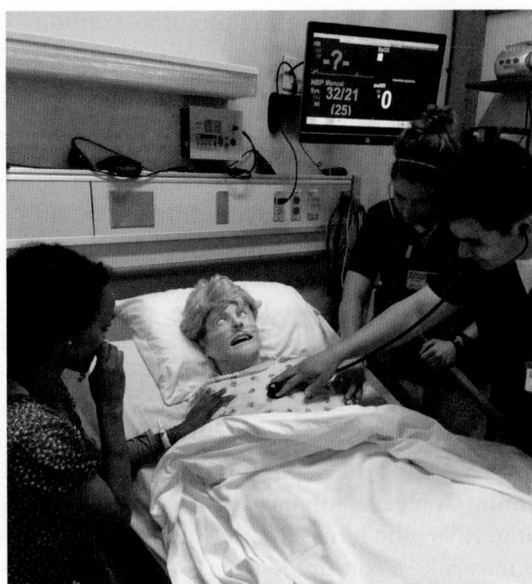

FIGURE 1.7 Students in modern day simulation lab.

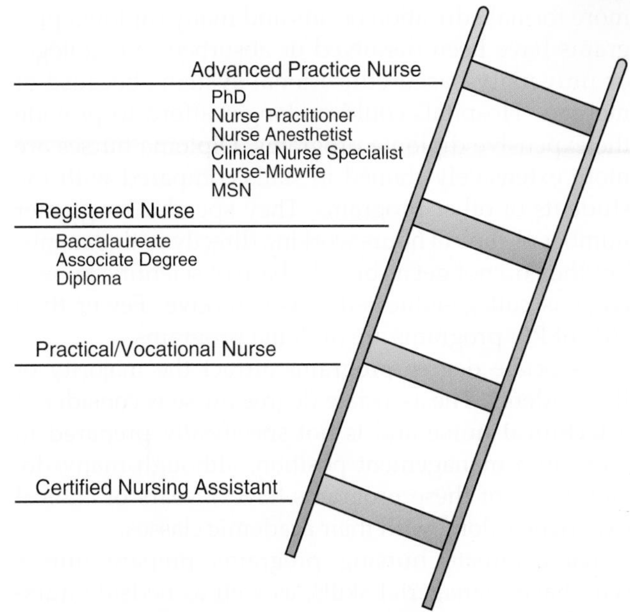

FIGURE 1.8 Nursing education ladder.

health care needs and strengths of the patient, establishes and implements a plan of action to meet those needs, and evaluates the outcomes of the plan. It is a circular process involving ongoing assessment, nursing diagnosis, planning, implementation, and evaluation. The nursing process is presented in depth in Unit II: The Nursing Process.

NURSING EDUCATION PATHWAYS

Formal education has been another way to build a professional image for nursing. Nursing education has been mostly moved from hospital training schools into institutions of higher learning. There are two levels of entry into nursing: practical (or vocational) nursing and registered nursing. Often a student studies to become a certified nursing assistant before going up the "ladder" to practical/vocational training. Each educational program produces graduates with skills for a particular level of entry into practice. A nursing assistant program is short, averaging 6 to 8 weeks. Basic personal care and basic nursing skills are taught. The practical nursing program generally takes 12 to 18 months to complete. The registered nursing program (RN) requires 2 to 5 years of education, depending on the type of degree sought (Fig. 1.7). If the student has already obtained a practical/vocational nursing license, the program may require only 1 more year to become an RN.

PRACTICAL NURSING

Practical nursing was created to fill a gap left by nurses who enlisted in the military services during World War II. Programs were developed to train practical nurses to care for well people and those who were mildly or chronically ill or past the acute stage of illness. RNs could then concentrate on the acutely ill. A need for practical nurses continued after the war, and NAPNES was formed to standardize practical nurse education and to establish licensure criteria for graduates. Practical nursing programs are offered in vocational schools, hospitals, proprietary schools, and community colleges. Graduates take the National Council Licensure Examination for Practical Nurses (NCLEX-PN) after program completion. Successfully passing the examination and obtaining licensure allows the use of the initials LPN or LVN after one's name. **Practical nurses provide direct patient care under the supervision of an RN, advanced practice RN, physician assistant, physician, dentist, or podiatrist.** Many community colleges have structured the practical nurse curriculum so that graduates can easily enter the second year of the registered nursing program. This type of curriculum is considered a "ladder program." Many LPN/LVN programs require that the entering student be a certified nursing assistant (Fig. 1.8).

After completion of an LPN/LVN curriculum and/or licensure, the graduate can seek certification by NAPNES in pharmacology, long-term care, and/or IV therapy. The pharmacology examination can be taken online. Each of the three certifications is valid for 3 years and can then be renewed.

REGISTERED NURSING

Graduates of three different educational programs are qualified to take the RN licensure examination (NCLEX-RN): a hospital-based diploma program, a 2-year associate degree program at a community college, or a 4-year baccalaureate nursing program at a college or university. RNs may provide bedside care or care in the community or supervise others in managing care of multiple patients.

Diploma schools continue to decrease as the desire to improve the professional image of nursing through more formal education occurs and many diploma programs have been dissolved or absorbed into college- or university-based educational systems because of mergers. Hospitals could no longer afford to provide the expensive diploma programs. Diploma nurses are more extensively trained in skills compared with the students of other programs. They spend a far greater number of clinical hours working directly with patients, but they do not get as broad a base of scientific knowledge as college-educated nurses receive. Fewer than 10% of RN programs are diploma programs.

Associate degree programs attract the majority of RN students. The associate degree nurse is considered a **technical** nurse and is not specifically prepared to work in a management position, although many do. Graduates of these programs have 2 years of clinical experience along with their academic classes.

Baccalaureate nursing programs prepare nurses who have managerial skills, as well as bedside nursing skills. The push toward **professionalism**, unification, and higher educational standards/consistencies for nursing has caused the ANA to propose that the baccalaureate degree be necessary for entry into professional nursing practice. There has been considerable controversy over this proposal because the many RNs who graduated from diploma or associate degree programs believe that their jobs may be threatened by such a proposal. To date, only some employers distinguish among the various educational programs of the RN. Magnet hospitals require that 100% of the nursing managers hold a Bachelor of Science in nursing degree (BSN), and although they make no specific recommendation for staff nurses, the typical hospital with Magnet designation tends to have about half of employed bedside RNs holding a BSN degree (Hawkins & Shell, 2012). In most facilities, however, graduates of all three RN programs are viewed the same. Another concern is that, if the more expensive and longer program were required to become a professional RN, employers would have to pay higher salaries. Differentiation of salaries based on educational degree primarily occurs only at the managerial level, not the bedside level. The nursing shortage tempered the push for all nurses to be baccalaureate prepared because the program is twice as long, but the ANA is again pressing for the BSN to be required for entry into RN practice.

? Think Critically

What are three educational differences between the practical nurse and the RN?

ADVANCED PRACTICE NURSING

Graduate programs are available in nursing for both master's and doctorate degrees. Nurses who pursue higher education are prepared as specialists in the various clinical branches of nursing, in research, or in administration. Another form of advanced education is the nurse practitioner program. RNs continue their training in a specialty such as family practice, pediatrics, maternity, psychiatry, adult health nursing, acute care, or geriatrics; once licensed, they can practice more independently than as an RN. Nurse practitioners (NPs) provide care in a hospital, outpatient, ambulatory care, or community-based setting. In many states, they can treat patients on their own and write prescriptions under the direction of a physician. NPs are one of the four types of advanced practice nurse. The other three include the titles certified nurse-midwife (CNM), certified registered nurse anesthetist (CRNA), and clinical nurse specialist (CNS). Each type of advance practice RN requires specific certification and training.

The ANA set up a separate American Nurses Credentialing Center to enhance the professional image of nursing. RNs who have experience in a particular specialty may take a comprehensive examination. Passing the examination provides the nurse with certification of expertise in that specialty. Certification is also available for the practical nurse under a program developed by NAPNES.

DELIVERY OF NURSING CARE

Various systems of delivering nursing care have been tried through the years. Today various adaptations are devised to meet the specific needs of the patients and nurses. **Functional nursing care** was the first care delivery system for the practical nurse. Practical nurses performed a series of tasks such as administration of medication and treatments. Care was rather fragmented; however, it was cost effective. **Team nursing** evolved in the 1950s and extended into the mid-1970s. An RN was the team leader who coordinated care for a group of patients. Work tasks were assigned to the other members of the team, the practical nurses and the nurses' aides. This system worked fairly well as long as there was excellent communication among the members and the team leader evaluated care delivered. **Total patient care** came next, in which one nurse carried out all nursing functions for the patient, including medication administration. This was an effort to provide less fragmented care for the patient. Of course, total patient care is more expensive.

Primary nursing appeared in the late 1960s and 1970s. In this system, one nurse plans and directs care for a patient over a 24-hour period. This method eliminated fragmentation of care between shifts. When the primary nurse is off duty, an associate nurse takes over the care and planning. Today, primary nursing is often modified with the use of cross-trained personnel assigned to help with duties. To increase the level of productivity, ancillary workers supervised by the RN are trained in multiple functions, such as clerical and housekeeping tasks, vital sign measurement, and phlebotomy. This system has not been entirely satisfactory.

Currently, because research is showing better patient outcomes with more of the care being delivered by nurses, there is a trend back to *total patient care.*

Relationship-based care appeared in the early 2000s (Koloroutis et al., 2004). It emphasizes three critical relationships: (1) the relationship between caregivers and the patients and families they serve; (2) the caregiver's relationship with him- or herself; and (3) the relationship among health team members (UCLA Department of Nursing, 2015). The motivation behind relationship-based care was to promote a cultural transformation by improving relationships to foster care for the patient. Some schools of nursing have adopted relationship-based care as the foundation of their nursing education curriculum.

Patient-centered care has been described since the 1950s, but it came to the forefront in 2001 when the Institute of Medicine (IOM) targeted six areas for improvement in the US health care system, including safety, effectiveness, patient-centeredness, timeliness, efficiency, and equitableness (Cliff, 2012). Patient-centered care has been fully embraced by the nursing community, and it is identified as one of the seven QSEN competencies (QSEN.org, 2015).

PRACTICE SETTINGS

Practical nurses work in health care organizations under the supervision of an RN, advanced practice RN, physician assistant, physician, dentist, or podiatrist. Traditionally, many LPN/LVN positions were found in the hospital setting, whereas community nursing, school nursing, and public health nursing were primarily the arena of the professional RN. Recent trends have changed, however, and expanded the employment landscape for the practical nurse. Hospitals now tend to hire primarily RNs, yet practice settings for the LPN/LVN remain plentiful and include the following health care organizations:

- **Hospitals:** Restorative care is provided to ill or injured patients.
- **Subacute and extended care facilities:** In facilities for subacute, intermediate, or long-term care; personal care and skilled care are provided for those requiring rehabilitation or custodial care.
- **Assisted-living facilities:** In facilities that provide housekeeping, prepared meals, and varying degrees of nursing care.
- **Physicians' offices:** Ambulatory patients receive preventive care or treatment of an illness or injury.
- **Ambulatory clinics:** Ambulatory patients come for preventive care or treatment of an illness or injury; often treatment by specialty groups is available on site. Numerous specialty clinics that employ LPNs/LVNs include cardiology, dermatology, allergy, immunology, pulmonology, and many others.
- **Renal dialysis centers:** Patients with kidney failure receive renal dialysis treatments.

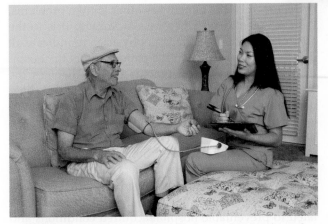

FIGURE 1.9 Home health nursing. (Photo copyright istock.com.)

- **Hospice and palliative home care:** Supportive treatment is provided for patients who are terminally ill, improving quality of life and ease of suffering.
- **Home health agencies:** In-home care is provided to patients by nurses who visit the home (Fig. 1.9).
- **Neighborhood emergency centers/urgent care clinics:** Minor emergency care is provided to patients within the community setting.
- **Correctional facilities:** Care is rendered to incarcerated individuals, assisting with physical examinations, administering medications, and performing medical treatments.
- **School nurse:** Triage, medication administration, first aid, and some care of students with diabetes.
- **Surgical centers:** These centers perform same day surgeries on typically healthier individuals than those found in a typical hospital operating room (OR). The LPN/LVN is often employed as the preoperative nurse in this setting.

As the role of the practical nurse expands, employment in other practice settings is possible.

TODAY'S HEALTH CARE SYSTEM

In times past, most medical care was provided by physicians in private practice. With the technological advances in medicine and the flood of new drugs on the market, health care costs have risen dramatically. Although the use of magnetic resonance imaging (MRI) and computed tomography (CT) provides much more data than a standard radiograph dose, both are very expensive. Microsurgical techniques allow procedures that would not have been possible 40 years ago. Older adults are living longer and needing more years of medical care and numerous prescription drugs.

Diagnosis-related groups (DRGs) were created by Medicare in 1983 as an attempt to contain rising health care costs. The DRG system means that a hospital receives a set amount of money for a patient who is hospitalized with a certain diagnosis. If a patient is admitted with pneumonia, only a certain number of days of hospitalization are allowed and will be paid for by Medicare. If the patient has other known problems, they are mentioned when he is admitted. It is to the advantage of the hospital and physician to indicate all possible diagnoses when the patient enters the hospital. If the patient with pneumonia also has diabetes, the length of stay is likely to be longer. Adding this diagnosis at admission provides an extra measure of money for the patient's care. Private insurance companies have adjusted their payments in many instances to be more in line with what Medicare will pay for the same problem. This system has created a large amount of paperwork for all health care agencies and caregivers. In 2008, Medicare stopped paying hospitals for care related to preventable hospital-acquired conditions and complications. This means that if a patient contracts an infection because of poor catheter care or poor aseptic techniques while in the hospital, for example, the hospital will not be paid for the care and extra days the patient is there to clear the infection. To clearly prove patient needs and proper care, nursing documentation of patient assessment and identified needs becomes very important.

In December of 2003, Congress passed the controversial Medicare Prescription Drug Improvement and Modernization Act, which took effect in 2007 as Medicare Part D. The aim of Part D was to supply financial relief to seniors who take multiple prescription drugs. There have been many problems. Although beneficial to low-income participants, it provides only modest relief for middle-income seniors. There is a gap, called the "donut hole," after a person's drug costs reach $2960. When someone is in the donut hole, they pay their medication costs until they reach $4700. Measures in the Affordable Care Act call for the donut hole to disappear by 2020 (Centers for Medicare & Medicaid Services, 2015).

There are six levels of care within the health care system (Fig. 1.10). The levels of care show the scope of services and settings where patients receive care across the spectrum of health and illness (Box 1.2). A **medical home** model within primary care is gaining momentum. A medical home is not a place; it is an *approach* to health care. The medical home is patient-centered, comprehensive, coordinated, accessible, and committed to quality and safety (Patient Centered Primary Care Collaborative, 2014). This approach focuses on holistic care of patients where care is coordinated among various providers.

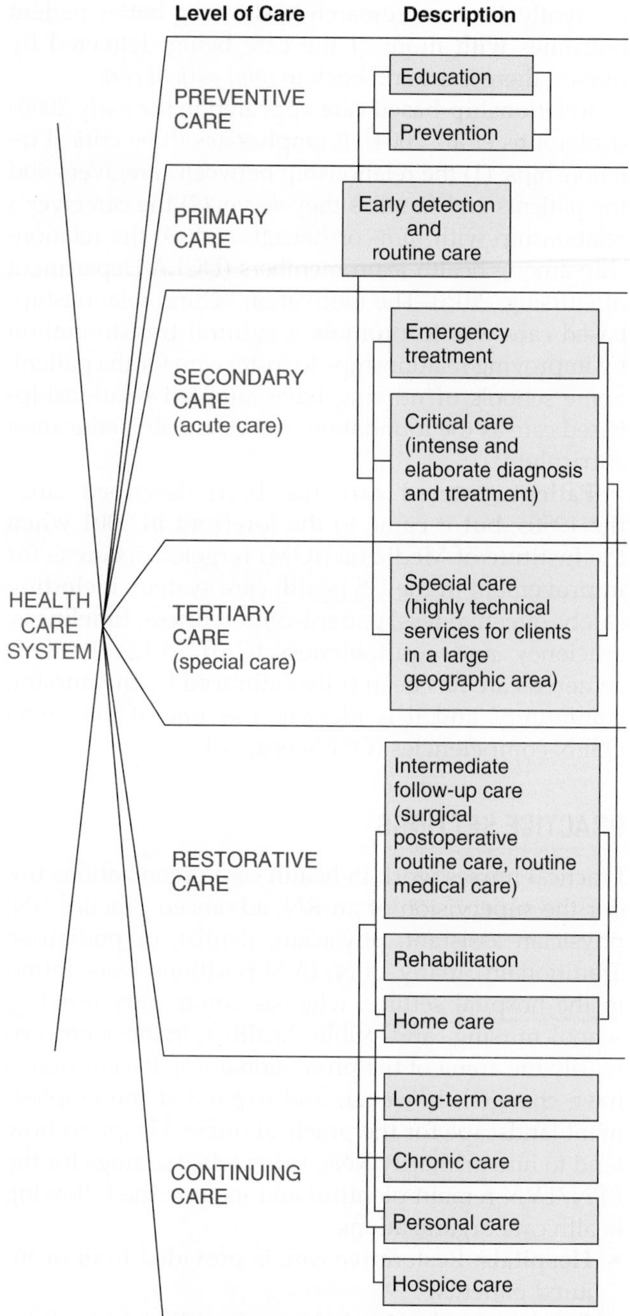

FIGURE 1.10 Levels of health care.

HEALTH MAINTENANCE ORGANIZATIONS

The need to decrease the high cost of medical care has caused health care providers to group together to provide services. **Health maintenance organizations (HMOs)**, a type of group practice, enroll patients for a set fee per month. They provide a limited network of physicians, hospitals, and other health care providers from which to choose. Two national HMOs are Kaiser Permanente and US Family Health Plan. The patient or employer pays a monthly fee for the insurance, and a small copayment may be required from the patient for each visit. Patients must be referred by their primary care provider for diagnostic tests, hospitalization (including emergency department visits), and consultation with a specialist. Part of the philosophy of the HMO is that because the patient does not pay the full cost for each visit, earlier treatment will be sought, and serious illness can be avoided. **One goal of the HMO is to keep patients healthy and out of the hospital.**

PREFERRED PROVIDER ORGANIZATIONS

Large businesses and insured groups may contract with **preferred provider organizations (PPOs)**. PPOs

Box 1.2 Examples of Health Care Services

PREVENTIVE CARE AND PRIMARY CARE
- Health promotion
- Prenatal care
- Well-baby care
- Nutrition counseling
- Exercise classes
- Family planning
- Meditation classes
- Emergency preparedness classes
- Fire prevention classes
- Mature driver courses
- Smoking cessation classes
- School physical examinations
- Illness prevention
- Immunization clinic
- Blood pressure screening
- Health fairs and screenings
- Mental health counseling and crisis intervention
- Child safety classes
- Annual physical checkups
- Vision screenings

SECONDARY CARE (ACUTE CARE)
- Radiologic procedures
- Laboratory and diagnostic procedures
- Surgical procedures
- Inpatient services
- Emergency care
- Restorative care
- Rehabilitation services
- Physical therapy
- Speech therapy
- Occupational therapy
- Home health care
- Cardiovascular and pulmonary outpatient rehabilitation

TERTIARY CARE (CONTINUING CARE)
- Extended (long-term) care
- Chronic disease management
- Assistive-living care
- Medical homes
- In-home personal care
- Hospice care
- Palliative home care

offer a discount on fees in return for a large pool of potential patients. This type of network performs these services for a set or **capitated cost**, meaning they are paid at a set fee for every patient enrolled in the network each year. Using PPOs allows insurance companies to keep their premium rates lower and in turn makes insurance coverage of employees less expensive for employers. Patients then choose a provider from the list of those associated with the PPO. There are usually a larger number of providers to choose from in a PPO than in an HMO.

There is considerable controversy about the effectiveness of this managed care approach to health care. Patients find that they cannot establish a long-term relationship with a care provider because employers' contracts with PPOs change as frequently as every year, and HMOs find that providers often leave for employment elsewhere. Patients resent having to see their primary care provider before seeing other specialists.

Cost Containment

Nurses must constantly think critically about cost containment while trying to give optimal care to patients. **Vigilant assessment with documentation is more important than ever to catch beginning complications before they become serious.** Budgeting issues for every department and unit in a health care agency concern each employee. The nurse who forgets to discontinue a heating pad the patient is no longer using, or forgets to charge for an item taken from the supply cart, is costing the nursing unit and the health care agency money. Documentation is exacting because every treatment and each use of equipment must be documented **with evidence showing it is needed.**

In an effort to cut costs, many hospitals have cross-trained personnel to fulfill more than one function. Unit secretaries may be trained to be electrocardiography (ECG) monitor technicians, or housekeeping staff may be trained to perform tasks usually done by nursing assistants, such as taking vital signs. Fewer nurses are found on nursing units than before (except in states with mandatory nurse-patient ratios), and they care for a larger number of patients. Nurses must learn to be good managers and to maximize use of ancillary personnel to accomplish their work.

Health care agencies are beginning to find that nurses are necessary to the agency and can provide more cost-effective and higher-quality care than ancillary workers can.

THE PATIENT PROTECTION AND AFFORDABLE CARE ACT

The Patient Protection and Affordable Care Act is being phased in over several years. There are positive and negative aspects to the Act, and many people have strong opinions about it. Since 2013, there have been insurance exchanges, along with requirements for uninsured people to purchase health insurance. Starting in 2015, people who have failed to purchase health insurance are being penalized on their income taxes. Provisions in the bill now prevent denial of insurance to those with pre-existing illnesses who formerly could not buy health insurance, and young adults have been allowed to remain on their parents' insurance through age 26. Starting in 2013, affluent people began paying an extra 3.8% tax on unearned income; drug manufacturers and the insurance industry are paying large annual fees to help cover the overall costs. Costs of the Medicare program will be contained by reducing payments to hospitals and health care providers. As coverage under the Affordable Care Act has expanded, the national uninsured rate has fallen from 16% to 11% of people under age 65 (people over age 65 generally have universal coverage by Medicare). People who have benefited the most from the Act include people ages 18 to 34, African Americans, Hispanics, and those living in rural areas (Quealy & Sanger-Katz, 2014). It is expected that the emphasis on prevention and coordinated care will produce a shift in nursing from the hospital to the community. There are many controversial parts of the bill, and the country is divided about whether the bill should be repealed and other health care legislation be written. What happens in the Congress in the coming years will determine if all parts of the legislation will remain.

Get Ready for the NCLEX Examination!

Key Points

- Providing comfort, tending to basic needs, and using herbal remedies were the functions of nurses in early civilizations.
- Florence Nightingale trained to become a nurse in the mid-1800s and started the first school of nursing in England.
- Nightingale's beliefs about nursing hold true today.
- Dorothea Dix organized volunteer "nurses" during the Civil War.
- Nurses' training became a way for women to obtain further education and a means of employment that could provide independence.
- In the early 1900s, US training school nurses staffed the hospitals, learned on the job, and worked without pay.
- Nurses moved from hospitals out into the community in the 20th century and provided midwifery services and patient education regarding prenatal, obstetric, and child care.
- Nursing expanded during World War II.
- Nursing is an art and a science.
- Evidence-based practice is used to help establish "best practices" based on research, patient values/preferences, and professional nursing expertise to employ for positive patient outcomes.
- The educational ladder in nursing progresses from the nursing assistant to the advanced practice nurse.
- The goals of nursing are to promote wellness, prevent illness, facilitate coping, and restore health.
- The roles of the practical nurse are caregiver, educator, collaborator, advocate, and manager. Practice settings are numerous for the practical/vocational nurse.
- Various nursing scholars have developed theories of nursing.
- *Standards of Nursing Practice* protect the nurse, the patient, and the health care agency where the nurse practices.
- The nurse practice acts define activities in which nurses may engage, and state the legal requirements and titles for organizations that enroll patients and supply all of their medical care. These organizations contract with care providers and facilities to provide medical care.
- There are six levels of care within the health care system.
- Health care costs have risen dramatically, and every effort is being made to cut costs.

Additional Learning Resources

SG Go to your Study Guide for additional learning activities to help you master this chapter content.

evolve Go to your Evolve website at http://evolve.elsevier.com/Williams/fundamental for additional online resources.

Online Resources

- *American Association for the History of Nursing*, www.aahn.org
- *Florence Nightingale Museum*, www.florence-nightingale.co.uk
- *National Association for Practical Nurse Education and Service*, www.napnes.org
- *National Council of State Boards of Nursing*, www.ncsbn.org
- *National League for Nursing*, www.nln.org
- *National Federation of Licensed Practical Nurses*, www.nflpn.org
- *American Nurses Association*, www.nursingworld.org
- *Nursing: Scope and Standards of Practice*, (for purchase) http://www.nursesbooks.org/Homepage/Hot-off-the-Press/Nursing-Scope-and-Standards-3rd-Ed.aspx
- *2015 ANA Code of Ethics for Nurses with Interpretive Statements* (online read-only document): http://nursingworld.org/MainMenuCategories/EthicsStandards/Tools-You-Need/Code-of-Ethics-For-Nurses.html

Review Questions for the NCLEX Examination

*Choose the **best** answer(s) for each question.*

1. The American Red Cross was founded by ____________________, as an outgrowth of service during the ____________________ War. *(Fill in the blanks.)*
   1. Dorothea Dix, First World
   2. Clara Barton, Civil
   3. Lillian Wald, Second World
   4. Florence Nightingale, Crimean
2. In setting up her nurses' training, Florence Nightingale carried out her belief that: *(Select all that apply.)*
   1. Fresh, clean air is beneficial to the sick.
   2. Sick people need adequate nutrition.
   3. Nursing should be taught by nurses.
   4. Proper nutrition is essential to recovery from illness.
   5. Any woman could be trained to be a nurse.

3. Inherent in any definition or philosophy of nursing are several core concepts. The core concepts include: *(Select all that apply.)*
   1. Promoting wellness.
   2. Restoring health.
   3. Facilitating coping.
   4. Sacrificing self for others.
   5. Preventing illness.
4. One main difference between a licensed practical/vocational nurse and an RN is that the licensed practical/vocational nurse:
   1. Usually is responsible for giving medications.
   2. Performs only noninvasive procedures.
   3. Cares for fewer patients than the RN.
   4. Is required to work in a supervised setting.
5. A student is deciding between different nursing educational programs for a future management role. Which would be the best choice?
   1. Nurse practitioner program
   2. Associate degree nursing program
   3. Baccalaureate nursing program
   4. Practical/vocational nursing program
6. Evidence-based nursing is based on: (*Select all that apply.*)
   1. Professional nursing expertise.
   2. Evidence from research that guides decision making.
   3. Patient values and preferences.
   4. Critical thinking, experience, and collaboration.
   5. Nursing values and preferences.
7. An advantage to the patient of a managed health care system is:
   1. Always receiving care from the same provider.
   2. Paying lower health insurance costs and smaller copayments.
   3. The ease of quickly seeing a specialist.
   4. Being able to walk into the clinic without an appointment.
8. The nurse is planning illness prevention activities for her patients. The best activity to choose would be: *(Select all that apply.)*
   1. Applying a dressing to a wound.
   2. Performing vision screenings.
   3. Referring a patient to a care provider.
   4. Promoting prenatal care.
   5. Performing nutritional education.

Critical Thinking Activities

Read each clinical scenario and discuss the questions with your classmates.

Scenario A
What type of employment do you think would appeal to you after graduation?

Scenario B
If you wish to continue your education after graduation from the practical nursing program, what path do you think would be best for you?

Scenario C
What are some ways that could be used to contain the high cost of medical care?

chapter 2

Concepts of Health, Illness, Stress, and Health Promotion

http://evolve.elsevier.com/Williams/fundamental

Objectives

Upon completing this chapter, you should be able to do the following:

Theory

1. Compare traditional and current views of the meanings of health and illness.
2. Describe what the word *health* means to you.
3. Define what *sickness* means to you.
4. Discuss why nurses need to be aware of any cultural, educational, and social differences that might exist between themselves and their patients.
5. Compare cultural/racial differences in disease predisposition and communication between the main cultures and different races.
6. List the components of holistic health care.
7. Identify the four areas of human needs, and give an example of each level of need.
8. Identify ways in which the body adapts to maintain homeostasis.
9. Explain why a particular stressor may be experienced differently by two people.
10. List the common signs and symptoms of stress.
11. Identify four ways in which a nurse can help decrease stress and anxiety for patients.

Clinical Practice

1. Observe patients during the data gathering and interview processes and determine their views on health and illness.
2. Recognize cultural differences in health care behaviors in the clinical setting and be able to share those observations with fellow students.
3. Determine a patient's position in Maslow's hierarchy during a clinical experience.
4. Describe alterations in homeostasis as observed in the clinical setting.
5. Document observations about stress-reduction techniques used by staff or patients during a clinical experience.

Key Terms

acute illness (p. 15)
adaptation (p. 16)
asymptomatic (ā-sĭmp-tō-MĂ-tĭk, p. 17)
autonomic (p. 22)
chronic illness (p. 15)
congenital (p. 15)
convalescence (kŏn-vă-LĔ-sĕns, p. 15)
coping (p. 17)
defense mechanisms (p. 26)
disease (p. 14)
etiology (ē-tē-Ŏ-lō-jē, p. 15)
health (p. 14)
health literacy (p. 19)
hierarchy (HĪ-ĕr-ăr-kē, p. 19)
holistic (hō-LĬS-tĭc, p. 19)
homeostasis (hō-mē-ō-STĀ-sĭs, p. 22)
idiopathic (ĭd-ē-ō-PĂTH-ĭk, p. 15)
illness (p. 15)
maladaptation (măl-ă-dăp-TĀ-shŭn, p. 16)
primary illness (p.15)
secondary illness (p. 15)
self-actualization (SĔLF ăk-tū-ăl-ī-ZĀ-shŭn, p. 22)
stress (p. 19)
stressor (p. 22)
subjective (p. 15)
terminal illness (p. 15)
wellness (p. 15)

Concepts Covered in This Chapter

- Collaboration
- Communication
- Patient education
- Stress
- Coping
- Health promotion
- Culture
- Homeostasis

HEALTH AND ILLNESS

The word *health* means many different things to people. For some health is the absence of **disease** (pathologic process that causes illness), whereas for others, it means optimum functioning on every level. The word *health* comes from a word that means wholeness. According to the Miller-Keane dictionary, **health** is "a relative state in which one is able to function well physically, mentally, socially, and spiritually in order to express the full range of one's unique potentialities within the environment in which one is living."

It is important to know your personal definition of *health* and **illness** (disease of body or mind) because your perception of these terms influences what you say and do when caring for patients. Because of cultural, educational, and social differences, you and the patient could have very different ideas about health and illness and what constitutes "good" health and effective health practices.

QSEN Considerations: Patient-Centered Care

Patient Beliefs

Before working with patients to accomplish health care goals, try to discover their beliefs about health and illness.

TRADITIONAL VIEWS OF HEALTH AND ILLNESS

The traditional view of health in Western culture was influenced by Plato, Aristotle, and other philosophers who were concerned only with biologic well-being. For many years, an acceptable definition of *health* was simply "the absence of disease." **The World Health Organization has defined *health* as "a state of complete physical, mental and social well-being and not merely the absence of disease or infirmity."**

In 1974, treatment of mental illness became recognized as a legitimate medical cost in the Federal Employees' Compensation Act. Following the lead of the federal government, other third-party payers (such as insurance companies) made similar changes. This willingness to pay for medical care for illnesses other than clearly defined physical diseases reflected a new and expanded understanding of the nature of health.

From birth to death, an individual's health status can vary from day to day or even hour to hour. People who are partially or completely paralyzed, suffering from a **chronic** (persisting for a long time) **illness**, deaf or blind, or living with an anatomic defect may think of themselves as fairly healthy and may lead full and productive lives. None of these people can be labeled as "sick," nor can they be called completely healthy. There are others who have no identifiable organic disease but who do not feel well and are not able to live their lives to the fullest.

Illness is a pronounced deviation from one's typical or "baseline" health status. Illness is an unavoidable, common part of life. We all occasionally have a cold or the flu. Illness is a personal thing; it is **subjective** (perceived only by the individual). **Only the person can tell you if she feels ill.** Illness may have a detectable basis in disease or trauma, or it may not. Disease is a pathologic process with a definite set of signs and symptoms; disease causes illness.

An **acute illness** is one that develops suddenly and resolves in a short time. Intestinal flu is an example of an acute illness. **Chronic illness,** such as hypertension, tends to develop slowly, can be controlled but not cured, and is long-lasting. A **terminal illness** is one for which there is no cure available; it ends in death. In the terminal phase of illness, death usually occurs within a short period, such as a few months, weeks, or days.

A **primary illness** is one that develops without being caused by another health problem. A **secondary illness** results from or is caused by a primary illness. Peripheral vascular disease resulting from diabetes is an example of a secondary illness, and it occurs because of the effect diabetes has on blood vessels.

Some diseases are inherited (genetic) or **congenital** (present at birth). Sickle cell anemia is an inherited disease. Fetal alcohol syndrome (FAS) is a congenital disorder caused by the intake of alcohol during pregnancy. An **idiopathic** illness is one for which there is no known **etiology** (cause).

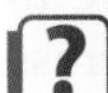
Think Critically

How is depression viewed? Is it considered an illness, a character weakness, or something else? How is it viewed by your family and friends? You may find many differences in how people view health as you explore the answers to the questions.

STAGES OF ILLNESS

Illness occurs in stages; there is a transition stage (onset), an acceptance stage (sick role), and a convalescence stage (recovery). When experiencing illness, people act in ways called **illness behaviors.** These behaviors include how people monitor the body, define and interpret symptoms, seek health care, and follow advice and self-care measures to regain **wellness** (physical and mental well-being). Illness behavior varies according to the stage of illness and the person's beliefs.

Transition Stage

The onset of illness may consist of vague, nonspecific symptoms. During this period, one may deny feeling ill but recognize that symptoms of an illness are present. Acknowledgment of a health problem occurs. As symptoms continue or worsen, self-medication may be used or medical assistance may be sought.

Acceptance Stage

Acceptance occurs as denial of illness stops and a "sick role" is assumed. This involves acknowledging illness and engaging in measures to become well. There is withdrawal from usual responsibilities and roles. Remedies from the pharmacy or home medicine cabinet may be used, or the person may go home and go to bed. If symptoms continue to worsen, medical treatment may be sought. Some people delay going to their primary care provider as long as possible. Fear of what the problem may be and of undergoing examination and diagnostic procedures often causes anxiety.

Convalescence Stage

Convalescence is the process of recovering after the illness and regaining health. If the illness or disease is chronic, a total recovery phase is replaced by **adaptation** (adjustment in structure or habits) to limitations and positive use of remaining capabilities, or by **maladaptation** (lack of adjustment).

Think Critically

What behaviors do different members of your family display when they assume the sick role?

CURRENT VIEWS OF HEALTH AND ILLNESS

Contemporary definitions of *health* and *illness* are more abstract and philosophical and, therefore, more vague than the precise definitions based on measurable criteria. **In general, being healthy means being able to function well physically and mentally and to express the full range of one's potentialities within the environment in which one is living.**

This concept takes health beyond the level of meeting basic physiologic needs and recognizes people's need to accept themselves as worthwhile, to live in harmony with others, and to express their personalities fully, thereby becoming more **self-actualized** (reaching one's full potential) and fulfilled. In the words of René Dubos, "Health is primarily a measure of each person's ability to do and become what he wants to become."

Current views of health and illness are based on the thoughts and ideas of men such as René Dubos and Halbert Dunn, who urged people to look at these concepts in a new way. Realizing that people are dynamic beings whose state of health changes daily and even hourly, they suggest that it is better to think of each person as being located somewhere on a continuum ranging from obvious disease through the absence of detectable disease to a state of optimum functioning in every aspect of life (Fig. 2.1). The phrase *high-level wellness* was first used by Dunn to signify the ideal state of health in every dimension of the human personality. Dunn does not consider high-level wellness to be the same as good health. He thinks of health as being a relatively passive state, one that a person enjoys because of hereditary and environmental factors that are essentially beyond her control. High-level wellness, on the contrary, is described as a dynamic and active movement toward fulfillment of one's potential (Dunn, 1973).

In Dunn's view, each person accepts responsibility for and takes an active part in improving and maintaining her own state of wellness. A person with a high level of wellness does so by virtue of her own efforts. A person who works at achieving high-level wellness improves her self-esteem, is able to accept and give love and concern for others, and lives each day of her life to its fullest insofar as possible.

In the contemporary view, *health* and *illness* are relative, rather than absolute, terms. This means that each person's state of health depends on many different things beyond biologic fitness (Fig. 2.2) Among the personal, psychosocial, and spiritual factors that influence a person's state of health at any given moment are the values and beliefs about what it means to be healthy and what it means to be sick, the image of oneself, and the ability to reach out and relate to others and to search for and find meaning and purpose in life. From this point of view, health is always dynamic.

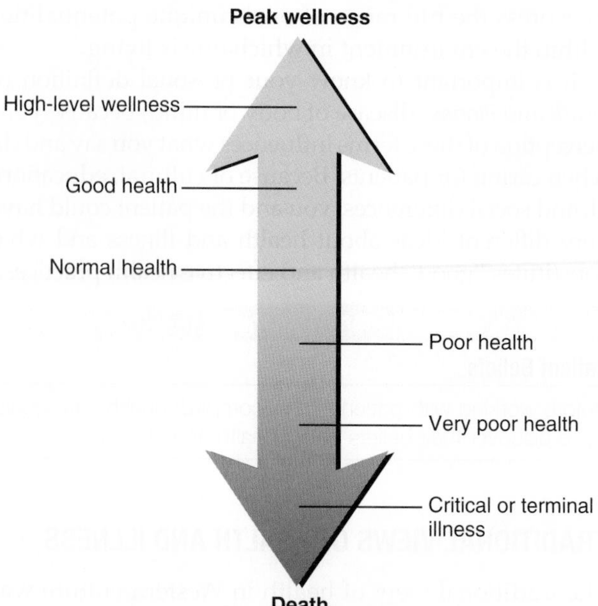

FIGURE 2.1 Health-illness continuum.

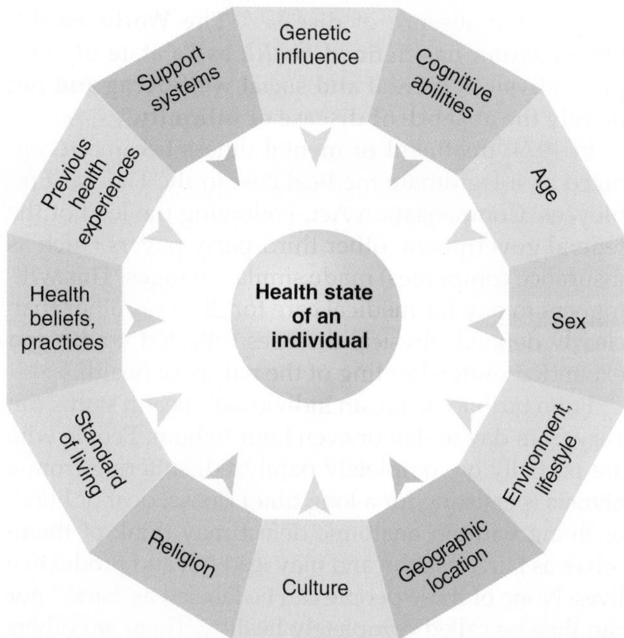

FIGURE 2.2 Multiple variables influence health and illness. (Modified from Ignatavicius, D. D., & Workman, M. L. (2002). *Medical-surgical nursing: critical thinking for collaborative care* (4th ed.). Philadelphia, PA: Saunders.)

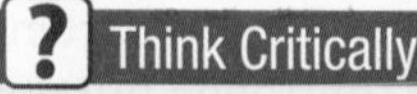
Think Critically

Where do you place yourself on Dunn's continuum?

IMPLICATIONS OF CURRENT VIEWS

These views of the nature of health and illness have greatly added to the complexity of health care. They challenge the traditional single-minded goal of curing disease. In the delivery of nursing care, current concepts of health and illness reinforce the value of nursing as primarily a caring profession.

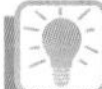
QSEN Considerations: Patient-Centered Care

Human Response to Illness

A common theme in all of nursing theory is that nursing is concerned with helping people cope with adverse physiologic, psychosocial, and spiritual responses to illness, rather than with treating the illness itself.

Although the nurse is involved in curing those who are ill or injured, this goal is primarily under the primary health care provider's control. Nurses have traditionally been concerned with promoting good health habits in their patients and giving them the support they need to cope with illness. Since Florence Nightingale, nurses have encouraged a wholesome environment in the home, hospital or other health care agency, and community.

Nurses seek to help patients use their **coping** (adjusting to or accepting challenges) abilities to best advantage and to adapt to conditions that cannot be changed. Nurses can help a patient with a chronic and incurable illness to minimize its harmful effects and encourage her to continue to set and attain goals in other dimensions of life.

THE CONSUMER CONCEPT OF HEALTH AND ILLNESS

Nursing places a high value on collaboration with people to help them become more independent and better able to meet their own health care needs. To achieve the goals of health promotion, disease prevention, and recovery from the effects of illness and injury, people must be both able and willing to accept responsibility for their health-related behaviors.

HEALTH AND ILLNESS BEHAVIORS

Health and illness behaviors are based on what a person knows and believes about health and illness and how one's own health is assessed.

Health behavior can be defined as any action undertaken to promote health, prevent disease, or detect disease in an early, **asymptomatic** (without symptoms) stage. ***Illness behavior*** is any activity a person takes to determine her actual state of health and to seek a suitable remedy for a health problem.

Some examples of health behavior include watching dietary intake to avoid becoming overweight, exercising regularly, obtaining available immunizations against communicable diseases, and having regular physical examinations. Health care providers encourage these behaviors because they perceive them as valuable. **If a patient does not undertake these behaviors when they have been recommended, then the nurse must consider whether there is a conflict in values between health care personnel and the patient.** Because of cultural and personal differences, not everyone views certain health practices and behaviors in the same way. What one eats or refuses to eat can be influenced by religious and cultural beliefs. Whether one allows oneself or one's children to be immunized can be dictated by religious convictions and restrictions. Early detection of disease can depend on a person's knowledge about normal physiology and psychology and signs of abnormal conditions of the body and mind.

Illness behavior is equally complex. Because it involves actions undertaken by an ill person, the underlying question the person must answer is "What does it mean to be ill?" or "How do I know I am ill?" The nurse must consider what the person knows about health and deviations from health, and what is believed to be an appropriate remedy for the health problems. Examples of illness behavior include consulting a physician or nurse, consulting the pharmacist, visiting a neighborhood health care clinic, and taking prescribed medications.

CULTURAL INFLUENCES ON CONCEPTS OF HEALTH AND ILLNESS

Great cultural diversity in the United States means there are many differences between the values and practices of various ethnic and minority groups. Effective nursing care, whatever the setting, depends on an appreciation of these differences and adjustments in care to accommodate them.

Some areas in which differences among racial and ethnic groups are most apparent are attitudes and practices related to birth, death, and general health care; susceptibility to specific diseases; responses to pain and suffering; personal hygiene and sense of privacy; and adjustment to life changes. Additionally, the words and concepts used to communicate feelings and behaviors related to health practices and remedies for sickness are different in each cultural group (Table 2.1).

The attitudes, beliefs, and practices of a cultural group may or may not conform to the nurse's idea of what is a productive and beneficial action of health promotion or illness prevention.

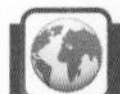
Cultural Considerations

TOUCHING

It is important to know your patient's cultural beliefs with respect to touching before beginning a hands-on examination. You may need to ask permission to touch or you may need a relative in the room. The patient may insist that someone of the same gender perform the examination.

Typically, health care professionals in the United States and other countries influenced by Western

Table 2.1 Cross-Cultural Examples of Cultural Phenomena Affecting Nursing Care

NATIONS OF ORIGIN	COMMUNICATION	SPACE	TIME ORIENTATION	SOCIAL ORGANIZATION	ENVIRONMENTAL CONTROL	BIOLOGIC VARIATIONS
Asian China India Hawaii Philippines Korea Japan Southeast Asia (Laos, Cambodia, Vietnam)	National language preference Dialects, written characters Use of silence Nonverbal and contextual cuing	Noncontact people	Present	Family: hierarchical structure, loyalty Devotion to tradition Many religions (e.g., Buddhism, Islam, Hinduism, Taoism, and Christianity) Community social organizations	Traditional health and illness beliefs Use of traditional medicines Traditional practitioners: Chinese physicians and herbalists	Liver cancer Stomach cancer Coccidioidomycosis Hypertension Lactose intolerance
African West coast (as slaves) Many African countries West Indian islands Dominican Republic Haiti Jamaica	National languages Dialect: pidgin, creole, Spanish, and French	Close personal space	Present over future	Family: many female, single parent Large, extended family networks Strong church affiliation within community Community social organizations	Traditional health and illness beliefs Folk medicine tradition Traditional healer: root worker	Sickle cell anemia Hypertension Esophageal cancer Stomach cancer Coccidioidomycosis Lactose intolerance
European Germany England Italy Ireland Other European countries	National languages Many learn English immediately	Noncontact people Aloof; Distant Southern countries: closer contact and touch	Future over present	Nuclear families Extended families Judeo-Christian religions Community social organizations	Primary reliance on modern health care system Traditional health and illness beliefs Some remaining folk medicine traditions	Breast cancer Heart disease Diabetes mellitus Thalassemia
American Indian 500 American Indian tribes Aleuts Eskimos	Tribal languages Use of silence and body language	Space very important and has no boundaries	Present	Extremely family oriented Biologic and extended families Children taught to respect traditions Community social organizations	Traditional health and illness beliefs Folk medicine tradition Traditional healer: medicine man	Accidents Heart disease Cirrhosis of the liver Diabetes mellitus
Hispanic countries Spain Cuba Mexico Central and South America	Spanish or Portuguese primary language	Tactile relationships Touch Handshakes Embracing Value physical presence	Present	Nuclear family Extended families *Compadragos;* godparents Community social organizations	Traditional health and illness beliefs Folk medicine tradition Traditional healers: *curandero, esperitista, partera,* and *señora*	Diabetes mellitus Parasites Coccidioidomycosis Lactose intolerance

Modified from Potter, P. A., & Perry, A. G. (2005). *Fundamentals of nursing* (6th ed.). St. Louis: Elsevier Mosby. Compiled by Rachel Spector, RN, PhD.

medical science have been taught according to the values and beliefs of a white, middle-class society. However, the cultural groups they care for may not necessarily share these values and beliefs. Unless this conflict is resolved, there may be a problem in communication and in meeting the goals of health care. The nurse's problem may lie in unrealistic expectations of what the patient can be convinced to do or of what can be done for her. The patient may experience problems because the quality and type of care desired may not be delivered. In addition, patients may have low **health literacy** (knowledge and skill making health care decisions). Low health literacy can adversely affect patient outcomes (Dickens, 2013).

Many cultural health beliefs are based on folk medicine passed down through the generations within a culture. Many cultures have their own healers: for example, a **medicine man, shaman,** or **curandero.** Those within the culture often seek the advice of this person before going to a licensed health professional. Beliefs in the various cures that the cultural healer suggests are powerful. Respect for the person's cultural beliefs in all areas is required to gain the patient's trust and for advice and patient education to be effective.

Assessment must be done without criticism, with an open mind, and with active listening. Judgmental terms such as *noncompliant, uncooperative, ignorant, lazy,* or *unmotivated* should not be used to describe another person's health behavior.

No conditions or strings should be attached to the unspoken contract between the nurse and the patient. The nurse need not condone what a patient is doing or not doing to maintain or restore health. The nursing point of view may be respectfully conveyed to the patient. Each patient must be dealt with as a unique individual whose concepts of health and illness and health care might be different from one's own.

THE HOLISTIC APPROACH

Nurses take a **holistic** approach to caring for the sick and promoting wellness. A holistic approach is one that considers the person's biologic, psychological, sociological, and spiritual aspects and needs. The current focus on holism was stimulated by Jan Smuts, a noted South African man who formulated a philosophical theory of holism. The value we place on human life, our ability to deal with sickness and death, and our decisions about how to behave toward other people are all profoundly influenced by our basic beliefs about other humans and our relationships with them. Some basic beliefs central to the holistic approach include the following:

- Each person is a unique integration of body, mind, and spirit, and the unified whole is more than the sum of the parts. A change in one aspect of a person's life brings about change in every aspect of her being and alters the quality of the whole.
- Each person has potential for growth in knowledge and skills and in becoming more loving toward herself and others.
- Humans are naturally inclined to be healthy; each of us has responsibility for our own well-being, self-healing, and self-care.
- The "person" of an individual belongs to herself; therefore, decisions about what happens to that person rightfully belong to the owner.
- The focal point of healing efforts is the person.
- Health care providers intervene on behalf of the adult patient only when their help is sought by the patient or when health needs cannot be met.

QSEN Considerations: Patient-Centered Care

Focus on the Patient

The focal point of healing efforts is patient-centered care, not the disease or injury.

QSEN Considerations: Teamwork and Collaboration

Patient as a Team Member

The relationship between health care professionals and their patients should be one of cooperation.

In holistic health care, traditional methods of surgical intervention and drug prescription are being combined with or replaced by acupuncture, acupressure, biofeedback, meditation to reduce tension and **stress** (biologic reactions to an adverse stimulus), and various relaxation techniques for the management of pain, to name some of the less traditional approaches. Chiropractic care, once looked on as questionable, is now covered by many insurance companies. Insurance companies are also becoming more inclined to pay for acupressure or acupuncture for treatment of pain.

MASLOW'S THEORY OF BASIC NEEDS

Nurses attempt to assist patients in meeting their needs and thereby achieving a higher level of health. People respond to needs as "whole" and integrated beings. Abraham Maslow, a psychologist, identified basic needs that must be met for existence and higher level needs for healthy integration of the whole being. He proposed a hierarchy of human needs as an explanation for the forces that motivate human behavior. **Hierarchy** is defined as the arrangement of objects, elements, or values in order of their importance (Maslow, 1970). Maslow's basic needs are the foundation of nursing practice, nursing education, and prioritization in the NCLEX-PN. Many nursing programs are built using Maslow's basic needs as the framework. Figure 2.3 shows Maslow's original hierarchy of needs and an adaptation of the hierarchy used to determine priorities of nursing care. Theoretically, the basic physical needs such as food, air, water, and rest must be satisfied before the higher emotional-level needs emerge. This is true in general, **but the order in which**

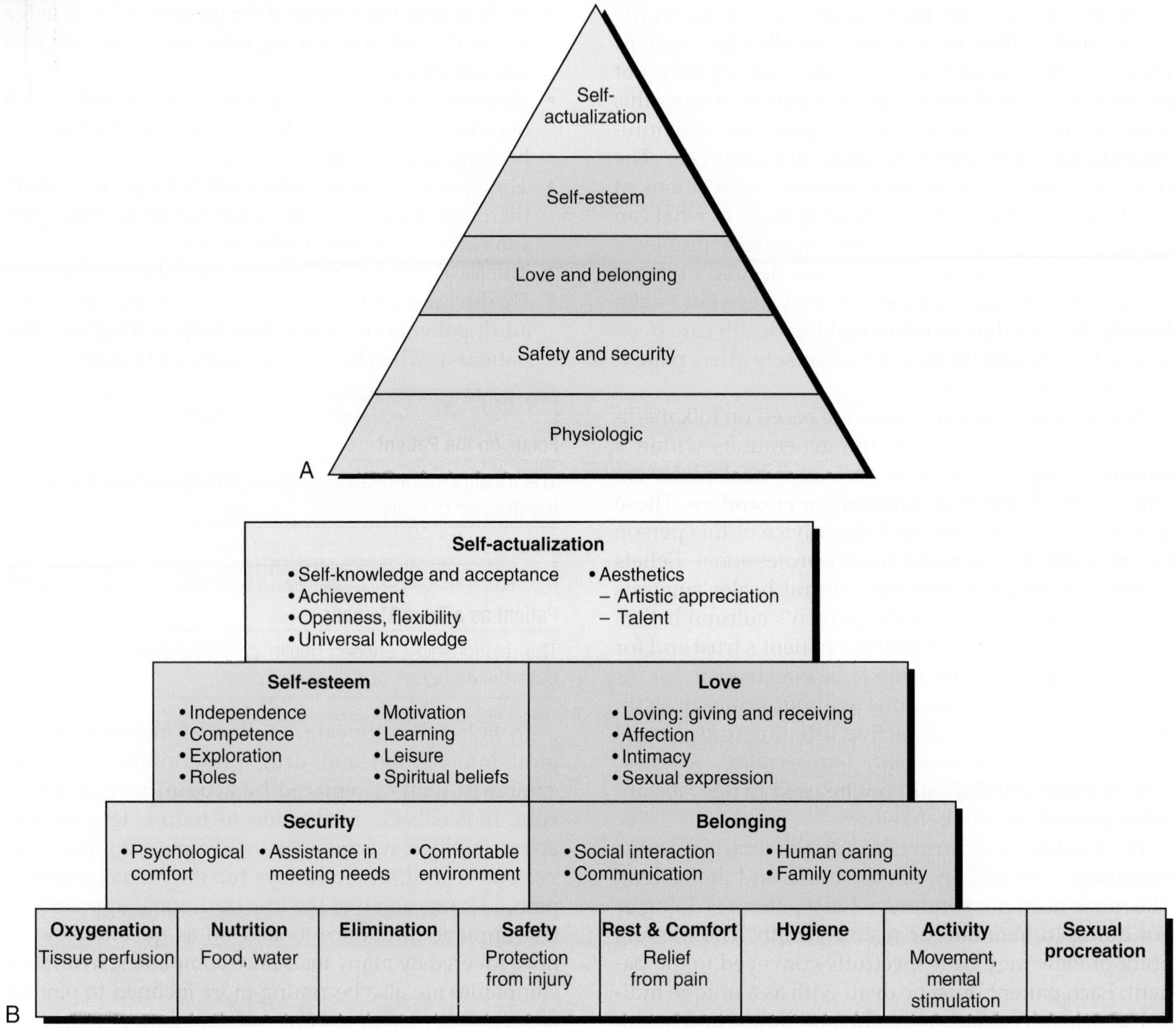

Self-actualization

Self-esteem

Love and belonging

Safety and security

Physiologic

A

Self-actualization
- Self-knowledge and acceptance
- Achievement
- Openness, flexibility
- Universal knowledge
- Aesthetics
  - Artistic appreciation
  - Talent

Self-esteem
- Independence
- Competence
- Exploration
- Roles
- Motivation
- Learning
- Leisure
- Spiritual beliefs

Love
- Loving: giving and receiving
- Affection
- Intimacy
- Sexual expression

Security
- Psychological comfort
- Assistance in meeting needs
- Comfortable environment

Belonging
- Social interaction
- Communication
- Human caring
- Family community

Oxygenation	Nutrition	Elimination	Safety	Rest & Comfort	Hygiene	Activity	Sexual procreation
Tissue perfusion	Food, water		Protection from injury	Relief from pain		Movement, mental stimulation	

B

FIGURE 2.3 (A) Maslow's hierarchy of needs. (B) Evolving hierarchy of needs adapted by nursing to help to determine priorities of care. (From deWit, S. C. [1998]. *Essentials of medical-surgical nursing* [4th ed.]. Philadelphia, PA: Saunders.)

needs are felt and become important to an individual is different from person to person and from situation to situation.

Once a human need is met, it does not remain satisfied forever. This is obviously true about food, water, air, and other basic first-level physiologic needs. In addition to continually needing food, people need assurance that they are important, held in esteem, and safe and secure from harm. The patient who is receiving medications and treatments for her illness also needs personal contact with loving and caring people.

Physiologic Needs

Fundamental physical needs are essential to maintaining life. The first physiologic need is for oxygen; this is immediately followed by the need for adequate cardiovascular function to supply the tissues with blood. The needs for adequate nutrition and for elimination come next.

Basic safety needs are almost as important as physiologic needs. If the patient cannot be protected from the dangers of being burned or a severe fall, attending to her physiologic needs is useless.

QSEN Considerations: Safety

Protect from Harm

Protection from physical harm, from a nursing standpoint, is often equivalent in importance to physical needs.

The need for rest comes next, and this includes freedom from pain, which can greatly interfere with rest. Hygiene needs follow the need for rest because good hygiene is a part of providing comfort, and it adds a measure of safety and protection against the invasion of bacteria.

Musculoskeletal activity is also a basic physiologic need because without activity of the muscles and joints, atrophy and deformity will occur, preventing normal function of the muscles and joints. Nurses therefore assist the patient with movement and ambulation or perform passive range-of-motion exercises for immobile patients.

Sexual expression is a physiologic and psychological need. Survival of a group in society clearly depends on sexual intercourse as a means of procreation to extend the existence of the group. Gratification of sexual needs fits best in the areas of self-esteem and love.

Security and Belonging

Once basic physiologic needs are satisfied, the needs for security and belonging demand attention. Security for patients mainly depends on the reassurance that their physiologic and safety needs will be met. Security also includes protection from psychological harm; freedom from anxiety and fear; and the need for structure, order, and a peaceful environment. The hospitalized child and the older adult are particularly susceptible to stress created by an unfamiliar, disorderly, or hazardous environment. People value order, routine, and rhythm in their daily lives and thrive more readily in an environment in which they believe that these things are present, although it should be remembered that orderliness and routine are much more important to some people than to others.

Adults who suddenly become ill might be anxious about finances, loss of control, change in their body image, continuation of employment, and what will happen to them in the future, if they must cope with the effects of a permanently disabling illness or injury. Therefore, emotional support from the nurse is very important. **Active listening on the part of the nurse is essential in meeting patients' security needs because, to feel secure, they must feel that their needs are being accurately perceived.**

Each person needs to feel that she belongs or is attached to others. People need to feel cared about, and they function best if they feel a sense of community with others. Some social interaction is essential to a sense of well-being and psychological balance (Fig. 2.4).

Communication is the method by which human interaction takes place and is therefore very important. Providing a means of communication, encouraging sharing of thoughts and feelings, and therapeutically interacting with the patient are at the core of good nursing practice. One can perhaps meet the patient's basic physiologic needs without communication, but it is impossible to meet other needs if good communication is not present. **Adequate feedback, clarification, and validation of communication are essential.**

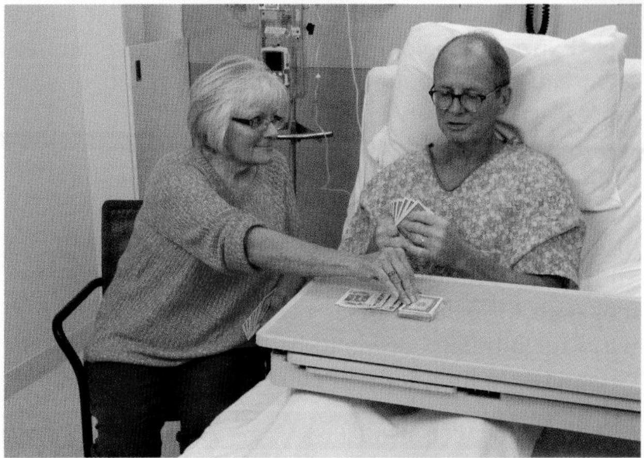

FIGURE 2.4 Spouse sharing leisure time with patient.

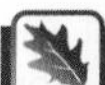 **Life Span Considerations**

Older Adults

Familiarity helps establish secure feelings. If someone comes into an older adult's room or house and rearranges that person's belongings, it threatens the older adult's feelings of security because she no longer knows where things are located.

Self-Esteem and Love

Self-esteem and love are interrelated because one cannot truly love others until one first loves or accepts oneself. Self-esteem develops from feelings of independence, competence, and self-respect and from recognition, appreciation, and respect from others. One's employment, or work, and various roles (e.g., as husband/wife, father/mother, brother/sister, child, or community leader) all contribute to self-esteem. For many, spiritual belief systems are an integral part of the sense of self and of one's relationship to the universe. Gratification of sexual needs contributes to the individual's feeling of wholeness and identification and behavior as a male or a female.

Freedom from boredom, mental stimulation, motivation to seek knowledge, and learning also play a role in self-esteem. People have a desire and a need to explore the environment and universe around them. Illness often brings about the need for new knowledge to provide for adequate self-care. Without this necessary learning, self-esteem will decrease. The nurse must become the teacher, helping the patient meet these needs.

Balance in a person's life is brought about by the ability to enjoy leisure activity, to play, and to seek things that bring a measure of happiness.

Illness and adversity, particularly physical adversity, often damage the patient's self-esteem. Nurses can be instrumental in helping to rebuild feelings of competence, independence, and self-respect.

Love consists of both giving and receiving. Without love and attention, an infant will withdraw and gradually die despite having her physiologic needs met. Extreme, prolonged deprivation of love and esteem can bring about neurotic behavior and organic illness.

Intimacy—the greater degree of connectedness, of feeling that one understands and is understood by another—is one of the fibers of love. The achievement of intimacy is the developmental task of the teenager and young adult. However, illness can greatly interfere with intimacy. Nurses need to help patients find ways for intimacy needs to be fulfilled, especially for patients with long-term or chronic illnesses.

 Life Span Considerations

Older Adults

An older adult who no longer has a mate or family, and whose close friends have all died, may become discouraged and depressed. Depression may progress to the degree that the person feels there is no reason to keep on living. This person needs psychological support and social integration to make new friends who will provide a measure of caring and attachment.

Self-Actualization

Self-actualization (reaching one's full potential) is a stage to which people do not advance until the physiologic, security and belonging, self-esteem, and love needs have been met. Self-actualization occurs when individuals are comfortable with themselves and are certain of their beliefs and values. These people are self-reliant, flexible, and open to new ideas; have sought knowledge and truth; and function close to their full potential. Creative expression, whether in an area of performance or appreciation, is part of the self-actualization process. Self-actualization is an ongoing process, not something reached at a particular time. Nursing actions that facilitate self-actualization are pertinent mainly during rehabilitation periods, when the nurse assists the patient in striving to achieve full potential.

Humans are rational, decision-making beings. A person is believed to want to have control over her life, even when choosing dependence over independence. Although a person is free to choose, there is no guarantee that every choice will be a wise one. Patients can and do decide not to take prescribed medications, to continue drinking alcohol to excess, to continue smoking, or to ignore advice of any kind offered by health care professionals. Nurses must understand that behavior is based on what a person perceives to be a need and how highly that person values satisfaction of that need.

 Think Critically

If you were ill and hospitalized, how would you prioritize the basic needs for yourself? Which areas would be most important to you in that situation?

HOMEOSTASIS

Homeostasis is a term first coined by W. B. Cannon in 1939 to describe a tendency of biologic systems to maintain stability of the internal environment by continually adjusting to changes necessary for survival. The suffix *-stasis* indicates a static or balanced state, involving continual adaptation, movement, and change. The term implies a steady state or equilibrium in which there are variations within set limits. These variations take place in a predictable manner: for example, variations in body temperature, changes in the acidity and alkalinity of body fluids, hormonal production and release, and other changes that occur during every 24-hour period. In health, continuous adaptation and change must take place in the internal environment to maintain its steady state (equilibrium). Another word for homeostasis is *equilibrium* (Cannon, 1967).

To enjoy some degree of health and sense of well-being, one must adapt to factors in the **external** environment. In other words, one needs to be in harmony with elements outside oneself by interacting with and integrating various elements into one's life. These elements include the physical, biologic, and psychosocial factors in the world in which one lives and works.

Living in harmony with external environmental factors requires both adaptability and stability.

Wellness is maintained or regained, at least in part, when one is able to keep a sense of balance while adapting to factors that can upset that balance. These factors include life experiences such as socialization, education, mental and physical stress, satisfaction, and rewards. Perhaps one of the most crucial factors in today's world is change. When change is required, additional stress is put on a person's inner resources, and this in turn can increase susceptibility to illness. When the body's equilibrium is disturbed, stress occurs. Stress is the sum of biologic reactions that take place in response to any **stressor** (adverse stimulus). The stressor may be physical, mental, or emotional and can come from within the body or from the environment. **Stress disturbs the organism's homeostasis and causes the body to attempt to adapt.** Physical or psychological illness may result from excessive stress or ineffective coping mechanisms. Adaptation that results in illness is considered maladaptation.

ADAPTATION

To adapt is to respond to change. The systems of the body have self-regulatory mechanisms to maintain homeostasis. These mechanisms require pathways of communication between the brain and the various body systems. Coordination of the central nervous system, the **autonomic** (not subject to voluntary control) nervous system, and the endocrine system is required for the body to adjust, adapt, and maintain equilibrium.

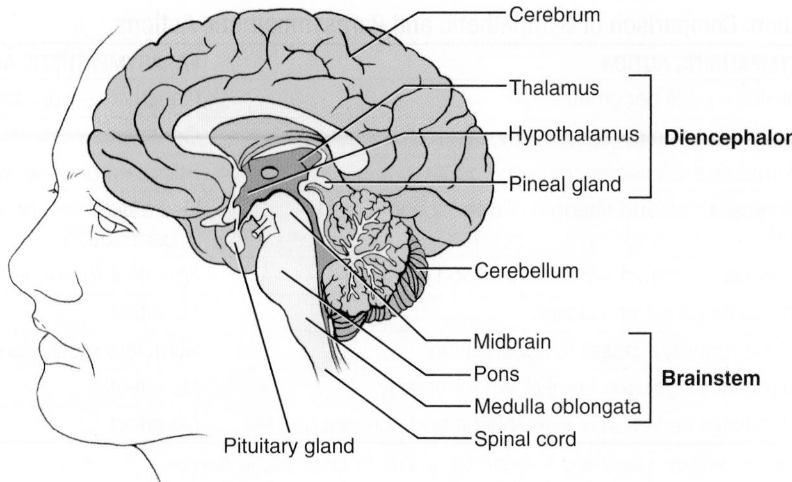

FIGURE 2.5 Central nervous system structures.

The central nervous system, consisting of the brain and spinal cord, coordinates adaptation within the body. The cortex, the thinking part of the brain, communicates with the midbrain and brainstem, which contain many of the structures involved in adaptation and maintenance of physiologic functions. Along with the action of the endocrine glands, these structures regulate breathing, heart action, blood pressure, body temperature, hunger, and sleepiness (Fig. 2.5).

The reticular activating system, a bundle of nerve fibers in the brainstem, transmits messages to the cortex from the sensory receptors of the body and carries messages back to the hypothalamus in the midbrain to regulate physiologic functions. The hypothalamus helps regulate the autonomic nervous system and the secretion of hormones by the endocrine system.

The autonomic nervous system regulates physiologic functions that are essentially automatic and beyond voluntary control. It is divided into the sympathetic and parasympathetic nervous systems. These two divisions act like the gas and the brake pedals of a car as they increase or decrease physiologic response of the body's systems and organs. For example, during vigorous exercise the sympathetic nervous system sends messages to the bronchi of the lungs to dilate so that more oxygen can be delivered. In contrast, when stepping out into bright sunlight, the parasympathetic system relays messages to the muscles controlling the iris of the eye to constrict the pupil so that less light is allowed to hit the retina.

When the brain perceives a situation as threatening, the sympathetic nervous system stimulates the physiologic functions needed for **fight or flight.** This type of reaction occurs when a person is suddenly confronted by a large, snarling dog on a walking path. The alarmed individual becomes more alert, breathes more deeply, and has muscles poised for fight or flight, and the heart pumps harder. Once the threatening situation is over, the parasympathetic nervous system works to restore equilibrium. In certain situations, the parasympathetic system may be stimulated to slow systems down as a protective measure against a perceived threat.

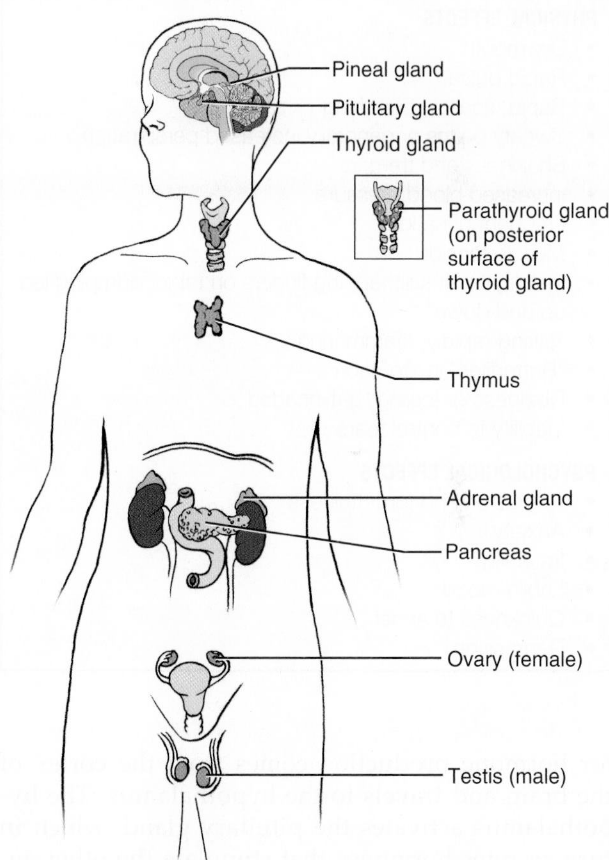

FIGURE 2.6 Major endocrine glands.

Although the autonomic nervous system reacts immediately to a perceived threat, the endocrine system must become involved to sustain the fight-or-flight state. The glands of the endocrine system produce hormones that act on other organs or systems of the body (Fig. 2.6). Initiation of a stimulus

Table 2.2 Alarm Reaction: Comparison of Sympathetic and Parasympathetic Actions

ORGAN	SYMPATHETIC ACTION	PARASYMPATHETIC ACTION
Iris of eye	Dilates—pupil becomes larger	Constricts—pupil becomes smaller
Bronchial tubes	Dilate—provide greater air flow	Constrict
Salivary glands	Stimulate thick secretions—dry mouth	Stimulate profuse, watery secretions
Heart	Increases rate and strength of contraction	Decreases rate; no effect on strength of contraction
Blood vessels	Generally constrict—increased blood pressure	No effect for many
Sweat glands	Stimulate sweat production	No effect
Intestines	Inhibit mobility—possible constipation	Stimulate motility and secretion
Liver	Stimulates glycogen breakdown for energy	No effect
Adrenal medulla	Stimulates secretion of epinephrine and norepinephrine	No effect

Modified from Herlihy, B. (2011). *The human body in health and illness* (4th ed., p. 216). St. Louis: Elsevier Science.

Box 2.1 Common Signs and Symptoms of Stress

PHYSICAL EFFECTS

- Dry mouth
- Rapid pulse
- Rapid, shallow breathing
- Sweaty palms or generally increased perspiration
- Shakiness and tremors
- Increased blood pressure
- Frequent urination
- Muscle tension
- Inability to sit still; tapping fingers on table, pumping leg up and down
- Talking rapidly; stammering
- "Butterflies" in stomach
- Dizziness or feeling light-headed
- Inability to control tears

PSYCHOLOGICAL EFFECTS

- Confusion and forgetfulness
- Anxiety
- Irritability
- Labile moods
- Quickness to anger
- Depression

for hormone production comes from the cortex of the brain and travels to the hypothalamus. The hypothalamus activates the pituitary gland, which in turn secretes hormones that stimulate the other endocrine glands. As long as the body's capacity is not overtaxed, the central nervous system, autonomic nervous system, and endocrine system regulate body systems to maintain homeostasis. Table 2.2 presents body responses when a fight-or-flight reaction occurs. Common signs and symptoms of stress are listed in Box 2.1.

? Think Critically

What signs and symptoms of stress do you exhibit when you face the threat of a major test, such as a final examination?

The General Adaptation Syndrome

In 1950, Hans Selye, a Canadian physician, published his research-based theories on stress. He found that no matter what the nature of the stressor was, the same nonspecific physical response occurred. The body attempted to deal with stressors by secretion of hormones that caused adaptive responses. Selye concluded that stress plays a role in every disease process because of faulty adaptation (maladaptation) by the body. If the body overreacts in defending itself, a surplus of hormones that are favorable to the development of inflammation and problems such as allergy, arthritis, and asthma may develop. When the body underreacts, too many anti-inflammatory hormones are circulating, body defenses are reduced, and serious infection may result.

Selye stated that a general adaptation syndrome (GAS) occurs in response to **long-term** exposure to stress. The stages are the **alarm stage,** the **stage of resistance,** and the **stage of exhaustion.** Brief stress responses result in adjustment by homeostatic mechanisms, and equilibrium is restored. During the alarm stage, hormone release mobilizes the body's defenses. Nonspecific signs of illness such as a slight rise in temperature, a loss of energy, decreased appetite, and a general feeling of malaise occur. During the second stage, the stage of resistance, the body is battling for equilibrium. If this stage is excessive or prolonged, the response becomes maladaptive and a pathologic condition occurs, which may be in the form of a stress-related disorder (Selye, 1974). Box 2.2 lists diseases and disorders considered stress related.

The stage of exhaustion occurs if the stressor is severe enough or is present over a long enough time to deplete the body's resources for adaptation. Critical illness or death results (Fig. 2.7). Examples of stressors that cause the GAS include trauma, burns, infection, severe cold, and emotional upsets.

Selye believed the body adapts to local stressors in similar ways. The local response is called the **local adaptation syndrome** (LAS). This takes place within

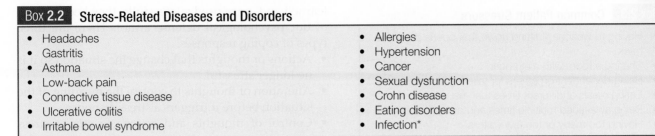

Box 2.2 Stress-Related Diseases and Disorders

- Headaches
- Gastritis
- Asthma
- Low-back pain
- Connective tissue disease
- Ulcerative colitis
- Irritable bowel syndrome
- Allergies
- Hypertension
- Cancer
- Sexual dysfunction
- Crohn disease
- Eating disorders
- Infection*

* Excessive stress weakens the immune system, making the person more vulnerable to invasion by pathogens

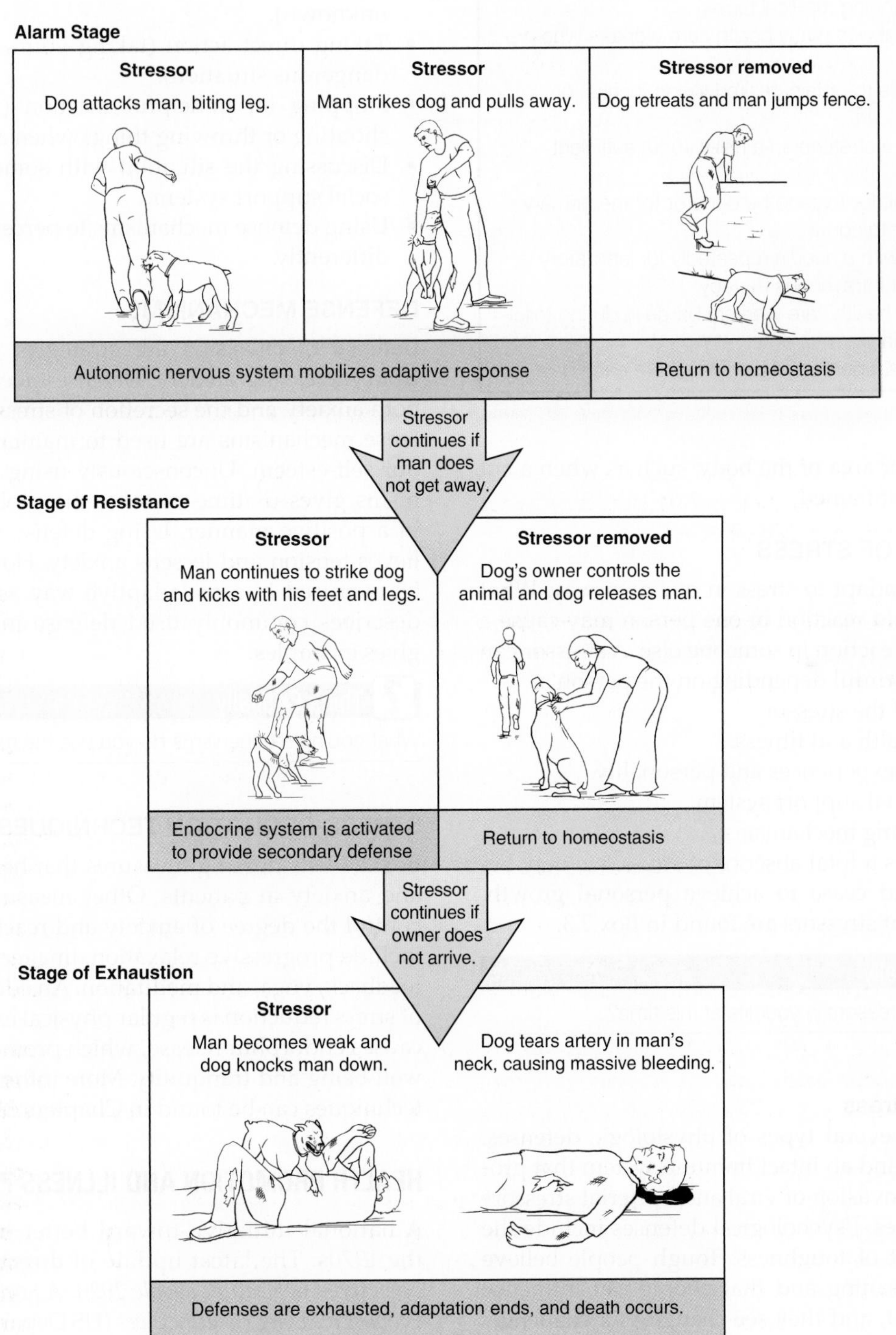

Alarm Stage
Stressor
Dog attacks man, biting leg.
Stressor
Man strikes dog and pulls away.
Stressor removed
Dog retreats and man jumps fence.
Autonomic nervous system mobilizes adaptive response
Return to homeostasis
Stressor continues if man does not get away.
Stage of Resistance
Stressor
Man continues to strike dog and kicks with his feet and legs.
Stressor removed
Dog's owner controls the animal and dog releases man.
Endocrine system is activated to provide secondary defense
Return to homeostasis
Stressor continues if owner does not arrive.
Stage of Exhaustion
Stressor
Man becomes weak and dog knocks man down.
Dog tears artery in man's neck, causing massive bleeding.
Defenses are exhausted, adaptation ends, and death occurs.

FIGURE 2.7 Stages of the general adaptation syndrome.

Box 2.3 Common Patient Stressors

- Having to wear an ill-fitting gown that opens down the back
- Sharing a room with a stranger
- Being dependent on others for toileting or bathing
- Eating meals at different times than usual
- Being awakened multiple times and at odd hours
- Having too many or too few visitors
- Worrying about medical costs, home bills, and family needs
- Being uncertain of the diagnosis and what will happen
- Not understanding medical terms
- Having to deal with many health care workers who are strangers
- Not being able to obtain desired foods, drinks, or objects
- Being left on a stretcher in a hall without sufficient warm covers
- Having to wait for tests to be done or for the primary care provider to come
- Being stuck with a needle repeatedly for laboratory specimens or intravenous therapy
- Having other health care workers barge in during toileting or cleansing
- Having different personnel providing care each day

a single organ or area of the body, such as when a cut finger becomes inflamed.

THE EFFECTS OF STRESS

We all react or adapt to stress in our own way. What may cause a mild reaction in one person may cause a much stronger reaction in someone else. A stressor can be helpful or harmful depending on the person's:

- Perception of the stressor.
- Degree of health and fitness.
- Previous life experiences and personality.
- Available social support system.
- Personal coping mechanisms.

When there is a total absence of stress, we may become bored and cease to achieve personal growth. Common patient stressors are found in Box 2.3.

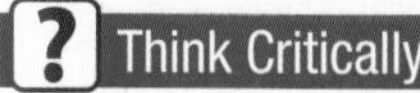

Think Critically

Can you list the stressors in your life at this time?

Coping With Stress

The body has several types of physiologic defenses. Unbroken skin and an intact immune system that protect us against invasion of viral and bacterial stressors are two examples. Psychological defenses include the personality trait of toughness. Tough people believe that life has meaning and that people can influence the environment, and they see change as a challenge. Hardy people cope well. **Coping** means adjusting to or solving challenges. Coping mechanisms help us to resist and master stressors. Coping mechanisms are learned and, once used successfully, they become part of our psychological defense armor. There are three types of coping responses:

- Actions or thoughts that change the situation so it is no longer stressful.
- Alteration of thoughts to control the meaning of the situation before it triggers a stress response.
- Control of thoughts and actions to stop a stress reaction.

Ways to achieve these responses are:

- Seeking information (eliminates fear of the unknown).
- Taking direct action (taking yourself away from a dangerous situation).
- Stopping an unhelpful reaction (refraining from shouting or throwing things when angered).
- Discussing the situation with someone from your social support system.
- Using defense mechanisms to perceive the situation differently.

DEFENSE MECHANISMS

Defense mechanisms are strategies that protect us from increasing anxiety. Defense mechanisms reduce both anxiety and the secretion of stress hormones. Defense mechanisms are used to maintain and improve our self-esteem. Unconsciously using defense mechanisms gives us time to solve the problem and adapt in a positive manner. Using defense mechanisms relieves tension and lessens anxiety. However, they can be overused in a maladaptive way as well. Table 2.3 describes commonly used defense mechanisms, and gives examples.

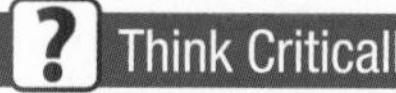

Think Critically

What coping mechanisms do you use the most?

STRESS-REDUCTION TECHNIQUES

Box 2.4 lists nursing measures that help reduce stress and anxiety in patients. Other measures that help to control the degree of anxiety and reaction to stressors include progressive relaxation, imagery, massage, biofeedback, yoga, and meditation. An additional method of stress reduction is regular physical exercise. Exercise causes endorphin release, which promotes a feeling of well-being and tranquility. More information on these techniques can be found in Chapters 31 and 32.

HEALTH PROMOTION AND ILLNESS PREVENTION

A national initiative toward better health began in the 1970s. The latest update of direction, goals, and objectives is *Healthy People 2020: A Society in Which All People Live Long Healthy Lives* (US Department of Health and Human Services, 2010). It is a comprehensive set of objectives for disease prevention and health promotion for the nation, created by scientists. Every nurse

Table 2.3 **Common Defense Mechanisms**

DEFENSE MECHANISMS	CHARACTERISTICS	EXAMPLE
Repression	The unconscious blocking of a wish or desire from conscious awareness.	You forget the name of someone for whom you have intense negative feelings.
Denial	Escaping unpleasant, anxiety-causing thoughts by refusing to acknowledge their existence. There is a persistent refusal to be swayed by evidence.	A woman whose husband died a year ago still speaks of him in the present tense and keeps his wardrobe in the closet.
Projection	Attributing an unconscious impulse, attitude, or behavior to someone else (blaming or scapegoating).	A man who is attracted to his friend's wife on an unconscious level accuses his own wife of flirting with his friend.
Reaction-formation	An intense feeling regarding an object, person, or feeling is out of awareness and is unknowingly acted out consciously in an opposite manner.	You treat someone whom you unconsciously dislike intensely in an overly friendly manner.
Regression	Returning to an earlier level of adaptation when severely threatened.	A child resumes bedwetting, after having long since stopped, after the birth of her baby brother.
Rationalization	Unconsciously falsifying an experience by giving a contrived, socially acceptable, and logical explanation to justify an unpleasant experience or questionable behavior.	A student who did not study for an examination blames his failure on the teacher's poor lecture material and the unfairness of the examination.
Identification	Modeling behavior after someone else.	A 6-year-old girl dresses up in her mother's dress and high-heeled shoes.
Displacement	Discharging intense feelings for one person onto another object or person who is less threatening, thereby satisfying an impulse with a substitute object.	A child who has been scolded by her mother hits her doll with a hairbrush.
Sublimation	Rechanneling an impulse into a more socially desirable object.	A student satisfies sexual curiosity by conducting sophisticated research into sexual behaviors.

Modified from Halter, M. J. (2014). *Varcarolis' foundations of psychiatric mental health nursing: a clinical approach* (7th ed., p. 284). St. Louis: Elsevier Saunders.

Box 2.4 **Measures to Help Reduce Stress and Anxiety in Patients**

- Explain everything: hospital routine; how the TV, lights, and curtains work; procedures; and diagnostic tests.
- Listen carefully to the patient; answer questions.
- Provide privacy; always knock before entering the room.
- Treat the patient with respect.
- Answer call lights promptly.
- Protect confidentiality.
- Check on the patient frequently.
- Make certain that dietary needs and wants are satisfied as much as possible.
- Return to the patient's bedside when you say you will.
- Bring requested as-needed (PRN) medication promptly; do not allow pain to go untreated; better yet, anticipate and offer PRN medications before the patient needs to request them.
- Provide uninterrupted rest and sleep periods; coordinate care and treatments.
- Keep visitors within acceptable numbers and time limits per patient's desire.
- Keep noise to a minimum.
- Insist that roommates respect each other's rights.
- Try to advise patient as to when to expect diagnostic tests to be performed and when the primary care provider usually makes rounds.
- Allow the patient some control: for example, give choices for time of bathing and ambulating.
- Keep the room temperature adjusted to patient's comfort.

has a responsibility to patients to promote better health through patient education about illness prevention; periodic diagnostic testing for hypertension, cancer, and diabetes; and safe health practices. Encouraging achievement of a healthy weight, regular exercise, adequate sleep, proper nutrition, quitting use of tobacco products, refraining from recreational drug use, and moderation of alcohol intake should be a standard part of nursing care. Nurses should model these behaviors for their patients. Specific practices to prevent back injury, latex allergy, spread of infectious agents, and needlestick injury help safeguard the nurse's health.

Illness prevention practices are related to health promotion. They consist of voluntary actions that an individual takes to decrease the potential or actual threat of illness. Such actions are divided into primary, secondary, and tertiary prevention. **Primary prevention** avoids or delays occurrence of a specific disease or disorder. **Secondary prevention** consists of following guidelines for screening for diseases that are easily treated if found early or for detecting return of a disease. **Tertiary prevention** consists of rehabilitation measures after the disease or disorder has stabilized. Following such health practices has been associated with a greater degree of health for people of any age, sex, or economic status. The United States and Canada

Box 2.5 *Healthy People 2020*

The overall goals are:

- Attain high-quality, longer lives free of preventable disease, disability, injury, and premature death.
- Achieve health equity, eliminate disparities, and improve the health of all groups.
- Create social and physical environments that promote good health for all.
- Promote quality of life, healthy development, and healthy behaviors across all life stages.

There are 42 focus areas and many objectives with a target for improvements to be achieved by the year 2020.

have published goals that are for essential health care services *and* involve patient education for disease and accident prevention, health promotion, and self-care behaviors (see Chapter 9). While caring for patients in different settings, nurses assist patients to mobilize and maintain appropriate coping mechanisms and provide patient education practices that promote good health. The overall goals of *Healthy People 2020* can be found in Box 2.5.

 **Health Promotion/Health Promotion Points**

Health Promotion Behaviors

PRIMARY PREVENTION

- Wearing seat belts and helmets
- Eating well-balanced meals
- Not smoking
- Avoiding dangerous behaviors
- Consuming no or minimal alcohol
- Getting scheduled immunizations and an annual flu vaccine
- Maintaining ideal body mass index
- Wearing sunscreen and sunglasses; avoiding tanning beds

SECONDARY PREVENTION

- Having regular Papanicolaou (Pap) smear tests
- Performing a monthly testicular self-examination
- Having mammograms and a colonoscopy as recommended
- Getting skin tests for tuberculosis screening
- Having routine tonometry tests to detect glaucoma

TERTIARY PREVENTION

- Following a cardiac or respiratory rehabilitation program
- Pursuing rehabilitation programs for stroke, head injury, or arthritis

Get Ready for the NCLEX Examination!

Key Points

- Cultural, educational, and social factors affect how people view health and illness.
- The World Health Organization redefined health as “a state of complete physical, mental, and social well-being and not merely the absence of disease or infirmity.”
- Illness occurs in stages: a transition stage (onset), an acceptance stage (sick role), and a convalescence stage (recovery).
- A contemporary definition of being healthy means being able to function well physically and mentally and to express the full range of one’s potentialities within the environment in which one is living.
- Dubos and Dunn promoted the philosophy that health and illness are dynamic states of being, constantly altering, and that each person moves up and down within a spectrum ranging from obvious disease through the absence of detectable disease and on to a state of optimum functioning in all aspects of life.
- Nursing is concerned with helping people cope with adverse physiologic, psychosocial, and spiritual responses to illness, rather than treating the illness itself.
- The essential task of nursing is to enhance and support patients’ healing strengths by helping them to use coping abilities to best advantage and to adapt to conditions that cannot be changed.
- A major goal of nursing is to get people to take charge of their own health and take positive steps to preserve or enhance it through positive health promotion or illness prevention actions.
- Different cultures have different values and beliefs about health and illness; cultural practices must be understood and respected by the nurse.
- A holistic approach considers the person’s physiologic, psychological, sociological, and spiritual aspects and needs.
- Maslow described a hierarchy of needs that nursing has adopted for prioritizing patient problems and care. The five areas of need established by Maslow are physiologic, safety and security, love and belonging, self-esteem, and self-actualization.
- Homeostasis is the tendency of the body’s biologic systems to adjust continually to maintain constant conditions that are optimal to maintaining life and health. It involves continual adaptation (response to change).
- Stress disturbs homeostasis and causes the body to attempt to adapt.
- When the body receives a threat, the sympathetic nervous system stimulates the physiologic functions needed for fight or flight. Once the threat is over, the parasympathetic nervous system mediates to return the physiologic functions to normal.
- Hans Selye developed the theory of the GAS, which occurs in three stages: the alarm stage, the stage of resistance, and the stage of exhaustion.
- Coping mechanisms are learned to help in the defense against stress. Defense mechanisms are unconscious strategies that protect us from increasing anxiety.
- Health can be promoted by personal practices regarding diet, exercise, rest, and refraining from risky health behaviors.

- Illness may be prevented by voluntary actions regarding health care practices, screening tests, and participation in treatment regimens.

Additional Learning Resources

SG Go to your Study Guide for additional learning activities to help you master this chapter content.

evolve Go to your Evolve website at http://evolve.elsevier.com/Williams/fundamental for additional online resources.

Online Resources

- *Hans Selye's General Adaptation Syndrome,* www.essenceofstressrelief.com/general-adaptation-syndrome.html
- *Culture Clues (cultural information),* http://depts.washington.edu/pfes/CultureClues.htm
- *Maslow's Hierarchy of Needs,* www.businessballs.com/maslow.htm

Review Questions for the NCLEX Examination

*Choose the **best** answer(s) for each question.*

1. Which statement *best* describes health? Health is:
   1. A relative state of being.
   2. The total state of physical and psychological well-being.
   3. The state of functioning well physically, mentally, and socially.
   4. Being free of sickness or infirmity.
2. It is important that the nurse understand that certain cultural traits should be assessed in patients. Patients of Asian, African, and Hispanic descent should be assessed for:
   1. Stomach cancer.
   2. Retinopathy.
   3. Sickle cell anemia.
   4. Lactose intolerance.
3. It is important to assess a patient's *actual* cultural beliefs because:
   1. A patient may not adhere to the usual health beliefs of her culture.
   2. Cultural beliefs play a major role in how the patient perceives herself.
   3. The family's beliefs are inherent in the patient.
   4. Cultural diversity is present in all parts of the United States.
4. When setting priorities of patient needs according to Maslow's hierarchy, you should: *(Select all that apply.)*
   1. Only consider physiologic needs.
   2. Consider airway status first.
   3. Consider safety a high priority.
   4. Place self-esteem needs before security needs.
   5. Place activity needs before belonging needs.
   6. Consider elimination needs before rest and comfort needs.
5. A patient had major surgery and says she is worried about what is happening at home, is worried about not being there to coach the soccer team tomorrow, is feeling pain, and wants to see her husband. Which action would you take *first?*
   1. Tell her not to worry about things at home.
   2. Allow her to call the children at home.
   3. Administer pain medication.
   4. Check to see who might be able to coach the soccer team.
   5. Put in a call to her husband so she can obtain information and have him arrange for someone to coach the soccer team.
6. Which is the *best* description of homeostasis?
   1. It is the tendency of the body to adjust constantly to changing conditions.
   2. It occurs when the equilibrium of the body is disturbed.
   3. It is the biologic reaction that takes place in response to a stressor.
   4. It is a static condition of the body during health.
7. The effects of stress on a person partially depend on:
   1. The presence of prior illness.
   2. The time of day it occurs.
   3. The surrounding environment.
   4. The perception of the stressor.
8. Common sympathetic reactions to a stressor that occurs suddenly include: *(Select all that apply.)*
   1. Constriction of the pupils in the eyes.
   2. Increase in saliva and tear production.
   3. A "weak in the knees" feeling.
   4. Pounding of the heart with rapid pulse.
   5. Dilation of the pupils.
   6. Increased blood pressure.

Critical Thinking Activities

Discuss the following questions with your classmates.

1. Share some of your family's values and beliefs that contribute to your own definition of health.
2. What does *illness* mean to you?
3. What are your most effective coping techniques? How can you increase your ability to cope effectively with stress?
4. How would you go about helping a patient mobilize personal coping mechanisms?

chapter

3 Legal and Ethical Aspects of Nursing

http://evolve.elsevier.com/Williams/fundamental

Objectives

Upon completing this chapter, you should be able to do the following:

Theory

1. Explain the legal requirements for the practice of nursing and how they relate to a student nurse.
2. Identify the consequences of violating the nurse practice act.
3. Examine the issue of professional accountability, professional discipline, and continuing education for licensed nurses.
4. Compare and contrast the terms *negligence* and *malpractice.*
5. Discuss what you can do to protect yourself from lawsuits or the damages of lawsuits.
6. Differentiate a code of ethics from laws or regulations governing nursing, and compare the similarities of the codes of ethics from the NFLPN, NAPNES, and ANA.
7. Describe the NAPNES standards of practice.

Clinical Practice

1. Reflect on how laws relating to discrimination, workplace safety, child abuse, and sexual harassment affect your nursing practice.
2. Discuss the National Patient Safety Goals and identify where these can be found.
3. Interpret rights that a patient has in a hospital, nursing home, community setting, or psychiatric facility.
4. Describe four elements of informed consent.
5. Explain advance directives and the advantage of having them written out.
6. Consider the relationship between the HIPAA and use of social media.

Key Terms

accountability (ă-kŏwn-tă-BĬ-lĭ-tē, p. 33)
advance directive (p. 39)
assault (ă-SĂLT, p. 40)
assignment (p. 33)
battery (p. 40)
competent (p. 38)
confidential (cŏn-fĭ-DĔN-shŭl, p. 36)
consent (p. 38)
defamation (dĕ-fă-MĀ-shŭn, p. 40)
delegation (p. 33)
discrimination (p. 34)
do-not-resuscitate (DNR) orders (rē-SŬ-sĭ-tāt, p. 39)
ethical codes, ethical principles, and ethics committee (p. 31)
ethics (p. 43)
euthanasia (yū-thă-NĀ-zhē-ă, p. 45)
false imprisonment (p. 41)
health care agent (p. 39)
incident report (p. 43)
invasion of privacy (p. 40)
laws (p. 31)
liability (lī-ă-BĬL-ĭ-tē, p. 39)
libel (LĪ-bŭl, p. 40)
living will (p. 39)
malpractice (măl-PRĂK-tĭs, p. 39)
negligence (p. 39)
nondisclosure agreement (p. 41)
nurse licensure compacts (p. 32)
nurse practice act (p. 32)
Occupational Safety and Health (OSH) Act (ŏ-kū-PĀ-shŭn-ŭl, p. 33)
Occupational Safety and Health Administration (OSHA) (p. 33)
patient advocate (ĂD-vō-kăt, p. 39)
privilege (PRĬ-vĭ-lĕj, p. 31)
protective devices (p. 41)
prudent (p. 39)
Quality and Safety Education for Nurses (QSEN) project (p. 35)
reciprocity (rĕ-cĭ-PRŎ-cĭ-tē, p. 32)
release (p. 39)
sentinel event (p. 35)
sexual harassment (hă-RĂS-mĭnt, p. 34)
slander (p. 40)
standards of care (p. 33)
statutes (p. 32)
tort (p. 32)
whistle-blowing (p. 45)

 Concepts Covered in This Chapter

- Communication
- Ethics
- Health care law
- Professionalism
- Quality

An understanding of legal and ethical codes is essential for nurses to practice safely and to protect the rights of patients and co-workers. Nurses work in situations that give them **privilege** (permission to do what is usually not permitted in other circumstances) in respect to a patient's body and emotions. Laws define the boundaries of that privilege and make clear the nurse's rights and responsibilities. **Ethical codes** (actions and beliefs approved of by a particular group of people) are different from laws; they are important because not all situations are covered by a law, and there may not be one *right* action. In these situations, **ethical principles** (rules of right and wrong from an ethical point of view) are applied, often by an **ethics committee** (a committee formed to consider ethical problems).

SOURCE OF LAW

Laws are rules of conduct that are established by our government (Box 3.1 lists specialized vocabulary). In the United States, law comes from three sources: the Constitution and Bill of Rights, laws made by elected officials, and regulations made by agencies created by elected officials. Constitutional laws, both federal and state, provide for basic rights and create the legislative bodies (senate and assembly) that write laws governing our lives.

Judicial law results when a law or court decision is challenged in the courts and the judge affirms or reverses the decision. This is called "establishing a precedent" because in the future other judges will base their decisions on the preceding, or earlier, decision. Our federal Supreme Court is the highest court to which an appeal of a court decision can be brought. One well-known health care issue that has been ruled on by the Supreme Court was *Roe v. Wade* (1972), which established a woman's right to obtain an elective abortion. More recently, state courts are hearing cases challenging laws that deal with abortion, euthanasia, and assisted suicide.

Box 3.1 Legal Terms and Definitions

Advance directive: Written statement expressing the patient's wishes regarding future consent for or refusal of treatment if the patient is incapable of participating in decision making.

Appeal: Challenge to a court decision; a higher court will judge whether the original decision is affirmed or reversed.

Civil rights, civil law: Personal or individual conditions (e.g., life, liberty, and privacy) guaranteed by the Constitution, the Bill of Rights, and federal or regulatory law.

Competent: Mentally and emotionally able to understand and act (make choices); able to appreciate consequences of actions.

Controlled substance: Specific drugs with a potential for abuse, such as narcotics, tranquilizers, stimulants, and sedatives. Laws regulate how these are prescribed, dispensed, and stored.

Crime: Violation of public law.

Damages: The monetary award to an injured plaintiff when the defendant is found responsible for the injury.

Defendant: Person accused of violation of public law (crime) or civil law (tort).

Emancipated minor: Person under 18 years of age who is legally considered an adult, usually because of marriage, parenthood, or enlistment in the armed services.

Felony: A serious crime that may result in a prison term of more than 1 year.

Health care agent: Person designated by the patient to make health care decisions when the patient is incapacitated (not able to make those decisions). Usually part of an advance directive.

Liability: Responsibility to pay or compensate for a loss or injury resulting from one's negligence.

Litigation: Lawsuit; legal process to prove the facts of a dispute.

Malpractice: When a professional causes harm by failing to meet the standard of care; failure to do what a reasonable and prudent person in a similar situation would do.

Malpractice insurance: Policy that protects a nurse from the expense of defending herself from lawsuit; will pay the amount awarded up to policy limits if a nurse is found guilty of malpractice.

Medical power of attorney: Legal assignment of the ability to make health care decisions for another person; similar to a health care agent.

Misdemeanor: Less serious crime than felony; may result in fines, imprisonment of 1 year or less, or both.

Negligence: Departure from the standard of care, which, under similar circumstances, would have ordinarily been exercised by a similarly trained and experienced professional.

Plaintiff: Person who believes he or she has been injured by the actions of another and seeks to prove it in a court of law.

Power of attorney: Legal action to allow a person to conduct business matters for another.

Precedent: A judicial decision that is used as a guide in interpreting the law and deciding cases afterward.

Privileged relationship: One that requires confidentiality; trust that information gained in the relationship will not be made public.

Statute: Legal term for a law.

Tort: Violation of a civil law; a wrong against an individual.

Administrative law comes from agencies created by the legislature. In health care, agencies such as the Department of Health and Human Services or the Office of Professional Licensing oversee nursing and the other health care professions. An individual state board of nursing is also an example of an agency that enforces administrative law. These agencies write regulations or rules that control the profession and its practice. Administrative law governs schools of nursing; licensure; hospitals, nursing homes, and home health agencies; and health care insurance such as Medicare, Medicaid, or private insurance company policies.

CIVIL AND CRIMINAL LAW

Statutes (laws) may be either civil or criminal. Civil law deals with potential wrongdoing of a person against another person. Civil law guarantees individual rights, and a **tort** is a violation of civil law. You may be guilty of a tort if you harm a patient, for example, by administering the wrong dose of medication. A lawsuit may result, and, if the **defendant** is found guilty, a monetary award may be given to the **plaintiff.**

Criminal law deals with potential wrongdoing of a person against society. A **crime** is a wrong against society, and imprisonment and/or fines may result if one is convicted of a crime. Criminal action charges in nursing could result if a nurse were involved in drug diversion, patient abuse, intentional death, or mercy killing. Serious crimes are called **felonies** and are punished with prison terms of a year of more, or even the death penalty; less serious crimes are **misdemeanors** and may result in prison terms of less than a year, monetary fines, or both.

LAWS RELATED TO NURSING PRACTICE AND LICENSURE

NURSE PRACTICE ACT

State licensure is required to practice nursing in the United States, and each state writes its own laws and regulations regarding licensure, in what is called a **nurse practice act.** These laws define the scope of nursing practice and provide for the regulation of the profession by a state board of nursing. ***It is important to know the nurse practice act of the state in which you work because these can differ from state to state.***

SCOPE OF PRACTICE

The scope of practice includes the definition of nursing for the registered nurse (RN) and the licensed practical or vocational nurse (LPN or LVN) and may include definitions for advanced practice nurses such as nurse practitioners or nurse anesthetists. Nurse practice acts regulate the degree of dependence or independence of a licensed nurse working with or under other nurses, physicians, and health care providers. For example, an LPN/LVN practices under the direction of an RN, advanced practice RN, physician assistant, physician, dentist, or podiatrist. Nurses must follow the lawful order of a physician (or other health care providers, as stipulated by the state's nurse practice act) unless it is harmful to the patient, and must have an order to perform certain functions, such as administering prescription drugs or placing a patient in a protective device. It is important to maintain competence in your area of employment so that you can determine whether an order may be harmful to a patient.

LICENSURE

Eligibility for licensure is determined by each state's board of nursing, usually involving completion of an approved educational program. The National Council of State Boards of Nursing, which develops the National Council Licensure Examination (NCLEX), has a representative from each of the state boards of nursing who has input on the examination. A passing score on this test is accepted by the states for initial licensure when all other state requirements for eligibility are met. A current trend regarding licensure involves the creation of **nurse licensure compacts**, whereby certain participating states allow nurses to be licensed in one state and practice in any state belonging to the compact. Nurses living in a noncompact state can apply for **reciprocity** (recognition of one state's nursing license by another state).

Student Nurses

Student nurses are held to the same standards as a licensed nurse. This means that although a student nurse may not perform a task as quickly or as smoothly as the licensed nurse would, the student is expected to perform it as effectively. In other words, she must achieve the same outcome without harm to the patient. The student is legally responsible for her own actions or inaction, and many schools require the student to carry **malpractice insurance.** The instructor who supervises a student is responsible for proper instruction and adequate supervision and evaluation of a student. Instructors are responsible for assigning students to patients of an appropriate level of complexity so that they do not jeopardize patient safety. A student's responsibility is to consult with the instructor when she is unsure in a situation, or when a patient's condition is changing rapidly. **Student nurses need to know the nurse practice act and its definition of nursing in the state where they are practicing, and they must not exceed the scope of practice. It is not legal to do something beyond the scope of nursing practice just because you were told to do so.** Hospitals or health care agencies may impose limitations on student practice, but they may not add duties or responsibilities beyond the scope of practice in that state.

 QSEN Considerations: Safety

Self-Awareness and Safety

It is important for you as a student to have self-awareness of your knowledge and clinical abilities. If there is any doubt of your competence to perform a task or care for a particular patient, double-check with your instructor.

PROFESSIONAL ACCOUNTABILITY

Accountability is taking responsibility for one's actions. Professional accountability is a nurse's responsibility to meet the patient's health care needs in a safe, effective, and caring way. To do so, students must prepare themselves in the classroom with **theory**—the textbook description of patient needs and nursing interventions—and then apply that information in the clinical setting. Accountability involves behaviors such as asking for assistance when unsure, performing nursing tasks in a safe manner, reporting and documenting assessments and interventions, and evaluating the care given and the patient's response. Accountability also includes a commitment to continuing education to stay current and knowledgeable.

Delegation

Delegation is the assignment of duties to another person. Some states differentiate between delegation (only to another licensed person) and **assignment**, which can be done to an unlicensed person, such as a nursing assistant. An LPN may supervise nursing assistants, technicians, or other LPNs. The nurse is responsible for ensuring patient safety and observing patient rights. It is the delegating nurse's duty to supervise and evaluate the care that a licensed or unlicensed person provides.

 Assignment Considerations

Nurse's Responsibilities

When a licensed nurse gives an assignment to another person, the nurse is responsible for ensuring that the person has the skills and abilities to perform the assignment safely, and that an unlicensed person is not performing acts that are legally restricted to nursing. The person delegating remains ultimately responsible to ensure that the task was completed, to learn any results or outcomes from the task, and to determine if any follow-up is necessary. When duties are delegated or assigned, effective communication between all parties is essential to ensuring quality in patient care (Saccomano & Zipp, 2014).

Standards of Care

Legally, you are responsible for your actions under the nurse practice act and according to the **standards of care** approved by the profession. These standards are defined in nursing procedure books, institutional policies, procedures or protocols, and nursing journals. On a national level, standards of care have been identified and published for clinical practice and specialty areas by professional nursing organizations. These standards provide a way of judging the quality and effectiveness of patient care and in legal cases determine whether a nurse acted correctly (see Box 1.1). Standards of care are continually being revised as treatments and techniques are updated and improved with nursing research. What is the standard today may not be the standard next year; it is crucial to keep current with continuing education.

PROFESSIONAL DISCIPLINE

State boards of nursing are also responsible for discipline within the profession. When a licensed nurse is charged with a violation of the nurse practice act, there will be an investigation and hearing to determine whether the charges are true. The most common charges brought against nurses include substance abuse, incompetence (doing something that can or did harm a patient), and negligence. **It is considered negligence not to report another professional's misconduct.** When a nurse is found guilty of professional misconduct, the penalties may result in a temporary suspension or loss of licensure.

CONTINUING EDUCATION

Many states have adopted laws that require evidence of continuing education after a nurse has passed the licensing examination. Once licensed, you are expected to function safely in any nursing situation. Therefore, it is necessary to continue your education about changes in health care practice, pharmacology, and technology. You may stay current by attending educational programs provided by your employer or professional organizations, reading nursing journals, taking college courses, or attending Internet webinars.

LAWS AND GUIDELINES AFFECTING NURSING PRACTICE

When a licensed nurse accepts employment with an agency or individual, the nurse is required to work within the laws and regulations governing nursing in that state. There are also federal laws that regulate safety and health in the workplace and forbid discrimination and sexual harassment. Although not law, the "Patient Care Partnership: Understanding Expectations, Rights, and Responsibilities" provides ethical guidelines for nursing practice (Box 3.2).

OCCUPATIONAL SAFETY AND HEALTH ADMINISTRATION

The **Occupational Safety and Health (OSH) Act** was passed in 1970 to improve the work environment in areas that affect workers' health or safety. It includes regulations for handling infectious or toxic materials, radiation safeguards, and the use of electrical equipment. With the passage of the OSH Act, Congress created the **Occupational Safety and Health Administration (OSHA)**, whose mission is to keep working conditions

Box 3.2 Patient Care Partnership: Overview*

When you need hospital care, your health care professionals at our hospital are committed to working with you and your family to meet your health care needs. Our goal is for you and your family to have the same care and attention we would want for our families and ourselves.

The sections below explain some of the basics about how you can expect to be treated during your hospital stay.

WHAT TO EXPECT DURING YOUR HOSPITAL STAY

- High-quality hospital care
- A clean and safe environment
- Involvement in your care
- Discussing your medical condition and information about medically appropriate treatment choices
- Discussing your treatment plan
- Getting information from you
- Understanding your health care goals and values
- Understanding who should make decisions when you cannot
- Protection of your privacy
- Help preparing you and your family for when you leave the hospital
- Help with your bill and filing insurance claims

Modified from American Hospital Association (2003). Patient Care Partnership: Understanding Expectations, rights, and responsibilities.
*Available at: http://www.aha.org/advocacy-issues/communicatingpts/pt-care-partnership.shtml

safe for all workers. Health care agencies, because of OSHA requirements, provide mandatory orientation and continuing education regarding a wide range of topics, from isolation procedures and blood-borne pathogen exposure, to fire or bomb threats, workplace violence and active shooter training, and lifting and evacuation procedures.

Safe storage and handling of toxic chemicals and drugs are important parts of the OSH Act. Each facility is required to keep a record of hazardous substances, including bleach, disinfectants, and other chemicals. The facility must store them properly in designated areas and maintain material safety data sheets (MSDSs), which outline the hazard the substance can pose. Employees must be updated on these workplace hazards and know the location of the MSDS collection.

CHILD ABUSE PREVENTION AND TREATMENT ACT

The Child Abuse Prevention and Treatment Act (CAPTA) is a federal law. It was enacted in 1974 and most recently amended and reauthorized in 2010 by the CAPTA Reauthorization Act of 2010. The Reauthorization additionally contains language designed to eliminate barriers to the adoption of foster children (often the victims of child abuse) and includes the Abandoned Infants Assistant Act, which provides grants to support families and prevent abandonment of infants and children (Children's Bureau, 2012). CAPTA defines child abuse and neglect as **"Any recent act or failure to act on the part of a parent or caretaker, which results in death, serious physical or emotional harm, sexual abuse, or exploitation, or an act or failure to act which presents an imminent risk of serious harm"** (Child Welfare Information Gateway, 2015). A child is a person under the age of 18 unless state law specifies a younger age. Many children who are victims of abuse are too young to speak for themselves. **CAPTA states that licensed health care personnel are required to report suspected child abuse.** Each facility usually has guidelines on how to report child abuse. Reporting suspected child abuse is an emotional event for everyone involved; however, the health and safety of the child must remain the primary focus.

Clinical Cues

In cases of child abuse, the account of the injury or accident given by the caregiver is often inconsistent with the physical signs and symptoms. A student should bring any suspicions of child abuse to the attention of the instructor.

DISCRIMINATION

Discrimination is making a decision or treating people based on a class or group to which they belong, such as race, religion, or sex. In 1964, federal legislation made it illegal for employers to **discriminate** (to hire, promote, or fire employees) because of race, color, religion, sex, or national origin. The law has been amended to prohibit discrimination related to a person's disabilities, age, pregnancy, childbirth, and related medical conditions. Discrimination laws protect people with human immunodeficiency virus (HIV) infection or acquired immunodeficiency syndrome (AIDS) and those recovering from drug or alcohol addiction. It is not legal for employers to ask questions on an employment application that would indicate race, other protected categories, or health status. Laws also require employers to make reasonable accommodations for people with a disability.

SEXUAL HARASSMENT

Sexual harassment is defined by the Equal Employment Opportunity Commission (EEOC) as "unwelcome sexual advances, requests for sexual favors, and other verbal or physical conduct of a sexual nature." Sexual harassment is illegal when used as a condition of employment or promotion or when it interferes with job performance. Sexual harassment prohibition has been further applied in schools and in the clinical setting. Student nurses and their instructors need to recognize what sexual harassment is; refrain from conversation or actions that create a hostile, intimidating, or offensive atmosphere; and report actions that are sexually harassing in the classroom or clinical setting. In our society, in which sexual comments and activities are commonplace on television and in movies, we must be aware of the right time and place for sexually suggestive or explicit words or touch. It is appropriate to state, "I am offended by your language (or conversation or inappropriate touch)." If the sexually explicit or harassing behavior continues, report it to your supervisor.

GOOD SAMARITAN LAWS

Good Samaritan laws protect a health care professional from liability if she stops to provide aid in an emergency. In most states, there is no legal requirement for a nurse to help in an emergency, but if a nurse does provide care, liability is limited unless there is evidence of gross negligence or intentional misconduct. In other words, you must not exceed your level of competence nor act recklessly. The Good Samaritan laws do not apply to employed emergency response workers.

PATIENT'S RIGHTS

In 1972, with revision in 1992, the American Hospital Association (AHA) developed the "Patient's Bill of Rights," a list of rights the patient could expect and responsibilities that the hospital must uphold. In 2003 this document was revised to "The Patient Care Partnership: Understanding Expectations, Rights, and Responsibilities" (see Box 3.2). This document is available in eight languages at www.aha.org. Although this is an ethical and not a legal document, state legislators have written laws that prohibit certain actions or guarantee particular rights. Since the first patient bill of rights, which was hospital oriented, many others have been published, particularly for residents of nursing homes and those in psychiatric units. These documents emphasize that patients continue to have rights even if they are helpless and sick. They seek to preserve the patient's dignity, privacy, freedom of movement, and information needs.

Under some legally specified conditions, certain rights may be suspended, such as in an emergency when the patient is unconscious or unable to communicate. Other conditions include the patient who is in danger of injury and cannot protect himself from harm, or when it is necessary to protect the public from harm. However, patients with psychiatric disorders in most states cannot be held against their will for more than 3 days, unless they are a distinct danger to self or others or are gravely disabled (unable to provide for basic needs). As long as someone is deemed harmless, the current principle is to protect the individual's right to be different, to disagree with the majority, to live one's own life, and to seek one's own solutions to private difficulties.

NATIONAL PATIENT SAFETY GOALS

The Joint Commission has developed goals to promote specific improvements in patient safety. The goals attempt to provide evidence- and expert-based solutions to areas that have caused problems with patient safety, for example improving staff communication and preventing mistakes in surgery. The Joint Commission's National Patient Safety Goals are updated every year and are available on its website (www.jointcommission.org). All nurses should review these goals annually.

A **sentinel event** is an unexpected patient care event that results in death or serious injury (or risk of such) to the patient. The Joint Commission tracks and reports sentinel events to improve hospital safety. One of the National Patient Safety Goals is to improve staff communication because communication is The Joint Commission's most frequently cited cause of a sentinel event.

QSEN Considerations: Safety

Communication and Safety

Safe and effective patient care depends on complete communication between caregivers. **"Handoff" communication** describes times when information is passed from one caregiver to another, such as a change-of-shift report, patient transfer to another unit or facility, or contact with the primary care provider.

One form of communication, termed the *SBAR method of communication,* is a strategy that reduces the likelihood of critical patient details being lost. SBAR is an acronym that stands for *S*ituation, *B*ackground, *A*ssessment, and *R*ecommendation. SBAR is useful when communicating with physicians because nurses and physicians are taught different ways to communicate patient information. Nurses are taught to communicate in narrative form and to include every possible detail, whereas physicians are taught to communicate using brief "bullet" points. This SBAR format encourages caregivers to communicate in a way that is concise, yet complete. The American Association of Colleges of Nursing (AACN) and the **Quality and Safety Education for Nurses (QSEN) project** advocate adding the letter *I* at the beginning of the acronym (*I*ntroduction of yourself and your patient, including your role and unit) and the letter *R* at the end of the acronym (for *R*eadback, to encourage verification) when communicating with people over the telephone or from different departments. The resulting acronym is ISBAR-R.

Communication

Example of ISBAR-R Communication: Handoff Report

Introduction: Hello, I'm Donna, the day-shift nurse. Are you ready for the shift report on Mrs. Smith in room S21?

Situation: You are communicating the 3:00 pm change-of-shift report for a 65-year-old patient who was admitted 3 days ago with pneumonia.

Background: Mrs. Smith is a 65-year-old patient who was admitted 3 days ago with pneumonia and shortness of breath. She has completed 3 days of antibiotic therapy, nebulizer treatments every 4 hours, and continuous supplemental oxygen therapy.

Assessment: Mrs. Smith has clear lung sounds, and her pulse oximeter reads 98% on 2L of oxygen. Vital signs: T 98.8°, P 86, R 22, and BP 128/72. She ambulated twice this shift down the length of the hall and denies shortness of breath. She has an occasional cough, productive of yellow sputum.

Recommendation: Monitor pulse oximeter readings with vital signs once a shift; administer antibiotics and nebulizer treatments on time, ambulate one more time this evening; consider administering PRN ("as needed") cough medicine at bedtime.

Readback: Ask receiving nurse if there are any questions and to read back notes for clarification.

BP, Blood pressure; *P,* pulse; *PRN,* as needed; *R,* respirations; *T,* temperature.

Communication

Example of ISBAR-R Communication: Calling the Health Care Provider

Introduction: Hello, I'm Donna caring for your patient Mrs. Smith on the Medical-Surgical floor.

Situation: I have results from the sputum culture and sensitivity ordered 3 days ago.

Background: Mrs. Smith was admitted 3 days ago with shortness of breath and has been taking cefazolin IV. A sputum culture was obtained before antibiotic therapy was started.

Assessment: The lab results from the culture and sensitivity indicate that the bacteria are resistant to cefazolin. She continues to be short of breath and has crackles in bilateral lower bases. Her temperature is 100.4 orally.

Recommendation: Prescribe another antibiotic that the organism is resistant to.

Readback: Readback any orders given by the health care provider.

The National Patient Safety Goals and requirements apply to nearly 15,000 hospitals and health care organizations accredited by The Joint Commission. There are specific goals for numerous types of patient care areas, such as ambulatory care, assisted living, behavioral health, home care, long-term care, hospitals (Box 3.3), and others. The QSEN project is a movement funded by the Robert Wood Johnson Foundation (RWJF) to educate future nurses in developing the knowledge, skills, and attitudes (KSA) needed to improve the quality and safety of our future health care systems (QSEN Institute, 2014).

Box 3.3 2015 Hospital National Patient Safety Goals

GOAL: IDENTIFY PATIENTS CORRECTLY
- Use at least two ways to identify patients.
- Make sure the correct patient receives the correct blood when they receive a transfusion.

GOAL: IMPROVE STAFF COMMUNICATION
- Get important test results to the right staff person on time.

GOAL: USE MEDICINES SAFELY
- Before a procedure, label medicines that are not labeled.
- Take extra care with patients who take medications to thin their blood.
- Record and pass along correct information about a patient's medicines.

GOAL: USE ALARMS SAFELY
- Make improvements to ensure that alarms on medical equipment are heard and responded to on time.

GOAL: PREVENT INFECTION
- Use the hand cleaning guidelines from the Centers for Disease Control and Prevention or the World Health Organization.
- Use proven guidelines to prevent infections that are difficult to treat.
- Use proven guidelines to prevent infection of the blood from central lines.
- Use proven guidelines to prevent infection after surgery.
- Use proven guidelines to prevent infections of the urinary tract that are caused by catheters.

GOAL: IDENTIFY PATIENT SAFETY RISKS
- Find out which patients are most likely to try to commit suicide.

GOAL: PREVENT MISTAKES IN SURGERY
- Make sure that the correct surgery is done on the correct patient and at the correct place on the patient's body.
- Mark the correct place on the patient's body where the surgery is to be done.
- Pause before the surgery to make sure that a mistake is not being made.

LEGAL DOCUMENTS

THE MEDICAL RECORD

When a person enters the health care system to visit a primary care provider, clinic, hospital, or emergency department or to receive home health care, a record is begun (or continued) that documents that person's health status or problem and the care given. The record is a legal document that includes records of all assessments, tests, and care provided. The medical record, is **confidential** (kept private), meaning that only people directly associated with the care of that patient have legal access to the information in the medical record. **The medical record is the property of the hospital, agency, or primary care provider—not the patient.** However, the patient does have the right of access to the medical record, and the patient may authorize his caregivers to provide copies of information in the medical record to other agencies—for example, if a patient transfers from one primary care provider or health care facility to another. Health care researchers and insurance companies may also gain access to medical information with the patient's permission.

Student nurses must protect their patients' confidentiality. Medical records may not be copied. Reports or notes on patients used for school purposes (case studies, nursing care plans, and task lists) should not identify the patient by name. Case discussion should indicate "a 67-year-old man" rather than "Mr. Joe Morales."

As a legal document, the medical record is used to determine the truth of what happened—what was

Box 3.4 Rights Provided by the Health Insurance Portability and Accountability Act

HIPAA covers six patient rights and provider responsibilities:

Consent: Written consents must contain a clause that says the patient agrees to allow the provider to use and disclose his information for treatment, payment, and health care operations. A notice must be attached to the consent form.

Notice: The provider's obligations are outlined regarding the privacy of the patient's health care information. It includes the six patient rights and the responsibilities of the provider. It details how the patient information will be protected, as well as a process for filing a complaint if the patient believes privacy rights have been violated.

Access: The patient has the right to inspect and copy his medical record.

Amendment: A patient has the right to amend his record for the purpose of accuracy.

Accounting for disclosures: Providers are held accountable for how patients' medical information is handled. Tracking of any disclosures of information not related to treatment, payment, or health care operations, or that were not authorized by the patient, must occur.

Restriction of disclosure: The patient can request that the provider restrict the use and disclosure of his information. However, the provider does not have to grant the request.

done or not done—to a patient during a period. Therefore, its contents always need to be accurate, pertinent, and timely. Changes to a patient's medical record may suggest dishonesty. Documentation should focus on the patient and the nursing care provided in objective terms, stating only the facts. Avoid using subjective terms or conclusions. For example, rather than documenting "patient depressed," instead document, "patient answers questions in a low tone of voice, using one word answers, and asks to be left alone." The medical record may be introduced as evidence in a court case. Documentation guidelines are discussed in Chapter 7.

HEALTH INSURANCE PORTABILITY AND ACCOUNTABILITY ACT

The Health Insurance Portability and Accountability Act (HIPAA) of 1996 required the creation of regulations regarding patient privacy and electronic medical records. Failure to comply with these rules may lead to civil penalties. Intentional violation of the regulations can lead to sizable fines and jail time. Box 3.4 presents the six patient rights covered in these regulations.

A considerable amount of information about patients is shared among health care professionals each day. HIPAA privacy rules took effect in 2003. These rules protect the way that patient information is conveyed and stored, and to whom information may be revealed. These rules state that disclosing medical information to family members, close friends, or other individuals identified by the patient *is* permitted if *the patient does not object.* It is important to make certain you have the patient's consent to relay information about his health care to family members. It is also important to know and follow the hospital's privacy policies.

The HIPAA rules also give patients the right to the information in their medical records and the right to amend an erroneous record. Privacy and confidentiality of patient information have always been part of the ethical code of nurses, physicians, and health care facilities; the new rules have simply increased awareness of the need for confidentiality and imposed new guidelines. Medical records and flow sheets must be secured and not left where they may be viewed by others. Public displays of patient information (e.g., on a white board in the nurse's station or computer screen with patient data) are not acceptable. It is important to log out when leaving a computer unattended. Nurses must be careful with printouts and other patient data and shred them when the shift is over. Patients must sign a specific release form if they want information to be sent to another agency, primary care provider, or insurance company.

Legal and Ethical Considerations

Social Media and HIPAA

Social media use has increased greatly since the implementation of HIPAA. Health care agencies and institutions have had to become more diligent in protecting personal health information (PHI) as a result. It is imperative that no PHI be disseminated, either intentionally or unintentionally, over social media. Posting of pictures, discussions (even those that do not use patient or hospital names), and images of X-rays all violate HIPAA and place the nurse in a serious legal situation. It is generally best to separate one's personal and professional life when dealing with social media. The National Council of State Boards of Nursing (2011) provides guidelines and suggestions for nurses in dealing with social media and nursing practice.

Legal and Ethical Considerations

Protecting Patient Privacy

- Keep interactions with patients as private as possible. If your patient is not in a private room, lower your voice to keep others from hearing what is said.
- Remember that any discussions about patients in clinical postconference are for educational purposes only and not for gossip. These discussions should never contain identifying information, and the cases should not be discussed outside the clinical conference or classroom setting.
- Do not leave patient information on display. If you use a clipboard, place a cover sheet to shield patient data.
- Before providing any information about your patient to anyone not directly involved in the patient's care (such as patient's family), check for authorization to release health-related information.
- Never photocopy the patient's medical record for any purpose.

- Remove all identifying information from personal notes or assignments. Maintain such notes in a secure and confidential manner, even if they contain no identifying patient information. They must not be left unattended at school, at home, in your car, or on your computer. Shred or destroy all such documents once the purpose has been fulfilled (e.g., once your assignment has been graded).

CONSENTS AND RELEASES

A **consent** is permission given by the patient or his legal representative. Consents and **releases** are legal documents that record the patient's permission to perform a treatment or surgery or to give information to insurance companies or other health care providers (Box 3.5).

Informed consent indicates the patient's participation in the decision-making process. The person signing must have knowledge of what the consent allows and be able to make a knowledgeable decision. Informed consent for surgery or treatment must include four elements. The patient must be told, in terms he can understand, (a) the risks and benefits of the proposed treatment, (b) the possible consequences of not having the procedure done, (c) alternatives to the treatment, and (d) the name of the health care professional who will perform the procedure. Obtaining informed consent is the responsibility of the health care provider performing the procedure or treatment. The nurse's role is witnessing of the signature, providing comfort and support to the patient, and explaining nursing care expected after the procedure. However, if the patient has questions or seems confused about the procedure or treatment, the nurse, as the patient's advocate, should not obtain the patient's signature until the patient's questions have been answered (Brent, 2013). **It is important to determine that proper consent has been obtained, both *legally* and *ethically*. Failure to obtain a valid informed consent may lead to charges of assault and battery or invasion of privacy** (explained later in this chapter).

To be valid, a consent must be signed by the person or the legal agent for that person. Consents must be freely signed without threat or pressure and must be witnessed by another adult. **Consent can be withdrawn at any time before the procedure or treatment is started**. When a person is older than 18 years and **competent**, he must sign the consent for treatment. A competent person is one who is legally fit (mentally and emotionally). A person is considered incompetent if he is unconscious, under the influence of mind-altering drugs (including narcotics used as "premedication" for the procedure), or declared legally incompetent. In these situations a next of kin, appointed guardian, or one who holds a durable power of attorney (discussed later) has legal authority to give consent. Minors (younger than 18 years) may not give legal consent; their parents or guardians have this right. If a child's parents are divorced, the custodial parent is the legal representative. Stepparents usually cannot give consent unless they have legally adopted the child. **An emancipated minor, or one who has established independence by moving away from parents or through service in the armed forces, marriage, or pregnancy, is considered legally capable of signing a consent form.**

Box 3.5 Types of Consents

Admission agreement: Commonly obtained at the time of admission to a hospital, this form delineates the hospital's or facility's responsibility to the patient. The hospital agrees to provide room, meals, basic nursing care, and medical care prescribed by the primary health care provider. The patient consents to diagnostic services, such as radiographs, medication administration, and nursing treatments. The patient acknowledges responsibility to pay for the services. Consent to bill insurance companies and provide medical information about the patient to receive payment is usually part of the admission agreement.

Operative consent: All surgical or invasive procedures, such as repair of a hernia or removal of the appendix, **biopsies** (taking a piece of tissue to examine), and many diagnostic tests that are **invasive** (involve an incision or cutting of the patient's body or the introduction of an instrument into a body cavity) require an operative consent. It may be called a surgical consent or permission for surgery or anesthesia. **The physician, surgeon, or anesthesiologist who performs the procedure is responsible for explaining the procedure, its risks and benefits, and possible alternative options.**

Consent to receive blood: A consent to receive a blood transfusion would indicate that the patient was informed of the benefits and risks of transfusion, as is done for surgical or invasive procedures. Some patients hold religious beliefs that would prohibit transfusions, even in life-threatening situations.

Research consent: Clinical research is carried out only with the patient's informed consent about the possible risks, consequences, and benefits of the research. A patient always has the right to refuse to participate in a research study, and no patient may be given a research drug or treatment without his informed consent.

Consent to release information: A specific consent to release confidential patient information to other agencies or people is required before the information may be released. An exception is that information may be shared between consulting or referring physicians without a specific consent.

Other consents: Special consents are required to perform an autopsy, donate organs after death, or be photographed, and for the disposal of body parts during surgery.

Implied consent is assumed when, during a life-threatening emergency, consent cannot be obtained from the patient or family. Consent may be obtained by telephone if it is witnessed by two people who hear the consent of the family member.

A **release** is a legal form used to excuse one party from **liability** (responsibility). A commonly used release is a **leave against medical advice (AMA)** (discussed later in the chapter). The term *release* may also refer to forms used to authorize an agency to send confidential health care information to another agency, school, or insurance company.

WITNESSING WILLS OR OTHER LEGAL DOCUMENTS

Occasionally, nurses may be asked to witness a will or other legal document. Although it is legal, most hospitals and health care agencies have policies against this. Wills or legal documents may be contested, and the nurse who witnessed the document can be called to court to testify regarding the patient's health, mental condition, or relationship to visitors. To avoid this conflict, hospitals often provide business office personnel or a notary public to witness the signature. To witness the signing of a legal document, you need not know the content of the document. Legally, it is necessary only that the witness confirms that the signature or mark is made under no influence (drug or otherwise) and that the person knows what he is signing.

ADVANCE DIRECTIVES

An **advance directive**, sometimes called a **"living will,"** is a consent that has been constructed before the need for it arises. It spells out a patient's wishes regarding surgery and diagnostic and therapeutic treatments. Clear direction for making decisions is then present if the patient suffers an accident or illness that renders him unresponsive or incompetent. This has become important because health care technology allows the prolonging and maintaining of life with sophisticated treatments that may cause conflict among family members or between the health care professionals and the family as to how the patient would want to live (or die) in this situation. When a person puts in writing his wishes regarding life support and the use of medical technology, both the medical community and the family have clear direction. A **durable power of attorney** is a document that gives legal power *to* a **health care agent** (surrogate decision maker), who is a person chosen by the patient to follow the patient's advance directives and make medical decisions on his behalf.

All 50 states recognize advance directives, but each state regulates advance directives differently, and an advance directive from one state may not be recognized in another, depending on the differences in their laws. Advance directives do not expire; it is a good idea for the patient to review his advance directive periodically to be certain it still reflects his wishes. Historically, emergency medical technicians (EMTs) have not been able to honor advance directives. Therefore, if a patient had an advance directive limiting the types of care he wanted and a loved one called 911, the EMTs had to perform any or all procedures to stabilize the patient and bring him to the hospital. More recently, however, many states have enacted provider orders for life-sustaining treatment (POLST) laws to allow EMTs to honor do-not-resuscitate (DNR) orders and/or advance directives, provided documentation is available at the scene.

Do-not-resuscitate (DNR) orders are written by a physician when the patient has indicated a desire to be allowed to die if he stops breathing or his heart stops. In this situation, no cardiac compressions or assisted breathing (cardiopulmonary resuscitation [CPR]) would be started. **It is very important for nursing personnel to know who is to be resuscitated and who is NOT.** Many facilities have implemented a color-coded wristband for the patient to allow quick determination of code status. A nurse who attempts to resuscitate a patient who has a physician's DNR order would be acting without the patient's consent and committing battery.

VIOLATIONS OF LAW

A nurse needs to know about a number of civil laws to practice safely and within the legal system. A nurse needs to know not only the law about her own practice but also how to act as a **patient advocate**, one who speaks for and protects the rights of the patient.

NEGLIGENCE AND MALPRACTICE

Negligence is failing to meet the standard of care; failing to do something that a reasonable and **prudent** (sensible and careful) person would do or doing something a reasonable and prudent person would *not* do.

Malpractice is negligence by a professional person. The person does not act according to professional standards of care as a reasonable and prudent professional would. **In nursing malpractice, a reasonable and prudent person is a similarly educated, licensed, and experienced nurse.** An example of nursing malpractice would be if a nurse did not check the patient's vital signs and condition after surgery, there was hemorrhage, and the patient went into shock and died.

To prove malpractice, four elements must be present: duty, a breach of duty, causation, and injury (Box 3.6). If even one of these four elements was not present, the nurse is not guilty of malpractice. For example, if a nurse made a clinical error that did not result in harm to the patient, the event would not be considered malpractice; however, it would be a deviation from the standard of care, and as such could be grounds for discipline by the employer, the licensing board, or both.

Box 3.6 Elements of Malpractice

Duty: The obligation to use due care (e.g., a nurse has a duty to monitor the condition of the patient for whom she is caring).
Breach of duty: Failure to use due care (e.g., a nurse fails to check the vital signs or condition of the patient after surgery or a nurse begins cardiopulmonary resuscitation on a patient who has a do-not-resuscitate order).
Causation: The nurse's action or inaction causes injury or harm to the patient. There must be a direct link between the breach of duty and the injury (e.g., the nurse's failure to check the patient's condition led to an undetected loss of blood that caused the patient's death).
Injury or damages: The actual harm or disorder that results from the negligence. Injury or damages may be physical, emotional, or financial. Pain and suffering, loss of the ability to continue in a job, physical or emotional disability, extended hospitalization, or death would all be considered injury or damage in a negligence action.

COMMON LEGAL ISSUES

Nurses have access to private information and personal contact that is permitted by their professional caregiver role. With that right to information and touch come legal responsibilities to respect the patient's privacy, to protect the patient's safety, and to ensure the patient's right to make decisions. When legal boundaries are violated and injury occurs, nurses may be subject to **litigation** (a lawsuit).

Assault and Battery

Assault is the threat to harm another or even to threaten to touch another without that person's permission. The person being threatened must believe that the nurse has the ability to carry out the threat. **Battery** is the actual physical contact that has been refused or that is carried out against the person's will. An example of assault would be the nurse who says, "If you don't let me give you this injection, two other nurses will hold you down so I can give it to you." Battery would occur when a patient is held down to receive an injection he has refused. It would also include the rough physical handling of an excited, confused, or psychotic patient in ways that would be described as angry, violent, or negligent.

Adults who are alert and oriented have the right to refuse medications, baths, treatments, dressing changes, irrigations, insertion of a catheter, and diagnostic tests, as well as surgery. Even if the test or procedure is necessary for the patient's well-being or comfort, the patient has the legal right to refuse. **It is the nurse's responsibility to explain why a particular drug or treatment is important. However, if the patient still refuses, the nurse should obtain a release from liability because the treatment is not done or the drug is not taken.** Performing a procedure without the proper consent is battery (except in emergencies when the patient is unable to give consent).

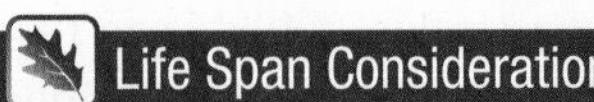

Older Adults

Although an older adult may be forgetful and require supervision of activities of daily living, he still has rights of privacy and self-determination (the right to consent to or refuse treatments). Nurses need to document carefully any explanations given and the patient's ability to understand the benefits, risks, and consequences of decisions.

Defamation

Defamation is when one person makes remarks about another person that are untrue, and the remarks damage that other person's reputation. There are two forms of defamation: **slander** (oral) and **libel** (written). Two nurses may be overheard talking about a physician in a way that holds the physician up to ridicule or contempt. If another person decides never to use that physician because of the derogatory comments, the physician's reputation is damaged and the nurses may be guilty of slander. An example of libel is a letter or newspaper article quotation stating that a person is incompetent or dishonest. The loss of respect for and trust of the person may result in damage to his reputation and loss of business. A person sued for slander or libel may be found innocent if the statements made were true or were said or written with no intent to harm the person, but for a justified purpose.

Invasion of Privacy

Invasion of privacy occurs when there has been a violation of the confidential and privileged nature of a professional relationship. When patients entrust themselves to our care, it is with the expectation of confidentiality—that what is told to the health care professional and what is learned about the patient's health and personal history are private information to which no one else should have access.

Invasion of privacy occurs when unauthorized persons learn of the patient's history, condition, or treatment from the professional caregiver. It might include the nurse's giving information over the telephone to a caller who asks about the patient's condition. It occurs when health care workers are overheard carelessly discussing their patients in the elevator or cafeteria. It occurs when a next-door neighbor asks about another neighbor who is in the hospital and the nurse tells him about the patient's condition. It occurs when a nurse, out of curiosity, reads the medical record of a public figure who has been admitted to her unit, but to whom the nurse is not assigned or responsible. Releasing information to a newspaper, another health care agency, an insurance company, or a person without the patient's valid consent is invasion of privacy. However, **nurses are required by law in most states to report information regarding child or elder abuse, sexual abuse, or violent acts that may be crimes (e.g., stab or gunshot wounds).** When such reporting is done in good faith, the nurse cannot be held liable for invasion of privacy. Be knowledgeable of the required reporting procedures for abuse or crime where you work.

Invasion of privacy extends to leaving the curtains or door open while a treatment or procedure is being done, or to leaving patients in a position that might cause them loss of dignity or embarrassment. Exposing the patient's body more than necessary, or leaving a confused and agitated patient in a hallway where he might behave in ways that would be embarrassing if he were in his normal state, are also examples of invasion of privacy. Interviewing a patient or family member in a room with only a curtain between the patients, or where conversation can be overheard, allows confidential information to be heard by unauthorized persons. **The reasonable and prudent nurse does for the patient what the patient cannot do for himself: covers the patient's body, protects him from public exposure, and preserves his dignity.**

A growing area of concern regarding privacy has to do with computerized data banks and the Internet. Many health care agencies are computerizing their records, and nurses (and other personnel) can enter and retrieve information about patients in that facility. It is important to remember that accessing information about someone who is not your patient (e.g., a celebrity or a neighbor) is an invasion of privacy, and can lead to losing your job, being named in a lawsuit by the victim, and disciplinary action on your nursing license. Audits of hospital electronic medical records can easily pinpoint what medical records are viewed by exactly which employees.

 QSEN Considerations: Informatics

Safeguard the Electronic Medical Record

Always safeguard patient privacy when entering or using data in a computer network.

HIPAA, discussed earlier, sets rules governing transmission of patient data (electronic, telephone, and fax), including the requirement that the sending facility must have reasonable safeguards in place to ensure the data are sent to the intended place and are treated in a confidential manner. Some hospitals require employees and individual nursing students to sign a **nondisclosure agreement** (NDA), also known as a confidentiality agreement, when they are hired or begin a clinical rotation, which gives the hospital legal recourse if they can prove the person broke confidentiality. A national data bank is envisioned in the future that could allow health care practitioners to access a patient's medical record wherever that patient sought care—from California to New York, from a clinic to a major medical center, and from a private practice physician to a pharmacist at the local drugstore. However, the need for safeguards to prevent unauthorized access, as well as the reluctance of many people to have confidential health information so readily accessible, may prevent this from becoming a reality soon.

False Imprisonment

Just as a patient has the right to refuse medications or tests or treatments, a patient has the right to leave a hospital or health care facility or to move about in it. Preventing a person from leaving or restricting his movements in the facility is **false imprisonment**. When a person wants to leave the hospital against the advice of the primary care provider, a release to leave AMA is used. The patient, by signing the form, releases the hospital and staff of responsibility for any consequences that occur because of the patient's leaving. It is also important to follow your facility's policies regarding a competent adult who wishes to leave AMA. The policy may include finding out why the patient wishes to leave, informing the primary care provider, informing the patient of the risks of refusing treatments, and carefully documenting all aspects of the situation.

People who have psychiatric disorders may be admitted to a psychiatric unit on a voluntary or involuntary basis. A person who is admitted voluntarily agrees to the admission, can refuse or accept any treatment, and can leave the facility as a regular discharge. If the primary care provider believes the patient should not be discharged, the patient can sign an AMA release.

An involuntary admission is made against the patient's wishes to protect him from self-harm or from harming others. There is a limit to the time (usually 72 hours) a person can be detained without consent. During that time, if the patient does not agree to a voluntary admission and health care personnel remain convinced that the person is a threat to self or others, two psychiatrists can petition a judge to issue a court order for the patient to be held in the psychiatric facility for a specific period.

Protective devices. The inappropriate use of devices that limit a person's mobility is a nursing action that can result in charges of false imprisonment. **Protective devices** may be mechanical, such as locks, rails, belts, or garments that prevent a person from getting out of a room, bed, or chair, or they may be chemical: drugs such as sedatives or tranquilizers that sedate the patient so that he is unable to move about. **An order by an authorized health care provider is necessary for any protective device, mechanical or chemical.** Typically, restraint orders must be renewed daily. Creative nurses and health care facilities have developed ways of allowing for mobility while protecting the confused or agitated person from danger. Nurses must try less restrictive techniques before resorting to the use of restraints. A reasonable and prudent nurse will carefully assess a patient's potential for falls or other harm and document the need for and proper application of provider-ordered protective devices to ensure the patient's safety. Consult with your supervisor about using protective devices in an emergency when no order is available. When using any protective device on a patient, be sure to follow facility policy for providing toileting, hydration, and mobility for the patient. Document the need to protect the patient from harm, and secure an order as soon as possible to protect yourself from liability for charges of false imprisonment or malpractice.

Life Span Considerations

Older Adults

Careful assessment of an older adult's mental status, medications, potential for orthostatic hypotension, balance, and mobility can identify the patient with a risk for falls and injury. Specific nursing interventions can then be identified and used to protect the patient from injury.

DECREASING LEGAL RISK

Nursing Competence

Although nurses cannot prevent a lawsuit from being filed, several actions can reduce the likelihood of a suit (Box 3.7). **First and most important is competent and well-documented nursing care.** Nursing **competence** is defined as possessing the suitable skill, knowledge, and experience necessary to provide adequate nursing care. Establishing rapport and effective communication skills can create a relationship in which patient anger or misunderstanding can be resolved rather than grow to lawsuit proportions. Competence in nursing also includes following the proper policies and procedures and upholding the standards of care. Sometimes in nursing you may observe another nurse "bending the rules" in an unsafe way to save time; as a novice in the field, you may feel peer pressure to follow "the way things are done on this unit." Rule bending might appear to be the only solution on a unit that is chronically understaffed, but it only provides a temporary solution. What is more likely needed is a permanent change in the situation that will make rule bending unnecessary (see QSEN: Teamwork and Collaboration). If hospital rules are out-of-date or unrealistic, it is important to get involved (e.g., on the hospital's policy committee) to change these rules, rather than work around them.

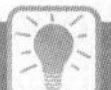
QSEN Considerations: Teamwork and Collaboration

Teamwork and Collaboration Knowledge

- Identify system barriers and facilitators of effective team functioning
- Examine strategies for improving systems to support team functioning

Sometimes a patient believes he has suffered an injury or loss. Documentation is the key element in proving that the nursing actions used were appropriate, thus protecting the nurse from liability.

Potential lawsuits may be avoided by early identification of dissatisfied patients. Many facilities have risk-management teams composed of people specially trained to deal with situations that may put the facility

Box 3.7 Guidelines to Reduce Legal Risk

1. **MAINTAIN COMPETENCE**
- Learn skills thoroughly.
- Know your state's nurse practice act.
- Know and follow your employer's institutional policies.
- Develop the ability to evaluate your knowledge and performance; identify areas in which you are weak and work to improve these.
- Attend continuing education programs and keep abreast of changes in health care.
- Keep records of workshops or seminars you attend.
- Identify experienced nurses whose competence you respect, and seek their assistance when you are unfamiliar with equipment or a technique.

2. **DOCUMENT FULLY: THERE IS AN EXPRESSION IN NURSING, "IF YOU DIDN'T DOCUMENT IT, IT DIDN'T GET DONE"**
- Accurate, factual, and timely documentation of the nursing assessment, plan, interventions, and evaluation is essential to prove that nursing care that meets standards of care was carried out.
- Anecdotal records are a tool for nurses to use in assisting their memory. Anecdotal records are the nurse's recollection or notes of an incident written as close to the time of the incident as possible, and kept by the nurse in a secure place. Relying on memory is a poor way to prove what a nurse did or did not do. Lawsuits often take years from the date of occurrence of an event to the filing and notice of a lawsuit.

3. **ESTABLISH RAPPORT**
- Develop rapport and treat each patient with respect: identify yourself, smile, listen attentively, and address patients by their preferred name.
- Be careful of damaging the relationship between the patient and his primary care provider or other staff by engaging in critical or negative conversation with the patient.
- Listen to patient complaints and communicate professionally to attempt to resolve problems.

4. **COMMUNICATE EFFECTIVELY**
- Therapeutic communication techniques can allow the patient to express feelings without the nurse agreeing or supporting charges of incompetence or negligence.
- Notify your supervisor of any situation in which a patient or family members are dissatisfied with the nursing care received or with another health care professional.
- Follow the procedure for communication with the risk management team.

5. **TAKE CARE OF YOURSELF**
- Be at your best for every clinical day.
- Follow the principles of proper nutrition and regular exercise and obtain adequate, restful sleep.
- Recognize that fatigue is a significant factor in making clinical errors: refrain from working hours in excess of what you can safely do, even though the money may be tempting.

at risk for a lawsuit. Part of a comprehensive risk-management program would include in-service programs to promote safety, preventive maintenance for equipment and the physical plant, and counseling and interventions in situations that pose a potential for lawsuits.

? Think Critically

How would you respond to a patient who complains to you that the nurse on the night shift ignored his call for assistance for 45 minutes, and that the nurse said that the unit was short staffed and the patient should not bother them unless it was absolutely necessary?

Incident or Occurrence Reports

If an occurrence is out of the ordinary, an **incident** (occurrence) **report** is often used to document what happened, the facts about the incident, and who was involved or who witnessed it. The incident report is a tool used by the risk-management department (see Chapter 10). This report is useful for several reasons. It allows the facility to note dangerous patterns: for example, if several visitors or staff have tripped and fallen in the same location or if a change in the appearance of a medication might have been a factor in several recent similar medication errors. The incident report also serves as an immediate recall of an occurrence that may result in injury or damages and future lawsuit. Some examples of when an incident report might be written include when a medication error is made, a patient falls out of bed, or a visitor faints in the hall (Fig. 3.1). **Incident reports are generally not filed as part of the patient's medical record; no reference to the incident report is made in the patient's medical record,** although the medically relevant details about the incident, if they relate to patient care, should be included in the progress notes. Incident reports should be timely, factual, and concise and should not contain unnecessary details, such as explanations about why the event might have occurred.

Liability Insurance

Liability insurance does not provide protection from being sued. However, it can protect the nurse's livelihood and assets should the nurse be sued. If a nurse is sued, liability insurance pays for the expenses of a lawyer to defend the nurse and pays any award won by the plaintiff up to the limits of the policy. It may also pay for attorney costs and related costs if the nurse is subjected to review by the state board of nursing. Having liability insurance does not increase your chances of being sued, and most authors agree that it is unwise to rely on the employer's liability insurance policy because there may be situations in which the institution's interests are at odds with your legal interests. Nursing liability insurance is relatively inexpensive and is available through nursing organizations and private insurance companies.

ETHICS IN NURSING

Ethics or **ethical principles** are rules of conduct that have been agreed to by a particular group. They are based on the consensus (agreement) of the group that these rules are morally right or proper. Professionals such as physicians, nurses, and lawyers have developed codes of ethics that provide a set of guidelines outlining the behavioral expectations of the profession. Ethics are different from laws: they are voluntary. There are nonprescribed legal penalties for violating a code of ethics; although in many instances, it may result in disciplinary action by a licensing or regulating agency. In some cases, ethics and the law overlap: for example, in dealing with issues of confidentiality. Nevertheless, in many cases, ethics deal with ideals or situations in which there is no right or wrong solution to a problem, and about which thoughtful, caring people may hold opposing views. Debate continues about life-and-death issues such as abortion, life support, and euthanasia. Common ethical terms that are important in practice are defined in Box 3.8.

Ethics are closely linked with **values,** the worth or importance of an action or belief to an individual. An ethical **dilemma** (problem or conflict) may result when people hold differing values. Codes of ethics attempt to provide a framework for making professional decisions.

Think Critically

How would you react to a patient who refuses surgery that might prolong and perhaps enhance his life? What values do you hold regarding quality of life, right to die, and self-determination? Is there a difference if the patient is 23 years old or 87 years old?

CODES OF ETHICS

The International Council of Nurses (ICN), the ANA, the NAPNES, and the NFLPN have developed codes of ethics for nurses (Box 3.9). Although the codes are worded differently, they have many commonalities. They all indicate the following:

- A respect for human dignity and the individual, and provision of nursing care that is not affected by race, religion, lifestyle, or culture
- A commitment to continuing education, to maintaining competence, and to contributing to improved practice
- The confidential nature of the nurse-patient relationship, outlining behaviors that bring credit to the profession and protect the public

In addition, NAPNES has set standards for nursing practice since 1941 (Appendix B). The standards represent the foundation for the provision of safe and competent nursing practice. Competence implies knowledge, understanding, and skills that transcend specific tasks and is guided by a commitment to ethical/legal principles. Box 3.10 presents the NFLPN Code for Licensed Practical/Vocational Nurses.

BASSETT HEALTHCARE

COMPUTER LOG # ______

INCIDENT/VARIANCE REPORT

#1001 4/88 rev. 8/94; 4/98; 6/98; 7/98; 8/98;11/98;9/03;11/03;1/04;10/04 (f:\riskmgt\.doc)

Instructions: Complete form immediately after an incident occurs. Send original to PI/RM within 24 hours of incident and keep copy for department use.

INCIDENT DATE: ______ TIME: ______

IDENTIFICATION: ☐ PATIENT ☐ VISITOR ☐ VOLUNTEER ☐ OTHER ☐ EMPLOYEE; DEPT ______

LAST NAME: ______ FIRST NAME: ______

CHART #: ______ AGE: ______ SEX: ☐ MALE ☐ FEMALE

Incident Location

☐ Inpatient Services Unit/Room: ______
☐ MIBH ☐ O'Connor ☐ Cobleskill Regional Hospital
☐ Tri Town Regional Hospital ☐ Little Falls Hospital
☐ Emergency Services
☐ Health Center: ______
☐ Food Services
☐ Laboratory: Section: ______
☐ Operative Services; Unit: ______
☐ Other
☐ Outpatient Services
Clinic: ______
☐ Outside Property
List: ______
☐ Pharmacy
☐ Radiology
☐ Rehabilitative Services

Category:

☐ Fall (Inpatient Units–STOP. Use fall analysis tool #6647)
☐ Fracture/Dislocation
☐ Burn
☐ Chemical Burn
☐ Contusion/Laceration
☐ Back/Muscle Strain
☐ Blood/Body Fluid Exposure (describe event thoroughly below)
    ☐ Blood ☐ Other body fluid ______
    ☐ Clean needle ☐ Contaminated needle
    Source patient chart #: ______
☐ Patient Care Equipment
    Equipment type/tag #: ______
    ☐ Equipment not available
    ☐ Electrical problem/shock
    ☐ Mechanical problem
☐ Security Variance
    ☐ Hospital property loss
    ☐ Personal property loss
    ☐ Suspected crime/assault
☐ Medical Gas
    ☐ Wrong source
    ☐ O_2 not connected
    ☐ Wrong O_2 % / flow
    ☐ Other:
☐ Patient left AMA without signing AMA form
☐ Medication and IV variance - STOP
Use medication variance report (#2308) and medication variance evaluation worksheet (#5610) to report
☐ Transport
☐ Procedural Variance
    ☐ Laboratory specimen/testing error
    ☐ Unlabeled specimen
    ☐ Mislabeled specimen
    ☐ Other
☐ Other

Brief Description: ______

Seen by provider?
☐ No ☐ Yes Date: ______
Outcome: ______

Investigation Outcome / Corrective Action (Must Complete) ______

Copy sent and referred to ______ for investigation and response.
(Attention receiving department: Send response to PI/RM)

SIGNATURE AND TITLE OF PERSON COMPLETING THIS FORM | DATE | SIGNATURE OF MANAGER/SUPERVISOR | DATE

FIGURE 3.1 Sample incident report. (Courtesy of Bassett Healthcare, Cooperstown, New York.)

Box 3.8 Ethical Terms in Nursing

- *Beneficence*: to do good; taking positive action to help others
- *Nonmaleficence:* to avoid causing harm to someone
- *Veracity*: being honest and truthful
- *Fidelity*: keeping promises
- *Autonomy*: respecting someone's self-determination
- *Justice*: treating people with fairness
- *Privacy* and *confidentiality*: respecting patient privacy and confidential information

Box 3.9 NAPNES Code of Ethics

The licensed practical/vocational nurse shall:

1. Consider as a basic obligation the conservation of life and the prevention of disease.
2. Promote and protect the physical, mental, emotional, and spiritual health of the patient and his family.
3. Fulfill all duties faithfully and efficiently.
4. Function within established legal guidelines.
5. Accept personal responsibility (for his/her acts) and seek to merit the respect and confidence of all members of the health team.
6. Hold in confidence all matters coming to his/her knowledge, in the practice of his/her profession, and in no way and at no time violate this confidence.
7. Give conscientious service and charge just remuneration.
8. Learn and respect the religious and cultural beliefs of his/her patient and of all people.
9. Meet his/her obligation to the patient by keeping abreast of current trends in health care through reading and continuing education.
10. As a citizen of the United States of America, uphold the laws of the land and seek to promote legislation that will meet the health needs of its people.

Box 3.10 NFLPN Code for Licensed Practical/ Vocational Nurses

1. Know the scope of maximum utilization of the LP/VN as specified by the nurse practice act and function within this scope.
2. Safeguard the confidential information acquired from any source about the patient.
3. Provide health care to all patients regardless of race, creed, cultural background, disease, or lifestyle.
4. Uphold the highest standards in personal appearance, language, dress, and demeanor.
5. Stay informed about issues affecting the practice of nursing and delivery of health care and where appropriate, participate in government and policy decisions.
6. Accept the responsibility for safe nursing by keeping oneself mentally and physically fit and educationally prepared to practice.
7. Accept responsibility for membership in NFLPN and participate in its efforts to maintain the established standards of nursing practice and employment policies, which lead to quality patient care.

ETHICS COMMITTEES

Many health care facilities have ethics committees that are composed of people from various departments such as nursing, medicine, surgery, psychiatry, pharmacy, legal, economics, spiritual, and social work. Together they develop policies, address issues in their facility, and come to a better understanding of ethical dilemmas from different viewpoints.

ETHICAL DILEMMAS

The nurse may face many ethical dilemmas. A current issue revolves around life-and-death decisions. When a patient is diagnosed with a terminal illness, family members and even the health care team may often have conflicting opinions about seeking life-prolonging treatment versus refusing such treatment. Patients have the right to information about alternative, as well as conventional, treatment options, with their risks, consequences, and benefits. Nurses must honor the patient's right to choose or refuse any treatment or procedure, even if it would not be the nurse's choice.

Perhaps even more difficult is the choice to initiate or terminate life support or treatment. Questions of whether to allow a patient to stop artificial feedings or not to treat an infection with antibiotics in a terminally ill person often raise uncomfortable feelings in nurses. Respecting the patient's right to self-determination means respecting and supporting a patient's informed choice regarding treatment. Providing compassionate care at the end of life honors the person's decision to live his remaining time in the way he chooses.

Another ethical issue involves **assisted suicide,** which is aiding a person (providing the means) to end his life. The Supreme Court in June 1997 held that there was no constitutional right to physician-assisted suicide. Legally, at this time, physician-assisted suicide is legal in Oregon, Washington, and Vermont, but it is illegal in most other states, although some do not specifically address assisted suicide in their statutes. The laws are often challenged, resulting in changes, therefore nurses should be aware of the status of such legislation in their state (Patients Rights Council, 2012). Assisted suicide is often confused with **euthanasia,** sometimes called mercy killing. Euthanasia is the act of ending another person's life, with or without the person's consent, to end actual or potential suffering. It is not legal in any state. Participation in assisted suicide is a violation of the ANA *Code for Nurses,* as well as the ethical tradition of "do no harm." The issue remains very controversial, with intelligent and caring people holding different values.

Daily, nurses face personal ethical decisions involving honesty, **whistle-blowing** (reporting illegal or unethical actions), and provision of care. Our professional code of ethics dictates that we act as patient advocates and safeguard our patients from harm. Who will know if a nurse gives a wrong medication or fails to assess an unconscious patient? Should a nurse report suspected incompetence or impairment of a fellow nurse or physician? What care can be omitted in a short-staffed unit where all the needs are urgent? How does a nurse treat difficult patients, those who are abusive or who arouse feelings of anger or hatred, such as a person convicted of brutal crimes?

Nursing codes of ethics provide guidelines for behavior that promote excellence in patient care and the profession. They promote values such as dignity, honesty, integrity, and compassion.

On an institutional level, the ethics committee may be occupied with end-of-life issues such as withholding or withdrawing life-sustaining treatments. On a state and national level, legislators choose where to spend money and write laws that affect health care. Those decisions are influenced by ethics and values, and nurses can have an influence by sharing their ethical concern for patients and speaking up for patients' rights.

Nurses can consciously consider what is right or wrong for them, in light of personal values. When a nurse feels confused or conflicted about the right course of action in a situation, talking with other nurses, the unit supervisor, or the ethics committee in the agency can assist the nurse in solving the problem from an ethical viewpoint.

QSEN Considerations: Patient-Centered Care

When Your Beliefs Differ From Those of Your Patient

There may be times when the patient makes medical decisions that conflict greatly with your values and beliefs. In this case, the appropriate action would be to ask that another nurse care for the patient if possible.

Get Ready for the NCLEX Examination!

Key Points

- Legislators, agencies, and courts create laws; codes of ethics are written by professional organizations. Laws are civil (private) or criminal (public). A civil wrong is a tort; a public wrong is a crime.
- Nursing is governed by state nurse practice acts, which define the scope of practice. State boards of nursing administer the law. Standards of care are developed by professional organizations. Students are held to the same standards and laws as the professionals are.
- Professional accountability means taking responsibility for one's own actions. Nurses may delegate patient care to unlicensed personnel, but they remain responsible for safe, effective patient care.
- Continuing education to keep knowledge and skills current and safe is an ethical responsibility. In many states, it is a legal requirement for continuing licensure.
- OSHA monitors the workplace for the health and safety of its employees.
- CAPTA requires licensed nurses and other health care professionals to report child abuse.
- The "Patient Care Partnership" recognizes that patients do not lose their civil rights when they are hospitalized.
- Consent is necessary to perform invasive procedures, to divulge confidential information, or to conduct research. Consent must be legally obtained to show the patient's permission.
- Types of advance directives include living wills and a medical power of attorney. A living will allows a patient to express his wishes about medical treatment; a medical power of attorney gives legal power to a person to make decisions when the patient is unable.
- HIPAA regulations strictly guard the privacy of patient information. They require a specific signed consent for release of information.
- Negligence and malpractice are common torts in health care; assault, battery, defamation, invasion of privacy, or false imprisonment may result in malpractice torts.
- A successful lawsuit requires the following four elements to be proven: duty, breach of duty, causation, and injury.
- Competent nursing practice, careful documentation, development of a caring relationship with patients, and professional communication can reduce one's likelihood of being named in a lawsuit. Patient safety, medication or treatment errors, and failure to assess are frequent areas of lawsuits for nurses.
- Malpractice insurance protects nurses from financial damages in the event of a lawsuit and pays for legal assistance.
- Codes of ethics have been developed by nursing organizations and provide principles to guide behavior in situations in which there may be no "right" answer.
- Ethical dilemmas result when people hold differing views on issues. Ethics committees can provide an interdisciplinary approach to solving ethical dilemmas.

Additional Learning Resources

SG Go to your Study Guide for additional learning activities to help you master this chapter content.

evolve Go to your Evolve website at http://evolve.elsevier.com/Williams/fundamental for additional online resources.

Online Resources

- *Brent's Law,* www.nurse.com/AskTheExperts/BrentsLaw
- *American Hospital Association: Patient Care Partnership,* www.aha.org/advocacy-issues/communicatingpts/pt-care-partnership.shtml

Review Questions for the NCLEX Examination

*Choose the **best** answer(s) for each of the following questions.*

1. Which action(s) violate the HIPAA? *(Select all that apply.)*
   1. Discussing the comatose patient's condition with his father-in-law
   2. Discussing the outcome of a patient's test with another nurse from the unit while in a crowded elevator
   3. Relaying information about the patient's concerns to the nurse who will care for him on the next shift
   4. Relaying a complaint about the quality of nursing care by the patient's wife to the charge nurse
   5. Updating your social media site about a difficult clinical day, including hospital and patient's diagnosis, but NOT the patient's name
2. You witness a nursing assistant force a patient who is trying to stand into a chair saying, "Don't keep trying to get up or I will restrain you." The nursing assistant's behavior is an example of:
   1. Assault
   2. Battery
   3. Assault and battery
   4. Negligence
3. Your patient has experienced severe complications during surgery and remains on life support. Decisions about care can be more easily made if the patient has which documents in place?
   1. A power of attorney over financial affairs
   2. An advance directive
   3. A will
   4. No special documentation is needed.
4. The visitor of one of your patients stops you in the hall and says, "I hope you will not try to revive my neighbor if her heart stops." The correct response is:
   1. "That decision is up to the physician."
   2. "We are all trained in CPR."
   3. "I understand your concern, but I can't discuss your neighbor's care with you."
   4. "There is a 'do-not-resuscitate' order in her medical record."
5. The student neglects to raise the head of the bed of a patient receiving continuous tube feedings. The patient aspirates and develops pneumonia. Which correctly describes the student's liability in this situation?
   1. The charge nurse is responsible because she did not delegate care appropriately.
   2. The LPN caring for the patient is solely responsible because she is licensed.
   3. The student is expected to provide the same standard of care as the LPN.
   4. Both the nursing instructor and the student are equally liable.
6. A patient confides that her broken arm is the result of her husband's abuse of her. In this instance, the nurse is required to:
   1. Get a second nurse to witness her statement.
   2. Report the abuse to the authorities.
   3. Assure the patient that the information will be kept private.
   4. Confirm the abuse with another family member and then notify the charge nurse.
7. Your patient asks you, "What do you think of my physician?" You mention that the physician does not seem to care about her patients or how well their symptoms are managed. As a result, the patient switches to another physician. The physician may have grounds to sue you for:
   1. Malpractice.
   2. Slander.
   3. Libel.
   4. Invasion of privacy.

Critical Thinking Activities

Read each clinical scenario and discuss the questions with your classmates.

Scenario A

José Morales is a 46-year-old husband and father of two grown children. He has painful metastatic bone cancer. He is being discharged with a pain management program that still does not completely ease his pain. He tells you that he plans to "end it all" once he is at home and asks you to help him with information about what kind and how much medication it would take so his death will not look like suicide. He also warns you not to tell anyone of his plans because of "confidentiality."

1. Describe how you would answer his questions about assisted suicide.
2. Discuss the issue of confidentiality among the health care team versus invasion of privacy. How would you handle his request not to tell anyone?

Scenario B

You are a staff nurse at a skilled nursing facility on the evening shift. A 66-year-old woman who is very confused and agitated is pacing in the halls, entering other residents' rooms, and attempting to leave the building. Another nurse grabs the patient roughly and shouts at her, "If you don't stay in your room, I'm going to tie you in that bed." The nurse escorts the patient to her room, pushes her into a chair, and ties a sheet across the patient's lap to prevent her from getting out of the chair.

1. Identify the legal and ethical violations the nurse has committed.
2. What is your legal and ethical responsibility in this situation?

Scenario C

How would you respond to a provider at the clinic where you work who asks you embarrassing questions about your sexual experience and suggests that you would benefit in your job if you entertained him at your home?

chapter

4 The Nursing Process and Critical Thinking

http://evolve.elsevier.com/deWit/fundamental

Objectives

Upon completing this chapter, you should be able to do the following:

Theory

1. Explain the use of the nursing process.
2. Identify the components of the nursing process.
3. Compare and contrast the terms *critical thinking*, *clinical reasoning*, and *clinical judgment*.
4. Identify the steps of the problem-solving process.
5. List the steps used in making decisions.
6. Identify ways to improve clinical reasoning skills.
7. Apply the critical thinking process to a real-life problem.
8. Discuss the use of critical thinking in nursing.
9. Explain the principles of setting priorities for nursing care.
10. List factors to be considered when setting priorities.

Clinical Practice

1. Apply the nursing process to a patient care assignment.
2. Use clinical reasoning to prioritize the care of a patient assignment.

Key Terms

assessment (data collection) (p. 49)
clinical judgment (p. 50)
clinical reasoning (p. 50)
critical thinking (p. 50)
decision making (p. 50)
evaluation (p. 49)
implementation (p. 49)
nursing diagnosis (p. 49)
nursing process (p. 48)
outcomes (p. 48)
planning (p. 49)
priority (prī-ŌR-ĭ-tē, p. 53)
scientific method (sī-ĕn-TĬ-fĭk, p. 48)

 Concepts Covered in This Chapter

- Caregiving
- Care coordination
- Clinical judgment
- Collaboration
- Communication
- Coping
- Development
- Ethics
- Evidence
- Functional ability
- Glucose regulation

THE NURSING PROCESS

The **nursing process** is a way of thinking and acting based on the **scientific method** (a step-by-step process used by scientists to solve problems). The nursing process is a tool for identifying patients' problems or potential problems and an organized method for meeting patients' needs. It was developed in the 1950s to describe the nurse's independent role in providing patient care. Nurses are taught to use this framework consistently and methodically (Fig. 4.1).

The five components of the nursing process are assessment (data collection), nursing diagnosis, planning, implementation, and evaluation. Box 4.1 provides a brief explanation of each component. The goals of this systematic, dynamic process are to explore patients' health status, identify actual or potential health care problems, determine desired **outcomes** (results of actions), deliver specific nursing interventions that will solve the problems and promote health, and evaluate caregiving and determine whether outcomes have been achieved. The components often overlap as the nurse continually assesses and evaluates the effects of actions. The licensed practical nurse (LPN)/licensed vocational nurse (LVN) role in the nursing process is shown in Table 4.1, as set by the LPN/LVN Standards described by the National Federation of Licensed Practical Nurses (NFLPN) (see Appendix B). The LPN role is explained more fully in Chapters 5 and 6.

Creating a patient care plan involves collaboration with the nurse, the patient, and other health team members. **Patient input during the planning stage**

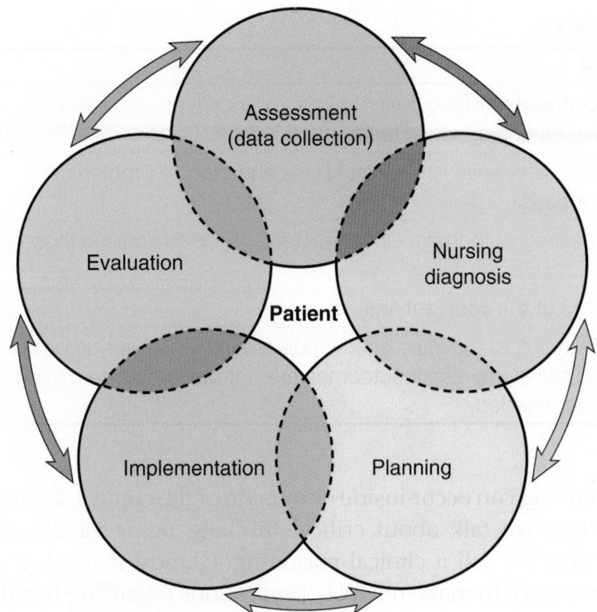

FIGURE 4.1 The nursing process: a dynamic, overlapping, continuous process encompassing patient-centered care.

Box 4.1 Components of the Nursing Process

Assessment (data collection): Collecting, organizing, documenting, and validating data about a patient's health status. Assessment data are obtained from the patient, the family, the primary care provider, diagnostic tests, and information about the patient from other health professionals.

Nursing diagnosis: The process by which the assessment data are sorted and analyzed so that specific actual and potential health problems are identified. The factors contributing to the problems are considered, and specific nursing diagnoses are chosen for the patient's care plan.

Planning: A series of steps by which the nurse and the patient set priorities and goals to eliminate or diminish the identified problems. The goals are stated as specific expected outcomes. The nurse and the patient collaborate and choose specific interventions for each nursing diagnosis. The interventions assist the patient in meeting the expected outcomes. The expected outcomes and nursing interventions are listed on the patient's nursing care plan.

Implementation: Carrying out the nursing interventions in a systematic way. The nurse carries out (or appropriately delegates) the interventions. The patient's response to the care given is documented.

Evaluation: Assessing the patient's response to the nursing interventions. The responses are compared with the expected outcomes to determine whether they have been achieved. The entire care plan is reassessed, and any changes needed are made.

Table 4.1 Correlation of Nursing Process and NFLPN Nursing Practice Standards for the Licensed Practical/Vocational Nurse

	STANDARD
	Shall know and utilize the nursing process in planning, implementing, and evaluating health services and nursing care for the individual patient or group.
1. *Assessment*	*RN function*
2. *Nursing diagnosis*	*RN function*
3. Planning	1. Assessment/data collection of health status of the individual patient, the family, and community groups. 2. Reporting information gained from assessment/data collection. 3. The identification of health goals.
4. Implementation	The plan for nursing care is put into practice to achieve the stated goals and includes: 1. Observing, recording, and reporting significant changes that require intervention or different goals. 2. Applying nursing knowledge and skills to promote and maintain health, to prevent disease and disability, and to optimize functional capabilities of an individual patient. 3. Assisting the patient and family with activities of daily living and encouraging self-care as appropriate. 4. Carrying out therapeutic regimens and protocols prescribed by personnel pursuant to authorized state law.
5. Evaluation	The plan for nursing care and its implementations are evaluated to measure the progress toward the stated goals and will include appropriate person and/or groups to determine: 1. The relevancy of current goals in relation to the progress of the individual patient. 2. The involvement of the recipients of care in the evaluation process. 3. The quality of the nursing action in the implementation of the plan. 4. A re-ordering of priorities or new goal setting in the care plan.

Table 4.2 Comparison of Scientific Method and the Nursing Process

SCIENTIFIC METHOD STEP	NURSING PROCESS STEP
Define the problem. Gather information.	**Assessment (Data Collection)** Take patient history, perform physical assessment, and gather results of diagnostic tests.
Analyze the information (data).	**Nursing Diagnosis** Consider assessment database and identify problems; choose nursing diagnoses.
Develop solutions. Make a decision.	**Planning** Determine desired outcomes. Choose interventions to achieve those outcomes.
Implement the decision.	**Implementation** Carry out the interventions.
Evaluate the decision.	**Evaluation** Assess the result of the interventions; determine whether outcomes have been achieved; revise the plan if outcomes are not being met; terminate interventions no longer needed.

results in greater success with the care plan and care coordination. Registered nurses (RNs) are officially responsible for the initiation of nursing care plans, but the LPN/LVN assists with each part of the care plan. The LPN is often responsible for data collection to assist the RN with the assessment phase. The nursing process allows for constant alterations in the care plan as patients' conditions change.

The nursing process is similar to other methods used to organize tasks in daily life. In planning a week's meals at home, the goal is to supply each family member with good nutrition. The *assessment*, or data collection, phase involves surveying the supplies on hand needed for food preparation. These data are analyzed to determine what must be purchased at the store; to *plan* specific menus; and to plan for deviation from normal meals, such as school lunches or quick dinners before a child's basketball game. *Implementation* includes shopping, preparing and serving the meals, and cleaning up afterward. *Evaluation* is performed to determine whether the plan was successful: Did the family members eat what was served? Was there too much left over? Was the expected outcome of balanced nutrition for each family member met? If not, should the plan be altered for next week? This is not a new way of thinking and doing; the process is just being applied in a nursing context.

? Think Critically

What activities do you do frequently in which you use this type of process for thinking and accomplishing things?

CRITICAL THINKING

Using critical thinking and the nursing process can help you develop good **clinical reasoning** skills that result in solid **clinical judgment.** What does this mean? ***Critical*** means requiring careful judgment. **Thinking,** in this context, means to reason. **Critical thinking is directed, purposeful, mental activity by which you create and evaluate ideas, analyze data, anticipate problems, use expansive thinking, reflect on experience, construct plans, and determine desired outcomes.** Critical thinking can occur inside or outside of the clinical setting. When we talk about critical thinking *inside the clinical setting* we call it clinical reasoning. Clinical reasoning is necessary to make reliable observations regarding health status and to draw sound conclusions from the data obtained from the patient and from other sources. Critical thinking and clinical reasoning are needed to creatively problem solve and to produce new ideas and solutions. Clinical reasoning is the keystone of good clinical decision making and the development of clinical judgment. **Clinical judgment** is the *outcome* of clinical reasoning: the conclusion or decision (sometimes a nursing diagnosis) you arrive at by exercising your clinical reasoning skills.

PROBLEM SOLVING AND DECISION MAKING

Nursing is a discipline that incorporates scientific knowledge and research methods. To solve problems, scientists use a consistent, logical method called the scientific method. The scientist first defines the problem, and then gathers information, analyzes the information, and develops solutions. The scientist makes a decision about which solution to use, implements the decision, and then evaluates the outcome of the decision. The nursing process has many similar characteristics to the scientific method. Table 4.2 compares the scientific method with the nursing process.

The **problem-solving** process has the following steps:

1. Define the problem clearly.
2. Consider all possible alternative solutions to the problem.
3. Consider the possible outcomes for each alternative.
4. Predict the likelihood of each outcome occurring.
5. Choose the alternative with the best chance of success and the fewest undesirable outcomes.

Decisions are necessary to solve problems. Nurses make decisions in each step of the nursing process. Good **decision making** is choosing the best actions to meet a desired goal and is part of the critical thinking process. Nurses often have to make quick decisions in moments of crisis; they also assist patients in making decisions. Nurses must problem solve continually. Critical thinking improves the outcomes of the problem-solving process.

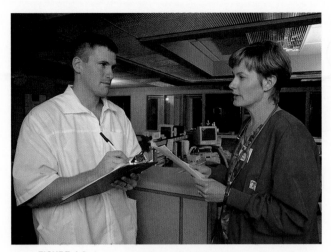

FIGURE 4.2 Student listening attentively to the staff nurse.

SKILLS FOR CRITICAL THINKING

Critical thinking involves a variety of skills. Foundation skills are effective reading, effective writing, attentive listening, and effective communication.

Effective reading involves reading material in a way that helps you pick out the main ideas and relevant data. Reading a paragraph and then restating the main ideas to yourself is one way to read critically.

Effective writing consists of writing thoughts coherently and concisely, yet clearly. Writing clearly, logically, and concisely is a learned skill that takes practice. Evaluating what you write helps improve this skill.

Attentive listening means consciously focusing on the topic of discussion. Attentive listening also takes practice. With our busy lives, we tend to rush ahead to form an answer or ask a question rather than wait until the speaker has finished. Pay attention to each word and the meaning the speaker is trying to convey (Fig. 4.2). To practice attentive listening, work with a partner. Have your partner tell you about something of interest. When she is finished, repeat back the main ideas of what was stated. Confirm with the speaker that you heard correctly.

Effective communicating requires speaking in a disciplined manner. The disciplined speaker thinks about what to say and how to state it clearly and concisely in a logical way before speaking. Effective speaking follows attentive listening. Much communication in our fast-paced society results in spontaneous response without conscious thought, and misunderstanding often occurs. Take time to consider your response before beginning to speak. Group interactions that provide feedback will help you assess and improve your speaking skill. Other skills and attributes found in the critical thinker are listed in Box 4.2.

A technique that nursing students have found helpful to promote critical thinking is **concept mapping.** Concept mapping helps students learn to synthesize pertinent assessment data, develop comprehensive care plans, link nursing interventions with health problems and nursing diagnoses, and effectively implement the care plan. It can help you see relationships within a concept or relationships between concepts. Concept mapping will help you gather data in a logical manner and then group those data in a meaningful way. Concept Map 4.1 shows the possible demands and responsibilities in a nursing student's life. Although this map does not show the interrelationships between the items depicted, try to visualize how one area may be affected by another. For example, study hours and work hours will probably affect the time available for sleep. Multiple lines could be drawn to show the interrelationships. Concept mapping is helpful in learning about the pathophysiology of a disease and how it affects the body. You will find many concept maps throughout this text.

Box 4.2 Skills and Attributes of the Critical Thinker

The critical thinker has the ability to:

- Maintain an open mind and a questioning attitude.
- Be confident, flexible, creative, and insightful.
- Recognize one's own biases and limitations.
- Be persistent in seeking solutions.
- Separate relevant from irrelevant information.
- Recognize inconsistencies in gathered data.
- Identify missing information.
- Consider all possibilities with curiosity.
- Anticipate potential problems.
- Use an organized and systematic approach to problems.
- Verify accuracy and reliability of data.
- Consider all possible solutions before making a decision.
- Admit what one does not know.
- Reason logically and reflect on experience.
- Strive for excellence and improvement.
- Draw valid conclusions from the evidence or data.
- Set priorities and make carefully considered decisions.
- Be empathic, humble, honest, and realistic.

? Think Critically

What critical thinking skills do you already use? Give some examples. Which critical thinking skill do you think is most important?

CRITICAL THINKING IN NURSING

Critical thinking in nursing requires skills and experience, as well as knowledge. Studies demonstrate that nursing professionalism influence a nurse's critical thinking ability. A positive self-concept is also linked to problem-solving and critical thinking ability. The QSEN project identifies evidence-based practice (EBP) as one of the major areas where prelicensure knowledge, skills, and attitudes (KSAs) are important for nursing students to acquire (Table 4.3).

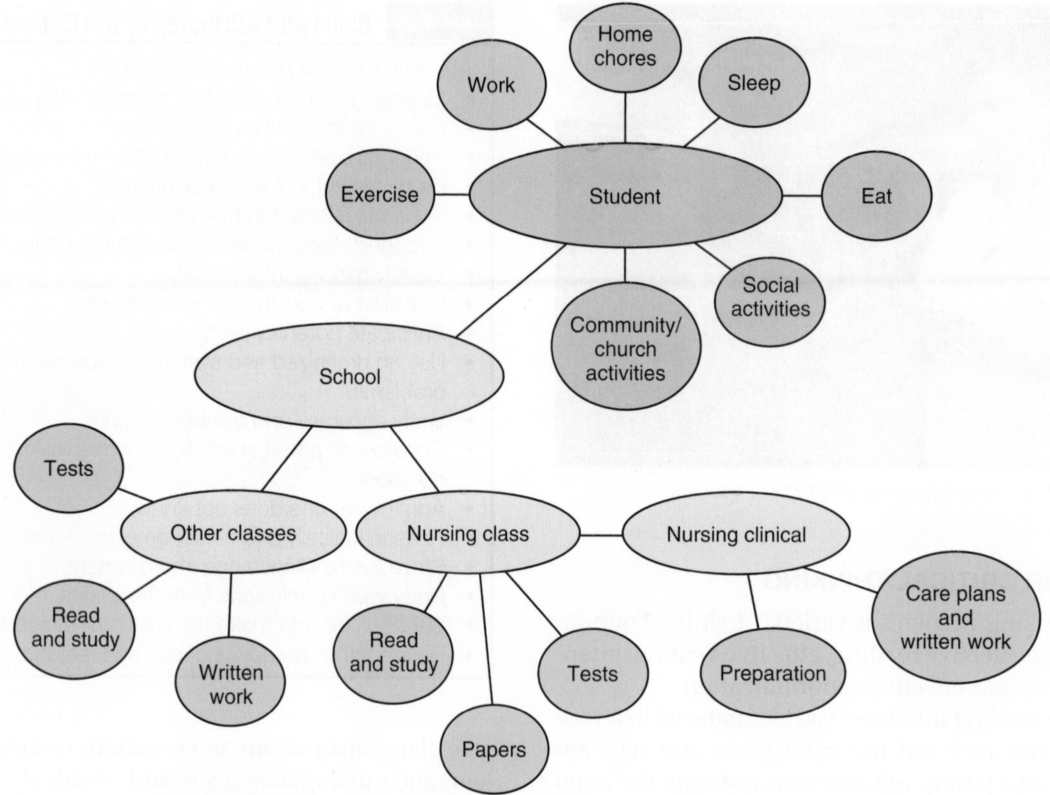

CONCEPT MAP 4.1 Demands on a nursing student's life and associated responsibilities.

Table 4.3 Evidence-Based Knowledge, Skills, and Attitudes for Prelicensure Licensed Practical Nurse/Licensed Vocational Nurse Students

KNOWLEDGE	SKILLS	ATTITUDES
• Knowledge of the scientific method • Knowledge of evidence-based practices in use at your clinical facilities • Distinguish between clinical opinion and evidence • Knowledge of reliable sources for evidence-based practice and clinical practice guidelines	• Participate in data collection or research activities • Implement the individualized plan of care as directed by registered nurse • Participate in structuring the work environment when integrating new evidence into standards of practice • Consult with clinical experts • Question rationale of interventions that lead to adverse outcomes	• Value the concept of evidence-based practice • Value the need for quality improvement • Value the need for ethical research • Appreciate the need for reading current nursing journals • Value the need for continuous improvement in practice based on new knowledge

Adapted from: http://qsen.org/competencies/pre-licensure-ksas/

 QSEN Considerations: Evidence-Based Practice

EBP Tools and Procedures

In health care facilities, access to current documented standard procedures and evidence-based reference tools at the bedside can contribute to improved patient outcomes and critical thinking skills. Nurses can access (hard copy) procedure manuals or (soft copy) electronic resources and apply evidence-based knowledge to their nursing practice. One such resource is the American Association of Critical-Care Nurses (AACN). The AACN publishes evidence-based resources such as Practice Alerts, evidence-based ranking systems, and protocols on how to apply scientific research findings to specific patient populations.

Critical thinking, clinical reasoning, and clinical judgment are applied to the nursing process in many ways. **Assessment (data collection)** is carried out in an organized, systematic way. Data are gathered to determine and eliminate or manage actual or potential health problems. The data are accurately recorded. Ways of helping patients obtain optimum wellness and independence are identified.

Nursing diagnosis requires analysis of data gathered during assessment, clustering related information, identifying problem areas, and choosing appropriate nursing diagnoses.

Planning involves determining specific interventions and desired outcomes for each nursing diagnosis.

While planning interventions, consider ways to promote optimum wellness and independence and the most efficient, cost-effective way to achieve the desired outcomes.

Implementation is the process of preparing and performing the interventions. Equipment and supplies are gathered and procedures are thought through before beginning them. Interventions are performed and responses to them are assessed. Changes in interventions are instituted as needed. Accurate documentation of interventions and patient response occurs.

Evaluation is carried out by gathering data to determine whether expected outcomes have been achieved. When interventions are not leading to expected outcomes, what needs to be done is reconsidered. Aspects of the care plan are modified or terminated as appropriate.

PRIORITY SETTING AND WORK ORGANIZATION

Critical thinking is used to set priorities for patient care. Nurses must also prioritize the tasks assigned to them. A **priority** is more important than something else is at the time. **Prioritizing involves placing nursing diagnoses or nursing interventions in order of importance.** Life-threatening problems are of **high priority.** Problems that threaten health or coping ability are of **medium priority. Low-priority** problems are ones that do not have a major effect on the person if not attended to that day or even that week. Prioritizing patient problems is usually based on the adaptation of Maslow's hierarchy of needs. Prioritizing will be discussed in Chapter 5.

Prioritizing to organize your work requires considering several factors. As a student, you begin by prioritizing care for one patient. After graduation, you will prioritize caregiving for many patients. When beginning your clinical day, go over your patient assignment worksheet, the Kardex, or the computer patient care plan and determine what needs to be done in the next hour. These items are of high priority. Some tasks may include vital signs, daily weights before breakfast, blood glucose readings before eating, morning insulin injections, preoperative assessments, and administration of medication for pain control.

When prioritizing such tasks, you must consider what will happen if the task is not done on time. The recovering patient whose vital signs have been stable for the past 24 hours will probably not suffer a bad consequence if you do not take her vital signs exactly at 8 am. Checking the blood glucose and administering insulin for a patient with diabetes are more time-critical tasks, as she may suffer an alteration in her health status if the tasks are not completed on time.

Other factors to consider are the surgery schedule, stability of each patient, amount of time to perform each task, availability of help, medication orders, unforeseen problems, and primary care provider making rounds. Knowledge, clinical reasoning, and clinical judgment will help you prioritize your workload.

When all tasks have a rather high priority and there is no way you can do them all alone, you must assign some tasks to others. After prioritizing your tasks for the first hour, consider priorities for the rest of the shift. Figure 4.3 shows one type of work organization sheet.

? Think Critically

How would you respond if you are about to check a patient's blood glucose and administer her insulin, and a primary care provider asks you to perform a wound dressing for a patient who is not assigned to you?

Priorities constantly change because patient needs and conditions change frequently. To maintain organization with your workload, you must be flexible and frequently re-order your tasks. Try to review your work organization plan at least every 2 hours during your shift, reprioritizing as needed.

APPLICATION OF PROBLEM SOLVING AND CLINICAL REASONING

The emergency department is a good place to observe how nurses prioritize caregiving and problem solving. When the emergency department nurse is faced with three patients seeking help, how does the nurse decide who is treated first? The first patient complains of severe chest pain; the second has a fever and a very bad cough; the third has a bleeding laceration on her chin.

There are six possibilities for the order of treatment. When considering the possible outcome of choosing each alternative, the nurse looks at the consequences of placing each patient first, second, or third. If the woman with the laceration is chosen to be first, the outcomes might be (1) she will stop bleeding; (2) the man with chest pain may be having a heart attack and may die, or he may be diagnosed with severe indigestion; and (3) the woman with the fever and cough may become angry and cause a commotion. If the man with the chest pain is prioritized to be treated first, the outcomes might be (1) his life may be saved, or it may be determined that he has severe indigestion; (2) the woman with the laceration may lose more blood, or the bleeding may stop by applying pressure while she is waiting to be treated; and (3) the woman with the cough and fever may cause a commotion or may be courteous about waiting.

Considering the likelihood of each outcome occurring is the next step. The nurse looks at the three patients and estimates that the man with chest pain has at least a 65% chance of it being a life-threatening heart attack and a 35% chance that he has indigestion; the chance of the woman with the fever and sore throat causing a commotion is about 5%, and the chance of this woman courteously waiting about 95%. If you

ASSIGNMENT/WORK ORGANIZATION SHEET

Patient/ Room #	7:30	8:00	9:00	10:00	11:00	12:00	1:00	2:00	3:00
J. G. 526	V. S. Quick Assess	Shower Δ dressing	Meds Chart	Full Assess Chart		V. S.	Pre-op Teaching Chart	I+O Tape report	Close Chart
G. H. 528A	V. S. ✓Feed Pump	Quick Assess	Meds Full Assess	Chart	Teaching ✓Feed Pump	V.S.	meds	I+O	Close Chart ✓Feed Pump
S. S. 528B	V. S. ✓IV Quick Assess	med ✓IV	Full Assess Chart	✓IV	✓IV	V.S. Teaching	✓IV Δ dressing	I+O	Close Chart

FIGURE 4.3 One example of a work organization sheet for a shift.

choose the man with the chest pain to be treated first, the chance of the woman with the laceration losing a serious amount of blood is about 20%, while the chance of stopping the blood with pressure while awaiting treatment is about 80% or better. Since the chance of a bad outcome is highest for the man with the chest pain, you choose to have him treated first. **The goal is to avoid having your clinical judgment cause injury to anyone.**

Besides ordering treatment for emergency department patients, you must decide many things each day, such as what size needle is best to use for an injection, what to tell the patient or her family about her prognosis, which tasks to assign and which to do yourself, which staff to assign to which patients, and which nursing diagnosis has the highest priority for a patient on a particular day. **With critical thinking skills, you can weigh many factors and skillfully solve problems, making good nursing care decisions most of the time.** No one makes perfect decisions all the time. Learning to apply the nursing process well will assist you in developing sound clinical judgment and following logical processes automatically when solving problems and making decisions. **Operating in a critical thinking mode while pursuing your nursing studies will help you develop the clinical judgment necessary for safe nursing practice.**

The nursing process is a way of thinking, as well as organizing. In this dynamic process, the nurse is constantly gathering data and evaluating. The next two chapters explain the components of the nursing process more thoroughly. The chapter bibliography identifies resources to enhance learning by improving critical thinking skills.

Get Ready for the NCLEX Examination!

Key Points

- The nursing process is a way of thinking and acting based on the scientific method. It is a framework for planning, implementing, and evaluating nursing care.
- RNs are officially responsible for the initiation of nursing care plans, but LPN/LVNs assist with the care plan, evaluate care, and help revise through collaboration with other health team members.
- The components of the nursing process are assessment, nursing diagnosis, planning, implementation, and evaluation.
- Formulating a care plan is a collaborative process among the nurse, the patient, and other health team members.
- The nursing process is similar to the scientific method.
- The steps to problem solving are (1) define the problem clearly, (2) consider all possible alternatives, (3) consider the possible outcomes for each alternative, (4) predict the likelihood of each outcome occurring, and (5) choose the alternative with the best chance of success and the least undesirable outcomes.
- Critical thinking is directed, purposeful mental activity by which you create and evaluate ideas, analyze data, anticipate problems, use expansive thinking, reflect on experience, construct plans, and decide on desired outcomes; it is needed to make reliable observations and draw sound conclusions. It can occur inside or outside of the clinical setting.
- Clinical reasoning is critical thinking in the clinical setting. Clinical judgment is the result or outcome of clinical reasoning.
- Critical thinking involves a variety of skills, including effective reading, writing, communication, attentive listening, and problem solving. It is applied in each phase of the nursing process.
- Practicing careful consideration of problems and purposeful thinking increases critical thinking skills.
- Priority setting involves placing tasks, nursing diagnoses, or nursing interventions in order of importance.
- Nurses use priority setting for work organization and care coordination. Priorities constantly change as patient needs change.
- With critical thinking, nurses can weigh factors, skillfully solve problems, and make good decisions a majority of the time.

Additional Learning Resources

SG Go to your Study Guide for additional learning activities to help you master this chapter content.

evolve Go to your Evolve website http://evolve.elsevier.com/deWit/fundamental for additional online resources

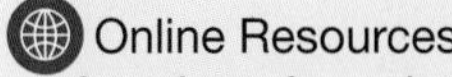

- American Association of Critical Care Nurses: www.aacn.org.

Review Questions for the NCLEX Examination

*Choose the **best** answer for each question.*

1. Input from the ______________________________ during the planning stage of the nursing process results in greater success. *(Fill in the blank.)*
2. Priorities of caregiving change constantly because: *(Select all that apply.)*
   1. The nurse's workload may change as patients are admitted.
   2. Primary care providers' orders may change throughout the shift.
   3. A patient's condition may deteriorate.
   4. Tests or therapies involve scheduled time off the unit.
   5. Many visitors are in the room to assist the patient.
3. Clinical reasoning is most important when:
   1. Planning wound care for a pressure injury.
   2. Organizing nursing care for several patients.
   3. Collaborating with other health team members.
   4. Drawing sound conclusions from assessment data.
4. Attributes of critical thinkers include: *(Select all that apply.)*
   1. Admitting what you don't know.
   2. Consulting with primary care providers.
   3. Anticipating problems.
   4. Reflecting on experience.
   5. Accepting others' decisions.
   6. Being confident about your decisions.
   7. Recognizing inconsistencies in gathered data.
5. Critical thinking will help you in the clinical setting to:
   1. Delegate work more efficiently.
   2. Make good decisions most of the time.
   3. Identify the best nursing diagnoses.
   4. Write care plans more effectively.
6. How do concept maps assist critical thinking? *(Select all that apply.)*
   1. They help point out relationships among the data.
   2. They link interventions, health problems, and nursing diagnoses.
   3. They provide a timeline pattern to improve planning.
   4. They help students synthesize pertinent data.
   5. They identify care coordination roles using color codes.
7. Which principle is most important when setting priorities for patient care?
   1. Classifying nursing diagnosis and interventions as high, medium, and low.
   2. Reevaluate and assess your priorities every 45 minutes.
   3. Respond to the loudest, most difficult patient first so the others can rest.
   4. Keep patients with visiting family well informed, but delay treatments.

8. Which is an example of clinical judgment?
   1. Weighing the pros and cons of which school to send your children to.
   2. Deciding which nursing midterm examination to study for first.
   3. Prioritizing which call light to answer first.
   4. Answering the primary care provider's question in a diplomatic manner.

Critical Thinking Activities

Read each clinical scenario and discuss the questions with your classmates.

Scenario A

As a student, you have several tasks to complete. There is an Anatomy and Physiology test in 4 days. You just collected the library materials you need for a comprehensive paper due in 1 week. A 50-page reading assignment needs to be completed for a lecture the day after tomorrow.

1. How would you organize to accomplish these tasks?
2. In what order of priority would you place each of these tasks? Explain why you placed each task in the order chosen.

Scenario B

Your clinical area does not have sphygmomanometers (blood pressure cuffs) on the wall by each patient; portable ones are used. You need to take 8 am vital signs (temperature, pulse, respiration rate, and blood pressure) quickly, and there is no portable unit available right now. How would you solve this problem?

Scenario C

Your clinical assignment is for:
M.H., age 72; diagnosis: pneumonia
F.S., age 52; diagnosis: leg ulcer
J.P., age 78; diagnosis: abdominal hernia repair

1. It is 9:45 am. If J.P. needs to be ambulated three times a day, M.H. needs his antibiotic given at 10 am, and F.S. needs her dressing changed this morning, in what order would you do these tasks?
2. How did you make this decision?

chapter 5

Assessment, Nursing Diagnosis, and Planning

http://evolve.elsevier.com/Williams/fundamental

Objectives

Upon completing this chapter, you should be able to do the following:

Theory

1. Identify the purpose of assessment (data collection).
2. Discuss the three basic methods used to gather a patient database.
3. Differentiate objective data from subjective data.
4. Use sources of data for the formulation of a patient database.
5. Correlate patient problems with nursing diagnoses from the accepted NANDA-I list.
6. Select appropriate outcome criteria for selected nursing diagnoses.
7. Plan goals for each patient and write outcome criteria for the chosen nursing diagnoses.

Clinical Practice

1. Collect assessment data for a patient and document it.
2. Analyze the data collected to determine patient needs.
3. Identify appropriate nursing diagnoses from the NANDA-I list for each assigned patient.
4. Prioritize the nursing diagnoses.
5. Write specific goal/outcome statements.
6. Plan appropriate nursing interventions to assist the patient in attaining the goals/expected outcomes.

Key Terms

cues (KĔWS, p. 63)
data (p. 57)
database (p. 57)
defining characteristics (p. 65)
etiologic factors (ē-tē-ō-LŌ-jĭk, p. 65)
expected outcome (p. 67)
goal (p. 66)
inferences (ĬN-fĕr-ĕn-sĕs, p. 64)
interview (p. 58)
nursing diagnosis (p. 64)
objective data (p. 58)
signs (p. 65)
subjective data (p. 58)
symptoms (p. 65)

 Concepts Covered in This Chapter

- Care Coordination
- Clinical judgment
- Collaboration
- Communication
- Patient education

ASSESSMENT (DATA COLLECTION)

The first three steps in the nursing process—assessment and data collection, nursing diagnosis, and planning—are discussed in this chapter. **Assessment** consists of gathering information about patients and their needs using a variety of methods. During the assessment phase of the nursing process, **data** (pieces of information on a specific topic) are systematically obtained, organized into a logical **database** (all of the information gathered about a patient), and documented. Data collection is a large part of assessment. Assessment for the licensed practical nurse/licensed vocational nurse (LPN/LVN) is guided by the National Federation of Licensed Practical Nurses (NFLPN) Standard 4 under the *Planning* area of the nursing process: "The planning of nursing includes assessment/data collection of the health status of the individual patient, the family and community groups" (see Appendix B). A registered nurse (RN) is designated as the staff must perform the initial admission assessment of each patient. However, the **LPN/LVN is often asked to assist with this task and participate in carrying out the plan by continuing to collect data.**

 QSEN Consideration: Teamwork and Collaboration

Collaboration With the Registered Nurse

Collaboration between the LPN/LVN and RN is imperative to ensuring that the patient's health care needs are met. This means that the LPN/LVN must communicate effectively, both verbally and in writing, with the RN and other members of the health care team.

 Assignment Considerations

Assigning Admission Tasks

If unlicensed assistive personnel (UAP) are available to help, you may assign the tasks of weighing, measuring, and obtaining a urine specimen for the newly admitted patient. The assistant could open the admission supplies and set up the patient's room. Be certain to alert the assistant of any safety measures needed for the patient.

The practice of nursing is concerned with how a patient *responds*, physiologically and psychologically, to their disease or disorder, treatment(s), life situation, and environment. To determine this, a database containing information about the patient must be established. It is in this capacity that LPNs/LVNs contribute, via data collection, to the assessment stage of the nursing process.

There are various approaches to data collection. One is a structured format to obtain a comprehensive database based on the 11 functional health patterns, as formulated by Mary Gordon (Box 5.1). After data in all 11 areas are collected, a review is performed to see if there are patterns indicating problems. The assessment data are then compared with the patient's baselines, such as usual blood pressure, heart rate, weight, and so forth. The functional patterns represent the interaction between the patient and the environment. The 11 patterns are each part of a whole, and any one pattern is understood only in conjunction with the other ten patterns. The analysis and comparisons help identify patient strengths and weaknesses. Many nursing schools teach this approach.

Box 5.1 Gordon's 11 Health Patterns

- Health perception–health management pattern
- Nutritional-metabolic pattern
- Elimination pattern
- Activity-exercise pattern
- Cognitive-perceptual pattern
- Sleep-rest pattern
- Self-perception–self-concept pattern
- Role-relationship pattern
- Sexuality-reproductive pattern
- Coping-stress-tolerance pattern
- Value-belief pattern

For each pattern, the following are assessed:

FUNCTIONAL

- Present function
- Personal habits
- Lifestyle and cultural factors
- Age-related factors

DYSFUNCTIONAL

- History of dysfunction
- Diagnostic test abnormalities
- Risk factors related to medical treatment plan

All problems identified within a pattern are considered according to their relationship to the other functional patterns. Nursing focus is aimed at improving the patient's functional status in each pattern area.

A second method of data collection is to begin with areas in which problems are evident, such as pain. Factors causing or affecting the pain are explored. This is a **focused assessment** because it is concerned with one very specific problem. The assessment and data collection then progress to how the problem affects other areas of the patient's life. If the patient is in acute distress, a focused assessment may be performed before a total assessment and data collection are completed.

A third method is to assess every area in Maslow's hierarchy of basic needs (see Fig. 2.3). Whatever method is used, assessment and data collection must be comprehensive, covering all aspects of the patient: physical, psychosocial, and spiritual.

An admission assessment and data collection **interview** (conversation in which facts are obtained) is usually performed when patients are assigned to the nursing unit, enter the care of a home health agency, or become residents in a long-term care facility. The nurse interviews the patient to find out his major complaints, performs a physical examination, and determines the patient's overall health status. Information is also gathered by observing the patient, reading the medical record or other sources of written information, and consulting with the family, significant others, and other health professionals.

Data obtained from the patient verbally that only the patient can describe or verify are called **subjective data.** A headache, tingling in the feet, or pain in the shoulder are examples of subjective data. Information obtained through the senses and hands-on physical examination is **objective data.** Objective data are signs that are seen, heard, measured, or felt by the person carrying out the assessment. The observed inabilities of a patient to grasp a glass in his left hand or to support his body when standing are examples of objective data. Vital signs, physical examination findings, and results of diagnostic tests are also objective data (Table 5.1).

Table 5.1 Examples of Subjective and Objective Data

SUBJECTIVE DATA EXAMPLES	OBJECTIVE DATA EXAMPLES
"I have a headache."	Temperature 101.4°F (38.6°C)
"I am nauseated."	135 mL emesis at 08:20
"The sharp pain is in my hip."	Bruise on right hip
"I've been feeling really blue lately."	Eyes downcast, flat affect
"I've been lonely since my husband died."	Only one visitor seen in the room all day
"I'm tired all the time."	Hgb 10.5 mg/dL, HCT 31%
"I'm afraid I have cancer."	Pathology report states tissue is adenosarcoma

Hgb, Hemoglobin; *HCT*, hematocrit.

Other sources of data include the primary care provider's history and physical, ancillary staff notes, and the admission note. Radiology and laboratory results also provide information for the database, as well as information provided by the patient's family or companions. Data collection in health care facilities is guided by a printed form (or computer screen) that is completed and entered into the patient's medical record. The nursing student may be assigned to interview patients using a more comprehensive form as part of a learning experience (Fig. 5.1). Other sections of the form include skin, nutrition, personal habits, pain, education, and psychological/spiritual assessments.

Think Critically

Can you think of two other pieces of information that might be obtained during an assessment that would be subjective data?

THE INTERVIEW

The interview is focused on gathering data and is not a social interaction. Good communication is vital to adequate assessment. Communication may be verbal (talking and listening) or nonverbal (facial expressions, body posture, movement, and gestures).

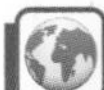

Cultural Considerations

Be Attentive to Cultural Needs

If your patient is of a different culture, recall the specifics of cultural differences in communication, personal space, and expected courtesies. Obtain an interpreter if there is a language barrier to good communication.

The course of the interaction is directed to elicit specific information concerning the patient's health status or feelings about her health. The interview contains three basic stages: (1) the opening, when rapport is established with the patient; (2) the body of the interview, when the necessary questions are presented; and (3) the closing segment of the interview. After establishing rapport, discuss the purpose of the interview. Indicate the closing of the interview by stating, "Do you have any questions?" or "I would be glad to answer any questions you have." Another way of closing the interview is to say something like, "Well, I guess that's all I need for now." Thank patients for their time, express some concern for their welfare, and tell them what will happen next. Summarize their problems and tell them when you will be back (see Chapter 8).

After the initial assessment, continue to gather data about the patient each time there is an encounter. **Assessment is an ongoing process.** If you are assigned to a patient in the days after the admission, a quick review of the medical record can provide data needed to provide adequate care.

Life Span Considerations

Older Adults

When interviewing an older adult, allow more time because the person will probably have a more extensive history and may take a little longer to recall the needed information.

MEDICAL RECORDS (CHART) REVIEW

A medical records (chart) review is a data collection tool that assists in obtaining the information needed to interview the patient intelligently or to prepare adequately for the day's patient assignment. To perform a medical records review, methodically look through the medical record, checking the sections listed in Box 5.2. Of course, if the patient has just been admitted, you can seek information only from the face sheet and the primary care provider's orders. If it is an electronic medical record, you will need to go to the various screens on the computer.

To do a review in preparation for your clinical assignment, look first at the face sheet and then at the most current primary care provider's orders, as well as those of the previous 2 days. Check the medication profile (medication administration record [MAR] or electronic medication administration record [eMAR]) to find out what medications the patient is receiving and whether the MAR or eMAR contains current orders. This will provide information about concurrent chronic conditions that may not be initially evident. Read the primary care provider's admitting history and physical assessment if they are included in the medical record. Scan any surgical procedure reports and accompanying pathology reports, paying particular attention to the conclusions. Note the psychosocial data on the face sheet. Does the patient live with family or a significant other? This information gives some idea of available support systems. Next, check the nurse's notes from the previous 24 to 48 hours, and then scan the current diagnostic test results. Read the nursing care plan or care map. Finally, read the nurse's admission assessment for data concerning events leading up to this hospitalization, previous hospital and illness experiences, other chronic health problems, and a history of allergies.

To visualize the nursing process in action, consider the following scenario:

> *Victoria Torres, age 76, room 728, bed A, suffered a stroke 3 days ago and has left-sided weakness (hemiparesis). She has difficulty with bladder control and urinary incontinence. She is left-handed, cannot firmly grasp objects, and, therefore, needs assistance with all personal care. She is receiving physical therapy to strengthen the muscles in her left arm and leg and is learning to walk with a walker, but she tires very easily.*

This information alone can help you begin to plan care for the patient. Concept Map 5.1 shows the

ADMISSION DATE & TIME	PRIMARY LANGUAGE IF NOT ENGLISH	ADMITTED FROM: ❑ ED ❑ ECF ❑ HOME ❑ DIRECT ❑ OTHER	HT. IN.	WT.	VITAL SIGNS
ROOM NUMBER:	❑ SIGN LANGUAGE	MODE OF TRANSFER: ❑ W/C ❑ BED ❑ GURNEY ❑ AMBULATED	❑ STATED ❑ MEASURED	❑ STANDING ❑ BED SCALE ❑ CHAIR SCALE	T R /min.
Patient Statement / Complaint:					R L P BP

Instruction of Routine and Services to Patient /Family

- ❑ Nurse Call System/Intercom
- ❑ Bed Controls
- ❑ Fall Prevention Program
- ❑ Patient Identification (Name & Date of Birth)
- ❑ Bedside Shift Report/Hourly Rounding
- ❑ Patient Care Handbook
  - Visitor Guidelines (Pg.5)
  - Patient Safety/How to Report Concerns (Pg.8)
  - Infection Prevention (Pg.9)
  - Pain Management (Pg.22)
  - Condition HELP

SIGNATURE & TITLE

The valuables/personal effects policy has been explained, and, I understand that Marian Medical Center does not assume responsibility for valuables (money, jewelry, or other personal effects) not secured in the Marian Medical Center safe.

________________ Signature
Patient or Responsible Person

La poliza tocante objectos de valor ha sido explicada, y yo entiendo que Marian Medical Center no asume responsibilidad por estos objectos (alhajas, dinero, etc.) o cualquier otra prenda personal que no sea asegurada en la caja fuerte de Marian Medical Center.

________________ Firma
Paciente o persona responsible por el paciente

DISCHARGE PLANNING

Environmental Concerns at home (i.e., stairs, lack of running water) ________

❑ Case Management notified (Discharge Planner)

Living situation: (home, B&C, SNF, living alone) ________

Anticipated Post Hospital Care issues: ________

Care Partner: Name: ________

Relationship: ________ Phone: ________

Other contact: ________

Relationship: ________ Phone: ________

Anticipated Ride Home ________ Phone: ________

MEDICAL HISTORY

	YES	NO
Diabetes	❑	❑
Asthma	❑	❑
Epilepsy / Seizure Disorder	❑	❑
Family Bleeding Tend.	❑	❑
Glaucoma	❑	❑
Cardiac	❑	❑
CHF	❑	❑
Pneumonia	❑	❑
AMI	❑	❑

Any other Medical/Surgical Conditions:

Marian Regional Medical Center
A Dignity Health Member

PATIENT ADMISSION ASSESSMENT

PAGE 1

ACCESS

6010-08(10/11)

PATIENT ID

FIGURE 5.1 Example of a patient admission assessment form. This is the first page of a four-page form.

NEUROLOGICAL STATUS

PUPIL SIZE CHART

1mm 2mm 3mm 4mm 5mm 6mm 7mm 8mm 9mm

R Reactive S Sluggish NR Non-Reactive

LEVEL OF CONSCIOUSNESS: ❑ ALERT ❑ ORIENTED
❑ Confused ❑ Slow to respond/Comprehend
❑ Disoriented ❑ Lethargic ❑ Vertigo
❑ Pupils: Size & reaction: Right ______ Left: ______

SENSORY LIMITATIONS:		❑ WNL			If Pt. Uses	If with Patient
❑ Taste	❑ Speech	❑ Sight	Glasses		❑	❑
❑ Touch	❑ Smell	❑ Hearing	Contact Lenses	❑ R ❑ L	❑	❑
			Hearing Aid	❑ R ❑ L	❑	❑

FUNCTIONAL STATUS (LEVEL OF SELF CARE)

MOBILITY: ❑ WNL ❑ Decreased mobility over last month
Limitations:
❑ Walking ❑ Stairs
❑ Transfer ❑ Standing
❑ Turning in bed ❑ Generalized Weakness
ASSISTANCE REQUIRED:
❑ Hygiene/Grooming ❑ Dressing ❑ Meals ❑ Other

	If PT Uses	If with Patient
Cane/Crutches/Walker	❑	❑
Artifical Limbs ❑ R ❑ L	❑	❑
Brace	❑	❑

WEAKNESS PARALYSIS/TRAUMA/SURGERY: ______
MOTOR FUNCTION CODE: 5 (Normal Strength)
RUE ______ 4 (Mild Weakness)
LUE ______ 3 (Moves Against Gravity)
RLE ______ 2 (Moves Not Against Gravity)
LLE ______ 1 (Some Movement)

❑ Request Rehab. Services consult
❑ Acute onset
❑ Changes in mobility in the last month
❑ ______

SAFETY RISK

		Score		Score
1. History of falling	No	0	5. Gait	
	Yes	25	Normal/bedrest/wheelchair	0 ______
2. Secondary diagnosis	No	0	Weak	10 ______
More than 1 medical dx	Yes	15 ______	Impaired	20 ______
3. Ambulatory Aid:			6. Mental Status:	
None/Bedrest/Nurse assist	No	0	Oriented to own ability	0 ______
Crutches/Cane/Walker	Yes	15 ______	Overestimates/forgets limitations	15 ______
Furniture	Yes	30 ______		
4. IV therapy/Saline lock	No	0		
	Yes	20 ______		

Total Score ______
❑ > 51 Initiate Safety Risk Protocol Care Plan Identified at High Risk for Fall
❑ Request PT evaluation

RESPIRATORY

❑ WNL BREATH SOUNDS RATE
❑ Accessory Muscles ❑ Secretions ❑ Nasal Flaring
❑ Dyspnea ❑ Tracheostomy ❑ Orthopnea
❑ Abnormal Breath Sounds ❑ Tachypnea ❑ Cough
❑ Oxygen ❑ Type ______

CARDIO VASCULAR

❑ WNL REGULAR RHYTHM, RATE
❑ Abnormal Pulses Apical/Radial/Pedal ❑ Abnormal Heart Sounds ❑ Pedal Edema
❑ Jugular Vein Distension ❑ Pacemaker

GASTRO INTESTINAL

❑ WNL
❑ NAUSEA-VOMITING
❑ TUBES
❑ N/G ❑ GT ❑ J/T
❑ OTHER ______
❑ BLOODY STOOL
❑ LAST BOWEL MOVEMENT: ______
❑ OSTOMY/ELIMINATION AIDS

❑ INCONTINENT OF BOWEL
❑ OCCASIONAL ❑ FREQUENT
❑ BOWEL SOUNDS
❑ NORMAL ❑ HYPO ❑ HYPER ❑ ABSENT
❑ CONSTIPATION ❑ DIARRHEA
❑ ABDOMINAL DISTENSION
❑ ABDOMINAL TENDERNESS/PAIN
LOCATION ______
❑ OTHER ______

GENITOURINARY / GYN

❑ Anuric ❑ WNL
❑ Nocturia ❑ Other: ______
❑ Burning ❑ Catheter
❑ Urgency Date Placed ______
❑ Urinary Incontinence
❑ Urinary Frequency
❑ Stress Incontinence

GYN

❑ Not Applicable
❑ Vaginal Discharge ______
❑ Unusual Bleeding
Pad Count ______
❑ Pregnant
❑ LMP ______

❑ If pregnant and over 20 weeks, complete OB Assessment.
Obtain prenatal record from L&D or Obstetrician

ACCESS

PAGE 2

FIGURE 5.1, cont'd Example of a patient admission assessment form. This is the second page of a four-page form. (Courtesy Marian Medical Center, Santa Maria, California.)

Box 5.2 Quick Medical Records Review

Look for the following information:

Face sheet: Age, sex, marital status/significant other, religion, occupation, residence, next of kin, address, allergies, insurance status

Primary care provider's orders: Admitting diagnosis; date of admission; current orders regarding diet, activity, frequency of vital signs measurement, daily weight, treatments, medications, diagnostic tests ordered, IV fluids, therapies ordered

Nurse's notes: Status during the last 24 hours

Primary care provider's progress notes: Findings from last 2 days status of problems

Medication administration record (MAR) or **Electronic medication administration record (eMAR):** Medications received, frequency of PRN medications, allergies

Primary care provider's patient history and physical: Current complaint, chronic problems, physical finding abnormalities, allergies, impressions

Surgery operative report: Procedure done, organs removed, type of incision, drains or equipment in place, blood loss, problems during surgery

Pathology report: Presence of malignancy or infection

Current diagnostic tests: Check for any abnormal findings: CBC, UA, blood chemistries, x-ray films, culture and sensitivity, other tests

Nursing admission history and assessment: Reason for hospitalization, average number of cigarettes smoked per day, average amount of alcohol consumed per day, last bowel movement, special diet requirements, use of aids or prostheses (e.g., hearing aids or eyeglasses), medications taken regularly, identification of significant other, previous hospitalizations or surgeries, baseline vital signs, physical abnormalities

Fall risk assessment: Risk factors to consider safety measures to provide

Skin assessment: Risk factors to consider areas needing inspection and care

Nursing care plan or problem list

CBC, Complete blood count; *IV,* intravenous; *PRN,* as necessary; *UA,* urinalysis.

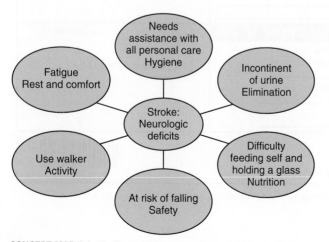

CONCEPT MAP 5.1 Health problems and needs of patient Victoria Torres from data given.

relationships between Mrs. Torres' identified health problems and Maslow's areas of basic need for which nursing assistance is indicated. However, you need to gather data systematically to obtain a full picture of the patient's problems and needs.

PHYSICAL ASSESSMENT

The RN obtains a health history and is responsible for the physical assessment. However, parts of this assessment may be delegated to the LPN/LVN. To conduct the assessment, use techniques of inspection (looking), auscultation (listening, usually with a stethoscope), palpation (using hands and the sense of touch), and percussion (tapping with fingertips to produce vibration and sound). (These techniques are discussed in Chapter 22.) An assessment should be carried out in a systematic manner. It begins with measuring height, weight, and vital signs. Record a history of what medications the patient is taking and any medication allergies. The list should include any over-the-counter medications the patient uses, including herbal preparations, and prescription drugs. Take a brief medical history. Ask about special assistive devices needed, such as hearing aids, glasses, a cane, a prosthesis, or dentures. Then perform a review of systems. Usually the assessment and data collection form contains a section for a psychosocial history and often one regarding needed assistance for self-care. Gather a nutrition and skin assessment and note the findings. A risk screening for falls may be required, and a determination of educational or discharge planning needs is appropriate so planning can begin.

Conduct a complete physical examination, paying particular attention to any system in which the patient is expressing a problem. If the patient has abdominal pain, auscultate and palpate the abdomen. If the patient complains of a joint hurting, examine the joint and check the range of motion of the extremity. If a urinalysis has been ordered, obtain a urine specimen before leaving the patient.

After the admission assessment, each patient should be visited and assessed during the first hour of each shift. Perform a head-to-toe examination, which should take approximately 10 minutes. Box 5.3 presents areas to cover for this assessment and data collection procedure. Later in the shift, explore particular problem areas for each patient in greater depth by conducting a *focused assessment*. Listen to the heart and lungs of patients with respiratory or heart problems; examine the abdomen of the patient with gastrointestinal tract problems or abdominal pain; and perform a neurologic examination on the patient with a neurologic disorder.

At the time of the initial data collection and assessment, determine what supplies and equipment will be needed for the patient for the shift. Ongoing nursing data collection and examination focus on the body systems in which there is a problem or potential problem. Concept Map 5.2 shows how data should be gathered

Box 5.3 Quick Head-to-Toe Assessment

INITIAL OBSERVATION
Breathing
How patient is feeling
Appearance
Affect
Skin color

HEAD
Level of consciousness
Ability to communicate
Mentation status
Appearance of eyes

VITAL SIGNS
Temperature
Pulse: rate rhythm
Respirations: rate, pattern and depth; oxygen saturation
Blood pressure: compare with previous readings

HEART AND LUNG ASSESSMENT, NEUROLOGIC CHECK
Auscultation of heart and lungs done to determine a baseline
Neurologic check done now if ordered or indicated

ABDOMEN
Shape
Soft or firm
Bowel sounds
Appetite
Last bowel movement
Voiding status

EXTREMITIES
Normal movement
Skin turgor and temperature
Peripheral pulses
Edema

TUBES AND EQUIPMENT PRESENT
Oxygen cannula: liter flow rate; chest tube functioning correctly
Nasogastric tube: suction setting, amount and character of drainage; percutaneous endoscopic gastrostomy (PEG) tube; jejunostomy tube
Urinary catheter: character and quantity of drainage
Intravenous catheters: type, condition of site(s), fluid in progress, rate
PEG: intact skin condition
Dressings: location, character and amount of drainage, wound suction device, drains
Pulse oximeter: intact probe; readings
Traction: correct weight, body alignment, weights hanging freely
Sequential compression device: correct application, turned on
Continuous passive motion: machine set and applied correctly, turned on
Cardiac monitor: leads placed correctly, alarm parameters set

PAIN STATUS
Use a pain scale (e.g., 0 to 10)

for every basic need and then analyzed to define Mrs. Torres' problems and attach the appropriate nursing diagnosis label. This map includes the next nursing process step, planning.

Think Critically

From the information about Victoria Torres that has been given, which areas do you think would need in-depth assessment?

ASSESSMENT IN LONG-TERM CARE

An extensive initial assessment is performed when a patient enters a long-term care facility. Reassessment is done at fixed intervals and with any change in patient condition. For Medicare patients, reassessment by an RN is necessary every 90 days, and the care plan is reviewed and revised at that time. In addition to the physical assessment, health history, and medication history, a functional assessment is performed. The functional assessment supplies a picture of the activities of daily living (ADLs) with which the patient will need assistance. An assessment of personal preferences regarding routines for bathing, sleeping, daytime activities, food likes and dislikes, hobbies, and so forth is completed. A fall risk assessment (see Fig. 20.3) and a comprehensive skin assessment (see Fig. 19.2) are part of the admission procedure. A mental status assessment completes the admission process. **Usually the LPN/LVN collects data for the RN, who finalizes and validates the assessment.**

ASSESSMENT IN HOME HEALTH CARE

The initial patient assessment in the home is performed by the RN. The family is assessed regarding attitude and ability to help with patient, their ability to provide emotional support for the patient, their ability to cope with the situation, and patient education that will need to be provided for them. The nurse must work within the patient and family's territory, and that requires a shift in attitude and perspective as compared with working in a health care facility. The LPN/LVN, when doing private duty in a home, performs daily assessments and maintains the necessary documentation. Changes found on assessment are reported to the RN supervisor.

ANALYSIS

Once the information has been gathered, the database is analyzed for cues that indicate deviations from the norm. **Cues are pieces of data or information that influence decisions.** Problems are identified so that nursing diagnoses can be synthesized and written by the RN as required by the American Nurses Association (ANA) Standard II: **Diagnosis** (available at: http://www.nursingworld.org/MainMenuCategories/ThePracticeofProfessionalNursing/NursingStandards). The LPN/LVN may assist in this process.

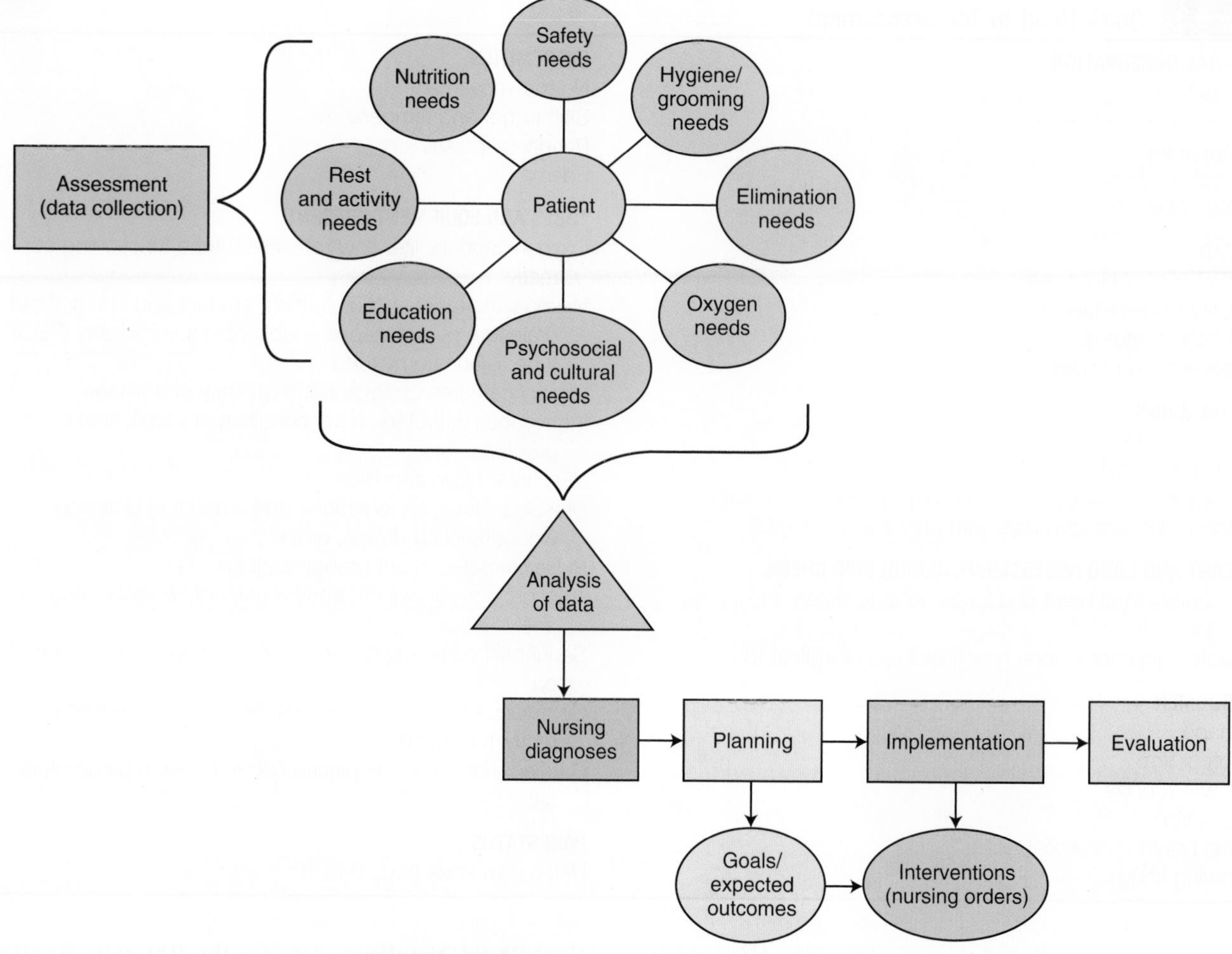

CONCEPT MAP 5.2 Basic needs and the nursing process.

As the database is analyzed and pieces of data are sorted, related data are grouped (clustered), and missing data are identified. An example of a cluster of data would be a need to void frequently, occasional incontinence of urine, and some burning on urination. These data are all related to a urinary system problem and describe how the patient is responding, physiologically, to their medical condition. Diagnosis depends on the nurse's knowledge base and previous experience. Typically, the nursing student uses reference material to read about the underlying condition, including signs, symptoms, and causes, to assist in this process. The database is reviewed for signs and symptoms of abnormalities. Once cues are identified, they are grouped, and inferences can be made regarding the patient's problems. While clustering the data, the nurse should interpret the possible meaning of the cues.

From Mrs. Torres' situation, cues suggesting that a problem exists include the following: she cannot firmly grasp objects with her left hand, she will need to use a walker to support herself when ambulating, and she is incontinent of urine. Factors contributing to the problem are also important. In Mrs. Torres' case, the fact that she has suffered a stroke and has some neurologic impairment is pertinent. Nursing diagnosis statements are used to state the specific problems.

Inferences (conclusions made based on observed data) made from the data above include that Mrs. Torres' mobility is decreased, she cannot perform self-care unassisted, she has left-sided weakness and is at risk of injury from a fall, and she is incontinent of urine. All these describe the ways in which she is responding to her disease process. Regarding care coordination, she will need encouragement and reinforcement for her physical therapy program.

Concept Map 5.2 shows how the assessment data collected by all techniques are analyzed. The map indicates the next steps to be completed in the nursing process: nursing diagnosis, planning with goals and expected outcomes, implementation with the selection of interventions to help the patient meet the expected outcomes, and evaluation to see if the outcomes have been met.

NURSING DIAGNOSIS

The second step of the nursing process results in the development of a diagnostic statement or **a nursing diagnosis. A nursing diagnosis statement typically involves three parts, indicating the patient's problem or potential problem (how the patient is responding); the causative or related factors, which can include the**

pathophysiology; and specific defining characteristics or the signs and symptoms. The medical diagnosis (e.g., stroke) is never included in the construction of the nursing diagnosis. Although RNs formulate nursing diagnoses, LPNs/LVNs are expected to be able to complete a care plan after the nursing diagnoses have been designated.

The diagnostic labels are formulated by the North American Nursing Diagnosis Association–International (NANDA-I) and are revised every 2 years. Research is ongoing to validate the current diagnostic labels and to support new nursing diagnoses, which are then added to the official NANDA-I list (NANDA International, 2015). Language changes to simplify the diagnoses are considered every 2 years. Most care facilities use a problem statement in care planning that may (or may not) conform to the NANDA-I terminology. Whatever the terminology used, the nursing diagnosis reflects the nurse's clinical judgment regarding the patient's response to an actual or potential health problem, and is the basis for the nurse's plan of care for the patient. Diagnoses may be actual or related to a risk, syndrome, or to promote wellness.

Once the nursing diagnoses are identified, the planning phase occurs. The NANDA-I list of diagnostic labels is used to form the first part (stem) of the nursing diagnoses used in nursing care plans. The nursing diagnosis describes a health problem amenable to nursing intervention. The current list of approved NANDA-I nursing diagnoses is inside the back cover of this book. The stem label (the problem) is combined with the cause or causative factors. An example of a nursing diagnosis for Mrs. Torres might be "Reflex urinary incontinence related to neurologic impairment, as evidenced by the inability to retain urine." "Reflex urinary incontinence" is the stem. Another nursing diagnosis appropriate for Victoria Torres is "Impaired physical mobility related to decreased motor function and left-sided muscular weakness, as evidenced by the inability to bear weight on the left leg." Because of her left-sided weakness, Mrs. Torres is at high risk for falling. This potential problem should be included on the care plan. The appropriate nursing diagnosis is "Risk for injury related to neurologic impairment" and "Muscular weakness as evidenced by inability to support body weight." It is acceptable to use standard abbreviations in the nursing diagnosis—for example, "Pain r/t injury to right ankle AEB discomfort and swelling" instead of "Pain *related to* injury to the right ankle *as evidenced by* discomfort and swelling." Sometimes nursing diagnoses are shortened on the hospital care plan by leaving off the defining characteristics (the "as evidenced by" part). Handbooks are available that present each of the approved nursing diagnosis labels, their possible etiologic factors, defining characteristics, and possible nursing interventions.

Table 5.2 Construction of a Nursing Diagnosis

Nursing diagnosis = Problem + Etiology (cause) + Signs and symptoms	
Problem	Nursing diagnosis label (stem)
Etiology	Related to (etiologic or causative factors)
Signs and symptoms	As evidenced by (defining characteristics)

? Think Critically

Do the nursing diagnoses with the problem related to a basic need described in the preceding paragraph apply to Concept Map 5.1?

ETIOLOGIC FACTORS

Etiologic factors are the causes of the problem. These are often the result of some pathophysiology. In Mrs. Torres' case, the etiologic factor for her decreased mobility is neurologic impairment.

DEFINING CHARACTERISTICS

Defining characteristics are those characteristics (signs and symptoms) that must be present for a particular nursing diagnosis to be appropriate for that patient. These supply the evidence that the nursing diagnosis is valid. **Signs** are abnormalities that can be verified by repeat examination and are objective data. A bruise on the arm would be a sign. **Symptoms** are factors the patient has said are occurring that cannot be verified by examination; symptoms are subjective data. A headache would be a symptom. You cannot see or verify that the patient actually has a headache; you must trust what the patient tells you.

Nursing diagnoses differ from medical diagnoses in that the nursing diagnosis **defines the patient's response to illness,** whereas the medical diagnosis **labels the illness.** Table 5.2 shows how a nursing diagnosis is constructed.

PRIORITIZATION OF PROBLEMS

Priorities of care are set so that the most important interventions for the high-priority problems for each patient are attended to first. Then, as time permits, the lower-priority problems are considered.

Once the nursing diagnoses have been formulated, they are ranked according to their importance. This order can be guided by the hierarchy of needs adapted from Maslow (see Fig. 2.3), by the patient's beliefs regarding the importance of each problem, and by what is most life threatening or problematic for the patient. **Physiologic needs for basic survival take precedence.** One of the first rules concerning priorities of care is that the **airway always comes first.** Without an adequate airway, the patient will die very quickly. Circulation usually is the next priority: Failure of the heart and loss of too much blood will also quickly cause death. Thereafter the nurse consults with and involves the patient in determining the priority of needs. A patient in considerable pain will usually give pain relief a higher priority than the need for food, at least on a short-term basis.

After physiologic needs are met, safety problems take priority. For a patient at risk for injury related to increased intracranial pressure as evidenced by decreased level of consciousness, safety is the priority need. Increasing intracranial pressure can be lethal. Nursing judgment is crucial in setting priorities. Nurses draw on their knowledge of the disease or disorder in question, the database, and their experience with similar patients. Critical thinking is used to make astute judgments regarding priorities.

After physiologic and safety needs have been met, the psychosocial needs of love and belonging, self-esteem, and self-actualization are given attention. **Every nurse must attempt to look at each patient holistically, keeping psychosocial needs in mind while working on physical problems.** Calling patients by their correct names, giving them opportunities to make some decisions about their care, protecting their privacy, and showing respect help meet psychosocial needs.

NURSING DIAGNOSIS IN LONG-TERM CARE

In a long-term care facility, the care planning process begins when a patient is admitted, often by the LPN/LVN. The supervising RN reviews the care plan, modifies it as needed, and finalizes it for the medical record. The same process is used to analyze data, identify problems and safety concerns, and choose nursing diagnoses appropriate for the new resident. Box 5.4 shows some of the more common nursing diagnoses found for residents in long-term care facilities. Once the nursing diagnoses are chosen, the plan is individualized for the resident.

NURSING DIAGNOSIS IN HOME HEALTH CARE

In addition to the patient's problems, nursing diagnosis in the home health care setting must include any problems identified in the family's ability to cope with the illness or situation and any patient education needs. The care plan encompasses the whole family rather than just the patient.

PLANNING

The third step of the nursing process is planning, and it correlates with the fourth NFLPN Standard, part 3, "the identification of health goals" (see Appendix B) (Fig. 5.2).

EXPECTED OUTCOMES (GOALS)

A **goal** is a broad idea of what is to be achieved through nursing intervention. **Short-term goals** are those that are achievable within 7 to 10 days or before discharge, whereas long-term goals take many weeks or months

Box 5.4 Selected Nursing Diagnoses Commonly Found for Long-Term Care Residents

- Impaired swallowing r/t weakness or paralysis of the swallowing muscles
- Risk for aspiration r/t impaired swallowing, depressed gag reflex, or decreased level of consciousness
- Impaired verbal communication r/t changes in the cerebral hemispheres
- Self-care deficit r/t impaired mobility, disturbed thought processes, or sensory impairment
- Chronic confusion r/t damage to cerebral tissue
- Impaired urinary elimination: incontinence r/t decreased ability to control elimination
- Risk for injury r/t falls, weakness, or altered thought processes
- Self-esteem, situational low r/t change in appearance, loss of self-control, role changes, or dependence on others to meet basic needs
- Imbalanced nutrition: less than body requirements r/t decreased oral intake
- Readiness for enhanced fluid balance r/t inadequate fluid intake or excessive fluid loss
- Chronic pain r/t chronic disease process
- Impaired skin integrity r/t damage to skin associated with friction, pressure, or shearing
- Impaired physical mobility r/t loss of muscle mass, tone, or strength, or paralysis
- Risk for constipation r/t medication side effects, decreased GI motility, loss of nervous control over defecation reflex, or decreased activity
- Impaired social interaction r/t depressed mood, withdrawal, or impaired communication
- Ineffective coping r/t inability to function at previous level, poor problem solving, or poor cognitive function
- Wandering r/t decreased cognition, anxiety, and agitation

GI, Gastrointestinal; *r/t*, related to.

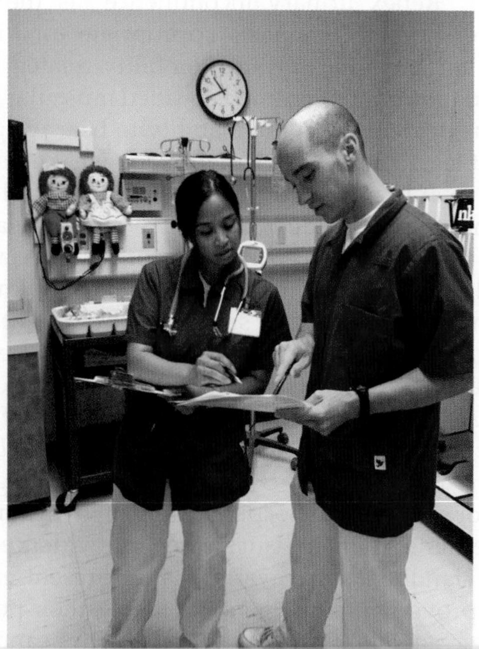

FIGURE 5.2 Nursing students collaborating on the plan of care.

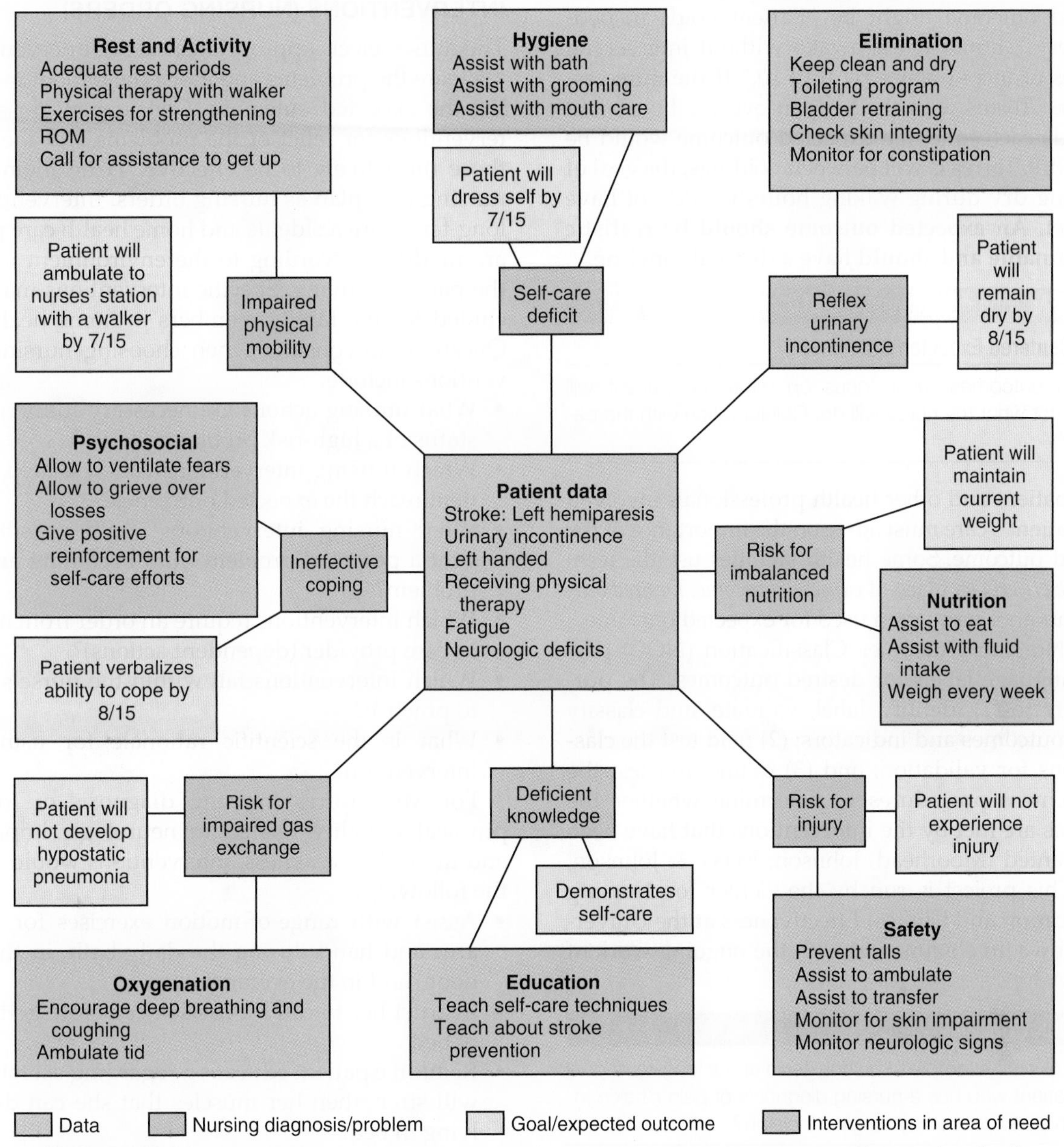

CONCEPT MAP 5.3 Correlating assessment data with nursing diagnoses, expected outcomes, and interventions for all basic needs for Mrs. Torres. *ROM,* Range of motion; *tid,* three times a day.

to achieve. **Long-term goals** often relate to rehabilitation. When goals are written as expected outcomes, it is easier to evaluate whether interventions have helped the patient meet them. Questions that the nurse considers in this part of the planning process are as follows:

- What are the goals for this patient? How can they be expressed as expected outcomes so that the success of nursing care can be easily evaluated?
- Should the goals for this patient be both short term and long term?
- What are the priorities of care?

A short-term goal regarding Mrs. Torres' incontinence might be that she stays dry for 2 hours at a time between toiletings. A long-term goal for this problem would be that she achieves total urinary continence.

Concept Map 5.3 shows how data for every basic need area have been collected and analyzed to identify problems and nursing diagnoses for Mrs. Torres. Goals have been formulated and converted into expected outcomes, and interventions have been chosen. Expected outcomes are derived from the goals. An **expected outcome** is a specific statement regarding the goal the patient is expected to achieve because of nursing intervention. An expected outcome for Mrs. Torres' nursing diagnosis of impaired physical mobility related to left-sided muscular weakness, as evidenced by inability to bear weight on the left leg, might be "Patient uses a walker to ambulate to the nurses' station without assistance by July 10." The expected outcome should also contain measurable criteria that can be evaluated to see whether the outcome has been achieved. For example, for Mrs. Torres' nursing diagnosis of reflex urinary incontinence related to neurologic impairment as evidenced by inability to retain urine, an appropriate expected outcome might be "Patient voids in bedpan every 2 hours while awake without intervening episodes of incontinence by July 10." If the nurse assists Mrs. Torres with the bedpan every 2 hours and she voids each time, the expected outcome would be met. If Mrs. Torres is wet between voidings, the goal of remaining dry during waking hours would not have been met. **An expected outcome should be realistic and attainable and should have a defined timeline.**

QSEN Considerations: Patient-Centered Care

Patient-Centered Expected Outcomes

Expected outcomes must focus on what the patient will achieve, not what the nurse will do. Collaboration with the patient is key.

The patient and other health professionals involved in the patient's care must agree on the importance of the expected outcome. Some health facilities use the term *discharge criteria* in place of *expected outcome. Desired outcome* is another term often used for expected outcome.

The Nursing Outcomes Classification (NOC) provides language labels for desired outcomes. The purposes are to (1) identify, label, validate, and classify patient outcomes and indicators; (2) field test the classifications for validation; and (3) define and test the measurement procedures to determine whether the outcomes are met by the interventions that have been implemented (Moorhead, Johnson, Maas, & Johnson, 2013). This project is run by the Center for Nursing Classification and Clinical Effectiveness at the University of Iowa, in conjunction with the ongoing work of NANDA-I.

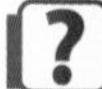
Think Critically

Can you give an example of a short-term and a long-term goal for the patient who has a nursing diagnosis of pain r/t skin interruption as evidenced by surgical incision?

PLANNING IN LONG-TERM FACILITIES

The planning process in long-term care facilities is the same as for any other facility. Expected outcomes are written for each nursing diagnosis. Maslow's hierarchy is used to determine priorities of care. Emotional and psychosocial needs must be addressed. Safety of the resident is a high priority. Family members are usually invited to the care planning session so that they provide input into the care of their loved one. They are also invited to periodic reviews of the care plan.

PLANNING IN HOME HEALTH CARE

Nurses collaborate with family members concerned with care of the patient when choosing the expected outcomes. This helps the family feel involved and gives a feeling of some control over what will be occurring in their home and for their loved one. Needs of the family are considered throughout the care planning process.

INTERVENTIONS (NURSING ORDERS)

The nurse selects appropriate nursing interventions to alleviate the problems and assist the patient in achieving the expected outcomes. Consider all possible interventions for relief of the problems and then select those most likely to be effective. Write them on the nursing care plan as nursing orders. Interventions for long-term care residents and home health care patients are modified according to the environment in which the patient is living. Specific interventions may be included for the family members in home health care. Questions to consider when choosing nursing interventions include:

- What nursing actions are necessary to monitor the status of a high-risk problem?
- Which nursing interventions can best help the patient reach the expected outcomes?
- What nursing interventions could possibly prevent a potential problem from becoming an actual problem?
- Which interventions require an order from a primary care provider (dependent actions)?
- Which interventions fall within the nurse's license to practice?
- What is the scientific rationale for using each intervention?

For Mrs. Torres' nursing diagnosis of impaired physical mobility related to neurologic impairment and muscular weakness, interventions would include the following:

- Assist with range-of-motion exercises for her left arm and hand during the daily bath, in the afternoon, and in the evening.
- Instruct her to call for assistance before getting out of bed.
- Reinforce patient education regarding exercises that will strengthen her muscles that she can do while lying in bed.

Interventions listed should include giving medications and performing ordered treatments. Concept Map 5.3 lists interventions that will be implemented for Mrs. Torres.

The Iowa Intervention Project is linking nursing interventions to nursing diagnoses. The project has developed a Nursing Interventions Classification (NIC) taxonomy. The nurse must still individualize the interventions to the patient's needs. The nurse uses critical thinking to link the correct interventions to the nursing diagnosis for a specific patient. There are seven domains in the NIC taxonomy: Physiological, Basic; Physiological, Complex; Behavioral; Safety; Family; Health System; and Community (Wilkinson, 2014).

Concept Map 5.3 shows the nursing diagnoses, goals, and interventions appropriate for Mrs. Torres. The nursing care plan in Fig. 5.3 shows further development of the concepts for four nursing diagnoses to meet Mrs. Torres' individual needs based on the assessment data.

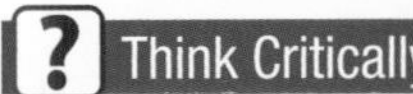

Can you support each nursing diagnosis in Concept Map 5.3 with the corresponding assessment data?

DOCUMENTATION OF THE PLAN

The nursing care plan is initiated by an RN, though the LPNs/LVNs often construct a plan of care, which is approved by the RN. The planning process is not finished until the nursing care plan is documented in the patient's medical record. If the LPN/LVN has constructed the care plan, the RN reviews it before it is placed into the record. Many health care facilities now use computerized programs to assist in constructing the nursing care plan. The nurse chooses the appropriate nursing diagnoses and then is presented with computer screens from which to choose the expected outcomes and the nursing interventions. The nurse can change or modify outcomes and interventions to individualize the plan. Some facilities use a standardized care plan, and the nurse adds and deletes items to individualize the plan. Once the entire plan is constructed, it is reviewed and placed in the medical record.

The nursing care plan should be constructed right after the admission database is collected. It must be readily available to each nurse who is assigned to the patient. **Once every 24 hours, the care plan is reviewed and updated.** Necessary changes can be made to it at any time. The new plan must be placed in the patient's record. Implementation and evaluation of the care plan are discussed in Chapter 6. Many hospitals are using a collaborative "care map" or "clinical pathway" type of plan that incorporates all interventions by the various members of the health care team (see Chapter 6). In such cases the nursing care plan is incorporated into the total collaborative plan.

Interventions for the long-term care resident are chosen in the same manner and individualized. There are generally more long-term goals and expected outcomes than there are short-term ones on the care plan because the resident will most likely remain in the facility for an extended time.

Nursing Care Plan — **Sample Nursing Care Plan**

SCENARIO Victoria Torres suffered a stroke and has left-sided paresis (muscle weakness). She is unable to bear weight on her left leg and cannot grasp items with her left hand. She is incontinent of urine. The following is the nursing care plan written for her. Date of initiation: 6/16.

PROBLEM/NURSING DIAGNOSIS Impaired physical mobility related to decreased motor function and muscular weakness, as evidenced by inability to bear weight on left leg.

Goals/Expected Outcomes	Nursing Interventions	Selected Rationale	Evaluation
Patient will ambulate to nurse's station using walker, unassisted, by 7/1.	Encourage active ROM to right leg and arm q 4 hr while awake.	Active ROM works muscles and prevents atrophy as well as helping them maintain strength.	*Is patient ambulating unassisted?* Yes, but only for a short distance.
	Assist patient in walking with walker in room tid.	Using the walker promotes confidence and helps build stamina for walking.	Continue plan.
	Encourage patient to walk with walker in hall at least once daily; assist as needed.	Positive reinforcement encourages the desired behavior.	
	Reinforce instructions from physical therapist for exercises and walker use.	Reinforcing instructions helps patient remember them and to perform exercises and use walker correctly.	

PROBLEM/NURSING DIAGNOSIS Reflex incontinence related to neurologic impairment, as evidenced by inability to retain urine.

Goals/Expected Outcomes	Nursing Interventions	Selected Rationale	Evaluation
Voids in bedpan q 2 hr while awake without intervening episodes of urinary incontinence by 6/30.	Collaborate on voiding schedule times. Keep schedule at bedside.	Patient knows her usual pattern for voiding.	*Have there been episodes of incontinence?* No.
	Assist patient to use bedpan.	Conserves energy and prevents spilling.	Expected outcome met 6/18.
	Praise patient for each 2-hr period of continence.	Positive reinforcement encourages the desired behavior.	
	Discuss patient's feelings about bladder problem and progress with retraining.	Allows patient to ventilate feelings; reduces anxiety.	

FIGURE 5.3 Example of a hospital-style nursing care plan. *ROM,* Range of motion; *tid,* three times a day.

Nursing Care Plan Sample Nursing Care Plan—cont'd

PROBLEM/NURSING DIAGNOSIS Risk for injury related to neurologic impairment and muscular weakness, as evidenced by inability to bear weight on left leg.

Goals/Expected Outcomes	Nursing Interventions	Selected Rationale	Evaluation
Will not suffer injury from fall at any time.	Keep walker positioned by bed for ease of use.	Object close at hand encourages use.	*Has patient suffered any injury?* No.
Will compensate for neurologic impairment with use of aids for ambulation by 7/1.	Encourage to use walker whenever out of bed.	Encouragement prompts desired action.	*Is patient using a walker?* Yes.
	Ask to use call bell for assistance whenever she needs to get up.	Assistance helps prevent falls.	Continue plan.
	Assess muscular strength, balance, and ability to walk safely with walker daily.	Patient must have sufficient muscle strength to safely use walker.	

PROBLEM/NURSING DIAGNOSIS Self-care deficit, hygiene and grooming, related to muscular impairment, as evidenced by inability to grasp items with dominant left hand and inability to walk without assistance.

Goals/Expected Outcomes	Nursing Interventions	Selected Rationale	Evaluation
Will assist with bath by bathing left extremities by 6/26.	Assist with hygiene and grooming activities; encourage patient to participate.	Encouragement prompts desired action.	*Is patient performing some part of ADLs using the right extremities?* Not yet.
Will attempt to brush hair with right hand by 6/26.	Collaborate with patient regarding daily goals; praise all accomplishments and attempts at self-care.	Goals are more likely to be achieved if the patient helps set the goals.	*Is patient attempting to wash left arm?* Not yet.
Will brush teeth with right hand by 6/30.	Assist patient in attempts at brushing teeth and combing hair using right hand.	Undue fatigue prevents successful achievement of the activity.	Continue plan.
Will learn to put clothes on right extremities before discharge.	Reinforce occupational therapist's instructions for dressing self; supervise practice and give encouragement.	Positive reinforcement encourages the desired behavior.	
	Prevent patient from becoming overtired when attempting own hygiene activities; space activities.		

FIGURE 5.3, cont'd

Get Ready for the NCLEX Examination!

Key Points

- Assessment, the first step of the nursing process, begins at admission with the admission interview, history, and physical assessment.
- Subjective data are pieces of information that are apparent only to the patient and can be described or verified only by the patient.
- Objective data are facts that are obtained through using the senses and hands-on physical assessment.
- A database is compiled through the interview, physical assessment, conversation with family and significant others, communication with other health professionals, and a medical records review that includes surveying results of diagnostic tests. The database is all the information obtained.
- Assessment is a continual, ongoing process.
- A medical records review is useful for gathering information for the nursing database and for obtaining information for a student assignment.
- A nursing history and assessment are performed at admission.
- The nurse should perform a quick head-to-toe assessment of each assigned patient at the beginning of each shift (see Box 5.3).
- The practice of nursing is concerned with how a patient responds to their disease or disorder, their treatments, and their life situation and environment, whereas the practice of medicine is concerned with the diagnosis and treatment of disease.
- A functional assessment is performed on patients being admitted to a long-term care facility.
- Emotional and psychosocial concerns are always considered when formulating a care plan for the long-term care resident.

- Analysis is used to sort and group assessment data so that nursing diagnoses can be chosen and priorities can be set.
- A nursing diagnosis statement indicates the patient's actual health status or a potential problem, the causative or related factors, and specific defining characteristics (signs and symptoms).
- Nursing diagnoses should be chosen from the NANDA-I approved list (see inside back cover).
- Expected outcomes are written based on the nursing diagnoses and problems.
- An expected outcome should be realistic, attainable, and measurable; have a defined timeline; and be easily evaluated.
- Planning is the third step of the nursing process, and it involves choosing appropriate nursing interventions and documenting the plan.
- Nursing orders are the interventions chosen that will best assist the patient in achieving the expected outcomes.
- A concept map can be constructed showing the areas of need, nursing diagnoses, goals, and nursing interventions. A complete nursing care plan can be constructed from the assessment data and the concept map.
- A nursing care plan should be documented in the medical record soon after the admission assessment.

Additional Learning Resources

SG Go to your Study Guide for additional learning activities to help you master this chapter content.

evolve Go to your Evolve website at http://evolve.elsevier.com/Williams/fundamental for additional online resources.

Online Resources

- *Concept Mapping,* www.snjourney.com/ClinicalInfo/CarePlans/CarePlanN.htm
- *Nursing Concept Map,* www.ehow.com/how_5526833_make-nursing-concept-map.html
- *Clinical Concept Care Map Format,* http://nursing.unm.edu/common/docs/teaching-learning-strategies/concept-map.pdf
- *Medical vs. Nursing Diagnosis,* www.wisc-online.com/Objects/ViewObject.aspx?ID=nur2803

Review Questions for the NCLEX Examination

Choose the **best** *answer for each question.*

1. A postoperative patient is having incisional pain. As part of the nurse's assessment, the nurse notes that the patient is grimacing when he or she changes position. The patient's grimace can be useful in the assessment and can be described in what manner?
   1. Nursing diagnosis
   2. Cue
   3. Diagnosis
   4. Inference
2. Which is the etiologic factor in the nursing diagnosis decreased mobility r/t left-sided muscular weakness, as evidenced by the inability to use the left arm for ADLs?
   1. Decreased mobility
   2. Left-sided muscular weakness
   3. As evidenced by
   4. Inability to use the left arm
3. What is the purpose of the initial health history and assessment?
   1. To collect data about a specific health problem
   2. To identify life-threatening problems
   3. To compare current health status to baseline data
   4. To establish a database to identify the patient's current health status
4. The patient's temperature is 100.4°F (38°C). The skin on her forehead is warm and dry. She has been incontinent, and her bed is wet. She complains of being very tired. Which data are subjective? *(Select all that apply.)*
   1. Temperature is 100.4°F (38°C).
   2. States, "I'm very uncomfortable."
   3. Bed is wet.
   4. Complains of being very tired.
   5. States, "I have a headache."
5. The patient's temperature is 100.4°F (38°C). The skin on her forehead is warm and dry. She has been incontinent, and her bed is wet. She complains of being very tired. Which nursing intervention would be the *highest* priority?
   1. Allow patient to rest.
   2. Change the bed linens and gown.
   3. Medicate for headache pain.
   4. Apply lotion to skin.
6. The role of the LPN/LVN in the patient admission procedure differs from that of the RN and might include: *(Select all that apply.)*
   1. Writes nursing diagnoses for the patient's care plan
   2. Obtains an ordered urine specimen
   3. Takes the patient's history
   4. Assists with physical data collection
   5. Orients the patient to the unit
7. Which statement correctly describes a nursing diagnosis when compared with a medical diagnosis?
   1. Nursing diagnoses and medical diagnoses are essentially the same.
   2. A nursing diagnosis supports a medical diagnosis.
   3. Medical and nursing diagnoses are not related to one another.
   4. The nursing diagnosis describes a patient response to the medical diagnosis.
8. Which is a correctly stated expected outcome?
   1. Sit in the chair three times a day.
   2. Patient will walk to the end of the hall this week.
   3. Use the incentive spirometer every 2 hours for 3 days.
   4. Patient will respond to pain medication.

Critical Thinking Activities

Read each clinical scenario and discuss the questions with your classmates.

Scenario A

The primary care provider's admitting diagnosis for Rachel Himmel is pneumonia. Her nursing diagnosis is impaired gas exchange r/t excessive lung secretions AEB crackles in both lungs. Discuss the difference between nursing diagnoses and medical diagnoses.

Scenario B

From the NANDA-I list of approved nursing diagnoses, select the one that best fits the following patient assessment data: Patient is unable to walk around house without becoming short of breath. Patient becomes fatigued after bathing and dressing in the morning. Patient had a severe case of the flu 2 weeks ago.

Scenario C

Develop a short-term and a long-term goal for Leora Chang, who fell, fractured her hip, and had a hip pinning surgery 3 days ago.

Scenario D

Choose nursing interventions for Leora Chang (patient in Scenario C) for the nursing diagnosis impaired skin integrity related to surgical procedure AEB incisional wound on left hip.

chapter 6

Implementation and Evaluation

http://evolve.elsevier.com/Williams/fundamental

Objectives

Upon completing this chapter, you should be able to do the following:

Theory

1. Set priorities for providing care to a group of patients.
2. Identify factors to consider in implementing the care plan.
3. Describe the Standard Steps commonly carried out for all nursing procedures.
4. Determine the steps a nurse uses to evaluate care given.
5. Discuss the evaluation process and how it correlates with expected outcomes.
6. Explain the term *quality improvement* and how it relates to the improvement of health care.

Clinical Practice

1. Develop a useful method of organizing work for the day.
2. Use the Standard Steps for all nursing procedures.
3. Revise the nursing care plan as needed.
4. Write an individualized nursing care plan for an assigned patient.
5. Implement a nursing care plan and evaluate care provided.

Key Terms

clinical pathway or care map (p. 74)
dependent nursing action (p. 74)
document (p. 76)
documentation (p. 76)
evaluation (p. 74)
implementation (p. 73)
independent nursing action (p. 74)
interdependent action (p. 74)
interventions (p. 73)
nursing audit (ĂW-dĭt, p. 77)
outcome-based quality improvement (OBQI) (p. 77)
quality improvement (p. 79)
time-fixed (p. 74)
time-flexible (p. 73)

 Concepts Covered in This Chapter

- Care coordination
- Clinical judgment
- Collaboration
- Patient education

IMPLEMENTATION

Implementation follows the assessment, nursing diagnosis, and planning stages. The standards for the licensed practical nurse (LPN)/licensed vocational nurse (LVN) concerning implementation are listed in Box 6.1. During the **implementation** (giving care) phase, the nursing **interventions** or nursing orders (actions) listed on the nursing care plan are carried out. Implementing care for a group of patients requires good work organization. There are many ways of organizing the shift's work, but in all instances, priority setting for tasks comes first.

PRIORITY SETTING

Tasks for the shift must be determined and then prioritized. The handoff report gives clues about high-priority tasks and imminent deadlines for certain tasks to be accomplished. Using a worksheet as discussed in Chapter 4, write down important information from the handoff report. Sequential, time-related tasks should be entered for each assigned patient. For example, write the intravenous (IV) flow rate, the fluid that will be used when the IV container is changed, and the expected time for changing the fluid.

 Safety Alert

Intravenous Fluid Orders

Whether or not your state allows you to hang IV fluids, you should know which fluid the patient is currently receiving and which fluid is to be started during your shift. Do not rely solely on the information from the handoff report. Check the container in progress yourself and verify it with the health care provider's order. Check the order for the fluid that is to follow the present one as well.

Note the time of the last administered dose of pain medication. If a patient is to have preoperative medication at 8 am, the preoperative routine must be completed before that time. **Time-flexible** (can be done any time) tasks are entered onto the worksheet schedule

Box 6.1 NFLPN Nursing Practice Standards Regarding Implementation and Evaluation

Standard 4 b states:

"Implementation: The plan for nursing care is put into practice to achieve the stated goals and includes:

(1) Observing, recording and reporting significant changes which require intervention or different goals.

(2) Applying nursing knowledge and skills to promote and maintain health, to prevent disease and disability and to optimize functional capabilities of an individual patient.

(3) Assisting the patient and family with activities of daily living and encouraging self-care as appropriate.

(4) Carrying out therapeutic regimens and protocols prescribed by personnel pursuant to authorized state law."

Standard 4 c states:

"Evaluation: The plan for nursing care and its implementations are evaluated to measure the progress toward the stated goals and will include appropriate person and/or groups to determine:

(1) The relevancy of current goals in relation to the progress of the individual patient.

(2) The involvement of the recipients of care in the evaluation process.

(3) The quality of the nursing action in the implementation of the plan.

(4) A re-ordering of priorities or new goal setting in the care plan."

between **time-fixed** (must be done at a set time) tasks. Critical thinking is essential to formulate a good work plan.

Note patient needs, such as tissues, on the worksheet so you can bring the items the next time you visit the patient. When planning time for uninterrupted care, consider:

- Whether visitors will be coming.
- When diagnostic tests are scheduled.
- What time the primary care provider may come to see the patient.
- Medication administration schedules.

You may need to revise the work schedule after the initial shift assessment. If the patient's condition becomes more acute, your nursing care priorities may need to change. Review the work organization sheet in Figure 4.3. It takes practice to set priorities correctly for multiple patients.

CONSIDERATIONS FOR CARE DELIVERY

Before carrying out the specific interventions listed on the care plan, identify the reason for the intervention, the rationale for the intervention, the usual standard of care, the expected outcome, and any potential dangers. A danger might be the possibility of introducing microorganisms during an invasive procedure.

Each intervention is either an independent nursing action or a dependent nursing action. An **independent nursing action** does not require a primary care provider's order, but it does require critical thinking and clinical judgment. Clinical judgment is derived from experience and knowledge. Each time you think critically about a patient problem, you build the knowledge base that will contribute to your ability to make accurate clinical judgments. The more experience you gain working with patients, the more reliable your clinical judgment will be. Performing patient education about the side effects of a medication is an independent nursing action. In contrast, administering a medication is a **dependent nursing action** because it requires a primary care provider's order. Giving a back massage is an independent nursing action; ordering a heating pad and applying it to a patient is a dependent nursing action. Assisting the speech therapist by helping the patient practice speech exercises is an **interdependent action**. Interdependent actions are those that come from collaborative care planning.

There is often controversy about whether a dressing change requires a primary care provider's order. The general rule is that the initial dressing placed at the end of surgery is changed only by the surgeon unless there is a direct order to change it. If drainage is extensive, the dressing is reinforced with sterile materials. After the surgeon has changed the dressing, there is usually an order to change the dressing as needed or every day or two. Some hospitals have standard protocols for subsequent dressing changes. **Check the facility's policy.** Another topic that is often questioned is whether a hot pack or cold pack can be applied without an order. Generally, applying a warm, moist pack to an inflamed IV area without an order is accepted practice. Again, some hospitals have standard protocols for this situation. Usually cold packs are applied to a sprain or strain in the emergency department even before the patient sees the primary care provider when an injury has occurred. There should be a written standard protocol for this situation. Technically, no dressing should be changed nor any hot or cold pack applied unless there is a standard protocol or order in place.

? Think Critically

Can you think of other instances in which a question has arisen about whether an order is needed? What about on night shift when a patient develops a high fever? Can the nurse use cold packs to bring the temperature down?

INTERDISCIPLINARY CARE

Many hospitals and health care agencies use a collaborative care plan referred to as an interdisciplinary care plan, a **clinical pathway, care map,** or a collaborative care plan. It is a step-by-step approach to the total care of the patient. This multidisciplinary approach to patient care is an example of care coordination. All disciplines involved in the care of the patient engage in collaboration to provide input to the plan. **The nursing care plan is not part of the patient's medical record when an interdisciplinary care plan is used; however, the nursing process is still used.** **Evaluation** is judgment of the effectiveness of the intervention or plan and is a collaborative process. Such pathways are standardized for particular medical diagnoses and then customized for the patient at the time of admission. A case manager, usually a registered nurse (RN), is in charge of reviewing the patient's progress along the path to see that actions are carried out and to determine whether the patient will achieve the expected outcomes in the predicted amount of time. These plans have been shown to be cost-effective in the delivery of health care.

IMPLEMENTING CARE

When a nursing intervention on the care plan calls for a procedure to be performed, review the hospital procedure manual regarding the steps involved. Each hospital has particular requirements for the way a procedure is to be carried out. Employees and students are expected to perform at the designated standard of care listed in the procedure manual.

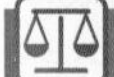 Legal and Ethical Considerations

Standards of Care

Legally, standards of care are set by the nurse practice act of your state, the professional association standards, and the agency's policies and procedures. Each agency has a policy and procedures manual. It is important to review the procedures you will be performing to make certain that nothing differs from the procedure you learned at school. Differences might be in the type of antiseptic solution used or in the steps to perform the procedure. If anything untoward happens to the patient because of the procedure, such as a health care–associated infection, you will be held accountable according to the procedure described in the agency manual.

For efficient use of time, consider which interventions for a particular patient can be combined. This is referred to as clustering of care. Generally, baths and bed making are clustered, and the time in the room is used to gather more assessment data or to begin implementing the patient education plan. Range-of-motion exercises may also be incorporated into the bath routine. Critical thinking helps with organization. Every patient interaction should be used as an opportunity to gather further assessment data.

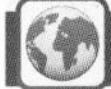 Cultural Considerations

Honor Cultural Practices

Inquire about cultural practices related to bathing, touching, touching by the opposite sex, attitudes toward teaching, and other nursing care activities you will be providing. In certain cultures or religions, it is not acceptable for people other than relatives or close friends to touch one another. This is particularly true for many people from the Middle East. Muslim women and those from Mexico and Central and South America are typically very modest, and there are often taboos about having someone of the opposite sex assist with intimate tasks. Older Japanese men may not listen to the instructions or patient education provided by a younger person or a woman.

Some Standard Steps are always followed when performing a nursing procedure. These steps are introduced in Box 6.2 and are included in Appendix A. The steps are based on the standards of clinical practice, the rights of patients, and safe nursing practice.

Implementation in Long-term Care

Most of the routine care of the residents in a long-term care facility is assigned to nursing assistants. Baths and personal care are done by nursing assistants. Exercise interventions are provided by nursing assistants, physical therapy aides, or restorative aides. Medications are administered by licensed nurses or by nursing assistants with certification in medication administration. The licensed nurse on duty who is assigned to a group of patients is responsible for assigning and overseeing the work of the nursing assistants. **The nurse performs any invasive procedure and any sterile procedure.** It is wise to spot-check the documentation of nursing assistants, because the nurse is ultimately responsible for adequate documentation on care of the patient. Assignment guidelines are provided in Chapter 10.

 Assignment Considerations

SAFELY ASSIGNING TASKS

The licensed nurse is responsible for knowing the capability of the person to whom a task is assigned. Each assistive person should have documentation of the tasks that he can safely perform in his personnel file. Be certain that the person to whom you assign a task for a particular resident or patient knows any safety requirements particular to that person and any precautions that must be taken while performing the task. For example, is the patient hearing impaired, and does she need a hearing aid turned on? Does the patient have weakness on one side? (If so, state which side.)

Implementation in Home Health Care

Although nurses make periodic visits to the home, unless a private-duty LPN/LVN is required, the family or patient will be implementing the interventions on the care plan. Perform patient education to ensure that the family member or patient can administer medications safely, change dressings properly, perform range of motion or help with other exercises safely, and perform treatments and other care activities correctly. Perform any procedure for which strict sterility is mandatory or any invasive procedure that could cause serious harm to the patient. Ask the patient or family member to keep track of care given and to call if the patient's condition changes. At each visit, review the documentation to see that the care plan is being carried out properly. The family should have a telephone number for the nurse and should be encouraged to call with questions or concerns.

DOCUMENTATION OF THE NURSING PROCESS

Each time a procedure is performed, a medication is administered, vital signs are measured, or something

Box 6.2 Standard Steps for All Nursing Procedures

AT THE BEGINNING OF THE PROCEDURE

- **Step A: Perform the task according to protocol.**

Mentally review the steps of the task beforehand. If you are uncertain how to do a task, check the agency's policy and procedure manual for the accepted method of performing the procedure. If you are uncertain, ask your instructor.

- **Step B: Check the order, collect the equipment and supplies, and perform hand hygiene.**

Verify that the procedure is to be done for the patient. Process equipment and supply charges. Take all equipment and supplies to the patient's room.

- **Step C: Identify and prepare the patient.**

Greet the patient, introduce yourself, and check the patient's identification using two identifiers such as the armband and asking the birth date. Explain what you are going to do in terms the patient can understand. Elicit questions and answer questions clearly. Provide necessary patient education related to the procedure to be performed.

- **Step D: Provide privacy and institute safety precautions; arrange the supplies and equipment.**

Close the door or curtains and drape the patient before beginning the procedure or discussing information the person might want kept confidential. Check equipment for breaks or wear and for safety. Set up the equipment and supplies in an orderly, methodical fashion. Raise the bed to an appropriate working height. Raise the side rail before turning the patient, and be certain that the wheels are locked. Perform hand hygiene to prevent contaminating the patient with organisms from the computer, the nurses' station, and the supply room.

DURING THE PROCEDURE

- **Step E: Use Standard Precautions and aseptic technique as appropriate.**

Protect yourself from blood and body fluids by wearing gloves. If there is a danger of splashing blood or body fluids, wear protective glasses or goggles and an impermeable cover gown or apron. Be careful with sharp instruments and needles so as not to nick your skin. (See Appendix D.)

AT THE END OF THE PROCEDURE

- **Step X: Remove gloves and other protective equipment.**

After making certain the patient is clean and dry, dispose of used supplies, and remove goggles and other protective equipment and discard or store appropriately. To remove gloves without contaminating yourself, begin by pulling one glove off without touching your skin; hold the removed glove in the palm of the remaining gloved hand and then reach to the inside of the other glove and roll it down the hand. Dispose of the gloves in the trash. Perform hand hygiene immediately.

- **Step Y: Restore the unit. Collect the used equipment; dispose of, clean, or store items in the proper places.**

Make the person comfortable, tidy the bed and unit, place the call light and personal items within reach, and provide for safety by lowering the bed and lowering side rails. Remove used equipment. Place soiled linens in a soiled-linen hamper. Clean reusable items and return them to the storage or processing area (central supply). Note on the computer that use of equipment is discontinued so no further charges will be made. Remove unsightly, odorous, or potentially infectious trash from the room. Inquire if anything else is needed. Perform hand hygiene before leaving the room.

- **Step Z: Record and report the procedure.**

Document assessment findings and the details of the procedure performed, or care given, in the medical record. Include any problems encountered and the patient's response to the care or treatment. The recording should be accurate, specific, concise, and appropriate and should include the specific time the procedure was performed and how it was done. Report abnormalities encountered to the charge nurse or primary care provider.

is done that is a planned part of nursing care, a notation must be made in the medical record. **Nursing documentation must indicate that the nursing care plan has been carried out.** If an intervention on the care plan is not documented, it is considered not done. **Review the nursing care plan before beginning care to have a clear idea of all of the areas that need documentation** (recording of pertinent data in the clinical record). Many hospitals require that nurses **document** on each patient at least every 2 hours and make some note about each problem or nursing diagnosis at least once every 24 hours. Long-term care facilities have unique documentation requirements, including specific requirements in the event of a significant change in patient condition (Centers for Medicare and Medicaid Services, 2012). **Care is documented on flow sheets daily.** After implementing care for the patient, document that care in the patient's medical record. Routine tasks such as bathing are recorded on care flow sheets (see Fig. 7.1). If a new problem is encountered, such as beginning skin breakdown, a nurse's note is required to document the assessment findings, the nursing diagnosis, and the plan to correct or alleviate the problem. The sooner care is documented after it is given the better. Guidelines for documentation are given in Chapter 7.

? Think Critically

Look at the sample hospital-style care plan in Chapter 5 (see Fig. 5.3). Can you identify which actions are independent, dependent, and interdependent?

EVALUATION

The fifth and final step of the nursing process is based on National Federation of Licensed Practical Nurses (NFLPN) Standard 4 c: **Evaluation** (see Box 6.1). Once the interventions have been carried out, you must determine whether they are effective in helping the patient reach the expected outcomes. If the expected outcomes have been reached, then goals have been met. Compare actual outcomes to the expected outcomes to determine whether progress has been made. For example, patient Victoria Torres (from Chapter 5) should be assessed throughout the day to see if she remains dry, uses the bedpan, and empties her bladder every 2 hours. If, for example, Mrs. Torres is assisted with the bedpan every 2 hours but at 11:30 pm she soiled the bed because she could not hold her urine any longer, then you should consider why this happened. Did she drink an excessive amount of fluid at dinner? Was there a considerable delay between the time Mrs. Torres called for assistance to urinate and the time someone entered her room to assist her? Progress has been made toward the expected outcome, but does the plan need to be changed by helping her urinate more frequently or by providing prompt assistance? When an expected outcome is not met, it may need to be rewritten. **Evaluation is a continual process.** The patient should provide feedback, when possible, about whether the expected outcome is being met.

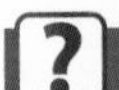 Think Critically

How might you evaluate whether the medication you are giving a patient for pain is effective?

EVALUATION IN LONG-TERM CARE

Evaluation is based on data obtained from assessment, analysis of the data, and determination as to whether the specific expected outcomes are being met. The resident and family should be consulted to find out whether the care plan is meeting needs adequately. The nurse considers whether the interventions on the plan are the best to meet the expected outcomes for those outcomes not yet met. If not, the plan is revised.

EVALUATION IN HOME HEALTH CARE

The nurse periodically assesses the results of the interventions and analyses to see whether the expected outcomes are met. The patient and family are included in the process for input as to whether the care plan is meeting their needs. If expected outcomes are not being met, the interventions are revised.

REVISION OF THE NURSING CARE PLAN

Ineffective interventions must be revised. If the interventions have been so effective that the problem is resolved and the nursing diagnosis is no longer appropriate, it is marked "resolved" on the nursing care plan. **If the expected outcomes are considered met, the nurses' documentation must contain data to support this.** Nursing care plans in the hospital are revised as often as every 24 hours, with resolved problems inactivated, new problems added, interventions revised, and progress toward outcomes evaluated. This

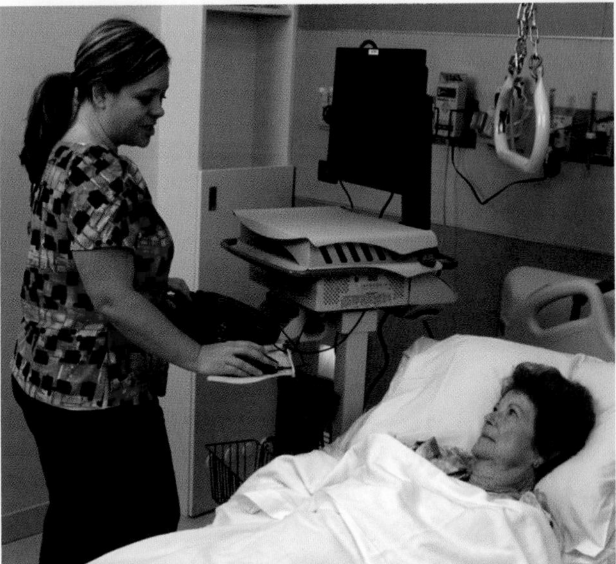

FIGURE 6.1 Nurse revising the nursing care plan.

is frequently done directly on the unit computer (Fig. 6.1). The LPN/LVN collaborates with the RN during this process.

Each nurse determines whether there is a better, more efficient intervention to help the patient achieve the expected outcomes. Constant evaluation is an integral part of every aspect of nursing. Concept Map 6.1 includes the last step of the nursing process. It depicts how, if an expected outcome is not met, the plan is revised with different interventions.

QUALITY IMPROVEMENT

Evaluation of nursing practice includes determining whether the nurse's actions were carried out with consideration for the patient's safety. Safety for the nurse and other workers is evaluated. A determination is made as to whether nursing practice has been performed in a cost-effective, time-efficient manner.

Outcome-based quality-improvement (OBQI) (improvement of the quality of performance) programs are used to evaluate nursing care delivered to patients.

 QSEN Considerations: Quality Improvement

Outcome-Based Quality Improvement

The goal of an outcome-based quality-improvement program is to improve nursing practice. Program goals are usually agency-wide, incorporating nursing audits and evaluation regarding compliance with standards for every department.

A **nursing audit** is the examination of a series of patient records to determine whether nursing care for those patients met particular standards and particular outcomes. For example, if IV cannulas are to be changed every 72 hours, the medical records are examined to see if there is a notation every 72 hours that the cannula was changed. The outcome is usually

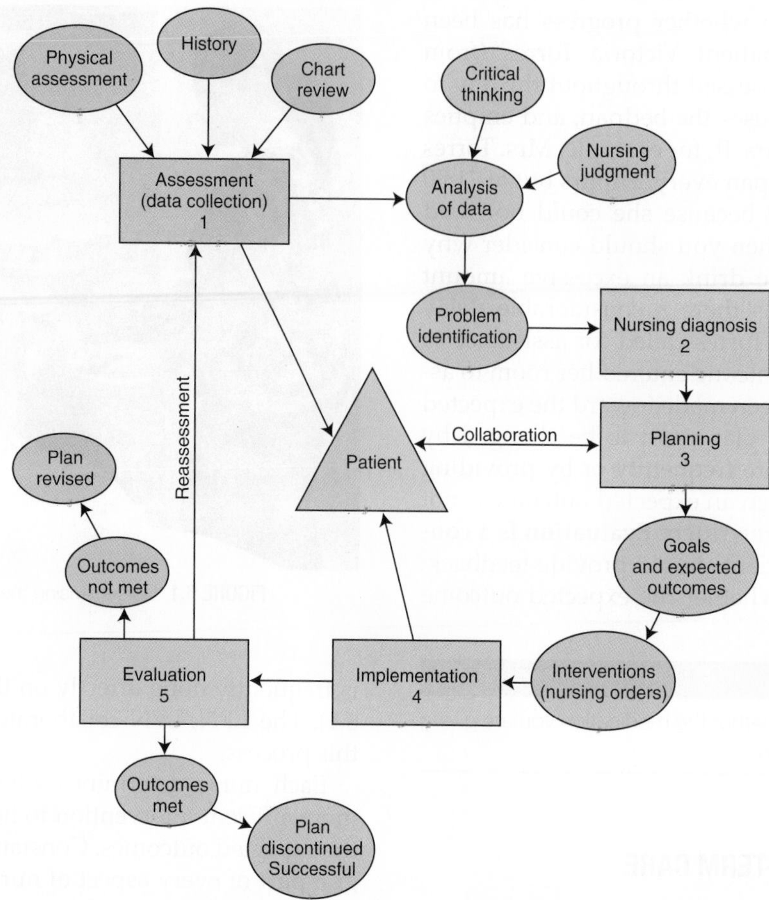

CONCEPT MAP 6.1 The nursing process in action.

expressed as a percentage of compliance (e.g., 98% of IV cannulas were changed every 72 hours over a specific period). If the standard of care is that each nursing diagnosis will be addressed in documentation every 24 hours, then a set number of medical records might be audited to see whether the nurses on that unit are meeting this standard. An audit is most often performed on medical records of patients who have been discharged. Every hospital must perform both medical and nursing audits to achieve and maintain accreditation. **Process** evaluations look at the activities of the nurses and what they have done to assess, plan, implement, and evaluate nursing care. Process evaluation criteria are the Standards of Clinical Nursing Practice developed by the American Nurses Association.

The purpose of evaluating nursing care is to achieve **quality improvement** by identifying specific areas that need changes. Evaluation is not performed to blame someone for carelessness, incompetence, or inefficiency. Quality improvement is a unit responsibility; therefore, nurses on a unit usually rotate as the quality management person for the unit to involve everyone in the process.

CONSTRUCTING A NURSING CARE PLAN

The RN may construct the initial nursing care plan, or, if the patient is admitted to a long-term care facility when an RN is not available, the LPN/LVN may construct a preliminary nursing care plan that an RN will review and modify as needed the next day. Most instructors require students to come to the clinical experience with a nursing care plan, or concept map, in hand for their assigned patients (Concept Map 6.2). Box 6.3 provides guidelines for the care planning process. Figure 6.2 shows a sample student nursing care plan for patient Victoria Torres (discussed in Chapter 5).

Having studied the parts of the nursing process and how the process as a whole is applied to care planning and to the practice of nursing, you should begin to incorporate the principles into your thinking. **The nursing process is inherent in every aspect of nursing and is a tool for success as a nurse.**

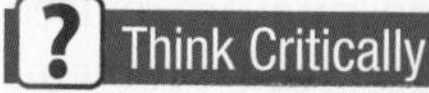

Think Critically

What do you think is the rationale for explaining a procedure to a patient before doing it?

Situation:
A 38-year-old female in otherwise good health is hospitalized with pneumonia. She had a respiratory infection that kept getting worse. After a week, she went to the doctor. Her chest radiograph showed she has pneumonia. She is short of breath, and her SpO_2 reading was 89 in the office. She was admitted to the hospital for antibiotic and respiratory therapy. A sputum culture showed pneumococci.

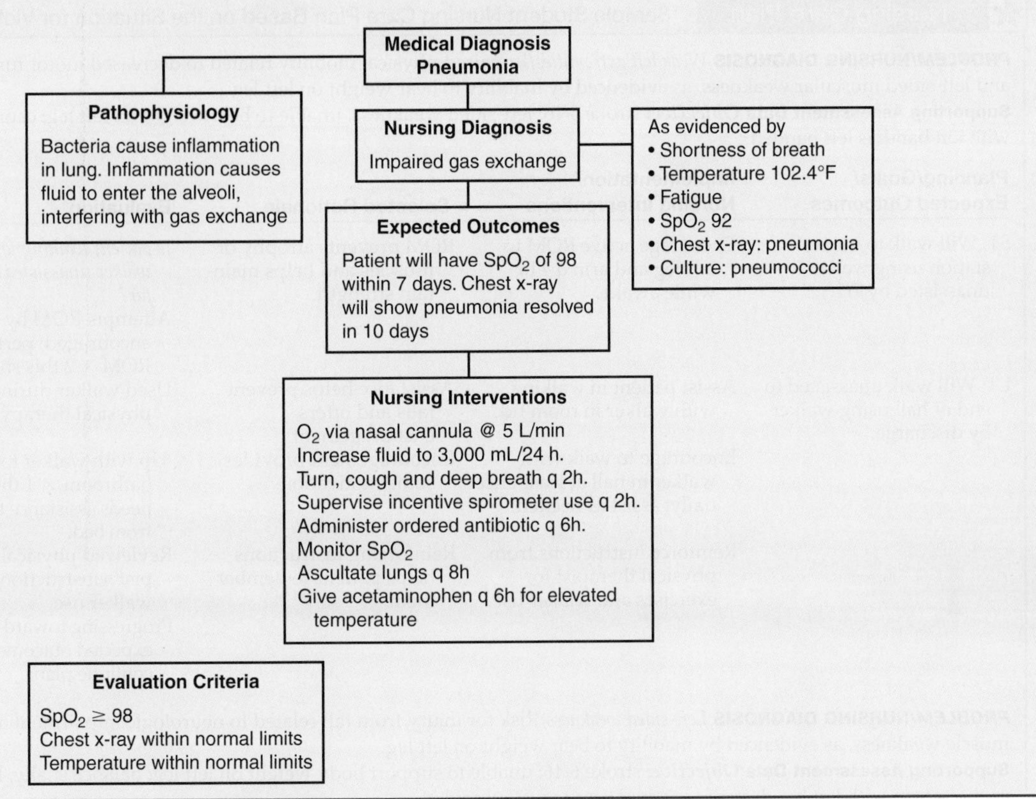

Medical Diagnosis
Pneumonia
Pathophysiology
Bacteria cause inflammation in lung. Inflammation causes fluid to enter the alveoli, interfering with gas exchange
Nursing Diagnosis
Impaired gas exchange
As evidenced by
• Shortness of breath
• Temperature 102.4°F
• Fatigue
• SpO2 92
• Chest x-ray: pneumonia
• Culture: pneumococci
Expected Outcomes
Patient will have SpO2 of 98 within 7 days. Chest x-ray will show pneumonia resolved in 10 days
Nursing Interventions
O2 via nasal cannula @ 5 L/min
Increase fluid to 3,000 mL/24 h.
Turn, cough and deep breath q 2h.
Supervise incentive spirometer use q 2h.
Administer ordered antibiotic q 6h.
Monitor SpO2
Ascultate lungs q 8h
Give acetaminophen q 6h for elevated temperature
Evaluation Criteria
SpO2 ≥ 98
Chest x-ray within normal limits
Temperature within normal limits

CONCEPT MAP 6.2 Nursing care plan as a concept map.

Box 6.3 Steps for Construction of a Nursing Care Plan

1. Collect data for the patient database.
   Obtain a patient history and perform a physical assessment (gather physical data). Review the medical record, noting data and current laboratory values relevant to the patient's problems or admitting diagnosis.
2. Analyze the database to determine current and potential problems.
   Group data according to body system and review for areas of abnormalities or problems. Identify problems and collaborate with the patient to see that she also considers each one a problem.
3. Choose appropriate nursing diagnoses based on defining characteristics of the patient's problems.
   Collaborate with the RN in choosing nursing diagnoses from the NANDA-I accepted diagnoses list: terminology = problem + cause + defining characteristic (signs and symptoms).
4. Rank the nursing diagnoses in order of priority.
   Confer with the patient about the priorities of the patient's problems and needs. Physiologic needs for oxygen and circulation must be met first. Number the diagnoses according to priority.
5. Plan the nursing care by defining goals and writing expected outcomes.
   Define the overall goals and write specific expected outcomes that will be easy to evaluate to determine whether they have been achieved. Include a time frame for each outcome to be achieved.
6. Plan nursing care by choosing appropriate nursing interventions that will assist in achieving the outcomes.
   Consider all nursing interventions known to be useful for the type of problem; choose those that can be expected to help this patient meet the goals and expected outcomes most quickly. Do this for each nursing diagnosis on the patient's list.
7. Implement the nursing interventions.
   Place the nursing care plan in the medical record. Communicate the care plan to staff members on other shifts. Carry out the nursing interventions using the Standard Steps for all nursing procedures.
8. Evaluate the actual outcomes of each nursing intervention; determine whether progress toward achieving the expected outcomes has been made.

Nursing Care Plan **Sample Student Nursing Care Plan Based on the Situation for Victoria Torres**

***PROBLEM*/NURSING DIAGNOSIS** *Weak left extremities*/Impaired physical mobility related to decreased motor function and left-sided muscular weakness, as evidenced by inability to bear weight on left leg.
Supporting Assessment Data *Objective:* stroke 6/16; left-sided weakness, unable to bear weight on left leg; cannot grasp with left hand; is left handed.

Planning/Goals/ Expected Outcomes	Implementation/ Nursing Interventions	Selected Rationale	Evaluation*
ST: Will walk to nurses' station using walker, unassisted by 7/1.	Encourage active ROM to left leg and arm q 4 hr while awake.	ROM prevents atrophy of muscles and helps maintain strength.	*Is patient walking with walker unassisted? How far?* Attempts ROM by self when encouraged; performed ROM × 2 this shift.
LT: Will walk unassisted to end of hall using walker by discharge.	Assist patient in walking with walker in room tid.	Assistance helps prevent falls and offers encouragement.	Used walker during physical therapy × 2.
	Encourage to walk with walker in hall at least once daily; assist as needed.	Encouragement provides some motivation.	Up with walker to bathroom × 1 this shift; needs assistance to get up from bed.
	Reinforce instructions from physical therapist for exercises and walker use.	Reinforcing instructions helps patient remember them.	Reviewed physical therapist's instructions for walker use. Progressing toward meeting expected outcomes; continue plan.

***PROBLEM*/NURSING DIAGNOSIS** *Left-sided weakness*/Risk for injury from fall related to neurologic impairment and muscle weakness, as evidenced by inability to bear weight on left leg.
Supporting Assessment Data *Objective:* stroke 6/16; unable to support body weight on left leg; balance shaky, lists to side; cannot grasp with left hand; staggers when tries to walk unaided.

Planning/Goals/ Expected Outcomes	Implementation/ Nursing Interventions	Selected Rationale	Evaluation
LT: Will not suffer injury from fall at any time.	Keep walker positioned by bed.	Object close at hand encourages use.	*Has patient suffered any injury from a fall? Is patient using aids to ambulation?* Walker is placed within reach toward foot of bed.
LT: Will compensate for neurologic impairment with use of aids to ambulation by 7/15.	Encourage to use walker whenever out of bed.	Encouragement prompts desired behavior.	States willingness to use walker at all times; is afraid of falling.
	Ask to use call bell for assistance whenever fatigued and needs to get up.	Assistance helps prevent falls.	Rang for assistance to get up this P.M.; states she is tired from all the visitors.
	Assess muscular strength, balance, and ability to walk safely with walker q 3 d.	Helps prevent falls should condition deteriorate.	Right arm and leg still weak; cannot fully support self without walker. Balance seems to be improving with walker use. Becoming more adept at moving walker and judging how to get around furniture; meeting expected outcomes; continue plan.

*Evaluation statements are examples of documentation indicating interventions have been carried out and the patient's response to them. The results of the actions reflect whether expected outcomes are being met.

Key: *d*, day; *hr*, hours; *LT*, long term; *q*, every; *ROM*, range of motion; *ST*, short term; *tid*, three times a day; *UA*, urinalysis.

FIGURE 6.2 Sample student nursing care plan.

Nursing Care Plan — Sample Student Nursing Care Plan Based on the Situation for Victoria Torres

PROBLEM/NURSING DIAGNOSIS *Wetting the bed*/Reflex incontinence related to neurologic impairment as evidenced by inability to retain urine.

Supporting Assessment Data *Objective:* Unable to control bladder consistently since stroke; frequent urinary incontinence; UA normal; no foul odor to urine.

Planning/Goals/ Expected Outcomes	Implementation/ Nursing Interventions	Selected Rationale	Evaluation
ST: Will void in bedpan q 2 hr while awake without intervening episodes of urinary incontinence by 6/30.	Collaborate on voiding schedule times. Keep schedule at bedside. Remind patient to ask for bedpan. Assist with bedpan.	Patient knows her usual pattern for voiding.	*Has patient had episodes of incontinence?* 2-hr schedule beginning after breakfast instituted.
LT: Will experience no episodes of incontinence by discharge.	Praise patient for each 2-hr period of continence.	Positive reinforcement encourages desired behavior and helps self-esteem.	Used bedpan at designated times; praise given. One soiling of bed at 11:30 pm Patient upset about bed soiling; states does see some progress. Achieving expected outcomes; continue plan.

PROBLEM/NURSING DIAGNOSIS *Unable to use left extremities*/Self-care deficit, hygiene and grooming, related to muscular impairment, as evidenced by inability to grasp items with dominant left hand and inability to walk without assistance.

Supporting Assessment Data *Objective:* States, "I can't seem to do anything with this arm and leg." *Objective:* stroke 6/16. Left-sided weakness of both extremities.

Planning/Goals/ Expected Outcomes	Implementation/ Nursing Interventions	Selected Rationale	Evaluation
ST: Will assist with bath by bathing left extremities by 6/26.	Assist with hygiene and grooming activities; encourage patient to participate.	Demonstrates caring.	*What hygiene and grooming activities has patient performed independently?* States she wishes to bathe herself without assistance; will attempt to do more of bath as fatigue decreases. Willing to do more than wash face tomorrow.
ST: Will attempt to brush hair with right hand by 6/26.	Collaborate with patient on daily goals; praise all accomplishments and attempts at self-care.	Participation in goal setting helps patient "own" the goal and desire to suceed in achieving it.	Attempted to brush hair; unable to do more than three strokes.
ST: Will brush teeth with right hand 6/30.	Assist patient in attempts at brushing teeth and combing hair using right hand.	Encouragement and praise help reinforce positive behaviors and increase self-esteem.	Occupational therapy scheduled for Friday. Will attempt to brush her own teeth tomorrow.
LT: Will learn to put clothes on left extremities before discharge.	Reinforce occupational therapist's instructions for dressing self; supervise practice and give encouragement.	Reinforcement helps patient recall how to efficiently dress; supervision helps prevent frustration.	Praised for use of hairbrush.
LT: Will perform her own hygiene and grooming within 3 mo.	Prevent patient from becoming overtired when attempting her own hygiene activities; space activities.	Neurologic damage to the brain causes easy fatigue. Fatigue will interfere with success and cause frustration.	Beginning to achieve expected outcomes; continue plan.

Critical Thinking Questions

1. While helping the patient with ROM excerises, she says to you, "Will I ever be able to walk normally again?" What would be the most therapeutic reply to this question?
2. How would you explain to the patient why it is important for her to use the call bell and ask for assistance when she desires to get up from the bed?
3. What is the rationale for praising the patient for each 2 hour period of continence?

FIGURE 6.2, cont'd

Get Ready for the NCLEX Examination!

Key Points

- During the implementation step of the nursing process, the planned nursing interventions are carried out.
- Priorities of care are set when developing a well-organized work plan for the shift.
- Before carrying out interventions, you need to understand the reason for the intervention, the usual standard of care, the expected outcome, and any potential danger.
- An independent nursing action is one that the nurse can perform without a primary care provider's order.
- A dependent nursing action requires a primary care provider's order before it can be legally carried out.
- An interdependent action is one derived from collaborative planning between two or more health care professionals.
- A clinical pathway or interdisciplinary care map contains the actions to be carried out by all of the health professionals involved in the patient's care. It is a managed care tool and is used to speed a patient to recovery as quickly and cost-effectively as possible.
- The family and resident are invited to the care planning conference in the long-term care facility.
- The care plan for the home health patient encompasses the needs and concerns of the family as well as those of the patient.
- Documentation of nursing care is essential and should be done soon after an action has been completed.
- Documentation must show the progress toward attainment of outcomes.
- Evaluation involves reassessment of data to determine whether the expected outcomes have been achieved.
- After evaluation, the nursing care plan is revised.
- The goal of a quality improvement program is improvement of nursing practice and patient care.
- Construction of a nursing care plan involves assessing the patient, analyzing the data, identifying nursing problems, prioritizing the problems, deciding on goals, writing expected outcomes, and choosing interventions. After the plan is implemented, the outcomes of the interventions are evaluated and the plan is revised as needed.

Additional Learning Resources

SG Go to your Study Guide for additional learning activities to help you master this chapter content.

evolve Go to your Evolve website http://evolve.elsevier.com/deWit/fundamental for additional online resources.

Review Questions for the NCLEX Examination

*Choose the **best** answer for each question.*

1. You assist a patient with her bath, change her dressing, rub her back, give her medication, review her dietary needs, and assist with physical therapy exercises. Which are examples of interdependent nursing actions? *(Select all that apply.)*
   1. Reinforcing dietary education
   2. Changing her dressing
   3. Assisting with her exercises
   4. Giving her a back rub
   5. Giving a bath
   6. Administering medication
2. Before carrying out a dependent nursing action, the nurse: *(Select all that apply.)*
   1. Makes certain the family is in agreement with the order.
   2. Verifies that the primary care provider's order is in the medical record.
   3. Considers whether there is any contraindication for the action.
   4. Reviews agency policies and procedures manual as needed.
   5. Gathers all equipment and supplies needed for the action.
3. The nurse evaluates the care provided to the patient by determining:
   1. Whether she is beginning to improve.
   2. Whether all planned interventions were carried out.
   3. Whether expected outcomes have been achieved.
   4. Whether she is well enough for discharge.
4. A patient who is 14 hours postoperative complains of shortness of breath. Which action should be implemented first?
   1. Auscultate the lungs.
   2. Question about previous shortness of breath.
   3. Check for an order for oxygen therapy.
   4. Reassure the patient.
5. A difference in the assessment of the patient entering a long-term care facility versus that of a hospital patient is that the long-term care resident is assessed for:
   1. Functional abilities.
   2. Psychosocial concerns.
   3. Emotional concerns.
   4. Skin problems.
6. An example of a dependent nursing action would be:
   1. Starting the continuous passive motion (CPM) machine.
   2. Providing a back massage.
   3. Encouraging the consumption of more fluid.
   4. Changing the patient's linens after an episode of incontinence.
7. When evaluating a patient admitted with a lower respiratory tract infection, which data are most important for the nurse to obtain?
   1. Level of pain or discomfort
   2. Medications taken at home
   3. Duration of the illness
   4. Bilateral lung sounds

Critical Thinking Activities

Read each clinical scenario and discuss the questions with your classmates.

Scenario A

Construct a nursing care plan from the following scenario: Mark Hansen, a 45-year-old man, is admitted with a fractured femur. He is placed in skeletal traction. His nursing diagnoses are impaired physical mobility r/t immobilization by traction and self-care deficit, bathing, grooming, and toileting, r/t immobilization.

Scenario B

Discuss and compare dependent and independent nursing actions on your care plan for Mr. Hansen.

Scenario C

What Would You Need to Know About the Order for Traction to Care for This Patient Properly?

chapter 7

Documentation of Nursing Care

http://evolve.elsevier.com/Williams/fundamental

Objectives

Upon completing this chapter, you should be able to do the following:

Theory

1. Identify three purposes of documentation (charting).
2. Correlate the nursing process with the process of documentation.
3. Discuss maintaining confidentiality and privacy of paper and electronic medical records.
4. Compare and contrast the six main methods of documentation.
5. List the legal guidelines for documenting on medical records.
6. Explain the approved way to correct errors in medical records.

Clinical Practice

1. Correctly make entries on a daily care flow sheet.
2. Demonstrate a systematic way of documenting **that ensures** all pertinent information has been included.
3. Document the characterization of signs or symptoms in a sample documentation situation.
4. Apply the general documentation guidelines in the clinical setting.
5. Navigate electronic medical records and document care correctly.

Key Terms

case management system charting (p. 87)
charting (p. 86)
charting by exception (p. 86)
computer-assisted charting (p. 86)
computerized provider order entry (CPOE) (p. 92)
electronic health record (EHR) (p. 90)
focus charting (p. 86)
medical record (p. 84)
PIE charting (p. 89)
problem-oriented medical record (POMR) charting (p. 86)
protocols (PRŌ-tō-kŏlz, p. 90)
source-oriented (narrative) charting (p. 86)

Concepts Covered in This Chapter

- Care coordination
- Communication
- Health literacy
- Patient-centered care
- Accountability
- Health care systems
- Patient care technology
- Patient education
- Informatics
- Health care quality
- Quality improvement

PURPOSES OF DOCUMENTATION

Documentation provides a written record of the history, treatment, care, and response of the patient while under medical and nursing care. It justifies claims for reimbursement, may be used as evidence of care in a court of law, shows the use of the nursing process, and provides data for quality-assurance studies. Each person who provides care for the patient adds documentation to the **medical record (sometimes referred to as a chart).** The medical record contains all orders, tests, treatments, and care that occurred while the person was under the care of the health care provider. The medical record is a communication tool for the professionals involved in patient care. Health team members use documentation to communicate what has been done, how the patient responded, and the current plan for care. Many different forms are used for documentation, and the most common forms are shown in the chapters specific to their content; for example, an intravenous (IV) flow sheet (parenteral infusion record) is shown in Chapter 36. The Joint Commission sets the standards for documentation. Common types of forms in patients' medical records are listed in Table 7.1.

Insurance companies and Medicare rely on documentation to determine actual length of stay, procedures performed, and diagnoses established and to

Table 7.1 Forms Used for Hospital Documentation

FORM	TYPE OF INFORMATION
General Forms	
Face sheet	Patient data, including the patient's name, address, phone number, next of kin, hospital identification number, religious preference, place of employment, insurance company, occupation, name of admitting health care provider, and admitting diagnosis.
Provider orders	The provider's directives for patient care.
Graphic sheet	Record of serial measurements and observations, such as temperature, pulse, respiration, blood pressure, and weight.
Nursing care plan	Care plan for the patient, including nursing diagnoses, goals and expected outcomes, and nursing interventions.
Nursing notes	Documentation of the nursing process (i.e., assessment, nursing diagnosis, planning, implementation, and evaluation); a record of interventions implemented and the patient's response to them.
Care flow sheet	Form on which check marks or short entries are made to indicate dietary intake, type of bath, wound dressing changes, oxygen in use, health care provider visits, equipment in use, level of activity, and so forth.
Medication administration record (MAR)	Documentation of all medications ordered, doses given, and doses not taken by the patient.
History and physical examination forms	Primary care provider's record of the patient's medical history and findings of the current physical examination.
Nurse's admission history and assessment	Nurse's current history, including usual habits, medications usually taken, and physical assessment findings at admission.
Progress sheet	Primary care provider's notes regarding the patient's progress.
Laboratory reports	Results of laboratory tests.
Radiology reports	Results of x-ray examinations.
Admission forms	Information on patient identification, conditions for admission, and consent for general medical and nursing care.
Intake and output (I&O) record	Serial record of 24-hr intake and output.
Miscellaneous Forms	
Ancillary staff sheets	Records of treatments by physical therapists, occupational therapists, respiratory therapists, and so forth.
Consultation sheet	Record of another health care provider called in to consult by the primary care provider.
Diabetic flow sheet	Record of blood glucose determinations and amounts of insulin administered.
Discharge form	Information about instructions given regarding wound care, medications, rest, activity restrictions, needed exercises, diet, and signs and symptoms to report to the primary care provider; also includes when to see the provider next.
Discharge planning sheet	Records by social services, home health agencies, case managers, and clinical nurse specialists regarding the discharge plans and patient's needs.
Fall risk assessment	Information regarding the patient's potential fall risk; particularly used for frail patients, older adults, or patients with neuromuscular impairments.
Frequent observations sheet	Used when frequent measurements of vital signs or neurologic assessments are needed (e.g., after surgery or after head trauma).
Intravenous (IV) flow sheet	Record of IV fluids and additives infused, type of IV catheter in use, date tubing was changed, and date dressing was applied.
Pain assessment	Record of pain level, when assessed, measures to reduce it, and effectiveness of treatment.
Preoperative checklist	List used to verify that the patient is ready to go to surgery.
Skin risk assessment	Data from thorough skin assessment on admission; evaluation of risk factors for skin breakdown; diagrams showing areas of redness, breaks in the skin, or pressure injuries.
Surgical or treatment consent form	Patient authorization for surgery or treatment.
Time-out form	Patient verification, site-mark verification, and time out performed before surgical procedure.
Transfer form	Information pertinent for the transfer of the patient to another unit or facility.

calculate charges due for reimbursement. Each piece of equipment in service must be documented. Medical records must display data that support the medical and nursing diagnoses. Evaluation data indicating that the treatment was successful or unsuccessful must be present to justify the duration of the hospital stay. Documentation of this type is also necessary for accreditation of the health care agency. Medical records are also used for research data collection. For example, statistics may be compiled for the number of cases of pneumonia treated, the average age of the patients, and treatment results, to see which treatments are most effective.

The medical record is a legal record and can be used as evidence of events that occurred or treatment that was given. When documentation is thorough, the record provides a way to show that standards of care have been met.

Documentation, also called **charting**, is used to track the application of the nursing process. The nurse writes down observations made about the patient, notes the care and treatment that was delivered, and adds the patient's response. Documentation shows progress toward the expected outcomes listed on the nursing care plan.

Documentation is useful for supervisory purposes to evaluate staff performance.

 QSEN Considerations: Quality Improvement

Medical Record Audits

Documentation in the medical record is audited as part of the health care agency's quality-improvement program. Evidence that care adheres to accepted standards should be present in the nurse's notes. The results of audits of the medical records tell nurse managers where improvement may be needed.

DOCUMENTATION AND THE NURSING PROCESS

The nursing care plan or interdisciplinary care plan provides the framework for nursing documentation. Documenting in the medical record is organized by nursing diagnosis or problem. An initial assessment is recorded for each shift. Standard areas of assessment are usually noted on flow sheets, and a note is added if an abnormality exists. Nursing diagnoses or problems are entered on the care plan, which is created soon after the admission assessment is complete. The plan is reviewed and updated every 24 hours. Implementation of each intervention is documented on a flow sheet or within the nursing notes. The specifics of what was done and how, plus the patient response, are documented. Evaluation statements are entered in the nurse's notes, and they indicate progress toward the stated expected outcomes and goals. Evaluation data must be documented showing that expected outcomes have been achieved before a nursing diagnosis is marked "resolved" or deleted from the care plan. When expected outcomes are not being met, the care plan is altered to better represent the patient's needs.

? Think Critically

If evaluation data are not showing progress toward expected outcomes, what part of the nursing care plan needs to be altered? Where in the medical record would this be done?

THE MEDICAL RECORD

The **medical record** contains data on a patient's stay in the health facility or while under the care of a health care provider. Each type of facility has a particular set of forms used to record information about the patient.

As a legal record, the medical record's contents are **confidential;** this means you can only give out information with the patient's written consent because the medical record contains personal information regarding the patient. **Only health professionals caring directly for the patient, or those involved in research or education, should have access to the medical record.** Protecting the patient's privacy is of prime importance. Do not discuss patient information with others not directly involved in the patient's care.

The medical record is the property of the health facility or agency, not of the patient or primary care provider. Patients do have a right to information contained in the medical record under certain circumstances (see Chapter 3). Keeping the patient and the family informed in a clear and timely manner usually satisfies their need for information. After the patient has been discharged, the medical record is sent to the medical records or health information department for safekeeping. It can be retrieved if the patient is admitted to service again within a 10-year span. Electronic records may be kept for longer periods, ranging from 10 years to indefinitely, depending on the state where the patient resides (Shepard, 2015).

? Think Critically

What would you say to your neighbor, who sees you working on the unit on which her sister's husband is a patient, if she asks you to check and see what her brother-in-law's primary care provider has documented about his condition?

METHODS OF DOCUMENTATION (CHARTING)

Different methods of documentation are used in various health care agencies. The six main methods of documentation are (1) **source-oriented (narrative) charting,** which is organized by "source" or author of the documentation entry; (2) **problem-oriented medical record (POMR) charting,** which focuses on the problems the patient experiences as a result of being ill; (3) **focus charting,** which centers on the patient from a positive perspective; (4) **charting by exception,** which focuses on deviations from predefined norms, using preset protocols and standards of care; (5) **computer-assisted**

Doe, John B.
Neverland Hospital
From 10/10/17 to 10/11/17
Room 645-1 ADM 10/09/17
Age 63Y Sex M
MD Sawbucks, Jackson
ID 4620958 MR 102756

FLOWSHEET	10/10	10/11	
ADLs—cont'd	11-7	7-3	3-11
Ambulate		done RN FR 10:00 done self FR 14:00	
Activity response		tolerated well FR 08:00 tolerated well FR 10:00 tolerated well FR 14:00	tolerated well FR 16:00 tolerated well RJK 20:00 tolerated well RJK 22:00
Feeding		self assist FR 08:00 self assist FRI 12:00	
Diet		regular FR 08:00 regular FR 12:00	
Ate %		80% FR 08:00 80% FR 12:00	
Hygiene		assist bath perineal care skin care back rub linen change FR 10:00	
Standard prec		yes FR 08:00 yes FR 10:00	yes RJK 20:00 yes RJK 22:00
SKIN	11-7	7-3	3-11
Skin assmnt	WNL RJK 00:00	WNL FR 08:00	WNL RJK 20:00
Braden sc	21 RJK 00:00	21 FR 08:00	21 RJK 22:00
INC/WDS UPPER	11-7	7-3	3-11
L shoulder			
Wound type	incision RJK 00:00	incision FR 08:00	incision RJK 20:00
Wound appearance	dry clean RJK 00:00	dry clean FR 08:00	dry clean RJK 20:00
L shoulder Wound dressing	dry intact checked RJK 00:00	dry intact checked FR 08:00	dry intact checked RJK 20:00
IV LINES	11-7	7-3	3-11
R subclavian			
Line type	triple RJK 00:00	triple FR 08:00	triple RJK 20:00
Rutken, Frances (FR) RN		Kahn, Roland J. (RJK) LPN	

FIGURE 7.1 Computer activity flow sheet. (Created by Susan C. deWit [SCD] RN; Carolyn Sims [CJS] LPN.)

charting, where data are input to the computer; and (6) **case management system charting,** which tracks variances from the clinical pathway.

Whatever method of documentation is used, you are required to document the patient's progress periodically during the shift or at the time of a home health visit. The medical record entries are either in your notes or on flow sheets (Fig. 7.1). Flow sheets track routine assessments, treatments, and frequently given care. The specific time frame required for documentation is found in the agency's policy and procedure manual. Some agencies require one note per patient contact; others require documentation every 1 to 3 hours during the shift.

Date	Time	Problem	Nurse's Notes
6/25/18	2015	#1	States has "sharp throbbing" pain at a 7 on a 1-10 pain scale.
			Started at 2000 when amb down hall. T 99, P 88, R 24, BP
			146/82. Unrelieved by change in position or rest.----R. Hill, LVN
	2020		Meperidine 75 mg IM RUOQ.------------------R. Hill, LVN
	2045		Resting quietly in bed. P 86, R 20, BP 146/78. States pain "has
			decreased considerably."------------------R. Hill, LVN

FIGURE 7.2 Example of source-oriented (narrative) charting.

Table 7.2 Major Components of the Problem-Oriented Medical Record

AREA	CONTENTS
Database	Initial assessment, general health history, findings of the physical examination, results of diagnostic and laboratory tests, psychosocial information, nursing assessment, and patient's response to the illness or problem.
Problem list	A list of problems derived from the information in the database. The list is continually updated with resolved problems deleted and new problems added. Problems are listed in the chronologic order in which they were identified, not by priority. Both actual and potential problems are listed.
Plan	A three-part plan of care is devised based on the identified problems. For each problem, there is a plan for diagnostic studies, a therapeutic plan, and a patient education plan. The primary care provider orders therapies for medical problems, and the nurse orders care for nursing problems.
Progress notes	Contain the assessments, plans, and orders of the physicians, nurses, and other therapists involved in the patient's care. Notes are organized by problem number from the problem list, and each problem is addressed in the SOAP format: S: Subjective data that include symptoms and patient's description of the problem O: Objective data based on health care team's observations, physical examination, and diagnostic tests A: Assessment or analysis of the meaning of the data obtained P: Plan to resolve the problem It is not essential to write a progress note on each problem every day.
Discharge summary	A summary of the problems the patient had, how they were resolved, and the plan for care after discharge.

SOURCE-ORIENTED OR NARRATIVE CHARTING

These records are organized according to the source of information. There are separate areas for physicians (focusing on medical problems), nurses (focusing on nursing diagnoses), dietitians, and other health care professionals to document their assessment findings and plan the patient's care. Narrative notes are phrases and sentences written without any standardized structure, content, or form. Narrative documentation used in source-oriented records requires documentation of patient care in chronologic order. Assessments usually follow a body systems format. The content is similar to a set of dated and timed journal entries (Fig. 7.2).

Advantages of the source-oriented (narrative) method:

- It gives information on the patient's condition and care in chronologic order.
- It indicates the patient's baseline condition for each shift.
- It includes aspects of all steps of the nursing process.

Disadvantages of the source-oriented method:

- It encourages documentation of both normal and abnormal findings, making it difficult to separate pertinent from irrelevant information.
- It requires extensive documentation time by the staff.
- It discourages physicians and other health team members from reading all parts of the medical record because of the lengthy descriptive entries in it.

PROBLEM-ORIENTED MEDICAL RECORD CHARTING

POMR charting focuses on patient status, emphasizing the problem-solving approach to patient care and providing a method for communicating what, when, and how things are to be done to meet the patient's needs. The POMR contains five basic parts: the database, the problem list, the plan, the progress notes (in which *all* members of the health care team document), and the discharge summary (Table 7.2). The precise form these records take varies greatly between agencies, but the essentials of documentation are the same.

As this documentation method evolved, the original *SOAP* format for progress notes (for *S*ubjective information, *O*bjective data, *A*ssessment data, and *P*lan) was modified to *S*ubjective, *O*bjective, *A*ssessment, *P*lan, *I*mplementation, *E*valuation (*SOAPIE*) and

Date	Time	Problem		Nurse's Notes
7/18/18	0800	#2 Pain, Abd	S.	States having RUQ pain radiating to right shoulder. Is "like
				a knife is poking me." States is a 6 on a scale of 1-10. "It
				started after I ate the bacon." States feels nauseous, but no
				vomiting.--
			O.	Pale, diaphoretic and shaky. Splinting abd c̄ hands.
				T 100° F, P 112, R 22, BP 134/88.
			A.	Abd pain.
			P.	Institute NPO status; medicate when IM order received.
				Notify physician.-----------------------------------J. Sims, RN

A

Date	Time	Problem		Nurse's Notes
6/25/18	1620	#1 Hypertension	S.	States feeling "warm and restless."----------------------------
			O.	Face flushed; skin hot to touch. T 103° F, P 120, R 26,
				BP 160/90.--
			A.	Hyperthermia r/t wound infection.
			P.	Medicate for ↑ temp.--
	1625		I.	Acetaminophen 500 mg PO c̄ full glass of H_2O. Gown
				changed. Heat turned down, blanket removed.-----------------
	1700		E.	T 101.6°F, P 95, R 24; temp falling. States is feeling better.
				Skin cooler to touch.---------------------------M. Bailey, LPN

B

FIGURE 7.3 (A) Example of POMR charting. (B) Example of SOAPIE charting.

SOAPIER. The additional letters stand for *I*mplementation, *E*valuation, and *R*evision. It is not necessary to use each component of the SOAPIER format each time you make an entry. If there are no subjective data, the *S* can be omitted or labeled "none." If there is no revision, the *R* can be left out (Fig. 7.3).

Advantages of the POMR method of documentation:

- It provides documentation of comprehensive care by focusing on patients and their problems.
- It promotes the problem-solving approach to care.
- It improves continuity of care and communication by keeping data relevant to a problem all in one place so that it is more available to all who are providing care.
- It allows easy auditing of patient medical records in evaluating staff performance or quality of patient care.
- It requires continual evaluation and revision of the care plan.
- It reinforces application of the nursing process.

Disadvantages of the POMR method of documentation:

- It results in loss of chronologic documentation.
- It is more difficult to track trends in patient status.
- It fragments data because of the increased number of flow sheets required.

Problem Identification, Interventions, and Evaluation Charting

Another offshoot of this method is **PIE charting,** which stands for *P*roblem identification, *I*nterventions, and *E*valuation. This type of documentation follows the nursing process and uses nursing diagnoses while placing the plan of care within the nurses' progress notes. It differs from SOAP notes because it does not use a traditional nursing care plan or require narrative documentation of the assessment data as long as they are normal. The problems, patient education, and discharge needs are listed under the *P* of the PIE format. Nursing diagnoses are kept on a problem list *(P)*, and each entry is marked with the problem number and title. With this method, the daily assessment information is placed on special flow sheets, and duplication of the information is avoided. Interventions performed are documented under *I*. The outcomes of the interventions are evaluated and documented under *E* (Fig. 7.4). When assessment data are abnormal, an *A* is added (APIE).

FOCUS CHARTING

Focus charting is similar to the POMR system, but it substitutes **focus** for the **problem,** eliminating the negative connotation attached to "problem." Focus charting is directed at a nursing diagnosis (e.g., pain), a patient problem (pressure injury), a concern (decreased food intake), a sign (fever), a symptom (anxiety), or an event (return from surgery). The note has three components: *D*ata, *A*ction, and *R*esponse (DAR) or *D*ata, *A*ction, and *E*valuation (DAE) (Fig. 7.5). The data component contains subjective and objective information that describes or supports the focus of the note. The action component includes interventions performed or to be

Date	Time	Problem		Nurse's Notes
7/18/18	1420	Pain r/t ROM	P.	Reinstruct in use of PCA and measures for distraction.
		exercises of rt	I.	Instructions for use of PCA given; encouraged to watch
		knee by CPM		TV movie for distraction. Knee position on CPM machine
		machine		OK; machine functioning at ordered settings. Repositioned
				upper body for comfort.
			E.	Using PCA as needed; pain decreased. States is tolerable at
				3 on a scale of 1-10. Watching movie.--------C. Harris, LPN

FIGURE 7.4 Example of PIE charting.

Date	Time	Problem		Patient Progress
7/01/18	1300	Skin breakdown	D.	Slight serous drainage on dressing; wound 1x2 cm c̄ left red
		right ankle		border; no odor; states hurts slightly.---------------------------
			A.	Cleansed c̄ sterile saline. DuoDerm thin applied.
			R.	Wound clean; minimal drainage present.-----T. Harper, RN

FIGURE 7.5 Example of focus charting.

implemented. The response component describes the outcomes of the interventions and whether the goal has been met.

The advantages of focus charting:

- It is compatible with the use of the nursing process.
- It shortens documentation time by using many flow sheets and checklists.
- The focus is not limited to patient problems or nursing diagnoses.

The disadvantages of focus charting:

- If the database is not complete, patient problems may be missed.
- It does not adhere to charting with the focus on nursing diagnoses and expected outcomes.

CHARTING BY EXCEPTION

Charting by exception was developed in the early 1980s by a group of nurses in Wisconsin. The goal was to decrease the lengthy narrative entries of traditional documentation systems and reduce repetition of data. **Charting by exception is based on the assumption that all standards of practice are carried out and met with a normal or expected response *unless otherwise documented.*** Agency-wide and unit-specific **protocols** (standard procedures) and standards of nursing care are the heart of the system. The standards and protocols are integrated into flow sheets and forms, and the nurse needs only to document abnormal findings or responses correlated with the nursing diagnoses listed on the nursing care plan (Fig. 7.6). Charting by exception is the direct opposite of the adage, "If it wasn't documented, it wasn't done." Charting by exception assumes that, unless documented to the contrary, all standards and protocols were followed and all assessment values were within accepted limits. This type of documentation may present some problems with legalities when a medical record is called into court because only abnormalities are documented in written words.

The advantages of charting by exception:

- It highlights abnormal data and patient trends.
- It decreases narrative documentation time.
- It eliminates duplication of charting.
- It lends itself to computerized documentation systems.

Disadvantages of charting by exception:

- It requires development of detailed protocols and standards.
- It requires retraining staff to use unfamiliar methods of record keeping and documenting.
- Nurses become so used to *not* charting that important data are sometimes omitted.

COMPUTER-ASSISTED CHARTING

An **electronic health record (EHR)** is a computerized comprehensive record of a patient's history and care across all facilities and admissions. This type of record has been set up as a goal of the Stimulus Law that President Obama signed in 2009.

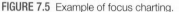

 QSEN Considerations: Informatics

Nursing Informatics

Nursing informatics is the "science and practice (that) integrates nursing, its information and knowledge, with management of information and communication technologies to promote the health of people, families, and communities worldwide" (American Medical Informatics Association, 2015). The electronic health record is a component of informatics.

GUIDELINES FOR USE OF THE NURSING/PHYSICIAN ORDER FLOW SHEET

1. Indicate the Nursing Diagnosis that relates to the nursing order in the far left-hand column of the category boxes. If the order is a physician order, indicate "D.O." ("Doctor Order") instead of the nursing diagnosis number.
2. Indicate the nursing or physician order. If the nursing order includes an assessment to be completed, use the following protocol:
   a. *NEUROLOGIC ASSESSMENT* - will include orientation, pupil movement, sensation, quality of speech/swallowing, and memory.
   b. *CARDIOVASCULAR ASSESSMENT* - will include apical pulse, neck veins, CRT, peripheral pulses, edema, and calf tenderness.
   c. *RESPIRATORY ASSESSMENT* - will include respiratory characteristics, breath sounds, cough, sputum, color of nailbeds/mucous membranes, and CRT.
   d. *GASTROINTESTINAL ASSESSMENT* - will include abdominal appearance, bowel sounds, palpation, diet tolerance, and stools.
   e. *URINARY ASSESSMENT* - will include voiding patterns, bladder distention, and urine characteristics.
   f. *INTEGUMENTARY ASSESSMENT* - will include skin color, skin temperature, skin integrity, and condition of mucous membranes.
   g. *MUSCULOSKELETAL ASSESSMENT* - will include joint swelling, tenderness, limitations in ROM, muscle strength, and condition of surrounding tissue.
   h. *NEUROVASCULAR ASSESSMENT* - will include color, temperature, movement, CRT, peripheral pulses, edema, and patient description of sensation to affected extremity.
   i. *SURGICAL DRESSING/INCISIONAL ASSESSMENT* - will include condition of surgical dressing and/or color, temperature, tenderness of surrounding tissue, condition of sutures/staples/steri-strips, appearance of wound including color, any exudate present, granulation tissue; approximation of wound edges, and presence of any drainage.
   j. *PAIN ASSESSMENT* - will include patient description, location, duration, intensity on a scale of 1 to 10, radiation, precipitating factors.
   k. *POST-MYELOGRAM COMPLICATION ASSESSMENT* - will include headache, nausea, and vomiting.
   l. *MYELOGRAM SITE ASSESSMENT* - will include presence of ecchymosis and drainage.

OR

Specify exactly which parts of assessment should be completed.

3. Top of sheet should be dated. Time should be indicated in the small box in upper right-hand corner of each category box.
4. Upon carrying out an order that has no significant findings, a "✓" in the appropriate category box is sufficient to indicate it was done. If the order includes an assessment, the following parameters will be considered a negative assessment and constitute the use of a "✓."
   a. *NEUROLOGIC ASSESSMENT* - Alert and oriented to person, place, and time. Behavior appropriate to situation. Pupils equal, round and reactive to light. Active ROM of all extremities with symmetry of strength. No paresthesia. Verbalization clear and understandable. Swallowing without coughing or choking on liquids and solids. Memory intact.
   b. *CARDIOVASCULAR ASSESSMENT* - Regular apical pulse, S_1 and S_2 audible. Neck veins flat at 45 degrees. CRT <3 sec. Peripheral pulses palpable. No edema. No calf tenderness.
   c. *RESPIRATORY ASSESSMENT* - Respirations 10-20/min at rest. Respirations quiet and regular. Breath sounds vesicular throughout both lung fields, bronchial over major airways, with no adventitious sounds. Sputum clear. Nailbeds and mucous membranes pink. CRT <3 sec.
   d. *GASTROINTESTINAL ASSESSMENT* - Abdomen soft. Bowel sounds active (5-34/min.) No pain with palpation. Tolerates prescribed diet without nausea and vomiting. Having BMs within own normal pattern and consistency.
   e. *URINARY ASSESSMENT* - Able to empty bladder without dysuria. Bladder not distended after voiding. Urine clear and yellow to amber.
   f. *INTEGUMENTARY ASSESSMENT* - Skin color within patient's norm. Skin warm and intact. Mucous membranes moist.
   g. *MUSCULOSKELETAL ASSESSMENT* - Absence of joint swelling and tenderness. Normal ROM of all joints. NO muscle weakness. Surrounding tissues show no evidence of inflammation, nodules, nail changes, ulcerations, or rashes.
   h. *NEUROVASCULAR ASSESSMENT* - Affected extremity is pink, warm and movable within patient's average ROM. CRT <3 sec. Peripheral pulses palpable. No edema. Sensation intact without numbness or paresthesia.
   i. *SURGICAL DRESSING/INCISIONAL ASSESSMENT* - Dressing dry and intact. No evidence of redness, increased temperature, or tenderness in surrounding tissue. Sutures/staples/steri-strips intact. Wound edges well-approximated. No drainage present.
   j. *PAIN ASSESSMENT* - If medication alone relieves pain and expected outcome is met, documentation on the Medication Profile is sufficient. No specific problem needs to be identified in the Nurses' Notes or Flow Sheet.
   k. *POST-MYELOGRAM COMPLICATION ASSESSMENT* - Absence of headache, nausea, and vomiting.
   l. *MYELOGRAM SITE ASSESSMENT* - Steri-strip dry and intact. No drainage present.
5. Upon carrying out an order that has significant findings, an asterisk is entered in the appropriate box. An asterisk (*) in the category box indicates to "See Significant Findings Section."
6. If status remains unchanged from previous asterisk entry, current entry may be indicated with an "→."
7. If an order no longer needs to be carried out, the next unused category box in that row indicates "order D/Ced," and a line should be drawn through the remaining boxes. Any unused rows can be left blank.
8. Each flow sheet is used for 24 hours.

FIGURE 7.6 Guidelines for the use of the nursing or physician order flow sheet. These guidelines appear on the reverse side of the first page of the flow sheet. (From Burke, L. J., & Murphy, J. [1995]. *Charting by exception applications: making it work in clinical settings*. Albany, NY: Delmar.)

QSEN Considerations: Informatics

KSAs for Prelicensure Licensed Practical Nurse/Licensed Vocational Nurse Students

KNOWLEDGE	SKILLS	ATTITUDES
• Knowledge of why information and technology skills are essential for safe patient care. • Identify essential information needed in a database to support patient care. • Describe examples of how computerized information is related to patient care quality and safety. • Recognize the time, effort, and skill needed for technology to become an effective and reliable tool for patient care.	• Learn how data are managed in the care setting before performing patient care. • Apply technology to support patient care. • Document patient care in an electronic health record. • Navigate the electronic health record. • Respond appropriately to clinical decision-making alerts, in collaboration with the RN.	• Appreciate the need to seek continuous learning of information technology skills. • Value technology that supports clinical decision making. • Protect patient privacy and confidentiality in electronic health records. • Value nurses' involvement in design of information technology systems for patient care.

KSA: knowledge, skills, attitudes; *RN:* registered nurse.
Adapted from http://qsen.org/competencies/pre-licensure-ksas/#informatics

In addition to knowing how to use information and communication technologies, such as EHRs to assist in providing care, it is also important to assure the information is secure and confidential. Within a hospital system, computer records are protected by passwords and a firewall. With the addition of wireless technology, the security issues have increased. Each user who has access to a patient record must have a secure password, which must be changed regularly to maintain security. Encryption and authentication software is used when reports are transmitted outside of the health care facility campus. See Box 7.1 for tips on computer documentation.

Legal and Ethical Considerations

Confidentiality and Security With Computer Documentation

You have a legal obligation to guard your password and not give it to anyone at any time for any reason. Be sure to shred any printed documents, such as report sheets or ISBAR-R communication sheets that may have any identifiable information before leaving the unit. In addition, keep them concealed while working. HIPAA requirements (see Chapter 3) mandate that all patient information be kept confidential.

Although your password gives you access to the records of patients on your unit, you will not be able to access patient records on other units. Only administrative personnel can view the record of any patient in the hospital.

ISBAR-R: introduction, situation, background, assessment, recommendation, readback; *HIPAA:* Health Insurance Portability and Accountability Act.

Box 7.1 Tips for Computer Documentation

- Attend a computer documentation orientation held by the facility. Obtain a "quick reference guide."
- Determine the "superuser" on your unit to be used as a resource.
- Refresh the computer screen often to keep track of the most current medical orders and other health care providers' entries.
- Document in a timely manner.
- Do not "copy and paste" anyone else's documentation.
- Do not share passwords or computer codes. Your code is your legal electronic signature.
- **Review your notes for accuracy before you select "confirm" or "save."**
- Never walk away from your terminal without logging off.

Computerized provider order entry (CPOE) provides for efficient workflow because, when orders are entered into the computer, they are automatically routed to the appropriate clinical areas for action. For example, an order for a new medication is entered on the computer and then automatically posted to the electronic medication administration record (eMAR) for that patient and to the pharmacy for the order to be filled. The order is always legible, and transcribing errors are eliminated.

In computerized documentation systems, it is important to have standard terminology appropriate for the entire interdisciplinary team. The Systematized Nomenclature of Medicine Clinical Terms (SNOMED CT) is a reference vocabulary developed for this purpose (International Health Terminology Standards Development Organisation, 2015). This is important in evidence-based practice for researchers to understand the relationships in the data to predict trends and consequences of care.

Health care agencies are mandated to use electronic documentation of patient care (Centers for Medicare and Medicaid Services, 2015).

Documentation can be done as interventions are performed with the use of a workstation on wheels (Fig. 7.7) or a hand-held terminal carried from room to room. Computer-assisted documentation can save nursing time. Entries can be made at the point of care, at the time a change in condition is observed or a treatment is given. The information is fresh, and no time has to be spent recalling details or organizing events in sequence. If the system uses a drop-down table or menu to select from, you can quickly choose the appropriate description or intervention and do not have to key in free text. Test and diagnostic results can be electronically added to the medical record as they are received, allowing for more rapid information flow between health care providers.

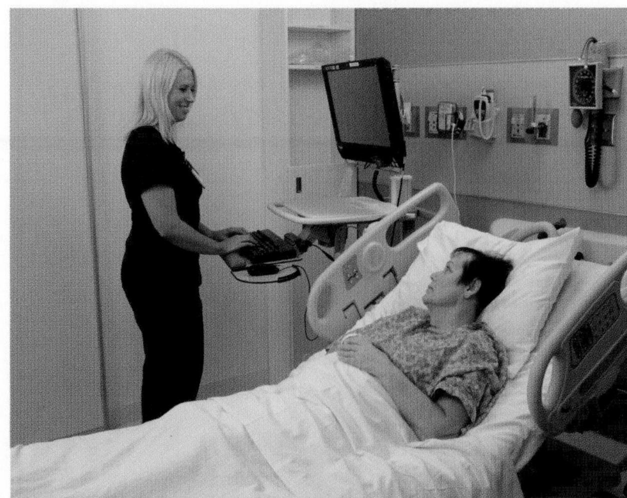

FIGURE 7.7 Nurse using a workstation on wheels at the bedside to do point-of-service documentation.

Computerized systems for documenting patient care vary. Any documentation system can be supported using electronic documentation. Some organizations use a combination of manual and electronic documentation. For example, some documentation systems produce a flow sheet with the expected patient outcomes and nursing interventions listed. The nurse initials those interventions that were implemented, writes a narrative note for other necessary information, and adds the printout page to the medical record. This adds some limited electronic functions to a manual system.

Other systems use the POMR format and produce a prioritized problem list. A care plan is constructed by selecting the diagnoses, expected outcomes, and nursing interventions from specific screens on the computer and keying in required information. A touch screen may be part of the system for choosing items.

A third type of system consists of selecting data from display screens to build the flow sheets and progress notes. The display screens are structured to allow documentation of current data and provide space for the addition of new findings. Much of the everyday care can be documented rapidly and completely in just seconds using such screens. Often the progress notes from all disciplines involved in the patient's care are integrated. A medical record of vital sign trends or laboratory value trends can be printed quickly. Figure 7.8 shows an example of a patient's electronic medical record.

In fully implemented EHRs, clinical information from all sources flow into the record. This results in a longitudinal medical record that contains documentation of all of a patient's health care through time. The record is divided into episodes of care. An episode of care can occur in the outpatient or inpatient setting, any time the patient received medical assessment and/or medical intervention. As mentioned earlier, laboratory results, diagnostic imaging results, pathology reports, medication administration, and other information from all care delivery settings are available via the EHR. This provides virtually instant access to a complete medical history.

At this time, fully integrated EHRs are not common. There are multiple vendors for EHR systems. Integration of these systems with an agency's current needs requires computer programming and interfaces, which can be expensive and time-consuming. Organizations must invest significant time and money to develop a true longitudinal EHR.

Most organizations using EHRs have a computer system that collects health care information while the patient is receiving either inpatient or outpatient services. The inpatient and outpatient systems may be integrated, allowing physicians to access all patient information in the computer system from their offices. However, the clinic medical record and the hospital system's medical record may still remain separate and require access to both computer systems to review.

A major consideration when using an electronic documentation system is confidentiality. Every individual who accesses the medical record has a password that is necessary for access to the assigned patient's medical record. Based on their position or job code, the person will be given a level of security that will allow access to only the specific information required for the job. When working on documentation at the computer, **never leave the terminal while part of a patient's medical record is on the screen.** Situate terminals so that passersby cannot view the information displayed. Organizations have specific policies outlining access, security, and use of the EHR. Organizations often require health care providers to sign nondisclosure agreements (see Chapter 3) regarding confidential patient information.

Electronic records provide vital information to health care personnel instantly so they can immediately review previous problems, treatments, and responses.

Cultural Considerations

Helpful Specific Cultural Information

Including the following patient information can enable the health care team with care coordination:

- Primary language spoken and communication needs (The Joint Commission requirement).
- Head of family or spokesperson.
- Dietary differences and foods not permitted in the diet.
- Ability to read and write in English.
- Beliefs about cause of illness.
- Special concerns related to religious/spiritual beliefs.
- Individual needs for uninterrupted time for meditation or prayer.

Advantages of computer-assisted documentation:

- The date and time of the notation are automatically recorded.
- Notes are always legible and easy to read.
- There is quick communication between departments about patient needs.

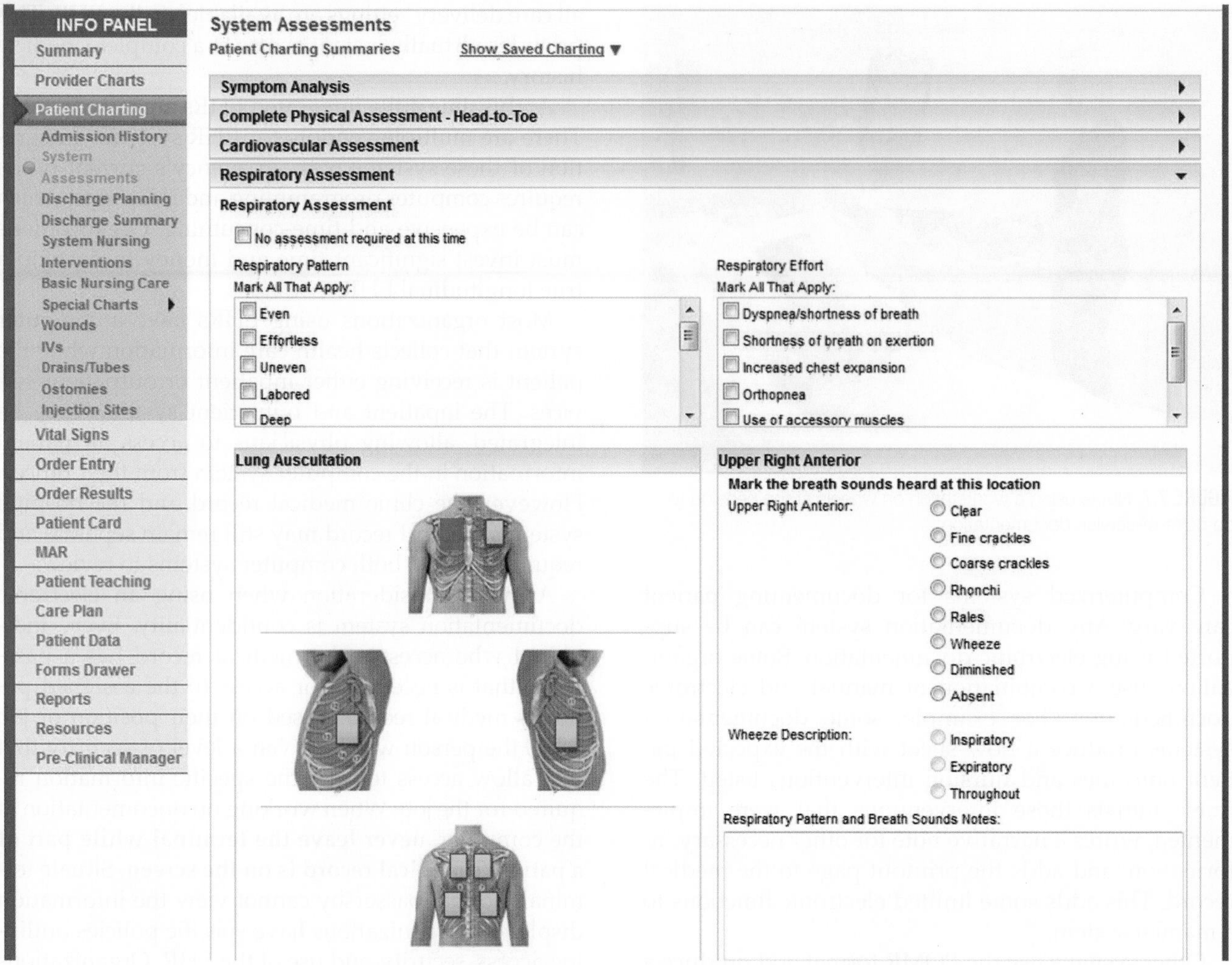

INFO PANEL
Summary
Provider Charts
Patient Charting
Admission History
System Assessments
Discharge Planning
Discharge Summary
System Nursing Interventions
Basic Nursing Care
Special Charts
Wounds
IVs
Drains/Tubes
Ostomies
Injection Sites
Vital Signs
Order Entry
Order Results
Patient Card
MAR
Patient Teaching
Care Plan
Patient Data
Forms Drawer
Reports
Resources
Pre-Clinical Manager

System Assessments
Patient Charting Summaries Show Saved Charting
Symptom Analysis
Complete Physical Assessment - Head-to-Toe
Cardiovascular Assessment
Respiratory Assessment
Respiratory Assessment
No assessment required at this time
Respiratory Pattern
Mark All That Apply:
Even
Effortless
Uneven
Labored
Deep
Respiratory Effort
Mark All That Apply:
Dyspnea/shortness of breath
Shortness of breath on exertion
Increased chest expansion
Orthopnea
Use of accessory muscles
Lung Auscultation
Upper Right Anterior
Mark the breath sounds heard at this location
Upper Right Anterior:
Clear
Fine crackles
Coarse crackles
Rhonchi
Rales
Wheeze
Diminished
Absent
Wheeze Description:
Inspiratory
Expiratory
Throughout
Respiratory Pattern and Breath Sounds Notes:

FIGURE 7.8 Example of portion of a patient's electronic medical record.

- Multiple health care providers can access the same patient's information at one time.
- It can reduce documentation time.
- Electronic records can be retrieved quickly.
- Reimbursement for services rendered can be faster and more complete because of complete and accurate documentation.
- A true electronic medical record can provide a complete longitudinal record of the patient's medical history at one point of access.
- Well-designed systems can reduce errors, having a positive effect on patient safety.

Disadvantages of computer-assisted documentation:

- A sophisticated security system is necessary to prevent unauthorized personnel from accessing patient records.
- Initial costs are considerable because many more terminals and an appropriate networking system must be purchased and interfaced for the system to work efficiently.
- Implementation of a full EHR system can take considerable time. This results in the need to use two systems, paper and electronic, during that transition.
- Significant cost and time are involved in training staff to use the system.
- Computer downtime can create problems of input, access, and transfer of information. Well-established backup plans (downtime procedures) must be developed.

CASE MANAGEMENT SYSTEM CHARTING

Case management is a method of organizing patient care through an episode of illness so that clinical outcomes are achieved within an expected time frame and at a predictable cost (see Chapters 1 and 2). A clinical pathway or interdisciplinary care plan takes the place of the nursing care plan. Documentation of variances is placed on the back of the pathway sheets. For example, a patient is admitted for abdominal surgery. The wound is healing well, but the patient develops pneumonia. The variance would be documented as in Figure 7.9.

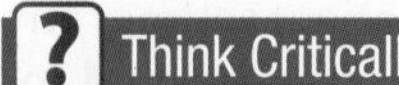

Think Critically

Which method of documentation seems easiest to you? Can you explain why?

Variation	Cause	Action Taken
Airway	Pneumonia	7/23 ↑ fluids to 2000 mL/day
Clearance	7/23	7/24 Proventil inhaler for wheezing
		7/24 Incentive spirometer use encouraged every 1° while awake
		7/26 Instructed in home O_2 use
		7/26 Unit Air contacted for oxygen delivery

FIGURE 7.9 Example of variance charting.

THE DOCUMENTATION PROCESS

When documenting patient care, present the patient's needs, problems, and activities in terms of **behaviors.** The notes focus on the immediate past and the present, never the future. In other words, only record what you have done for the patient, not what you plan to do. For example, after assisting a patient to ambulate, you might record, "Ambulated 20 feet down the hall and back."

Documentation should be accurate, brief, and complete. When documentation follows these guidelines, it presents a photographic view of the patient to anyone who reads the nursing notes.

ACCURACY IN DOCUMENTATION

Be specific and definite in using words or phrases that convey the meaning you wish expressed. Avoid using the words *appears to* or *seems* in phrases such as *appears to be resting*. Document the behavior; the patient either is or is not resting. Words that have ambiguous meanings and slang should not be used in documentation. For example, how much is "a little," "a small amount," or a "large amount"? What do phrases such as *ate well*, *taking fluids poorly*, and ***tolerated well*** mean? Although such words give a general idea of what is meant, they are not specific: they are subjective phrases. Someone else reading the notes will not know if the patient who "ate well" had a half a piece of toast, juice, and a cup of coffee or ate a bowl of cereal, scrambled eggs, two slices of bacon, 4 oz of orange juice, and two cups of coffee. Instead of documenting a conclusion such as "taking fluids poorly," record the behavior and the specific amounts of liquid taken in a particular amount of time, such as "given fluids at frequent intervals, but takes only a few swallows; intake from 0700 to 1000: 30 mL of coffee, 60 mL of orange juice, and 50 mL of water." Specific data about size, amounts, and other measurements provide a means for the reader to determine whether the condition is getting better, getting worse, or staying the same. Rather than use the term *tolerated well*, describe what happened, even if it is a statement such as "walked in hall without problems."

BREVITY IN DOCUMENTATION

When charting, sentences are not necessary. Articles (*a*, *an*, and *the*) may be omitted. Because the medical record is about a particular patient, the word *patient* is left out whenever it is the subject of the sentence. Each statement should begin with a capital letter and end with a period. Rather than stating, "Patient left for surgery via stretcher at 10:15," simply state, "To surgery via stretcher at 10:15."

Abbreviations, acronyms, and symbols acceptable to the agency are used in documentation to save time and space. Each agency has its own list of acceptable abbreviations and symbols. This list is usually found in the policy and procedures manual.

You must choose which behaviors and observations are noteworthy, or your nurse's notes will be lengthy and irrelevant. In most agencies, if data (such as patient voiding) are recorded on a flow sheet, they need not be documented again in the nurse's notes. No other notation is made in the nurse's notes unless there is a problem or some significant related data. A good way to learn what should and should not be documented is to read over the notes of experienced nurses who are known to document accurately and well. **A rule of thumb is that if the behavior or finding is abnormal or is a change from previous behavior or data, document it.**

LEGIBILITY AND COMPLETENESS IN DOCUMENTATION

Legibility is important in any handwritten documentation. The medical record may be called into court, and what you wrote may be scrutinized and evaluated. If the writing is not easily legible, misperceptions of what was written can occur.

Completeness is more important than brevity. You should record information about the patient's needs and problems and specify the nursing care given for those needs or problems. In other words, any time you document anything abnormal, also document what you did about it, or at minimum who you notified. If you document, "Skin at IV site reddened and slightly swollen," you must include a note about what you did about the problem. The full note should read, "Skin at right forearm IV site reddened and slightly swollen in 4-cm area. IV DC'd and warm moist pack applied for 20 minutes. Redness and swelling receding. IV restarted in left hand with 20 ga catheter."

What constitutes complete documentation may vary among hospitals, extended-care facilities, and other health care agencies. Home care documentation must particularly note safety factors in place and the need for continued care (Fig. 7.10). Long-term care facilities may require only a monthly summary for

Routine Home Health Assessment

Patient: Clifford-Oscar, Randall **Nurse:** Williams, Cerys
Visit Date: 3/19/2017; 4:26PM

Data/Safety/Dx - Patient Data

Source of information:	Patient
Residence	Patient's owned or rented residence
Lives with	Lives alone
Financial concerns	None
Assistance with care	Relatives
Main caregiver	Son
Caregiver availability	One to two times a week
Assistance type	Environmental support—home maintenance IADL assistance Facilitates patient participation in appropriate medical care Financial agent Health care agent Medical power of attorney Psychosocial support Shopping
Health risks	None of the above
Functional limitations (485)	*Bowel/bladder (incontinence)* *Endurance* *Ambulation* *Dependent ADLs*
Activity oders (485)	*Up as tolerated*

Data/Safety/Dx - Safety

Pt with Hx of falls	Yes

History/Vitals/Pain - Primary Pain Location Descript

Present pain	0
Acceptable pain (Phys)	*3*

History/Vitals/Pain - Vital Signs

Temperature	99.0
Radial pulse	60
Apical pulse	60
Pulse rhythm/quality	Regular
Respirations	20 Comment: O_2 sat 97% on RA
B/P sitting	130/70
Pedal pulses	Bilaterally equal and weak

Psychosocial/Skin/Ulcers

Skin S/S	Dry Friable/fragile Intact
Wound/pressure injury/ stasis ulcer	None present

HENT/Res/CV/Neu - Cardiovascular

Cardiovascular signs/sypmtoms	Consistently cold extremities Dysp after amb <20 ft: dress/use commode Endurance limitations
Heart (cardiac) sounds	S1 S2

HENT/Res/CV/Neu - Head/Ears/Eyes/Nose/Throat

HEENT S/S	Glasses
Status of vision	Impaired vision Partially impaired cannot see medication labels or newsprint
Hearing/understanding	No observable impairment can hear and understand complex instructions and abstract conversation
Expression ability	Expresses complex ideas, feelings, and needs clearly without visible impairment
Speech patterns	Spontaneous

Patient: Clifford-Oscar, Randall
Team: Home Care
Record #: 12345

FIGURE 7.10 Printout from home care agency electronic documentation. (Courtesy Mission Hospice and Home Care, San Mateo, California.)

Routine Home Health Assessment
Patient: Clifford-Oscar, Randall **Nurse:** Williams, Cerys
Visit Date: 3/19/2017; 4:26PM

HENT/Res/CV/Neu - Neurological	
Neuro S/S	No significant findings [Go to Mental Status]
Mental status (485)	Alert Oriented
Confusion occurrence	Never
Anxiety occurrence	None of the time
Depression identification	None of the above observed or reported
Behavior issues	None of the above behaviors observed
Behavior occurrence	Never

HENT/Res/CV/Neu - Respiratory	
Respiratory sign/symptoms	Diminished endurance/fatigue Dyspnea on exertion Endurance limitations Orthopnea Pursed-lip breathing
Lung fields right	Clear all lobes
Lung fields left	Clear both lobes
Dyspnea	With moderate exertion such as while dressing, using commode, walking distances less than 20 feet

Musc/ADLs/IADLs - Musculoskeletal	
Musculoskeletal S/S	Holds on to furniture

GI/GU/Endc/Plan	
Immune system	No signs of infection Potential for infection
Medication change since last visit	No

GI/GU/Endc/Plan - Gastrointestinal	
Last BM	Today
Present bowel pattern	Regular
Bowel incontinence occurrence	Very rarely or never has bowel incontinence

GI/GU/Endc/Plan - Genitourinary	
Genitourinary S/S	WNL for patient [Go to M1600]
Urinary incontinence	Patient requires a urinary catheter (i.e., external - indwelling - intermittent - suprapubic) (GO TO GASTRO INTESTINAL)

GI/GU/Endc/Plan - Medical Safety	
Med safety measures	*Stress body mechanics* *Universal/Standard precautions* *Label/Storage of medication*

GI/GU/Endc/Plan - Nutrition	
Nutritional S/S	No significant findings
Nutritional requirements	No added salt
Meal patterns	Eats alone most of the time Eats 3 meals a day
Skin turgor	Rebounds instantly

GI/GU/Endc/Plan - Planning	
Plan for next visit	Patient has not had any S/S of UTI since last visit. Changed 18 french 10ml catheter, patient tolerated procedure well. Able to fully insert catheter without feeling resistance or bladder limitation this visit. Patient reports catheter comfortable, pale yellow urine draining well.
Education/assist	Assistance need Diet/exercise Disease process Medication management Safety measures
Medications assessed for	Effectiveness
Instructed/copy to	Patient
Plan of care discussed with	Patient

Patient: Clifford-Oscar, Randall
Team: Home Care
Record #: 12345

FIGURE 7.10, cont'd

patients in stable condition or a note when their condition changes (Fig. 7.11), whereas hospitals caring for acutely ill patients require continual documentation of the patient's condition, with entries made every few hours. For completeness in documentation about the patient's signs or symptoms, note something about each of the seven factors listed in Box 7.2.

WHAT TO DOCUMENT

In addition to assessment data related to signs and symptoms, information on the topics in Box 7.3 is to be documented either on flow sheets or in the nurse's notes. The documentation examples included with the procedures throughout this book show how to describe different types of information.

General Documentation Guidelines

In addition to those mentioned above, there are several other general rules to consider when charting (Box 7.4). Figure 7.12 shows the use of regular versus military time for medical record entries.

Date/Time	Licensed Nurses Progress Notes
4/15/18	Pt asked both nurses at med carts for IM injection Cortisone and "could I have meds right
7-3 shift	now?" Instructed to take seat at breakfast table. Pt's roommate called nurse. Pt supine on
	floor no changes to LOC. Walker at side A/O. Answered all questions appropriately, no Δ in speech and
	mentation.--
	VS taken by this RN: T 98.6, P 76, R 16, BP 120/80.--
	Denies HA, no s/s CVA/TIA- clear conversation, no paralysis. C/O right knee discomfort
	when asked what heppened- why she fell. Assisted to chair. Denies pain. Neuro VS
	unremarkable: PERL hand grips strong- no s/s hypoglycemia, no sweating or lethargy, alert,
	gave complete date, answered questions appropriately. Reported to supervisor: Vivian Violet, RN DON.
	--M. Markham, RN

FIGURE 7.11 Example of long-term care facility documentation.

Box 7.2 Guidelines for Documenting a Sign or a Symptom

Location in the body: Describe the exact location.

Quality: Describe in patient's terms; for example, a person having a myocardial infarction (heart attack) might describe the chest pain as feeling as if the chest is being "squeezed in a vise."

Quantity: Document the intensity of the symptoms (i.e., mild, moderate, or severe). Use a scale of 0 to 10 for pain, with 10 being the highest. Indicate the degree of impairment and the frequency, volume, and size or extent of the sign or symptom. Note the number of times the patient has vomited, the amount each time, and whether nausea is constant or intermittent.

Chronology: Note the sequence of development:

1. Time of onset of the sign or symptom
2. Duration (minutes, hours, or days)
3. Pattern of variation and frequency and the course of the signs or symptoms (e.g., Do they stay the same, get better, or get worse over time?)

Setting: Where is the patient (e.g., at home, in bed, or in the car)? What is the patient doing (e.g., running, sleeping, or eating). Who is the patient with (e.g., mother, spouse, or boss) when the symptoms occur?

Aggravating or alleviating factors: What makes the signs or symptoms worse and what makes them better? Does a hot shower make a skin rash worse? Does eating cause more or less pain?

Associated manifestations: Signs and symptoms rarely occur singly. For instance, does the patient have nausea before vomiting? Has there been a weight change since the onset of vomiting?

Box 7.3 Types of Information to Be Documented

- Admission note
- Assessment data for all body systems
- Body care
- Death
- Degree of activity
- Diagnostic tests
- Diet and fluids
- Discharge from the facility
- Dressings and wound care
- Intake and output
- Intravenous infusions
- Medications
- Mental state and mood
- Mood, concerns, or discomfort
- Oxygen in use
- Primary care provider's visits and calls to provider
- Postoperative care
- Procedures performed
- Sleep
- Specimens obtained and their disposition
- Patient education
- Travel from the unit
- Tubes and equipment in use
- Visitors

Box 7.4 General Guidelines for Documenting

- Verify you are on the correct patient's computer screen *before* beginning to document in the medical record. Record the initial assessment at the beginning of the shift.
- Use a 24-hour clock (military time; see Fig. 7.12).
- Documentation is done only by the person who made the observation or performed the intervention and who is legally responsible for the accuracy and quality of care.
- Record objective data after completing each task. Never document before a task is actually done.
- Follow hospital policy for amending the record.
- Clearly identify care given by another health care team member.
- When a patient refuses a medication, record an explanation for the refusal in the medical record. Document the exact words the patient used when refusing to comply with the treatment regimen. Document any instructions given to the patient and any patient behaviors that are against the instructions.
- Spell medical record entries correctly. Use a dictionary or "spell check" to check words you are unsure how to spell.
- If you suspect that a medical order or progress note is incorrect, seek clarification from the person who wrote the order or the note. If you make an error when documenting, follow agency policy for correcting the error.

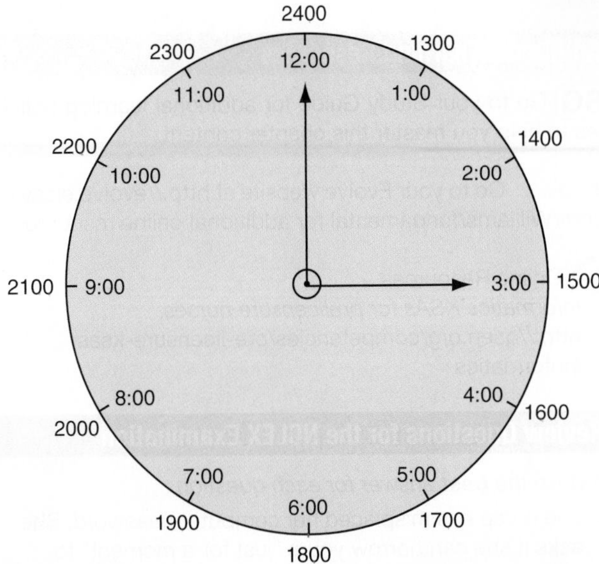

FIGURE 7.12 Military time versus civilian time. (From Potter, P. A., & Perry A. G. [2005]. *Fundamentals of nursing* [6th ed.]. St. Louis, MO: Mosby.)

Get Ready for the NCLEX Examination!

Key Points

- Documentation provides a communication tool for the health care team; maintains a record of the history, care, and treatment of the patient; is a legal record; is a quality assurance tool; and provides a basis for reimbursement of services.
- The nursing care plan is the framework for nursing documentation.
- Evaluation data that are documented must show progress toward expected outcomes.
- Information in the medical record must be kept confidential, and only those health professionals directly involved in the patient's care should have access to the record.
- There are six main methods of documentation: (1) source-oriented (narrative) style, (2) POMR style, (3) focus charting, (4) charting by exception, (5) computer-assisted charting, and (6) case management system charting.
- Besides nurses' and physicians' progress notes, many flow sheets are used to document patient information.
- An advantage of the source-oriented method is that information on the patient's condition and care is listed in chronologic order.
- An advantage of the POMR system is that it improves continuity of care by keeping data relevant to a problem all in one place.
- An advantage of focus charting is that it shortens documentation time by using many flow sheets and checklists.
- Although charting by exception highlights abnormal data and patient trends, it presents problems if called into court because only abnormal findings are documented in writing.
- Computer documentation is expensive to institute, but it saves considerable nursing time.
- Case management system documentation tracks variances from the care map.
- Documentation should show the application of the nursing process, and present a snapshot of the patient's condition and care.
- Documentation must be objective, accurate, brief, and complete.
- Document the patient's behaviors and statements, not your opinions or conclusions.
- The list of activities and data that must be documented about the patient each day is extensive.
- Tell the nurse when, what, and how to document patient assessments, activities, and interventions.

Additional Learning Resources

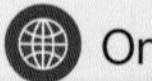 Go to your Study Guide for additional learning activities to help you master this chapter content.

evolve Go to your Evolve website at http://evolve.elsevier.com/Williams/fundamental for additional online resources.

Online Resources

- *Informatics KSAs for prelicensure nurses,* http://qsen.org/competencies/pre-licensure-ksas/#informatics

Review Questions for the NCLEX Examination

*Choose the **best** answer for each question.*

1. The nurse has misplaced her computer password. She asks if she can borrow yours "just for a moment" to view patient data and promises she will not document anything. Your best course of action is:
   1. Allow her to use your password, just this once.
   2. Sit with her and access the data together.
   3. Inform her to contact the IT Department to obtain a new password.
   4. Tell her you're busy, and to ask someone else.
2. Which is the most precise example of appropriate documentation?
   1. "Aggressive and combative during a.m. care."
   2. "Received 250 mL tube feeding during shift, tolerated well."
   3. "Ambulated 2× during shift, 50 ft with assistance of one. Preactivity vs: 85, 18, 110/70; postactivity vs: 95, 22, 120/76."
   4. "Ambulated to nurses station and back, tolerated well."
3. Patients frequently request copies of their medical records. You understand that: *(Select all that apply.)*
   1. Patients have a right to a copy of their medical record immediately after discharge.
   2. Only people directly associated with the care of that patient have legal access to the information in the medical record.
   3. The patient and family have a right to read the record, and should be given the medical record any time they ask for it.
   4. The medical record is the property of the hospital or agency, not of the patient.
   5. The patient does have right of access to the medical record but must follow the proper procedures for obtaining these.
4. When documenting, it is wise to always:
   1. Include the names of all visitors with the time of the visit.
   2. Ensure you are on the right medical record.
   3. Sign your full name, date, and time on each sheet.
   4. Use acronyms you are familiar with to shorten notes.
5. When a patient's medical record is needed as evidence for a legal action, you are aware that the record is the property of:
   1. The patient.
   2. The patient's lawyer.
   3. The court.
   4. The health care agency.
6. The assumption in charting by exception is that:
   1. If it was not documented, it was not done.
   2. Patient care is documented chronologically.
   3. Unless otherwise documented, all standards have been met.
   4. A SOAPIER format note must be made each shift.
7. An advantage of electronic medical records is that:
   1. Computers are always up, running, and available.
   2. Security of information is guaranteed with the computer system.
   3. Others can see what is being input as the nurse documents.
   4. It can save nursing time compared with writing out notes.
8. When documenting the patient's condition and nursing care, the nurse records: *(Select all that apply.)*
   1. Activities planned for later in the shift.
   2. Goals for the medical treatment and evaluation.
   3. Interventions performed and patient response.
   4. Patient statements and behaviors that are observed.
   5. Clinical data measurements.

Critical Thinking Activities

Read each clinical scenario and discuss the questions with your classmates.

Scenario A

Read the following scenario and then practice writing a POMR progress note and a focus charting note using the data given.

Marvin Barnes was admitted with the medical diagnosis of pneumonia. He has symptoms of problems with oxygenation because of his excessive pulmonary secretions. When you go to assess him, you discover that his temperature is 102.6°F (39.2°C); pulse 112 beats/min; respirations 26 breaths/min and shallow; and blood pressure 147/92 mmHg. He is coughing and produces yellow-green sputum. He is having difficulty stopping the cough. He has oxygen via nasal cannula running at 3 L/min. He has acetaminophen ordered for fever over 100.2°F (37.9°C). You tell him that you will be back with medicine for his fever and that you will call the primary care provider for an order for some cough medicine to relieve the cough.

Scenario B

Discuss the guidelines that will help you document so that you would be protected if there were a lawsuit involving a patient to whom you had given care.

chapter 8

Communication and the Nurse-Patient Relationship

http://evolve.elsevier.com/Williams/fundamental

Objectives

Upon completing this chapter, you should be able to do the following:

Theory

1. Describe the components of the communication process.
2. List three factors that influence the way a person communicates.
3. Compare effective communication techniques with blocks to communication.
4. Describe the difference between a therapeutic nurse-patient relationship and a social relationship.
5. Discuss the importance of communication in the collaborative process.
6. List three guidelines for effective communication with a primary care provider by telephone.
7. Identify four ways to delegate effectively.
8. Discuss five ways the computer is used for communication within the health care agency.
9. Describe how communication skills can affect the quality and safety of patient care.

Clinical Practice

1. Use interviewing skills to obtain an admission history from a patient.
2. Interact therapeutically in a goal-directed situation with a patient.
3. Communicate effectively with a patient who has a communication impairment.
4. Give an effective report on assigned patients to your team leader or charge nurse.
5. Be present and nonjudgmental when communicating with patients, and be mindful of their needs.

Key Terms

active listening (p. 101)
advocate (p. 103)
aphasia (ā-FĀ-zē-ă, p. 113)
being present (p. 103)
body language (p. 101)
communication (kŏ-myū-nĭ-KĀ-shŭn, p. 101)
confidentiality (kŏn-fĭ-dĕn-shē-ĂL-ĭ-tē, p. 111)
congruent (kŏn-GRŪ-ĕnt, p. 102)
delegate (DĔ-lĕ-gāt, p. 115)
empathy (ĔM-pă-thē, p. 111)
feedback (p. 101)
incongruent (ĭn-kŏn-GRŪ-ĕnt, p. 104)
input (p. 117)
ISBAR-R (p. 115)
mindful (p. 102)
nonverbal (NŎN-vĕr-bŭl, p. 101)
nonjudgmental (p. 103)
patient-centered care (p. 104)
perception (pĕr-CĔP-shŭn, p. 102)
personal space (p. 103)
rapport (ră-PŌR, p. 110)
shift report (p. 114)
therapeutic (thĕr-ă-PYŪ-tĭk, p. 106)
therapeutic communication (p. 104)
verbal (VĔR-bŭl, p. 101)
walking rounds (p. 114)

Concepts Covered in This Chapter

- Collaboration
- Communication
- Culture
- Patient education
- Professionalism
- Safety

THE COMMUNICATION PROCESS

Communication occurs when one person sends a message to another person who receives it, processes it, and indicates that the message has been interpreted (Fig. 8.1). The receiver must acknowledge that the message has been received and comprehended for communication to be complete. Good communication requires **active listening** (focusing on what is being said), timely **feedback** (return of information and how it was interpreted), and validation of assumptions about nonverbal cues.

By its nature, communication is a continuous, circular process that occurs in two ways: **verbal** (in words) and **nonverbal** (without words). Verbal communication consists of words either spoken or written. Nonverbal communication, also known as **body language,** is conveyed by gesture, expression, body

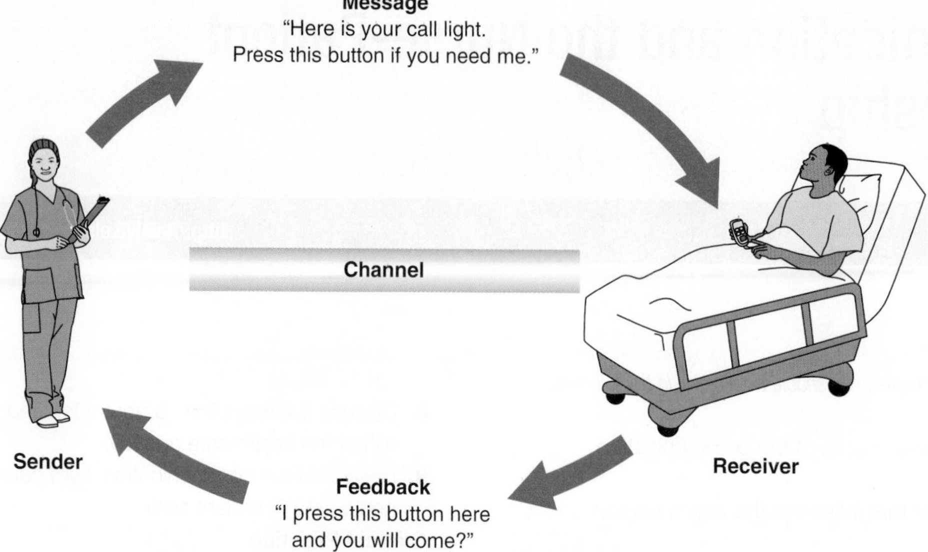

"Here is your call light.
Press this button if you need me."
Channel
Sender
Receiver

"I press this button here
and you will come?"

FIGURE 8.1 The communication process.

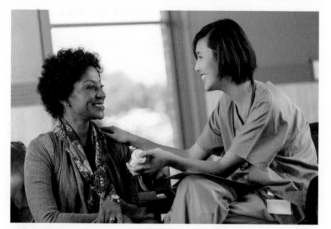

FIGURE 8.2 Nonverbal communication signals that the nurse is listening and interested in what the patient is saying. (Photo copyright istock.com.)

posture, intonation, and general appearance. Nonverbal communication conveys more of what a person feels, thinks, and means than is actually stated in words (Fig. 8.2). Sometimes the person's nonverbal communication is not **congruent** (in agreement) with the verbal communication. If you state that you want to sit and talk for a while and then sit with legs crossed and a foot bouncing rapidly during the conversation, the message is one of impatience rather than attentive listening.

Think Critically

Look at Fig. 8.2. Identify five messages the nurse is sending through nonverbal communication. What feedback is the patient giving to the nurse?

You can learn about patients by observing nonverbal behavior. **Anxiety, fear, and pain are often expressed by nonverbal cues.** Wincing when turning, a pinched expression, or picking at the bed covers may indicate what patients are really feeling, although they say they are fine. Rigid body posture or slow movements often indicate pain. Restless movements may indicate anxiety. Experience will increase your ability to assess nonverbal communication. Validate **perception** (recognition and interpretation of sensory stimuli) of nonverbal communication with the patient. This can be done by asking about feelings and thoughts. For, example, "Mrs. Lopez, you seem a little restless [and anxious] today. Would you like to talk about something?"

Clinical Cues

Giving positive feedback increases the likelihood that a desired behavior will be repeated. For example, you are trying to get Mrs. Panopoulos to perform activities of daily living independently. *"Mrs. Panopoulos, I saw you combing your own hair this morning.* (State the observed behavior.) *I really liked the way that you styled it.* (Give praise.) *Keep up the good work!"* (State the desired behavior.)

FACTORS AFFECTING COMMUNICATION

Culture, past experience, emotions, mood, attitude, perceptions of the individual, and self-concept all contribute to the way people communicate. Every culture has norms for appropriate communication. The norms include the distance between communicators, whether eye contact should be established, the tone of voice, and the amount of gestures used. The physical environment and the person's comfort level can also influence the ability to receive and process the information. It is important to be **mindful** (highly aware and alert) of each individual's style and needs.

Cultural Differences

The licensed nurse practitioner (LPN)/licensed vocational nurse (LVN) needs to be prepared to care for patients that do not speak or understand English. Facilities that accept federal funds (e.g., Medicaid) are legally required to provide language access to all patients. Most health care agencies have a list of interpreters that can be called for assistance. If not, follow your facility's guidelines for obtaining an interpreter (Fig. 8.3). Be accepting; do not show impatience with someone's lack of ability to speak English.

In the United States, 18 inches to 4 feet is the distance that individuals generally place between themselves and a new acquaintance. This distance is called **personal space**. There are cultural differences in the amount of personal space that patients need between them and the person with whom they are speaking. In general, American Indians, Northern Europeans, and Asians maintain more distance from others than do Hispanic, Southern European, or Middle Eastern people. For women, personal space will lessen based on the closeness of the relationship with other people. Men, on the contrary, do not vary their personal space in the same manner. Typically, men do not vary personal space based on the closeness of their relationships (Holt et al., 2014).

Cultural Considerations

Eye Contact

Most Americans expect direct eye contact when interacting with someone. Other cultures—for example Japanese, Chinese, Vietnamese, and Laotians—may consider it rude to look directly at someone. When a Japanese woman makes brief eye contact, she is being polite and respectful. She is not lacking self-confidence nor is she showing a lack of interest. For Jamaicans, direct eye contact toward an authority figure or between strangers may indicate a challenge. In Muslim cultures, only a brief moment of eye contact between a man and a woman is permitted.

Learn how eye contact is used in your patient's culture by observing how your patient interacts with others. Find opportunities to talk with colleagues from different cultures to learn about eye contact and other communication nuances.

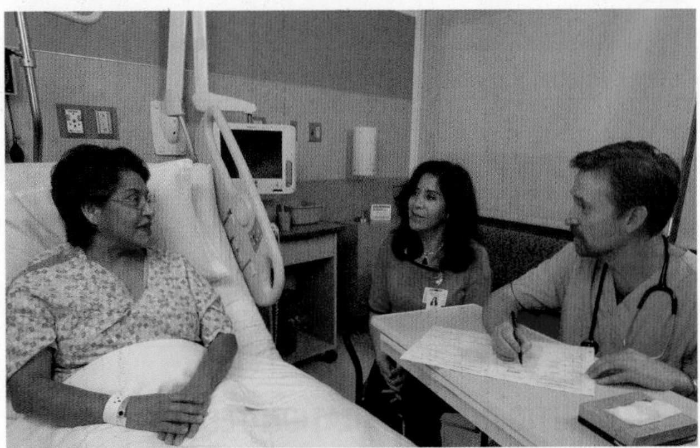

FIGURE 8.3 Communicating with the assistance of an interpreter.

Past Experience

All of our experiences affect how we perceive communication. Interpretation of messages is influenced by cultural values, education, familiarity with the topic, occupation, and life experiences.

Think Critically

You are with Mrs. Ito, and the physician walks in and says, "A cardiac catheterization needs to be done to see if the coronary arteries are blocked." The patient has limited experience with hospitalization and medical terminology. She shyly looks down at her hands. It is unclear if she understands. What could you do?

Emotions, Mood, and Environment

Emotions, mood, and even the environment can drastically affect the way messages are sent or interpreted. A highly anxious person may not correctly hear what is said or may interpret the message differently than the sender intended. A depressed person tends to use few words. A person who is upset or stressed may speak in a loud, harsh tone or be more abrupt than usual. Patients may be in a stressful hospital environment, away from home, sleep deprived, and perhaps in pain. By recognizing emotions and moods, keeping patients as comfortable as possible, communicating clearly, and frequently obtaining feedback, misunderstandings can be reduced.

Attitude, Perceptions, and Self-Concept

A person's attitude, perceptions, and self-concept affect both how a message is worded and the body language that accompanies it. When your attitude is one of acceptance of the patient, caring and concern are displayed by open, attentive body language. If you have a negative perception of and disapprove of the patient's behavior, you may use a closed body stance and stern expression and be somewhat distant during interactions. Someone with an accepting attitude will make an effort to understand what a person is trying to convey during the communication by **being present** (focused on the moment) and being an **advocate** (representative) for their needs.

Try to be open and attentive to patients' communications, to maintain a **nonjudgmental** (refraining from judgment) attitude, and to not take personally anything unpleasant a patient says when upset or frightened.

COMMUNICATION SKILLS

Some people are naturally more effective communicators than others are. Effective communication can, however, be learned by practicing and improving basic communication skills.

 QSEN Considerations: Patient-Centered Care

Communication

Nurses must have *knowledge* of the principles of effective communication, implement the *skill* of communicating effectively, and possess the *attitude* of wanting to improve communication skills. **Patient-centered care,** with the patient as the focus, is essential in providing compassionate and coordinated care based on respect for patient preferences, values, and needs (QSEN, 2014a, 2014b).

Active Listening

Active listening requires great concentration and focused energy. All of the senses are used to interpret verbal and nonverbal messages; attention is on what the speaker is saying; and the mind is focused on the interaction. Listen for feelings as well as words. It takes practice to tune out other thoughts that try to intrude, and to avoid formulating a response until the speaker is finished. When you are an active listener, you demonstrate interest, and a trusting relationship can be built. An active listener maintains eye contact without staring, gives the patient full attention, and makes a conscious effort to block out other distractions. An active listener does not interrupt, and waits for the full message before interpreting what is said. Responding to the content and feelings of the message by stating what you, as the listener, understand was said by the patient completes the process. Nonverbal cues that indicate active listening are leaning forward, focusing on the speaker's face, nodding slightly to indicate the message is being heard, and maintaining an open body posture (Giroux, 2013).

Interpreting Nonverbal Messages

The speaker's posture, gestures, tone, facial expression, and eye movements should be observed. A smile or frown, hunched-down posture, and hand-wringing all express feelings. When taking in nonverbal messages, remember that they must be interpreted in the context of the *speaker's* culture, not the listener's. The listener must decide whether the nonverbal messages are congruent with the spoken message. Mixed messages, in which the verbal and nonverbal messages are **incongruent** (do not agree), require the listener to explore what the speaker really wishes to communicate.

Clinical Cues

Laughing, smiling, and appropriate use of humor can decrease stress and anxiety and have a positive effect on the immune system. Encourage and support your patient's efforts to smile and be positive; however, be sensitive to incongruent behaviors. If you think your patient is smiling to cover her fears or anxieties, provide openings for her to express her true feelings.

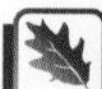 Life Span Considerations

Older Adults

When interacting with an older adult, try not to speak too quickly. Allow more time for the person to process your message and formulate a response. Many older adults have some degree of hearing loss, but do not assume that all older adults have hearing loss. Face the person so that your lips can be seen and she has the best chance of hearing your words. If the person wears a hearing aid, be certain it is in place and turned on. If the older adult has impaired hearing on one side, position yourself on the side with better hearing. Touch the patient's arm or shoulder gently to gain her attention before you start speaking.

Obtaining Feedback

A vital part of communication is checking to see if you interpreted a message correctly. You can do this by rephrasing the message or directly asking a feedback question, such as "Is your headache severe?" "Are you uncertain about having this surgery?" or "Does the idea of having anesthesia scare you?" The response received should verify whether the original message sent was interpreted correctly.

Focusing

Keeping the patient's attention focused on the communication task can save time. The effective communicator refocuses the other person gently to the issue when the focus has wandered. Occasionally the approach, "We'll come back to that later, but right now I need to know…" will quickly refocus the communication. At other times, commenting, "I think we were talking about…" is what is needed.

Adjusting Style

Consider the patient's style and level of usual communication when interacting. If the person is a slow, calm communicator, adjust to that pace. If a response is slow in coming, allow plenty of time for response; try not to display impatience. If it is comfortable for the patient to display feelings only in the context of telling a story about a related topic, allow enough time for full development of the topic so that the feelings can be adequately expressed.

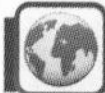 Cultural Considerations

Conversational Pace and Flow

Long pauses are a natural part of conversation in some cultures. This is often found among Native Americans. Do not be too quick to assume the speaker is finished. Among some cultural groups, giving a direct "no" answer is considered rude, so maintaining silence means "no." This may be true of those raised in a Japanese family. Often it is necessary to "give permission" to ask questions. Certain groups regard asking questions as rude or disrespectful.

THERAPEUTIC COMMUNICATION TECHNIQUES

Therapeutic communication (communication that is focused on the patient needs) promotes understanding between the sender and the receiver. Various phrases or cues may be used to promote understanding or facilitate an interaction between a patient and the nurse. These techniques should be used judiciously and in a varied manner or the interaction will feel stilted and uncomfortable (Table 8.1).

USING SILENCE

Appropriate use of silence is one of the hardest techniques for most students to develop. The new nurse is often uncomfortable with silence, and so tends to be too quick to end it. Silence gives the patient time to think and respond. Remaining attentive and using body language indicating patience and interest will encourage the patient to verbalize feelings or thoughts.

Clinical Cues

If you are having trouble using silence, remember you are not passively waiting for the patient to speak. Observe nonverbal behaviors during this silence. Note the patient's body position (e.g., relaxed or tense), expression on the face (e.g., thoughtful or sad), conditions of the environment (presence or lack of personal items), and indicators of emotional duress (picking at nails, restless movements, or looking down to avoid eye contact). These observations provide a significant amount of objective data.

ASKING OPEN-ENDED QUESTIONS

An open-ended question is broad, indicating only the topic, and it requires an answer of more than a word or two. An open-ended question allows the patient to elaborate on a subject or to choose aspects of the subject to be discussed. Open-ended questions or statements are helpful to open up the conversation or to proceed to a new topic. They usually cannot be answered with one word or just "yes" or "no." "Tell me about your day" versus "Did you have a good day?" or "How did you sleep?" versus "Did you sleep well?" are examples of open-ended versus closed questions. The closed question forces the listener to stick directly

Table 8.1 Therapeutic Communication Techniques

TECHNIQUE	EXAMPLE	RATIONALE
General leads	"Go on." "I see." "Uh huh." "Please continue."	Encourages patient to continue or elaborate.
Open-ended questions or statements	"Tell me more about that feeling." "I'd like to hear more about…"	Encourages patient to elaborate rather than answer in one or two words.
Offering self	"I'm here to listen." "Can I help in some way?"	Shows caring, concern, and readiness to help.
Restatement	Patient says, "I tossed and turned last night." Nurse says, "You feel like you were awake all night."	Restates in different words what the patient said; encourages further communication on that topic.
Reflection	Patient says, "I'm so scared about the surgery; anesthesia terrifies me." Nurse says, "Something scares you about anesthesia?" Patient looks scared. Nurse says, "You look scared."	Reflects received message back to patient. Also encourages further verbalization of feelings. Reflects feelings. Can also be used if patient is unable to verbalize or if nonverbal information is incongruent with verbal.
Seeking clarification	Patient says, "Having my little girl come to visit me was so hard. I'm so upset." Nurse says, "Something about your daughter's visit upset you?"	Seeks clarification about the source of the upset feeling. Helps the patient clarify thoughts or ideas.
Focusing	"Do you have any questions about your chemotherapy?"	Asking a goal-directed question helps the patient focus on key concerns.
Encouraging elaboration	"Tell me what that felt like." "I need more information about that." "Tell me more about that experience."	Helps the patient describe more fully the concern or problem under discussion.
Giving information	"The test results take at least 48 hours." "You will get a preoperative injection that will make you sleepy before you are taken to the operating room."	Provides patient education relevant to specific health care needs or situation.
Looking at alternatives	"Have you thought about…?" "You might want to think about…." "Would this be an option?"	Helps patients see options and consider alternatives to make their own decisions about health care.
Silence	Patient says, "I don't know if I should have chemotherapy, radiation, or both." Nurse remains silent, sitting attentively but quietly.	Allows patient time to gather thoughts and sort them out.
Summarizing	"You've identified your alternatives pretty clearly." "You are aware of the important signs and symptoms to report to your primary care provider; you plan to call to make an appointment next week."	Sums up the important points of an interaction.

to the topic and to be concise. **Open-ended questions create an inviting atmosphere for sharing thoughts, feelings, and concerns.**

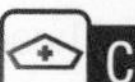 Clinical Cues

Closed questions are usually not considered part of the therapeutic communication process; however, at times, closed questions are appropriate: when you are gathering information ("Have you ever had a blood transfusion?"), if the patient is highly anxious ("Are you hurt?") or confused ("Do you need to go to the toilet?"), or if the patient is at a young developmental age ("Would you like the red one or the blue one?").

RESTATING

Listen for the basic message the patient is conveying and then rephrase the heart of the message. If the patient states, "My son hasn't been to see me in months," responses that restate the thought in different words might be as follows: "Your son hasn't been around much lately," or "You miss your son's visits." **Restating is used to encourage the patient to continue with information on a topic.**

Reflection is another way to restate the message. The same words the patient has said are reflected back. A patient says, "I'm worried about cancer," and the nurse replies, "You are worried about cancer." The idea is simply reflected back to the speaker in a statement to encourage continued dialogue on the topic. **Restating and reflection should be used sparingly and skillfully.** If overused, the patient will quickly recognize that you are repeatedly saying her words back to her, which is annoying.

CLARIFYING

Clarifying helps verify that the message heard is what the patient intended. It is particularly useful when the dialogue has rambled. If a patient says that family members visited and that they all sat around and drank coffee, and then says that sleeping was difficult last night, the nurse might say, "Are you saying that the coffee kept you awake?" This asks for confirmation that it was the caffeine in the coffee that prevented sleep, and not a problem brought in by the family that might have caused the sleeplessness.

USING TOUCH

Gentle touch indicates caring is **therapeutic** (effective or curative). It may be used to signify support for the person or when appropriate words are hard to find. Use touch judiciously, and take into consideration the patient's cultural and personal feelings about being touched by a stranger. You should have verbal or implied permission from the patient for touch to occur. Messages accompanied by touch can add a feeling of caring and comfort. Touching the patient warmly on the shoulder and saying, "I'm glad the medicine has relieved your pain" indicates caring. Touch must be beneficial for the patient; it should not be done to meet the nurse's needs. Consider how the patient will perceive and interpret touching before implementing it. Pay close attention to the patient's nonverbal feedback to determine if touch should be avoided moving forward.

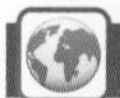 Cultural Considerations

Using Touch to Communicate

Some cultures are more accepting of touch within the health care setting. For example, a Portuguese patient may interpret touch as reassuring. For the patient from Mexico, it may be advisable to touch while you are giving a compliment to neutralize the power of the "evil eye." Koreans traditionally hug and touch family members or close friends, but touching from strangers is considered disrespectful unless for physical examination purposes. Touching during communication is also uncommon in the Japanese culture. In Muslim culture, touch between members of the opposite sex is generally inappropriate.

USING GENERAL LEADS

Use general leads to get the interaction under way. If a patient says, "I feel guilty for breaking my leg," a general lead would be, "Tell me more about that." General leads cannot be answered with "yes" or "no" and require more than a few words in response. "Perhaps you'd like to talk about your chemotherapy," "I noticed the doctor came after I left yesterday; perhaps you'd like to talk about what he said," and "I hear you are being discharged today; what do you think about that?" are other examples.

OFFERING OF SELF

Being available to the patient is one way of offering yourself. Answering call lights quickly or checking on something immediately states that you are available to the patient, but this is not always possible. Letting the patient know when you will return or when you will obtain the desired information conveys availability. Fulfilling such promises helps establish trust. Another form of offering yourself is to tell the patient, "I'll just sit here with you for a while," and remain with the patient.

ENCOURAGING ELABORATION

Statements such as "You said you have had a difficult time these last few months" or "Tell me more" encourage the patient to share feelings. "I'm not certain that I follow what you mean" is another way to encourage the patient to continue. **Encouraging elaboration is used when more information is needed about a topic.** This technique might be used rather than restatement or reflection.

PROVIDING PATIENT EDUCATION

Nurses must provide patient education about medications, procedures, diagnostic tests, and self-care.

Giving information concisely and allowing time for questions is therapeutic for the patient. Giving too much information can be confusing. Pay attention to nonverbal signals and ask for feedback to verify that the patient has understood the information given. It is vital that patient education is communicated effectively, and it may require the patient repeat the information or perform a return demonstration. The feedback you receive from the patient or family regarding the information communicated will determine whether the patient education needs to be repeated.

LOOKING AT ALTERNATIVES

Nurses help patients solve problems. To accomplish this, they are sometimes directive in assisting the patient in looking at alternative solutions to a problem. Some helpful leads for this purpose are "You might think about…," "Have you thought of your options?" or "What might be possible solutions?" The focus is on helping patients look at things from their point of view while you refrain from giving advice.

SUMMARIZING

Summarizing what has occurred during the interaction is helpful. A summary of alternative solutions to a problem, decisions made, plans for action, or feelings that have been expressed provides closure. "You've indicated that you have a choice between undergoing surgery and trying medication for your problem. We've discussed the potential side effects and benefits of both treatments, and now you'd like time to think about it" would be a summarizing statement.

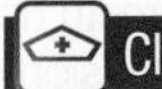

Clinical Cues

To improve your therapeutic communication skills, you have to practice. Your instructor may ask you to do a process recording. Practice your skills with a real patient, and then analyze and think about the patient's behavior and your response. (See Table 8.2 for a sample process recording.)

BLOCKS TO EFFECTIVE COMMUNICATION

Just as some phrases and cues encourage effective communication, other phrases or cues tend to block or terminate interaction. Table 8.3 summarizes blocks to effective communication.

CHANGING THE SUBJECT

When a patient is speaking and you change the subject, it indicates discomfort, disinterest, or anxiety on your part. You are avoiding listening to a patient's pain, distress, fear, or perception of problems. If you change the subject in an effort to keep the patient's thoughts off unpleasant things, you deny the patient's desire to express feelings. Sometimes the patient will talk about an experience that is similar to something

Table 8.2 Sample Process Recording: Communicating with the Patient Who Is Withdrawn

Setting and Brief Synopsis of Situation

Ms. Jake is a young woman with chronic renal failure. She frequently projects anger towards the staff, and she has been refusing her medication for several days. Several of the area dialysis centers have refused to treat her because of her "noncompliance." Most of the time she has the blanket over her head whenever anyone enters the room. As I enter the room today, she turns her back towards me. The television is on.

PATIENT'S NONVERBAL BEHAVIOR	PATIENT'S VERBAL BEHAVIOR	NURSE'S VERBAL AND NONVERBAL RESPONSE	THERAPEUTIC TECHNIQUE OR BLOCK	EVALUATION AND ANALYSIS OF NURSE AND PATIENT BEHAVIORS
Ms. Jake looks at me as I enter the room, then turns away and pulls the sheet up to partially cover her face.	None	"Ms. Jake, I am going to bring your medication in several minutes, but I wanted to check on you first and see how you were doing." I smile tentatively.	Offering self (therapeutic)	Ms. Jake rejects my attempts at communication by turning away. She is using the sheet to put up a physical barrier. Should I respect this as a sign that she wants privacy? Or should I try some other method to establish rapport?
Looks over at me as I speak, but turns away again.	None	Ms. Jake, I would like to spend a little time with you. If you don't want to talk, that's okay we can just sit together." I sit down where she can see me if she turns over. I try to let my body relax.	Offering self (therapeutic)	I feel really nervous and awkward. Am I doing the right thing? Ms. Jake continues to appear withdrawn. Maybe she just needs some time to think and rest, but I told her I would stay for a short time, so I will follow through.

Continued

Table 8.2 Sample Process Recording: Communicating with the Patient Who Is Withdrawn—cont'd

PATIENT'S NONVERBAL BEHAVIOR	PATIENT'S VERBAL BEHAVIOR	NURSE'S VERBAL AND NONVERBAL RESPONSE	THERAPEUTIC TECHNIQUE OR BLOCK	EVALUATION AND ANALYSIS OF NURSE AND PATIENT BEHAVIORS
Looks at me occasionally and then turns back.	Clears throat	I smile at her when she looks at me. I take a breath and try to let the tension go out of my shoulders. I see there are no personal items and the room is very dark. I look up at the television and say, "This is a very sad story."	Silence (therapeutic?)	The darkness of the room and the lack of personal items create an atmosphere of sadness and depression. I remember that no family has come to visit. There is a sad story on the television. Suddenly, I feel very sad. I am not sure if commenting about the television program is correct; however, the television seems symbolic for our generally feeling of sadness.
She turns over and sits up; looks at the television.	"I know. That woman on the show is crazy."	I sit a little straighter and look over at her. "So you've been following this news story?"	Closed question (nontherapeutic)	I am surprised and happy for her verbal response, but I am unprepared, so I ask the first question that pops into my head. A better response would have been to use a reflective statement (i.e., "So you think the story is sad.")
Ms. Jake is looking at the TV and watching a commercial about baby diapers.	"I always buy that kind for my nephew. I take care of him all the time."	"How old is he? Do you have any pictures of him?"	Asking two questions without allowing time for her to answer (nontherapeutic)	I am overly excited to have made some small connection with her. I hope that she will keep talking.
		I stand up and go over to the bed.	Moving closer (therapeutic)	Physically, I feel the need to get closer to her. Ms. Jake and I have used the television to make a connection. I think she is trying to express something personal about herself.
Ms. Jake points toward the closet. She is sitting upright and has moved the cover aside. She starts combing her hair as we talk.	"He's 2 years old. Pull my purse out of that closet. The pictures are in the side pocket."	We look at the pictures together. "He's really a cutie. So what do you two do together when you take care of him?" I am standing at the bedside, and I look as she points out features of the pictures.	Asking for elaboration (therapeutic)	Ms. Jake's body position is relaxed. It feels like she wants to make a connection. I am not exactly sure how to proceed. I am afraid that I might say something that will cause her to stop talking and withdraw. Also I need her to take her medication, but if I rush her will she get angry?
She stops combing her hair and looks down. She looks sad.	"We used to go to the park, but I have been sick and missing my dialysis. I just hate dialysis."	I watch her as she is speaking. I nod my head occasionally and I listen attentively.	Active listening (therapeutic)	At this point, Ms. Jake talks continuously for 4-5 minutes about dialysis and how difficult it has been for her to have this chronic health condition. My active listening is appropriate.

Table 8.2 Sample Process Recording: Communicating with the Patient Who Is Withdrawn—cont'd

PATIENT'S NONVERBAL BEHAVIOR	PATIENT'S VERBAL BEHAVIOR	NURSE'S VERBAL AND NONVERBAL RESPONSE	THERAPEUTIC TECHNIQUE OR BLOCK	EVALUATION AND ANALYSIS OF NURSE AND PATIENT BEHAVIORS
A tear rolls down her cheek as she speaks, but she continues to talk.		I hand her a tissue and I reach out and hold her hand as she speaks.	Gentle touch (therapeutic)	Her verbal and nonverbal behaviors are congruent.
She smiles at me and lightly taps me on the shoulder. She gets out of bed and opens the curtain to let the light in.	"I'll talk your ear off if you let me. I'm ready to take my medicine now, but I don't want the big yellow one; it makes me nauseated."	I smile back. "I'm really glad you told me so much about yourself. It helps me to understand what you are going through, and you have had a lot to cope with. Let me talk to the charge nurse about the yellow pill. Maybe there is something that we can do about the nausea, maybe not, but we can try. Let me get your other medications right now. I'll be back in a couple of minutes."	Giving feedback, expressing appreciation and providing information (therapeutic)	Commenting on the television program seems to have opened a dialogue. I would like to discuss this with my instructor, because I don't understand exactly why Ms. Jake started talking to me. Is opening the curtains a way of letting the outside world in? I feel very successful at this point. I understand more about her behavior and why she has been covering her head and turning away. Also she has expressed a concrete reason for refusing to take her medicine and now I can try and do something about it.

Table 8.3 Blocks to Effective Communication

TECHNIQUE	EXAMPLE	RATIONALE
Changing the subject	Patient says, "I'm so worried about my husband." Nurse says, "It is time for your bath now."	Deprives the patient of the chance to verbalize concerns.
Giving false reassurance	"I'm sure it will turn out fine." "You don't need to worry."	Negates the patient's feelings and may give false hope, which, when things turn out differently, can destroy trust in the nurse.
Judgmental response	"I don't think that was a good thing for you to do considering you have diabetes."	Nurse is judging the patient's action. Implies that the patient must take on the nurse's values and is demeaning to the patient.
Defensive response	Patient says, "My doctor never seems to know what is going on." Nurse says, "Dr. Smith is a very good doctor; he's here every day."	Nurse responds by defending the doctor. Prevents patients from feeling free to express their feelings.
Asking probing questions	"Why were you there at that hour?" "What did you intend to prove?"	Pries into the patient's motives and therefore invades privacy.
Using clichés	"Cheer up, you'll be home soon." "This won't hurt for long." "You have a long life ahead of you."	Negates the patient's individual situation; stereotypes the patient. This type of response sounds flippant and prevents the building of trust between patient and nurse.
Giving advice	"If I were you, I would…." "I think you should…." "Why don't you…."	Tends to be controlling and diminishes patients' responsibility for taking charge of their own health.
Inattentive listening	Turning your back when the patient is sharing feelings or pertinent information; showing impatience with body language (e.g., tapping your foot or having your hand on the door to go out).	Indicates that the patient is not important, that the nurse is bored, or that what is being said does not matter.

that happened to you. It is tempting to relate your experience, directing the conversation away from the patient. Students often make this mistake. Over time, you will learn to consider whether the information is of real value to the patient before sharing your personal experiences.

OFFERING FALSE REASSURANCE

Giving reassurance not based in fact is damaging because it discounts the patient's concerns and destroys trust. Saying "Don't worry; everything is going to be fine" when a patient has valid concerns indicates a lack of understanding. The nurse who tells a woman who has just had breast surgery that she should not think that her husband will find her scar distasteful because she is "still a beautiful woman" is offering inappropriate reassurance about someone else's feelings. This type of comment conveys the message that you do not care about the patient's fears and feelings about her new body image, which jeopardizes the professional relationship. Reassurance should be based on fact. Informing a patient that there will be some discomfort after a diagnostic procedure but analgesic medication will be available to relieve the discomfort is better than saying that it is a simple procedure and not to worry. A realistic approach helps maintain trust.

GIVING ADVICE

Giving advice is another area that prevents many novice nurses from being therapeutic. **Giving advice places the focus on the nurse rather than the patient.** In addition, many patients think that they must do what you say because you are the authority figure. Your role is to guide patients to alternatives for solving their own problems.

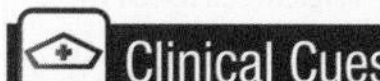
Clinical Cues

Do **not** use phrases such as "Why don't you...," "When that happened to me, I did...," or "I think you should..." Rephrase to help the patient explore various alternatives. For example, "Have you thought of your options?" or "You might want to think about...," or "Have you considered...?"

USING DEFENSIVE COMMENTS

Becoming defensive when a patient has a complaint interferes with effective communication. If a patient complains that the call light is not promptly answered in the evenings and you state, "You should realize how short-staffed we are in the evenings," the patient is denied the right to a valid view and complaint. By taking a position opposite to the patient's point of view, you take on the role of adversary rather than helper. Acknowledge the patient's feelings by saying something like, "It's upsetting when no one can get here promptly."

ASKING PRYING OR PROBING QUESTIONS

Probing questions may place the patient on the defensive. This occurs when you ask questions about the patient's private business, and these questions are not related to the treatment or clinical condition. Questioning why the patient did or did not do a particular thing makes the patient defensive about the action and causes feelings of discomfort. If you ask a patient who has been injured in an automobile accident, "Why were you driving so fast in the rain?" you are inappropriately probing.

USING CLICHÉS

A cliché is an overused expression that may be unrelated to the current situation. Comments such as "You'll be fine," or "Don't worry, it will turn out OK," are clichés. They show a lack of respect for the patient as an individual and discount the patient's feelings or experiences. It is better to express that you are available to listen to the patient's concerns and feelings and to be supportive as needed.

LISTENING INATTENTIVELY

Failing to listen to what the patient is saying is a communication block. If you continue to straighten the room and turn away while the patient is trying to express feelings or something of importance, your actions express that you are not interested. **Interrupting, or jumping in before the patient has finished speaking, or frequently changing the subject also indicates inattentive listening. Allow the patient to finish speaking before responding to what she has communicated.**

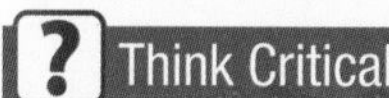
Think Critically

Observe nurses in the hospital as they communicate with patients. What types of blocks to communication do you see occurring? Speculate as to why these nurses are blocking communication with their patients.

INTERVIEWING SKILLS

An interview is more directed than a therapeutic communication interaction is. It is planned and has a definite purpose. It is important to establish **rapport** (a relationship of mutual trust) with the patient before beginning an interview. Introduce yourself and ask how the patient wishes to be addressed. Include the family in your greeting. Explain the purpose of the interview and provide privacy. Ask patients if they wish their family or friends to remain during the interview by saying, "Would it be better if we were alone for this interview?" Eliminate excess noise by turning off electronics. Be certain the patient is comfortable, draw up a chair to within 3 to 4 feet, and sit down facing the patient (Fig. 8.4). Chapter 5 contains more information about the interview.

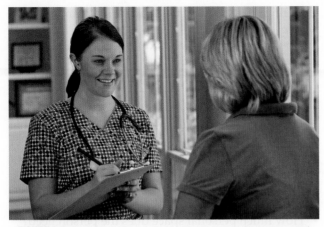

FIGURE 8.4 Interviewing the patient. (Photo copyright istock.com.)

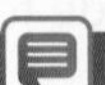 Communication

Establishing Rapport

To establish rapport with a patient so that you can proceed with the interview or therapeutic interaction, you might use a few of these phrases:

- "Hello, Mr. Sanchez, I'm John; I'd like to know more about you. Can you tell me a little about what you do for a living [or did before you retired]?"
- "Mrs. Jackson, I see that you live alone. Can you tell me a little about your friends and activities?"
- "Ms. Lee, you've had a lot happen to you over the past few weeks; it must be hard to have your life interrupted this way."
- "Janice, your mom says you play basketball. It must be hard not being able to play during this part of the season."
- "Joey, it's OK to be angry and cry when you've been hurt. Can you tell me how your leg feels now?"

When obtaining a health history during an admission interview, take control of the interaction and initially ask closed questions that call for specific data. This type of direct interview does not allow the patient to ask questions or discuss concerns until all the necessary information has been collected. Examples of questions might include:

- What medications did you take today?
- Do you have pain?
- Do you have any allergies?
- If you have been hospitalized before, what was the year of your hospitalization?

After taking the history, use open-ended questions to find out how the patient feels about the hospitalization. Examples of useful open-ended questions include "What brought you to the hospital?" "What are your concerns about this hospitalization?" and "Do you have any questions?" This last question indicates that the interview is ending. A brief summary statement, ending with "I think I have the information I need," closes the interview. Thank the patient for supplying the information collected before finishing. An example of the nursing admission history form is found in Chapter 5.

 Life Span Considerations

Older Adults

When taking a lengthy history from an older adult, it may be necessary to redirect the interaction frequently if the patient focuses too long on one illness or hospitalization.

THE NURSE-PATIENT RELATIONSHIP

The nurse-patient relationship focuses on the patient, the relationship has goals, and it is defined by specific boundaries. The relationship takes place in the health care setting, and boundaries are defined by the patient's problems, the help needed, and the nurse's professional role. When the patient is discharged, the relationship ends.

Good communication skills establish a therapeutic relationship between you and the patient that assists in the healing process. **In this relationship, you are in a helping role rather than a social role.** Interaction between you and the patient should build trust. Without trust, the patient will discount much of what you say.

A social relationship differs from a therapeutic one in that the focus is on both participants and the usual goal is to meet one's own needs. The social relationship is established for mutual enjoyment, with considerable sharing of experiences, life events, and thoughts.

Characteristics in the nurse that facilitate a therapeutic nurse-patient relationship include effective communication skills, **empathy** (ability to understand the situation from another's perspective), a desire to help, honesty, a nonjudgmental attitude, genuineness, acceptance, and respect. **Confidentiality, or keeping information private, must be maintained for trust to endure.**

EMPATHY

Empathy is the ability to place oneself in another's position. It involves being able to see situations from another person's perspective and perceive them as that person does. If empathy is present, the other person's feeling is understood. Empathy is different from sympathy. With sympathy, concern and perhaps sorrow are felt, indicating that the person is experiencing something difficult. Warmth, a nonjudgmental attitude, and a focus on the patient's feelings are present when empathy is expressed. Again, be careful when using clichés such as "I know how you feel" or "I understand what you are going through." No one can really know or feel what someone else is experiencing. State an interpretation of the patient's feelings and then seek validation that the interpretation is accurate.

 Think Critically

Why is empathy important in the nurse-patient relationship? Discuss incidents when you (or someone you observed) had trouble feeling empathy for a patient. What were the outcomes? What could have been done to alter the situation?

BECOMING NONJUDGMENTAL

Becoming nonjudgmental takes considerable practice and discipline, and it is directly related to the degree of empathy a person is capable of generating. It is far easier to accept people as they are if you can truly see things from their perspective. Patients come from all kinds of backgrounds and have many different sets of values. To be nonjudgmental, you must look at the patient in reference to *her* values rather than your own.

MAINTAINING HOPE

Maintaining hope is an important part of the nurse-patient relationship. There is always hope, even if the direction of hope changes. The dying patient can hope for less pain, peace, a pleasant moment, and a good laugh. A patient with cancer can hope for a positive prognosis, a healing outcome from surgery or therapy, or emotional growth from the illness experience. The nurse should help the patient establish realistic hopes, but even unrealistic hopes should not be totally dismissed. **Hope is what helps a patient cope in a difficult situation.**

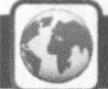 Cultural Considerations

Truth Telling

In the Jewish orthodoxy, doctors were historically discouraged from telling patients if they had a terminal illness, as crushing one's hope prematurely may cause unnecessary suffering. In the last century, however, this topic has become more complicated, with a shift away from a paternalistic ("doctor knows best") medical culture to a greater emphasis on patient autonomy (Gesundheit, Zlotnick, Wygoda, Rosenzweig, & Steinberg, 2015). Being culturally aware of your patient's beliefs will help you improve communication with them.

Application of the Nursing Process

Assess the patient's language ability during the first encounter. Consider the following questions when gathering data about the patient's communication needs:

- Does the patient speak and understand English, or is a translator needed?
- Is the vocabulary level equivalent to that of the average person of this age or will it be necessary to simplify language?
- Does the patient have a neurologic impairment that causes problems with the comprehension of oral or written communication or with the ability to hear or speak?
- What cultural factors affect how this patient interacts verbally?
- How much personal space does the person need?
- If the person is unable to speak but can communicate in writing, what provisions should be made to accommodate this?

Patients who have problems with communication are given the nursing diagnosis impaired verbal communication.

In addition to writing individual expected outcomes, you must plan appropriate amounts of time with the patient for a communication interaction. An assessment interview should not take more than 30 minutes. If the patient has communication impairment, varying amounts of time will be needed for each interaction. When a patient does not speak English, plan ahead and locate an interpreter before beginning an interaction with the patient.

NURSE-PATIENT COMMUNICATION

Trust and understanding are the keys to effective nurse-patient communication. When the nurse possesses knowledge, skills, and attitudes (KSAs) related to patient-centered care, successful nurse-patient communication can be achieved.

 QSEN Considerations: Patient-Centered Care

KSAs for Prelicensure Licensed Practical Nurse/Licensed Vocational Nurse Students

KNOWLEDGE	SKILLS	ATTITUDES
— Understanding there are many dimensions of patient centered care, including: • Patient/family preferences and values • Physical comfort • Emotional support • Involvement of family and friends — Knowledge of pain and suffering — Knowledge of how culture and ethnicity affects the patient and his/her values — Knowledge of strategies to empower families — Knowledge of principles of effective communication	— The ability to understand patient values and preferences and communicate these to the health care team — Provide nursing care with sensitivity to the individual patient — Gather and report data to the RN regarding patient pain and discomfort; implement measures to relieve such — Assess your own communication skills — Communicate care provided for the patient	— Value seeing the situation "through the patient's eyes" — Value the patient's knowledge of his/her own health — Recognize own attitudes about working with patients from different cultural, ethnic, and social backgrounds — Recognize own values and beliefs — Value active partnership with patient — Respect patient beliefs and practices — Value continuous improvement of own communication skills

Adapted from: QSEN's Patient Centered Care KSAs. Available at: http://www.qsen.org/ksas_prelicensure.php

COMMUNICATING WITH THE HEARING-IMPAIRED PATIENT

When a patient has a hearing impairment, determine how to interact with the patient to promote the best level of communication. If the patient has hearing aids, see that they are used, that the batteries are functioning, and that the device is turned on. A hearing aid does not guarantee that the individual will hear perfectly. The following techniques promote comprehension for a hearing-impaired person:

- Get the person's attention, making certain the person is aware that verbalization is going to take place. If the person is seated, sit down.
- Face the person directly. Speak slowly and distinctly. Do not cover your mouth, chew gum, or have food in your mouth when speaking.
- Do not shout because this can distort speech.
- Maintain voice pitch at midrange, neither low nor high.
- Maintain a distance for speaking to a hearing-impaired person of 2½ to 4 feet.
- Never speak directly into the person's ear. This can distort the message and hide all visual cues.
- Be aware of nonverbal communication.
- Use short, simple sentences. Try to limit each sentence to one subject and one verb.
- If the patient does not appear to understand or responds inappropriately, rephrase the statement.
- Give the person time to respond to questions.
- Ask for rephrasing to make certain the patient has understood important information.

COMMUNICATING WITH AN APHASIC PATIENT

The patient with **aphasia** (difficulty expressing or understanding language) will require specialized nursing interventions. Recruit the assistance of a speech therapist to determine methods to facilitate communication for these patients. A white erasable board is handy for aphasic patients who can write (Fig. 8.5).

Some techniques can be helpful when communicating with a patient who has aphasia because of neurologic damage from a stroke or head injury. The use of appropriate nonverbal gestures sometimes helps. Guidelines presented in Box 8.1 can assist you in communicating more effectively with the aphasic patient.

COMMUNICATING WITH OLDER ADULTS

Older adults vary greatly in their communication abilities, interests, and capabilities. Healthy older adults sometimes require more time to think and formulate a response. Other older adults may have hearing, sensory, or motor impairments that interfere with communication. Be certain you have the person's attention before beginning an interaction. Eliminate outside distractions. Introduce one idea at a time, and do not rush the person, as this may cause confusion.

It is especially important to obtain feedback from an older adult that the message has been clearly understood. If people have difficulty comprehending, they may just nod their head,

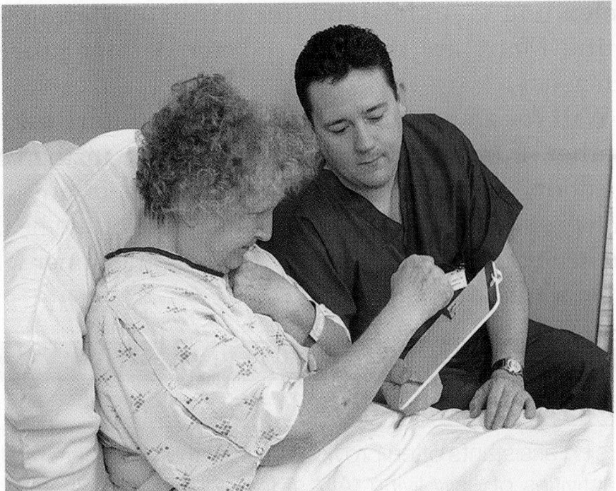

FIGURE 8.5 Communicating with an aphasic patient.

Box 8.1 Communicating With the Aphasic Person

- Make sure you have the person's attention before you start.
- Make the environment as relaxed and quiet as possible.
- Assume the patient can understand what is heard unless deafness has been diagnosed.
- Speak to the patient as an adult; do not act as if the patient is mentally incompetent.
- Talk to the patient; do not talk to someone else in the room about the patient.
- Include the patient in group conversation and decision making as much as possible. Face the patient, establish eye contact, and speak slowly and distinctly without dropping the voice level at the end of sentences; do not shout.
- Give directions with short phrases and simple terms; use gestures to enhance the words.
- Phrase questions so that they can be answered with a "yes" or "no," and look for nonverbal behavior that agrees with the patient's answer.
- Give the person time to respond to questions; processing may be slower than usual.
- Ask only one question at a time; be patient and wait for an answer. Resist the urge to finish sentences or offer words.
- If you need to repeat something, use the same words the second time. If there is still difficulty, phrase what was said differently.
- Use body language, drawings, gestures, and facial expressions to enhance the message.
- Allow one person to speak at a time.
- Praise all attempts to speak and downplay any errors. Avoid insisting that that each word be produced perfectly.
- Encourage independence and avoid being overprotective.

pretending to understand, for fear of appearing forgetful. Many are embarrassed about their hearing deficiency.

Wait for an answer to one question before asking another. Introduce one subject at a time in the conversation, and give only one instruction in any one sentence. It is important for all members of the health care team to communicate in a consistent manner with older adults.

Assignment Considerations

Sharing Communication Tips

Nursing assistants often provide much of the basic care related to activities of daily living (ADLs) for older adults. Share your knowledge about how to communicate with older adults and ask the assistants for their input. Ask them to share their communication success stories.

COMMUNICATING WITH CHILDREN

When communicating with children, consider the influence of development on language and thought processes. Young children are very responsive to nonverbal messages. A young child may become frightened by sudden movements or gestures. Approach children at their eye level and use a calm, quiet, friendly voice.

When interacting with an infant, keep the mother within the baby's view. With a toddler or a preschooler, focus on the child's needs and concerns. Use simple, short sentences and concrete explanations with familiar words.

For the school-age child, give simple explanations and demonstrate how equipment works. Allow the child to handle the equipment if possible. Listen carefully to the child's fears or concerns.

An adolescent needs time to talk. Use active listening, avoid interrupting, and show acceptance. Try not to give advice, and avoid embarrassing questions if possible.

Above all, with any child, be honest and tell the child what to expect.

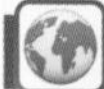

Cultural Considerations

Assisting Older Adults from Other Cultures

In some cultures, older adults are not accustomed to taking instruction from a young person. It may be necessary to enlist the aid of an adult family member who will learn the essentials of self-care for the patient, and then have that person perform the patient education. Provide printed materials and be available to demonstrate or answer questions.

If you are from your community's nondominant culture and your primary language is not English, it is important to work on your English language skills and correct pronunciation. Your patients depend on good communication with you. If you cannot communicate well in English, you may miss important signs and symptoms of a change in a patient's condition. When a patient is unable to communicate well with the nurse, it adds further stress to the patient's situation and leads to dissatisfaction with care. Most communities have classes for students who wish to improve their English.

COMMUNICATION WITHIN THE HEALTH CARE TEAM

Communication within the health care team occurs through writing and reading nurses' notes; care providers' orders; the dietitian's notes; and notes and orders of the respiratory, physical, speech, and occupational therapists, as well as listening to and giving a **shift report** (a verbal communication on the details of a patient's condition and treatment). Completing forms for the laboratory, radiology, and other departments is another method of communication. Entering information on the computer is an essential tool for communication among hospital departments. Communication boards can be helpful for reminding team members about patients at risk for falls or other problems to watch for (Fig. 8.6). Clear communication is necessary when consulting with care providers about orders and when delegating tasks to ancillary workers.

END-OF-SHIFT REPORT

Many different formats are used to give a report. Sometimes the report is given as the nurses from the off-going and oncoming shifts walk from room to room together; known as **walking rounds.** If the report is recorded on an audiotape or if computerized sheets are used, there must be an opportunity to ask and respond to questions. Whatever format is used, the same essential information is necessary for each patient. Get in the habit of organizing the report in the same way each day. A full report on each patient should take about 1 to 3 minutes. Give only essential information. It takes practice to give a logical, organized, concise report on a group of patients. Practicing at home with an audio recorder can help you gain confidence and

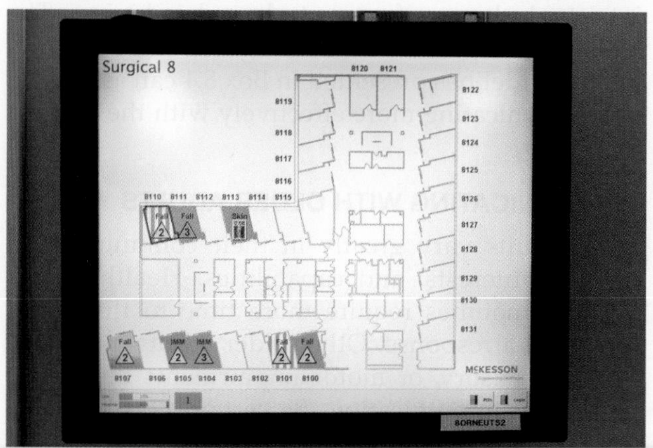

FIGURE 8.6 Communication board on a nursing unit.

present information more concisely. Box 8.2 presents the information usually given in an end-of-shift report. Styles of reporting include **ISBAR-R** (*I*ntroduction, *S*ituation, *B*ackground, *A*ssessment, *R*ecommendation, and *R*eadback) and SBAR-Q (*Q*uestions) formats. If the initial information is handed out on a computer printout, it need not be repeated. The room number and patient's name are sufficient as a starting point after introducing yourself. See Table 8.4 for an ISBAR-R template you can use in clinical practice for handoff reporting.

Safety Alert

ISBAR-R

In accordance with the National Patient Safety Goals and the QSEN program, an end-of-shift report should be conducted in a standardized manner to reduce the risk of patient injuries and errors during handoff communication. The ISBAR-R format gives caregivers the opportunity to ask and respond to questions concerning patient care. This format is borrowed from military communication models and has been successfully used in some health care settings.

Computerized documentation is now available in most hospitals that allow nurses to access an electronic or printed information sheet for each of their patients at the beginning of the shift. These sheets can be taken and used as a work organization sheet. If notes are added to the sheet during the shift, all the information needed for the report at the end of the shift should be readily at hand. This sheet is also useful when telephoning care providers.

Box 8.2 Information Included in End-of-Shift Report

- Room number; bed designation; patient name, age, and sex; date of admission; medical diagnoses; and name of primary care provider. (If a computer census sheet is used that contains some of this information, then only the room number, name, and any missing data are given.)
- Tests and treatments or therapies performed in the past 24 hours with patient response (e.g., computed tomography [CT] scans, surgery, and procedures); intake and output for past shift.
- Significant changes in patient condition.
- Scheduled tests; consults or surgery; current intravenous solution, flow rate, and amount remaining; next solution to be hung; oxygen flow rate; equipment in use and current settings (e.g., gastric suction on low).
- Current problems (e.g., dehydration, severe pain, anxiety, depression, insufficient rest, or abnormal laboratory values or test results); amount of assistance with activities of daily living (ADLs) needed.
- Scheduled treatments, PRN (as needed) medications given, times given, and patient response.
- Concerns, need for order changes, patient education, pertinent family dynamics, and emotional status.

QSEN Considerations

Improve Communication

Communicate patient values, preferences, and expressed needs to other members of the health care team during shift report to improve communication and patient outcomes (QSEN, 2014a, 2014b).

QSEN: Patient-Centered Care.

TELEPHONING PRIMARY CARE PROVIDERS

Primary care providers must be telephoned from time to time. Orders may be unclear; the patient's condition may change; the patient may have a particular request; or you may need further information about the patient.

If a primary care provider is called regarding a change in a patient's condition or in any situation in which new orders are anticipated, certain steps should be followed. Have current data on the patient at hand, including data from the last vital signs assessment, pertinent laboratory data, information on intake and urinary output, and medications received. Have the patient's work information sheet, medical record, and a pen ready, and anticipate the information that the primary care provider might need to make a decision. Know what allergies the patient has. Perform a quick assessment before calling, and prepare a concise statement of the problem or concern. Document the call in the medical record, and note the health care provider's statement that the order is read back correctly.

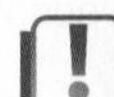

Safety Alert

Taking Telephone Orders

To apply the ISBAR-R format to a telephone order, you should introduce yourself (including the hospital unit), verify the patient's name and background, report the patient's current condition, listen to the order, write down the order, and then read it back to the provider to ensure accuracy (Box 8.3).

The student nurse should have an instructor or another registered nurse standing by to speak with the provider and take the order again, including readback, because **students cannot legally take telephone orders.**

ASSIGNMENT CONSIDERATIONS AND DELEGATING

You must communicate well when you assign tasks and **delegate** (authorize another person to do something) to others effectively. Give clear, concise messages and listen carefully to feedback. Include the desired results and the time constraints for completion of the task. It is better to say, "Let me know if Mrs. Hope's noon temperature is above 101.2°F" than to say, "Let me know if Mrs. Hope's temperature is high." Ask the person to whom you are assigning a task if there are

Table 8.4 ISBAR-R Tool

Date/Time: **Room:**

Patient Handoff Communication*		
I Introduction	Pt. Name: Age/Sex: Date of Admit:______	Sending unit/RN: Receiving unit/RN: Primary MD/Admitting: Consultants:
S Situation	Dx: Current Conditions: Postop Day#______	Interventions/Responses: Meds given: PRNs given:
B Background	Past Med/Surg hx:	Allergies: Code status: Isolation status: Fall risk: yes ____ no ____
A Assessment	VS: T____ P____ BP____ Pain level: ____ O_2sat Pertinent Labs: WBC ⟩ H / H ⟨ RBC NA / CL / BUN ⟨ Glucose K+ / CO_2 / Creat FSBG: Rad Results: Lines: I&O: Dressings/Appliances:	Neuro: Resp: Cardio: GI/GU: Diet: Musculoskeletal: PT/OT: Skin: Psychosocial: **Restraints:** Med/surg or Behavioral Where: ____ Rationale: ______ MD order due: ________
R Recommendations	STAT orders/urgent issues pending: Labs pending: Next due for PRN: What to watch for in this pt:	Planned tests/Procedures: Goals/Treatment plan: Consults: Discharge needs/Care coordination:
R Readback	Summarize the verbal information obtained above (done if handoff communication was done via telephone)	Ask if the receiver has any questions.

NOT A PERMANENT PART OF THE PATIENT RECORD

*Modified from the ISBAR Tool created by El Camino Hospital, Mountain View, California.

Box 8.3 Example of ISBAR-R Communication

I: Dr. Savoy, this is Nurse Lopez at ABC Extended Care Facility. I'm calling in regard to Mr. Tanglewood in room C12.
S: Mr. Tanglewood is an 85-year-old man with Alzheimer disease. He tripped in the bathroom and bumped his head on the toilet about 30 minutes ago. One of the nursing assistants saw him trip, and there was no loss of consciousness at any time.
B: He is normally alert and oriented to person, and he routinely ambulates independently.
A: His blood pressure is currently 140/83, pulse 75, respirations 16 per minute. He has a 3-cm laceration and hematoma just superior to his left eyebrow. The bleeding was readily controlled with direct pressure. We have applied an ice pack and pressure bandage over the wound. He is alert, and his speech is clear and appropriate to his baseline. Patient denies pain or tenderness to his head. He does appear to have bruising on his forehead. The patient extended his right hand to break his fall.
R: Could I get an order to have him transported to the emergency department for additional evaluation and treatment? And do you have any additional orders for Mr. Tanglewood?
R: Thank you, Dr. Savoy. Let me repeat that order. Mr. Tanglewood will be transported to the emergency department by ambulance. After the evaluation, he will be sent to radiology for x-ray examination of his right hand.

any questions about what is to be done, and ask for a summary of what is understood about the task to be done. Although a task may be delegated, the ultimate responsibility will remain with you.

COMPUTER COMMUNICATION

The computer is used to transmit requests for laboratory, dietary, radiology, physical therapy, respiratory therapy, and other services. The primary care provider enters medication orders into the computer, and the orders are communicated to the nurse on a patient medication administration record. Supplies for patient care are ordered on the computer, and patient care plans are updated using the keyboard or a touch screen (Fig. 8.7).

Legal and Ethical Considerations

Computer Usage and Safeguarding Patient Information

Computerized patient information requires extra vigilance to safeguard confidentiality. When you use the computer at the health care facility, never leave a computer screen open when you are finished. Always log out so that someone else cannot access information using your password, and never share your password with others. If your facility uses e-mail to communicate about patient care, you will likely receive training to prevent Health Insurance Portability and Accountability Act (HIPAA) violations (see Chapter 3).

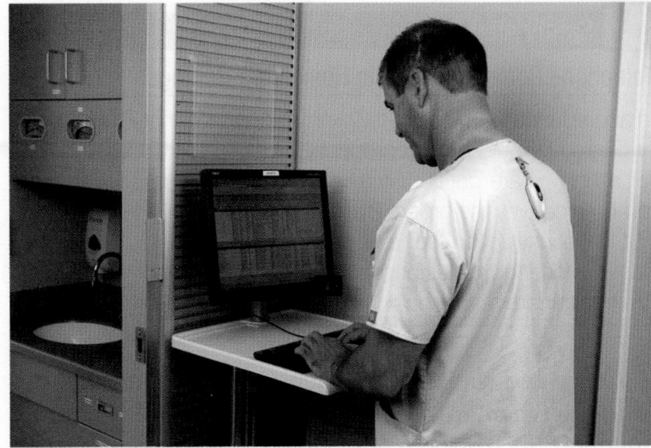

FIGURE 8.7 Using a computer to communicate patient information.

Many hospitals and home care agencies are converting to computer documentation. In some agencies, a hand-held computer is used to note medications given, **input** (put in information) vital signs, document assessment data, and record the nurse's observations. The Joint Commission historically stated that the texting of medical orders was not acceptable. Recently, however, they have reversed their decision, and now state that orders may be transmitted via text messaging under specific guidelines including secure sign-on process, encryption of messages, date/time stamping, and other specifications (The Joint Commission, 2016). Computer and technology skills are essential for today's nurse.

COMMUNICATION IN THE HOME AND COMMUNITY

Nurses who work in home care often have both a professional and a social relationship with their patients and families. Often, the nurse is the only person whom the patient sees on the day of a visit. Because of the social aspects of the visit, it is essential to state when instructions are about to be given so that active listening can occur.

Home Care Considerations

Tips for Efficient Interviewing

Before the initial home visit, ask the home care patient or family to list all medications the patient is taking, including over-the-counter medicines and herbal preparations, and to have the vials and bottles all in one place. Ask that a list of the patient's care providers with phone numbers be ready for you, plus the dates of any recent hospitalization or surgery. This will save you time when doing the interview, and you can take the lists with you for the later completion of your paperwork. Leave written step-by-step instructions with the patient whenever possible. The primary nurse will often call between visits to see how treatment is progressing and to assess for any problems.

Safety Alert

Telephone Communication in Home Care Settings

In accordance with the Joint Commission's National Patient Safety Goals, it would be inappropriate for a provider to leave orders for a home care patient on a voice-mail message or to ask the family to convey the orders to the nurse. Likewise, a nurse should not leave instructions for a nursing assistant in a voicemail message. Exchange of telephone information between members of the health care team should follow the ISBAR-R format.

Office and clinic nurses often assess patients who call in to see whether they have an urgent need for medical attention. Such assessment requires good communication to obtain the data needed to make such a decision (Fig. 8.8). The office nurse gives telephone instructions to patients on how to treat minor illnesses or injuries. It is important in these situations to obtain feedback so that there is no doubt that the patient understands the instructions.

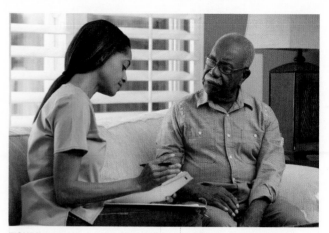

FIGURE 8.8 Nurse performing patient education. (Photo copyright istock.com.)

Get Ready for the NCLEX Examination!

Key Points

- Communication is a continual, circular process and occurs in two ways: verbal and nonverbal.
- Culture, experience, emotions, attitude, mood, and self-concept all contribute to the way people communicate.
- An active listener maintains eye contact without staring, gives the patient full attention, and makes a conscious effort to block out other sounds and distractions.
- Silence and therapeutic touch can be effective forms of communication.
- Asking open-ended questions, restating, clarifying, using general leads, offering of self, encouraging elaboration, giving information, looking at alternatives, and summarizing are all therapeutic communication techniques.
- Changing the subject, offering false reassurance, giving advice, making defensive comments, asking probing questions, using clichés, and inattentive listening are blocks to good communication.
- A therapeutic relationship focuses on the patient; helping the patient maintain hope is important.
- Empathy, a desire to help, honesty, a nonjudgmental attitude, genuineness, acceptance, and respect for the individual also facilitate a therapeutic nurse-patient relationship.
- Special communication techniques are needed for the patient experiencing aphasia, for patients with a hearing impairment, and for children.
- Be accepting and do not show impatience if a patient does not speak English; look for cultural cues regarding eye contact and distance between speaker and listener.
- Handoff report should include patient's name, age, and changes in condition; current concerns; treatments; and response to therapies, and should use the format ISBAR-R.
- When taking telephone orders, introduce yourself and verify the patient, listen, write, and read back what you have written.
- Protect passwords and log off when using the computer.

Additional Learning Resources

SG Go to your Study Guide for additional learning activities to help you master this chapter content.

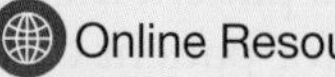 Go to your Evolve website at http://evolve.elsevier.com/Williams/fundamental for additional online resources.

Online Resources

- Review the case studies of a child who died (The Josie King Story) and two who nearly died (Chasing Zero: Winning the War on HealthCare Harm) because of medical errors. What can we learn about patient communication and empathy from these tragic events? Both are available at: http://qsen.org/faculty-resources/videos/
- Improving Patient-Provider Communication (Joint Commission Video): www.jointcommission.org/multimedia/improving-patient-provider-communication---part-1-of-4/

Review Questions for the NCLEX Examination

*Choose the **best** answer for each question.*

1. The nurse is using therapeutic communication to establish rapport. The nurse says, "How are you feeling this morning?" Which nonverbal behavior is congruent with the nurse's verbal question?
   1. Looks at patient; stands with a relaxed body position
   2. Nods head up and down; arms folded across chest
   3. Smiles at patient and makes the bed while patient answers
   4. Adjusts IV and evaluates equipment and environment
2. A patient expresses serious concerns about the outcomes of a scheduled surgical procedure. Which response indicates that the nurse is using active listening while the patient is speaking?
   1. Nurse tells the patient not to worry about the surgery.
   2. Nurse asks the patient to take her medication before continuing.
   3. Nurse asks the patient why she is afraid of the surgery.
   4. Nurse nods his head.
3. What is a correct beginning for an ISBAR-R communication with a physician?
   1. "Your patient, Mr. Leo, is agitated and combative."
   2. "Dr. Thomas, this is Patricia, the nurse caring for your patient, Mr. Leo."
   3. "Mr. Leo has demonstrated escalating inappropriate behavior ever since his dose of Lithium was reduced."
   4. "I need you to come and evaluate your patient, Mr. Leo."
4. The nurse enters the patient room to perform patient education. Which nonverbal communication by the patient is an indication that the education time should be rescheduled? *(Select all that apply.)*
   1. Wringing hands while the nurse is talking
   2. Maintaining eye contact with the nurse
   3. Looking down with shoulders slumped
   4. Arms crossed in front of the chest
   5. Patient is seated facing the nurse
5. The patient is aphasic. Which communication strategy would be appropriate in working with this patient? *(Select all that apply.)*
   1. Lean forward and say "Go on…."
   2. Face the patient, establish eye contact, and speak slowly.
   3. Use gestures to enhance the words.
   4. Help the patient by finishing her sentences.
   5. Explain procedures to the family member instead of the patient.
   6. Give directions with short phrases and simple terms.
6. Which observation might indicate the staff could benefit from an in-service training on the topic of patient-centered care KSAs?
   1. Nurses are seen consistently demonstrating principles of effective communication.
   2. Nurses are allowing family members to bring in home remedies "from the old country" after obtaining permission from the primary care provider.
   3. The unit implements a 24-hour visitation policy.
   4. The staff complains about admitting patients from a certain geographic region of the world because "they are always so loud."
7. A way to promote trust with a patient is to:
   1. Allow family members to visit whenever they want.
   2. Assure the patient that her physician is excellent.
   3. Follow through when you say you will do something.
   4. Talk with her at length, about her life, likes, and dislikes.
8. A nurse is assigning a task to the nursing assistant. Which is the best example of how to communicate the task to the assistant?
   1. "Please do all the vital signs for my patients, and pay special attention to Mrs. Hondo and Mr. Takeda."
   2. "Please report any abnormal vital signs throughout the day, and keep an eye on Mrs. Hondo and Mr. Takeda."
   3. "Please check Mrs. Hondo's and Mr. Takeda's blood pressure and pulse as ordered by the primary care provider. Call me if you have problems."
   4. "Please do vital signs at 8 am on Mrs. Hondo and Mr. Takeda, and if the pulse is more than 85 beats per minute, let me know."

Critical Thinking Activities

Read each clinical scenario and discuss the questions with your classmates.

Scenario A

You are working with a patient who is quiet and withdrawn. When you walk into her room, she appears tearful and upset, but she tells you that nothing is wrong. How would deal with this situation? What type of nonverbal communication would you expect this patient to exhibit?

Scenario B

Consider your own communication style. What three factors do you think have had the greatest influence on the way you communicate?

Scenario C

Develop your own checklist for giving a handoff report. Why is it important for the oncoming nurse to have an opportunity to ask questions?

chapter

9 Patient Education and Health Promotion

http://evolve.elsevier.com/Williams/fundamental

Objectives

Upon completing this chapter, you should be able to do the following:

Theory

1. Discuss the purposes of patient education.
2. Use patient education to promote the national goals of health promotion and disease prevention as listed in *Healthy People 2020* and the *Health Canada.*
3. Describe three ways in which people learn, and correlate the importance of these types of learning to patient education.
4. List and differentiate between conditions and factors that can affect learning.
5. Describe barriers to teaching and learning.
6. Identify adjustments to the patient education plan needed for teaching very young patients or older adults.
7. Discuss types of resources available to assist in patient education.
8. Name three things that must be included in the documentation of patient education.
9. Describe ways for patient education to be continued after hospital discharge.

Clinical Practice

1. Assess an assigned patient's learning needs.
2. Develop a patient education plan based on the patient's learning needs.
3. Implement the patient education plan at a prearranged time.
4. Evaluate the effectiveness of the patient education and the plan.

Key Terms

affective domain (dōw-MĀN, p. 121)
auditory learning (ăw-dĭ-TŌR-ē, p. 121)
behavioral objectives (bē-HĀV-yōr-ăl, p. 125)
cognitive domain (KŎG-nĭ-tĭv, p. 121)
feedback (p. 126)
kinesthetic learning (kĭn-ĕs-THĔT-ĭc, p. 121)
psychomotor domain (sī-kō-MŌ-tŏr, p. 121)
return demonstration (p. 126)
visual learning (p. 121)

 Concepts Covered in This Chapter

- Learning
- Health literacy
- Patient education
- Learning environment

PURPOSES OF PATIENT EDUCATION

The ultimate goal of patient education is the prevention of illness, promotion of wellness, and restoration of health. **Nurses teach patients about their disease or disorder, surgery, and self-care** (Box 9.1). Patient education is one of the most important roles of the nurse. Nurses perform patient education in every setting in which they practice. For example, preoperative education covers the various phases of the surgery, what will be experienced, what can be expected, and the exercises to be done afterward. With same-day surgery and hospital stays being so short, patient education has become an even higher priority. **Before discharge, the patient must be taught how to care for himself at home.** This requires collaboration on the patient education plan among the various health professionals involved in the care, as well as communication with the family and home care nurse, if any.

Patient education contributes to achievement of the goals of *Healthy People 2020,* a program of the US Department of Health and Human Services, and the objectives of *Health Canada.* An objective of *Healthy People 2020* is to "attain high quality, longer lives free of preventable disease, disability, injury, and premature death." Objectives speak to promoting healthy behaviors, protecting health, ensuring access to high-quality health care, and strengthening community health promotion programs. Canadian objectives include "Prevent and reduce risks to individual health and the overall environment," and "Promote healthier lifestyles" (Health Canada, 2014). Effective patient education is also linked to patient satisfaction, which,

Box 9.1 Topics for Patient Education

- The disease process
- Preoperative and postoperative care
- Diagnostic tests and procedures
- Information needed for self-care and restoration
  - Diet
  - Exercise
  - Medication purpose, schedule, and special considerations
  - Medication side effects
  - Symptoms to report to health care provider
  - Skills such as asepsis, dressing change, splint or brace attachment, injections, intravenous administration at home, use of mechanical or other aids
  - Prosthesis care
  - Working with a physical therapist
  - Working with a speech therapist
  - Working with an occupational therapist
- Prevention of illness and health promotion
  - Stress reduction and relaxation techniques
  - Proper cough technique
  - Smoking cessation
  - Immunizations
  - First aid
  - Hygiene
  - Safety (home, car, and workplace)
  - Prenatal care
  - Infant and child care
  - Parenting
  - Nutrition
  - Exercise benefits
  - Beneficial screenings (blood pressure, vision, cholesterol, mammography, prostate-specific antigen, blood glucose, skin for cancer, and colonoscopy)
  - Disaster preparedness

in turn has implications for facility reimbursement rates.

Discharge planning requires looking ahead to meet the patient's ongoing needs at home. **It is a process that begins at the time of admission.** This includes assessing for special needs, learning to identify appropriate education moments, and providing learning opportunities that are brief and focused on preparing the patient for self-care. A **teaching moment** occurs when the patient is at an optimal level of readiness to learn and apply a particular piece of information. Teaching, like discharge planning, is an ongoing process with opportunities that arise in many situations. Take cues from the patient's questions, or try to stimulate interest in what he needs to know. Saying, "You'll want to know things you can do to lower your risk of another heart attack" tends to stimulate interest in the recovering myocardial infarction patient.

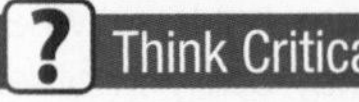

Think Critically

Can you list three general education topics that might be appropriate for most patients under your care?

MODES OF LEARNING

Research has shown that people learn in three ways: (1) visually, through what they see **(visual learning)**; (2) aurally, through what they hear **(auditory learning)**; and (3) kinesthetically, by actually performing a task or handling items **(kinesthetic learning)**. Although most people can learn by any of these routes, one route is usually dominant. For example, if a person is primarily a visual learner, **telling** him everything and not using any written materials or visual examples will make learning much more difficult. Many people do not know how they learn best. It is important to use a variety of teaching techniques so that the patient both sees and hears the information and performs the action being taught. Additionally, the material being presented (e.g., insulin self-injection) may dictate the method of patient education that will be best to use (kinesthetic), although it should be reinforced with other modes (auditory or visual).

QSEN Considerations: Patient-Centered Care

Learning Styles

It is important to determine and adapt to the patient's dominant learning style when performing patient education.

Think Critically

Which of the three routes of learning usually works best for you? How have you seen a child learn? How have you seen an older adult learn?

During the education sessions, listen to how the patient makes responses because the language used may give clues to the person's best learning mode.

Learning can also be categorized by domains. In the **cognitive domain**, the learner takes in and processes information by listening to or reading the material. For example, explaining how handwashing can break the chain of infection can give the spouse of an immunocompromised patient valuable information. In the **affective domain**, the material is presented in a way that is appealing to the learner's beliefs, feelings, and values. For example, people must value cleanliness before you can teach them to wash their hands frequently. In the **psychomotor domain**, the learner processes the information by performing an action or carrying out a task. For example, demonstrating proper handwashing technique can reinforce the desired behaviors. All three domains are important to the patient's translation of the learning to desired behaviors.

ASSESSMENT OF LEARNING NEEDS

To prepare a patient education plan, you must first know what the patient needs to learn. What does the person need to know about the disease or condition, diet, activity, medication, wound care, treatment, or self-care? This information establishes the learning needs.

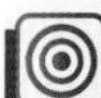 Focused Assessment

Assessment for Teaching and Learning

Assess the following:

- Barriers to learning
- Ability to learn
- Cultural factors to be considered
- Language level and literacy; need for interpreter
- Patient's health beliefs
- Emotional and physical readiness to learn
- Patient's learning goals
- Patient's dominant learning style
- Family support and availability
- Concerns about learning skills
- Concerns about care after discharge
- Materials available for patient education
- Location for patient education with appropriate environment
- Times when patient education could take place

Patients may require far more complex education than can be accomplished in the short time before discharge. In such cases, the basic survival skills are taught first, and after discharge the advanced skills are taught in group or private sessions. Often, a home health nurse continues with the patient education plan. Make a list of the learning needs and then prioritize them so that you can concentrate first on teaching the essential knowledge needed for safe care at home. Place the identified learning needs on the patient's care plan.

 Think Critically

How would you assess the patient's current understanding to determine where he has knowledge deficits related to his health or self-care?

FACTORS AFFECTING LEARNING

Before beginning to teach, you must assess for factors that might interfere with the patient's ability to learn. Conditions that can affect the learning process include poor vision or hearing, impaired motor function, illiteracy, and impaired cognition. Age may interfere with the strength or dexterity for performing certain tasks. Personal stress, illness, low literacy, and lack of support are other examples of barriers to learning. Consider all barriers to learning before beginning to teach. Physical, occupational, or speech therapists can be helpful in helping the patient overcome these types of problems so patient education can begin. Barriers for the teacher (you) might include limitations on time, limited time to prepare for patient education, and lack of space and privacy.

Situational factors that interfere with learning include pain, nausea, fatigue, a sense of being overwhelmed by all that is happening, and multiple interruptions. Attempt to reduce such situational factors before beginning patient education by doing the following: (1) offer pain or nausea medication as needed, and then wait for the pain or nausea to be reduced before performing patient education; (2) present material in a calm, unhurried manner; and (3) place a "do not disturb, patient education in progress" sign on the door to avoid unnecessary interruptions.

Box 9.2 NANDA-I Diagnoses Related to Teaching and Learning

Examples of NANDA-I diagnoses that indicate the need for patient education include:

- Deficient knowledge
- Ineffective health maintenance
- Readiness for enhanced health management
- Readiness for enhanced parenting
- Readiness for enhanced self-care

Readiness to Learn

Assess the patient's readiness to learn. Motivation plays a large role in effective learning. The desire to return to independence or to return to the comfort of home is often the motivating factor. **Work with patients to show them the advantages of learning what they need to know.** Patient education sessions will be more successful if the patient is comfortable and rested and there are a minimum of interruptions.

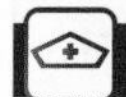 Clinical Cues

If the patient is in a double room and the roommate has several visitors who are making noise, take the patient to the conference room or other location for the patient education session, to promote better communication and reduce distractions.

Begin by establishing rapport and developing trust, and maintain a warm, sincere attitude.

Although several nursing diagnoses can be used for learning needs, the most commonly used one is *Deficient knowledge;* the specific need finishes the statement (Box 9.2).

Cultural Values and Expectations

The patient's cultural values and personal expectations regarding treatment and recovery may differ from those of the nurse and other health care providers. This can interfere with the patient's ability to cooperate and learn needed skills for self-care.

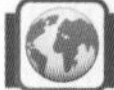 Cultural Considerations

Acceptance of Patient Education

While planning patient education for male patients of other cultures, find out if the man will be receptive to your patient education. Traditional older Japanese men may not heed what a younger female is trying to teach. This may apply in other cultures as well. Interaction with the family or with the patient himself can provide the needed information.

 QSEN Considerations: Patient-Centered Care

Working Within the Patient's Values and Cultural System

The patient may wish to use herb poultices on a wound rather than the medication the primary care provider prescribes. Often a compromise can be worked out, such as alternating the poultice with the medication prescribed (as long as the poultice is not harmful). As an aid to healing, patients may practice religious rituals with which the nurse is unfamiliar. In hospitals on American Indian reservations, it is common to see a physician and a tribal shaman working side by side, honoring the strong belief that physical healing must be accompanied by spiritual healing. Such practices rarely conflict with medical treatment and may greatly benefit the patient.

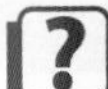 Think Critically

Can you think of a situation in which a patient's culture or value system might prevent his cooperation with learning self-care aspects of his treatment plan?

Confidence and Ability

Often patients express a lack of self-confidence, saying, "I'll never be able to do that." In such instances, you must explore these feelings, being careful to enhance rather than harm the patient's self-esteem. Praise and encouragement go much further than negativity in promoting needed learning. Patient education may need to be broken down into small steps.

 Communication

Teaching the Patient Who Lacks Self-Confidence

Mrs. Dunn, age 72, is to be discharged tomorrow. She has a wound on her left thigh that needs to be cleaned and dressed daily after discharge.

Nurse: "Mrs. Dunn, I've brought the supplies we need to do your dressing change."

Mrs. Dunn: "Oh, I don't think I can do it myself; it seems so complicated."

Nurse: "We'll work on it a step at a time. By the time you go home tomorrow, you will feel much better about it."

Mrs. Dunn: "Well, I'm willing to try. I do want to go home."

Nurse: "The first step is easy, we just wash our hands."

Mrs. Dunn: "Oh, good, I already know how to do that!"

Nurse: "Now, I use gloves here in the hospital, but you won't need to do that."

Mrs. Dunn: "I'm glad. Gloves make me so clumsy."

Nurse: "Are you right-handed? OK, remove the old dressing by gently holding the skin smooth with your left hand while pulling the tape up with your right hand."

Mrs. Dunn: "That was easy."

Nurse: "Good. Watch me open this package of gauze squares. Open the top and peel back the sides. Stop when you get to the bottom seam. Can you open that one for me?"

The patient picks up the package. She fumbles at first and then manages to grasp the edges and pull them apart as instructed. The nurse does not rush her.

Nurse: "Perfect. Now place it on the table with the paper side down, like this."

The patient places her pack as the nurse has shown her.

Nurse: "Now open the bottle of sterile water like this."

The nurse opens a bottle and sets the cap down on the table upside down.

Nurse: "By laying the cap down this way, the open side stays clean and will not contaminate the bottle when I put it back on. Now, you do it."

The patient picks up the bottle and twists it open, laying the cap on the table like the nurse did.

Nurse: "You're a fast learner, Mrs. Dunn. Now, pour a little on the gauze squares like this."

The patient watches and then pours some water in the middle of her gauze squares.

Nurse: "Now pick up one of the gauze squares and clean the wound just like the nurses have been doing it."

Mrs. Dunn: "I'll try, but this is the part that always hurts."

Nurse: "I know, but it usually hurts less when you do it yourself. And if it isn't cleaned out well, it won't heal. You can take some acetaminophen about an hour before you change the dressing. That will help. I'll do the first square, and then you do the second, OK?"

The nurse swabs out the wound gently.

Nurse: "Now you try it."

The patient picks up the gauze, squeezes out the excess water, and dabs a couple of times at the wound.

Mrs. Dunn: "Like that?"

Nurse: "Yes, that's the idea. See if you can go over the wound a little more slowly from top to bottom with a new gauze square. It's important to use a clean one each time you go back over the area."

Mrs. Dunn: "OK. Is this better?"

Mrs. Dunn cleans the area a little more thoroughly.

Nurse: "Yes. I'll give you some acetaminophen before we meet this afternoon and see if that makes it easier for you."

The nurse finishes cleaning the wound.

Nurse: "Now Mrs. Dunn, squeeze a bit of this antiseptic ointment into the wound."

Mrs. Dunn: "How much do I use?"

Nurse: "Just a line down the center. It will spread out when the dressing is applied."

The patient squeezes the ointment into the wound.

Nurse: "That's right. Now, for the dressing you want to use a non-adherent pad as the first layer. That way it won't stick to the wound. Cut the non-adherent pad in half. You can cut right through the closed package, and the second half will be in a wrapper waiting for next time."

Mrs. Dunn: "Oh, good. I hate to waste things."

Mrs. Dunn cuts the non-adherent pad in half.

Nurse: "Now, let's get the tape ready before you take the wrapper off the non-adherent pad. We will be putting gauze over the non-adherent pad and you will need to tape all the way around the edges. If you tear the four pieces of tape and gently stick one end to the table edge, they will be easy to get when you're ready for them."

Mrs. Dunn: "OK. This is what I do when I'm wrapping packages."

Nurse: "Then you are a tape pro, Mrs. Dunn. Now, lay the non-adherent pad on the wound and gently press it down. That spreads the ointment and the pad will stick and stay in place while you finish the dressing."

She watches while the patient places the non-adherent pad.

 Communication—cont'd

Nurse: "Great. Now open another pack of gauze squares like I showed you. Put those on top of the non-adherent pad and tape everything down."

Mrs. Dunn: "It's really important to get the tape ready first. Otherwise, you'd run out of hands!"

Nurse: "Exactly. Now, after each dressing change, you wash your hands again, and then you are done. See how well you did? Do you feel better about doing this now?"

Mrs. Dunn: "Quite a bit. I still feel all thumbs, though, and I worry about getting the sore clean enough by myself."

Nurse: "I think having some pain medicine will help. I'll bring your acetaminophen around 1:00, and we'll do the dressing again about 2:00."

Mrs. Dunn: "OK, and thank you. My husband will be here then. Is it okay if he watches?"

Nurse: "Absolutely. He can help you when you get home."

It is essential that the patient education plan be developed collaboratively, with input from all of the disciplines involved in the patient's care. The specifics of the plan should be discussed and agreed on. Each knowledge deficit is listed as it is identified, and the date is included. The person responsible for providing patient education in each area is also noted. The teacher may be the nurse, physical or occupational therapist, dietitian, speech therapist, or respiratory therapist. The nurse is responsible for overseeing the plan specifics. Even when another person is performing the patient education, the nurse reinforces it. For example, a patient who has undergone a traditional hip replacement surgery will be taught by the physical therapist to avoid crossing the legs or flexing the hip beyond 90 degrees. The nurse will reinforce this information, so it is important to know exactly what is being taught. Consistency in teaching is important if the patient is to master and retain new information.

Play techniques can be successful when teaching younger children. The use of dolls and play equipment is appropriate and helpful. Teaching must be done in short segments to allow for the child's limited attention span. Language must be tailored to the child's level of understanding. Children interpret language literally, so avoid idioms because they can be easily misunderstood.

When teaching older adults, the pace is slowed to allow more time for processing the information.

 Patient Education

Special Considerations When Teaching Older Adults

When preparing to teach older adults, consider the following:

- Provide good lighting; a light source coming over the shoulder of the patient is excellent.
- Provide written materials to reinforce the patient education.
- Use large type, black printing on nonglare paper for printed materials.
- Be certain the patient is wearing glasses, if needed, and that the lenses are clean.
- If the patient wears a hearing aid, be certain it is turned on and adjusted.
- Use short sentences and speak slowly; pause frequently to allow time for mental processing.
- Keep medical terms to a minimum and explain those you do use. Use specific terms when giving directions.
- Ask questions at frequent intervals to check for comprehension.
- Allow time for questions.
- State the most important points first, and repeat them at the end of the session.

Never assume that patients are literate. Many adults have completed schooling without learning to read adequately, and they may have spent a lifetime hiding this fact from others. A patient education plan that incorporates visual and kinesthetic techniques will often be the most effective for these individuals.

Some patients who speak English as a second language may not be able to read English, even if they are fully literate in their original language. When working with a patient for whom another language is primary, offer printed and audiovisual materials in their native language, if available. If English is limited, use an interpreter for patient education sessions.

When printed materials are used, review them with the patient and ask questions to determine whether the information has been understood. Be aware of the patient's educational level so that you can tailor your vocabulary and patient education materials, but avoid talking down to people. **Assess what patients already know about the information or skills they need to learn so that you can build on their current knowledge base.** Do they have a basic knowledge of anatomy and how the body works? What do they already know about their medications? If they are going to give their own injections, have they ever handled a needle and syringe before? These are all examples of health literacy, or the ability to understand basic health information and services that the patient needs in order to make the best decisions they can regarding their healthcare. Patient education is most effective when you can relate the material to a subject that patients already understand. It can also be helpful to determine whether they have a relative or close friend who is knowledgeable about their health issues and willing to help them after discharge.

THE PATIENT EDUCATION PLAN

Preparing a patient education plan involves analyzing the assessment data, establishing behavioral objectives or goals, and creating a plan for assisting the patient in achieving these goals in the most timely and effective manner. **Behavioral objectives** represent the desired changes or additions to current behaviors and attitudes, and should be meaningful for the patient. They state what you are trying to teach the patient to do. "Patient will change the wound dressing using aseptic technique" is a behavioral objective. Behavioral objectives should be stated in terms that make their achievement easy to evaluate. The above objective would be evaluated by watching the patient change the wound dressing and determining whether aseptic technique was used.

The patient education plan is part of the care plan. Some agencies use a separate form for the patient education plan so that there is plenty of room to note the specifics. Specialty areas may have a standardized patient education plan. An example would be postpartum patient education plans for self-care after delivery or for basic infant care.

RESOURCES FOR PATIENT EDUCATION

Many books and articles provide suggested methods and patient education aids for particular topics. Audiovisual materials, pamphlets, and hands-on equipment are also good resources. Become familiar with what is available in your facility. Many agencies have closed-circuit TV patient education modules available on the room televisions. Community agencies may also provide educational tools. Local government agencies often provide printed and online listings of community public service programs. Nursing specialists may be available to assist with information and patient education plans or to do the actual teaching. Hospital social workers and patient representatives are also good sources of information about what is available.

Some instructional materials are designed to assist the medical professional, and others are directed to the patient. The Internet has a wide variety of resources available for patient education, but not all are medically sound. You must ensure reliability of the source and not rely on blogs or opinion. For example, for up-to-date medical recommendations on vaccinating children, the advice of the American Academy of Pediatrics will be medically sound advice, whereas the opinion of a famous actor will not necessarily be based on scientific best evidence. An Internet search by topic will provide links to myriad resources. Leading medical centers and universities across the United States and Canada, as well as governmental agencies such as the National Institutes of Health (NIH), the Centers for Disease Control and Prevention (CDC), and the National Institute of Mental Health (NIMH), have websites with excellent patient education resources.

IMPLEMENTING THE PLAN

Begin by establishing a time with the patient to begin the teaching. Patient education should be done at a time when visitors, physician rounds, and treatments will not cause interruptions. Patient education can be done one-on-one or in a group setting. Be certain that the room temperature is acceptable and the patient is comfortable. Medicate the patient before the teaching session if pain control is needed. Provide good lighting. Be certain he can hear and see you adequately.

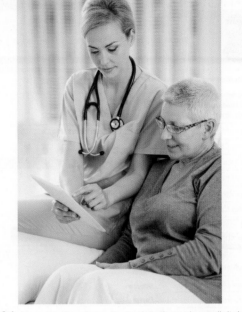

FIGURE 9.1 Nurse performing patient education using a digital tablet. (Photo copyright istock.com.)

Keep the patient education session short. Involve the patient in the process; call him by name, and ask for feedback as you progress. If teaching a group, establish eye contact frequently with each person in the group. Pause at intervals and ask if there are questions. When teaching a procedure, discuss the steps of the procedure, demonstrate the procedure, and then talk patients through each step while they perform it (Fig. 9.1). Have them write down the steps, or provide them with a written guide they can follow.

Performing daily care for your patient is a perfect time for patient education. Although there will be specific patient education sessions, view every nurse-patient interaction as an opportunity for patient education. Teaching is not a "one-time" item to check off your daily task list; rather, it is a continuous process. Teaching patients to perform range-of-motion exercises on their weak extremities can be done while bathing them. Teaching about wound care can accompany the process of changing the dressing. Reinforcing information about a medication can be done when administering the medication.

The patient needs to receive written or printed information about what has been taught to take home: for instance, a pamphlet or clearly written list of steps to accomplish a procedure, such as performing a blood glucose determination. When possible, this should be in the patient's primary language.

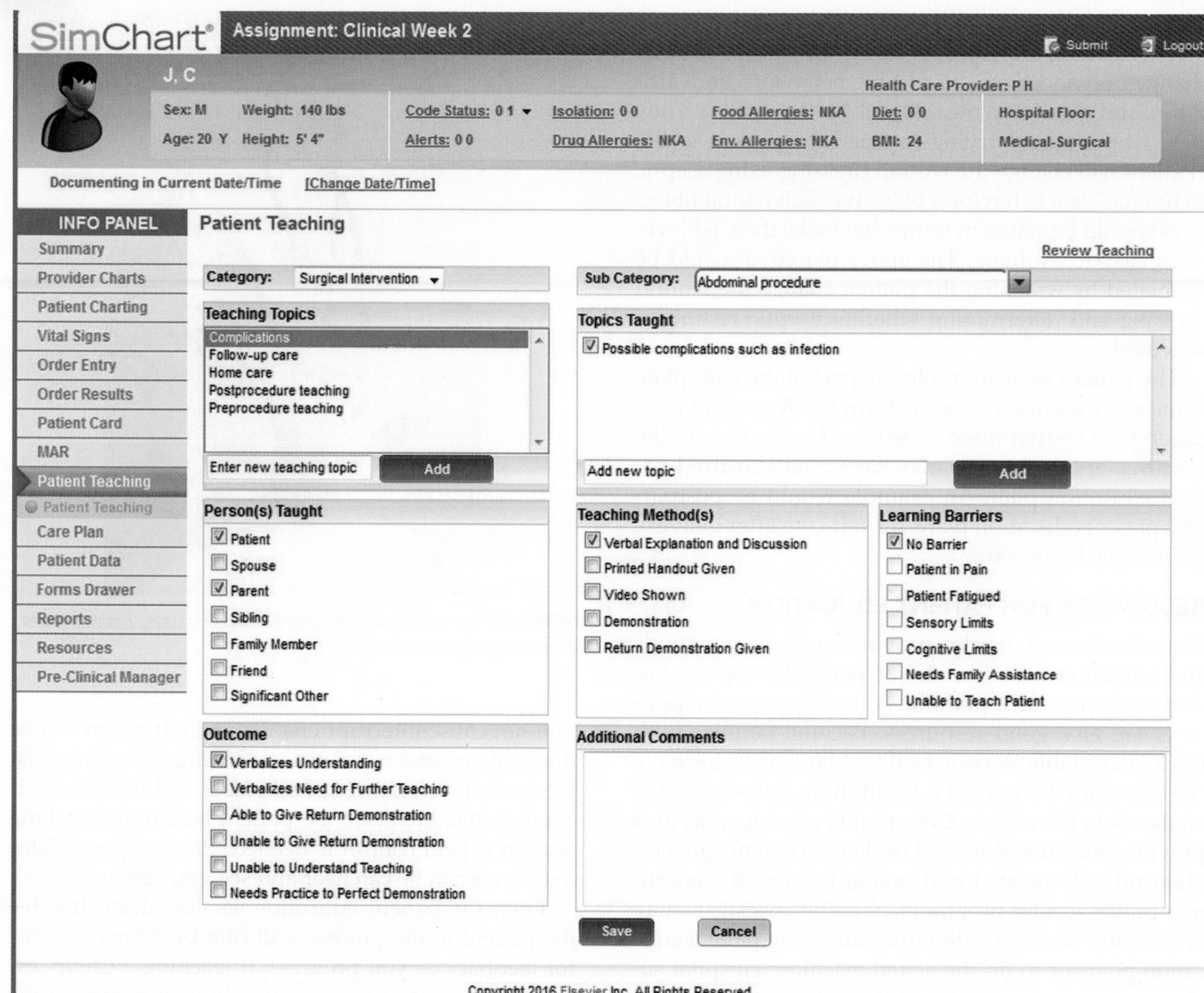

FIGURE 9.2 SIM chart patient education screen shot.

Legal and Ethical Considerations

Use of an Interpreter

Health care facilities must use an interpreter or a telephone interpretation service when obtaining a history or providing necessary patient instruction to someone who does not have a language in common with the health care staff.

Allow patients to perform at their own speed. The first step is learning to do the skill correctly. Performance will become more rapid with practice. Learning is a process of many steps, and rushing these steps can cause confusion, frustration, and a sense of failure for both the patient and the nurse. Plan a time to review what has been taught. If patient education occurs over several sessions, each patient education session should begin with a review of what was previously learned. If the patient was taught a specific skill, such as drawing up insulin, have the patient demonstrate that skill. This is called a **return demonstration.**

EVALUATION

Evaluating the effectiveness of patient education is critical to the success of the process. It involves giving and obtaining **feedback** (return of information about the process) from the patient regarding what was taught, then using this feedback to determine whether effective learning has in fact taken place. A return demonstration of a skill is one way of evaluating the patient's learning. Point out what steps were done correctly and gently make suggestions about needed corrections in the procedure. When the patient is learning information rather than a skill, ask questions to obtain feedback about retention and comprehension of the material taught. Allow the patient time to think through the answers. Let the patient use any printed materials handed out. This shows you that the patient can appropriately use the resources you provided. Make positive comments about the retained information.

 Life Span Considerations

Older Adults

Writing down the steps of a procedure helps all learners focus. It is particularly helpful for assisting older adults in increasing and integrating the information. It also aids recall of the information and assists in diminishing any sensory distraction such as background noise.

If the return demonstration or the review questions indicate that the patient has not mastered the skill or material taught, you would need to repeat the instruction and reevaluate performance before going on to a new area of patient education. It may also be necessary to alter the method of teaching to use the patient's strongest learning strategies more effectively. The patient education plan should be adjusted and updated according to the evaluation data obtained. New learning needs may also be identified during the teaching and evaluation sessions. These need to be included in the patient education plan.

DOCUMENTATION

Patient education often occurs informally while performing a nursing task such as administering medications. This makes it a challenge to document patient education consistently. Each nurse is legally responsible for providing patient education, and documentation is essential. The following information should be documented: Specific content taught, the method of teaching used, and evidence of evaluation with specific results of the teaching. This allows nurses providing continuing care for the patient to follow up and reinforce the patient education (Fig. 9.2).

COORDINATION WITH DISCHARGE PLANNING

Patients may be discharged home before necessary learning is complete. Information regarding the patient's education needs to be communicated to the primary care provider's office. If the patient is being referred for home health services, it is also necessary to communicate the information to the home care nurse. In addition, the family or significant others who will be caring for the patient should be included in the patient education sessions. When the patient lives alone, it is important to assess accurately whether he has the motor skills necessary to care for himself. Specific learning needs that remain should be discussed with all involved parties, including the patient, and the plan for teaching shared. Send a printed plan home with the patient. A telephone call to the home health agency or to the primary care provider's office helps provide continuity of teaching.

Get Ready for the NCLEX Examination!

Key Points

- Nurses continually teach patients about aspects of their disease or disorder, diet, medications, treatment, and self-care.
- Patient education is a major part of patient care.
- There are three methods of learning: visual, auditory, and kinesthetic.
- The first step in patient education is to assess what the patient needs to know (learning needs and knowledge deficits).
- Many factors can affect learning: physical limitations, situational factors (including pain), readiness to learn, personal values and expectations, age, attitude, and ability to comprehend.
- Environmental factors such as room temperature, noise level, lighting, and interruptions by others can affect learning.
- Establishing rapport and mutual trust are essential to effective patient education.
- A patient education plan is devised and documented based on the patient's learning needs.
- Learning needs must be prioritized to ensure that patients learn those things most important to safe self-care before discharge.
- Books, articles, pamphlets, audiovisual materials, and demonstration equipment are good resources for patient education. Nursing specialists are another resource.
- Including the patient in the development of the plan will help keep the patient involved in the education process.
- Patient education may occur one-on-one or in a group setting.
- Evaluating the effectiveness of patient education is critical to the success of the process.
- To evaluate, obtain feedback from the patient either by question and answer or ask for a return demonstration.
- Documentation of patient education and the learning achieved is a legal responsibility and should be done consistently.
- Collaboration with other health care professionals involved in the patient's care is essential for uniformity and continuity of teaching.

Additional Learning Resources

SG Go to your Study Guide for additional learning activities to help you master this chapter content.

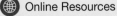

evolve Go to your Evolve website at http://evolve.elsevier.com/Williams/fundamental for additional online resources.

 Online Resources

- *Health Canada*, www.hc-sc.gc.ca/ahc-asc/activit/about-apropos/index-eng.php
- *Healthy People 2020 Goals and Objectives*, www.healthypeople.gov/2020/topicsobjectives2020/default.aspx

Review Questions for the NCLEX Examination

*Choose the **best** answer for each question.*

1. Evidence that the primary purpose of patient education has been achieved is that patients:
   1. Share with others what they have learned.
   2. Reduce the time they are hospitalized.
   3. Follow the treatment plan prescribed.
   4. Provide correct and safe self-care after discharge.
2. A patient who underwent an appendectomy asks the nurse about caring for his incision. He states that he is an auditory learner. The nurse determines that he will best learn by:
   1. Watching the nurse perform the care.
   2. Reading a pamphlet on how to perform incision care.
   3. Listening to the nurse's verbal instructions about care of the incision.
   4. Opening the packaging and placing the dressing on his wound himself.
3. A patient newly diagnosed with diabetes has stated that he doesn't understand why he needs insulin. His statement indicates a learning need regarding:
   1. The disease process of diabetes.
   2. The types of insulin available.
   3. The diet a diabetic needs to follow.
   4. The role weight management plays in treatment.
4. When starting the second teaching session for a patient, the nurse should first:
   1. Present the new material to be covered in this session.
   2. Question the patient about learning from the first session.
   3. Briefly review what was taught in the first session.
   4. Review the entire patient education plan.
5. When first teaching a young child about insulin injections, an appropriate approach would be to:
   1. Teach in a group setting.
   2. Use a needle, a syringe, and an insulin vial.
   3. Use a doll to demonstrate an insulin injection.
   4. Set firm limits on behavior while teaching.
6. To overcome barriers to learning for a hearing impaired person: *(Select all that apply.)*
   1. Make certain there is adequate light in the room.
   2. Be certain the hearing aid is turned on and adjusted.
   3. Eliminate other noise in the room as much as possible.
   4. Provide colored pictures of the steps of the procedure being taught.
   5. Speak loudly, repeating each statement.
   6. Gain the patient's attention and speak in a normal low tone while facing him.
7. A nurse is caring for a patient who can speak and understand some English but is not fluent. The nurse should:
   1. Use a professional or certified interpreter from the hospital's list of available interpreters.
   2. Ask one of the patient's children to help with interpretation.
   3. Ask a family member to help with the interpretation.
   4. Ask an employee from another department to assist with the interpretation.

Critical Thinking Activities

Read each clinical scenario and discuss the questions with your classmates.

Scenario A
Identify factors that you think might interfere with learning for a patient.

Scenario B
Discuss cultural or religious beliefs that you think might have a direct effect on the patient's patient education plan.

Scenario C
Assess the learning needs of three patients, and then share commonalities of those needs with your clinical group.

chapter 10

Delegation, Leadership, and Management

http://evolve.elsevier.com/Williams/fundamental

Objectives

Upon completing this chapter, you should be able to do the following:

Theory

1. Differentiate between the three different leadership styles discussed in the chapter.
2. Compare and contrast examples of effective and ineffective communication.
3. Describe four characteristics of an effective leader.
4. List four considerations for delegating tasks to UAPs.
5. Explain why interpersonal relationships are important when delegating and managing others.
6. Compare and contrast the skills and functions of the team leader with those of the charge nurse.
7. Identify management functions of the LPN/LVN working in a long-term care facility, home care, or an outpatient clinic.
8. Discuss techniques of effective time management.
9. Explain the importance of the readback for verbal or telephone orders.

Clinical Practice

1. Determine the leadership style of the charge nurse on the unit to which you are assigned.
2. Appropriately delegate three tasks to a nursing assistant or UAP.
3. Create a time-efficient work organization plan for a shift.
4. Demonstrate proficient use of the hospital computer.
5. Accurately and carefully acknowledge orders per facility policy.
6. Document accurately for reimbursement.
7. Know your facility's policies and procedures, and uphold the standards of nursing practice.
8. Find a mentor who can coach you on improving your delegation and management skills.

Key Terms

accountable (p. 132)
authority (p. 132)
autocratic (aw-tō-KRĂ-tĭk, p. 130)
collaboration (p. 130)
competence (p. 132)
confidence (p. 132)
conflict resolution (p. 132)
constructive criticism (p. 133)
delegate (p. 130)
democratic (p. 130)
interpersonal relationships (p. 130)
laissez-faire (LĔS-ā-FĂR, p. 130)
mediate (MĒ-dē-āt, p. 132)
mentor (p. 138)
responsibility (p. 130)
risk management (p. 138)
self-esteem (p. 132)
stat orders (p. 137)
unlicensed assistive personnel (ŭn-LĪ-sĕnst ă-SĬS-tĭv pĕr-sŏ-NĔL, p. 130)

 Concepts Covered in This Chapter

- Care coordination
- Caregiving
- Clinical judgment
- Collaboration
- Communication
- Culture
- Evidence
- Family dynamics
- Infection
- Leadership
- Pain
- Professionalism

The licensed practical nurse (LPN) and licensed vocational nurse (LVN) are taking on more and more leadership functions, particularly in the skilled nursing facility. Leadership is a comprehensive process that includes the guidance of staff and the effective use of resources to meet patient needs. Leadership requires a good understanding of one's self and a good grasp of basic management techniques. This chapter discusses management skills and leadership qualities that the LPN/LVN needs to be effective beginning during the first year after graduation.

THE CHAIN OF COMMAND

Once you are hired, become familiar with the organizational structure of the facility where you work. This information is provided during your formal orientation. Be certain you know the chain of command for your area. Who is your immediate supervisor? From whom do you take orders? To whom does your supervisor report? To whom should you report changes in patient condition or signs of complications? To whom do you go with concerns or complaints? Who is in charge of scheduling? What is the procedure for calling in sick?

LEADERSHIP STYLES

Most leaders employ a blend of leadership styles. A permissive or **laissez-faire** leader does not attempt to control the team and offers little if any direction. This leader assumes that team members are competent and self-directed and will do what needs to be done correctly and efficiently. This leader may have a need to be liked by everyone and therefore avoids any blame for things that go wrong by allowing members to function completely independently. Although this leadership style usually is not effective in the day-to-day management of patient care operations, it can be effective in certain situations involving a highly motivated, highly creative group that works well with minimal guidance—for example, a committee.

The authoritarian or **autocratic** leader tightly controls team members. Staff members are rarely consulted when decisions are being made. Rules are set without input from the staff, and directives and orders are given out constantly. This type of leadership style has been described as "my way or the highway." **The leader closely supervises the work of each staff member.** When mistakes are made, they are quickly pointed out. The leader's goal is accomplishment of tasks efficiently without regard to people.

The **democratic** leader consults with staff members and seeks staff participation in decision making. The team members' skills and knowledge are readily used to ensure efficient team functioning. Team members are respected as individuals, and there is an open and trusting attitude. The democratic leader is part of the team, not above it, and accepts **responsibility** for the team's actions.

There is no one set of qualities that makes a good leader. Box 10.1 lists responses that nurses have given when asked what they think makes a good leader. Such a leader instills confidence, trust, and spirit in the team. Appropriate leadership fosters growth among the team members.

? Think Critically

Consider what leadership qualities you have and what qualities you would aspire to achieve. With what type of leader would you prefer to work? Why? When would autocratic leadership be important? Why?

Box 10.1 Attributes of a Strong Nursing Leader

- Ability to teach
- Active listener
- Articulate
- Assertive
- Calm
- Considerate
- Consistent
- Decisive
- Excellent clinical skills
- Excellent problem solver
- Fair
- Flexible
- Good role model
- Good sense of humor
- Objective
- Open minded
- Organized
- Responsible
- Sensitive
- Strong character
- Tactful

KEYS TO EFFECTIVE LEADERSHIP

As an LPN/LVN, you will be expected to work with other members of the health care team. **Collaboration (working together) is essential for patient care.** Collaborative practice includes learning to work effectively with **unlicensed assistive personnel** (UAPs). UAPs include unit secretaries, nursing assistants, homemaking aides, housekeeping personnel, and technicians.

QSEN Considerations: Teamwork and Collaboration

Delegation

To collaborate with unlicensed assistive personnel, you must learn to **delegate** (entrust to another) tasks appropriately and effectively.

EFFECTIVE COMMUNICATION AND RELATIONSHIPS

Strong nursing leaders use good communication skills and recognize that every team member has a valuable role in patient care. Communicating in direct, concise terms in a tactful, friendly, nonthreatening way is essential to create a supportive and healthy work environment. Obtaining feedback about directions given and listening actively and mindfully (see Chapter 8) to reports, suggestions, and complaints establishes a pattern for two-way communication. This helps the leader stay in tune with the atmosphere, attitudes, and problems of others on the health care team. Showing care and concern for team members can help develop positive **interpersonal relationships** that promote team cooperation. Relationships and trust develop over time through conversations and interactions. The Joint Commission emphasizes the importance of communication by health care providers in one of its National Patient Safety Goals.

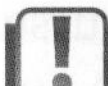
Safety Alert

National Patient Safety Goal 2

The Joint Commission has set the following goal for health care facilities: **"Improve staff communication."**

One component of this goal is to, "Get important test results to the right staff person on time."

Introduction, situation, background, assessment, recommendation, and readback (ISBAR-R) communication (see Chapter 8) is a communication tool that many institutions are adopting to improve communication among staff.

QSEN Considerations: Safety

Safety and Communication

Your role as patient advocate is one of your most important nursing roles. There are times when you must speak up when you disagree with the decisions or actions of others. Speaking up can be intimidating, especially to someone with more experience than you. Tools you can employ:

1. **The Two Challenge Rule**: voicing your concern at least twice to promote acknowledgment by the receiver. The first challenge is usually in the form of a question ("Doctor, the patient is having blood pressure problems, should she still be discharged?"). The second challenge should provide support for the concern and may be presented by the person making the initial challenge or by another team member ("The patient has had a drop in blood pressure of 20 mmHg, and her heart rate has increased by 30 beats per minute. I am concerned that she is too unstable to be discharged home."). The two challenge rule ensures that the concern has been heard, understood, and acknowledged.
2. **The CUS Technique**: **c**oncern, **u**ncomfortable, **s**afety. State your concern. State why you are uncomfortable. State the safety issue involved.

Source: Agency for Healthcare Research and Quality (2014). Pocket guide: TeamSTEPPS. www.ahrq.gov/professionals/education/curriculum-tools/teamstepps/instructor/essentials/pocketguide.html#communication

Communicating effectively includes taking the time to attend to the person by stopping what you are doing, establishing eye contact, being polite by saying "please" and "thank you," and using a warm tone of voice (Fig. 10.1). A smile adds warmth to the interaction. Saying, "I would like you to take vital signs on the right side of the hall, please," rather than "Go and take vital signs on that side of the hall," usually enlists better cooperation and a more pleasant attitude toward the task. Your style of communication and actions also reflect your trust and respect toward others. Consider the other person's culture and how it may affect verbal and nonverbal communication (see Chapter 8). **Treat others how you would like to be treated.**

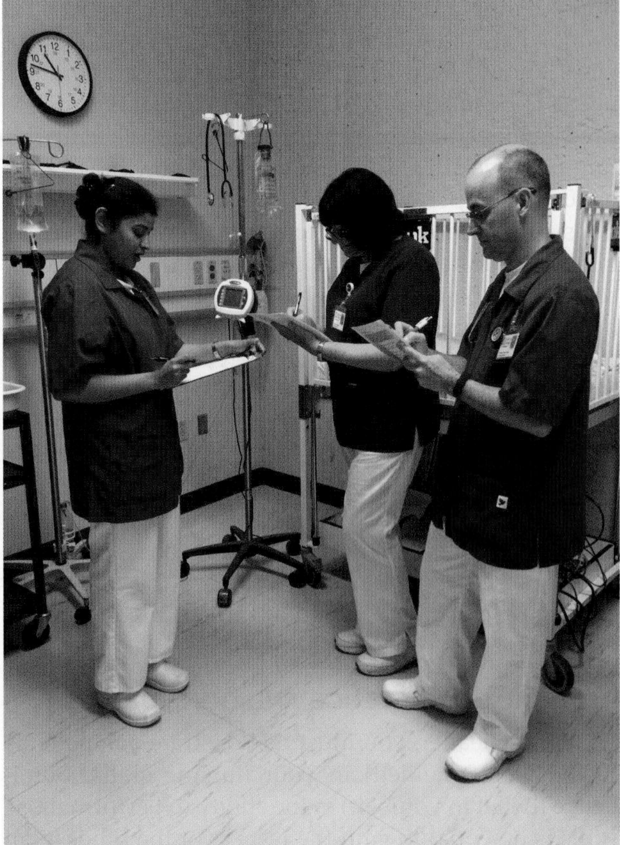

FIGURE 10.1 Charge nurse delegating a task to staff nurses.

QSEN Considerations: Teamwork and Collaboration

Strategies for Communicating Information With the Team

1. Briefing: often used when there is new information to be shared. The Team Leader initiates the briefing. Included in a briefing: (a) who is in charge, (b) lines of communication, and (c) member responsibilities and expected behaviors.
2. Call-Out: a strategy for communicating important information during an urgent or emergent patient situation to keep everyone informed about what is happening (example: "patient's BP is falling: from 100/60 down to 80/40").
3. Check-back: used to make sure information was received correctly. (a) Sender communicates a message; (b) receiver acknowledges that message was received and states it back; (c) sender verifies that the message was received correctly.
4. Huddle: an impromptu meeting held when the need arises. A huddle is a chance for team members to touch base with each other, evaluate changes in the plan that might be needed, and reorganize the work flow.
5. Debrief: an informal meeting held after a situation or event to discuss the event; usually including what went well, what didn't work, and how the situation might be handled differently next time.

Source: Agency for Healthcare Research and Quality (2014). Pocket guide: TeamSTEPPS. www.ahrq.gov/professionals/education/curriculum-tools/teamstepps/instructor/essentials/pocketguide.html#communication

When assigning tasks, be specific about what is to be done, how it is to be done, and when the task is to be completed. It is better to say, "Please take Mrs.

Jones' temperature at 2:00 pm and let me know right away what it is so that I can let her primary care provider know," than to state, "Mrs. Jones' temperature needs to be taken at 2:00 pm." Likewise, it is better to say, "Tell me immediately if Mr. Hernandez's temperature is above 101.2°F," than "Let me know if Mr. Hernandez's temperature is high." Ask if there are questions before ending the interaction, and follow up to make certain the task was completed on time. Avoid conflict by being thorough when giving directions, making a request, or assigning a task. If a conflict does arise, try to remain calm and open and actively listen to the problem. Accept responsibility for any part you played in development of the conflict. Focus on the issue rather than on the feelings of those involved. **Mediate** (settle differences) by communicating openly. Sort out the issues involved by identifying key themes in the discussion. Consider the options and weigh the consequences of each option. Choose the option for **conflict resolution** (resolving a conflict) that offers the best outcome.

CLINICAL COMPETENCE AND CONFIDENCE

As a nurse leader, you must demonstrate **competence** (being well qualified) in your nursing skills. **Confidence** (belief in yourself) in the ability to perform those skills is essential to gain the respect of the other team members. Along with this competence and confidence should be sufficient **self-esteem** (pride in yourself) to readily admit when a mistake has been made or when you don't know something. Announcing "I don't know, but I will find out" is the best way to handle these situations. Others will respect you more if you admit that you don't know everything. This shows that you are human and provides an atmosphere in which others can admit what they do not know and can ask for help.

ORGANIZATION

Being a leader requires good organization. Organizing the work of a unit requires strong time management skills. Plan each day carefully with some built-in flexibility for unforeseen events. Knowing the strengths of each member of the health care team helps you more effectively divide the workload. Decision-making ability is needed to quickly divide up patients and assign tasks to various personnel.

Problem-solving skills provide the means for making difficult decisions. The problem-solving process is much like the nursing process. The good problem solver first defines the problem (assessment) and then looks at the alternatives. The outcomes of using each of the alternatives are estimated (planning), and then one of the alternatives is chosen to be tried as the solution to the problem (implementation). If the alternative chosen does not solve the problem, then the whole process is repeated (evaluation). See Chapter 4, Critical Thinking.

DELEGATION

In beginning the discussion of delegation, it is helpful to contrast it with the term *assignment*. Assignment of tasks is a method of distributing the unit's workload, usually by the charge nurse. In assignment, the nurse directs the UAPs to complete tasks within their job description—tasks for which they are hired and paid to perform. This always occurs at the start of the shift, but may also occur at any time during the shift. In contrast, delegation occurs when a licensed nurse transfers the **authority** to perform a selected nursing duty in a selected patient situation. In delegating a task to a UAP, you are, in essence, "sharing" power with your UAPs. **Many states do not allow LPNs/LVNs to delegate,** and even in a state where it is allowed, you must also be certain that delegation is allowed in your facility.

Delegation is done with careful thought; for example, it is not appropriate to delegate a nursing duty simply because you dislike it. Furthermore, you must be certain that the individual to whom you are about to delegate is competent to perform such a duty (written evidence of competence is best, to be described shortly), that the patient situation is stable, and that the task has a predictable outcome.

You are accountable (must answer) for the tasks you delegate, if in fact you are permitted by law to delegate. Legally, you are responsible and accountable for the outcome of any task you delegate to another. Delegating appropriately means that you must (1) know the capabilities and competencies of the person to whom you are delegating, (2) know whether or not the task falls within the domain of tasks that can legally be delegated by you, (3) communicate effectively with the person to whom you are delegating, and (4) understand the patient's needs.

Before any tasks are delegated to a nursing assistant or other UAP, that person should be thoroughly oriented to the facility and the unit. **Competencies of unlicensed personnel must be documented before tasks are delegated to them.** This requires evidence of a training program and **written evidence by a qualified nurse or instructor that the person has demonstrated competence in the task or skill.** If you do not have access to such written documentation, it is best to observe the UAP perform the task or skill the first time you delegate it to verify that a level of competence has been reached. If the task has not been a part of the UAP's formal training program, then you should demonstrate how the task should be done and ask for a return demonstration. Within the area of general competencies, the UAP should be assessed for competence in patient safety issues such as infection control and moving and positioning patients.

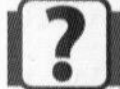 **Think Critically**

How would you tactfully tell a unlicensed assistive personnel that you would like to see him perform a particular task before assigning him to do it on his own?

Box 10.2 Tasks That Can Be Delegated to Unlicensed Assistive Personnel[a]

- Applying a condom catheter
- Applying a hearing aid
- Applying cold packs
- Applying elastic stockings
- Applying warm compresses
- Assisting to deep breathe and cough
- Assisting with ambulation
- Giving a bath
- Making a bed
- Performing fingerstick blood glucose monitoring
- Collecting specimens
- Emptying drainage containers
- Feeding patients
- Filling water pitchers
- Giving a sitz bath
- Administering an enema
- Giving a vaginal douche
- Measuring weight and height
- Measuring vital signs
- Performing oral hygiene
- Performing range-of-motion exercises
- Providing hair care
- Providing skin care
- Recording intake and output
- Removing a urinary catheter
- Repositioning patients
- Stocking supplies
- Taking specimens to the laboratory
- Toileting patients
- Transferring patient to a chair or bed
- Turning patients

[a]May vary from state to state or facility to facility.

Be familiar with your state's nurse practice act so that you know what tasks and skills fall within your legal domain. This tells you what you must *not* delegate. In addition, some professional nursing organizations, such as the American Association of Critical-Care Nurses (www.aacn.org), have documents that outline examples of tasks that might be appropriate for delegation; however, you must ensure that this matches what is allowed in your state. Your agency should have a job description that spells out what the UAPs can and cannot do. Be certain that you are familiar with the UAP job descriptions before you delegate a task. **It is up to you to know what the UAP cannot do.** The agency's policies and procedures and the standards of practice for your area of nursing help to define what the UAP is allowed to do (Box 10.2). **Assessment or aspects of the analysis, planning, or evaluation phases of the nursing process must be performed by the registered nurse (RN). These functions cannot be delegated to unlicensed personnel.** Most tasks that are delegated to UAPs are technical, repetitive skills that have a predictable patient outcome. **Interventions that require clinical judgment should not be delegated.**

It is important to remember the goal and purpose of delegation. Nurses delegate to complete more work in the same time frame; however, delegated work must be done safely, correctly, and cost-effectively. Effective delegation includes giving feedback on how the task was performed. Give praise where it is due; share favorable comments from patients about the UAP's work and interactions. If the delegated task did not go as expected, communicate exactly what went wrong in a supportive manner. **Provide privacy before giving criticism.** Be tactful. You might share that the patient was upset that it took three tries for the UAP to obtain an accurate blood pressure. Asking, "Do you think you need some more supervised practice and suggestions on how to take blood pressures smoothly? Would you like me to demonstrate it again?" allows the UAP a face-saving way to admit that more instruction is needed. Ask what might help the UAP perform better the next time.

When giving **constructive criticism**, begin by tactfully acknowledging feelings or expressing empathy. Statements such as, "I understand that we are one aide short today," begin the interaction on a less threatening note. Next describe the behavior. An example would be, "I've noticed that on three mornings this week it has been 9:30 am before vital signs you took were recorded." Then state the expectation for future compliance such as "The vital signs need to be recorded no later than 8:30 am from now on." Finally, state the consequences if the expected action does not occur. This can be done by stating something like, "The primary care providers and medication nurses have to track you down when the vital signs are not posted on time. This can affect patient safety and care. If vital sign recording is late again, I will have to document your inability to complete the task on time." **When performance by a UAP has been poor, document the specific facts (not your opinions).** The unit manager should also be made aware of the performance problem.

When delegating a variety of tasks, help the UAP prioritize the order in which they should be done. It takes many months for most UAPs to be able to discern which tasks take priority over others.

The patient must be told when an unlicensed person will be performing some tasks that were formerly only performed by nurses. This is within the domain of a patient's rights. Simply tell the patient that you, the nurse, have primary responsibility for the care given, but that the UAP is your assistant and will be doing certain tasks.

LEADERSHIP ROLES

BEGINNING LEADERSHIP ROLES

Initially, the new LPN/LVN performs leadership functions in working with UAPs, including delegation of tasks and supervision of the UAPs' work. Later, after being thoroughly oriented to the facility and its

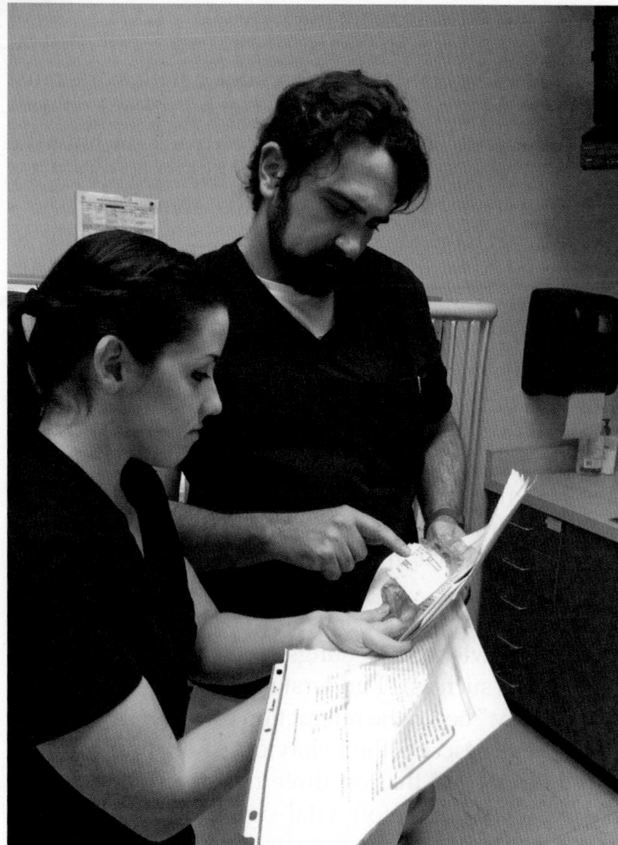

FIGURE 10.2 Charge nurse discussing a new procedure with a staff nurse.

policies and demonstrating competence, team leading may be required. A team leader coordinates and makes assignments for other personnel, assists with patient care, helps resolve conflicts, assists in writing policies and procedures, contributes information for evaluation of UAPs, and collaborates with physicians and other health team members.

When working in a medical clinic, the LPN/LVN team leader is often responsible for overseeing the scheduling of patients, performing quality improvement audits, training staff, evaluating staff, coordinating team members to accomplish the daily work, assisting in writing policies and procedures, attending staff meetings, and resolving staff conflicts (Fig. 10.2).

? Think Critically

What leadership functions do licensed practical nurses/licensed vocational nurses perform in the facility in which you are assigned for clinical experience?

ADVANCED LEADERSHIP ROLES

Eventually the LPN/LVN may become a charge nurse or a supervisor of UAPs in settings such as home care or outpatient clinics. A charge nurse must have training and experience in nursing administration and supervision plus additional preparation in a specialized area in many states. A minimum of 1 year of staff nurse experience is often required before taking on charge nurse duties. Sometimes, however, life experience in other roles can speed up the assumption of the leadership role.

The ability to recognize significant changes in patient condition and to take necessary action is a primary quality in a charge nurse. The charge nurse is the manager's designee and has all of the manager's authority for the shift; he is **responsible for the total nursing care of the patients on the unit during the shift.**

In a long-term care facility, the charge nurse receives the report from the previous shift, makes patient assignments, makes rounds and assesses all patients, directs the administration of medications and treatments, confers with team members throughout the shift, and reports to the oncoming shift on patient status. Charge nurses may also oversee training of UAPs and evaluate the unit's health team members. Charge nurses must be skilled at conflict resolution.

? Think Critically

Tips for Conflict Resolution

Conflict may arise for various reasons: different priorities, different values, varying perception of events. The following are some strategies to remember in conflict resolution:

1. Choose a private location away from others. This gives everyone the best chance of speaking honestly, rather than posturing.
2. Focus on the issue at hand, not the personalities involved.
3. Focus on an observable goal that can be achieved, whether a large one (e.g., "I'd like to see a harmonious work place where everyone wants to deliver excellent patient care") or a smaller one ("I'd like to see you two work together as a team").
4. Begin by discussing the positive aspects you observe before discussing the negative aspects.
5. Use "I" statements, not blaming.
6. Try to get to the heart of the conflict. It may take time and effort to expose. For example, one nurse may have "excellent patient care" as her main objective, and the other nurse's primary goal is to "get out on time." As the facilitator of the conflict resolution, you must point out that these goals are not incompatible, and can both be achieved with careful thought ("win-win").
7. Strive for "win-win" rather than "win-lose" outcome. Win-win takes more time and effort, and may require more than one conflict resolution session to achieve.

Sources: Agency for Healthcare Research and Quality (2014). Pocket guide: TeamSTEPPS. www.ahrq.gov/professionals/education/curriculum-tools/teamstepps/instructor/essentials/pocketguide.html#communication; Covey, S. R., (2004), Collins, J. (2013), Covey, S. (2013). The 7 habits of highly effective people. Powerful lessons in personal change (25th Anniversary ed.). New York, NY: Simon & Schuster; and Zerwekh, J., & Garneau, A. Z. (2015).Nursing today: transitions and trends (8th ed). Philadelphia, PA: Elsevier Saunders.

MANAGEMENT SKILLS FOR THE LICENSED PRACTICAL NURSE/LICENSED VOCATIONAL NURSE

All nurses are expected to be able to manage time, use a computer, order supplies, acknowledge orders, place telephone calls to primary care providers and families, process verbal orders, and document care appropriately, including for reimbursement of patient costs.

An LPN/LVN working in a home care agency may be asked to assign and supervise nursing assistants and home health aides, including making patient care assignments, assisting with orientation and evaluation, verifying that documentation for reimbursement is correctly completed, and giving and receiving reports on assigned patients.

TIME MANAGEMENT

Leaders need to use time efficiently. Learning certain techniques will help with your time management. Begin each workday by making a "to-do" list before the shift starts, providing a loose structure for the day. Formulate one or two broad goals for the day.

The goal for the home care nurse might be "to complete four visits by lunchtime." This would involve organizing and planning the most efficient order for patient visits, gathering all needed supplies, notifying each patient of the approximate time of the visit, organizing paperwork to be completed, and making certain the car has gas.

Organizing for the workday in a medical clinic varies depending on the type of clinic and the nurse's assigned duties. The goals for a clinic nurse might be to "ensure rooms are stocked and set up for treatments, and patients are roomed in an efficient manner." Obtain history and initiate documentation in the electronic medical records (EMR) for patients scheduled to be seen, update medication list in EMR, anticipate and perform specimen collection, replenish supplies in examining rooms, and other duties.

For the staff nurse in the hospital, the shift's goal might be to "ensure that all assigned patients are kept comfortable and safe and that all scheduled treatments and medications are given." After you receive the shift report and obtain patient assignments, set your priorities. Identify the patients with the most urgent or life-threatening problems. Which patients are physically unstable and need to be checked frequently? Which patients have frequently scheduled treatments? Which patients are at highest risk for complications? Which patients are at risk for injury because of confusion? Set priorities according to patient need. Unstable patients take precedence over stable patients. Administer scheduled medications and treatments before tasks that are ordered "three times per day."

The goal for the long-term care nurse might be to "delegate and ensure care coordination of assigned patients to finish all scheduled tasks on time and keep the patients safe and comfortable."

Take a few minutes before making rounds to devise a time schedule for the work of the shift (Fig. 10.3). Use a grid or the computer interface that shows each hour of the shift and each patient and room number. Note times you will delegate tasks, assess patients, check intravenous (IV) lines, administer treatments, turn patients, document care, perform patient education, and prepare for handoff report. **Documentation is a critical task in all settings and must be considered a priority to be done as soon as possible when organizing to accomplish the daily workload.**

Monitor the electronic medication administration record (eMAR) or use a separate grid to note when medications are due for each patient, including as needed (PRN) medications. As you work throughout the day, you can make small notes on your work organization sheet that will provide data and a guide for documenting and giving handoff report.

Next consider tasks that need to be done sometime during the shift, such as checking the "crash" cart. Note on your work schedule when you think you will have time to do that. Finally, consider activities that you would like to do if time permits, such as spending time talking with a lonely patient, giving a back rub, or making a phone call to a patient's family. Note these at the bottom of the worksheet.

Once the work is organized, begin your patient assessment/data collection rounds. Do this early in the shift. Patient status can sometimes change dramatically during shift change. Quickly gather data regarding each patient's area of greatest problem (usually their admission diagnosis). Check all tubes and equipment attached to the patient. You will be able to do more in-depth observations later in the shift. Right now you just need to determine whether there are any emergencies, get a feel for the patients' status and needs, and determine what equipment and supplies you will need for each patient during the shift. Inquire about the need for pain medication or other PRN medication while initially in the room. These then can be brought back during early morning medication rounds unless the medication is a badly needed analgesic; this should be administered immediately.

At the end of the workday, evaluate the effectiveness of your time management. Did your schedule help? Did it work as well as you had planned? What took more time to complete than you thought it would take? What would you do differently if you could have a "do over"? This analysis helps you to create a more workable plan the next time. Keep in mind that work plans must be flexible. Even the best plans can be derailed if one patient's status deteriorates markedly. This happens to all nurses from time to time.

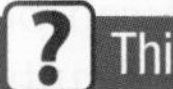

Think Critically

Can you design a shift time management sheet that suits your work style and needs?

USING THE COMPUTER

Computers have become a vital communication, documentation, and information management tool in all health care facilities. The proficient use of computers

Shift Worksheet

Room #______ Patient initials_____ Age_____ Admit Date______ Dx______________________

MD Name________________________ Call MD for_____ Code Status_______ Allergies_________

Activity_______ Diet_______ I/O_______ Labs_________________________

IV (site/fluid/rate)____________ Foley___ tubes/drains:__________ dressing_______ O2_____

Handoff Report:

	Assessment	Vitals/pain	New orders	Meds	Treatments	Procedures	Misc
0800							
0900							
1000							
1100							
1200							
1300							
1400							
1500							

PRN meds: pain______________ dose/freq_____________ last given______________

PRN meds: nausea____________ dose/freq_____________ last given______________

PRN meds: other_____________ dose/freq_____________ last given______________

Be sure to tell next shift:____

FIGURE 10.3 Sample time management tool. Use one page per patient or create your own tool and put several patients on one page.

will assist the nurse in performing everyday functions for patient care and unit administration. The computer is used to place orders to the various departments for supplies, medications, diets, laboratory and diagnostic tests, and engineering and housekeeping needs. Real-time documentation of patient care and current status is shared with team members electronically. Surgery and procedures are scheduled by computer. Staffing patterns may also be monitored by computer. Nursing care plans are constructed on the computer. Evidence-based practices (EBPs) and nursing resources can be easily accessible through computers (Fig. 10.4). Acuity levels for patients are tracked. The agency census is compiled on the computer. Laboratory results are sent to the unit via computer.

To be a team leader or charge nurse, you must be adept at using computers and various programs to efficiently perform all necessary job tasks. The computer is used for most communication and coordination within the agency. The Health Insurance Portability and

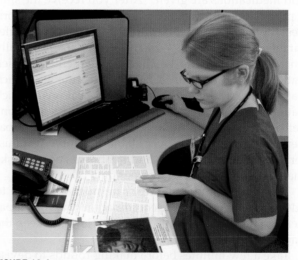

FIGURE 10.4 Nurse using computer for EBP research. (From Yoder-Wise, P. *Leading and managing in nursing* [5th ed.]. St. Louis, MO: Mosby; 2013.)

Accountability Act (HIPAA) privacy rule (see Chapter 3) mandates that we take special precautions and safeguard all electronic patient data, just the same as we do with written patient documentation.

RECEIVING NEW ORDERS

Most facilities have moved towards EMR and computerized provider order entry (CPOE). There may still be a few instances where nurses still work with paper medication administration record (MARs) such as procedural areas, emergency situations, or when computers are off line. In those cases, the nurse would follow the facility policy for documentation and acknowledging for computer downtime situations. When receiving new orders from the computer (or written orders), first read all of the orders. Then acknowledge them as received as dictated by the CPOE system protocol. Verbally communicate the **stat orders** immediately to the nurse responsible for carrying them out. Enter the orders into the computer care plan and eMAR (or paper MAR if used). Each medication order must include the patient's name and room number, the name of the medication (preferably both generic and trade name), ordered dosage, route of administration, the times the doses are to be given, the date the order was written, and the date it is to be discontinued and/or renewed. Acknowledge each medication as it is ordered by the health care provider and verified by the pharmacist. Narcotics, anticoagulants, hypnotics, and antibiotics must be renewed every 48 to 72 hours, depending on agency policy and state laws. Notify the person who will be administering the medication. Dietary orders are transmitted to the dietary department and entered on the computer care plan along with notations for any fluid restrictions or requirements for intake and output (I&O) recording. A list of patients on I&O may be kept at the nurses' station. Clarify any unclear orders directly with the ordering provider. Because of frequent changes in orders, all medication orders on the MAR should be verified with the medical record orders once every 24 hours.

Note any positioning, I&O, treatment requirements, and use of special equipment on the computer care plan for each patient. **Note all allergies at the beginning of your shift, acknowledge them on the eMAR, and alert all personnel.**

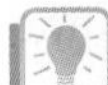
QSEN Considerations: Safety

Allergy Wristbands

Many facilities have wristbands for patients with allergies to improve communication and promote medication safety. Check that all safety protocols are in place to protect your patient.

When a medication is discontinued, notify the nurse administering the medications. Alert the pharmacy to the discontinuation order, and follow facility protocol for returning leftover doses of the medication to the pharmacy for proper crediting to the patient's account. Acknowledge the discontinue order.

Orders for laboratory and diagnostic tests must be transmitted to the appropriate department by telephone or computer with the correct requisition slip filled out. Print the forms and label the specimen containers with the patient's identifying information. Perform this task at the bedside for proper patient verification. If blood samples are to be drawn when the patient is in a fasting state, then an NPO (nothing by mouth) status must be transmitted to the dietary department, to the nurses, and to the patient. Post an NPO sign on the door to the patient's room. The test must be ordered to be drawn before the breakfast hour. Laboratory and diagnostic test orders are recorded in the computer care plan along with dietary restrictions and pretest medications.

Preoperative orders should include diet or NPO status desired, necessary preoperative treatments, a notation regarding the operative consent and the exact procedure to be performed, laboratory and diagnostic tests to be completed, patient education required, and orders for sedatives or preoperative medications. There may also be orders for the type of surgical preparation to be performed and when, insertion of an IV cannula and what solution is to be started, insertion of a urinary (Foley) catheter, or application of elastic hose. **All orders written preoperatively are considered canceled at the time the patient enters surgery.** Brand new orders must be entered in their entirety for the postsurgical patient. "Resume previous orders" is not acceptable by most institutional policies.

Postoperative orders should include a schedule for vital sign measurement; directions for care of tubes, suction, and dressings; IV solutions to be infused; medications to be administered; diet permitted; measurement of I&O; directions for positioning, activity, turning, coughing, and deep breathing; and time to catheterize if the patient is unable to void and does not have an indwelling catheter. Additional orders may request circulation checks or monitoring of neurologic status.

TAKING VERBAL ORDERS

Taking verbal and telephone orders can be unsafe unless carefully performed. The individual giving the order can misspeak, and the individual receiving the order can mishear, misunderstand, or misinterpret the order due to numerous factors such as distractions, background noise, different pronunciations or accents, or cell phone noise. If the prescribing care provider is present on the unit, he or she should enter the orders into the computer rather than giving verbal orders. If implementation of an order is time critical and the care provider is not available in person, a telephone or text order may be the most appropriate and efficient way to provide expedient care to the patient. When taking verbal, text, or telephone orders, the nurse is expected to enter the orders in the computer for the prescribing care provider to verify later.

Safety Alert

Readback

The Joint Commission discourages the use of verbal and telephone orders, but there are some clinical situations in which time is of the essence and the nurse may need to take a verbal, telephone, or text order and enter it into the computerized provider order entry system. Facilities typically have policies and procedures for accepting and entering verbal or telephone orders that follow earlier developed Joint Commission guidelines. According to the guidelines, institutions must verify verbal or telephone orders by having the person receiving the order "read back" the order to the prescribing care provider. This **readback** requires that the person accepting the order actually enter the order into the CPOE system in order to read it back. There are specific guidelines by the Joint Commission for text messaging of orders (Chapter 8). In some facilities, providers must enter the orders, and verbal, telephone, or texted orders are not accepted.

The ability of the LPN/LVN to legally take verbal orders depends on state laws and the written policies of the employing agency. **Verbal orders can only be taken by licensed nurses, and in some states only by an RN.** Some institutions stipulate that verbal orders not be taken except in emergencies.

If your state and agency allow you to take a verbal or telephone order, follow the guidelines in Box 10.3. The nurse enters it into the electronic health record (EHR) with the date, time, electronic signature, and notation of the provider who dictated the order. **The provider must authenticate the order by electronically signing the written form of the verbal order as soon as possible.**

Box 10.3 Guidelines for Taking Telephone Orders

- Have the patient's medical record open to the appropriate screen to accept a new provider order. Know the provider's name.
- Enter the order verbatim (word for word) as it is given to you by the provider.
- Read it back to the provider as entered; verify spelling of medications or diagnostic tests. Do this every time with every provider. Ask the provider to confirm that the order is correct.
- Document the date and time, the name of the ordering provider, and your electronic signature.
- Ensure that the provider signs off on the order when making rounds; this must be done within 48 hours in most agencies.
- If a telephone order is requested during the hours from midnight to 6 am, have another person, preferably a nurse, on an extension to verify the order. Providers awakened from a sound sleep sometimes do not recall the exact order. Have the other nurse verify the order.
- Make an entry in the nurse's notes describing the circumstances that prompted a telephone order. Include the statement that the orders were read back to the provider and that they were confirmed to be accurate by the provider when read back, and the name of any other nurse verifying the order.

DOCUMENTING FOR REIMBURSEMENT

All nurses must document care delivered and equipment used for a patient; otherwise the hospital may not be reimbursed. A charge nurse or supervisor makes certain that all staff are documenting correctly. Each type of agency has guidelines regarding the details of care that must be documented and how often each must be noted.

In long-term care facilities that receive Medicare or Medicaid reimbursement, the Minimum Data Set (MDS) 3.0, a comprehensive resident assessment tool, must be completed as accurately as possible for the facility to receive the maximum Medicare or Medicaid payment for services rendered. Many facilities use a special MDS coordinator to ensure that these computerized forms are completed correctly and transmitted to state and federal agencies by the deadlines. Poor or incomplete documentation may lead to fines imposed by the US Department of Health and Human Services, as well as decreased reimbursement.

RISK MANAGEMENT

The increasing occurrence of lawsuits against health care facilities, physicians, and nurses has focused attention on **risk management** (management of areas to decrease risk of harm to patients, occurrence of lawsuits, or excessive damages awards by juries). Risk management practices attempt to prevent unfavorable events or to reduce the agency's liability. A key risk management tool is to practice nursing following accepted professional standards and the agency's policies and procedures. The unit leader must insist that all workers adhere to the facility's written policies and procedures. Nurses must uphold the standards of practice for the area in which they work. Attending to patient complaints and showing concern when patients are upset can help decrease the risk of a disgruntled patient suing if something goes wrong. It is important to advise your supervisor when a significant problem has occurred on the unit, along with writing an incident report when there has been cause for a patient or the patient's family to be upset with care (see Chapter 3 for a discussion on incident reports). Understanding family dynamics and mediating patient and family complaints is part of the leadership role.

Leadership and management skills develop with practice and continued learning. Professional growth is an important aspect of an evolving career in nursing. Each nurse should seek his own direction and pursue growth opportunities. Reading nursing journals, joining professional organizations, volunteering, taking classes to improve skills or finding an experienced nurse to be a **mentor** (teacher or coach) are a few examples. After a year of experience in direct patient care, enough confidence may have been gained to take on greater responsibility in a leadership role.

Get Ready for the NCLEX Examination!

Key Points

- Leadership is a learned skill that requires a good grasp of management techniques, effective communication skills, clinical competence, knowledge of the agency's organizational structure, and an understanding of yourself and the effect of your leadership and communication styles on others.
- Laissez-faire leaders offer little, if any, direction; autocratic leaders tightly control team members; and democratic leaders frequently consult other staff members and seek participation in decision making.
- Organization of work tasks for the unit is essential; delegation is necessary to accomplish the workload.
- To safely and effectively delegate, you must know the capabilities and competencies of the person to whom you are delegating, understand which tasks you can legally delegate, avoid delegating interventions that require clinical judgment, and provide feedback.
- Delegation and team leading are beginning leadership functions of the LPN/LVN.
- The charge nurse is responsible for the total nursing care of the patients on the unit during the shift. This position requires training and experience in administration and supervision of other personnel.
- Computer expertise is necessary for work efficiency and safe patient care.
- Risk management techniques include following policies and procedures and showing care and concern for patients.

Additional Learning Resources

SG Go to your Study Guide for additional learning activities to help you master this chapter content.

evolve Go to your Evolve website at http://evolve.elsevier.com/Williams/fundamental for additional online resources.

Review Questions for the NCLEX Examination

*Choose the **best** answer for each question.*

1. Which is an example of democratic leadership?
   1. The manager explains new rules for staff scheduling, and then asks for a vote on how to implement them.
   2. Will, the charge nurse, directs others during an emergency situation without asking for input or feedback.
   3. The nurse manager asks advice from her staff nurse friends as she determines the unit holiday schedule.
   4. The charge nurse does not address staff nurses' failure to follow unit policies and procedures.
2. A good way to handle conflict is to: *(Select all that apply.)*
   1. Speak sternly to those involved.
   2. Tell those involved to solve the problem.
   3. Quickly impose a resolution to the problem.
   4. Remain calm and open and listen to all sides.
   5. Focus on the issues, not the personalities involved.
3. Delegation of a specific task to a UAP requires: *(Select all that apply.)*
   1. Knowledge of the UAP's competencies.
   2. Understanding of the nurse practice act.
   3. Direct supervision of the performance of the task.
   4. Documentation that the task was delegated.
   5. Follow-through by verification that the task was completed.
4. When managing your time during your shift, what should you do first?
   1. Make patient rounds.
   2. Delegate tasks.
   3. Set priorities.
   4. Create a time schedule.
5. The nurse manager is selecting the next nurse she wants to promote to the charge nurse position. Which candidate would be the best choice?
   1. A young new graduate with a bubbly personality who gets along with everyone
   2. A recent graduate, out of school for 9 months, who is articulate and highly organized and once held leadership positions in another field
   3. An experienced nurse of 20 years with a sarcastic disposition, who knows the unit better than anyone
   4. A traveling nurse who often ignores provider orders that are different from what he thinks is best for the patient
6. According to The Joint Commission, there are safety concerns about: *(Select all that apply.)*
   1. Use of abbreviations.
   2. Computerized medical records.
   3. Handoff communication.
   4. Delegating tasks to UAPs.
   5. Use of verbal orders.
7. One risk management technique that is known to often be effective is to:
   1. Call family members by their given names.
   2. Assign the same nurse to care for the patient all week.
   3. Listen empathetically to complaints or concerns.
   4. Tell the patient the physician knows best.
8. Which tasks can you delegate to a UAP who has the appropriate training? *(Select all that apply.)*
   1. Administering an enema
   2. Applying a condom catheter
   3. Giving vitamins with breakfast
   4. Assisting with first ambulation after surgery
   5. Obtaining a fingerstick for blood glucose monitoring

Critical Thinking Activities

Read each clinical scenario and discuss the questions with your classmates.

Scenario A

You are assigned eight medical-surgical patients on the day shift. You have one nursing assistant who can help you but who also is assigned to help another nurse. What tasks should you consider delegating to this UAP? How would you verify that the tasks you have delegated have been done and done correctly? Would this method help build team spirit?

Scenario B

You are team leader on one hall. Two of your staff begin to bicker about who should answer the call light that keeps coming on. How would you handle the situation?

Scenario C

A patient needs to have her blood glucose checked before breakfast. You want the nursing assistant to perform this task, and she has been trained to do it. The nursing assistant approaches the patient to perform the procedure, and the patient refuses. How would you handle this refusal?

chapter 11

Growth and Development: Infancy Through Adolescence

http://evolve.elsevier.com/Williams/fundamental

Objectives

Upon completing this chapter, you should be able to do the following:

Theory

1. Describe prenatal development.
2. Compare the development of the male and the female.
3. Describe the physical development of children.
4. Discuss Freud's theory of personality and the mind.
5. Discuss moral development according to Kohlberg.
6. Explain the stages of Erikson's theory of psychosocial development.
7. Explain the stages of Piaget's theory of cognitive development.
8. Identify the principles of growth and development.
9. Discuss age-appropriate discipline measures for children.
10. Identify two advantages of early childhood education.
11. Explain the male and female physical changes of puberty.
12. Identify developmental tasks of adolescence.
13. Discuss at least three concerns related to adolescence.

Clinical Practice

1. Explain the importance of regular prenatal health care.
2. Discuss recommended feeding patterns for newborns and older infants.
3. Provide health promotion teaching to parents and school-age children.
4. Explain the importance of screening young children for physical development.
5. Explain how parents and other caregivers can encourage age-appropriate cognitive and psychosocial development.

Key Terms

abortion (p. 145)
autonomy (ăw-TĂ-nō-mē, p. 151)
bonding (p. 148)
cephalocaudal (cĕ-făl-ō-KĂW-dăl, p. 147)
cognitive (p. 142)
conception (p. 142)
ego (p. 143)
egocentric (ē-gō-SĔN-trĭk, p. 150)
embryonic (ĕm-brĭ-Ŏ-nĭk, p. 145)
fetal (p. 145)
gender (p. 145)
gender roles (p. 151)
genes (JĒNS, p. 145)
germinal (JĔR-mĭ-nŭl, p. 145)
id (p. 143)
ideology (ī-dē-Ŏ-lō-jē, p. 156)
initiative (ĭ-NĬ-shă-tĭv, p. 151)
intelligence (p. 153)
libido (lĭ-BĒ-dō, p. 143)
morals (p. 151)
Moro reflex (p. 147)
neonate (NĒ-ō-nāt, p. 146)
peers (p. 151)
prepuberty (prē-PĔW-bĕr-tē, p. 152)
psychosocial (sī-kō-SŌ-shŭl, p. 142)
puberty (p. 152)
reflexes (RĒ-flĕx-ĕz, p. 147)
self-concept (p. 153)
sensorimotor (sĕn-sŏr-ē-MŌ-tŏr, p. 148)
sexual orientation (p. 156)
siblings (p. 145)
social competence (KŎM-pĕ-tĕns, p. 153)
superego (p. 143)
theory (p. 143)
time-out (p. 151)
trimesters (TRĪ-mĕs-tĕrz, p. 145)
vernix caseosa (VĔR-nĭx kă-sē-Ō-sa, p. 147)
viable (VĪ-ă-bŭl, p. 145)
zygote (ZĪ-gōt, p. 142)

Concepts Covered in This Chapter

- Anxiety
- Caregiving
- Cognition
- Communication
- Coping
- Culture
- Development
- Elimination
- Ethics
- Functional ability
- Health promotion
- Immunity
- Nutrition
- Pain
- Patient-centered care
- Patient education
- Reproduction
- Sexuality
- Stress

The study of human development is fascinating. It is the study of how people change, and stay the same, over time. Each of us is a unique person who continues to develop throughout life. The more you learn about human development, the more you will appreciate the complexity of life. Studying human development may help you better understand yourself and others.

In some ways, people show consistency from one stage of life to another. Some personality traits, for example, appear early in childhood and persist through life. In other ways, such as physical development, people change as they get older. The chapters in this unit focus on three aspects of human development: physical, **cognitive** (knowledge and thinking processes), and **psychosocial** (personality and getting along in society). The physical aspect is easy to understand; we can see children grow. Physical development begins at **conception** (union of ovum and sperm), continues into young adulthood, and includes the normal changes of later adulthood. Cognitive and psychosocial development also begins early in life and continues throughout the life span.

In caring for pediatric patients and their families, your understanding of human growth and development will allow you to recognize normal expected behaviors and development and, over time, anticipate potential problems that may require nursing interventions. It is also important to customize your care to individual patient needs via patient-centered care.

These three facets of human development—physical, cognitive, and psychosocial—are not separated. Each interacts with the others. Every person is a combination of all three. They are discussed separately for the purposes of study and observation.

People do change over time. **We influence our own development through choices that we make.** Only humans can do that! We are resilient and flexible; we can bounce back, adapt, and get stronger.

OVERVIEW OF STRUCTURE AND FUNCTION

PRENATAL DEVELOPMENT

WHAT HAPPENS IN THE GERMINAL STAGE OF PRENATAL DEVELOPMENT?

- Rapid cell division begins within 36 hours of fertilization. The growing **zygote** travels through the fallopian tube to the uterus. It is now called a **blastocyst.** During the second week, it attaches itself to the uterine wall.
- Supportive tissues essential to the pregnancy are also developing. The **placenta** develops to attach the blastocyst to the uterine wall. The **umbilical cord** carries fetal blood to and from the placenta. Nutrients and oxygen pass from the mother's bloodstream through the placenta to the bloodstream of the fetus. The blastocyst is surrounded by amniotic fluid and contained in a strong, double-walled membrane called the **amniotic sac.**
- The germinal stage lasts for 2 weeks after fertilization.

WHAT HAPPENS IN THE EMBRYONIC STAGE OF PRENATAL DEVELOPMENT?

- For the next 6 weeks, the embryo continues to grow rapidly.
- The beginnings of all systems and organs are formed. The nervous system develops most rapidly. The heart begins beating about 3½ weeks after conception.
- Arm and leg buds appear in the fifth week. Eyes and ears begin to take shape.
- Fingers and toes begin developing in the sixth week. The spinal cord is visible on ultrasound at 7 weeks.
- About 95% of body parts are formed by the eighth week.

WHAT HAPPENS IN THE FETAL STAGE OF PRENATAL DEVELOPMENT?

- Organs and systems become refined and begin functioning. Rapid growth continues. This stage lasts until birth.
- External genitalia appear in the third month. Long bones are visible on radiograph in the fourth month. By the fifth month, the fetus is 11 to 12 inches long and may weigh 1 pound.
- The remaining months are the maturation time for all systems.

WHAT CAUSES MULTIPLE BIRTHS?

- Most multiple births occur when more than one ovum is fertilized; these babies are called **fraternal siblings.** They are like other siblings, who share only some genetic similarities.

- Use of fertility medication increases the number of ova released, often leading to multiple fraternal siblings.
- **Identical siblings** (one fourth to one third of twin births) occur when a single zygote separates in the early stage of cell division into two or more individual blastocysts.

ADOLESCENT DEVELOPMENT

HOW DOES A GIRL MATURE INTO A WOMAN?

- Girls may begin puberty as early as 9 or as late as 17 years of age; the average age is around 12 years. These changes may occur over several years.
- The pituitary hormone **follicle-stimulating hormone** (FSH) stimulates the ovaries to begin producing estrogen hormones.
- Estradiol, from the ovary, is responsible for the appearance of secondary sex characteristics. These include breast development, widening of the hips, the appearance of axillary and pubic hair, and growth of the reproductive organs.
- FSH also stimulates the development of ova, and menstruation begins.

HOW DOES A BOY MATURE INTO A MAN?

- Boys usually begin puberty a little later than girls do; the average age for boys is 14 years.
- The pituitary hormone **interstitial cell-stimulating hormone** (ICSH) activates the testes to produce testosterone. FSH, also from the pituitary, stimulates the testes to begin producing sperm.
- Testosterone is responsible for the development of male secondary sex characteristics. These include enlargement of the reproductive organs; lowering of the voice; growth of facial, pubic, and axillary hair; thickened bones; and increased size of skeletal muscles.
- Nocturnal emissions occur. For the first year, the concentration of sperm in semen is quite low.

AGE GROUPS

The growth and development of children and adolescents can be divided into these common age groups:

- **Prenatal:** conception to birth
- **Infancy:** birth to 18 months
- **Early childhood:** 18 months to 6 years
- **Middle and late childhood**: 7 to 11 years
- **Adolescence:** 12 to 18 years

Each individual's development and functional ability is unique. You cannot judge someone's development without considering physical, cognitive, and psychosocial aspects. Family and cultural factors must also be examined when making an assessment. Boundaries of each group should be considered flexible when assessing an individual.

THEORIES OF DEVELOPMENT

A **theory** (an idea formed by reasoning from facts), especially about human development and behavior, is based primarily on observations. Theories are attempts to explain something; they are always being adapted to new information.

Sigmund Freud (1856–1939) contributed to the understanding of personality development. His psychoanalytic theory has three parts: (1) levels of awareness, (2) components of the personality or mind, and (3) psychosexual stages of development. The **levels of awareness** consist of the conscious, subconscious, and unconscious mind. The conscious mind is based in reality and what is sensed, perceived, and thought. The subconscious stores thoughts, feelings, and memories. These are easily brought into the conscious mind. The unconscious level is the part of the mind that is not accessible to one's awareness. The unconscious mind stores memories that are usually painful, thus shielding the person from anxiety and stress.

Freud stated that there are three **functional components of the mind**. The first is the **id** (body's basic primitive urges). The id is concerned with satisfaction and pleasure. The pleasure principle, or **libido**, is the main force driving human behavior. At birth, we are all id. Second is the **ego**, considered the "executive of the mind." It emerges in the fourth or fifth month of life. It is the problem solver and reality tester, and it develops with the person's interaction with the environment and the demands of the id. In this way, the child learns to delay immediate satisfaction of needs. Third, the **superego** is a further development of the ego. It represents the moral component, the portion of the mind that judges, controls, and punishes. It dictates what is right and what is wrong and acts like a conscience. According to Freud, these three components of the mind are constantly in conflict with each other. Unrestrained id dominance can lead to a personality breakdown in which the person demonstrates childlike behavior throughout adult life. A harsh superego can block reasonable needs and drives and prevent full development of the personality in a healthy way. Table 11.1 shows Freud's stages of psychosexual development.

Erik Erikson (1902–94) was a psychologist interested in the psychosocial aspect of development. He defined eight psychosocial stages, each identified by a psychosocial task that must be successfully mastered before the person can progress to the next stage. This growth aids development of a healthy ego. Erikson also believed that cultural, social, biologic, and environmental factors contribute to development. Table 11.2 summarizes this theory for children, adolescents, and adults.

Jean Piaget (1896–1980) was a psychologist who developed a theory about how children learn. He said that all people are born with a need to adapt to the environment, and the ability to use knowledge increases as a child grows. Piaget stressed two principles that allow this to happen: (1) organization, through which we

Table 11.1 **Freud's Psychosexual Stages of Development**

STAGE AND AGE	MAJOR DEVELOPMENTAL TASKS	DESIRED OUTCOMES/FUNCTIONAL ABILITY
Oral (0-1 years)	Beginning of ego development Relief from anxiety through oral gratification of needs	Realization that needs can be met and development of trust in the environment
Anal (1-3 years)	Learning independence and control; focus on the excretory functions Ability to delay gratification	Control over impulses
Phallic (oedipal) (3-6 years)	Development of sexual identity Beginning of superego development Focus on genital organs	Identification with parent of the same sex
Latency (6-12 years)	Focus on relationships with same-sex peers Growth of ego functions (social, intellectual, and mechanical) and the ability to care about and relate to others outside the home	Development of skills needed for coping with the environment and others
Genital (12 years and beyond)	Emancipation from parents Planning of life goals Development of personal identity Focus on relationships with members of the opposite sex	Ability to find pleasure in love and work and to be creative

Adapted from Varcarolis, E. M., & Halter, M. J. (2014). *Essentials of Psychiatric Mental Health Nursing* (2nd ed.). Philadelphia: Elsevier Saunders and Polan, E., & Taylor, D. (2011). *Journey Across the Life Span: Human Development and Health Promotion* (4th ed.). Philadelphia: F.A. Davis.

Table 11.2 **Psychosocial Development According to Erikson**

AGE	PSYCHOSOCIAL CRISIS	TASK	RESOLUTION OF CRISIS: SUCCESSFUL	RESOLUTION OF CRISIS: UNSUCCESSFUL
Infancy (birth-18 months)	Trust vs. mistrust	Attachment to the mother	Trust in people; faith and hope about the environment and future	General difficulties relating to people effectively; suspicion; trust-fear conflict; fear of the future
Early childhood (18 months-3 years)	Autonomy vs. shame and doubt	Gaining some basic control over self and environment	Sense of self-control and adequacy; willpower	Independence-fear conflict; severe feelings of self-doubt
Late childhood (3-6 years)	Initiative vs. guilt	Becoming purposeful and directive	Ability to initiate one's own activities; sense of purpose	Aggression-fear conflict; sense of inadequacy or guilt
School age (6-12 years)	Industry vs. inferiority	Developing social, physical, and learning skills	Competence; ability to learn and work	Sense of inferiority; difficulty learning and working
Adolescence (12-20 years)	Identity vs. role confusion	Developing sense of identity	Sense of personal identity	Confusion about who one is; identity submerged in relationships or group memberships
Early adulthood (20-35 years)	Intimacy vs. isolation	Establishing intimate bonds of love and friendship	Ability to love deeply and commit oneself	Emotional isolation and egocentricity
Middle adulthood (35-65 years)	Generativity vs. stagnation	Fulfilling life goals that involve family, career, and society	Ability to give and to care for others	Self-absorption and inability to grow as a person
Later adulthood (65 years-death)	Ego integrity vs. despair	Looking back over one's life and accepting its meaning	Sense of integrity and fulfillment	Dissatisfaction with life

Adapted from Varcarolis, E. M., & Halter, M. J. (2014). *Essentials of Psychiatric Mental Health Nursing* (2nd ed.). Philadelphia: Elsevier Saunders.

try to make sense of our world; and (2) adaptation, the process of discovering new information and adjusting our thinking patterns. The four stages of Piaget's theory are given in Table 11.3. As children develop, each stage helps them understand the world more thoroughly.

Lawrence Kohlberg (1927–87) developed a theory of moral development. He defined three levels of moral development occurring along with cognitive growth:

1. **Preconventional reasoning:** Young children obey rules to avoid punishment. Moral values are not internalized. Most children are in this stage until about age 9.
2. **Conventional reasoning:** At this level, children and adults conform to social standards to avoid

Table 11.3 Cognitive Development According to Piaget

DEVELOPMENTAL STAGE	AGE	DEVELOPMENTAL TASK	DESCRIPTION
Sensorimotor	Birth-2 years	To recognize permanence of objects	Unable to do things or distinguish self from environment; reflexes evolve into repeated actions that become coordinated movements; learns that objects in environment are still present even when they are not seen, touched, tasted; begins goal-directed and imitative behavior
Preoperational	2-7 years	To develop symbolic mental abilities	Thinking limited; centered on self; learns to use language as tool; establishes routines; thought focused on only one part of situation; cannot understand more than one dimension of object; justifies own behavior at all costs
Concrete operations	8-11 years	To develop logical, objective thinking	Understands numbers, length, mass, area, weight, time, and volume; can see interrelations; able to reflect and discover relationships in environment
Formal operations	12-15 years	To learn to think abstractly	Able to consider all possibilities of situation; can think in terms of probability and proportions; uses problem-solving approach to conflicts

From Morrison-Valfre, M. (2013). *Foundations of Mental Health Care* (5th ed.). St. Louis: Elsevier Mosby.

disapproval or to avoid guilt. Decisions are based on understanding the social order, laws, justice, and duty. Children begin using conventional reasoning at around 11 and may remain in this stage throughout life.

3. **Postconventional reasoning:** People at this level have internalized moral principles. They are generally law abiding and follow their conscience. Kohlberg believes that only a minority of adults operate at this level.

PRINCIPLES OF GROWTH AND DEVELOPMENT

Many factors influence growth and development. Heredity and environment are major factors. Some developmental psychologists have tried to determine which is more important. So far, there is not much agreement.

Family structure is also important. Are there two parents in the home? What is the parenting style? What is the socioeconomic situation? Some people think that birth order plays a part. **Gender** (being male or female) can influence how a child is raised.

Even with numerous variables affecting growth and development, some basic principles exist:

- Growth occurs in orderly and predictable ways. Patterns and stages can be anticipated.
- The rate of growth and development is individual. Even **siblings** (brothers and sisters) develop at different rates.
- Development is lifelong. Physical growth is seen in childhood, but normal changes continue throughout life.
- Development is multidimensional. It involves many processes, including physical, cognitive, and psychosocial aspects.
- A person's development is continual, but the rate of development varies. At times development seems static.

PRENATAL DEVELOPMENT

Prenatal development begins at the time of conception, when the mother's ovum is fertilized by the father's sperm. A new and unique cell, the **zygote** (fertilized egg), is formed, and under healthy circumstances, it will become a baby.

Among the many influences on prenatal development is genetics. **Genes** (segments of DNA carrying the blueprints of development) pass from parents to child through the sperm and the ovum. The nucleus of the individual cells contains 23 unpaired chromosomes, which are filled with tightly coiled strands of DNA. The zygote contains 23 chromosomes from the father and 23 chromosomes from the mother; thus, once joined, the human cells contain 46 chromosomes. These 46 chromosomes become a unique combination that will almost certainly never occur again (except in the case of identical twins). That is why each of us is different from everyone else.

EVENTS IN PRENATAL DEVELOPMENT

Prenatal development occurs in three stages: **germinal** (initial), **embryonic** (early formation), and **fetal** (late). An overview of prenatal development is provided here.

Pregnancy is divided into three **trimesters** (periods of 3 months). A full-term pregnancy lasts 40 weeks. Birth within 2 weeks on either side of the estimated date is considered normal. If the baby is delivered earlier than 38 weeks of gestation, the infant is called **premature.** Premature babies can survive if their systems are mature enough to support life and if the delivery occurs in a safe place. When a pregnancy ends before the fetus is **viable** (able to survive outside the womb), it is called an **abortion.** A naturally occurring abortion is often called a **miscarriage.**

MATERNAL INFLUENCES

The single most important factor in maintaining a healthy pregnancy is early and regular prenatal health care. Visits with health professionals help expectant mothers understand what is happening and how they can contribute to healthy fetal growth. This care also allows the health professional to detect signs of potential problems and intervene before the problems become serious. A healthy outcome for both mother and child is always the goal. Lack of prenatal care is a serious problem for some women, and maternal mortality rates in the United States have been rising. Lack of care can occur because of economics, fear, ignorance, lack of access, or other reasons. *Healthy People 2020* addresses the health and well-being of women, infants, children, and families. The risk of infant (and maternal) mortality and pregnancy-related complications can be decreased by proper care before conception and between pregnancies, it is imperative to refer pregnant women to an agency that can provide prenatal care regardless of their economic position.

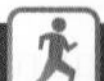 **Health Promotion/Health Promotion Points**

Prenatal Care

- A female should seek prenatal care as soon as she suspects she is pregnant.
- If planning to become pregnant, she should be certain that her intake of folic acid is at least 400 mcg/day and her immunizations are up to date for those diseases that could harm the fetus (rubella in particular), and seek control of any chronic disease.
- Fathers should be encouraged to participate in prenatal care and planning decisions to promote early family bonding.

A second influence in prenatal development is the mother's health. Women with a chronic illness who are pregnant are usually considered high risk. This especially includes women with diabetes or rheumatic heart disease. Obesity also places a pregnant woman in the high risk category. Contracting a communicable disease during pregnancy also presents a risk to fetal health. German measles (rubella) is one communicable disease known to harm a fetus.

A third influence can be the mother's age. Pregnancy before the mother reaches her adult growth, at about age 16, can be a high risk situation. At the other extreme, a woman experiencing her first pregnancy after age 35 is considered high risk. Any pregnancy when the mother is over 40 is also high risk.

A fourth influence is the mother's nutritional state. **Women need to be well nourished before pregnancy begins and throughout the pregnancy.** The mother's nutrition is vital for healthy fetal development. A woman who begins a pregnancy at a healthy weight should gain approximately 25 to 35 lb; prepregnancy weight may either increase or decrease this recommendation (typically, 11 to 20 lb for obese women, 15 to 25 lb for overweight women, and 28 to 40 lb for underweight women). Excessive weight gain can complicate the delivery and make it harder to lose weight later.

Emotional stress is a fifth influence on the pregnancy. Women who experience severe emotional stress may put the fetus at risk. This is because stress affects the physiology of blood flow and may restrict blood flow to the placenta, interfering with fetal nutrition and oxygenation. The American Congress of Obstetricians and Gynecologists recommends screening pregnant women for depression during each trimester and in the postpartum phase.

The sixth influence is the use of chemicals. Chemicals known to interfere in some way with fetal development include alcohol, nicotine, caffeine, some medications, and street drugs. As scientists study babies with problems, it is becoming apparent that even casual use of any of these chemicals may be risky.

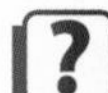 **Think Critically**

You have a friend who suspects she is pregnant for the first time but is postponing seeing a care provider. What will you say to her?

INFANTS

For the first month of life, the baby is a **neonate** (newborn). This month is a period of adjustment for the infant and the new parents. Infancy extends through the first 18 months.

 **Health Promotion/Health Promotion Points**

Infant Health Care

- Regular checkups with the infant's health care provider should occur at 2 months, 4 months, 6 months, 9 months, and 1 year after birth.
- Immunizations for hepatitis B, diphtheria, tetanus, pertussis, *Haemophilus influenzae*, rubella, measles, mumps, polio, pneumococcus, varicella, influenza, and hepatitis A are recommended at birth, 2 months, 4 months, 6 months, and between 12 and 18 months for the infant. The current immunization schedule can be found at: www.cdc.gov/vaccines/schedules/index.html.

NUTRITION

Healthy newborns can manage without calories for the first 12 to 24 hours, but usually are breastfed or bottle fed sooner. After that, they need to have caloric intake to survive. Most pediatricians recommend breastfeeding; breast milk is perfectly designed for the newborn's digestive system. It also provides the newborn with protective antibodies for the first few months. Babies who are breastfed longer than 6 months may learn how to stop eating when they are full, reducing the risk of being overweight when they are older. Increasing the number of women who breastfeed their infants is a *Healthy People 2020* objective.

Parents who choose to use infant formula either initially or later should know that it closely resembles human milk. The primary care provider will recommend the type of formula. Cow's milk is not advised for babies until 11 to 12 months of age because of possible allergic reactions.

The stomach of newborns holds only an ounce or two at first; that is why they need to eat often. Babies grow rapidly; by age 1 month, they are eating larger amounts. Feeding time should provide emotional closeness. Infants should be held and talked to while being fed. Bottle-feeding is a good way to involve fathers and other family members in the infant's care.

For the first 6 months, babies need only breast milk or infant formula. The first solids are usually baby cereals, strained vegetables, and strained fruits. It is best to add new foods slowly (one at a time) to see how well the baby tolerates them. Most babies can eat table food by 1 year of age. Older infants enjoy finger foods, but they should not be given pieces of sausage, hot dogs, peanuts, popcorn, or hard candies that could be aspirated (inhaled into the respiratory tract).

APPEARANCE AND CAPABILITIES OF NEWBORNS

At birth, the newborn's skin and scalp are often covered with **vernix caseosa** (a cheesy, waxy substance that protects the skin in fetal life). This wears off in a day or two. Babies' heads appear large in comparison to their bodies and may be temporarily misshapen. They move their arms and legs aimlessly; the hands and feet may appear slightly cyanotic for a while. Newborns should cry spontaneously after birth. They usually are quiet when wrapped tightly in a blanket and held, because this provides a feeling of security.

A newborn may appear helpless but really has many capabilities. **Reflexes** (instinctive protective actions) present at birth include blinking, yawning, grasping, stepping, hiccoughing, sucking, and swallowing. The **Moro reflex** (startle response) can be elicited by making a loud noise near the baby, who will react by arching his or her back and assuming a typical posture with flexion (bending) and adduction (midline movement) of the extremities and fingers fanned initially.

Newborns can also express themselves by crying; parents quickly learn the meaning of the different cries they make. Newborns watch everything and everyone. Their response to people and surroundings is the way they communicate.

A typical newborn sleeps from 16 to 20 hours each day. This time is important for growth and development. Eating and being loved and cared for usually fill the waking hours. Wakefulness increases as they get older. By 1 year of age, most infants need only a morning and afternoon nap.

PHYSICAL DEVELOPMENT

The average newborn weighs 7 to 7½ lb and is 20 to 21 inches long. Less than 5.5 lb is considered low birth weight and more than 8.8 lb is considered high birth weight. There are two categories of low-birth-weight babies. The first is **preterm babies** who are born before 37 weeks of gestation and weigh less than 5 lb. The second category is **small-for-dates babies.** These infants are born at term but weigh less than 90% of what they should weigh.

All babies should double their birth weight at 5 to 6 months and triple it by 1 year. They should also grow ½ to 1 inch/month during the first 6 months and ⅜ inch/month from 6 to 12 months. At well-baby visits, the baby's growth is measured and documented on standard growth charts.

Health Promotion/Health Promotion Points

Indications for Pediatric Evaluation

If a baby is not gaining weight or growing within normal percentiles on the growth chart or is showing definite developmental delays, further evaluation should be done by a pediatrician.

The newborn's eyes are dark blue or gray. The permanent eye color develops by age 9 to 11 months. Newborns can see light and darkness and seem to prefer bright colors. Their vision is focused best at 8 to 15 inches from their eyes, or about the distance to the face of the person who is feeding them. Visual acuity increases in harmony with their growing awareness of their surroundings.

Newborns can hear well and are afraid of loud noises. Infants prefer their mother's voice to those of other women, and they often recognize voices of other family members.

The sense of touch is not well differentiated at birth, but babies need to be touched and held. They can feel pain, although it is more generalized than specific for the first few months. Try to involve both mothers and fathers in the handling and care of the child. Positive reinforcement is important for new parents.

The baby's first teeth, the bottom incisors, usually appear between ages 5 and 11 months. By 12 months, many babies have six to eight temporary teeth.

The brain grows rapidly in infancy and early childhood. Neurons present at birth are not fully developed. As the baby grows, the neurons continue to extend, grow, and make connections. A newborn's brain weighs 25% of the adult brain weight; this increases to 66% in the first year. By age 2 years, the brain weighs 80% of the adult brain weight. Infants and young children need a healthy diet, including fats, for brain growth to occur. They also need stimulation for neuron connections to form.

MOTOR DEVELOPMENT

Motor development occurs in a typical pattern called **cephalocaudal** (proceeding from head to tail) development. This means that babies can lift their head before they can lift their chest. They can sit before they can stand. Development also proceeds from the center of the body toward the outside. They control their shoulders before they control their arms and fingers. Large muscles develop coordination before smaller ones do. For example, they can walk before they can draw. **The pattern is consistent, although the rate may vary from one child to another.**

Milestones in motor development are shown in Box 11.1. Parents may need reassurance if one child develops more slowly than another does. Children perform motor skills only when they are developmentally ready.

Several environmental factors influence a child's motor development. Children need good nutrition, health care, emotional support, and the opportunity to practice motor skills. Deprivation of any of these factors may cause developmental delay.

Safety for the helpless infant is a primary concern.

 QSEN Considerations: Safety

Infant Safety Factors

- Never leave an infant alone in a house or car.
- Place the infant on his or her back for sleep, propping slightly on one side or the other for variation. Do not place the infant on his or her stomach to sleep.
- Never leave an infant alone on a surface that does not offer protection against falls.
- When traveling in automobiles, always restrain infants in a rear-facing car seat in the back seat until age 2.
- Always test bathwater to make sure it is not too hot before putting an infant into the water.
- Keep small objects out of reach to prevent entry into the infant's mouth and choking. "Button" lithium batteries, often found in children's toys, cause numerous child injuries and deaths.

COGNITIVE DEVELOPMENT

According to Piaget's theory of cognitive development, babies actively construct their own cognitive world. They organize experiences and observations and then make adaptations in thinking when new situations occur. Newborns display this process by eagerly sucking on everything that comes near their mouth. Later, they learn that some things, such as a nipple or thumb, are suitable for sucking. These items provide satisfaction, either nutritionally or emotionally. Sucking on a blanket or a toy does not provide the same satisfaction.

The first cognitive stage is **sensorimotor.** This begins with babies experiencing things about themselves: for example, becoming aware of the sensations of their body and discovering their toes. Then babies move on to learn about other people and objects in their world.

By the time babies are about 8 months old, they realize that an object still exists even when they cannot see it. This is called **object permanence.** It is demonstrated when an infant is shown an object and then looks for it after it is hidden.

Most infants begin babbling at 3 to 6 months; this is the cooing, gurgling stage. Babies learn language by listening to people around them and imitating the sounds they hear. Parents who talk to their babies and spend time with them stimulate language development. Babies often say their first word at 11 to 13 months and begin using two-word sentences at 18 to 24 months. The same sequence exists all over the world.

An infant's efforts at discovery depend on the assistance and guidance of adults. **Caregivers can stimulate cognitive development by spending time with the baby, talking, singing, playing, and loving.** Many kinds of experiences should be provided. Babies thrive on receiving lots of attention and being part of family activities (Fig. 11.1).

PSYCHOSOCIAL DEVELOPMENT

Infants learn to interact with other people by experience with their caregivers. **Bonding** (sense of attachment between two people) occurs with one or two primary caregivers first, usually the mother and father. The infant's need for stimulation and love grows during the first 3 months. Physical contact, caring, and familiarity are important aspects in bonding. By 5 or 6 months, the baby is ready to include other people in relationships.

Bonding gives babies the security they need to develop the sense of trust. Erikson believed that

Box 11.1 Milestones in Infant Motor Development

- **4 to 6 weeks:** Stops crying when held
- **2 months:** Lifts and turns head
- **3 months:** Reaches for and tries to grasp objects
- **4 months:** Sits with support; coos
- **5 months:** Recognizes people; holds own bottle; splashes in water
- **6 months:** Rolls over; sits alone; plays peek-a-boo
- **9 months:** Crawls; knows own name; understands "no"
- **10 months:** Some walk with help
- **12 months:** Most walk alone

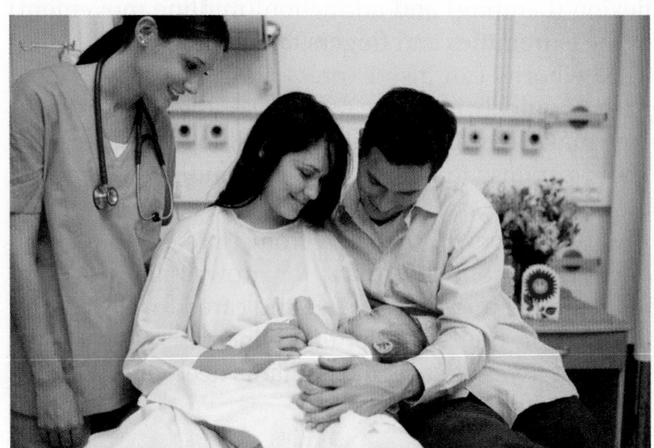

FIGURE 11.1 Every newborn arrives with great potential. (Photo copyright istock.com.)

infants learn to trust others when they receive warm, consistent care. To develop trust, infants need to feel comfortable and secure and believe that the caregiver will always meet their needs. Infants who have a sense of trust will have confidence to explore new situations and can usually handle short separations from parents. This will help the infant develop relationships with other people throughout life.

A healthy baby recognizes family members and shows insecurity with strangers by 6 to 7 months of age. Studies show that infants with a secure attachment to another human are happier and less frustrated at 2 years of age than infants with a less secure attachment are.

Think Critically

Can a baby develop trust in a foster-care situation?

YOUNG CHILDREN

Young children are defined as those between 18 months and 6 years of age. This group is sometimes divided into toddlers (1 to 3 years) and preschoolers (4 to 5 years). Many developmental milestones occur in these years.

PHYSICAL DEVELOPMENT

The rate of growth in early childhood is slower than in infancy. Young children lose baby fat and appear slimmer as the trunk lengthens. Most young children grow 2 to 3 inches in height and gain 4 to 6 lb each year. Boys are slightly larger than girls are during this period. The size of muscles and bones increases, which can lead to greater strength. The heart and lungs become more efficient, and the child's immunity improves.

Heredity and the environment have been shown to influence physical development. The primary environmental influence is nutrition. Children 4 to 13 years of age need 1200 to 1800 calories/day. Sometimes when the child eats very little, it concerns parents; at this age, some children are fussy eaters. Children 2 to 3 years of age only need 1000 calories/day and need less fat and sugar in their diets than they are usually fed. This means that young children who eat too many high-calorie foods and are not physically active can be at risk for obesity-related illness if interventions are not taken early.

Vision improves during the early childhood years. By age 2, visual acuity is usually 20/40. Vision may be checked during a preschool physical examination in the primary care provider's office, but this is usually done during the kindergarten physical examination or at the beginning of the first grade. Visual screening may be performed by the school nurse.

Health Promotion/Health Promotion Points

Health Care for Young Children

- Regular checkups are recommended at least every 2 years to assess growth and development.
- Immunization boosters are recommended between 4 and 6 years of age, and again at 11 or 12 years (Fig. 11.2).
- Caution should be used when treating children with antiviral drugs for influenza. Studies have shown only minimal shortening of symptoms with possible exposure to unneeded side effects.
- Parents should be taught to recognize the signs of pain in children who are ill or recovering from surgery, and to understand how to manage pain with medications or nonpharmacologic means to prevent undue suffering or discomfort.
- A test for iron deficiency may be appropriate for the child who is not eating well.
- Nutrition and healthy childhood weights are being evaluated at earlier ages because obesity rates are increasing nationally for preschoolers and children ages 6 to 11 years.
- When a child enters preschool, a physical examination that will include a urinalysis and vision test is often required. The examination may reveal health problems that are not obvious so that early intervention can occur.
- Children should be physically active at least 60 minutes/day.
- The American Academy of Pediatrics guidelines recommend no television, smartphones, or computers for children under age 2, and less than 2 hours of screen time per day for children and teens. These activities have been linked to an increase in attention problems, development of unhealthy eating habits, higher body mass index, and obesity.

During early childhood, new teeth continue to erupt. A full set of 24 deciduous teeth should be present by age 3 years. Tooth brushing and flossing should begin as soon as a child has teeth, and the child should be taught/supervised as soon as motor skills allow. The first dental visit may be made when a child is 2 to 3 years old.

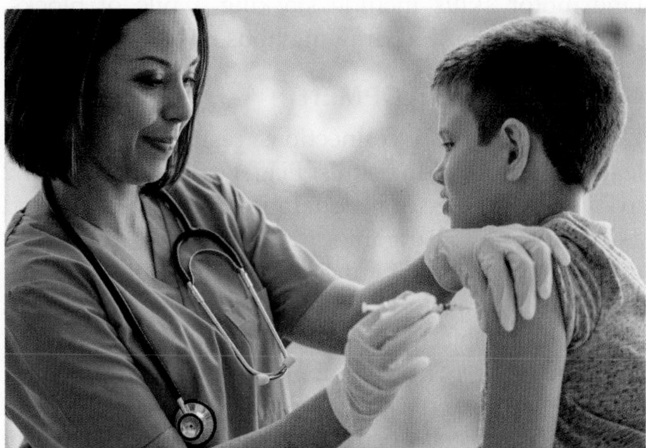

FIGURE 11.2 Prekindergarten immunizations help ensure a healthy start to school. (Photo copyright istock.com.)

A growth chart can monitor the child's physical growth. Height and weight are plotted on the graph and compared with those of the average child. Most children fall within the guidelines of the curve. A child who falls below the 5th percentile or above the 95th percentile may need further evaluation because something physical may be wrong. **It is important to monitor the child's growth so that any problems can be treated before they become serious.** Growth progress should be steady.

MOTOR DEVELOPMENT

Motor development proceeds as growth occurs. Neuromuscular maturation is needed for motor skills to develop. A milestone of this age group is toilet training, the age for which varies from culture to culture. Most children are physiologically ready to be bowel trained between 1½ and 2 years, but successful toilet training also depends on psychological readiness. Regarding elimination, daytime bladder control usually occurs later than bowel control; nighttime bladder control occurs later still.

Young children also learn to feed and dress themselves, and become independent in many activities. Improving neuromuscular skills lead to better coordination. For example, at age 2 years, children usually hold someone's hand to go up a stairway and take only one step at a time. At 3 years, they can climb stairs using alternate steps, although they may still need to hold on. By age 4 years, they can climb a stairway alone. At 5 years, they run upstairs without even thinking about it.

A commonly used assessment tool is the **Denver Developmental Screening Test,** also known as the Denver II. It is a simple and rapid way to assess the functional ability and developmental maturity of young children before they start school. The test giver observes gross and fine motor skills, language, and social ability. Gross motor skills measured include walking, jumping, using a tricycle, throwing and catching a ball, hopping on one foot, and balancing on one foot. Fine motor skills include stacking a pile of blocks, drawing people, and drawing houses.

COGNITIVE DEVELOPMENT

Expanding neuron connections result in increasing learning and thinking skills. Piaget called the ages of 2 to 7 years the stage of **preoperational thought,** defined as learning how to organize thoughts. This stage is subdivided into symbolic function and intuitive thought.

In the **symbolic function substage,** children can think about objects, people, and events in their absence by using mental symbols of them. Watch a child draw a picture or play a game of pretend. The child can think about objects even though they are not currently present.

Some interesting normal occurrences happen during these years. Children have vivid imaginations, and many cannot easily distinguish between reality and fantasy. Cartoon characters are real to the young child, and stuffed toys are alive. Young children engage in magical thinking. Because they do not understand cause and effect, they may think that their thoughts influence events.

Another phenomenon is the child's **egocentric** (I am the center of the world) belief. Young children believe they are the most important people in the world. They think that their desires should be fulfilled on demand, and they cannot grasp another person's viewpoint.

In the **intuitive thought substage,** thinking abilities expand, thoughts are better organized, and early problem solving occurs. Abstractions such as time and numbers often remain hazy.

One highlight in young children's cognitive development is their curiosity. This often surpasses their caution, making safety a concern. Children lack the experience and knowledge to understand possible dangers. Childproofing a home (keeping cleaning supplies, medicines, and other hazards out of reach) is essential. Children at this age need instruction about dangers: cars, crossing streets, strangers, and acceptable ways to touch and be touched. The home and play environment should be free of lead contamination to protect against lead poisoning. **Parents and other caregivers are primary safety teachers by example and concern.**

QSEN Considerations: Safety

Safety Guidelines for Infants and Young Children

- Use a crib with correct spacing between spindles or slats.
- Never leave an infant alone on an elevated surface or in a high chair, stroller, walker, infant carrier, or other equipment.
- Secure stairways with a safety barrier and keep exit doors closed and possibly locked.
- Check toys for loose buttons, long strings, small parts, and rough edges.
- Do not use plastic bags within an infant's reach.
- Remove toxic plants from the home; supply chewable objects such as teething rings.
- Do not leave an infant alone in the bathtub at any time.
- Add safety locks on the doors of appliances, cupboards, and drawers where dangerous, caustic, or toxic items are kept.
- Prevent the child from chewing on old windowsills or furniture that might have been painted with lead paint.
- Display the number for the poison control center close to the telephone.
- Avoid using tablecloths that hang over the table within an infant's reach.
- Cover electrical outlets and keep wires and cords out of the reach of a child.
- Keep household cleaners and medications in childproof containers out of a child's reach.
- Avoid giving a child hard candies, nuts, popcorn, or small pieces of food that could be easily aspirated.
- Do not drink hot liquids while holding an infant.
- Keep the child away from hot surfaces.

- Dress the child in flame-retardant sleepwear.
- Use plastic eating and drinking utensils rather than glass or ceramic.
- Supervise all activities around animals.
- Correctly use approved safety seats and restraints for infants and children.
- Supervise children at play and teach them about street dangers.
- Instruct children never to talk to or go anywhere with strangers.
- Keep knives out of the reach of children; keep power tools and guns locked up.
- Keep matches out of the reach of children.
- Turn pot handles toward the back of the stove.
- Ensure swimming pools are fenced with a locked gate.
- Teach children to swim if they are often near water. Young children are 88% less likely to drown if they have taken swimming lessons.
- Use an automatic garage door opener that is programmed to rise if the door strikes an object.
- Keep clotheslines above the level of the adult head.
- Mark glass doors with decals.

Attention spans begin to lengthen during these years. A 5-year-old can sit still for a story much longer than can his or her 2-year-old sibling can. This makes conversations interesting. A child's memory also improves with age.

Language develops rapidly during childhood. Most 6-year-olds know 8000 to 14,000 words. Sentence length usually increases proportionately to age. The speed with which a child learns to talk is not necessarily indicative of intelligence. Girls often begin to talk sooner than boys do, and firstborn children may talk at a younger age than their siblings do.

Young children have lively imaginations. Some develop an imaginary friend who accompanies them everywhere. This friend can conveniently be blamed for minor problems, too. The playmate usually disappears when the child is 5 or 6 years old. Pretend play is also imaginative. Pretending is important between 3 and 8 years, as the child experiments with various roles.

PSYCHOSOCIAL DEVELOPMENT

Erikson's second stage of development occurs from 18 months to 3 years. **Autonomy** (independence) develops as children learn to feed themselves and to do other things without help. Children are also highly verbal and can say "no," often with great conviction.

Caregivers who are impatient and do everything for the child may cause feelings of shame and doubt to develop. If parents are overprotective and critical, for example, children may be ashamed of themselves and doubt their ability to accomplish things.

Erikson's stage for ages 3 to 6 years is called **initiative** (willingness to try). Young children are energetic, eager, and curious. They know no fear and want to explore the world. They are also beginning to develop a conscience and to learn what is right and wrong. Will the child be successful in this stage of initiative or will he or she be plagued by guilt by not doing the right thing? Parents can aid children through this stage by giving them freedom to explore within safe limits, by encouraging their questions and ideas, by supporting successes, and by helping the preschooler develop self-esteem.

Young children do need to learn discipline. Many parents find that enforcing **time-out** (quiet time alone without toys) is often effective. Experts recommend that 1 minute be used for each year of age. This must occur immediately after the offense or the child will not relate the behavior to the punishment.

Children learn **gender roles** (behaviors and attitudes a culture expects and approves for males or females) during this stage. They observe the behaviors expected of boys and girls and how they differ. By age 3, children know their own gender, and by 6 years, they can usually identify another person's gender by watching appearance and behavior. Some psychologists believe that sex hormones, even in young children, strongly influence a child's behavior. Others believe that the gender roles children adopt are more influenced by their environment. Parents and other adults provide strong influences in the child's gender role adaptation. This occurs through their examples, the toys they provide, and the way they treat children.

? Think Critically

Are there gender stereotypes? What examples support your answer? Should gender roles be encouraged? Why are stereotypes a concern to some?

A new sibling often arrives in a family during an older child's early years. There is a natural rivalry when children think they must compete for their parents' attention. Parents should make every effort to give adequate attention to each child and to treat each as an individual. A young child can be somewhat prepared for the arrival of a new baby through talking with the parents, reading storybooks about babies, and participating in special sibling classes. Older children continue to need reassurance that they are still loved.

Morals (values of right and wrong) are developed during young childhood. Young children are developing a conscience. They start to understand other people's feelings, which is the beginning of empathy.

The importance of **peers** (others of similar age and background) increases as children get older. The young child is first influenced in the home by parents and family members. By age 3 years, the child needs exposure to other children. Children naturally begin to seek friendships and experiences outside the home by age 6.

Play contributes to cognitive and psychosocial development. Children's play helps them learn and understand the world around them. Several types of

Box 11.2 Types of Play

- **Onlooker play:** A child watches others playing, but does not interact (ages 1 to 2 years).
- **Solitary play:** Children play alone (age 1 year on).
- **Parallel play:** Children play next to each other but with little interaction (18 months to 3 years).
- **Associative play:** Children play together, sharing toys and activities and communicating (ages 2 years on).
- **Cooperative play:** Children play together. Games have rules and goals. Groups may have a leader (ages 5 years on).

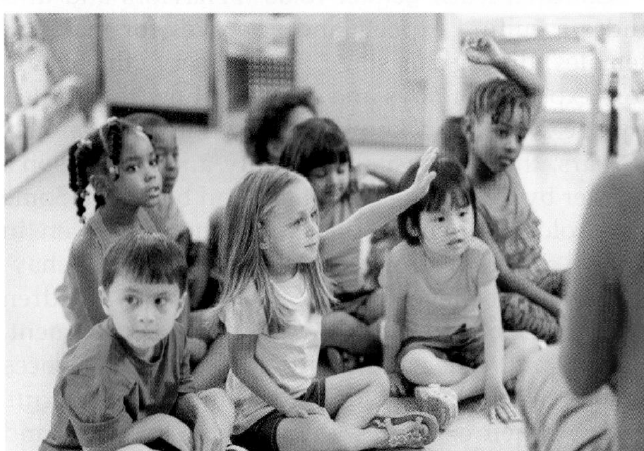

FIGURE 11.3 Preschool children enjoy story time. (Photo copyright istock.com.)

play are shown in Box 11.2. Play should be spontaneous and voluntary. Most preschoolers prefer playing with same-gender children. Children also enjoy playing with adults.

DAY CARE AND EARLY EDUCATION

Many young children in the United States are cared for by adults other than their parents some of the time. Over 64% of mothers with children under the age of 6 years are working (Bureau of Labor Statistics, 2016). Childcare may be provided in a home or group setting. Topics to consider when choosing care are the approach to discipline, general child-rearing practices and beliefs, activities available for the child, attention to safety and health, and a nurturing atmosphere. Parents should carefully check a day care situation before entrusting their child to it.

Group settings provide stimulation for the child in areas that may not be available in the home setting. The day care center or preschool provides an opportunity for the child to adjust to leaving home for a time before the beginning of regular school years (Fig. 11.3). The child also learns socialization skills. The government provides funds for Head Start, a preschool program for children in lower-income families. The child's behavior should be monitored for signs of stress when in a childcare setting because some children are too young and not mature enough to adapt.

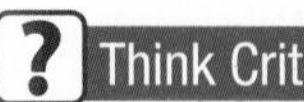

Think Critically

How would you counsel parents regarding proper assessment of a day care situation?

MIDDLE AND OLDER CHILDREN

Middle and older children are those from ages 7 to 11 years. Children move through elementary school, join group activities, and become more grown up. They are filled with energy and enthusiasm. They begin to express their own ideas with confidence and are interesting people.

PHYSICAL DEVELOPMENT

Growth continues to be slow and steady. Children grow an average of 2 to 3 inches in height and gain 3 to 5 pounds in weight each year. Periods of several months may pass without apparent growth, followed by periods of rapid growth. Change is most noticeable in leg length, and the body trunk becomes slimmer. By age 11 years, some children begin to show signs of **prepuberty** (beginning sexual development).

Children can run, hit a baseball, swim, and perform many other physical activities. This demonstrates increasing coordination skills.

One health concern for this age group is regular dental care because permanent teeth are erupting. Children in this age range often need orthodontic treatment. Getting adequate sleep is another concern; a child at this age is often energetic and busy. Parents should monitor schedules so that children do not become overly busy. Education about healthy nutrition is also important because habits formed now will influence future diet and health. The rate of obesity among children has grown, related to fast food, calorie-laden juices and sodas, and large servings. **Young people who are properly nourished throughout their childhood tend to be healthier as adults.** Numerous *Healthy People 2020* objectives are directed at increasing the consumption of healthful diets and maintaining a healthy weight.

COGNITIVE DEVELOPMENT

Piaget called this stage of cognitive development **concrete operational thought.** Children think in concrete ways about real things, and they draw conclusions based on what they see and know. Ideas are organized and fixed. This demonstrates early problem-solving skills. Children think in black and white; they may have trouble accepting "maybe" situations. They are able to classify things and identify relationships (for example, they can organize their friends by height). Children often enjoy collecting items and can spend hours organizing their dolls, rocks, or baseball cards.

Cognition is also apparent in **intelligence** (a combination of verbal ability, reasoning, memory, imagination, and judgment). No one knows whether heredity or environment is the greater influence on intelligence; certainly both are important. Children may be given some type of group-administered intelligence test during their elementary school experience, but these are not used for making important educational decisions. Scores are given as an **intelligence quotient (IQ)**. IQ tests often emphasize language and mathematical skills. The average person has an IQ of 110, with ranges of 80 to 120 considered normal. **Children and their parents need to understand that IQ measurements are only estimates of academic abilities and are not measures of a person's worth or potential for academic success.**

The field of psychology is moving away from the use of a single IQ score. Other tests may be used to measure aspects of intelligence. Most people probably possess many kinds of intelligence and should be encouraged to discover and nurture their individual strengths and talents. Kinds of intelligence and talent include linguistic, mathematic, spatial, musical, bodily kinesthetic, interpersonal, and intrapersonal.

Often during the early school years, children with learning problems are identified. Special programs can be helpful for children whose mental development is delayed. Children who have an IQ below 70 and problems adapting to everyday life are often considered to have special learning needs. This may be an inherited, organic problem, or it may be a result of illness, malnutrition, or lack of mental stimulation.

Numerous types of learning disabilities can be identified through testing and screening procedures. Many children can be helped to develop study habits and alternative learning methods to reach their full potential in the education experience.

The other extreme in the range of intelligence is the gifted child, who has an IQ well above average (140+) and/or possesses superior talent. Gifted children also need individualized programs. Traditional educational systems may not provide adequate challenge. Important decisions, such as the need for specialized instruction for a gifted student or placement in special education for a child with learning difficulties, are made by individually administered intelligence tests given by specialized professionals (Kaufman, 2013).

Studies of successful adults have led to the concept of emotional intelligence. Components of emotional intelligence can be found in Box 11.3. Parents need to model healthy emotional skills. Adults should help children learn to talk about feelings. When children's feelings are acknowledged and taken seriously, helping them find healthy ways of coping with their feelings becomes easier.

Box 11.3 Components of Emotional Intelligence

- Knowing one's own feelings and using them to make good decisions
- Managing feelings to keep distress from interfering with the ability to think
- Motivating oneself despite persistent setbacks
- Staying hopeful
- Delaying gratification
- Empathizing with others
- Developing rapport with others

Box 11.4 Functions of Children's Friendships

- **Affection:** Providing an emotional relationship outside of the family
- **Companionship:** Sharing activities
- **Ego support:** Supplying emotional support and encouragement
- **Physical support:** Spending time together
- **Social comparison:** Practicing social behaviors
- **Stimulation:** Thinking of new ideas

PSYCHOSOCIAL DEVELOPMENT

Children in the middle years continue to develop their **self-concept** (the way one views oneself). Children need to feel that they are valuable and important. **A comfortable relationship with parents and other adults is vital for development of a healthy self-concept.**

They also begin developing **social competence** (ability to get along with others). They learn coping skills for dealing with minor stressors. They learn that their behavior may influence others, and they become aware of how they appear to other people.

Erikson called the middle to late childhood psychosocial development stage **industry versus inferiority.** Children are energetic and capable; they want to accomplish things. They are interested in how things are made and work. Parents and teachers can aid the child through this stage by encouraging ideas, complimenting accomplishments, and helping a little at times. Every child can be complimented on some accomplishment; positive reinforcement helps them thrive. Children need support in facing their problems; they learn that problems can be managed.

The importance of peers increases as children grow. Middle and older children often organize clubs or teams. Belonging to a group builds self-esteem. Group activities are usually with same-gender children. Friendships are vital. Many children have one best friend with whom they share secrets and special times (Box 11.4).

PARENTING

Parents of middle and older children must adjust their expectations and degree of control. It is natural for children to begin spending more time with friends and

Table 11.4 Parenting Styles and Outcomes

STYLE	PARENT BEHAVIORS	CHILD MAY BECOME
Authoritative	Firm, in control; has rules; warm, loving, and encouraging	Self-reliant, responsible, socially competent
Authoritarian	Firm, in control; has rules; emotionally distant	Socially anxious
Permissive	Rules, if present, are flexible; may be emotionally warm or not	Impulsive, aggressive, and lacking self-control

less with family. Yet parents should remain interested in and involved with their children.

Children at this age can be given more responsibility, including household chores. They need to have opportunities to make decisions. Parents may need guidance in gradually decreasing the amount of supervision.

Some children must spend time alone before or after school because of their parents' schedules. The decision of when this is advisable depends on the length of time involved, the child's age and degree of responsibility, and the living situation. Most children under 11 years should not be left alone for more than an hour. Each family makes this decision, when necessary, on its own.

? Think Critically

How old were you when you were left alone at home? Do you remember how you felt about it? Does your community, state, or province have regulations or laws about this?

Middle and older children can no longer be disciplined by a time-out. Denial of privileges is often a better tool. Because of the importance of friends and social events, restricting those activities is often effective.

Psychologists have identified three parenting styles: permissive, authoritarian, and authoritative (Table 11.4). The authoritative parent is often considered the ideal. The reality is that most parents do not use only one style. Two parents in the family may use different styles. Styles may also change with additional children in the family and as the parents mature.

? Think Critically

What parenting style do you think your parent(s) used? Was it the same for your siblings? Will you use the same style in raising children? How do people learn to be parents?

CHILD ABUSE

Abuse of children by parents or others can occur at any age. There are many types of abuse: physical, sexual, emotional, neglect, and verbal. Each is damaging to the child's development.

Psychologists have determined that many abusers were themselves victims of abuse and have poor self-concepts. They may not know how to maintain a healthy relationship. This does not excuse his or her behavior but it serves as a warning that the cycle may continue unless someone intervenes. **Health care workers are required, in most states, to report signs of abuse to social agencies or law enforcement authorities** (see Chapter 3).

ADOLESCENTS

The adolescent years begin at age 12 and continue to age 18. The actual years are less significant than the experiences and development that occur. Because development is different for each individual, some 12-year-olds appear more physically mature compared with their peers. Another person may be 18 and still behave in adolescent ways at times.

Young children often talk about growing up, and older children may express eagerness to become teenagers. Many changes occur, and this can be a confusing time in the young person's life.

PHYSICAL DEVELOPMENT

Adolescents experience major physical changes with the onset of **puberty** (sexual maturation), which occurs gradually over several years. Normal development of the reproductive system depends on the health of the entire body, especially the endocrine system. **Genetics and nutrition are the primary influences on the age at which puberty occurs.**

Puberty also stimulates a growth spurt in adolescents, and growth periods may lead to fatigue. Both boys and girls usually continue to gain weight while they are growing in height. Girls usually reach their adult stature by the time they are 18 years old; boys may continue to grow taller well into their 20s.

The difference in the rate of physical development is often a concern to adolescents. Two friends may be the same age, but one may be more developed than the other is. Because girls mature earlier, they are often taller than boys are their age. Adolescents seldom think they compare favorably to their peers. They are preoccupied with their bodies and pay a lot of attention to their appearance.

Safety is a concern as adolescents expand their social networks and activities.

QSEN Considerations: Safety

Safety Guidelines for Adolescents

- Teach proper warm-up and stretching maneuvers to use before playing sports. Bones are growing more rapidly than muscles and tendons are at this stage, and injuries from sports activities are frequent.
- Encourage use of appropriate safety equipment for sports. Safety helmets must be worn when riding a bicycle or scooter. Elbow- and kneepads and a helmet should be worn when skateboarding or in-line skating.
- Teach all aspects of water safety, particularly that one should not swim alone or dive into shallow water or water of unknown depth.

- Once the adolescent is ready to drive, provide education on automobile safety along with the dangers of driving under the influence of alcohol or another drug.
- Reinforce the need for caution and appropriate behavior as the teen increases Internet communication and social networking.
- Provide education about the dangers of drug and alcohol use.
- Encourage good nutrition, physical activity, and limited use of television and video game playing to avoid obesity risks.

SEXUALITY

Because the sex hormones influence thoughts and desires, it is natural for adolescents to seek sexual activity. The media and entertainment industries also encourage sexual thoughts. The Centers for Disease Control and Prevention (CDC) reported in 2013 that 47% of US high school students had experienced intercourse, and 41% had not used a condom the last time they had sex (CDC, 2015a, 2015b). Although the body is capable of intercourse in adolescence, many young people are not prepared for the emotional aspects of sexual activity. Early sexual activity is associated with high risk of sexually transmitted infections, pregnancy, and emotional pain (Wisnieski & Matzo, 2013).

Health Promotion/Health Promotion Points

Counseling for Adolescents

- If an adolescent is or intends to become sexually active, responsible sexual behavior and birth control need to be addressed.
- Provide information on contraception options, sexually transmitted infections, and prevention of transmission.
- Although AIDS is transmitted in other ways, transmission through sexual intercourse is a real danger, and its incidence by this mode is rising. Even though deaths from AIDS are declining, quality of life is greatly affected by it, and deaths do occur.
- Nurses in the school, the clinic, and the physician's office have many opportunities to provide appropriate teaching and counseling regarding sexual behavior.

AIDS, Acquired immunodeficiency syndrome.

Studies show that adolescents actually know much less about sexuality than they pretend or think they know. Sex education is direly needed to prevent pregnancy and sexually transmitted infections (STIs). Parents remain the best teachers, but they often avoid that role. Schools are often expected to teach about sex and reproduction. Adolescents need information about physical changes and sexual development. Even when adolescents have been taught the basic facts about sexual behavior, they often do not think that such facts will apply to their own circumstances. The United States has a high rate of adolescent pregnancy. Parents, churches, and other organizations can help adolescents develop strategies for saying "no" to sexual activity.

COGNITIVE DEVELOPMENT

Adolescents are learning to think in creative, abstract, logical, and idealistic ways. They begin to examine their own thoughts and try to analyze the thoughts of others. Piaget labeled this stage **formal operations.** Beginning between ages 11 and 14, thought becomes more abstract; the adolescent can think about ideas. Some enjoy becoming philosophical. Communication skills improve as adolescents better organize their thoughts in logical ways.

Young people may analyze how they want to be, how their parents should be, and how the world should be in the future. Sometimes this idealism becomes frustrating for them as they encounter reality. Adolescents also become more aware of other people and of what others think about them. They want to fit into society. They also become egocentric again. Adolescents tend to believe that others are as interested in them as they are in themselves. They may indulge in attention-seeking behavior.

Another part of egocentrism is the belief that one's own experiences are unique. Adolescents may not realize that other people have faced disappointments and problems, too. They may also believe that they are immortal. They cannot imagine that anything bad would happen to them, so they may avoid using contraception and take risks with drinking and driving.

The role of schools in the cognitive development of adolescents remains significant. **Schools that address students' individual learning needs can aid young people in their search for meaning and identity.** Teachers who understand adolescents can help them figure out the world and stimulate their intellectual growth. School and extracurricular activities are also important for social activity.

PSYCHOSOCIAL DEVELOPMENT

The psychosocial development of adolescents can be turbulent. Emotions may be erratic when hormones are newly released. The young person has to learn how to handle those emotions and how to get along with other people.

Change continues in the relationships between adolescents and their families. Teens seek to be autonomous and free of parental control, yet many adolescents also yearn to have rules and to know that parents care about them. Parents should gradually allow young people to make more of their own decisions; both parents and teens also have to learn to live with the consequences.

Time spent as a family unit often lessens when the child becomes an adolescent. It is natural for the teen to want to spend more time with peers. Parents should allow more freedom for peer interaction, but should monitor the teen's activities and friends. Trying to hold the teen too closely may lead to estrangement. Many people admit only later in their lives that family relationships are important during adolescence.

Serious conflict between parents and teens is most common, when it occurs, during early adolescence. This corresponds to the time of major hormonal shifts and helps explain why the junior high or middle school years may be difficult. When conflict exists, it usually becomes less acute as the adolescent matures. By age 17 or 18, relationships with parents often become smoother. The daily negotiations and minor conflicts that occur are natural results of development that help adolescents find their own identity.

Adolescents continue to learn about the world and other people during time spent with their peers. In early adolescence, young people have a strong need to conform to a peer group. They often want to dress alike, behave alike, and do the same things that their group does.

Dating is an important adolescent experience that also helps young people discover their individual identity. Dating serves many other purposes such as recreation, status, and achievement. Most adolescents become interested in the opposite sex early in puberty (Fig. 11.4). The interest grows as they mature. Young people's groups include both boys and girls, gradually evolving into group-dating events.

Erikson's stage for adolescence is **identity versus role confusion.** The adolescent struggles with questions: Who am I? What am I about? What will I do with my life? The teen who is successfully coping with these questions develops an acceptable sense of self. The teen who is not successful may remain confused, withdraw from society, or passively follow the crowd. Some teens conquer this challenge during adolescence, whereas others struggle longer. A healthy identity is open to change as time goes on.

Some adolescents experiment with a variety of roles in society. This may cause conflicts with parents, as teens explore alternative lifestyles or value systems. The types of jobs that adolescents may try can also aid them in discovering who they are. Contemporary theorists agree that the resolution of this identity search may extend into adulthood. This is especially true with young people who continue their education after high school.

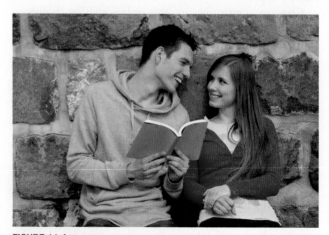

FIGURE 11.4 Dating provides opportunities to help establish values. (Photo copyright istock.com.)

Parents of adolescents can aid them in successful psychosocial development by supporting their decisions, acknowledging their struggles, and respecting them as they mature. Parents and teens who have had open communication and mutual respect during their earlier years should navigate this challenging time with less trouble compared with those whose prior relationship was shaky.

TASKS OF ADOLESCENCE

Discovering their identity is a primary psychosocial task for adolescents. They begin making decisions that will affect the rest of their lives. One of these is choosing a vocation. Although teens are seldom expected to decide on a lifetime vocation, they should have some ideas about the kind of work they would enjoy.

Ideology (a belief or value system) should be fairly well established by the end of adolescence. A moral code begins to be incorporated. One's **sexual orientation** (sexual preference) should also be set. According to the 2013 National Health Interview Survey, studies estimate that 1.6% of the population is homosexual and 0.7% is bisexual. However, according to 2015 Gallup polls, Americans who were surveyed estimated that 23% of the population is gay, lesbian, bisexual, or transgender, which is substantially higher than the 3.8% of the population who identified themselves in the early results of the survey. All people need to accept and understand their own preference. Adolescence can be a difficult time for people who are unsure of their orientation.

Some theorists claim that mate selection is also part of adolescent development. In the United States, many young people prefer to postpone marriage until later in their lives.

CONCERNS IN ADOLESCENT DEVELOPMENT

Pregnancy

When an adolescent becomes pregnant, she needs assistance in discussing options. It is difficult to decide whether to place the child up for adoption, to keep the child and remain single, to keep the child and marry, or to abort the pregnancy. Often the father contributes little to the financial and emotional support of the infant of an adolescent mother. Sometimes adolescents who are unmarried keep the baby, and the grandparents end up with the responsibility of raising the child. This is becoming a significant burden for the older generation. Often the adolescent mother does not continue her education and then has trouble becoming a self-sufficient adult.

In 2014, the birth rate for US girls ages 15 to 19 fell to a record low of 24.2 births per 1000 girls (CDC, 2016). An adolescent pregnancy is a high-risk pregnancy because the young expectant mother is still physically growing. Younger mothers are more likely than older mothers are to have premature babies with low birth weight. Pregnant adolescents must be guided toward early prenatal care, parenting classes, and psychosocial counseling. The social problems generated by adolescent pregnancy are significant as many become single mothers and end up needing public assistance for themselves and their child.

Employment

Many adolescents seek part-time work. Most authorities agree that there are positive and negative aspects of adolescent employment. First jobs can be valuable in teaching a strong work ethic and money management. Some adolescents work to help supplement the family income or to pay for special clothes or a car. However, depending on the number of hours worked, school grades may suffer. Sleep may also suffer, just when the body needs more sleep for growing. Family interactions may also be affected.

Chemical Abuse

According to the U.S. National Library of Medicine, alcohol is the substance most abused by youth and young adults, followed by marijuana and inhalants (CDC, 2013). Prescription drug abuse by teens is also on the rise, accompanied by the false belief by some that these drugs are safe because a provider prescribed them for someone. Young people do not achieve positive development in cognitive and psychosocial aspects when they abuse chemicals. Alcohol and use of other drugs can contribute to risky sexual behavior and is often a factor in teen pregnancy. Ecstasy, a popular drug for some teens, can shrink the hippocampus (the part of the brain important for memory storage) by 10%. Depression may become a problem as the teen becomes isolated from usual activities and school because of the chemical abuse.

Eating Disorders

Adolescents (particularly girls) who are obsessed with body image may develop severe eating disorders. **Anorexia nervosa** is a disorder in which food intake is severely limited and strenuous exercise may be used to control body weight. The body becomes emaciated, and sexual development is delayed. Anorexia nervosa may result in death if untreated. **Bulimia nervosa** is characterized by binge eating followed by inducing vomiting or using laxatives to eliminate the foods from the body. Bulimia nervosa may accompany anorexia nervosa or be a disorder by itself. Bulimic individuals tend to maintain a more normal weight. Both disorders are psychological illnesses that manifest with physical symptoms, and both can have long-term negative physical effects. Growing up in a dysfunctional family may contribute to the development of eating disorders.

Depression

Mental health disorders are sometimes undiagnosed in adolescence. Untreated depression may be the cause of attempted or successful suicide. At other times, depression seems to be a sudden reaction to a change in one's life. Many factors can contribute to depression in the adolescent, including the feeling of not "fitting in" and being bullied. Bullying can even intrude on the safety of the home via the Internet ("cyberbullying"). According to The Cyberbullying Research Center, 26% of middle school and high school students have been victims of cyberbullying, and 16% have been involved in bullying. Studies demonstrate decreased substance use and mental health problems when youth view the family as a resource for support and advice (Ackley & Ladwig, 2014).

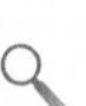

 QSEN Considerations: Safety

Depression in Adolescents

- Any adolescent who exhibits signs of depression should be evaluated by a mental health professional skilled in working with young people.
- Suicide is a far too frequent occurrence among depressed teens.
- Signs of adolescent depression include declining school grades, chronic melancholy, alcohol or other drug use, and expressions of feeling down or blue.

 QSEN Considerations: Safety

Smoking in Adolescents

Exposure to any nicotine can adversely affect adolescent brain development and result in nicotine addiction. Smoking rates are on the decline in most states; however, there has been an increase in the use of e-cigarettes. If this trend continues, 5.6 million young people will die prematurely (Potera, 2015).

Early Deaths

Causes of death among adolescents in the United States, in order of frequency, are accidents, homicide, and suicide.

Get Ready for the NCLEX Examination!

Key Points

- Growth and development begin at conception and continue throughout life. Development includes physical, cognitive, and psychosocial aspects.
- Development of children is commonly divided into five stages: prenatal, infancy, early childhood, middle and late childhood, and adolescence.
- Freud's theory has three parts that include levels of awareness, components of the personality or mind (the id, ego, and superego), and psychosexual stages of development.
- Erikson's theory of psychosocial development identifies certain tasks that should be accomplished at each stage.
- Piaget's theory of cognitive development identifies ways that children learn to think and to understand the world.
- Kohlberg's theory of moral development identifies stages in the development of moral behavior.
- Early and regular prenatal health care is essential for optimal development of the fetus.
- Newborns have many capabilities at birth, but depend on caregivers to meet their needs.
- An infant's cognitive and psychosocial development is enhanced by adults who provide a variety of appropriate stimulation and bonding.
- Growth should be monitored regularly to detect any concerns as early as possible.
- Young children are naturally curious but are not aware of possible dangers in their world.
- Health promotion and safety are important throughout childhood and adolescence.
- Parents who use day care providers should be selective about choosing caregivers. Preschool can help prepare a child for school and teach socialization skills.
- Good childhood nutritional habits will contribute to health throughout life.
- Children in the middle years are industrious; success in activities increases their self-worth.
- Childhood friendships provide important stimulation and help children learn to get along with other people.
- Three different parenting styles have been identified: permissive, authoritarian, and authoritative. Children develop differently with different parenting styles.
- Discipline measures change as a child grows. Young children are often given time-outs. Older children may need to be denied an activity.
- The physical and emotional changes of puberty can be upsetting for the adolescent; sexual thoughts and desires increase.
- Adolescents' cognitive development becomes abstract, idealistic, and more adultlike.
- Adolescents are concerned about discovering their own identity, finding their place in the world. Dating is an adolescent ritual important in psychosocial development.
- Conflicts between adolescents and their parents are common as teens experiment with adult roles and behaviors.
- Adolescents should determine their ideology and sexual orientation, and they should have some ideas about vocation, by the end of this stage.
- Concerns of adolescence include pregnancy, employment, chemical abuse, eating disorders, depression, and early death.

Additional Learning Resources

SG Go to your Study Guide for additional learning activities to help you master this chapter content.

evolve Go to your Evolve website at http://evolve.elsevier.com/Williams/fundamental for additional online resources.

Review Questions for the NCLEX Examination

*Choose the **best** answer for each question.*

1. A mother brings her 9-month-old baby into the clinic for a well-baby check. While gathering data, you notice that the baby appears to be communicating in two-word sentences. The mother affirms your observation when you ask her about her baby's language development. You inform the mother that:
   1. The baby's language development seems to be occurring more quickly than expected.
   2. The baby might be experiencing developmental delays.
   3. The baby's language development seems to be right on track.
   4. It is part of the required information on the well-baby checkup form.
2. The single most important factor in maintaining a healthy pregnancy is:
   1. Early and regular prenatal care.
   2. High nutritional consumption during pregnancy.
   3. Finding an obstetrician that you trust.
   4. Planning to do the right thing for the baby.
3. Which adolescent is an example of a current trend?
   1. A high school athlete is taking his grandmother's Vicodin to self-treat a recent back injury.
   2. A 16-year-old girl is expecting a baby in 2 months.
   3. A 17-year-old high school student has withdrawn from school because he is in the end stages of AIDS.
   4. A high school senior has begun taking amphetamines to help increase her study time.
4. Parents of children ages 3 to 6 years may need guidance in:
   1. Making the child feel secure when a newborn arrives.
   2. Helping the child cope with peers.
   3. Effective methods of toilet training.
   4. Allowing the child to make more of his or her own decisions.
5. A parent who insists that the child stay in his or her room for the full 4-minute time-out and then smiles and hugs the child when the time is up is showing a parenting style that is:
   1. Authoritative.
   2. Passive.
   3. Authoritarian.
   4. Punitive.

6. Growth and development should be monitored regularly for every child to:
  1. Provide statistics needed for proper research.
  2. Detect abnormal growth patterns so that early care and treatment of problems can begin.
  3. Provide data to establish norms for growth and development at various ages.
  4. Reassure parents that their children are healthy.

7. An effective discipline measure for an adolescent is: *(Select all that apply.)*
  1. Restricting social activities for a limited time.
  2. Grounding them to the house for several weeks.
  3. Assigning extra chores.
  4. Fining them a portion of their allowance.
  5. Taking away the cell phone for 1 week.

8. The adolescent who is thinking in logical and abstract ways as he completes a term paper shows:
  1. Aspects of industry.
  2. Identity confusion.
  3. Appropriate cognitive development.
  4. Appropriate psychosocial development.

Critical Thinking Activities

Read each clinical scenario and discuss the questions with your classmates.

Scenario A

A single mother brings her 7-year-old daughter to the clinic where you are working because of a bad cold. The child is smaller than average. As you interview them, you learn that because of the mother's work schedule, the girl is home alone every school morning for 2 hours and does not always eat breakfast. What concerns about this situation might you have?

Scenario B

The math teacher at the high school told the parents of a 17-year-old student that he is unpleasant in class, falls asleep often, does not consistently hand in homework, and made a D on the last test. The mother asks you what to do. When she tried to talk with her son, he became sarcastic and walked out. He has a part-time job at a local fast-food restaurant.

chapter

12 Adulthood and the Family

http://evolve.elsevier.com/Williams/fundamental

Objectives

Upon completing this chapter, you should be able to do the following:

Theory

1. List three stages of adulthood.
2. Explain Schaie's theory of cognitive development in young and middle adults.
3. Discuss Erikson's stages of psychosocial development in young and middle adults.
4. List at least three functions of families.
5. Describe the effects of divorce on involved persons.
6. Describe the physical and psychosocial development and changes of young and middle adults.

Clinical Practice

1. Design an educational program to help adults maintain a healthy lifestyle.
2. Identify at least three health concerns of young adults.
3. Identify at least four health concerns of middle adults.
4. Explain how caring people can nourish the cognitive and psychosocial development of adults.

Key Terms

achievement stage (p. 161)
andropause (p. 167)
baby boomers (p. 166)
boomerang children (BŪ-mĕr-ăng, p. 165)
career (p. 161)
empty nest syndrome (SĬN-drōm, p. 168)
executive substage (ĕx-Ĕ-kĕw-tĭv, p. 161)
generativity (jĕn-ĕr-ă-TĬ-vĭ-tē, p. 161)
intimacy (ĬN-tĭ-mă-sē, p. 161)
maturity (mă-TŬR-ĭ-tē, p. 163)
menopause (MĔ-nō-păwz, p. 167)
mentors (p. 169)
patient-centered care (p. 161)
presbycusis (prĕz-bē-KŪ-sĭs, p. 166)
presbyopia (prĕz-bē-Ō-pē-ă, p. 166)
responsibility stage (rĕ-spŏn-sĭ-BĬ-lĭ-tē, p. 161)
sandwich generation (p. 169)
stagnation (stăg-NĀ-shŭn, p. 161)
vocational (p. 164)

 Concepts Covered in This Chapter

- Caregiving
- Cognition
- Communication
- Coping
- Culture
- Development
- Ethics
- Family dynamics
- Health promotion
- Infection
- Mobility
- Pain
- Reproduction
- Sexuality
- Stress

ADULTHOOD AS CONTINUING CHANGE

Adulthood usually begins at age 18 years, although people may continue adolescent behaviors into their 20s. Adults continue to grow and develop throughout the life span. As the body continues to change with age, it becomes increasingly susceptible to health disorders, and the person must work harder to maintain health. Thinking patterns and life goals also change as the person acquires more life experiences.

Erik Erikson describes three stages of adulthood. The first stage is young adulthood, ages 18 to 35 years. The second stage is middle adulthood, ages 35 to 65 years. Older adulthood is the third stage, starting at age 65 to death. As with younger people, the age ranges should be regarded as flexible when considering an individual.

THEORIES OF DEVELOPMENT

SCHAIE'S THEORY OF COGNITIVE DEVELOPMENT

Piaget thought that adolescents and adults think in the same ways (see Chapter 11). Contemporary theorists, on the contrary, believe that formal operational thinking becomes more refined during adulthood. Several stages of cognitive development in adults were identified and defined by K. Warner Schaie, who expanded on Piaget's ideas.

Schaie called the young adult stage of cognitive development the **achievement stage** (needing to learn and use your abilities successfully). He believed that young adults are optimistic and strive to improve themselves. They want to apply what they have learned, continue to learn, prove their competence, and increase their **career** (work that requires specific training) choices.

The **responsibility stage** (concerned with real-life problems; being in charge of self and others) occurs in middle adulthood. At this stage, adults are responsible for themselves, a job, often a family, and perhaps some aspect of the community. This includes attention to the needs of a spouse, children, co-workers, and others.

For some middle adults, Schaie identified the **executive substage** (being responsible for major corporations or the country). He states that many middle adults with multiple responsibilities learn to function as executives in their lives. They delegate appropriately, juggle roles, and manage complex situations.

ERIKSON'S STAGES OF ADULT PSYCHOSOCIAL DEVELOPMENT

Erikson called the young adult stage **intimacy** versus isolation. *Intimacy* refers to close, meaningful relationships. Young adults want to give of themselves and to be committed to others. They establish intimate, intense relationships with other people. Maintaining close family ties is another positive example.

Generativity (guiding the lives of the next generation) versus **stagnation** (inactivity, self-absorption) is the psychosocial stage of development seen in middle adults. Many are willing and eager to help young members of their family or community. Middle adults are productive people who accept the interdependence necessary for satisfactory living. People who are stagnant may have trouble keeping a job, are not interested in volunteering, and are self-involved.

FAMILIES

Because people are social beings, one cannot study an individual's development without knowing about the family environment that influences it. ***Family*** is defined as a group of individuals who care about and for each other (Fig. 12.1).

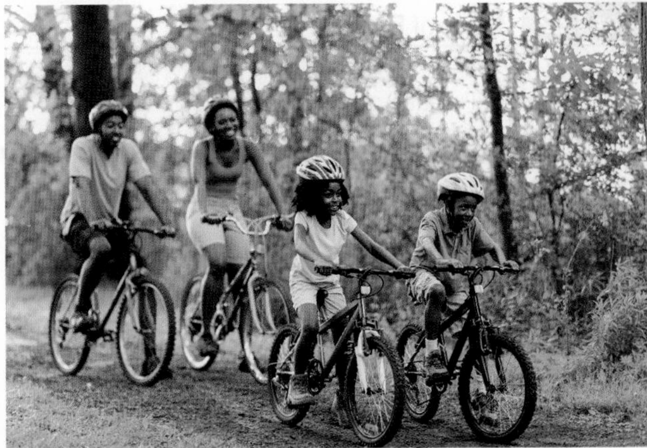

FIGURE 12.1 Exercising together helps keep everyone healthy. (Photo copyright istock.com.)

Box 12.1 Functions of the Family

- **Physical maintenance:** Providing essentials for life
- **Protection:** Creating an atmosphere for health and safety
- **Nurturance:** Providing loving care and guidance
- **Socialization:** Interacting appropriately with others
- **Education:** Teaching about values and the world
- **Reproduction:** Continuing the species
- **Recreation:** Having fun together
- **Support:** Helping and caring for each other

Families provide an important environment for children to learn basic values and how to relate to other people. Functions of families are listed in Box 12.1. A family's cultural and ethnic background also influences children. **The family's support remains important throughout life.**

 QSEN Considerations: Patient-Centered Care

The Family in Health Care

In the health care setting, **patient-centered care** is an important concept, which includes the family as an integral piece. Family members are considered more than visitors are; health care providers share important information, as appropriate (but not in violation of the Health Insurance Portability and Accountability Act [HIPAA], see Chapter 3), and make decisions with the patient's best interest in mind. Being respectful of family values and communication is part of patient-centered care.

TYPES OF FAMILIES

There have always been different kinds of families, but awareness of differences is greater now than it was in the past. Some types of families are defined in Box 12.2.

 Think Critically

What kind of family did you have as a child? Did you ever wish it were different? What kind of family do you have now?

Box 12.2 Types of Families

- **Nuclear:** One or two parents and child(ren).
- **Extended:** Parent(s), child(ren), grandparent(s), and other relatives.
- **Step:** One parent and child(ren) and a new parent.
- **Blended:** Mom and her children and dad and his children.
- **Single parent:** Woman or man in a separate household with child(ren) because of divorce, death, desertion, or individual preference.
- **Partner:** Parents of the same gender. Children are from previous relationships, artificial insemination, or adopted.
- **Cohabitation:** Couples who live together with their children but remain unmarried.
- **Foster parent:** Temporary adult caregiver(s) providing for child(ren)'s care, while waiting for child to be adopted or for natural parent situation to improve.
- **Adopted:** Caregiver(s) obtaining legal guardianship over children and becoming parent(s). Grandparents may adopt grandchildren if young parents are not able to provide for their care, or couples unable to conceive may adopt children.

HISTORICAL CHANGES IN FAMILIES

Sociologists have identified many changes in family life in the past 50 years. Varieties of families are one example. Other changes include:

- **Urbanization:** Rural families of the past were more self-sufficient than today's city dwellers. Only a small percentage of the population now lives on farms.
- **Mobility:** Many families do not stay in one community, usually because of a changing job market. Some children attend four or five schools before they finish high school. This also affects relationships among the extended family.
- **Size:** The average size of families is decreasing. As living expenses increase, people realize they cannot afford as many children as their parents or grandparents did.
- **Use of paid caregivers:** Most two-parent families have two or more wage earners. Most single parents are employed. Children are cared for by others for part of every workday.
- **Fathers' roles:** Since the 1980s, men are taking a greater role in their children's lives. Whether married or single, many men enjoy participating in child care. It is also more common for single fathers to be custodial parents than it was in earlier decades.
- **Increased longevity:** Health care advances contribute to longer life spans. Some families have four or five living generations.

DIVORCE AND FAMILIES

According to the Centers for Disease Control and Prevention/National Center for Health Statistics (2015), the number of divorces reported each year is 50% of the total marriages. People expect a great deal from marriage; partners expect each other to be best friends, confidantes, and perfect lovers. Some factors that increase the risk of divorce are listed in Box 12.3.

Box 12.3 Risk Factors for Divorce

- Bride and groom younger than 20
- Lower economic status
- Cohabitation before marriage
- Premarital pregnancy
- Having children from a previous marriage
- Either partner having been previously divorced
- Knowing each other for only a short time before marriage
- One or both not finishing high school
- No religious affiliation or practicing different faiths
- One or both having divorced parents

Divorce early in a marriage, especially before there are children, may seem the least harmful. However, the people involved may be deeply affected. There may have been abuse or infidelity. Counseling may be necessary for people ending a difficult relationship.

Divorce can be especially hard on young children, who may believe they are to blame for the family breakup. The children often harbor guilt and may fantasize about reuniting the family.

Older children and adolescents can sometimes understand that their parents' marital problems are not their fault, but they are still affected by the divorce. It may influence the way they relate to other people, especially as they begin dating, and may affect their ability to trust others.

Some couples discover that they have little in common after their children are grown, and they may divorce at that point. The adult children often have trouble understanding why this happens.

Divorce also affects the parents and other relatives of the divorcing couple. Sometimes grandparents lose opportunities to be with their grandchildren. The increasing incidence of divorce in the latter half of the 20th century is viewed as a major cause of poverty because so many divorced women have low incomes. **Divorce occurs between two people, but the effects ripple into their extended families and their community.**

YOUNG ADULTS

Millennials (people born between 1982 and 2000) now outnumber the baby boomers. There are now over 83 million millennials, making up over one quarter of the US population (United States Census Bureau, 2015). Millennials are also more ethnically diverse compared with previous generations. The decade after high school is a time of transition for young people. Most are completing adolescent developmental processes and moving into the roles and responsibilities of young adults. Several major events usually occur during this

Box 12.4 Behaviors Indicating Maturity

The ability to:
- Acknowledge and express feelings with restraint
- Laugh at yourself
- Accept responsibility for your own actions
- Tolerate frustration
- Accept diversity and individuality in others
- Trust others
- Display self-confidence
- Cope with stress
- Discipline yourself
- Handle problems without losing sight of goals

time. Decisions young adults make during these years influence the rest of their lives.

In our culture, two significant milestones signal young adulthood. The first is **economic independence,** which usually happens when a person is employed full time. Many young people in college or technical education programs cannot reach this milestone until later. The second is **independent decision making.**

Some theorists say that **maturity** (being fully developed) is a significant marker of reaching adulthood. It is probably more accurate to say that we are all growing toward maturity. **Mature people have established a philosophy of life based on their own belief system and personal ethics** (Box 12.4).

PHYSICAL DEVELOPMENT

Most young adults are physically at their peak. Their strength, endurance, and energy are at high levels. Most report their general health as good; few have chronic health concerns. Young adults usually have fewer colds and minor illnesses than when they were children. Good physical health at age 30 is considered an indicator of good physical health in later years as well.

Patient Education

Health Habits for Young Adults

Provide health teaching to young adults on the following topics:
- Developing healthy dietary and exercise habits to promote a healthy weight.
- Exercising to increase endurance, strength, flexibility, and muscle tone. The US government recommends a weekly routine of 75 minutes of vigorously intense aerobic activity, OR 150 minutes of moderately intense aerobic activity, OR an equivalent mix of moderately and vigorously intense aerobic activity, PLUS performing muscle-strengthening activities that work all major muscle groups two times a week.
- Maintaining weight within normal limits and reducing fat to less than 30% of calories.
- Recognizing that muscle development and fat accumulation contribute to changes in body shape.

Skeletal development is completed when young adults reach their full stature. For women this often occurs by age 18 or 19; men can continue to grow until their late 20s. The physical differences between men and women are significant. Generally, men are taller, heavier, and stronger than women are. They have broader shoulders, narrower hips, and larger hands and feet.

Dental maturity is achieved with the eruption of wisdom teeth. Regular dental care is important to maintain healthy teeth and gums.

Physical growth of the brain continues into the mid-20s, peaking during these years, and memory is acute, making learning easier. Growth of neural connections continues into later years. Middle and older adults continue to learn but often at a slower pace.

The ages of 19 to 26 are physically the best years for reproduction. Many young adults choose to delay childbearing until they are economically and emotionally prepared for parenting.

The validity of studies about sexual behavior is often questioned because the results are based on self-reporting. During young adulthood, sexual preferences are identified, and there may be numerous partners. Promiscuity increases the risk of sexually transmitted infections (STIs), especially HIV infection.

HEALTH CONCERNS OF YOUNG ADULTS

Risky Behavior

Because young adults are generally healthy and feel well, they may feel invincible and engage in risky behaviors, such as chemical abuse, overeating, inadequate sleep, an inactive lifestyle, and sexual promiscuity. Abuse of chemicals often contributes to other risky behavior.

Young adults die primarily because of accidents, homicide, or suicide. Accidents are the primary cause of death for white males; homicide is the leading cause of death for African American males (Centers for Disease Control and Prevention, 2015b).

Stress-Related Illness

Young adults over age 30 begin to be affected by stress-related health problems such as obesity, diabetes, headaches, gastrointestinal problems, and hypertension. The incidence of these conditions increases as people get older. People may use alcohol or other drugs in unhealthy attempts to relieve stress.

Early Disease

The third health concern for young adults is development of diseases, especially cancer. Women should have annual pelvic examinations, including a periodic Papanicolaou (Pap) smear to screen for cervical cancer. According to the American Cancer Society (2015), women in their 20s and 30s should have a breast examination every 3 years by a health care provider and a screening mammogram annually starting at age 45 (or age 40 if desired), then every 2 years after age 55 as long as the woman remains in good health. Women determined to be at higher risk for breast cancer should have annual mammograms and magnetic resonance imaging (MRI) scans.

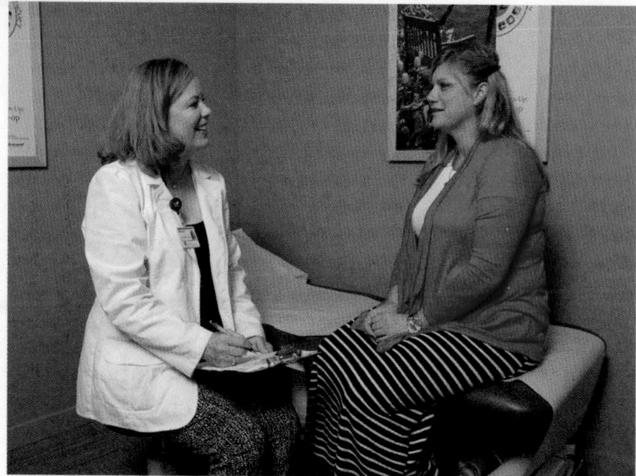

FIGURE 12.2 Regular physical checkups monitor health status.

Some providers recommend that young men learn how to perform monthly self-examination of the testicles beginning at age 15. They should see their primary care provider if they detect any growths or changes.

Both men and women should have annual physical examinations to screen for cardiovascular disease, hypertension, diabetes, and high cholesterol and to assess weight management (Fig. 12.2). Periodic Mantoux tests are advised to screen for tuberculosis. Immunizations should be kept current.

COGNITIVE DEVELOPMENT

In the achievement stage of Schaie's theory, young adults apply their intelligence to higher education and to early career development. Young adults are no longer egocentric. They are more able to reason, solve problems, and set reasonable goals.

Patient Education

Teaching Young Adults

Keep in mind the following points when teaching young adults:

- Build on previous knowledge and skills.
- Make the goals of patient education clear.
- Indicate how the new knowledge can be applied and how it is of personal benefit.
- Use interactive, problem-oriented methods that relate to daily tasks at home, work, or school.

Cognitive development of young adults is aided by the support of others. Young adults may need guidance to identify their goals clearly and continue striving toward them.

Continuing Education

Many young adults continue their education after high school. Higher education can help people understand their world, learn to manage their time, and prepare for a career.

It is generally believed that 1 or 2 years of higher education, even if career goals are unclear, can help young adults learn more about themselves and the world. For those who do not want to continue school beyond high school, many careers are best learned on the job or in vocational/technical schools.

Careers and Work

The ability to earn a living is an important accomplishment of young adulthood. Working provides the means of personal, social, and financial survival. It can also give someone a sense of identity and increase self-worth and respect. Some view their work as a service to others.

Exploration of **vocational** (trade, profession, or occupation) choices is expected in late adolescence and early adulthood. Some counselors encourage young adults to try several kinds of jobs to determine what type of work might provide the most satisfaction. It is common for individuals to have up to seven different jobs throughout their work life. Disillusionment about the ideal job is frequent as realities of the work world are identified.

Think Critically

How many kinds of jobs have you had? What jobs have you left in the past? What are you looking for in a career? How is a career different from a job?

What do young adults want from their work? Adequate money must be considered, but it is not always most important; the priority is finding interesting work. They also want the opportunity to use their skills and abilities, and a chance for advancement.

Unemployment can be the result of many factors, but it is often viewed as personal failure, even if it is the result of a weak economy. In tough economic times, even jobs that are historically plentiful, such as nursing, can be difficult to find. Prolonged and unwanted unemployment can cause financial crisis, loss of self-esteem, and depression.

The roles of employed women in the United States continue to stimulate discussion. **Gender equality** is the movement for equal opportunity and equal pay for women and men. Young women often have a dilemma when choosing a type of work. Some may prefer to be full-time homemakers and mothers. That option may be impossible because of the economic pressures facing young families.

Concerns about career versus family may cause personal or family conflict. Family-friendly employment policies benefit both women and men. The kinds of work available to women remain restricted in some fields. According to the Institute for Women's Policy Research (2015), women with full-time, year-round employment still only earn 78 cents on the dollar when compared with men.

PSYCHOSOCIAL DEVELOPMENT

Independence from the parental family is a primary achievement during young adulthood. This is interpreted as living on your own and making your own decisions. The trend toward young adults being **boomerang children** (children who return to the parental home temporarily) has grown considerably as children find it difficult to make sufficient money to establish a home of their own. Sometimes returning young adults bring their children along, commonly because of economic hardship.

Erikson called the young adult stage of psychosocial development **intimacy versus isolation.** It is important that people continue the development of meaningful relationships with others. If this task of developing intimacy is not accomplished, the young adult might not trust others and may be hesitant to develop close relationships. This could lead to withdrawal and depression.

According to Erikson, adolescents should find identity, which helps them become more independent. Independence precedes the need for developing intimacy and sometimes may conflict with it. A secure and independent person is ready to be intimate with another and can allow the other person to be independent.

Personality development continues throughout the life span. Most theorists agree that your early life is significant in forming your basic personality. Major personality changes in adulthood are not likely to occur. The person who is usually happy will remain so; the opposite is also true. **Changes that a person wants to make require self-analysis and a lot of work.**

DEVELOPMENTAL TASKS

Marriage

Deciding whether to marry is a major concern in young adulthood. Ninety percent of Americans do eventually try marriage. The average age at first marriage is 27 for women and 29 for men (United States Census Bureau, 2014). These ages are increasing as more people choose to delay marriage, often for higher education. Selection of a marriage partner is a critical decision; there are no foolproof rules for mate selection. **Although opposites may attract, successful marriages often involve partners who share basic values and philosophies about life.** Young love is romantic and intense. Marriage requires mutual respect, sharing, and commitment. The fear of making a poor choice is one reason people decide to cohabit before or instead of marrying. Married people are generally healthier and happier throughout their lives.

Single adults include those who have never been married and those who are widowed, separated, or divorced. In the United States people who live alone make up approximately 27% of US households (Henderson, 2014), an increase from previous years. Many singles live full, happy lives. There are positive and negative aspects to living alone. Single people can be independent with their time and money; they do not have to be concerned about a partner's ideas or desires. However, they have no one to depend on when trouble occurs. They have to be responsible for their own decisions. Many single adults report that they are often lonely.

? Think Critically

What are some of the challenges facing a young adult who is also a single parent? What kinds of guidance might be needed from a health care provider?

Parenting

Many people become parents during young adulthood. Some couples carefully discuss and plan decisions about having children. Others choose not to use birth control measures. The National Center for Health Statistics reports that the average age of first-time mothers is 26. The birth rates are declining for teenagers aged 15 to 19, as well as for women in their 20s. In contrast, rates are increasing for women in their 30s and late 40s (HealthProfessional/National Vital Statistic Report, 2015).

Some women delay having children in favor of career development. They might then have trouble with conceiving after age 30 as fertility declines. The option of in vitro fertilization is available but expensive. By age 40, a pregnant woman is statistically considered a high risk pregnancy. Technological developments have made it possible for some women to become pregnant into their 50s. **Childbearing, however, is only the beginning of parenting.** The issues of day care, discipline, and other child-rearing decisions continue for years. Most people learn about parenting from the examples seen in childhood.

? Think Critically

If you have a child, are you aware of your parenting style? Is it similar to or different from the way your parents raised you? If you do not have a child, what kind of parent do you think you would be? Would you want to use the model of your parents?

In the past, young families were often geographically near older relatives and had the emotional support of extended family. Many young families today do not live near other family members and may struggle with child-rearing issues. Some areas have developed Early Childhood and Family Education (ECFE) programs through schools or community organizations, where young adults can share concerns and learn about successful parenting. Tips and resources are also available for parents coping with the challenges of raising adolescents.

Home Management

The tasks involved in making life run smoothly need regular attention. Having groceries on hand, keeping the house in order, managing money, doing laundry, having the oil changed in the car, and cleaning the refrigerator are examples of tasks involved in home management.

Developing a Social Group

Having friends who share values is vital for socialization. Friendships beyond the extended family are valuable. For young adults, this can be a challenge when they go away to school or take a job in a new locale. They may have always lived in one area until this stage, and now have to make new friends in a different part of the world. Young adults who are confident, outgoing, and willing to be active in their community have a good chance of succeeding.

Community Responsibility

Beginning involvement in community affairs is another mark of young adulthood, as people begin to think about the world beyond their family. Examples of this include joining a service organization, being involved in a religious community, or becoming active in local government. Young adults with healthy psychosocial development begin to reach beyond their own needs to be concerned with others. Sharing your expertise by volunteering is good for society as a whole.

MIDDLE ADULTHOOD

Middle adulthood is from ages 46 to 64. Middle adults are often viewed as in the best years of their life, the wise, powerful leaders. However, stereotypes about people growing older begin to appear: life is "downhill" and unhappy. Some people are reluctant to admit they are middle aged because of such negative views. These can be challenging years, too, as people expand their personal and social involvement.

The oldest **baby boomers** (people born between 1946 and 1964) reached middle age in the 1990s. This large group of people (estimated at 79 million) has had a major effect on US society at every stage of their development. They have challenged traditional beliefs and forged new ways of thinking about and living at every developmental stage.

PHYSICAL DEVELOPMENT

Physical changes begin to appear during the middle years of life, and some people seek ways to slow the aging process. **The rate of change, even changes of aging, varies among individuals.** Not every person will experience every change; most changes occur so gradually that they may be unnoticed for years. Individuals who exercise regularly, eat sensibly, and take care of their bodies can often delay some of these changes.

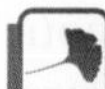
Complementary and Alternative Therapies

Herbs and Supplements to Help Slow Various Problems of Aging

- **Black cohosh (*Cimicifuga racemosa*):** To lessen signs and symptoms of menopause
- **Garlic (*Allium sativum*):** To reduce blood pressure and cholesterol and to prevent blood clots
- **Vitamin E:** To possibly prevent or slow dementia; may help prevent heart attacks
- **Glucosamine and chondroitin sulfate:** To help maintain cartilage and decrease arthritis
- **Evening primrose (*Oenothera biennis*):** To treat signs and symptoms of dry skin and menopause
- **Ginkgo (*Ginkgo biloba*):** To improve blood flow to the brain and decrease forgetfulness

These remedies have been used for the various problems, but they are not Food and Drug Administration (FDA) approved. They may work in some patients, but not others, and can interact with many prescription medications.

During the middle adult years, there is a natural redistribution of body weight, which changes the contours of the body, even if weight remains constant. Men commonly add inches around the waist as body fat increases by about 30%. Women's body fat increases by nearly 40% and is often added to hips and thighs. It becomes more difficult to lose weight.

One common occurrence is **presbyopia** (decreased flexibility of the eye lens). This makes near vision more difficult, leading to the need for reading glasses. By age 60, some people may have retinal damage because of lessened blood flow, leading to visual problems. Cataracts may develop during the middle years. Regular eye examinations and the use of corrective lenses can help maintain vision.

Presbycusis (loss of hearing) begins in early adulthood, but rarely becomes apparent until later. The ability to hear higher-pitched sounds is lost earlier than the ability to hear lower sounds is. Men seem to lose this sense at younger ages than women do. **Noisy work settings and loud music can contribute to eventual hearing loss by damaging auditory nerve endings.**

Health Promotion/Health Promotion Points

Hearing Loss in Middle Adults

- The person who thinks hearing acuity is decreasing should be tested for hearing loss.
- It is much easier to adapt to a hearing aid when hearing loss is in the early stages.

Health Promotion/Health Promotion Points

Bone Health in Middle Adults

- Women with a family history of osteoporosis should begin regular bone density screening at age 45.
- Anyone who has experienced a loss of height of 2 inches since age 20 should be screened for osteoporosis.
- Women should consume 1000 mg of calcium each day, increasing it to 1200 mg/day after age 50; men should

consume 1000 mg of calcium each day, increasing it to 1200 mg/day after age 70 (National Institutes of Health, 2013).
- Obtaining sufficient vitamin D from sunlight or supplementation is also important.
- Assessment of hormone levels in aging women and men can aid in finding interventions to improve quality of life during menopause and andropause.

Gradual compression of the spinal column occurs as intervertebral disks shrink; this can cause the loss of up to 1 inch of height by age 60.

Muscles throughout the body lose tone and elasticity during these middle years. Fatigue arrives earlier with physical labor. Reaction time may also slow. Muscle changes also affect internal muscles; heart and lungs become less efficient. Blood pressure increases because arteries become less elastic. The skin becomes less resilient, and wrinkles appear. Changes in the muscles of the digestive system may cause disturbances and food intolerances.

Many people in middle age begin to have graying hair. Thinning of scalp hair can occur in both genders. Increased hair growth in men is seen in bushier eyebrows and hair occasionally in noses and ears. These changes may be hereditary.

Both males and females produce sex hormones. Women produce greater amounts of estrogen, and men produce greater amounts of testosterone. As middle age proceeds, this balance shifts slightly. This is most obvious in women; the decrease in estrogen production in the mid to late 40s causes menstrual changes and eventually **menopause** (cessation of menstruation). The average age of menopause is 51. This ends the reproductive years and may be accompanied by minor physical and psychological signs and symptoms (Box 12.5). Some women see menopause as a natural event and the beginning of new freedoms and choices; other women have a negative view. Women can learn about their bodies and the natural changes from a variety of sources. They can discuss their feelings with others to better understand and cope. Many women seek new ways to contribute to their profession or their community.

The shift in hormone balance also occurs in men, but more gradually. Symptoms of male **andropause** (low testosterone levels) may include loss of muscle strength, decreased bone density, fatigue, reduced libido, depression, fatigue, and mood changes. A blood test of hormone levels can determine whether testosterone therapy should be considered. Sexual ability does not decline in either sex.

Box 12.5 Signs and Symptoms That May Occur With Menopause

- Decreased vaginal lubrication
- Emotional lability
- Fatigue
- Flushing and hot flashes with heavy sweating
- Headache
- Heart palpitations
- Insomnia

HEALTH CONCERNS

Health status becomes a greater concern in middle adulthood. Lifestyle, heredity, and use of the health care system are major influences on the state of health. People who make efforts to take care of themselves are generally healthier than those who do not. This includes controlling one's diet and remaining physically active. Health screening for diabetes, risk factors for heart disease, hypertension, and colon cancer should occur at regular intervals.

Health Promotion/Health Promotion Points

Blood Pressure Control in Middle Adults

Adults should keep their blood pressure below 120/80 mm Hg; adults with prehypertension 120 to 139/80 to 89; and adults for stage 1 hypertension 140 to 159/90 to 99—by:

- Decreasing sodium intake
- Drinking minimal alcohol
- Participating in regular aerobic exercise
- Promoting an overall healthy lifestyle

Data from Mayo Clinic Staff (2015) High blood pressure. www.mayoclinic.org/diseases-conditions/high-blood-pressure/in-depth/blood-pressure/ART-20050982

Leading causes of death in the 50s and 60s are heart disease, cancer, chronic lower respiratory disease, accidents, and stroke (Centers for Disease Control and Prevention, 2015a). The major health problems of middle adults include accidents, alcohol abuse, obesity, diabetes, heart disease, hypertension, and mental illness. Healthy stress management at all ages contributes to improved general health.

COGNITIVE DEVELOPMENT

Schaie's stage of responsibility is seen as middle adults manage the complexities of their lives. Studies show that, despite many variations of peak and decline, intellect generally remains stable in middle adulthood (Schaie, 1996). Early signs of illnesses may cause the impression of slight mental decline. People who are active and use their intellect remain bright and interested in life.

Creativity is believed to peak during middle adulthood. However, many people are creative and productive in their older years as well. Creative people are often creative throughout their lives. Men and women are equally creative and intelligent.

One aspect of cognition that may change in midlife is memory. Middle adults often need to work harder at remembering things, and many find lists and notes helpful. Older people should not be overly concerned about forgetfulness; it is more likely related to a busy life than to cognitive problems.

 Health Promotion/Health Promotion Points

Cognitive Stimulation in Middle Adults

Working crossword or Sudoku puzzles, working jigsaw puzzles, playing bridge, playing board games that require strategy, studying some new subject, using computer programs such as "Brain Age," and other activities that stimulate the mind all help maintain mental crispness.

Work Life

Satisfaction with work is a part of cognitive development. It increases throughout life for most men and women. Many people spend more time in work-related activities during the middle years. Increased income and responsibilities accompanying career growth explain increased satisfaction. Most career advancement occurs during the 50s.

Middle adults may make a conscious decision to make a midlife career change. Some begin evaluating their desires and accomplishments. If a dream is unfulfilled, perhaps a change will help it come true. Middle adults begin to realize that their own life spans are limited and may want to try new areas of interest while they have time. Some adults are willing to change their lives entirely by starting a new career. Midlife changes are handled best when the person has a good support system.

Some middle adults are forced to change careers because of labor market demands, and they may have a difficult time adjusting. Job loss resulting from downsizing, and the need for retraining, are serious concerns. Changes in technology and informatics may create new work opportunities for some or take opportunities away from others.

? Think Critically

Do you know anyone who has made a midlife career change? Was it by choice? Was the result satisfactory?

People often choose a career path with the hope and expectation of advancement and promotion in their fields. In recent decades, it has become more common for women to take advantage of numerous career choices perceived to be unavailable to their mothers and grandmothers. Although women's earning power still lags behind men's, women who choose not to have children enjoy nearly the same career advancement as men (Houghton, 2013). Both women and men who choose to place family concerns ahead of career goals may find their career advancement is slowed.

Many baby boomers are finding that as retirement age approaches, they do not have the financial reserves necessary to support themselves and must continue working. Some do retire, run short of money, and have to reenter the job market.

The use of leisure time is also important. Middle adults should develop interests outside their work. Leisure activities can be healthy ways to reduce stress. Hobbies can also help people prepare for retirement by providing fulfillment.

Lifelong Learning

Many adults discover that returning to college is rewarding and challenging. They may enroll in one or two classes or may undertake an entire program of study. This may fulfill a lifelong goal, it may be necessary to keep a job, or it may help them prepare for a career change.

Women who chose to raise a family before developing a career are especially likely to prepare for new jobs and new lives in midlife. Rather than think of this stage as downhill, they think of it as an opportunity to try another path.

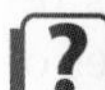 Think Critically

Do you know anyone who returned to or began college after the age of 40? How did they feel about it? What kind of support did they need?

PSYCHOSOCIAL DEVELOPMENT

Relationships with other people remain the focus of psychosocial development in middle adults. People in these years also begin to think more globally about life and their roles.

Marriage

The marital relationship often grows from romance and passion into the affectionate love of middle adults. The steady companionship of a partner is important for social and psychological support. Some marriages improve as children leave home and child-rearing responsibilities lessen. Couples may find more time for each other. It is vital that they have and develop mutual interests and activities.

A couple who has been unhappy for years may decide to divorce when the children are gone. A woman who had been at home when children were younger may discover a new world if she begins a job or returns to school. Changing roles and responsibilities can create or intensify marital problems.

The **empty nest syndrome** (children have left home, causing a sense of loss) affects some middle adults who have centered their lives on their children. They may need guidance in finding additional interests. Conversely, many adults look forward to more freedom when children are no longer dependent on them.

Friendships

Whether single or married, middle adults need to have close friends. Friendships that have endured for years continue to be vital. Many middle adults find new importance in relationships with siblings. Friends and siblings find more time for each other once the time-consuming work of parenting is past.

Parenting

Most studies of middle adults involve those whose children are leaving or have left the parental home. Couples who had children later in life will enter midlife with younger children. Therefore, parenting concerns vary.

Those with adult children can find this stage rewarding. Parents gain satisfaction in realizing that their child is a responsible young adult. If grandchildren arrive in the family, another dimension is added. Grandparents usually enjoy baby-sitting at times and inclusion in the younger family's life (Fig. 12.3).

Caring for Parents

The relationship with aging parents is another concern in midlife. If the relationship has been mutually supportive, these can be satisfying years. As adults mature, they may become more appreciative of the struggles their own parents experienced. Family dynamics may improve as children realize the sacrifices and guidance their parents provided.

Some middle adults find themselves in the **sandwich generation** (with dependent children at home and dependent older adults needing care). As longevity increases, older adults may need assistance and support. Daughters and daughters-in-law often become primary caregivers for older adult parents.

Caring for aging parents can be stressful when combined with personal careers and family responsibilities. Families must make important decisions. Open communication within the family can ease the adjustments. Community resources are available to assist families who need support and help with caregiving.

Generativity

Erikson's middle adult psychosocial stage of **generativity versus stagnation** is most easily seen in parents whose children have become young adults. However, people who are not parents, or those whose children live far away, often get involved in nurturing younger people. Most middle adults are confident regarding the knowledge they have accumulated. They are concerned for others and want to contribute to the community. They may do this through social activities, leadership roles in community or religious organizations, and career involvement. Middle adults are often **mentors** (teachers or coaches) to younger adults in these settings.

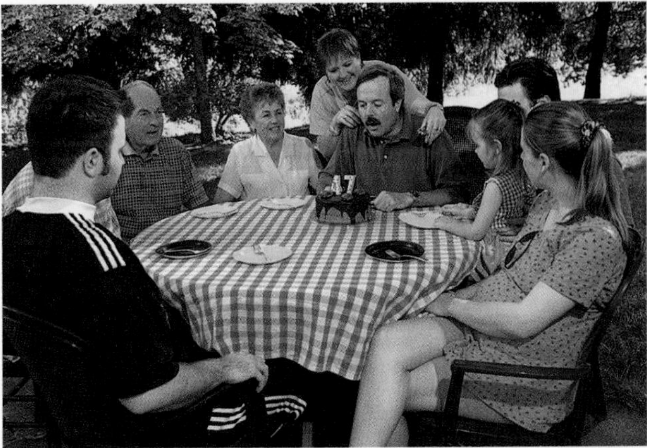

FIGURE 12.3 Family gatherings contribute to our sense of belonging.

Think Critically

Do you have a mentor? Are you a mentor? How did that relationship develop?

Some adults are said to experience a midlife crisis, but most psychologists say that is not a common issue. There are many changes in midlife, and some of them may create a crisis for some people, but no single event causes a crisis for all middle adults.

Middle adults realize that they are no longer young. They begin to evaluate their self-concept and their role in the world. There may be times of pain or stress because of physical decline or financial problems. They must explore many questions to continue healthy development. **Middle adults accept that life is not simple and that circumstances occur over which they have little control.**

Sincere listening and caring by other people can help individuals develop to their full potential. Education about life changes helps understanding and aids in coping with challenges. There are support groups for people in crises. Learn about such groups in your locality and make referrals when needed.

Get Ready for the NCLEX Examination!

Key Points

- Adulthood is a time of continuing change and growth. Young adulthood is ages 18 to 35; middle adulthood is considered to include ages 35 to 65. Older adulthood starts at age 65 and lasts until death.
- Schaie's theory of cognitive development calls the young adult stage that of achievement. Middle adults are in the stage of responsibility.
- Erikson's theory refers to the young adult stage as that of intimacy versus isolation. Middle adults are in the stage of generativity versus stagnation.
- Families are groups of interacting individuals who care about and for each other. Families are how children learn basic values.
- Approximately 50% of marriages end in divorce. Divorce affects many people besides the couple involved.
- Maturity is a goal. Mature people demonstrate responsibility, confidence, trust, and self-discipline.
- Young adults are generally healthy and in the best years for reproduction.
- Health promotion practices help adults achieve and maintain health.
- Career exploration is common during early young adulthood. Work provides many benefits economically, socially, and developmentally.
- Personality does not change significantly during the life span. People who want to change must work hard at it.
- Marrying and establishing a family are typical goals of young adults, although they may be postponed until a career is established. Married people are generally happier throughout their lives.
- Young adults expand their concern for other people and for the community.
- Gradual physical changes related to aging begin in the 30s and continue during middle adulthood.
- Menopause means the end of the reproductive years for women. Andropause is a low testosterone level that can gradually happen to men, and although reproductive ability is not lost, physical and cognitive changes occur.
- A person's lifestyle, especially diet, exercise, and stress management, is a major influence on health. Heredity and use of the health care system also contribute.
- Leading causes of death in the 50s and 60s are heart disease, cancer, vascular disease, and accidents.
- Work satisfaction typically increases through life. Middle adults have greater responsibilities and may earn more money. Many become mentors.
- Many adults find returning to school challenging and rewarding. Learning should be a lifelong activity.
- Relationships with others remain the focus of psychosocial development. Marriage, extended family, and friendships are valued.
- Some middle adults become involved in caring for their older adult parents. This can be stressful for families; open communication and community support can help.

Additional Learning Resources

SG Go to your Study Guide for additional learning activities to help you master this chapter content.

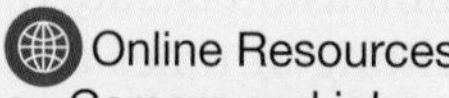

Go to your Evolve website at http://evolve.elsevier.com/Williams/fundamental for additional online resources.

Online Resources

- Careers and jobs
  - *FREE High School Career Test*, http://www.yourfreecareertest.com/index.html
  - *Career Aptitude Test*, http://www.whatcareerisrightforme.com/career-aptitude-test.php
  - *Job/Career Hunting Article*, http://jobsearch.about.com/od/careeradviceresources/a/careermanage.htm
  - *Midlife career change*, www.career-tests-guide.com/midlife-career-change.html
- Parenting and family
  - *Family Strengths:* http://extension.missouri.edu/bsf/strengths/index.htm
  - *Family Strengths: Handouts and worksheets:* http://extension.missouri.edu/bsf/strengths/fshandouts.htm
  - *Parenting styles:* www.verywell.com/parenting-styles-2795072
  - *American Academy of Pediatrics:* www.healthychildren.org
- Returning to school as an adult
  - *Facing your fears of returning to school as an adult:* www.educationcorner.com/fear-of-returning-to-school.html
  - *Tips for adults going back to school:* http://singleparents.about.com/od/homelife/a/back_to_school.htm
- Mentoring
  - *How can a mentor benefit your career?* http://careerplanning.about.com/od/workplacesurvival/a/mentor.htm
  - *Mentoring: A mutually beneficial partnership:* www.mindtools.com/pages/article/newCDV_72.htm
- Weight management
  - *Body Mass Index Table,* www.nhlbi.nih.gov/health/educational/lose_wt/BMI/bmi_tbl.htm
  - *Dietary Guidelines for Americans,* www.cnpp.usda.gov/DietaryGuidelines
  - *Physical Activity Guidelines for Americans,* http://health.gov/paguidelines/
  - *Academy of Nutrition and Dietetics,* www.eatright.org

Review Questions for the NCLEX Examination

*Choose the **best** answer for each question.*

1. Young adults are likely to spend leisure time in activities that are:
   1. Calm and quiet, alone or with only one or two others.
   2. Inclusive of their parents and grandparents.
   3. Physically and mentally demanding and competitive.
   4. Ways to earn extra money.

2. The cognitive development of young adults is aided by:
   1. Peers who are experiencing similar problems.
   2. Support of mentors to help identify goals and provide encouragement.
   3. Interactive games and computer-based training.
   4. Providing new learning experiences that are unrelated to past knowledge.
3. Failure to develop through Erikson's stage of young adulthood will cause the person to be:
   1. Unable to form meaningful relationships.
   2. Unsuccessful in further education.
   3. Unable to keep a job.
   4. Unsure of how to raise children.
4. Which health screenings are most appropriate in the middle years of life? *(Select all that apply.)*
   1. HIV
   2. Colon cancer
   3. Hypertension
   4. Diabetes
   5. Memory decline
5. When working with depressed middle-aged adults, and following Erikson's theory, you encourage them to find meaning in life by:
   1. Developing intimate relationships with spouses.
   2. Caring for their older adult parents.
   3. Contributing to the development of younger people.
   4. Volunteering as a hospital aide.
6. A 58-year-old man complains that he has difficulty remembering everything he wanted to buy when he gets to the store. Your best response would be:
   1. "Forgetting some things is a common occurrence with aging."
   2. "Do your siblings have similar problems?"
   3. "You should always take a list with you to the store."
   4. "Life is so busy that everyone forgets things now and then."
7. Successful coping with midlife changes are likely when the individual:
   1. Has children still at home.
   2. Has a good support system.
   3. Is married.
   4. Is established in a career.

Critical Thinking Activities

Read each clinical scenario and discuss the questions with your classmates.

Scenario A

As a clinic nurse, you are interviewing a new patient, a 34-year-old high school French teacher who complains of irregular menstrual periods. She has been married for 2 years and has no children.

1. What are some of the health concerns this patient might have? How can you help her understand the workings of her reproductive system?
2. What kinds of questions can you ask to help determine whether this patient is within the parameters of expected cognitive and psychosocial development?

Scenario B

Another clinic patient is a 52-year-old man who has recently been diagnosed with type 2 diabetes mellitus. He is 5 feet, 11 inches tall and weighs 245 lb. His blood pressure is 160/100 mmHg at this time. He works as a computer consultant and travels about 3 days each week.

1. How will you begin exploring any health concerns he may have? What will you say to determine how much of his diagnosis he understands? How can you encourage him to follow the prescribed regimen for maintaining or improving his physical health?
2. What is his expected stage of cognitive development? Where would you expect him to be in the occupational cycle? What are some questions you might ask?
3. You learn that he is divorced and shares custody of three adolescent children. How can you tactfully determine whether he is at the appropriate stage of psychosocial development?

chapter

13

Promoting Healthy Adaptation to Aging

http://evolve.elsevier.com/Williams/fundamental

Objectives

Upon completing this chapter, you should be able to do the following:

Theory

1. Compare the biologic theories of aging.
2. State how a person might behave in light of the psychosocial theories of aging.
3. Identify four factors that contribute to longevity.
4. Discuss physical changes that occur as adults age.
5. Explain Schaie's theory of cognitive development in the older adult.
6. Explain Erikson's stage of psychosocial development in the older adult.

Clinical Practice

1. Identify at least six signs and symptoms of normal aging.
2. Design an educational program to help older adults maintain physical health.
3. State three ways the nurse could help older adults maintain cognitive health.
4. Identify nursing problems related to changes in psychosocial health.
5. Guide the older adult's family members regarding signs that the older adult needs assistance.

Key Terms

ageism (Ā-jĭsm, p. 178)
aging (p. 172)
benign senescence (bē-NĪGN sĕ-NĔ-sĕns, p. 174)
biologic theories (p. 173)
centenarians (sĕn-tĕn-ĀR-ē-ănz, p. 174)
dementia (dē-MĔN-shē-ă, p. 176)
demographic (dĕ-mō-GRĂ-fĭk, p. 174)
ego integrity (p. 178)
elder abuse (p. 179)
gerontologists (jĕr-ŏn-TŎ-lŏ-jĭsts, p. 173)
individualized aging (p. 172)
life span (p. 173)
longevity (lŏng-JĔ-vĭ-tē, p. 173)
psychosocial theories (SĪ-kō-SŌ-shăl, p. 173)
reminiscence (rĕ-mĭ-NĬ-sĕns, p. 178)
wisdom (p. 177)

Concepts Covered in This Chapter

- Caregiving
- Cognition
- Communication
- Coping
- Development
- Health promotion
- Infection
- Inflammation
- Learning
- Nutrition
- Safety
- Stress
- Teaching

OVERVIEW OF AGING

Aging (a continual process of biologic, cognitive, and psychosocial change) begins at conception. Although there is no way to escape it, we can learn to live with it. As a nurse, you will care for people of all ages, and many of your patients will be older adults. You are also aging, as are your family members and friends. Knowing about normal development in the later years of life will help you in many ways.

Older adults are not all alike. Some are active, busy, and healthy; others are inactive because of illness and may be dependent on others. Being an older adult means different things to different people; **it is your perception of aging that influences your definition of being old.**

QSEN Considerations: Patient-Centered Care

Viewing the Older Adult as an Individual

Individualized aging describes how older adults should be viewed as individuals, not as a stereotypical member of the group; for example, an older adult who has a chronological age of 85 may have a physiologic age of 65 because of healthy lifestyle habits and choices.

Scientists are interested in learning how people can maintain a healthy body into advanced years. Research about healthy aging is ongoing, and results are changing our ideas. Many older adults have the potential for

Box 13.1 Myths About Older Adults

- Older adults are sick.
- Older adults cannot learn new things.
- It is too late for lifestyle changes to improve health.
- Genetics are the main factor in longevity.
- Older adults are not sexual.
- Older adults are a drain on society.
- Older adults are senile.
- Older adults are typically isolated from their families.
- Older adults usually live in nursing homes.
- Older adults are poor.
- Old people are unhappy.

years of interesting and productive life. The later years of life can be exciting and rewarding. Most people do not mind growing older, especially if they are relatively healthy. Others fear that the later years of life will be painful, boring, and filled with illness. Overcoming the myths about aging (Box 13.1) can be a challenge for nurses when working with middle and older adults.

Health Promotion/Health Promotion Points

Healthy People Objectives: Older Adult

- Increase the proportion of older adults who use the Welcome to Medicare benefit.
- Increase the proportion of older adults who are up to date on a core set of clinical preventive services.
- Increase the proportion of older adults with one or more chronic health conditions who report confidence in managing their conditions.
- Increase the proportion of older adults who receive Diabetes Self-Management Benefits.
- Reduce the proportion of older adults who have moderate to severe functional limitations.
- Increase the proportion of older adults with reduced physical or cognitive function who engage in light, moderate, or vigorous physical activities.
- Increase the proportion of the health care workforce with geriatric certification.
- Reduce the proportion of noninstitutionalized older adults with disabilities who have an unmet need for long-term services and supports.
- Reduce the proportion of unpaid caregivers of older adults who report an unmet need for caregiver support services.
- Reduce the rate of pressure injury-related hospitalizations among older adults.
- Reduce the rate of emergency department (ED) visits due to falls among older adults.
- Increase the number of states and the District of Columbia that collect and make publicly available information on the characteristics of victims, perpetrators, and cases of elder abuse, neglect, and exploitation.

Source: www.healthypeople.gov/2020/topics-objectives/topic/older-adults/objectives

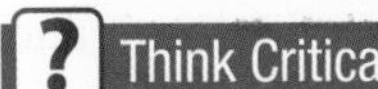

When are people considered old? What does it mean to be old? How do older adults view life? What are the concerns of older people?

THEORIES OF AGING

There are numerous theories about aging. Some **gerontologists** (specialists in the study of aging people) claim that aging is primarily determined by genetics, whereas others are certain that environment and lifestyle play important roles. These factors seem to interact with other things to determine how long a person lives.

Biologic theories (theories based on cellular function and body physiology) provide ways to look at the physical aging process. The *biologic clock* is one of these theories; this states that body cells are programmed to function for a specific length of time after which they break down and die. When too many cells quit functioning, the person eventually dies.

Advocates of the *free-radical theory* believe that cells are damaged by toxins, ions break off from ion pairs, and the resulting free radicals are unstable. This occurs in the environment, in waste products of metabolism, and from disease. These toxins are causes of free radicals, or oxidizing substances in the body. The use of antioxidant vitamins and lotions is supposed to counteract the harmful chemicals.

The *wear-and-tear theory* states that body cells and organs eventually wear out, like machinery.

In the *immune system failure theory*, the system loses its ability to protect the body from disease. Older people become more susceptible to diseases such as influenza, which may kill them. The *autoimmune theory* is similar; here the body no longer recognizes itself and begins to attack itself and break down, as occurs in some types of arthritis.

Think Critically

Can you think of any health problems that could serve as examples of the biologic theories of aging?

There are also **psychosocial theories** (theories related to socialization and life satisfaction). The *disengagement theory* suggests that it is normal for older people and society to withdraw from each other. Most gerontologists, however, no longer give credence to this concept. In contrast, the *activity theory* states that people who remain interested and active will continue to enjoy life and to live longer. Conversely, people who make no effort to contribute become less and less involved and shorten their life as a result.

In the *continuity theory*, each individual continues to live and develop as the unique person he or she is. Individuals' basic personalities do not change, and they cope with aging in ways similar to how they coped with other stages of life.

LONGEVITY

The **life span** (maximum years one is capable of living) for humans is 115 to 130 years. **Longevity** (length of life) has been increasing. In 1900, the average length of life in the United States was 47 years. The US Census

Bureau (2012) projects the average life span to be 78.9 years. What is causing this increase?

A major contributor to longer life is that people are healthier throughout their lives now than they were 100 years ago. Principles of hygiene have helped eliminate many illnesses. Health care and nutrition have improved, and anti-infective drugs are commonly used. Technology allows surgeons to perform intricate procedures and replace body parts.

Education also contributes to longevity. People who are better educated practice preventive health care, and they may seek treatment earlier in the course of an illness.

Lifestyle makes a significant difference in longevity. A healthy diet and lifestyle, including stress management and regular exercise, are crucial. Nonsmokers usually live longer than smokers do; people who abuse chemicals risk shortening their lives. Married people tend to live longer.

A person's personality seems to affect the length and quality of life. **The optimistic, happy person generally lives longer.** This is true even when a chronic illness is present.

Gender has been a contributing factor to longevity in the past; women in the 20th century lived 6 to 7 years longer compared with men. Women continue to outlive men, and the duration varies by country: by about 4 years in the United States and by about 5 years in Canada (Central Intelligence Agency, 2014). This female-longevity advantage seems to disappear after age 90 (Jacobs, 2014).

The final factor in longevity is genetics. Studies of twins have suggested that heredity determines 20% to 30% of longevity in people who live to age 85. For **centenarians** (people 100 years old or older) genetics may be even more important perhaps because of differences in the T cells (Pellicano et al., 2014).

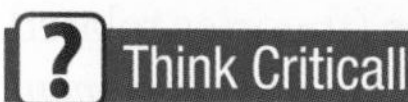

Think Critically

How long did your ancestors live? Has the longevity of your family been increasing? How long do you think you will live?

DEMOGRAPHICS

Demographic (statistics about populations) studies show that the number of older people in the United States grows every year. In 2013 nearly 45 million people were over age 65—14% of the total population. The number of older adults grew at a faster rate than the total population. Older women outnumber older men, but according to the US Census Bureau life expectancy is projected to increase more for men than for women in the coming years (Velkoff et al, 2014). The Administration on Aging (2014) predicts that we will have 98 million older adults by 2060.

For purposes of study, the older adult population is often divided into three distinct groups: the "young old" are 65 to 74 years of age; the "middle old" are 75 to 84; and the "very old" are 85 and beyond. The federal Social Security system originally used age 65 as a marker for retirement. Today, seniors born in the years 1943–59 will qualify for full coverage at 66 years, and those born after 1960 will qualify at age 67. The qualification age may extend further in the coming years. The young old are those who remain fairly healthy and active. You may not even recognize them as old when you see them in the shopping mall or restaurant. Many contribute to their community and may remain employed, at least part time. They are not much different from middle adults.

The middle old are in a transition time. As people approach 80, they may become frail and are less able to be as active. The very old are the most rapidly growing group, and this group will continue to increase in the future. These are also the most dependent older adults.

Centenarians are becoming more common. According to the last census taken, there were 53,364 centenarians in 2010 (US Census Bureau, 2015), with 20 men for every 100 women over age 100.

Living a long and better life is everyone's goal. The ancient Greeks were the first to say they wanted to "die young, as late in life as possible." Most centenarians enjoyed good health at least into their 90s. To live to be very old, you have to be healthy for most of your life. **People are becoming healthier, better educated, and actively involved in their own health care and therefore are living longer.**

? Think Critically

Do you know any centenarians? What are they like? What does this mean for nursing and other health care providers?

PHYSICAL CHANGES

Physical declines happen to everyone. **Benign senescence** (normal physical changes of aging) begins early in adulthood, but often goes unnoticed until a problem develops. Changes mentioned in Chapter 12 continue. Table 13.1 summarizes the physiologic changes of aging. Heart and lungs gradually become less efficient. Bones become more fragile, and posture becomes bent.

The skin is thinner and more fragile; a reduced amount of subcutaneous tissue causes older adults to complain of feeling cold. Older people often have smaller appetites. Vision continues to deteriorate; night driving becomes difficult.

Hearing deficits may become more pronounced. Nearly half of the population over age 75 has some hearing loss. Various types of hearing aids can be helpful. The earlier a person with hearing difficulty obtains a hearing aid, the better the brain can adjust to it and provide a good quality of hearing.

Changes in the brain also occur with normal aging. There may be less blood flow. Neurotransmitters may be imbalanced. Any loss of brain cells caused by injury

Table 13.1 **Typical Changes of Aging, Potential Health Problems, and Helpful Nursing Responses**

BODY SYSTEM	SOME TYPICAL CHANGES	POSSIBLE HEALTH PROBLEMS	HELPFUL NURSING RESPONSE
Cardiovascular	Increased heart size Decreased cardiac output, causing less blood flow to all organs; thickened heart valves and blood vessels; less elasticity of blood vessels; slower blood cell production and immune response	MIs, stroke, hypertension, and infection	Assess for signs and symptoms of MI, stroke, or other circulation or organ problems. Monitor for infection and encourage good hygiene and frequent hand washing.
Respiratory	Thickened alveolar walls, causing less elasticity Weakened respiratory muscles Decreased vital capacity and tidal volume Decreased number of cilia	Respiratory failure, shortness of breath; lack of oxygen to meet body needs	Monitor BP, respiratory function, oxygen saturation levels, and shortness of breath. Educate on oxygen therapy and the importance of exercise.
Musculoskeletal	Thinned intervertebral disks, decreased bone calcium, and smaller muscle mass Less elasticity of ligaments and tendons Degeneration of cartilage	Osteoporosis, osteoarthritis, tendonitis, and rheumatoid arthritis	Encourage exercise, range of motion, good diet high in calcium, and nutritional supplements as needed.
Integumentary	Thinner, drier skin Loss of subcutaneous fat Slowed rate of hair and nail growth	Pressure injuries, resulting from friction/tears	Educate on good skin care, use of moisturizers, and prevention of pressure injuries.
Urologic	Decreased bladder capacity and tone Loss of nephrons, slowed function of remaining nephrons Decreased sphincter control	Urinary incontinence	Assess and monitor for bladder control and need for medications.
Neurologic	*Vision:* presbyopia, slowed accommodation, cataract development, and decreased peripheral vision and depth perception *Hearing:* presbycusis, thicker eardrum, increased wax production, and decreased hair cells in inner ear *Taste, smell, and touch:* decreased number of receptors *Balance:* may be affected by decreased circulation *Reflexes:* slowed reaction time Slowed autonomic system responses	Decreased sensory perceptions: safety risk, fall risk, and decreased appetite	Educate on normal aging expectations and safety issues to prevent falls and other injuries.
Endocrine	Slowed production of all hormones Decreased metabolic rate Delayed insulin response	Diabetic response, hyperthyroidism or hypothyroidism	Monitor labs for abnormal hormone levels and need for hormone therapy.
Gastrointestinal	Decreased secretion of saliva and other digestive enzymes Slowed peristalsis Slowed liver and pancreatic functions Reduced absorption of nutrients	Constipation, malnutrition, and anemia	Educate patient on need for healthy diet and nutritional supplements.
Reproductive	Decreased hormone production; atrophy of ovaries, uterus, and vagina; benign prostatic hypertrophy Slowed sexual responses	Menopause, andropause, infertility, decreased libido, and sexual dysfunction	Monitor labs and symptoms to determine need for hormone therapy or other medications.

MI: myocardial infarction.

or illness will affect the body's functions. The brain can adapt by growing more dendrites up to age 90 if the person is reasonably healthy. Brain changes are also important in trying to understand cognitive changes in older adults, such as sensory and memory losses.

Think Critically

What health problems might be associated with the changes identified in Table 13.1? What nursing responses could be helpful?

HEALTH CONCERNS

Most people over 75 have at least one chronic health problem. Hypertension is the most common, affecting more than half of older adults, followed by arthritis and heart disease. Obesity contributes to joint problems by causing increased stress on joints; it also contributes to hypertension. For many older adults, these conditions do not prevent living active and full lives.

Other common concerns include cancer, diabetes, asthma, chronic bronchitis or emphysema, stroke, and influenza. The leading causes of death are heart disease, cancer, chronic lower respiratory disease, stroke, Alzheimer disease, diabetes, influenza, and pneumonia (Federal Interagency Forum on Aging Related Statistics, 2012). Older people are often concerned about falling, especially about breaking a hip, and about being dependent on others.

QSEN Considerations: Safety

Accident Prevention

Accidents may happen because of changes in depth perception, changes in gait, and slower reaction times. It is important to teach older people safety measures to prevent falls (see Chapter 40). Resistance training can improve balance and help prevent falls.

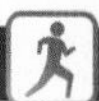

Health Promotion/Health Promotion Points

Fitness for the Older Adult

- A fitness program to promote strength and balance is an excellent way to decrease the risk of falls and to promote the ability to stay independent.
- Many communities have special fitness programs for older adults.

Mental health in the older adult may be difficult to evaluate. Many treatable physical conditions, such as malnutrition, dehydration, infection, and misuse of medications, can lead to impaired cognition. A thorough examination should be done to make an accurate diagnosis. It is estimated that more than one million older adults experience depression, and older adults who have suicidal thoughts are more likely to act on them successfully compared with younger people with similar thoughts (Aziz & Steffans, 2013). Signs and symptoms of depression in the older adults are listed in Box 13.2. Depression can often be treated successfully with medications and counseling.

Depression is a risk factor and possibly an early sign of **dementia** (degeneration of brain tissue). Dementia occurs in a small percentage of older adults, yet the incidence rises with age. Confusion, memory loss, and disordered thinking are early signs. This problem has numerous causes, from malnutrition to mini-strokes to Alzheimer disease (see Chapter 41). Between 5% and 15% of older adults have dementia; 60% to 80% of these people have Alzheimer disease (Alzheimer's Association, 2015).

HEALTH PROMOTION BEHAVIORS

Eating a healthy diet helps delay physical aging. Encourage older adults to learn about nutrition and meal planning. Additional seasonings can counter the loss of taste buds. Some providers encourage a daily multivitamin. Eating is a social experience for many, so they should find opportunities to share meals with others. Many communities offer communal dining; prepared meals can also be delivered to a home.

Physical activity also postpones many effects of aging. Daily activity, whether walking, biking, or swimming, keeps the body functioning. Benefits from weight training include reduced risk of osteoporosis, hypertension, and diabetes, and increased ability to perform activities of daily living (ADLs). *Exercise and Physical Activity: Your Everyday Guide from the National Institute on Aging,* in English or Spanish, is available free online. It describes appropriate exercises to keep fit and promote good balance.

Another positive behavior is having regular physical examinations to monitor chronic conditions and to screen for new problems. Older adults may need encouragement to participate in their own health care management. The cost of health care is a concern to some, but programs designed for older adults help provide regular care.

Older adults who smoke should be encouraged to quit. They may have been smoking for years, but the health benefits of quitting are significant, even in advanced years. Individual counseling, support groups,

Box 13.2 Signs and Symptoms of Depression in Older Adults

- Feeling sad or "empty"
- Feeling hopeless, irritable, anxious, or guilty
- Loss of interest in favorite activities
- Feeling very tired
- Not being able to concentrate or remember details
- Not being able to sleep or sleeping too much
- Overeating or not wanting to eat at all
- Thoughts of suicide, suicide attempts
- Aches or pains, headaches, cramps, or digestive problems

Source: National Institute of Mental Health, 2015. www.nimh.nih.gov/health/publications/older-adults-and-depression/index.shtml

and nicotine replacement have been shown to be effective. Alcohol use should also be limited because its effects may be greater in older adults and it may interfere with prescribed medications and supplements. Some adults may need guidance in taking prescribed medications correctly.

Health Promotion/Health Promotion Points

Medication Regimen Aids for Older Adults

- Using a weekly pill-minder box with compartments for each day, or for different times of each day, is a useful tool for helping the older adult take medications on time.
- The pillbox is refilled weekly, and a list can be made to aid the person when filling the box.

COGNITIVE ASPECTS OF AGING

Schaie's stage of cognitive development for older adults is called the *reintegrative stage*. This states that older adults are more selective about how they spend their time. They take time for interesting activities, but not for things that seem irrelevant. A woman who hosts family meals on special occasions may try new recipes and enjoy a cooking class; however, someone who lives alone and rarely entertains may not be interested in such activities. Discovering the interests of older people can provide clues to ways to stimulate and maintain their cognitive abilities. One person may enjoy crossword puzzles, and another may enjoy reading mysteries (Fig. 13.1).

Healthy adults can maintain intelligence into advanced years. The speed of thinking may slow, but thinking processes remain intact. Many older adults who are ill or who have vision or hearing deficits do not suffer cognitive dysfunction. They should be certain that glasses or hearing aids are in place before interacting with other people.

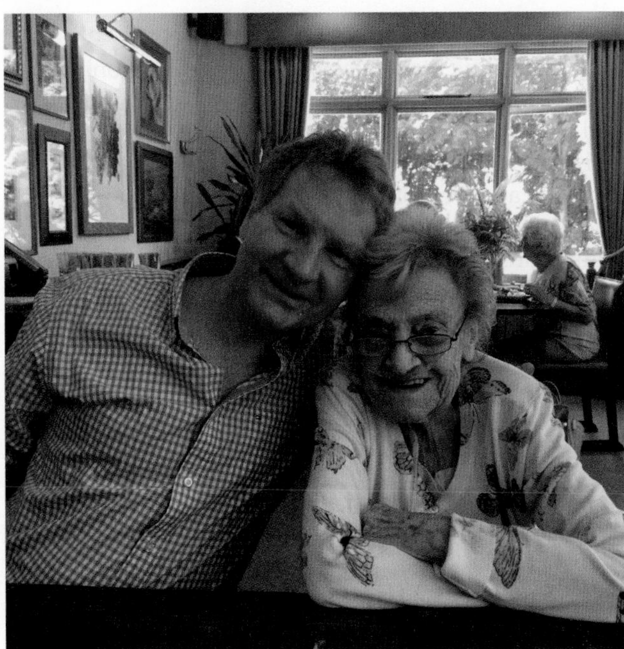

FIGURE 13.1 Going out with family provides cognitive stimulation.

WISDOM AND LEARNING

Wisdom (having good judgment based on accumulated knowledge) is often credited to older adults because of their wealth of life experiences. Younger people can benefit by listening to the advice of older people.

Some people assume older adults can no longer learn. This is not true. Subjects of interest can fascinate the older learner. They have more patience for learning. Many have learned to operate computers and enjoy using that technology. Elder hostel programs provide stimulating opportunities to learn and sometimes travel with other older adults.

 Patient Education

Teaching the Older Adult

Keep these points in mind when performing patient education for the older adult:

- Provide motivation for the content to be learned.
- Keep the topic relevant to the learner.
- Assess readiness to learn and take advantage of "teaching moments" (when the learner is most receptive).
- Use visual aids in large print and bright colors.
- Provide good lighting in the room and on the materials.
- Ensure the learner has reading glasses (clean) and hearing aid (turned on) if used.
- Speak clearly, distinctly, and slowly in a normal tone.
- Obtain feedback at intervals about what has been taught.
- Relate learning to better autonomy, health, and activity.

MEMORY ISSUES

Some older adults have problems remembering recent events; this is short-term memory loss. They may not recall much of yesterday; however, long-term memory remains intact. They can remember many details of their younger life. Memory aids such as making lists or notes on a calendar can help keep life orderly.

 Health Promotion/Health Promotion Points

Cognitive Stimulation in Older Adults

Regular exercise of at least 30 minutes five times a week helps decrease mental decline. Encourage older adults to engage in some sort of exercise program, even simply walking in the neighborhood. Exercise classes at the senior center or parks and recreation department are available in many communities. Even moderate activity and resistance training (for bed-bound older adults) has been shown to be beneficial.

The more severe memory losses and dementias of aging are often the result of circulatory changes. People experiencing memory changes and their family members should not assume that such changes are inevitable. The older adult should be evaluated for nutritional status, hypertension, arterial health, endocrine disorders, and specific neurologic problems. Sometimes underlying conditions can be treated and the memory problems will be resolved.

EMPLOYMENT AND RETIREMENT

The ability and desire to keep a job vary, depending partially on the older adult's cognitive ability. Some types of work maintain a mandatory retirement age, particularly if the work involves public safety. In other situations, retirement is a matter of preference.

? Think Critically

What suggestions could you give older adults to help them remain active after retirement?

Some people are eager to leave a regular job and may retire in their 50s or early 60s. Some continue to work because they need the income or desire the social outlet. Retiring early requires planning for finances and other concerns. Other people enjoy working and want to continue beyond a traditional retirement age. About 9% of older adults are at poverty level according to income, and 26% are in the low-income group (Federal Interagency Forum on Aging Related Statistics, 2012). The percentage of older adults in the workforce continues to rise, and is expected to exceed 30% by 2022 (Pew Research Center, 2014).

Workers who lose their jobs a few years before retirement may find it hard to obtain other employment at similar wages. **Ageism** (discrimination because of age) is illegal in the United States. A worker who has lost a job in favor of a younger person simply because of age has recourse through the government and the courts.

? Think Critically

Do you know anyone who lost a job in his or her 50s or early 60s? Were they able to find other employment at a comparable income? How did they feel about that experience?

Retirement brings with it major changes in many aspects of lifestyle: no alarm clock, no set schedule, no coffee break with co-workers, no need to dress neatly, no paycheck. People who have adequate finances may feel comfortable about retiring. Some travel extensively if health and finances permit.

Many early retirees decide to begin a second career. Older adults may continue to work in family businesses. Others volunteer to keep themselves busy and involved. The contributions of older adults should not be underestimated. According to the Pew Research Center (Livingston, 2013), approximately 3 million children in the United States are being raised primarily by a grandparent. Again, attitude is important. People whose lives revolved around their work may have difficulty adjusting to retirement. Some become disillusioned with retirement and find another job. Others become depressed, withdraw, and die. Recent retirees should be encouraged to set small daily or weekly goals until the adjustment has been made.

HEALTH PROMOTION BEHAVIORS

Behaviors that help with successful cognitive aging are the same behaviors that are encouraged throughout life. Having a positive attitude remains important. Some people are unhappy with their lives and unwilling to try to change. Encouragement is always appropriate. For example, you can remind them of their accomplishments, of their success in raising children, or even the accomplishment of living a long life.

Active involvement in a job and community during earlier adulthood often carries into continuing involvement in hobbies, religious and service groups, and volunteerism in older adulthood. Remind older adults how much they have to offer their community.

Using the brain by reading, doing puzzles, using a computer, and writing keeps the neural connections active and healthy. A computer game called "Brain Age" has been shown to improve cognition in older adults. The brain, like a muscle, should be exercised regularly. Even the physically limited older adult can maintain mental stimulation with a little effort.

PSYCHOSOCIAL ASPECTS OF AGING

Erikson's stage of development for older adults is called **ego integrity** (state of being complete) versus despair (see Table 11.2). Older people naturally spend time thinking about their lives. If they find their lives have been good, then they are satisfied and have ego integrity. However, if they are unhappy about the way life has evolved, they will despair. Resolution to ego integrity may occur if you can help the person find enough areas of satisfaction to outnumber the areas of regret.

LIFE REVIEW

This is the time for **reminiscence** (reviewing one's life). If individuals accept that they have had good lives and that they have contributed to others, then they are satisfied. People who were not successful at working through a developmental stage when younger may find unhappiness with the way their lives progressed. Sometimes it is enough to realize that one did the best one could under the circumstances.

Many psychologists consider this stage of life review important as a person faces mortality. **Being content with accomplishments is important for self-worth at any stage of life.** The older adult simply has more years about which to reflect.

FAMILY RELATIONSHIPS

Families continue to be important in older adulthood. Married people seem to live longer than those who are alone do (Fig. 13.2). Widows usually adjust better than do widowers. According to the Federal Interagency Forum on Aging Related Statistics (2012), 39.9% of all women

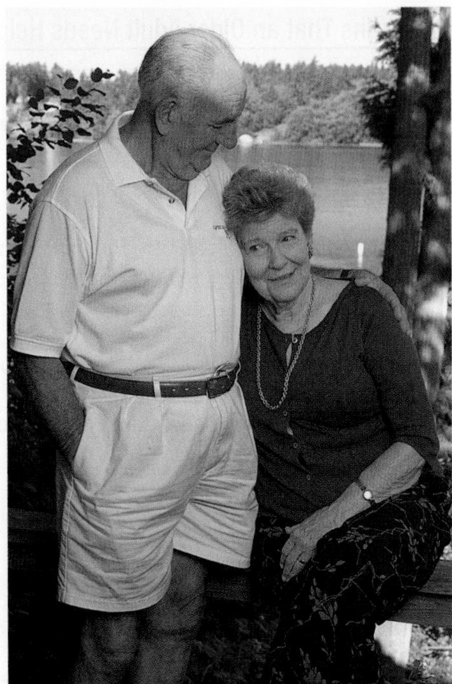

FIGURE 13.2 Romance can exist in later life.

over age 65 are widows; 12.7% of men in that age group are widowers. Many widowed, divorced, or single older adults continue to date, and some will remarry.

Think Critically

Widowers frequently die within 1 year of their wife's death. Why do you think that is true?

The majority of older adults who have children live within 40 miles of one child. Contact with that child usually occurs at least weekly. This is important because the older parent may need assistance with one or more aspects of daily life.

The active older adult may contribute to extended family life by helping with childcare of grandchildren or great-grandchildren. Sometimes retired adults end up raising grandchildren. Adult children may have died or may be imprisoned, hospitalized, or otherwise unable to care for the children. This arrangement can bring both benefits and problems for the children and for the older adults.

Approximately one out of every ten older adults is affected by **elder abuse** each year (Hoover & Polson, 2014). Those over age 80 have the greatest incidence, with the primary type being neglect. When it occurs in a family, it is for many of the same reasons abuse happens to children or spouses. Elder abuse may also occur in a long-term care setting.

Legal and Ethical Considerations

Reporting Elder Abuse

All licensed professionals are required to report any signs of or suspected abuse to a law enforcement agency. Social services personnel or law enforcement officials will conduct an investigation.

SOCIAL ACTIVITY

Community involvement was discussed earlier relative to cognitive development; it is also important for psychosocial health. **Older adults need to feel needed; this contributes to their self-concept and emotional health.** Some volunteers and part-time workers choose those activities primarily for the social activity.

Older adults experience a gradual loss of their peer group as friends and siblings die. These can be difficult times for the survivors; they continue to need support from their family and community. Those who have cultivated friendships with younger people fare best.

LIVING ARRANGEMENTS

Many older adults prefer to live in their own homes as long as they are physically able. Others choose to rent an apartment when they cannot maintain a house and yard. More than half of older adults lived with a spouse in 2014 (Administration on Aging, 2014). About 28% of noninstutionalized older adults lived alone (more women than men); many of these older adults need some assistance at times. About 2.2 million grandparents age 65 or over lived in households with grandchildren present in 2014. That number continues to grow. One recent trend in living arrangements is an increase in the number of multigenerational households where a grandparent and another generation live under the same roof (Pew Research Center, 2013).

A small number of adults over age 65 live in institutional settings (3.4% overall); however, with each decade of life, this number increases, reaching about 10% for those over age 85 (Administration on Aging, 2014).

As more people live to be older adults, it is important for them to remain healthier longer. Although this is beginning to happen, people over age 85 remain the frailest and will probably continue to need help with daily activities. As that group grows, more nurses and other health care workers will be needed to give care.

HEALTH PROMOTION BEHAVIORS

Older adults have several psychosocial challenges to face. They need to accept and adjust to a changing body. Family roles change, especially if one spouse becomes ill or dependent on the other or dies. There are changes in the use of time because of retirement. Finally, older adults have to face their own mortality.

The helpful behaviors for these adjustments continue to revolve around maintaining an optimistic outlook, staying as physically fit as possible, and remaining involved with others. **Those who face the future with a hopeful, positive attitude will cope better with aging.**

Older adults should be encouraged to make a living will and to designate someone to make health care decisions for them in case they cannot. Completing a durable power of attorney for financial arrangements is recommended. Each state has guidelines and forms that can be obtained from lawyers or health clinics. The office of the patient's primary care provider should be given a copy of the documents.

Older adults with children should involve them in planning. If there are no children, another relative, a younger friend, or a trusted lawyer can be named as their trustee.

WHEN A PARENT NEEDS HELP

It is not easy for adult children to admit that a parent needs their assistance. Sometimes the nurse can help stimulate a conversation about the future and offer resources for the family.

Some older adults recognize that they need help and initiate discussion with their children or others. They may decide to move to a smaller apartment or into an assisted living facility. Others deny their aging and resist making any changes until a crisis arises. This denial is an understandable way of maintaining their dignity and self-esteem.

PLANNING AHEAD

Experts recommend adult children keep communication lines open with their parents. The parent may need encouragement to discuss alternative living arrangements or other needed changes. Adult children should try to:

- **Plan ahead:** Discuss possibilities and make plans with the parent before a crisis occurs. This way decisions will be mutually agreeable and less traumatic.
- **Include everyone:** Siblings should share in planning and decision making. No one adult child should feel wholly responsible.
- **Find important information:** This includes knowing about the parent's financial situation, current medical care and medications, and alternative housing possibilities. If parents are reluctant to discuss changes, they may need more time to think about it. Consider the choices and seek out resources.

Box 13.3 Signs That an Older Adult Needs Help

- Neglected personal hygiene, irregular dressing, and soiled clothing
- Altered eating habits in the past year resulting in weight loss; decreased appetite or missed meals
- Neglected home and less than desirable sanitary conditions
- Inappropriate behavior such as being unusually loud or quiet, being paranoid, being agitated, or making phone calls at all hours
- Frequent falls, burns, or injuries
- Social isolation and cessation of activities previously important
- Altered relationship patterns such that friends and neighbors express concern
- Inability to find the right words
- Forgetfulness resulting in unpaid bills, unopened mail, missed appointments, or hoarding money
- Confusion about medications
- Unusual purchases such as more than one subscription to the same magazine or increased buying from television advertisements

OBSERVING CHANGES

Safety is a basic need. Adult children must make decisions for parents who are no longer able to care for themselves safely. If older adults show signs of deteriorating behavior, it is time for adult children to make some of those decisions for them (Box 13.3).

RESOURCES FOR FAMILIES

Many communities provide services for older adults including adult day services, chore services, transportation, counseling, companionship programs, exercise and rehabilitation programs, and telephone reassurance services. To learn what is available in your community, begin with the yellow pages or the Internet. Your state agency on aging coordinates information. The federal Administration on Aging can also provide information. AARP has information about services for older adults.

Get Ready for the NCLEX Examination!

Key Points

- The majority of older Americans are in reasonably good health and living independently. Americans are living longer.
- There are biologic theories of aging and psychosocial theories of aging.
- Many factors contribute to longevity, including maintaining a healthy lifestyle, appropriately using the health care system, genetics, and education.
- Young old adults are ages 65 to 74; middle old adults are ages 75 to 84; very old adults are age 85 and beyond. Centenarians are people age 100 and older.
- Leading causes of death in older adults are heart disease, cancer, chronic lower respiratory disease, stroke, Alzheimer disease, diabetes, influenza, and pneumonia.
- Exercise for increasing strength and balance helps prevent falls and promotes longer independence.
- Older adults can benefit by improving their diets and increasing their physical activity. A positive attitude helps all aspects of aging.
- Schaie's stage for older adults is the reintegrative stage; older adults are careful about how they spend their time and take time only for things that interest them.
- Short-term memory may weaken with age, but memory aids can help. Although mental processing slows, given time, the older adult can do as well as a younger adult can.
- The age of retirement varies widely. Older adults are a growing segment of the US part-time labor force, whereas others engage in volunteering.
- Erikson's stage for older adults is ego integrity versus despair. Older adults reminisce, and if life has been satisfactory, they have ego integrity.
- Family relationships remain important. Role changes occur when a spouse becomes ill, dependent, or dies.
- Many older adults prefer living in their own home as long as possible. Multigenerational households are becoming more common.
- Adult children of older adults should remain aware of their parents' status and be prepared to help if the parents are no longer able to care for themselves safely.

Additional Learning Resources

SG Go to your Study Guide for additional learning activities to help you master this chapter content.

evolve Go to your Evolve website at http://evolve.elsevier.com/Williams/fundamental for additional online resources.

Online Resources

- *Administration on Aging*, www.aoa.gov.
- *AARP* (organization geared for people over age 50), www.aarp.org.
- *Centers for Disease Control and Prevention, Healthy Aging*, www.cdc.gov/aging.
- Site for, about, and by caregivers, www.caregiver.com.

Review Questions for the NCLEX Examination

*Choose the **best** answer for each question.*

1. Demographers in the United States predict increasing numbers of older people because: *(Select all that apply.)*
   1. The baby boomers are healthier with age than were previous generations.
   2. Medical technology is extending life for many, especially those with heart disease.
   3. Most people today are much happier than previous generations were.
   4. There are more wealthy people who can afford quality health care.
   5. More vitamins and supplements are available to delay aging.
2. Natalie and her parents live with Natalie's grandparents, second-generation Italian immigrants, on several acres of rural farmland. The family runs a pasta manufacturing plant on the property. This is an example of:
   1. An intergenerational household.
   2. A suburban household.
   3. A single-family household.
   4. Economic hardship.
3. To fulfill Erikson's psychosocial stage, older adults can be encouraged to:
   1. Play with their grandchildren.
   2. Continue with hobbies and light exercise.
   3. Remain employed as long as possible.
   4. Review their lives, recalling accomplishments.
4. The important behaviors that can help an older adult to age successfully include:
   1. Moving closer to a child.
   2. Remaining physically and mentally active.
   3. Limiting exercise to conserve strength.
   4. Eating at least 2000 calories daily.
5. To help parents plan for possible future changes, adult children should:
   1. Investigate alternative housing arrangements.
   2. Keep communication lines open within the family.
   3. Choose a nursing home for the parent.
   4. Consult with the parent's primary care provider.
6. Depression in older adults: *(Select all that apply.)*
   1. Is a natural part of aging.
   2. Has been linked to high suicide rates in seniors.
   3. Is best treated with medication and counseling.
   4. Can be easily diagnosed by a health care professional.
   5. May be the result of a chronic illness or loss of body function.
7. Signs of elder abuse include: *(Select all that apply.)*
   1. Fear of caregivers.
   2. Bruises and cuts in various stages of healing.
   3. Timid and withdrawn behavior.
   4. Forgetfulness.
   5. Disheveled appearance.

Critical Thinking Activities

Read the clinical scenario and discuss the questions with your classmates.

One of your home care patients is an 82-year-old woman with arthritis and type 2 diabetes. She had a hip replacement 3 months ago after a fall and has recently returned to her apartment after rehabilitation in a long-term care facility. You are to assist her with her hygiene needs and monitor her medications.

1. What are some observations you could make to assess her cognitive abilities and stage of development?
2. How might you assess her psychosocial development?
3. What could you do to assist her in adjusting to this stage of her life?

chapter 14

Cultural and Spiritual Aspects of Patient Care

http://evolve.elsevier.com/Williams/fundamental

Objectives

Upon completing this chapter, you will be able to do the following:

Theory

1. Develop a beginning understanding of transcultural nursing.
2. Learn to differentiate between culture, ethnicity, race, and religion.
3. Evaluate the influence of culture on the ways health care consumers manage their health and health care resources.
4. Critically evaluate the effect of poverty on the quality and accessibility of health care.
5. Develop an understanding of the nurse's role in providing culturally congruent care.
6. Identify the primary features of cultural competence.
7. Identify the major barriers to the development of cultural competence.
8. Plan patient-centered care with regard to patients' cultural needs.
9. Demonstrate cultural competence when caring for patients with diverse ethnic backgrounds.
10. Discuss boundaries of professional care for a patient whose cultural and religious beliefs are different from yours.
11. Identify signs of spiritual distress in a patient and plan three interventions to relieve it.

Key Terms

agnostic (ăg-NŎS-tĭk, p. 185)
atheist (Ā-thē-ĭst, p. 185)
baptized (p. 186)
beliefs (p. 185)
chi'i (CHĒ, p. 192)
circumcision (sŭr-kŭm-SĬ-shŭn, p. 188)
communion (p. 186)
cultural awareness (KŬL-chŭr-ăl a-WĀR-nĕs, p. 189)
cultural competence (KŎM-pĕ-tĕns, p. 190)
cultural sensitivity (sĕn-sĭ-TĬ-vĭ-tē, p. 189)
culture (p. 184)
curandero (kŭr-ăn-DĔ-rō, p. 193)
dialects (DĪ-ă-lĕkts, p. 191)
egalitarian (ē-găl-ĭ-TĂR-ĭ-ăn, p. 191)
enculturation (ĕn-kəl-CHə-rā-SHən, p. 184)
ethnic (p. 184)
ethnicity (p. 184)
ethnocentrism (ĕth-nō-SĔN-trĭsm, p. 190)
faith (p. 185)
generalization (jĕn-ĕr-ăl-ī-ZĀ-shŭn, p. 190)
holistic (p. 192)
kosher (KŌ-shŭr, p. 188)
matriarchal (MĀ-trē-ăr-kăl, p. 191)
patriarchal (PĀ-trē-ăr-kăl, p. 191)
prejudice (PRĔ-jŭ-dĭs, p. 190)
race (p. 184)
racism (p. 190)
religion (p. 185)
rituals (p. 185)
shaman (SHĂ-măn, p. 193)
spiritual distress (SPĬR-ĭ-tū-ăl, p. 195)
spirituality (p. 185)
stereotype (STĔR-ē-ō-tīp, p. 190)
subcultures (p. 184)
transcultural nursing (p. 184)
values (p. 184)
worldview (p. 184)
yang (p. 192)
yin (p. 192)

Concepts Covered in This Chapter

- Addiction
- Anxiety
- Communication
- Culture
- Evidence
- Family dynamics
- Professionalism
- Safety

TRANSCULTURAL CARE

Culture and spirituality permeate every aspect of life. People experience health and make lifestyle choices according to their cultural and spiritual beliefs. More importantly, culture and spirituality have a huge influence on the way patients manage their health and use their health care resources. Research has repeatedly demonstrated that nursing care based on patients' unique cultural and spiritual needs significantly improves patient outcomes and overall quality of care. This understanding has given rise to the discipline of **transcultural nursing**. Transcultural nursing was formalized as a practice area and a distinct field of scholarly inquiry by Leininger (2002, 2006), who described it as nursing care that recognizes cultural diversity and is sensitive to the cultural needs of the patient and family. Leininger's theory postulates that human caring is a universal aspect of every culture; it is present in all cultures although it may be expressed in culturally unique ways. It provides what every human needs to grow, remain well, avoid illness, and survive or face death.

QSEN Considerations: Patient-Centered Care

Transcultural Nursing

Transcultural nursing was a novel idea several decades ago. However, it is now a standard of nursing practice, and all nurses are expected to provide care that is congruent with patients' cultural needs.

WHAT IS CULTURE?

Culture is a collection of beliefs, values, and assumptions about life that is shared and maintained by a group of people and transmitted intergenerationally (Leininger & McFarland, 2002). Culture encompasses a variety of learned behaviors, beliefs, attitudes, and norms that regulate social conduct and define the worldview of the members of a particular group. A ***worldview*** is a comprehensive system of beliefs used by individuals and groups to explain and interpret reality. Cultural beliefs and norms are transferred from a group to the individual members of the group, who adopt them and incorporate them into their personal **values** and beliefs. This process is known as ***enculturation***. Personal values and beliefs are based on the messages communicated and reinforced within the person's sociocultural context from an early age.

There are four distinguishing features of culture:

- *Culture is learned and acquired* in a social context through the process of enculturation, which starts at birth and continues throughout life as a seamless and unconscious process. Members of a culture perceive their cultural norms as "normal" and "natural," even though culture is learned and is **not** genetic. The best example of this is language acquisition: infants adopt and learn the language of their adoptive families and primary caregivers regardless of their ancestry.
- *Culture is shared* by a group. Examples of cultural groups include families, tribal groups, regional populations, nations, professional groups, and distinct subgroups within a wider society.
- *Culture is incorporated into individuals' identity.* Through the process of enculturation, individuals adopt the identity of their cultural group and see it as an intrinsic part of self. Consequently, culture defines individuals' perception of self and others.
- *Culture is dynamic* and changes under the influence of shared experience. Cultural norms, however, tend to evolve at a slow pace. This can be a source of conflict within a cultural group. Examples of these include intergenerational conflicts, where an older generation resists cultural norms promoted by a younger generation.

Ethnicity and ***ethnic group***(s) are terms used to define a group of people who share the common and distinct culture based on shared ancestry, social experience, regional and/or national history. Examples of ethnicity include Japanese, German, and Armenian. ***Race*** is a social classification that assigns a group membership based on physical characteristics. For example, people are assigned racial labels based on skin color. *Race* and *ethnicity* are often used interchangeably on health care questionnaires. This is incorrect because they are essentially different categories. Two people can be of the same race but belong to completely different ethnic groups and vice versa. Nurses must understand these differences and avoid assigning ethnic and racial labels based on physical characteristics or their own beliefs about culture and race. When required to state patients' ethnicity or race, ask the patients to self-identify.

The modern history of North American societies is shaped by immigration. The United States and Canada continue to be top destinations for international migrants. Consequently, these two countries have culturally diverse populations with many ethnic groups. In addition to the traditional cultural groups, the United States and Canada are home to many **subcultures:** smaller groups within the culture whose members have similar views and goals in addition to or in place of those of the main culture. A subculture is based on characteristics such as socioeconomic status, education, occupation, political beliefs, sexual orientation, or residence in a rural versus urban area.

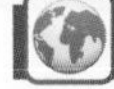

Cultural Considerations

People living in poverty constitute a subculture because of their shared beliefs and practices. The focus is day-to-day survival. People in poverty may have unstable family relationships, poor family dynamics, and higher prevalence of alcohol and drug abuse or addiction. Emotional and physical disorders can impair the ability to take care of basic needs for shelter, food, and clothing, leading to homelessness. People in poverty are more vulnerable to illnesses and diseases such as malnutrition and tuberculosis. Chronic conditions and disorders affecting them may become worse because they go untreated as a result of a lack of resources. Inadequate access to health care limits their ability to use preventive care services or seek care for acute illnesses. The net result is that this group has much worse health status compared with the general population.

! Safety Alert

Cultural Diversity and Medication Safety

- Patients from some Asian and Latino cultures may stop taking medications without telling their health care providers. This may be due to a reluctance to share personal information.
- African Americans and Native Americans may doubt the need for medications when symptoms ease and may discontinue drugs such as antibiotics or antidepressants.
- Vietnamese patients may take only half of the prescribed dose of a medication, believing it is too strong.
- All ethnic groups metabolize central nervous system (CNS) medications more slowly than do whites and, therefore, require smaller doses. Up to 10% of whites and 1% of Asians lack the enzyme that converts codeine to morphine in the body, making codeine an ineffective choice for pain medication in these people (Kaplow & Hardin, 2007).

UNDERSTANDING SPIRITUALITY

The terms *religion* and *spirituality* are often used interchangeably; however, these are two very different concepts. The word ***spirituality*** comes from Latin and can be translated as '"breath of life." It is a deeply subjective experience that tries to explain one's relationship to the wholeness of the physical and non-physical world, and the meaning of one's life. Although it is a central feature of religious experience, spirituality does not automatically imply religiosity. An individual can be spiritual but not religious. However, religion is commonly examined in the context of discussion about spirituality.

Religion is a formalized system of belief and worship. **Rituals** (ceremonial acts) are practices related to health, illness, birth, and death, and prescribed behaviors that are part of organized religion and sometimes spirituality. **Religious beliefs** are convictions or opinions derived from religious doctrine that one considers true. **Faith** is a belief that cannot be proven or for which no material evidence exists. A person who does not believe in God or does not subscribe to any religious doctrine is an **atheist**. This is quite different from an **agnostic**, a person who neither believes nor denies the existence of God in religious sense because it cannot be completely proved or disproved through the existing knowledge systems.

Humans begin acquiring their spiritual and religious beliefs from birth. This process typically occurs in the context of their immediate sociocultural environment through the processes of enculturation, and spiritual and religious indoctrination. Spiritual and religious beliefs mature in ways of thinking that influence lifestyle, behavior, attitudes, and convictions about life, health, illness, and death. Beliefs change over time and may be affected by personal experiences, including changes in health status. **During illness, and especially in the face of death, religious and spiritual beliefs may be strengthened, questioned, or rejected.** Health care decisions may be influenced by beliefs regarding health as a gift or illness and disease as a punishment. There also may be religious prohibitions or requirements for treatment. Some people with spiritual beliefs may see illness or disease as displeasure of the spirits that requires special rituals and ceremonies to appease. Many patients use prayer, meditation, and other spiritual practices along with medical treatment options.

MAJOR RELIGIONS IN THE UNITED STATES AND CANADA

The United States and Canada are civil societies that offer religious freedom to all. This means that they do not have an official religion, and individuals and groups are free to pursue their religious beliefs in a peaceful way that does not interfere with rights of other members of society. Consequently, there are many religious communities in both the United States and Canada, including (but not limited to) Christianity, Islam, Judaism, Buddhism, Hinduism, Confucianism, and Taoism. Religious beliefs are often incorporated into cultural beliefs. However, not all members of a particular cultural group are religious, even when the cultural identity of the group is closely tied to religion. Therefore, include questions about spiritual beliefs in the initial patient assessment and allow all patients to express their spiritual beliefs in the way they wish.

CHRISTIANITY

Christianity has three main branches: Roman Catholic, Eastern Orthodox, and Protestant. Each branch has multiple denominations with many subgroups within each denomination. Beliefs and religious rules of one denomination or group may differ and even contradict those of another group. The best way to find out the specifics of a particular group is by consulting a religious official from that group.

Regardless of the differences between various denominations, there are common themes and features:

- Strict monotheism expressed as a belief that there is only one God who is the creator of everything.
- The Bible is the primary text and resource.
- Most Christian churches have a specified and hierarchical organizational structure.
- Most Christian denominations have an organized set of rituals or sacraments to address life events such as marriage, holidays, and death.

Catholic and Eastern Orthodox beliefs related to health care are presented in Box 14.1.

Box 14.1 Roman Catholic and Eastern Orthodox Beliefs and Health Care

ROMAN CATHOLIC

Birth: Infants must be **baptized** soon after birth because of the belief that babies not baptized will not go to Heaven. Even aborted fetuses must be baptized. If a priest is not immediately available, the nurse may baptize by pouring holy water on the head and saying, "I baptize you in the name of the Father, of the Son, and of the Holy Spirit." Document the information in the nurse's notes, and inform the priest and the family.

Holy Eucharist: Patients receiving **communion** must not have anything to eat or alcohol to drink 15 minutes before receiving the consecrated wafer, if possible; however, if death is imminent, this fasting requirement is waived. Medicine and fluids may be taken any time.

Anointing of the sick: When the patient is ill, the priest is called to give this sacrament. He applies holy oil to the patient's forehead and hands. This sacrament may also be done after death. The nurse records this in the nurse's notes.

Diet: When hospitalized, the Catholic patient is excused from dietary rules.

Death: Catholics must receive the anointing of the sick, the Holy Eucharist, and make a confession. Although cremation is acceptable, ashes must not be kept in the home of a relative or friend. Scattering the ashes is considered an irreverent treatment of the human body. Ashes must be "committed to the sea or the ground in an urn, coffin, or other suitable container" (*Catholic Answers,* 2012).

Birth control: Natural family planning and abstinence are the only acceptable birth control methods. Nurses may teach family planning. Sterilization is forbidden unless needed for medical reasons.

Organ donation: Organ donation is acceptable if an individual is truly deceased, the person has given informed consent verified by a trusted source (consent of next of kin is acceptable if the individual did not previously make his wishes known), and the remains must be treated with respect (*Catholic Answers,* 2012).

Religious articles: Rosary beads are used to pray. Medals and other objects are important to the patient and should be kept visible and secure.

EASTERN ORTHODOX

Birth: The baby is baptized by immersion in water three times, followed by anointing with holy oil called chrism. Chrismation can only be performed by the patriarch or chief bishop of the local church.

Holy communion: Call the priest if the patient wants to receive communion.

Anointing of the sick: The priest will do this at the bedside.

Diet: Hospitalized patients are excused from fasting from meat and dairy products on holy days.

Holidays: Christmas is celebrated January 7, and New Year's Day on January 14.

Death: The priest must be called by the nurse while the patient is conscious for the patient to receive the last rites (anointing of the sick). The Orthodox Church discourages assisted deaths, autopsy, cremation, and organ donation.

Birth control and abortion: Not permitted.

Clinical Cues

Offer quiet time for reading scriptures or devotionals. Do not interrupt the patient for procedures during these quiet times.

Some Christian denominations oppose abortion and birth control, and may even oppose medical treatments and procedures such as blood transfusion and transplantations. They can forbid or limit the use of alcohol, tobacco, and other substances that are considered drugs. Practicing Christians may wish to see a cleric while hospitalized or, in some cases, they may want to use specific religious texts that are not readily available. Contact the pastoral care department to make the appropriate arrangements. Similarly, practicing Christians may want to fast when hospitalized before religious holidays. Communicate the patient's preferences to the dietitian to accommodate the patient's dietary preferences with the minimum negative effect on her recovery.

Some of the general protestant practices relevant to health care are presented in Table 14.1. However, because of the diversity of Christian denominations and their beliefs, always conduct a comprehensive spiritual assessment to identify the individual patient's specific spiritual needs.

? Think Critically

From the information in Table 14.1, you know that Jehovah's Witnesses will not accept a blood transfusion. How would you react if a 24-year-old female accident victim who is a Jehovah's Witness says that she refuses to accept a blood transfusion, even though she knows she is likely to die without it? How would you handle this situation?

ISLAM

Islam originated in the Middle East, where it is still the most common religion. It is also found in parts of Africa and Asia and increasingly in Europe and North America. The main place of worship is called mosque (Fig. 14.1). Islam includes a wide variety of groups that vary in the level of orthodoxy, but there are some shared features:

- Strict monotheism expressed as a belief in one God called Allah.
- Islamic teachings are summed up in the holy book, the Koran (*Qur'an*), which should not be touched by anybody who is considered ritually unclean.
- Religious officials are called *Imams* and are regarded as authorities on theological questions.
- Pork and its derivatives are prohibited, and alcoholic beverages and drug abuse are generally forbidden.
- Modesty for women, particularly in dress, is highly important.

Table 14.1 Protestant Beliefs Affecting Health Care

DENOMINATION	BELIEFS
Christian Science	• Do not normally seek traditional health care; have their own midwives and nurses. • Believe that sickness, evil, and sin are not of God but of the mind. Illness and sin can be changed by altering thoughts rather than by medical intervention. • Illness and sin are overcome through prayer, which alters thoughts. • A practitioner may be called to minister to the sick person to provide spiritual healing. May seek the services of an orthopedic surgeon to set a fracture. • Do not take medications.
Jehovah's Witnesses	• Abortion is forbidden. • Taking blood into the body is prohibited, and transfusion of blood or blood products is not permitted. Transfusion with dextran or blood expanders is permitted. • An organ transplant may be accepted, but the organ must be cleansed with a non-blood solution before transplantation. • Only meat that has been drained of blood may be eaten. • The body must be buried with all its parts, which prevents donation of tissues.
Church of Jesus Christ of Latter-day Saints	• A church elder should be notified in the event of death. • Natural means of birth control are recommended. • Cleanliness is vital. A sacred undergarment may be worn that should be removed only in an emergency. If removed, the garment should be put back on as soon as possible.
Seventh-Day Adventist	• The Sabbath is observed on Saturday. • Many are vegetarians, and most avoid eating pork.
Unitarian Universalist Association	• Strong belief in a woman's right of choice regarding abortion. • Advocate donation of organs and body parts for transplant and research.
Mennonite	• Women may wish to wear head covering while hospitalized.

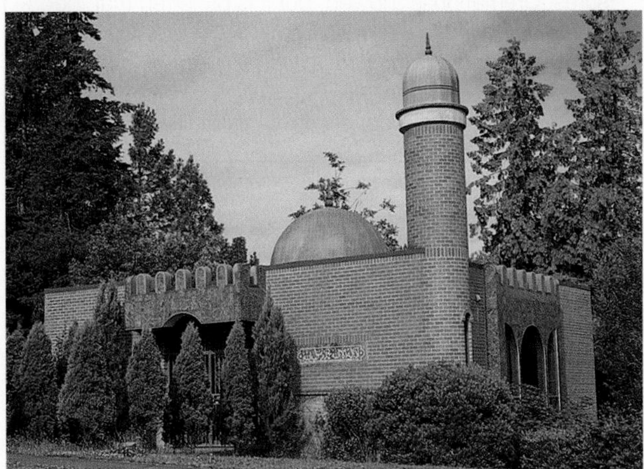

FIGURE 14.1 The main place of worship for Muslims, the mosque.

- The body is washed at the time of prayer, and privacy is required for prayer.

The Five Pillars of Islamic faith include (1) to proclaim the Shahadah (confession of the faith); (2) to perform the mandatory five daily prayers on time; (3) to fast during the month of Ramadan, the ninth in the lunar calendar, from dawn to sunset; (4) to pay Zakat religious tithes to the poor; and (5) to make a pilgrimage in Mecca, at least once in a lifetime.

Women in a traditional Muslim family may not enjoy the degree of independence and freedom assumed to be the norm in North America. They may have limited ability to make health care decisions, and sometimes the husband's presence is required when they sign health care documents. Beliefs and practices related to health care are listed in Box 14.2.

Box 14.2 Muslim Beliefs and Health Care

Birth: After birth, the baby is bathed immediately and then given to the mother. The father whispers the call to prayer in the infant's ears. Circumcision is recommended before puberty. A baby born prematurely but at 130 days of gestation or more is treated the same as a full-term infant.

Diet: No pork or alcoholic beverages are allowed. All meat animals must be killed and blessed in a special way.

Death: Patients must face Mecca, confess sins, and beg forgiveness in the presence of the family. If family is unavailable, any practicing Muslim can provide this support. After death, the body should not be touched until the family has washed and prepared it and positioned it facing Mecca. Burial is performed as soon as possible. Cremation and organ donation are forbidden. Autopsy is prohibited except for legal reasons.

Birth control and abortion: Many believe that artificial birth control interferes with God's will; others believe that women should have only as many children as the husband can afford, and contraception is permitted. Abortion is forbidden.

Other practices: Washing is required at prayer time. Privacy must be provided for prayer. The Koran should not be touched by anyone ritually unclean, and nothing is to be placed on top of it.

Care of women: Women are not allowed to sign a consent form or make decisions about family planning; therefore, the husband must be present. Muslim women are modest and usually wear clothing that covers all of the body. Muslim women prefer female care providers.

Box 14.3 Jewish Beliefs and Health Care

ORTHODOX JUDAISM

Birth: Babies are named by the father. Male children are named 8 days after being born, when circumcision is done. Female babies are usually named while the Torah is read in synagogue. Nurses need to be sensitive to the wishes of parents of an infant who has not yet been named.

Care of women: The woman is thought to be not in a state of purity during her menses or after the birth of a child until she has bathed in a pool called a mikvah. Nurses need to be sensitive to the woman's needs. The Orthodox Jewish man cannot help the woman with her care; the nurse will need to do so.

Dietary: Kosher rules include no mixing of milk and meat, using separate utensils for milk and meat, not eating any animal not slaughtered according to Jewish law, fasting during the Yom Kippur holiday (unless one cannot fast for medical reasons), not eating raised breads during Passover, and saying thanksgiving before and after meals. Nurses can help by giving the patient time and quiet for this practice.

Sabbath: From sunset Friday to sunset Saturday. The laws say to not ride in a car, smoke, or use lights, money, telephone, or television. Surgery or other medical treatments are postponed if possible.

Death: Death happens when respiration and circulation cease and cannot be corrected. Orthodox Judaism forbids assisted death. It is the duty of the family and friends to visit, and someone needs to be with the patient when she dies and when the soul leaves the body. The body should not be left alone until burial, usually within 24 hours. The body may only be touched or washed by an Orthodox person or the Jewish Burial Society. On the Sabbath, a body must not be handled. The nurse may do basic care while wearing gloves. Autopsy is not approved. If done, all body parts removed must be buried with the body.

Birth control and abortion: Birth control is discouraged, and vasectomies are forbidden. Abortion is allowed only to save the mother's life or in very dire circumstances.

Organ transplantation: This may be allowed with the rabbi's approval.

Shaving: The beard is a sign of holiness, and no blade must touch the skin. Scissors or an electric razor may be used.

Hats: Orthodox men wear skullcaps (yarmulkes) all the time, and women cover their hair after marriage.

Prayer: Prayer to God is required. Nurses need to allow a quiet environment for prayer.

REFORM JUDAISM

Birth: Orthodox practice may or may not be observed, but circumcision may be practiced.

Care of women: The beliefs do not follow the rules about not touching women.

Dietary: Kosher diets are usually not observed.

Sabbath: There is Friday evening worship in temples but no other rules.

Death: The beliefs allow life support but no heroic measures. Cremation is allowed, but it is preferred that the ashes be buried in a Jewish cemetery.

Organ transplantation: This is allowed with the rabbi's approval.

Hats: Praying is usually done without yarmulkes.

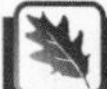
Life Span Considerations

Older Adults

The Muslim patient may insist on a same-sex caregiver because of the strong taboo regarding touching nonfamily members of the opposite sex.

JUDAISM

Judaism has several branches: Orthodox, Conservative, Reform, and Reconstructionist. The religious leader in Judaism is called a *rabbi*, and the primary place of worship is the synagogue. Judaism began when the one God revealed himself to the nomadic tribes of the Middle East at Mt. Sinai in Egypt thousands of years before the birth of Christ. Strict rules regarding hygiene, diet, ethical behavior, social justice for the powerless, and religious ceremony were passed down orally and later written down in the Torah, which is the basis for both the Hebrew Tanakh and the Christian Old Testament. Orthodox Jews follow the strictest interpretation of Jewish law. Food is prepared according to Jewish dietary laws during slaughter, processing, and packaging and is then labeled **kosher**. Jewish religious laws may be relaxed during illness, but it is still important to consult with the patient to be certain that nursing care does not cause spiritual distress. There are rituals regarding care of a dead body and burial, and the rabbi should be consulted.

Circumcision is a Jewish religious ritual performed by a man called a *mohel* on the eighth day of a boy's life. It involves the ceremonial removal of the penile foreskin. Box 14.3 presents the major Jewish beliefs to be considered when planning health care.

HINDUISM, BUDDHISM, AND TAOISM

Many Hindus are vegetarians because they believe that eating meat involves harming a living creature. Illness is seen as the result of the misuse of the body or a consequence of sin committed in a previous life. They strongly believe that life is controlled by God and that the individual has little control over what happens. Within the family, the oldest woman is considered the authority on health and healing matters. She should be consulted and included in any patient education. **Ayurvedic** medicine, founded in India, follows principles of "hot" and "cold" to balance the diet as needed for the season and the disease state.

Buddhists believe spiritual peace and liberation from anxiety through following Buddha's teachings

Table 14.2 Religious Dietary Practices

	SEVENTH-DAY ADVENTIST	BUDDHIST	EASTERN ORTHODOX	HINDU	JEWISH	MUSLIM
Beef	—	Avoided by most devout	—	Prohibited or strongly discouraged	—	—
Pork	Prohibited or strongly discouraged	Avoided by most devout		Avoided by most devout	Avoided by most devout	Prohibited or strongly discouraged
All meat	Avoided by most devout	Avoided by most devout	Permitted but some restrictions apply	Avoided by most devout	Permitted but some restrictions apply	Permitted but some restrictions apply
Eggs/dairy	Permitted but avoided at some observances	Permitted but avoided at some observances	Permitted but some restrictions apply	Permitted but avoided at some observances	Permitted but some restrictions apply	—
Fish	Avoided by most devout	Avoided by most devout	Permitted but some restrictions apply	Permitted but some restrictions apply	Permitted but some restrictions apply	—
Shellfish	Prohibited or strongly discouraged	Avoided by most devout	Permitted but avoided at some observances	Permitted but some restrictions apply	Avoided by most devout	—
Meat and dairy at same meal	—	—	—	—	Prohibited or strongly discouraged	—
Leavened foods	—	—	—	—	Permitted but avoided at some observances	—
Ritual slaughter of animals	—	—	—	—	Practiced	Practiced
Alcohol	Prohibited or strongly discouraged	—	—	Avoided by most devout	—	Prohibited or strongly discouraged
Caffeine	Prohibited or strongly discouraged	—	—	—	—	Prohibited or strongly discouraged

From *Kittler/Sucher Food and Culture*, 6th ed. © 2012 Brooks/Cole, A part of Cengage Learning, Inc. Reproduced by permission. www.cengage.com/permissions.

are important in promoting health and recovery. Taoists believe that illness or disease is due to an imbalance in yin and yang.

 **Life Span Considerations**

Older Adults

- Older adults may be particularly upset with interruptions in their religious practice caused by illness or hospitalization.
- Providing time for prayer, reading scripture to them, or contacting their religious leader may assist in decreasing spiritual distress.

Asian diets tend to consist of less meat and more vegetables than the typical American diet does. Meats are sliced, diced, or shredded and added in small quantities to vegetables. A variety of sauces and spices are used in cooking. "Hot" or "cold" foods are consumed during illness or disease to regain balance within the body. Many religions have dietary rules (Table 14.2).

DEVELOPING CULTURAL COMPETENCE

Nurses must develop cultural competence to deliver care that meets standards of culturally congruent care. Developing cultural competence is a lifelong process. It begins with the development of cultural awareness and cultural sensitivity. ***Cultural awareness*** involves developing understanding that health is expressed differently across cultures, and that culture influences an individual's response to health, illness, disease, and death. ***Cultural sensitivity*** is the ability to

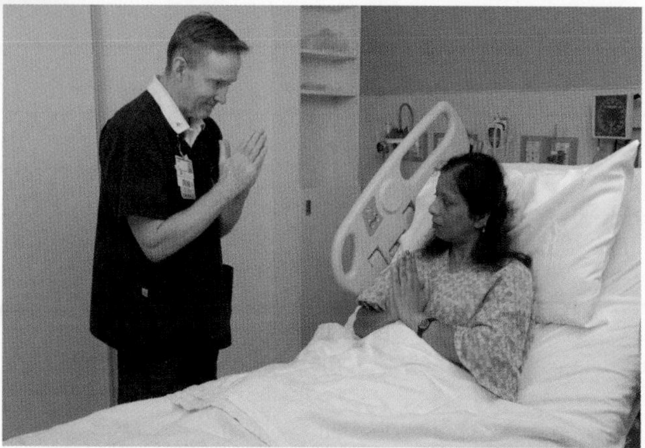

FIGURE 14.2 A nurse giving a traditional greeting to a Hindu patient. This method of greeting honors the spirit within each of us.

engage and communicate with an individual from another culture in a manner that demonstrates respect for their cultural norms and beliefs (Fig. 14.2). ***Cultural competence*** involves knowing yourself, examining your own values, attitudes, beliefs, and prejudices. It entails keeping an open mind and trying to see the world from a different cultural perspective. There are many ways to develop cultural competence. Literature written by authors from other cultures can provide a wealth of information and insight into others' views of the world. Respect differences among people, recognizing that every group has its strengths and weaknesses. Be open to experiential learning: each contact with an individual from another cultural group is a perfect learning opportunity. Learn to communicate effectively while being mindful of nonverbal communication such as body movements, use of personal space, and gestures (Holland, 2012). Be resourceful and creative in modifying nursing interventions in culturally competent ways. Consider your nursing actions carefully when interacting with a patient from another culture.

Cultural Considerations

Cultural Aspects to Consider

The following should be considered when caring for a patient from a different culture:

- Form of address considered appropriate within the culture
- Whether an interpreter is needed
- Whether eye contact is considered polite or rude
- Amount of space between speakers considered appropriate when conversing
- The meaning of nonverbal gestures such as head nodding, smiling, and hand gestures, as well as unacceptable gestures
- When, where, and by whom touch is acceptable
- Who the traditional decision makers are within the culture and family
- Manner and attire of a person considered a "professional," one whose instructions are valued

BARRIERS TO CULTURAL COMPETENCE

There are six major barriers to cultural competence: stereotyping, prejudice and racism, ethnocentrism, cultural imposition, cultural conflict, and cultural shock.

Stereotyping is applying certain beliefs and behaviors about a culture to an individual or group without assessing individual needs. Although stereotypes can be either positive or negative, they are problematic because they block nurses' ability to learn about specific individuals or groups. Stereotypes should not be mixed with **generalizations**, which identify common trends, patterns, and beliefs of a group. Whereas generalizations may be true for the group, they may not necessarily be true for an individual. Ask the patient to provide additional information to determine if a generalization is true. Failure to conduct that assessment may lead to stereotyping.

Prejudice can be defined as an emotional manifestation of negative stereotypes and deeply held beliefs about a group. ***Racism*** is a form of prejudice that takes place when individuals, groups, and/or institutions exercise power against groups that are judged inferior.

Ethnocentrism is the belief that one's own cultural group determines the standards by which other groups' behavior should be judged. *Cultural blindness* is an inability to recognize the differences between one's own cultural beliefs, values, and practices and those of another culture.

Cultural imposition is the act of imposing one's own cultural beliefs, values, and practices on individuals and groups from another culture. It is different from *cultural relativism*, which is an ability to recognize that each cultural group has its own set of beliefs and that each culture should be evaluated on its own merit. Nurses often impose their values on patients by forcefully promoting Western biomedical traditions while ignoring the patients' value of treatment forms.

Cultural conflict is a perceived threat arising from a misunderstanding of expectations when nurses are unable to respond appropriately to another individual's cultural practice because they are unfamiliar with the practice. Cultural conflicts are unavoidable, but nurses should do whatever is necessary to minimize their effect on the delivery of culturally congruent care.

Cultural shock is the feeling of helplessness, discomfort, and disorientation experienced by an individual attempting to understand or effectively adapt to a cultural group whose beliefs and values are radically different from the individual's culture.

CULTURAL DIFFERENCES

Particular areas in which cultural differences are evident include communication, view of time, family organization and structure, nutritional practices, issues related to death and dying, and health care beliefs (Purnell & Paulanka, 2014).

COMMUNICATION

Language is the most obvious component of cultural identity. It is considered one of the defining features of a cultural group. In addition to a shared primary language, a group can also develop multiple dialects. A ***dialect*** is an identifiable variation of a language specific to a particular group or region. In addition to language, cultural groups tend to develop unique nonverbal communication patterns, including degree of acceptable eye contact, appropriate amount of personal space, acceptable touching, and meaning of gestures such as head nodding. Prolonged eye contact may be unacceptable in some cultures. In European American cultures, 18 inches is the usual space between people that is comfortable when they are talking together. Asians, people from the Middle East, and Hispanics tend to stand closer together when they converse. In some cultures, it is considered impolite to disagree with a person in a position of power, such as health care providers. This may result in patients giving an outward appearance of agreement even though they disagree with what is being said or do not truly understand the presented information. Always evaluate patients' understanding of the information. Do not simply assume understanding based on verbal and nonverbal cues.

Learning key phrases in other languages frequently encountered or using translation lists of common questions or symptoms may foster communication. Certified health care interpreters are typically available either on-site at the clinical agency or by telephone via specialized agencies. Your facility may use an Interpreter on a Pole (IPOP) device, which consists of a portable telephone attached to a moveable unit (similar to a portable blood pressure machine). Using the speakerphone, you communicate with the patient with the help of a trained medical interpreter.

In exceptional situations, patients' family members may be able to provide translations. However, it is typically best to avoid using family members because the patient may be reluctant to share information in the presence of family. In addition, family members may not have adequate language skill themselves and may not be versed in the specialized language of health care.

VIEW OF TIME

Orientation to time and perceptions of timeliness vary from one culture to another. This can cause misunderstanding. Members of European American culture value time and tend to be future oriented. There is a sense of time urgency (not enough time), and importance is placed on punctuality and schedules. Other cultures, notably the Hispanic American and the African American, do not have this same view of time. These cultures focus on the here and now, without the feeling of urgency to be somewhere exactly on time. Generally, this applies to social occasions rather than business or health care appointments.

Some cultures tend to be past oriented and attach considerable importance to traditions. This often takes form of the Ancestor worship. Other cultures may have strong focus on the here and now as they see the past as irrelevant and the future as unpredictable. A balance of all three views is prevalent for many individuals. **It is important to know the patient's view of time.**

FAMILY ORGANIZATION AND STRUCTURE

Family households may be male dominated **(patriarchal)**, female dominated **(matriarchal)**, or **egalitarian** (equal share between spouses). The family dynamics and power structure often determine the way health care decisions are made. Some cultures have strict gender roles. For example, in patriarchal societies, men are typically assigned the role of primary breadwinner, whereas women are assigned the role of caregiver. Respect the cultural differences and do not impose egalitarian cultural ideas prevalent in North America.

Treatment of older adults varies widely across cultures. In some cultures, older adults are considered wise and are revered. In these cultures, children are expected to provide care for their parents and grandparents when necessary. In other cultures care of older adults might be provided by specialized agencies.

The family structure tends to be culture specific. In some cultures, the nuclear family consists of the spouses and their children as a norm. In other cultures, the basic family unit includes extended family members who live in the same household. Allow patients to define their family and respect their choices.

NUTRITIONAL PRACTICES

Choice of food and eating habits are culture specific. Besides providing nutrition, food also has symbolic and social meaning. People learn from their family culture what foods are "good for you," what foods should be avoided, and what foods are used for specific illnesses or diseases. Certain foods are associated with celebrations and others with comfort and nurture. When a patient is in a health care facility, food choices may be limited, and the usual time and rituals of eating may change. Foods are categorized in some cultures (Asian, Hispanic, and Middle Eastern) as "hot," "cold," or "cool," based not on their temperature but on their presumed effect in the body. Each culture has its own set of foods that are viewed as "hot" or "cold." That effect is used to counteract illness or disease—cold foods are used to treat "hot" illnesses or diseases, and hot foods are used to treat "cold" illnesses or diseases. Because of these beliefs, some patients would consider it inappropriate to drink ice water when ill. A comprehensive nutritional assessment is essential when it comes to the provision of culturally congruent nursing care.

 QSEN Considerations: Patient-Centered Care

Food and the Patient's Family

In some cultures, family members provide food for the patient. Allowing family to provide food for the patient may help meet the patient's nutritional needs. More importantly, it provides a sense of comfort and security for a patient who may feel frightened and isolated in the health care setting. Work with families to ensure that the food complies with the prescribed treatment and nutritional guidelines.

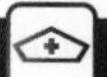 Clinical Cues

It is culturally sensitive to check with the patient before leaving a pitcher of ice water at the bedside.

 Think Critically

What food and drink do you seek or avoid when you have the following illnesses: nausea or vomiting, a severe cough and stuffy nose, or diarrhea? What foods calm you when you are stressed or upset?

DEATH AND DYING

Each culture has its own approach to death and dying. There is no "correct" way of expressing grief because manifestations of grief are very much culture specific. Some cultures encourage emotional expressions, whereas others consider it inappropriate. There are also considerable variations when it comes to informing the patients of a terminal illness. In many Asian cultures, face-to-face disclosure by a physician with privacy and time to absorb the bad news is important, although ideally, health professionals have first inquired about the patient's preferences for receiving this type of information (Larkin & Searight, 2014).

In some cultures, the body must be buried whole, whereas others prefer cremation. Organ transplantation may not be allowed. Learn cultural views about autopsy and organ donation before approaching a family on these issues. The family may have cultural rituals for preparing the body for burial. Become knowledgeable about rituals regarding death and bereavement.

HEALTH CARE BELIEFS

Beliefs about health, disease, illness, and treatment are culturally based. In cultural groups that believe the world is dominated by supernatural forces, people think that their fate depends on the action of a god or gods. They are at the mercy of spiritual forces. Religion is an integral part of culture, and it often plays an important part in the patient's treatment.

All cultures have an element of folk or home remedy medicine that is handed down through families to treat common illnesses. Folk medicine relies on home remedies and self-care practices. Folk medicine is often used first before consulting a health care professional or it may be used along with seeking professional assistance for an illness. Treating a cough with a particular type of tea with honey and lemon is an example of a folk medicine remedy. A person may continue to drink the tea even after going to the clinic and receiving a prescription for antibiotics. Knowing how a patient's family usually treats the type of illness the patient has is important in understanding a patient's reluctance to follow the prescribed regimen. Although the scientific view of health care is the majority view in the United States, it may not be the belief of a person raised in another culture or in a US subculture. Table 14.3 presents values, practices, and beliefs of various cultures.

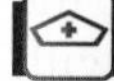 Clinical Cues

Not all people of a particular culture have the same values, beliefs, or practices. Because of the many variables in what people believe about health and illness, it is essential to assess what each patient believes about the cause of the present illness or disease, and the way to health.

Table 14.3 Common Cultural Values, Practices, and Beliefs

Asian/Pacific Islander Americans	• Value self-control, age, authority, and harmony (avoidance of conflict). • Maintain a **holistic** (attention to mental, social, spiritual, and physical aspects) view of health and illness in which nature is a dominant force. Health dependent on the flow of **chi'i** (universal life force or energy). If chi'i is out of balance or in disharmony, illness may result. • **Yin** (negative, dark, cold, and feminine) and **yang** (positive, light, warm, and masculine) are the names given other balancing forces affecting health; when they are out of balance with each other, illness may occur. • *Acumassage* (manipulating the energy flow), *acupressure* (compressing the flow), and *acupuncture* (inserting needles to interrupt the energy flow) are treatments used to restore balance between yin and yang. • May believe that a misdeed leads to illness or that disease or accident is due to misdeeds in a previous life. • Often are reluctant to express emotion to others. Tend to be stoic about pain. • Consider it disrespectful to disagree with those in authority. May be overly agreeable in attempt to maintain harmony. • Buddhism, Taoism, Hinduism, and Christianity are prominent faiths.

Table 14.3 Common Cultural Values, Practices, and Beliefs—cont'd

Hispanic Americans	• Value the family over the individual; family system is patriarchal (head of family is father). • Individuals must actively develop their potential through strength of will and volition. • Health is seen as a gift from God; maintaining health by achieving equilibrium is important. • Equilibrium is achieved through prayer, religious objects, rituals, and use of herbs and spices, and by treating others fairly and with respect. • Often seek help within the family first when ill. Some may seek the services of a **curandero** (folk healer). • May believe in use of "hot" and "cold" foods to restore equilibrium. (Certain foods have hot or cold properties unrelated to temperature of food.) • May be superstitious; some believe that staring at an infant or commenting on its beauty brings *mal de ojo* (the evil eye). May wear an amulet to ward off *mal de ojo.* • Wearing of religious objects and placing them in the home is common. • Expect a thorough examination when visiting a health professional. Often expect a prescription for treatment. • Consider it acceptable to be vocal about illness or pain. • Comforted by a touch on the arm, shoulder, or back; this helps promote rapport. • Expect health care personnel to dress professionally, exhibit professionalism, listen attentively, and answer questions patiently. • Consider the spiritual dimension of life to be very important. • Believe that health requires being in harmony with the supernatural forces and the Creator.
African Americans	• Among new immigrants or among lower socioeconomic families, health and illness may be intertwined with religion and with good and bad forces. • Families are often multigenerational, close, and supportive. Members of the church may also be considered "family." • Family structure is often matriarchal. (The mother is the head of the family.) • May believe that all illness is preventable if they are attentive to their relationship with God, nature, and other people. • Folk or home remedies and faith healers may be used, as well as professional health care. • Christianity and Islam are prominent faiths.
American Indians	• Majority of tribes share a present orientation, a respect for the aged, and an inclination to work cooperatively with avoidance of individual gain. • Believe in keeping a natural harmony between humans and the universe. The universe is made up of individual, family, community, tribe, environment, and spirit world. • Each individual has a physical and a spiritual dimension, each of which is governed by different laws. Living by both sets of laws results in a balanced, healthy, and happy life. • Believe illness occurs when there is disharmony in some aspect of the individual, the environment, or the spirit world. • Believe in the cyclic nature of birth, life, and death. • Periods of silence and avoidance of eye contact show respect. • Health care practices are linked to spirituality and living in harmony with the universe. • Harmony is achieved by respecting the earth and all living things, honoring the spirits, and appeasing them when they are angry. • Treatment of illness includes herbal medicines, rituals, fasting, massage, and consultation with the **shaman** (medicine man or woman). • The family and community provide strength and spiritual support in times of illness.
European Americans	• Value youth, attractiveness, cleanliness, order, punctuality, individualism, education, and hard work. • Future oriented. • Value self-care and self-improvement and use preventive health practices. • Maintain scientific view of health and illness in which life is controlled by physical and biochemical processes that can be altered by human intervention. • Often use home remedies before seeking professional health care. • Use medical technology and health care professionals to diagnose and treat illness. • Extended family support often disrupted by geographic distance. • Older adults may need care outside the family because of lack of family proximity or the demands of family's employment. • Christianity and Judaism are prominent religious faiths.
Arab Americans	• Value family and affiliation with others; may have daily gatherings of extended family. • Food plays a central role in life. Caring is shown by offering food. Muslims do not eat pork nor do they drink alcohol. • Common bonds of group are the Arabic language and the Islamic religion, although many Arab Americans are Christian. • Touch is generally only acceptable between members of the same sex except within the family. • Considered rude to pass things with the left hand, which is considered "unclean." • Considered rude to sit with the sole of the shoe within view of someone. • Professional occupations are favored, and most people are well educated. • Expect an effective cure from health care rather than personal care. • May be reluctant to disclose detailed information about themselves to strangers.

Methods of treatment of illness or disease from cultures that believe in holistic health care are increasingly becoming accepted in the Western science-based health practices. Complementary therapies such as massage, acupuncture, and chiropractic adjustment are being recommended along with the use of prescription medications and other standard treatments. Evidence is pointing to a connection between mind and body that influences health, and more emphasis on the use of prayer and meditation is beginning to occur.

Patient Education

Meditation

Meditation can be used as part of spiritual practice for clearing the mind and focusing, or simply as stress relief. There are various types of meditation. Here is a basic meditation technique that can be taught to patients. Meditation creates a relaxation response and has been demonstrated to reduce anxiety.

- Choose a quiet place in which to meditate.
- Plan a session of 20 minutes while learning: the time can be extended to an hour later if desired.
- Choose the floor, a portion of the bed, or a chair in which to sit while meditating.
- Assume a comfortable position with legs either crossed in front or flat on the floor. Try to keep your back straight. Position your hands so that the right index fingertip touches the tip of the left thumb. (Rationale: If you start to fall asleep, the pressure on the thumb will awaken you.)
- Close your eyes, but remain awake and relaxed.
- Begin slow, deep, abdominal breathing. Think of breathing in light and joy and breathing out troubles and stress.
- Focus on a low humming sound, a single thought of a bright light, or an image of a bright red-orange ball.
- Do not fight thoughts creeping into your mind, but dismiss them and return to your focus.
- You may have a clock close by and can slowly open your eyes to check the time toward the end of the meditation period.
- When the time is up, open your eyes and stay in position for a few minutes to adjust to the outer world again.
- Get up slowly and evaluate the positive effects of the experience.

Life Span Considerations

Older Adults

- The older patient is more likely to value long-held cultural patterns.
- Conflicts may arise among the generations when the children have adopted the modern cultural view and seek to impose it on their parents.

SUSCEPTIBILITY TO DISEASE

Some health conditions are more common in certain groups because of sociocultural factors and/or genetics. For example, people of African or Mediterranean ancestry (regardless of culture) have more prevalence of sickle cell trait or sickle cell anemia. Similarly, keloid formation (abnormal scar tissue formation) and sarcoidosis (fibrous nodules that can interfere with function) are also more common in patients of African ancestry. Patients of Eastern European Ashkenazy Jewish ancestry may carry the trait for a fatal neurologic disorder of infancy called Tay-Sachs disease. Lactase deficiency—the absence of an enzyme needed to digest lactose, a sugar found in milk and milk products—is more common in people of Latino, African, Chinese, Thai, and American Indian ancestry. Latino and American Indian populations have a greater susceptibility to diabetes. Hypertension is more prevalent among cultural groups that use a lot of salt in the diet. Certain health conditions are more common among members of traditionally disadvantaged groups with limited access to resources. For example, substance abuse is more common among the poor. Be aware of the conditions that are common to a particular group of patients.

❖ NURSING PROCESS IN TRANSCULTURAL NURSING

◆ ASSESSMENT (DATA COLLECTION)

Consider the general aspects of the patient's culture and spiritual orientation before beginning the assessment. What are the social customs? What are the nonverbal communication patterns? Is eye contact considered polite or rude? Is touch acceptable? What are the taboos regarding touch? What is the appropriate personal space between people when talking? Begin the introduction in English unless you speak the patient's language. Obtain an interpreter if one is needed, and then begin the general assessment.

The Joint Commission requires that every patient receive a spiritual assessment by a nurse. Observe for the presence of religious or spiritual objects such as a cross, Star of David, Bible, rosary beads, prayer shawl or cap, feathers or amulets, crystals, or books on spirituality. However, do not jump to conclusion based on the presence of overt cultural or religious symbols. Remember, the best sources of information about patients' cultural and religious beliefs are the patients themselves. Allow patients to self-identify and respect their choices.

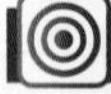

Focused Assessment

Cultural and Spiritual Assessment

To assess cultural aspects that may affect health care, ask the following questions:

- What do you think caused this illness?
- What problems has the illness created for you?
- What has been done to treat the illness so far?
- What do you fear about this illness or its treatment?
- What type of treatment do you think is appropriate?
- What benefits do you expect from treatment?
- What traditional remedies or rituals might be used in your culture to treat this illness?

Some simple questions can identify spiritual aspects that need further exploration or referral to a spiritual or religious counselor:

- Is there anything we (the nursing staff) should know about your cultural and spiritual practices and needs?
- How can we support your cultural or spiritual practices?
- Do you have any culture- or religion-specific food requirements?
- Do you need a quiet space or dedicated time for your spiritual practice?
- Is there a spiritual or religious leader (priest, rabbi, pastor, or imam) with whom you would like to meet? Would you like to talk with the chaplain?
- What helps you cope with this illness? What worries you or frightens you?

◆NURSING DIAGNOSIS

Some nursing diagnoses specifically related to cultural and spiritual problems or differences might be as follows:

- Impaired verbal communication
- Decisional conflict
- Spiritual distress

Spiritual distress may be related to feelings of guilt and unworthiness if the patient views illness as punishment for wrongdoing or sin. Other indications of spiritual distress are feelings of abandonment, anger, despair, or hopelessness as the patient questions the presence of God. Fear of death also causes spiritual distress. The need to seek forgiveness, either from significant people in the patient's life or from God, is often expressed. Spiritual distress may also be related to a conflict between one's religious or spiritual beliefs and medical treatment or the inability to attend or actively participate in religious services or spiritual rituals.

◆PLANNING

While planning care, consider the patient's family, social support system, and beliefs in culturally traditional health care practices. Write individual expected outcomes for the selected nursing diagnoses. Integrate the patient's cultural practices related to the illness and treatment into the planned interventions as much as possible. Expected outcomes related to the above-mentioned nursing diagnoses might be that the patient will:

- Express comfort with the designed care plan.
- Express needs and opinions through an interpreter.
- Cope with cultural differences of agency routines.
- Develop, reestablish, or continue the spiritual practices that nurture a relationship with God or a higher power.
- Express comfort with the patient's relationship to God and significant others.
- State that she feels at peace.
- Identify and employ spiritual supports: prayer, reading, visits from a religious/spiritual representative, or engagement in religious/spiritual rituals.

◆IMPLEMENTATION

Implement care with respect for the patient's cultural and spiritual practices. Enlist family members to assist with the patient's care if that is desirable within the culture (Fig. 14.3). Provide cultural information to other health team members. Show courtesy and respect for the patient as an individual.

Cultural Considerations

Culturally Sensitive Nursing Interventions

- Secure a skilled interpreter for history taking or important patient education.
- If needed, use "flash cards" or a communication board with common phrases or questions in the patient's language.
- Assist the patient and the family in developing a therapeutic diet with culturally indicated or preferred foods.
- If appropriate, involve the extended family in formulating the patient's treatment plan.
- Advocate for the patient's right to choose or refuse treatment.
- Provide quiet space and private time for spiritual practices.
- Contact the religious or spiritual leader if requested by the patient.
- Incorporate in the care plan religious or spiritual ceremonies that are significant to the patient.

Developing a therapeutic caring relationship permits patients to express their fears, concerns, and distress and allows the nurse to identify culturally and spiritually appropriate interventions. Be aware of your own cultural and spiritual beliefs and make sure they do not affect your ability to provide the care that meets patients' cultural and spiritual needs.

Religious objects may be important to the patient. Be certain that items such as a medal or crucifix, rosary beads, Bible, Koran, prayer shawl and cap, or prayer rug are respected and within reach (Fig. 14.4). If these

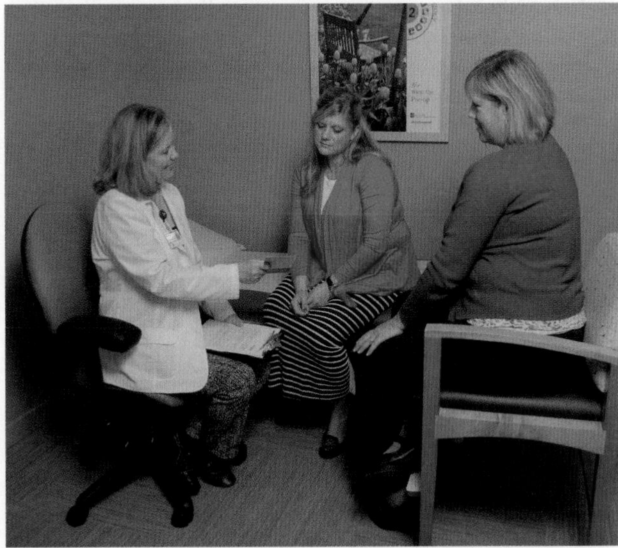

FIGURE 14.3 Observe and respect the way in which extended family members view being involved in the health care decision making.

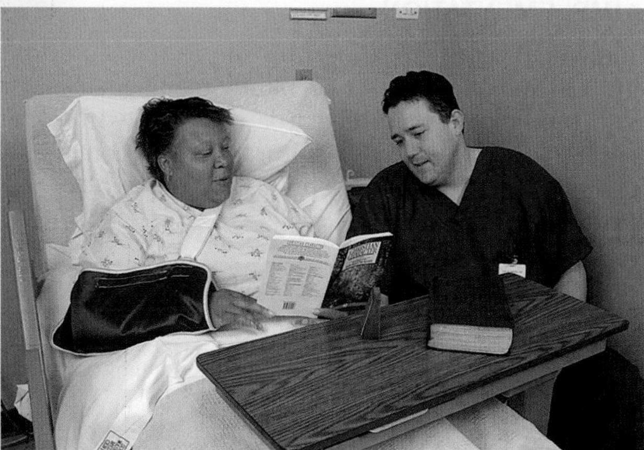
FIGURE 14.4 Attending to the patient's spiritual needs.

must be removed during surgical procedures, assure the patient that they will be restored as soon as possible after the surgery. In some clinical agencies, special arrangements can be made to keep the item with the patient throughout the surgery or procedure.

Think Critically

How would you respond if the patient asks you to participate in a cultural or religious practice that is in conflict with your own cultural and spiritual beliefs? What can you do to support the patient's cultural or spiritual beliefs in this situation?

◆EVALUATION

Evaluation is based on achievement of the expected outcomes, not whether treatment is successful from the standpoint of the nurse's cultural orientation. Transcultural nursing is successful when mutual understanding and trust develop between the patient and the nurse. Nurses must be sensitive to their patients' cultural and spiritual aspects to give holistic care. Nurses can contribute to a positive health care experience when they learn about the patient as a unique individual and advocate for the patient's rights to choose health care practices that fit with her cultural or spiritual background.

Get Ready for the NCLEX Examination!

Key Points

- Culture is a complex combination of the values, beliefs, social norms, and spiritual practices held by a majority within a particular social group.
- Ethnicity, nationality, race, spirituality, and religion are primarily sociocultural ideas.
- Culture affects the way individuals experience and manage their health.
- Cultural and spiritual practices play important roles in patients' recovery.
- Transcultural nursing is nursing care that recognizes cultural diversity and is sensitive to the cultural needs of the patients and families.
- Provision of culturally congruent care is one of the standards of nursing practice in the United States and Canada.
- Nurses are expected to engage in lifelong learning about cultural competence and culturally congruent care.
- Cultural awareness and cultural sensitivity are critical for the delivery of culturally congruent nursing care.
- Large groups can have distinct subgroups with their own unique health needs and challenges.
- People within the subculture of poverty may have a difficult time meeting their health care needs.
- Areas in which cultural difference is evident are communication, view of time,family organization and structure, nutritional practices, issues related to death and dying, and health care beliefs (see Table 14.3).
- Be aware of major health issues affecting specific groups.
- Always display respect for patients' cultural and spiritual needs and include them in the assessment.
- Choose nursing diagnoses based on the assessment data and develop plan of care specific to the identified nursing diagnoses.
- Include interventions that demonstrate cultural and spiritual sensitivity in the nursing care plan.
- Base evaluation on the achievement of expected outcomes.

Additional Learning Resources

SG Go to your Study Guide for additional learning activities to help you master this chapter content.

evolve Go to your Evolve website at http://evolve.elsevier.com/Williams/fundamental for additional online resources.

Review Questions for the NCLEX Examination

*Choose the **best** answer for each question.*

1. Your 45-year-old, mentally competent patient is having excessive blood loss from surgery. She is a Jehovah's Witness and refuses a blood transfusion. Her blood pressure has been falling, and she has a rapid heart rate. What would an appropriate nursing intervention be?
   1. Assist the RN in administering IV fluid boluses and medications to support the blood pressure.
   2. Make the patient comfortable with a warm blanket because she is avoiding lifesaving measures.
   3. Prepare to help the RN administer blood after the patient loses consciousness.
   4. Try to convince the patient that she should have the blood transfusion.

2. An older Japanese adult who does not speak English is admitted to the surgical unit after major abdominal surgery, with no family member present. The nurse cannot speak the patient's language. To assess for pain, the nurse should:
   1. Look for nonverbal indicators of pain: grimacing, moaning, or restlessness.
   2. Obtain the services of a translator to devise question-and-answer cards regarding pain.
   3. Wait for the family to come to ask the patient about pain.
   4. Use nonverbal gestures to get the patient to indicate his pain level.
3. An older Mandarin-speaking woman is grimacing and refusing to eat when served hospital food. What should the nurse do to meet the patient's nutritional needs?
   1. Contact the kitchen and order a rice or noodle dish.
   2. Continue serving hospital food until the patient decides to eat it.
   3. Contact the primary caregiver to assess the patient's dietary habits.
   4. Use the certified health care translator to explain to the patient that the kitchen will try to accommodate her nutritional request if possible.
4. A patient who is Roman Catholic asks to have the priest come to hear her confession and administer communion before she goes to surgery. The priest arrives the evening before the patient is scheduled for the operating room but after normal visiting hours. The nurse should:
   1. Suggest that the priest return after surgery because the patient has been medicated and is drowsy.
   2. Provide privacy for the priest to hear confession and administer communion.
   3. Inform the priest that the patient has not attended confession for a long time.
   4. Offer to stay with the patient and the priest during the visit to assist the priest.
5. Hindus believe that illness or disease is caused by: *(Select all that apply.)*
   1. A lack of piety and inattention to the rituals of Hinduism.
   2. Misusing the body in some way.
   3. Sin committed in a former life.
   4. Eating the wrong foods.
   5. Misusing natural resources.
6. The nurse is caring for a newly admitted homeless male patient who states that his last meal was 12 hours ago, but insists that he must talk to the pastor before he eats. Which statement would indicate that the nurse is providing culturally congruent care?
   1. "You should eat first. It'll be easier for you to talk to the pastor once you had some food."
   2. "I'll contact our pastoral care department to arrange the pastor visit, and the kitchen to order a meal for you. Your meal will be here for you when you are ready to eat."
   3. "I'll contact the pastor and ask him to come in as soon as possible. Would you like me to ask him to bring some food with him?"
   4. "The pastor doesn't mind if you eat before you see him. You should have some food. It will make you feel better."
7. When an Islamic Arab American dies in the hospital, you know: *(Select all that apply.)*
   1. To thoroughly wash the body before wrapping it.
   2. Not to touch the body before the family bathes it.
   3. To position the body facing north.
   4. To turn the bed so that the body faces Mecca.

Critical Thinking Activities

Read each clinical scenario and discuss the questions with your classmates.

Scenario A

Rosa Souza is a 76-year-old patient of Mexican origin preparing for surgery to treat an abdominal tumor for which she had previously been treated by a *curandero*. She is Roman Catholic, wears religious medals, and reads from her Spanish Bible. Her family (husband, two daughters, one son, and several grandchildren) is often present, surrounding the bedside. She will be having surgery in several days.

1. What assessments are important for Mrs. Souza from a cultural or spiritual viewpoint? What questions would you ask?
2. What religious activities might be important for Mrs. Souza? How can you determine these?
3. Discuss the dilemma of limiting visitors to allow Mrs. Souza to rest versus accommodating large numbers of family at the bedside.

Scenario B

Esther Sommes is a 33-year-old patient being treated for end-stage kidney failure and diabetes. She is aware that her disease is terminal. On her admission record, she indicated "none" for religion.

1. What is the difference between religion and the spiritual dimension of a person?
2. What assessment of Ms. Sommes's spirituality is indicated?

Scenario C

You are assigned an Arab American man as a patient.

1. In what ways could you provide culturally sensitive care for this Arab American patient?
2. How could you accommodate the family's need to visit in groups and to supply him with special food?

chapter 15

Loss, Grief, and End-of-Life Care

http://evolve.elsevier.com/Williams/fundamental

Objectives

Upon completing this chapter, you should be able to do the following:

Theory

1. Correlate the stages of grief and of dying with their associated behaviors and feelings.
2. Discuss the concept of hospice care.
3. Identify three common fears a patient is likely to experience when dying.
4. Describe common symptoms related to physiologic changes at end-of-life stages.
5. List the common signs of impending death.
6. Illustrate the difference between the patient's right to refuse treatment and assisted suicide.
7. Understand ethical guidelines in the *Code of Ethics for Nurses* regarding the patient's right to refuse treatment, euthanasia, and assisted suicide.

Clinical Practice

1. Identify ways in which you can support or instill hope in the terminally ill patient and his family.
2. Demonstrate compassionate therapeutic communication techniques with a terminally ill patient and/or his family.
3. Describe one nursing intervention for comfort care that can be implemented in a hospital or a nursing home for a dying patient for each of the following problems: pain, nausea, dyspnea, anxiety, constipation, incontinence, thirst, and anorexia.
4. Explain the reason for completing an advance directive to a terminally ill patient, as well as what "health care proxy" and "DNR/DNI".
5. Prepare to provide information regarding organ or tissue donation in response to family questions.
6. Assist with postmortem care for a deceased patient.

Skills & Steps

Key Terms

acceptance (p. 204)
advance directive (p. 209)
anticipatory grieving (ăn-TĬ-sĭ-pă-tō-rē, p. 200)
assisted suicide (SŪ-ĭ-sīd, p. 209)
autopsy (p. 211)
bargaining (p. 204)
bereavement (bĕ-RĒV-mĭnt, p. 200)
brain death (p. 4)
Cheyne-Stokes respirations (SHĀN-stōks rĕs-pĭ-RĀ-shŭns, p. 208)
closure (KLŌ-zhŭr, p. 208)
comfort care (p. 204)
coroner (KŎR-ō-nĕr, p. 210)
death (p. 201)
denial (p. 204)
durable power of attorney for health care (DŪ-ră-bŭl, p. 209)
dysfunctional (dĭs-FŬNK-shŭn-ăl, p. 200)
euthanasia (active, passive) (ū-thă-NĀ-zhē-ă, ĂK-tĭv, PĂ-sĭv, p. 209)
grief, grieving process (p. 200)
health care proxy (PRŎX-ē, p. 209)
hope (p. 204)
hospice (HŎS-pĭs, p. 202)
loss (p. 199)
obituary (ō-BĬ-chū-ĕr-ē, p. 209)
palliative (păl-ē-Ā-shŭn, p. 201)
postmortem (pōst MŌR-tĕm, p. 211)
rigor mortis (RĬ-gŏr MŌR-tĭs, p. 212)
shroud (SHRŎWD, p. 211)
thanatology (thăn-ă-TŎL-ō-jē, p. 204)

Concepts Covered in This Chapter

- Culture
- Palliation
- Family dynamics
- Ethics
- Health care law

Loss, grief, and death are inevitable parts of life. Some losses may be expected parts of development across the life span. For example, parents may experience a sense of loss when their children move out. Other losses require adjustment processes that are more complex and may elicit strong grief reactions. Examples of such losses are the unexpected or early death of an important person, abrupt decrease in functional capacity, and loss of independence. There is no single "right" way of responding to loss. The response depends on many factors such as culture, previous experiences, and personal meanings attached to the loss.

People in North America are living longer than ever before. Life expectancy in the United States increased by 1.7 years from 2003 to 2013. In 2013, life expectancy in the United States stood at 76.4 years for males and 81.2 years for females (Centers for Disease Control and Prevention [CDC], 2015). Canada has been experiencing the same trend; the latest data available indicate that life expectancy in Canada is 79 years for males and 83 years for females (Statistics Canada, 2012). This means that the proportion of older adults in total population will continue to increase. Nurses must be able to respond to these demographic changes and provide nursing services that reflect the unique needs of this population.

Death is a universally shared event. All cultures and religions have beliefs and rituals to explain and cope with death, loss, and grief. Avoiding discussions about death and dying is common in the mainstream North American cultures; death is often described using oblique expressions such as "passing away" and "passing on." Children are commonly kept away from funerals, and most people have little contact with the dying. Many adults can state that they have never seen a dead body, and more can say that they have not been present during a death. However, there has been a recent move away from silence and denial toward a willingness to examine death as an inevitable and intrinsic part of life.

NURSES' ATTITUDES TOWARD END-OF-LIFE CARE

Even nurses who provide care to critically ill or dying patients on a daily basis may have difficulty dealing with death and dying. Much like other health care professionals, nurses are primarily focused on cures and illness prevention, and they may perceive death as a professional failure rather than an intrinsic part of the life cycle. Reflect on your own attitudes, feelings, values, and expectations about death in order to provide the best end-of-life nursing care. Study the professional nursing literature and other resources that discuss legal, ethical, financial, and health care delivery issues related to this important topic. In addition, be ready to collaborate with other health care professionals to provide the dying persons with holistic care that meets their physical, psychological, social, and cultural needs.

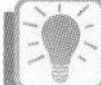 QSEN Considerations: Patient-Centered Care

Support for the Dying Patient

Providing support to the family, friends, and significant others is an integral part of end-of-life care that requires compassionate, excellent communication skills, and the ability to reflect carefully on your own feelings and beliefs about death and dying. Learn when and how to transition from the aggressive curative treatment to end-of-life care with palliative interventions designed to help the dying person and their loved ones through the experience of death.

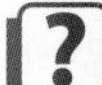 Think Critically

What are your earliest memories of death—a pet, a relative, a friend? How was the death explained to you? Was it frightening, confusing, reassuring? What is the most prominent memory of the event?

CHANGE, LOSS, AND GRIEF

CHANGE

Visionary family therapist Virginia Satir described loss, grief, and mourning as experiences intrinsically linked with life changes (Belvins, 2008). These are normal and often inevitable transitions over the life span. Satir further noted that, when people experience these changes, they progress through six stages: status quo, introduction of a foreign element, chaos, integration, practice, and new status quo. These are similar to the stages that Kübler-Ross, Maciejewski, and others have described as stages of grief and loss. Be aware of the processes used by patients to process change in order to support patients going through these transitions.

LOSS

Loss is to no longer possess or have an object, person, or capacity. It is a common occurrence in everyday life, for example, losing money, a job, one's health, or life. Death is often described as the most difficult loss for a person to accept. A loss can be physical, such as the amputation of a leg or the inability to speak or walk after a stroke. A loss can also be psychosocial. Disfiguring surgery or scarring from burns may result in an altered self-image and emotional problems. A person may lose the ability to carry out the role of homemaker or wage earner because of illness. A familiar environment and independence may be lost with a move to a nursing home. Often loss consists of both physical and psychosocial aspects.

Loss can be viewed as ranging from minor to catastrophic. A person's reaction to loss does not necessarily depend on the size of the loss; it is much more influenced by the person's perceived value of the loss. The experience of loss is deeply personal, and the value attached to it is a result of a complex interplay of emotional responses, personal experiences, and sociocultural influences. For example, the loss of a pregnancy may have a different meaning to a woman who has struggled with fertility issues for a long time than it would to a woman with many children who lost an unplanned pregnancy. **Only the person experiencing the loss can define the value of the loss;** set aside your own values, fully accept the patient's experience of loss, and provide adequate support.

GRIEF

Grief is an emotional reaction to loss. The time required for the **grieving process** varies from one individual to another. Dying persons and their loved ones experience loss and grief when faced with a terminal diagnosis. **Bereavement** is the state of having suffered a loss by death. A person who is grieving may experience physical and emotional symptoms, such as crying, fatigue, changes in appetite, sleep disturbances, loneliness, and sadness (Box 15.1). When a person thinks or knows that a loss is going to occur in the future, **anticipatory grieving** may occur. This happens when patients and their families face a serious or life-threatening illness, and it is believed to improve their ability to cope with the loss when it occurs.

Grieving may also be **dysfunctional** when it falls outside normal responses. In prolonged grieving, the person seems trapped in a stage and unable to progress. However, there is no actual time frame for completion of grieving, and a major loss may result in grieving for 1 to 2 years. Visible absence of grieving may be viewed by others as a good adjustment, but it often results in later psychosomatic illness.

STAGES OF GRIEF

Although every individual grieves in their own way, research has demonstrated that there are common themes. The grief process progresses through several distinct stages, each characterized by a set of identifying behavioral and emotional responses. Every individual moves through the stages at his own pace, and may skip a stage or return to an earlier stage. Nurses have always been taught to recognize the great individuality of the grieving person and offer supportive care for the symptoms or behavior the person demonstrates, rather than anticipating what grieving response is the right one.

Until recently, the hypothesis of these stages had not been investigated empirically. However, the stages of grief theory were put to the test by Maciejewski et al. (2007). Their examination of the stage theory of grief has revealed that denial is not the first grief indicator. Instead, the loss is readily accepted, and yearning is the dominant grief indicator. This is followed by anger and depression. The five grief indicators—denial, yearning, anger, depression, and acceptance—peak within 6 months after the loss. Reevaluate and create additional nursing plans for patients who continue to score high in these areas after 6 months.

You can assist people who are grieving by accepting their feelings and behaviors and validating their loss. To **validate** the loss is to reassure the grieving person that the loss was important and understood. Providing a quiet presence and having a warm, caring concern for the person's well-being and the ability to listen to the person speak about the pain and loss are supportive behaviors (Fig. 15.1). Recognize any cultural or religious rites and encourage grieving individuals to tell you what the person (or lost object) was like and what the loss means to him or her. Avoid clichés such as, "You'll forget all about this after a while," and never minimize the loss. Observe the patient's nonverbal communication, and use appropriate nonverbal language such as a smile or a gentle touch. Crying may be embarrassing for the patient. A simple act of handing the patient a tissue acknowledges the acceptability of weeping. You may be uncomfortable in a situation in which you feel like crying along with the patient. The patient will not be offended by your crying and may draw support from a shared experience. You

Box 15.1 Symptoms of Grief

- Depression, sadness, crying, and mood swings
- Fatigue, apathy, lack of interest and motivation, inability to concentrate, and inability to complete tasks
- Loneliness and isolation
- Sleep alterations: sleeping more or insomnia (inability to sleep)
- Loss of appetite, weight loss or weight gain, and nausea
- Change in sexual interest
- Anxiety, shortness of breath, chest pains, rapid heartbeat, sighing, and heaviness in the chest
- Feelings of helplessness, restlessness, anger, guilt, and irritability
- Forgetfulness, tendency to make mistakes, and accident proneness
- Confusion, disorientation (especially in older adults), and indecisiveness
- Symptoms of the same illness that the deceased suffered
- Sensing the loved one's presence, hearing the voice, seeing the face, and expecting the person to walk in the door
- A need to tell and retell and remember things about the loved one and the death experience

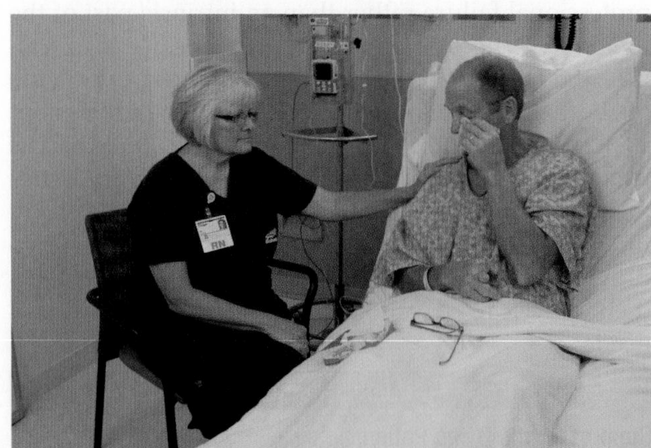

FIGURE 15.1 The nurse provides caring and comfort to the patient who experiences grief.

can acknowledge feelings of sadness and loss, but do not invalidate or minimize patients' feelings by making statements such as "I know just how you feel" or "Don't cry."

As a person moves through and adjusts to the stages of the grieving process, there is a continuing change in function. With the stage of acceptance, the level of daily function improves and stabilizes. Successful movement through the grieving stages allows the grieving person to emerge with realistic memories of the event and object of grief, rediscover the meaning of life, and begin experiencing pleasure, social relationships, and activities. The time it takes to move through the stages depends on the loss and its meaning to the person.

DEATH AND DYING

Death as a physiologic event is typically defined by the absence of spontaneous breathing and heartbeat. Life support technologies have significantly altered the process of dying, and it is now possible to support basic life functions externally using pharmaceutical and mechanical support (Perrin & MacLeod, 2013). Therefore, the definition of *death* is now centered on the concept of **brain death**, which is defined as the absence of brain activity as evidenced by the absence of electroencephalogram (ECG) waves. Brain death is characterized by three cardinal findings: coma, absence of brain stem reflexes, and apnea. A patient experiencing brain death whose physiologic functioning is supported by external means is a potential donor for organ transplantation. The time to process organ collection for transplantation is precious. Know the procedures and policies in your practice areas and act in a timely manner.

Death may be sudden, unexpected, and instant, as when a person is killed in an accident or dies of a sudden, unexpected health problem such as massive heart attack. It may also be the ultimate outcome of declining health over a period of time as in the case of chronic disease. Finally, death may be a result of overall loss of functional and physiologic capacities associated with normal aging. Nurses who work in an emergency department, intensive care unit, medical-surgical unit, nursing home, or hospice will each have different experiences of patients' death and dying. In these different cases and situations, the individuals who die and those who care about them will experience different emotions and physical reactions.

Cultural Considerations

Cultural Views About Disclosure

Many people think they have the right to know if they are dying, and nurses often do not like it if that fact is being hidden from a patient. However, always consider cultural factors that might influence the way disclosure is handled. For example, Mexican Americans and Korean Americans are less likely to want to be told if they have a terminal illness. They also believe that the family, not the patient, should make decisions about life-sustaining treatments. These beliefs need to be considered before speaking to a patient about a terminal prognosis.

Each death and dying experience is unique, although some commonalities can help you provide truly satisfying care to the patient and the family (Box 15.2).

END-OF-LIFE CARE WITHIN THE HEALTH CARE SYSTEM

The focus in our health care system has been one of cure and the development of diagnostic, technical, and chemical interventions to treat disease and injury that often have been fatal in the past. As a result, patients may be viewed as failures of the system if they die in spite of the health care team's best efforts. Those with terminal illness who refuse life-prolonging (or death-delaying) treatment may believe their needs will not be met in the acute care environment (Box 15.3).

HOSPICE AND PALLIATIVE CARE

According to the World Health Organization (WHO), the goal of **palliative** care is to reduce or relieve the symptoms of a disease without attempting to provide a cure (WHO, 2015a). It does not hasten or postpone death. Instead, it preserves life while accepting death

Box 15.2 Standards of Care for the Terminally Ill

1. Actively involve dying patients and their loved ones in the discussion of the end-of-life care within the acceptable cultural parameters.
2. Consider the terminally ill patient's preferences, personality, and lifestyle when planning care. Rigid rules, routines, and agency regulations should not be automatically applied.
3. Focus on the maintenance of functional capacity and alleviation of suffering through the control of symptoms, regardless of the expected length of time until death.
4. Maintain pain control as a major goal of treatment.
5. Allow the patient's preferences and intentions regarding health care as set out in an advance directive, or by durable power of attorney for health care, to take precedence as far as the law will allow.
6. Ensure that the patient feels safe and secure with the care that is provided and with the level of communication regarding this care.
7. Provide dying patients with opportunities to spend final moments in a personally meaningful way with people who are important to them.
8. Encourage family members and significant others to discuss the patient's imminent death and their emotional needs with nurses.
9. Provide family members and significant others with private time with the patient before and after death as desired.
10. Allow family members to perform rituals and carry out cultural customs regarding the body after death.

Box 15.3 Rights of the Dying Patient

The person who is dying has the right to:

- Be treated as a person until death
- Caring human contact
- Have pain controlled
- Cleanliness and comfort
- Maintain a sense of hope, whatever its focus
- Participate in his care or the planning of it
- Respectful, caring medical and nursing attention
- Continuity of care and caregivers
- Information about his condition and impending death
- Honest answers to questions
- Explore and change religious beliefs
- Maintain individuality and express emotions freely without being judged
- Make amends with others and settle personal business
- Say goodbye to family members and significant others in private or with the assistance of the nurse
- Assistance for significant others with the grief process
- Withdraw from social contact if desired
- Die at home in familiar surroundings
- Die with dignity
- Respectful treatment of the body after death

as a normal and expected outcome. Palliative care interventions are designed to optimize patients' ability to live as active and complete a life as possible until death. Competent adults suffering from incurable, life-threatening conditions may decide they no longer desire aggressive treatment such as chemotherapy, assisted ventilation, or dialysis. Instead of life-sustaining measures, the patients may choose treatment options that maximize the quality of life and improve symptom management. This does not imply that the patient will not receive any treatment. They will continue to receive treatments that support the goal of optimizing their quality of life, including complex medical and surgical interventions. The key difference is that the goal of the interventions is not to provide cure or to recover the lost function but to preserve the quality of life and alleviate suffering. Palliative care is now considered a specialty practice area in nursing, and the need for it is increasing (Mayer & Winters, 2016). Palliative care nurses are trained to provide care focused on symptom management, psychological and spiritual support, and specialized education for the patients and their families. The Hospice and Palliative Nurses Association (HPNA) offers education and specialty certification to licensed practical nurse/licensed vocational nurses (LPN/LVNs) interested in specializing in palliative care (HPNA, 2015). **Be aware that the concept of palliative care is not exclusive to the end-of-life care; it is used in a variety of practice areas when the focus of care needs to switch from the curative focus to the focus on quality of life.**

Hospice is both a distinct nursing practice area and a philosophy of care for the dying and their families. Care for the dying has been around as long as humans have. The modern concept of hospice care was developed in England in the early 1960s, as a reaction to the dying person's need for care and comfort (National Hospice and Palliative Care Organization [NHPCO], 2015). A hospice originally was a medieval guest house or stopping place for travelers. Hospice care was originally confined to institutional settings. However, the name *hospice* is also now used to describe the specialized care provided to the dying in small clinics, houses, long-term care facilities, or the patient's (or patient's family's) own home (Lakasing, Kulkarni, Sparkes, & RaviChander, 2014).

The intent of hospice care is to help patients in the end stage of life, and their families, to experience the process of death with the highest quality of life and least amount of disruption as possible. To receive the greatest support and most compassionate care possible, discussion of hospice should take place as soon as the patient or the patient's care team realizes that there is no cure for the patient's condition and the patient is in a dying process. Educate the patients and their families about hospice and palliative care, and advocate for your patients by initiating appropriate referrals as soon as possible.

The hospice philosophy is based on the acceptance of death as a natural part of life, and it emphasizes the quality of remaining life. Patients with incurable illnesses are faced with daily suffering. They not only suffer from the physical aspects of the disease, such as pain, but also from psychological, spiritual, and emotional discomfort as well. The needs of the patients and their significant others are met through a multidisciplinary team approach where the team provides palliative care (Nursing Care Plan 15.1). Nurses who care for dying patients have a unique opportunity to become an intimate part of their lives. Nurses can support dying patients physically and emotionally while maintaining a professional role.

Whether the nurse is assisting the patient in the hospital or at home, the primary goal of hospice and palliative care is to improve quality of life, alleviate suffering, and improve the end-of-life experience for the patients and their loved ones. To achieve satisfactory outcomes, certain comfort measures are required. Palliative care requires a specialized body of knowledge and skills that can be difficult to learn because it is not focused on a "cure." Family members are involved in this planning, and necessary support is provided to meet the needs of all those affected by the impending death (Fig. 15.2). Registered nurses (RNs) and LPNs or home health aides provide nursing and personal care; trained volunteers are used to provide a variety of respite (relief) or socialization services. Hospice care may be provided in the patient's home, nursing home, hospital, or hospice unit. Following up with the family during the year after the death provides assistance with the grieving process.

Nursing Care Plan 15.1 Care of the Dying Patient

SCENARIO Mrs. Rodney is in the palliative care unit, actively dying from breast cancer with metastases. She is receiving pain medication, complains of thirst, and is expressing considerable pain.

PROBLEM/NURSING DIAGNOSIS *Pain is not adequately controlled*/Pain related to breast cancer process and metastases.

Supporting Assessment Data *Subjective:* Pain at a level of 8/10. *Objective:* Grimacing with movement, holding body rigid; advanced breast cancer with metastases.

Goals/Expected Outcomes	Nursing Interventions	Selected Rationales	Evaluation
Patient and family will verify that patient has adequate pain control. Patient will verbalize relief or control of pain.	Assess characteristics of pain: location, severity on a scale of 0 to 10, frequency, precipitating factors, and factors that relieve the pain.	Pain management is most successful when the underlying cause of pain is identified and treated.	Is pain controlled adequately? Patient reports adequate control of pain and does not have increased BP, P, or R; diaphoresis, dilated pupils, guarding, facial mask of pain, crying or moaning, abdominal heaviness, or cutaneous irritation.
	Eliminate factors that precipitate pain (e.g., excessive noise, wrinkled bed sheets, joint discomfort from positioning, thirst, wet bed and gown, cluttered environment, and interrupted rest).	Pain may be aggravated by many factors.	
	Offer analgesics on a set, around-the-clock schedule per physician orders.	Scheduled dosing controls pain better than PRN dosing does.	Gave additional analgesia at 3:30 pm for escalating pain.
	Teach patient to request more analgesia before breakthrough pain becomes severe.	It is easier to prevent severe pain than to curtail it once the cycle begins.	
	Explore nonpharmacologic methods for reducing pain and promoting comfort: • Back rubs • Foot rubs • Slow, rhythmic deep breathing • Imagery exercises • Relaxation exercises • Repositioning • Diversional activities such as music, TV, and games • Restful intervals between care or treatments	Combination of analgesia and nonpharmacologic measures yields the best pain control.	Using imagery and breathing techniques. Refused back rub. Repositioned every hour. Watching TV. Body posture is more relaxed. Continue plan.

CRITICAL THINKING QUESTIONS

1. What are some ways to help Mrs. Rodney with her pain? Should she be given additional pain medication (opioids)?
2. Some of the family members are afraid that additional opioids will hasten Mrs. Rodney's death. What can you say to the family members?

BP, Blood pressure; *P,* pulse; *PRN,* as needed; *R,* respirations.

THE DYING PROCESS

Theories of Death and Dying and Emergence of Thanatology

Although dying is a personal experience that varies from one individual or group to another, the dying process has some universal themes. Multiple theories have identified commonly seen patterns and emotions experienced by the dying persons and their loved ones: fear of dying, yearning, guilt, hope, despair, and even humor. Some theorists believe that the grieving process associated with dying goes through distinct stages. Others point out that an individual's reaction to the threat of death is consistent with the way the person coped with difficulties in the past, and that the evolution of grief is fluid rather than a linear process. Coping with death takes many forms, affecting the dying person, as well as others connected to them, including family, friends, and caregivers. Coping with

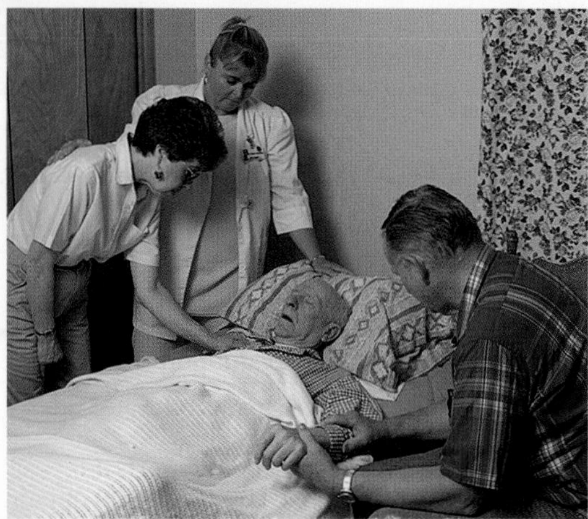

FIGURE 15.2 The hospice nurse assists the family in saying goodbye to the dying patient.

Table 15.1 Kübler-Ross Stages of Coping With Death

STAGE	DESCRIPTION
Denial	"No, not me." The person cannot believe the diagnosis or prognosis. Denial serves as a buffer to protect the patient from an uncomfortable and painful situation. A patient may seek other opinions or believe there has been an error.
Anger	"Why me?" The person looks for a cause or fixes blame. Displaced anger may target physicians, nurses, family, and even God. Powerlessness to control the disease and events is an underlying issue.
Bargaining	"If I'm good, then I get a reward." The wish is for extension of life, or later for relief from pain, and the person knows from experience that "good behavior" is often rewarded.
Depression	"It's hopeless." There is a sense of great loss, of the impending loss of being. People mourn losing family, possessions, responsibilities, and all they value.
Acceptance	"I'm ready." The pain is gone, the struggle is over, and the patient has found peace. There is withdrawal from engagement in everyday activities and interests. Verbal communication is less important, and touch and presence are most important.

death may also involve tasks or actions that the dying person must work on in the physical, social, psychological, and spiritual arenas. An example of a physical task would be to minimize physical distress such as pain. A social task might be to enhance or restore a relationship that is important to the dying person. Other examples would be updating a will, making amends, and saying goodbye to friends and loved ones.

One of the most influential theorists when it comes to exploration of death and dying was Elisabeth Kübler-Ross. In the late 1960s, she began talking with terminally ill patients and identifying their needs. She also began educating medical students, nurses, and physicians about death and the stages through which she saw terminally ill patients progress. She transformed the way the health care community and much of the public view death, and she promoted research into the areas of loss and death. Because of her pioneering work, nurses and physicians are much more sensitive to the needs of the dying patient and family. Other researchers have added to her work, and the field of **thanatology** (the study of death) continues to grow.

Kübler-Ross's identification of the stages a dying person moves through has been the foundation for understanding the dying process. Five stages, similar to those of the grief process, are described as being characteristic of dying: denial, anger, bargaining, depression, and acceptance (Kübler-Ross, 1969) (Table 15.1). The stages overlap, and as with the grieving process, the patient may move back and forth or even skip stages. In some cases the patient may "get stuck" in one stage and not move through to acceptance. Family members and patients are often at different stages. Nurses, too, move through the stages when they care for patients who are dying.

Cultural Considerations

Cultural Views About Death

Certain cultures believe that talking about death can bring it on. This belief is found in some people from Greece, China, Italy, Korea, Mexico, and the southern African nations. The nurse must consider the patient's cultural orientation before broaching the subject of death or terminal illness.

QSEN Considerations: Patient-Centered Care

Hope and the Dying Process

Hope is an inner positive life force, a feeling that what is desired is possible. It takes many forms and changes as the patient declines. At first, there is hope for a cure, then hope that treatment will be possible, next hope for prolonging life, and finally hope for a peaceful death. Open-ended questions such as, "What are you hoping for from this admission?" or "What are you hoping for today?" can allow patients to talk about their needs. You can always be supportive of hope by recognizing and affirming the wish the patient is expressing.

NURSING AND THE DYING PROCESS

Patients express many fears when they know they are dying, which may include fear of pain, loneliness, abandonment, the unknown, loss of dignity, and loss of control. There may also be unfinished business that occupies the patient's thoughts. The concept of **comfort care** focuses on identifying symptoms that cause the patient distress and adequately treating those symptoms. Prevention of many symptoms is possible by anticipating their likelihood. Use the nursing process to identify the existing and anticipated needs of dying patients and manage their care in accordance with their unique needs.

Therapeutic communication is a crucial skill for providing high quality end-of-life nursing care (Williams, 2016). Nursing students and novice nurses are often fearful of not knowing what to say or of saying the wrong thing. To master this skill, begin by becoming comfortable with your own beliefs, values, and attitudes about death and dying. Next, read and learn about the actual dying process and observe experienced nurses talking with dying patients and grieving relatives. Be open to the difficult questions of life and death that permit patients to discuss their feelings and needs. Patients are usually sensitive as to how caregivers (and family members) react to uncomfortable subjects. Often, a patient will not bring up a subject that can be anxiety-provoking or painful to think about with family or staff members. Time and experience are the best teachers. Chapter 8 discusses specific therapeutic communication skills in detail.

A trusting relationship with the patient can develop when you are able to meet the identified needs. Listening skills, observation, and use of nonverbal communication, touch, and presence all contribute to the patient's sense of acceptance. Fears of isolation or loneliness decrease with nursing care that seeks to treat the patient with compassion and individuality. The family's anxiety decreases as they see the patient responding to the care and attention of the team.

Think Critically

What questions that a dying person might ask would be most difficult for you to respond to? Think about what you might say in response to such questions.

❖ APPLICATION OF THE NURSING PROCESS

◆ ASSESSMENT (DATA COLLECTION)

A baseline assessment and continuing data collection are essential to identify the problems and needs of the patient and his family. An admission history should determine what they have been told by the primary care provider regarding the illness and its expected course. Asking clear, open-ended questions such as, "What has your doctor told you about your condition?" or "What have you learned so far about your disease?" may help identify knowledge the patient needs to make informed decisions. Questions about advance directives regarding treatment options, resuscitation, advanced life support, and organ donation can provide information about the patient's attitude toward death and the stage of his grief or dying reaction (e.g., denial or anger). Asking questions about religious beliefs and practices, as well as asking directly "What do you hope for during this admission?" and "What are your concerns?" elicits data for the provision of comprehensive comfort care. **At no time should the patient be pushed to discuss something he is obviously avoiding.** A question such as, "Is there anything else you would like to talk about?" opens the door for issues the patient may wish to discuss.

Use Analgesia Cautiously

Does your patient have renal or hepatic dysfunction? Administration of opioid pain medication may need to be altered to avoid respiratory depression, hypotension, or central nervous system (CNS) toxicity. Consider the dosage recommendations given when a patient with renal dysfunction is prescribed an opiate.

An assessment of the patient's **physical** condition includes such measures as weight (with attention to usual weight), mobility, and the ability to perform activities of daily living, weakness or energy level, appetite (nausea, indigestion, or gas), bowel and bladder function, and respiratory function. Perform a detailed assessment of pain, including location, nature, and what relieves it or makes it worse. Assess pain using a numeric scale or similar method of measuring the patient's report of pain. The frequency of pain assessment depends on many factors, such as the severity of pain and whether pain is increasing or well controlled on the current treatment regimen (see Chapter 31).

The patient's **emotional** condition can often be observed during the interaction, and symptoms such as anxiety, agitation, confusion, or depression may be obvious. Validating your observation with the patient allows them to speak about his feelings. Stating, "Tell me how you are coping with all this" begins to reveal strengths and needs. Begin **spiritual** assessment with questions that allow the patients to self-identify their spiritual beliefs and possible religious affiliations. If they identify a specific affiliation, ask if they would like to talk to a cleric or spiritual advisor from the identified religious or spiritual community. Even when a patient indicates "none" for religious affiliation, they may have spiritual needs. Be aware of clues and statements that may be indicative of spiritual distress such as "Why is God punishing me?" or questioning what the meaning in his life has been.

◆ NURSING DIAGNOSIS

Nursing diagnoses for the dying patient vary, depending on the disease process. For example, a patient dying of end-stage renal disease will have problems with fluid excess, whereas a patient dying of chronic obstructive pulmonary disease (COPD) will have problems with ineffective airway clearance.

◆ PLANNING

Both the patients and their loved ones must be included in the planning of care and in establishing goals or outcomes. Planning should be a team effort, with all team members aware of the patient's goals and needs.

QSEN Consideration: Patient-Centered Care

Care Planning

The care planning process for end of life should be driven and controlled by the patient whenever possible.

Agency rules and routines that are geared toward a cure should be relaxed to recognize that the goal of treatment is comfort. These would include relaxing restrictive visiting hours; eliminating routine vital signs and laboratory work; and flexible scheduling of the activities of daily living.

◆ IMPLEMENTATION

Promote self-care as long as the patient is able. The patient's loved ones can derive much satisfaction in learning to provide physical care when the patient is no longer able to be independent. Be sensitive to patient or family member reluctance to provide (or receive) what is uncomfortable for either one, such as performing perineal care for a parent.

Common Problems of the Dying Patient and Nursing Management

Anticipatory guidance. Anticipating death assists in preparing the family and patient by giving them guidance about physical changes, symptoms, and complications that may arise. This may also aid the patient and family in deciding about possible hospice care.

End-stage symptom management. Many expected symptoms, such as pain, gastrointestinal distress, dyspnea, fatigue, cough, "death rattle," and delirium, are related to metabolic changes at the end of life. The last few days of patient life have been studied extensively. Recognize the symptoms and be able to either alleviate them or help explain them to the patient and family.

Pain control. Although nursing research has demonstrated safe and effective principles of pain control, many terminally ill patients unnecessarily die without adequate pain control. Several myths still contribute to inadequate pain relief. There is great misunderstanding about the role and possible side effects of opioid analgesia. Research suggests that nurses may still be uncomfortable with aggressive pain management because they are afraid that increasing opioid dosage may hasten death (Coyle, 2014). Patients and their loved ones may have concerns about addiction and dependency. **A truly compassionate nurse studies and learns about pain management and applies those principles in daily practice.**

Health Promotion/Health Promotion Points

The WHO Three-Step Ladder for Pain Relief

The WHO (2015b) has developed a three-step ladder to follow for adequate pain relief. According to this ladder:

1. Start with nonopioid drugs + 1 adjuvant therapy.
2. If pain persists or increases, add an opioid designated for mild to moderate pain.
3. If pain persists or increases, change to an opioid designated for moderate to severe pain.

The pain ladder is additive to the first step. In other words, when changing from one step to the next, always continue the previous step(s) as well.

Pain can be controlled (eliminated) in almost all cases when the medical and nursing teams work together (see Nursing Care Plan 15.1). The best way to manage pain is by a regularly scheduled pain medication regimen, augmented with PRN (as needed) medications when regularly scheduled pain medications are inadequate to achieve pain control (Wagner & Hardin-Pierce, 2014). Carefully assess pain location, intensity, and response to medication every 2 to 4 hours, or more often if needed, to determine the necessity for increases in dosage. **There is no risk of becoming addicted or of reaching a safety or effectiveness limit when narcotics are increased in response to pain for the dying patient.** Patients with severe pain can receive huge doses of narcotics without respiratory depression or tolerance when the dose has been increased in response to increasing pain. Because comfort is the goal of palliative care, administering only oral medications, when feasible, is the preferred choice. However, this may not be possible as death draws near, and it is the goal to allow a pain-free death. In some cases, it may be possible to administer transdermal or rectal pain medications. The oral route and long-acting transdermal patches can also avoid the necessity of injections. Even when the patient is no longer taking fluids by mouth, small amounts of concentrated pain medication can be inserted in the buccal cavity (cheek) (Table 15.2). Transdermal fentanyl (patch) has helped eliminate the burden of pain at the end of life. You may have read that this method of pain relief carries high risk, but remember that patients in severe pain may receive higher doses of pain medication safely. Sometimes this regimen is supplemented with rescue doses of morphine if pain is not controlled.

Nonchemical approaches to pain relief include visualization and guided imagery, relaxation and breathing exercises, massage, music therapy, meditation, religious healing, biofeedback, hypnosis or self-hypnosis, transcutaneous electrical nerve stimulation (TENS), and hydrotherapy (e.g., whirlpool). Teach the patient one or more of these simple techniques as adjuncts to drug therapy. Provide a quiet environment and assist the patient as necessary (see Chapter 31). Some patients do not respond to the standard medicines or

Table 15.2 Opioid Use in Patients With Renal Impairment

DRUG	RECOMMENDATION
Morphine	Use cautiously with dose adjustment and careful monitoring
Hydrocodone	Use cautiously with dose adjustment and careful monitoring
Oxycodone	Use cautiously with dose adjustment and careful monitoring
Codeine	DO NOT USE
Methadone	Safe
Fentanyl	Appears safe; reduce dose
Meperidine	DO NOT USE
Propoxyphene	DO NOT USE

adjunct therapy. In these cases, radiation treatment, nerve blocks, implanted pumps, or surgery may be required.

Dyspnea and respiratory distress. Difficult breathing may be seen early in the dying process in certain lung or heart disorders. It is also seen shortly before death, when respirations may become noisy, irregular, or labored. Respiratory distress at the end of life is considered extreme suffering, and it requires an aggressive treatment (Perrin & MacLeod, 2013). Secretions in the lungs accumulate and block the airways to contribute to noisy or rattling respirations known as "death rattle." The patient is usually not responsive, or not aware of the dyspnea, but it is upsetting to family members. Suctioning is not effective in clearing the secretions, but medications such as a scopolamine patch or morphine can decrease secretions and ease breathing. Administering oxygen by nasal prongs may provide comfort.

Constipation and diarrhea. Constipation is predictable for a patient receiving opiates, experiencing decreased fluid intake and mobility, and having certain abdominal diseases. In addition to classic nursing measures for preventing constipation (see Chapter 30), consult with the primary care provider for orders for stool softeners and a standing laxative order. Suppositories and enemas, or manual disimpaction, can be avoided in most cases with careful monitoring and adherence to a laxative schedule.

Anorexia, nausea, and vomiting. **Anorexia,** or loss of appetite, may be due to nausea, drug side effects (especially a sore mouth), the disease process, or the slowdown that occurs naturally in the dying process. Antiemetic medications are the first choice to eliminate nausea and vomiting. Small servings, home-prepared food favorites, and attention to eliminating unpleasant sights and odors at mealtime may stimulate a poor appetite. A bad taste can be improved by frequent oral care, mouthwashes, or hard candies (sour balls). A nutritionist may be helpful in suggesting food choices that are appealing and easily digested. You can do a great deal to support the patient and the family with an explanation of the dying process: that decreased intake is more comfortable for the patient than having food to digest and move through a system that is slowing down. There is also some evidence to suggest that starvation decreases the patient's awareness of pain by producing chemicals that act as pain relievers. Weight loss is commonly seen in dying patients, but few patients complain of feeling hungry. **Dysphagia** (difficulty swallowing) may also be a problem. Moistening the mouth with fluids or artificial saliva may be helpful. Additional care of the dysphasic patient is presented in Chapter 27.

Dehydration. As death nears, patients spend more time sleeping or in a semiresponsive state. They take in fewer and fewer fluids until the question arises about providing intravenous (IV) fluids or tube feedings out of concern for dehydration. Research has shown that dehydration results in less distress and pain and that hydration does not improve comfort. Dry mouth and thirst are the most common complaints, which may be induced by the drugs being administered, and these can be alleviated by small sips of fluids, ice chips, lip lubrication, and moisturizing swabs when the patient is unconscious or unable to sip fluids. Resulting decreased urine output means less effort to use a commode or less incontinence. This issue is best discussed before it arises, at the time advance directives are being established. It is an emotional issue, and families often have a difficult time accepting that withholding fluids is more comforting than administering them. Comfort them with an explanation of how the dying person is indeed made more comfortable by withholding fluids. Educate the patient's loved ones about the benefits and burdens of hydration. Many times the course is for patients to choose what to take or to refuse further nourishment. This is referred to as "patient-endorsed intake."

Delirium. Dying patients may experience hallucinations or altered mental status. Search and address possible causes of delirium such as pain, positional discomfort, or bladder distention and address those physical problems. Discuss the delirium with the patient's loved ones and encourage the family to talk to the patient in quiet tones while remaining calm.

Impaired skin integrity. Weight loss, decreased nutrition, incontinence, and inactivity all contribute to the risk of skin breakdown. Turn and position the patient; use protective measures such as an air pressure mattress, heel or elbow protectors, and sheepskin or foam pads; and keep the skin clean and dry. An indwelling or condom catheter may be indicated to conserve the patient's dwindling energy and to prevent skin breakdown.

Weakness, fatigue, and decreased ability to perform activities of daily living. Increasing weakness eventually results in the patient's becoming bed-bound. Accept the patient's wishes regarding walking, sitting up in a chair, or remaining in bed. **The dying patient is not going to get stronger or better; they get weaker and weaker, not because they are lying in bed, but because they are dying.** Allow patients to do as much as possible for themselves, and provide physical care when they are no longer able.

Anxiety, depression, and agitation. Emotional or psychological symptoms may be treated with appropriate drugs with good effect. Listen and use good therapeutic communication skills to allow the patient to express his fears, feelings, and needs and convey nonjudgmental acceptance (see Chapter 8). Skillful assessment of these symptoms may identify physical pain or spiritual distress that can be treated.

Spiritual distress and fear of meaninglessness. Each person needs to believe that his life has had meaning; this is the spiritual nature of the dying process. A life review allows the patient to put his life in perspective. Reminiscing is one way of starting a life review. Encourage the patient to tell about family photographs or albums. Ask, "What was it like when you were a child [or worked on the farm, lived in the city, or met your wife]?" **It is more important to listen than to talk.**

◆ EVALUATION

Evaluation is based on the identified, patient specific outcomes. The desired outcomes depend on which nursing diagnoses are pertinent to the patient's situation. In most cases, the degree of comfort obtained for the patient by the nursing interventions needs to be evaluated. Was pain adequately controlled? Was tissue integrity protected? Were actions to facilitate the patient's and family's grieving process effective? Was the patient's fear alleviated? Did interventions for a self-care deficit make the patient more comfortable? Answers to these questions help determine whether expected outcomes have been met. If the care plan is not effective, the plan must be revised.

SIGNS OF IMPENDING DEATH

PHYSICAL SIGNS

As death approaches, the patient grows physically weaker and begins to spend more time sleeping. Body functions slow. Appetite decreases, and the patient may refuse even favorite foods and later fluids as well. Explain to the patient and the family what to expect. Moistening the patient's lips and mouth and providing oral hygiene will be more comforting than "pushing" food or fluids.

Urine output decreases, and urine becomes more concentrated. There may be edema of the extremities or over the sacrum. Incontinence may occur as patients become less aware of their surroundings. However, be alert to the possibility of urinary retention and the need for catheterization.

Vital signs change as death approaches. The pulse increases and becomes weaker or thready. Blood pressure declines, and the skin of the extremities becomes mottled, cool, and dusky. Respirations become shallow and irregular. Secretions may pool in the lungs, causing respirations to sound moist. Often at the time of death, a "death rattle" of those secretions occurs. **Cheyne-Stokes respirations**—respirations that gradually become shallower and are followed by periods of **apnea** (no breathing)—may be noted. Body temperature may rise, and the patient (if responsive) may complain of feeling hot or cold, although the extremities are cool to the touch as circulation slows. Blankets should be used as the patient desires.

PSYCHOSOCIAL AND SPIRITUAL ASPECTS OF DYING

As outlined in the Kübler-Ross stages of coping with dying, it is hoped that the patient will have reached the stage of acceptance as death draws closer. During this time, the patient will talk about making funeral arrangements and "putting my affairs in order." To die with **closure** is to say goodbye to those people and things that are important. It may also involve saying, "I'm sorry, forgive me," "I forgive you," and "I love you." It is a time when the patient may give to family and friends special memories or possessions. A life review can assist patients in telling their story and putting their life in perspective. Helping the patient write or share his life story with significant others allows them to keep special memories of their loved one.

 QSEN Consideration: Patient-Centered Care

Communication at the End of Life

Make sure that the communication is focused on the patient rather than the caregiver, and be mindful of cultural consideration. Allow the dying person and their loved ones to discuss the things that concern them the most, not the topics of concern to the caregivers.

As individuals approach death, their spiritual needs take on greater importance. As patients ponder the meaning of their life, their beliefs about what happens to them in death take on new meaning. Religious practices and rituals have great significance for some patients. It is important for you to be familiar with those beliefs (see Chapter 14). **Rather than impose your own religious beliefs on dying patients and family, you should assist patients in finding comfort and support in their own belief systems.** An assessment of the patient's spiritual needs is outlined in Chapter 14, and when indicated, you may collaborate with the patient's religious representative or hospital chaplain to provide spiritual care.

As life ebbs, the patient speaks less and is more withdrawn. Everyday activities and news are not of interest, and nonverbal communication becomes most important. Sitting with patients and using touch, such as holding their hand or stroking their hair, are most meaningful. Even when patients appear to be sleeping or nonresponsive, physical touch and presence are comforting. **Always be aware of remarks you make in the presence of an unresponsive patient because they DO hear. Hearing is believed to be one of the last senses to be lost before death, and "dying" patients have awakened to report conversations by family and health care workers that they were not meant to overhear.**

Dying patients may exhibit confusion and disorientation. They may report dreams or visions of deceased relatives, and they usually are not frightened by these experiences. Often this is comforting, and they may speak of preparing for a journey to join loved ones. At times patients may become restless and agitated. Adequate pain and anxiety medication can ease the distress of these symptoms. Keep soft lights on in the room. Assurance that it is "OK to go" and that family members will take care of each other may ease dying individuals' anxiety about leaving their responsibilities.

As death approaches, one or more family members or significant others may want to remain with the dying person. Most clinical agencies support this and provide special provisions for the families of dying patients. Be available to the family and explain what to expect as death approaches, as well as how to communicate with the patient and what to do to help make the end of life as peaceful as possible.

? Think Critically

What would you wish to include in your **obituary** (a notice of the death published in newspapers)? Write your own obituary, imagining at what age you would die, and what will have happened in your life (education, jobs, family) between now and the time of your death. What funeral arrangements will you make?

LEGAL AND ETHICAL ASPECTS OF LIFE-AND-DEATH ISSUES

Patients have rights to make decisions about their health. These rights apply to end-of-life situations, advance directives, and the designation of a health care proxy.

ADVANCE DIRECTIVES

An **advance directive** or **living will** is a legal document that outlines the patient's wishes for health care preferences at that time when they may be unable to communicate their choice. A **durable power of attorney for health care** is a legal document that appoints a person **(health care proxy)** chosen by the patient to make health care decisions if the patient becomes incompetent or incapable of communication. Discussing advance directives with patients opens the communication path to establish what is important to them and what they view as promoting life versus prolonging dying. Patients determine under which situations they would agree to **do-not-resuscitate (DNR)** or **do-not-intubate (DNI)** orders. Their choices regarding artificial feeding and fluids, ventilators, and administration of antibiotics are documented.

Life-Span Considerations

Older Adults

- When competent older adults have not completed an advance directive before admission, even though it may be difficult to communicate with them, they should be included in discussions and decisions about end-of-life care.
- Confusion about time or place does not automatically make patients incapable of expressing their wishes and preferences.

Patients with advanced chronic progressive illness can have a "Provider Orders for Life-Sustaining Treatment" (POLST) form initiated by their health care providers. The form provides orders for emergency medical personnel regarding end-of-life wishes and summarizes a person's advance directives.

Much of the debate in health care today deals with end-of-life decisions such as euthanasia, assisted suicide, adequate pain control, and death with dignity. Nurses must keep up to date on legal decisions related to these issues and continue to learn and apply new nursing theory and procedures regarding end-of-life care. They must also deal with their own feelings and values regarding patient choices to seek life-prolonging or death-seeking treatment.

EUTHANASIA

Euthanasia is the act of ending another person's life to end suffering, with (voluntary) or without (involuntary) his consent. It may be called "mercy killing." Some distinction is also made between active and passive euthanasia. **Passive euthanasia** occurs when a patient chooses to die by refusing treatment that might prolong life. An example would be withholding artificial feeding or parenteral (IV) fluids when the patient is unable to take them orally. It would also include not treating pneumonia with antibiotics. **Honoring the refusal of life-prolonging treatment of a patient with a terminal illness is legally and ethically permissible. Active euthanasia** is generally defined as administering a drug or treatment to end the patient's life. The arguments for legal and ethical considerations regarding euthanasia are presented in Table 15.3.

Assisted suicide is distinguished from active euthanasia. It is making available to patients the means to end their life (such as a weapon or drug) with knowledge that suicide is their intent. Assisted suicide has generated a great deal of debate and dialogue in health care. Nurses witness firsthand their patients' despair,

Table 15.3 Legal and Ethical Considerations for Euthanasia

VOLUNTARY EUTHANASIA	INVOLUNTARY EUTHANASIA
Arguments for	
• Respects individual liberty and rights • Provides more dignified death • Reduces suffering • Demonstrates mercy • Supports constitutional right to privacy • Demonstrates right of self-determination • Upholds right to autonomy	• Reduces depletion of financial resources • Allows the patient dignity • Reduces suffering • Demonstrates mercy • Supports right to die
Arguments Against	
• Exploits the terminally ill • Breaks the Hippocratic oath • Unnecessary—nature will take its course • Morally wrong	• Ignores informed consent • Violates right to life • Unnecessary • Morally wrong
Legal Considerations	
The courts have approved the withholding of treatment in both voluntary and involuntary euthanasia cases if the parties can demonstrate that it is in the best interest of the patient, and the family requests it. However, be aware that "assisted suicide" is illegal in most states, and legal consequences may follow. In addition, active euthanasia is never legal nor permissible.	

pain, and debilitation. Assisting the patient's death may be seen as a compassionate and humane response. Although an individual case may be compelling, there is a large potential for abuse of this solution for difficult care problems, especially for older adults, the disabled, and the poor. Oregon passed a law legalizing assisted suicide in 1998; Montana and Washington states also allow assisted suicide in limited cases. The courts in other states continue to decide cases involving assisted suicide and active euthanasia that may change the legal status of such acts. The discussion about legal and ethical aspects of euthanasia continues.

Although assisted suicide might be legally permissible in some jurisdictions, the American Nurses Association (ANA) strictly prohibits nurses' participation in these acts (ANA, 2013). **Both active euthanasia and assisted suicide are considered violations of the ANA's *Code of Ethics for Nurses*.**

ADEQUATE PAIN CONTROL

Adequate pain control continues to be one of the most problematic issues in the end-of-life care. Physicians may be reluctant to prescribe large enough doses of pain medication for fear of legal action under the Controlled Substances Act. They may also be concerned about being viewed as prescribing lethal doses in an assisted suicide effort.

Nurses must be advocates for compassionate end-of-life care. Knowledgeable and skillful symptom management; the relief of suffering; and the promise of presence, of not abandoning the patient, are the cornerstones of end-of-life care that can eliminate the person's desire to choose euthanasia or suicide.

ORGAN AND TISSUE DONATION

Many organs and tissues can be transplanted from one person to another. The need for organs and tissues for transplantation far exceeds the supply. People can indicate their wish to be donors on their driver's license or in advance directives, but the next of kin must give permission to remove the organs or tissues of a dead person. Organs such as hearts, lungs, and livers can only be obtained from a person who is on mechanical ventilation and has suffered brain death when perfusion has been maintained. Other tissues can be removed up to several hours after sudden death. The donor must be free of infectious disease and cancer. The United Network for Organ Sharing (UNOS) set the criteria and provides support for organ donation and transplantation procedures to the public and to health care professionals (UNOS, 2015).

The primary care provider is usually the person that requests organ donation from family members, but you may be in a position to answer questions the family raises about organ donation. You should know that donation of organs does not delay funeral arrangements; there is no obvious evidence that the organs were removed when the body is dressed; and there is no cost to the family for the removal of organs donated.

POSTMORTEM (AFTER DEATH) CARE

When the patient stops breathing, the heart may continue to beat for several minutes. The cessation of cardiac contraction is considered the onset of death. When a patient is being mechanically ventilated, brain death must be established to determine death. In a hospital or nursing home, a physician is usually designated as the person responsible for pronouncing the death. However, in some institutions, midlevel providers, such as physician assistants and nurse practitioners, may perform this function. When a patient dies at home, the pronouncement of death may be delegated to an undertaker, RN, or coroner. A **coroner** is a person with legal authority to determine cause of death. A coroner investigates any deaths that occur under suspicious circumstances, including deaths that result from injury, accident, murder, or suicide. Any death within 24 hours after admission to the hospital or during surgery, or death of a person who has not been under a physician's care, is reported to the coroner. In the health care setting, if a death is a coroner's case, no tube or line is removed from the body to prevent removal of evidence of wrongdoing. IV lines and associated tubing are simply cut and tied off, with the catheters left in place.

A death certificate is completed by the physician, the undertaker, and a pathologist if an autopsy is done. An **autopsy** is an examination of the body, organs, and tissues to determine the cause of death. Consent for autopsy must be obtained from the next of kin, except in a coroner's case, when no permission is needed.

As the nurse, you are responsible for **postmortem** (after death) care of the body. Family members may wish to assist with or perform the preparation of the body as their last service to the patient, especially if they have been present throughout the dying process. If family members were not present when the patient died, the body may be prepared for the family to come to say goodbye and for removal to the morgue or undertaker (Skill 15.1). Ask if the family wishes to be left alone with the body for their final goodbyes. Provide privacy and whenever possible, accommodate the family's cultural and religious needs. Return the patient's personal belongings to the family, especially jewelry or valuables. Dispose of or return unused drugs to the pharmacy according to agency policy. Unused drugs are never given to the family.

Nurses can gain a great deal of satisfaction in caring for the dying patient and his family. Helping patients attain their goal of dying with dignity, without pain, and with a sense of closure is a tremendous challenge, but one that is rewarding. You should realize that you will also grieve for the dying patient. Many hospitals and health care agencies provide for support sessions after a particularly difficult death or when a unit has a succession of unexpected or challenging losses. You need to take care of yourself in order to continue taking care of your patients, and this includes recognizing the normal feelings that occur with loss and allowing yourself to move through the grief rather than trying to avoid it. Talking with the chaplain, co-workers, and other experienced nurses can support and heal the grief. Seeking professional assistance may be indicated if grieving becomes dysfunctional.

Skill 15.1 Postmortem Care

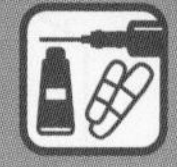
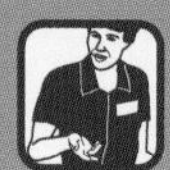
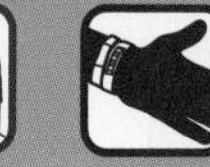
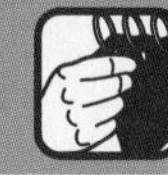
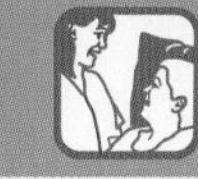

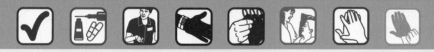

After death, you will prepare the body for transport to the morgue or funeral home. Always check records to see whether the patient is a designated organ donor. If so, initiate the organ donation process according to agency policy.

Supplies

- **Shroud** (sheet used to wrap body after death) pack or body bag (depending on your facility's preference)
- Death care kit (shroud/body bag, gauze 4 × 4 dressings, and protective pads if not in shroud pack)
- Gloves
- Bag for belongings
- Valuables list
- Bathing supplies
- Comb and brush
- Tape and large safety pins
- Body tags or labels
- Gurney or morgue cart

Review and carry out the Standard Steps in Appendix A.

ACTION *(RATIONALE)*

Assessment

1. Verify the patient's identification. *(Ensures that the patient is properly identified.)*
2. Determine whether an autopsy will be done; check for signed autopsy consent. *(Drainage or other tubes are not removed if an autopsy is planned.)*
3. Determine whether the family wishes to assist with bathing or caring for the body, or if they wish to view the deceased after the nurse prepares the body. *(Family may gain closure from this last act of care for their loved one.)*

Planning

4. Gather equipment, and prepare the working space by raising the bed to proper height and positioning the over-the-bed table for use. *(Promotes work efficiency and prevents back strain.)*

5. Close the door and/or privacy curtains. *(Protects privacy and dignity.)*

Implementation

6. Perform hand hygiene and don gloves. *(Protects you from contact with body fluids.)*
7. Position the patient in supine position with a pillow under the head and the head of the bed elevated 15 to 20 degrees. Close the eyelids, if necessary, by grasping the eyelashes and gently pulling lids down over the cornea. *(Raising the head prevents pooling of blood, which might discolor the face. Closing the eyelids protects the eyeballs.)*
8. Replace the dentures if they are out of the mouth if hospital policy requires it. Close the mouth. A small rolled towel may be placed under the chin if needed to keep the mouth closed. Depending on agency policy, dentures may be placed in a labeled denture cup without water and sent with the body so that the mortician does not have to remove the dentures again to embalm the body. *(Closing the eyelids and mouth protects the eyes and keeps the face in the most natural position during* ***rigor mortis*** *[rigidity of muscles that occurs after death].)*
9. Remove any jewelry and clothing. List all personal articles on the valuables list. Place in bag to be returned to the family and handle according to agency policy. *(This provides for return of personal property to the family.)*
10. Wash all areas of the body soiled with blood, feces, urine, or drainage. Place protective pads under rectum and between the legs to protect from drainage from the rectum, vagina, or urethra. *(After death, sphincter muscles relax, allowing leakage of stool, urine, or body fluids.)*
11. Comb the hair and arrange neatly. *(Combing the hair improves the appearance of the body and prevents matting or tangling.)*
12. Deflate any balloons and remove all tubes (IVs, catheters, and nasogastric) unless an autopsy is planned, if this is agency policy. Otherwise, convert IV catheters to intermittent locks. To secure tubes left in place, remove the drainage bag or IV fluid container, cut the tubing, and fold over twice. Secure with a rubber band. *(Properly deflating balloons before tube removal prevents tissue damage. Leaving the IV catheter in place prevents leaking during embalming and prepares the body for the coroner or undertaker.)*
13. Change any soiled dressings and remove adhesive marks with appropriate solvent. Place small dressings over wounds and secure with paper tape. *(Improves appearance of the body.)*
14. Dress the body in a clean gown if the family will be viewing the body, and remain with them unless they wish to be alone. The gown may be removed before wrapping the body. *(Dressing the body preserves dignity, and remaining with the family provides emotional support.)*
15. After the family leaves, attach identifying tags, usually on the big toe or ankle and the wrist. *(Proper identification ensures that the body will be transported to the correct mortuary.)*
16. Place padded ties around the ankles; crisscross the wrists over the abdomen and secure; and place a gauze tie or chin strap under the jaw to keep the mouth closed. Some mortuaries prefer that the limbs not be tied together. In this case, position the arms in a natural position at the sides of the body and keep the legs straight and together. *(Ankles and wrists are sometimes secured to prevent the arms and legs from being damaged during transport. However, the ties can damage the skin and make embalming more difficult.)*
17. Place the body on the shroud or in the morgue bag and check for placement of drainage pads. Fold the shroud according to agency procedure using the numerical order indicated. Secure the shroud at the chest, waist, and knees, and place an identification (ID) tag on the outside. *(The shroud covers the body and prevents unnecessary exposure. The ID tag ensures correct disposal of the body. Some mortuaries prefer the body not be shrouded.)*

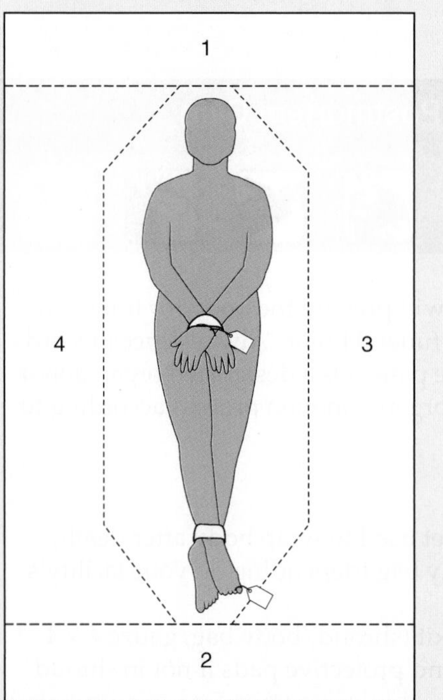

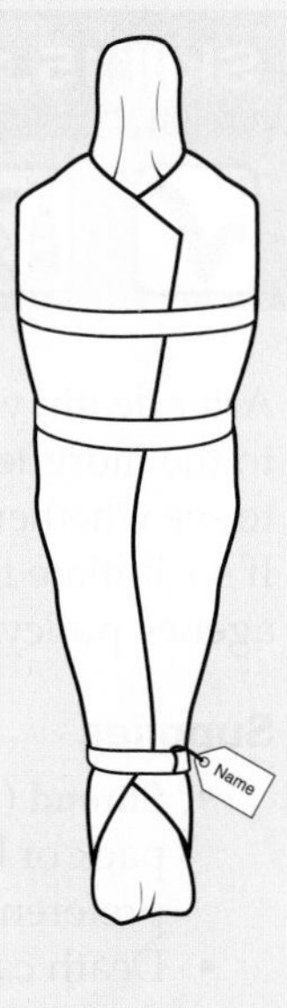

Step **17**

18. Transfer the body to the stretcher or morgue cart. Secure the body with straps that are secure but not so tight as to cause bruising. Remove gloves and perform hand hygiene. Transport the body to the morgue in the service elevator unless the mortuary will come to the room to transport it. *(Transport to*

the morgue is done quickly and with as little notice as possible, because it may upset other patients or visitors to see the body. Doors to patient rooms may be closed and the elevator held ready for transport. In some agencies, the face may be left uncovered so passersby think the person is just unconscious. Some mortuaries come directly to the room to transport the body.)

Evaluation

19. Ask yourself: Was the procedure carried out in a quiet, respectful way? Was the family supported and helped to say goodbye? Did the deceased appear clean, peaceful, and well cared for? *(Determines whether expected outcomes have been met. Indicates whether the way in which the procedure was carried out needs to be changed.)*

Documentation

20. Note the care provided in the medical record. *(Documentation is legal proof of the nursing care provided.)*

Documentation Example

2/17 1030 Pt stopped breathing. 1033 No apical pulse detected. Dr. Grover notified.

1040 Pronounced dead by Dr. Grover. Family present and assisted in washing and preparing the body for transport to morgue. Foley catheter removed. ID tags attached to right toe, right wrist, and outside of shroud. Transported to morgue at 1120. (Nurse's electronic signature)

? Critical Thinking Questions

1. Catherine Baumgartner has just died from complications because of extensive drug-resistant tuberculosis. The patient has been in isolation with minimal visitor contact, and the family has had to follow isolation precautions to visit the patient.
   a. Would you perform postmortem care differently than you would for a patient who died from cancer? If so, what would you do differently?

Get Ready for the NCLEX Examination!

Key Points

- *Loss* is to no longer possess or have a person, object, or situation. Grief is a normal reaction to loss. Death is the most difficult loss human beings experience.
- The grieving process consists of feelings and acts that move to eventual recovery. The symptoms of the grieving process include crying, depression, loss of appetite, changes in sleep, loneliness, and sadness. The grieving person may be the patient, loved one, or caregiver.
- Each person who grieves does so in a unique way that depends on the value of the loss to them, their previous experiences with loss, and their learned coping skills.
- Nurses assist the grieving person through validation of the loss, teaching of adaptive coping skills, and caring support.
- Therapeutic communication techniques—active listening, avoiding clichés, and attention to nonverbal communication—are invaluable in dealing with the person who is experiencing loss.
- Death may occur in different ways, and each person's reaction to death will also be different.
- Hospice is a concept of care for the dying and their families that focuses on symptom control, comfort measures rather than a cure, and a team approach to meeting the expressed needs of the patient and the family.
- Kübler-Ross theory of the stages of dying includes denial, bargaining, anger, depression, and acceptance.
- The dying person may experience fear of pain, of the unknown, and of loss of control, as well as guilt, hope, and despair.
- Hope is a positive life force that can be nurtured in different ways for the dying.
- Palliative care is a concept of providing care that relieves symptoms when a cure is not possible. This concept can be applied in any setting.
- The nursing process identifies the physical, emotional, social, and spiritual aspects of the dying patient's care and provides care using a comprehensive team approach.
- Patients may have tasks to complete before death, such as saying goodbye, making amends, reconciling with family or friends, and doing a life review.
- Research and practice provide effective ways of controlling pain and managing symptoms of nausea, constipation, anorexia, dyspnea, anxiety, or spiritual distress.
- Terminal dehydration has been shown to be palliative in reducing pain. IV hydration is not indicated unless it is a patient's choice.
- Signs of impending death include decreasing level of consciousness, decreasing urine output, mottling of skin, cool extremities, Cheyne-Stokes respirations, "death rattle," and incontinence. Hearing and touch are among the last senses to be lost before death.
- Nurses must be aware of patients' religious beliefs and assist them in the practice of the religious rituals that are important to them.
- Advance directives indicate a patient's choices about end-of-life decisions such as DNR orders and artificial hydration or tube feedings.

- Euthanasia and assisted suicide are legal and ethical issues for health care professionals.
- Assisted suicide is ethically not acceptable for health care professionals. Legally it is being tested in the courts, and new laws are constantly being proposed.
- Donation of organs from a dying person is possible if relatives give permission. Nurses have an important role in explaining the aspects of organ donation.
- Nurses are responsible for care of the body after death (except in some religions).
- Caring for patients in the final stage of life can be rewarding and satisfying. Nurses will recognize signs of grieving in themselves after a patient's death.

Additional Learning Resources

SG Go to your Study Guide for additional learning activities to help you master this chapter content.

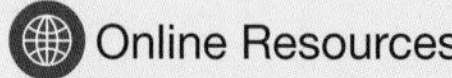
Go to your Evolve website at http://evolve.elsevier.com/Williams/fundamental for additional online resources.

Online Resources

- *Grace Happens,* www.Griefnet.org
- *NACC,* www.nacc.org/resources/links/death.asp
- *On Death and Dying,* www.WhatMattersNow.org

Review Questions for the NCLEX Examination

*Choose the **best** answer for each question.*

1. A patient recently diagnosed with cancer says to the nurse, "If I can just live until my son graduates from college, I'll donate 10% of my estate to the church." The patient is in a stage described by Kübler-Ross as:
   1. Acceptance.
   2. Denial.
   3. Bargaining.
   4. Anger.
2. A therapeutic response the nurse could make when a patient says, "I don't want to die" is:
   1. "I'm sure you don't want to die."
   2. "You have an excellent physician; maybe you won't die."
   3. "None of us wants to die."
   4. "I'm sorry you are going through this; would you like to talk about it?"
3. Comfort care for a terminally ill patient would include:
   1. Magnetic resonance imaging (MRI) to determine whether metastases are causing bone pain.
   2. Use of medication to relieve nausea.
   3. Insertion of an IV line to provide fluids.
   4. A gastrostomy tube to provide nutrition when the patient is unable to eat normally.
4. Which is the best pain control strategy for the unresponsive dying patient?
   1. Opioid q3h IV, with PRN breakthrough dose IV
   2. Opioid q4h PO, with a PRN breakthrough dose PO
   3. Opioids q3h IV, with a PRN breakthrough dose PO
   4. Opioids q3h IV and mindful meditation for breakthrough pain
5. The deceased patient's wife states that their religion requires that the family perform a special ritual and say a prayer at the bedside immediately after death "to help his soul leave the body." Which is the best response to the family's request?
   1. Tell the wife that the hospital has a nondenominational chapel where the family can say the prayer and perform the ritual.
   2. Provide the family with privacy and offer assistance as needed.
   3. Gently explain that they will be allowed to see the deceased after you verify whether you need to contact the coroner.
   4. Explain that they can stay with the deceased until the end of visiting hours.
6. An assigned patient has prostate cancer and is declining rapidly. He is frightened by the progression and asks you if there is any hope. What is the nurse's best response?
   1. "Your prostate cancer is incurable. We have exhausted our treatment measures, but I can discuss comfort measures with you."
   2. "Would you like me to call a chaplain for you? Maybe it's time to put your trust in a higher power."
   3. "There is always hope. Let's look at how we can address your issues together. What is it that you are hoping for at this point?"
   4. "You cannot give up! A positive attitude helps effect a cure."
7. After receiving palliative care for several months, your patient has died. The family is feeling deep grief. The nurse also feels saddened and knows that:
   1. Crying is inappropriate because you are not even a family member or a close friend.
   2. It is appropriate for the nurse to shed some tears, allowing movement through the grief rather than trying to avoid it. The nurse may also need to seek professional assistance.
   3. The nurse needs to ignore feelings and stay strong for the family in order to provide better nursing care.
   4. The nurse should avoid the family and allow them to grieve in private. The nurse is no longer needed, and the nurse's presence just reminds them of their loss.

Critical Thinking Activities

Read the clinical scenario and discuss the questions with your classmates.

Lynn Nuñez, a 45-year-old woman with advanced breast cancer that has spread to her lungs and bones, is admitted to your unit for terminal care and palliation. She has draining sores on her left breast. She is experiencing a great deal of pain when she moves, but she does not want sedation. Her wish is to spend her last days with her family, which includes her husband, mother and father, and two teenage daughters. The family is close and supportive, but is having a hard time seeing Lynn suffer. She is Roman Catholic, and the parish priest has visited daily. She has indicated she does not wish to have extraordinary measures, including feeding tubes, IVs, or antibiotics. She has a DNR order.

1. What do you think are Lynn's prioritized needs for care?
2. If she were assigned to you for care, what might you suggest for:
   - Frequency of vital signs measurement
   - Personal care: bathing, mouth care, and skin care
   - Feeding: what, when, and how much
   - Activity level
3. What might your response be if Lynn were to ask you, "Why do I have to suffer like this?"

chapter

16 Infection Prevention and Control: Protective Mechanisms and Asepsis

http://evolve.elsevier.com/Williams/fundamental

Objectives

Upon completing this chapter, you should be able to do the following:

Theory

1. List the types of microorganisms that can cause infection in humans.
2. Discuss the links in the infection process and give an example of each.
3. Discuss factors that make older adults more susceptible to infection.
4. Explain how the body's protective mechanisms work to prevent infection.
5. Explain how the inflammatory and immune responses protect the body.
6. Identify means for removal or destruction of microorganisms on animate and inanimate objects.
7. Compare and contrast medical asepsis and surgical asepsis.
8. Describe accepted methods of disinfection and sterilization.

Clinical Practice

1. Discuss the surveillance, prevention, and control of infections in hospitalized patients.
2. Demonstrate proper hand hygiene techniques.
3. Consistently demonstrate the application of the US Centers for Disease Control and Prevention (CDC) Standard and Transmission-Based Precautions while caring for patients.
4. Prepare to teach a home care patient with a wound infection how to prevent spread of infection to family members.

Skills & Steps

Key Terms

antibiotic (p. 218)
antimicrobial (ăn-tī-mī-KRŌ-bē-ăl, p. 218)
antiseptic (ăn-tĭ-SĔP-tĭk, p. 236)
asepsis (ā-SĔP-sĭs, p. 226)
aseptic (ā-SĔP-tĭk, p. 220)
bacteria (băk-TĒ-rē-ă, p. 217)
contaminated (p. 220)
debris (dĕ-BRĒ, p. 223)
disinfectants (dĭs-ĭn-FĔK-tănts, p. 236)
fungi (FŬN-jī, p. 219)
helminths (HĔL-mĭnths, p. 219)
immune response (ĭ-MŪN rē-SPŎNS, p. 224)
interferon (ĭn-tĕr-FĒR-ŏn, p. 224)
medical asepsis (p. 226)
microorganism (mī-krō-ŌR-găn-ĭz-ĕm, p. 217)
pathogens (PĂTH-ō-jĕnz, p. 217)
personal protective equipment (PPE) (p. 231)
prions (p. 219)
protozoa (prō-tō-ZŌ-ă, p. 219)
rickettsia (rĭ-KĔT-sē-ă, p. 219)
Standard Precautions (p. 231)
sterile (p. 220)
sterilization (stĕr-ĭ-lĭ-ZĀ-shŭn, p. 220)
surgical asepsis (p. 226)
viruses (p. 219)

Concepts Covered in This Chapter

- Infection
- Inflammation
- Immunity
- Safety
- Stress
- Tissue integrity

An **infection** is the entry of an infectious agent, a **microorganism** (organism only visible with a microscope), into the body that multiplies and disrupts tissue integrity. Left untreated, an infection may result in illness and disease. Health care professionals work to eliminate infection from the body and to prevent its spread to others. Careful hand hygiene is essential to prevent **cross-contamination.** Box 16.1 presents vocabulary related to infection. Microorganisms capable of causing disease are called **pathogens** (Fig. 16.1). Nonpathogenic organisms that are prevalent on and in the body are called **normal flora** (Table 16.1). Normal flora prevents more harmful microorganisms from colonizing and multiplying within the body. Normal flora accomplishes this by occupying receptor sites on cells, monopolizing the nutrients, and secreting substances that are toxic to other microorganisms. Some pathogenic microorganisms produce harmful **toxins,** and others release **endotoxins.** Endotoxins are responsible for the symptoms seen in diseases such as botulism, tetanus, diphtheria, and *Escherichia coli* infection.

INFECTIOUS AGENTS

BACTERIA

Bacteria are single-cell microorganisms lacking a nucleus that reproduce from every few minutes up to several weeks. Bacteria are classified according to their need for oxygen, their shape, and their Gram-staining properties. **Aerobic bacteria need oxygen to grow and thrive. Anaerobic bacteria grow only when oxygen is not present.** A laboratory technique called Gram staining is performed to help in classifying the bacteria's outer cell surface. This identification process also helps determine the most effective method to use in eliminating the microorganism. The specimen to be tested for bacteria is placed on a slide, stained, and then treated with a contrasting dye; those retaining the stain are **gram positive,** and those losing the stain and taking up the counterstain are **gram negative.** Many gram-negative bacteria are more dangerous than gram-positive bacteria because they may produce an endotoxin that can cause hemorrhagic shock and severe diarrhea and can alter resistance to other bacterial infection. Classification of bacteria according to their **morphology** (shape) places them into one of three main groups: **cocci** (round), **bacilli** (rod shaped),

Box 16.1 Vocabulary Related to Infection

Aerobic: Needs oxygen to live and grow.
Anaerobic: Able to live and grow only in the absence of oxygen.
Bactericidal: An agent that is able to kill or destroy bacteria.
Colonization: Microorganisms take up residence and grow.
Community-associated infection: An infection that was present or incubating before the patient came in contact with health care or had a medical procedure performed.
Cross-contamination: Transmission of infectious microorganisms from one person or object to another.
Culture: Propagation of living organisms or tissue in special media conducive to their growth.
Disinfectant: An agent that reduces the number of viable microorganisms.
Endotoxin: A heat-stable toxin associated with the outer membranes of certain gram-negative bacteria that is released when the cells are disrupted.
Exotoxin: An unstable, highly toxic by-product of select microorganisms that can be found in both gram-positive and gram-negative bacteria.
Exudate: Fluid in or on tissue surfaces that has escaped from blood vessels in response to inflammation and that contains protein and cellular debris.
Gram-negative: Bacteria that lose the stain in the Gram method of staining.
Gram-positive: Bacteria that retain the stain in the Gram method of staining.
Health care–associated infection: Infection that was not present or incubating on admission to a health care facility; acquired during hospitalization.
Host: An animal or plant that harbors and provides sustenance for another organism (a parasite).
Infection: Invasion and multiplication in body tissues of microorganisms that cause cellular injury.
Inflammation: Localized response caused by injury or destruction of tissues that serves to contain the injurious agent and injured tissue.
Leukocytosis: Increase in the number of leukocytes in the blood, resulting from infection or other causes.
Phagocytes: Cells (e.g., macrophages) capable of ingesting particulate matter.
Phagocytosis: The engulfing of microorganisms and foreign particles by phagocytes.
Spores: Oval bodies formed within bacteria as a resting stage during the life cycle of the cell; characterized by resistance to environmental changes (heat, humidity, or cold).
Toxin: A poison; a poisonous protein produced by certain bacteria.
Vector: Carrier that transports an infective agent from one host to another, such as animals, insects, and rodents.
Virulence: Degree to which a microorganism can cause infection in the host or invade the host.

and **spirochetes** (spiral). Some grow in chains (streptococci), some in pairs (diplococci), and some in clusters (staphylococci).

Final identification involves chemical testing of the bacteria by performing a **culture.** To do this, the body secretion or specimen is transferred to a medium in which it can grow. Sensitivity tests are then performed to determine which **antibiotic** (chemical substance that can kill or alter the growth of bacterial microorganisms) is most effective against the bacteria.

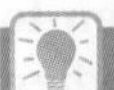

QSEN Considerations: Safety

Sensitivity Results

The sensitivity results, available 48 to 72 hours after the culture, typically show that the organism is (1) resistant, (2) susceptible, or (3) has intermediate resistance. The nurse must be sure the primary care provider is aware of the sensitivity results in case treatment needs to be altered.

When culture results show that a drug-resistant organism is responsible for an infection, extreme care must be taken to prevent the spread of the organism. The four most common multidrug-resistant organisms are (1) methicillin-resistant *Staphylococcus aureus* (MRSA), (2) vancomycin-resistant *Enterococcus* (VRE), (3) extended-spectrum beta-lactamase–producing (ESBL) pneumonia (*Klebsiella pneumoniae* or *E. coli*), and (4) *Clostridium difficile (C. diff)*. A quick test, the BD GeneOhm StaphSR assay, identifies MRSA bacterium in 2 hours by testing a blood sample. Another example of a drug-resistant organism is penicillin-resistant *Streptococcus pneumoniae,* which causes a form of pneumonia that can be difficult to treat. Another emerging threat to public health and safety is a group of resistant organisms called carbapenem-resistant Enterobacteriaceae, which are highly resistant organisms and can cause infections in the urinary tract, bloodstream, wounds, and lungs (Centers for Disease Control and Prevention [CDC], 2015a).

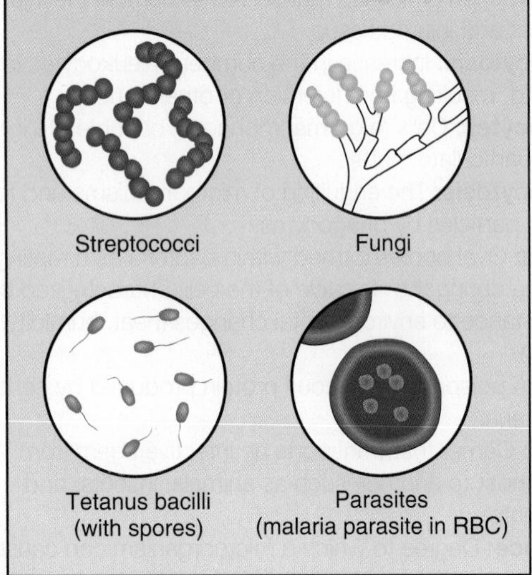

FIGURE 16.1 Pathogenic microorganisms. *RBC,* Red blood cell.

These organisms, especially MRSA, are being contracted outside the hospitals now and are an increasing problem. Patients must be educated about the correct use and possible misuse of **antimicrobial** (killing or suppressing growth of microorganisms) agents. Encourage each patient to take the entire antimicrobial prescription as ordered by the heath care provider to ensure full treatment of the infection. Incomplete treatment allows some microorganisms to live, giving them a chance to mutate and develop drug resistance. Consistent use of the US Centers for Disease Control and Prevention (CDC) Standard Precautions plus any Transmission-Based Precautions (e.g., Airborne Precautions, Contact, or Droplet Precautions) is essential, especially when a drug-resistant organism is present.

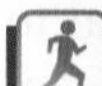

Health Promotion/Health Promotion Points

Preventing Spread of Drug-Resistant Organisms

Take the following precautions to prevent the spread of drug-resistant organisms in your community:

- Wash hands frequently; use an alcohol-based rub when soap and running water are unavailable.
- Keep any cut or abrasion clean and covered with a bandage until healed.
- Avoid sharing personal items such as razors, towels, and makeup.
- Avoid contact with other people's bandages or wounds.

Table 16.1 Normal Flora of the Body[a]

SITE	NORMAL FLORA
Upper respiratory tract (nose, mouth, throat)	*Corynebacterium* species *Enterobacter* species *Haemophilus* species *Klebsiella* species *Lactobacillus* species *Neisseria* species *Staphylococcus* species *Streptococcus* (*viridans* group) *Streptococcus pyogenes* (group A) Various types of anaerobes
Skin	*Acinetobacter* species *Corynebacterium* species *Staphylococcus aureus* *Staphylococcus epidermidis* Yeasts
Small bowel and colon	Anaerobes *Bacteroides* species *Clostridium perfringens* *Enterobacter* species (coliforms) *Streptococcus faecalis* (enterococci or group D)
Vagina	Alpha-hemolytic streptococci Enterobacteriaceae Enterococci *Lactobacillus* sp. Many types of anaerobes *Staphylococcus epidermidis*

[a]The lower respiratory tract, central nervous system, bladder, and upper urinary tract are normally sterile (no microorganisms present).

PRIONS

Prions are protein particles that lack nucleic acids and are not inactivated by usual methods for destroying bacteria or viruses. They do not trigger an immune response but cause degenerative neurologic disease such as variant Creutzfeldt-Jakob disease (a human version mad cow disease).

PROTOZOA

Protozoa are one-celled microscopic organisms belonging to the animal kingdom. Protozoa that are pathogenic to humans include the *Plasmodium* species that causes malaria; *Entamoeba histolytica,* which causes amebic dysentery; and other strains capable of causing diarrhea.

VIRUSES

Viruses are extremely small and can be seen only with an electron microscope (Fig. 16.2). They are composed of particles of nucleic acids, either DNA or RNA, with a protein coat and sometimes a membranous envelope. **Viruses can grow and replicate only within a living cell.** Once inside cells, viruses can trigger an immune reaction or damage cells in other ways. Their survival and multiplication depend on host tissue. Viruses are identified in the laboratory by fluorescent techniques, electron microscopy, and tissue culture.

RICKETTSIA

Rickettsia are small round or rod-shaped microorganisms that are transmitted by the bites of lice, ticks, fleas, and mites that act as **vectors.** They multiply only in host cells. Examples of rickettsial infection include Rocky Mountain spotted fever and typhus.

FUNGI

Fungi are tiny, primitive organisms of the plant kingdom that contain no chlorophyll. Examples include yeasts and molds. Fungi feed on living plants, animals, and decaying organic material. They thrive in warm, moist environments. Fungi reproduce by means of **spores.** In humans, fungal infections are called **mycoses.** When the balance of normal flora is altered by antimicrobial therapy, fungal infections such as vaginal candidiasis may occur.

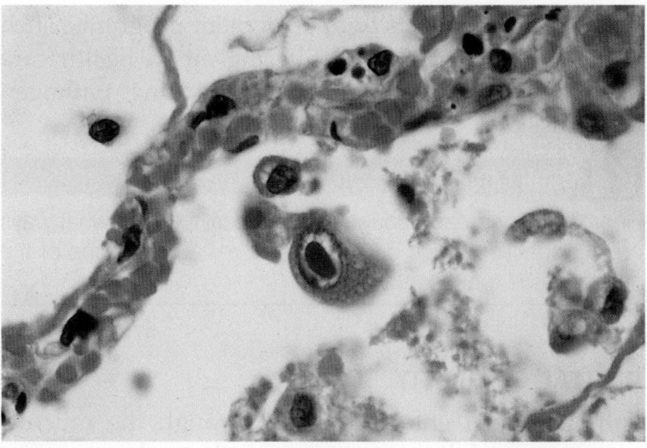

FIGURE 16.2 Electron microscope view of viruses. (From Kumar V, Cotran, RS, Robbins SL. *Basic Pathology.* 7th ed. Philadelphia, PA: Saunders; 2003.)

HELMINTHS

Helminths are parasitic worms or flukes belonging to the animal kingdom. Pinworms, which mostly affect children, are the most common helminths worldwide. Roundworms and tapeworms are other helminths.

OTHER INFECTIOUS AGENTS

Several types of organisms differ enough in structure to fall outside the above classifications. Mycoplasmas are very small organisms without a cell wall. They cause infections of the respiratory or genital tract. *Mycoplasma pneumoniae* is an example. *Chlamydia,* another type of organism, affects the genitourinary and reproductive tracts and has become more common in the past 20 years. In countries where hygiene is poor, *Chlamydia trachomatis* is responsible for trachoma, an eye disease that can cause blindness. In the United States, the same organism causes a significant amount of sexually transmitted infections.

PROCESS (CHAIN) OF INFECTION

The process by which an infection is spread from one person to another can be thought of as a continuous chain. Each link must be present in its proper order for the chain to remain intact and for the infection to spread. Figure 16.3 shows how the links of the chain connect and infection occurs. If just one link is broken, the transmission of the microorganism cannot occur. Nursing care focuses on breaking the chain of infection.

CAUSATIVE AGENT (LINK ONE)

A causative agent is any microorganism or biologic agent capable of causing disease. These agents include bacteria, viruses, protozoa, prions, rickettsia, fungi, and helminths.

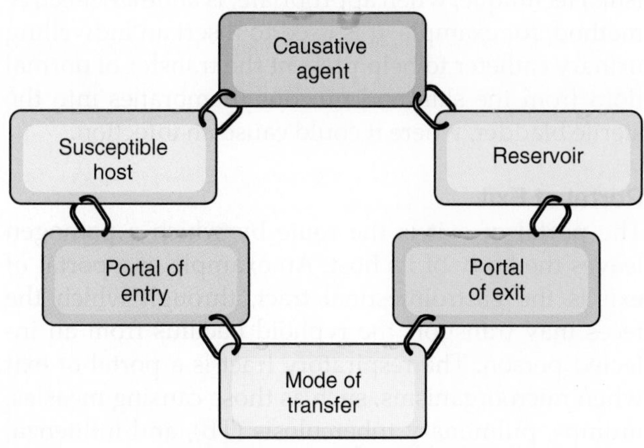

FIGURE 16.3 The infection chain.

Some microorganisms are more virulent than others. Characteristics that affect **virulence** are ability to (1) adhere to mucosal surfaces or cell walls, (2) penetrate mucous membranes, (3) multiply in the body, (4) secrete harmful enzymes or toxins, (5) resist **phagocytosis** (destruction by white blood cells [WBCs]), and (6) bind with iron (essential to bacterial growth). Microorganisms differ in structure and characteristics (see Fig. 16.1). If the pathogen is not contained, the patient may become ill. The four stages of the infection process are incubation, prodrome, illness, and convalescence and are discussed in more detail in Chapter 17.

Pathogenic microorganisms must be destroyed or rendered harmless to remove this link from the chain. Disinfection, which destroys or reduces infection-producing organisms, and **sterilization**, which removes all organisms, are methods used in the process of destroying microorganisms, pathogens, or pathogenic products. Procedures for disinfection and/or sterilization should be used in all areas where patients are receiving treatment.

The most effective means for destroying viruses and all other kinds of microorganisms is to expose them to a high temperature for a specified amount of time; the temperature should be at least 250°F (121°C) for 20 to 30 minutes if using a steam sterilizer, and at least 320°F (160°C) for 90 minutes to 3 hours if using dry sterilization. This can be accomplished by using a special machine called an autoclave.

The Centers for Disease Control and Prevention (CDC), a US government agency (http://www.cdc.gov), provides a wealth of information on all aspects of infectious diseases, including their prevention and control.

RESERVOIR

Reservoirs are places where microorganisms are found. Reservoirs can be infected wounds, human or animal waste, animals and insects, **contaminated** (made unclean) food and water, or a person with an infection. Standard Precautions are used to prevent the spread of infection from the reservoir. Good hand hygiene is one of the most effective ways to prevent the spread of microorganisms. Using **sterile** (free from all microorganisms) technique, when appropriate, is another effective method; for example, it is used to insert an indwelling urinary catheter to help prevent the transfer of normal flora from the skin and mucous membranes into the sterile bladder, where it could cause an infection.

Portal of Exit

The portal of exit is the route by which a pathogen leaves the body of its host. An example of a portal of exit is the gastrointestinal tract, through which the feces may transport the typhoid bacillus from an infected person. The respiratory tract is a portal of exit when microorganisms, such as those causing measles, mumps, pulmonary tuberculosis (TB), and influenza, are released with coughing or sneezing. The skin and mucous membranes can also serve as a portal of exit when an open or draining wound exists.

Portal-of-exit transmission can be interrupted by identifying and treating infected patients. Isolation techniques and barrier precautions that include the proper handling and disposal of secretions, urine, feces, and **exudate** can prevent pathogen transfer. CDC recommendations for Transmission-Based Precautions and isolation techniques are based on scientific evidence that has proven how various pathogens are transmitted. Chapter 17 outlines specific recommendations.

MODE OF TRANSFER

Modes of transfer of pathogens include (1) direct personal contact with body excretions or drainage such as from an infected wound; (2) indirect contact with contaminated inanimate objects (called **fomites**), such as needles, drinking and eating utensils, dressings, and hospital equipment; (3) vectors such as fleas, ticks, mosquitoes, and other insects that harbor infectious agents and transmit infection to humans through bites and stings; (4) droplet infection, or contamination by the aerosol route through sneezing and coughing; and (5) spread of infection from one part of the body to another.

The mode of transmission can be interrupted by effective hand hygiene, proper disinfection and sterilization of medical equipment, use of both surgical (sterile) and medical **aseptic** (free of microorganisms) technique in performing procedures and diagnostic tests, and use of Standard Precautions to prevent contamination. Teach patients to cover the mouth when sneezing or coughing, to dispose of soiled tissues correctly, to wash hands after contact with potentially contaminated items, and to avoid people who have an infection to reduce transmission of pathogens.

Clinical Cues

Current CDC recommendations are to sneeze or cough into the bended elbow rather than covering the mouth with the hands. This way, the spread of the respiratory droplets is prevented and hands are not contaminated.

Controlling insects with abatement programs, such as mosquito control, and filtering air in health care facilities are other methods of reducing pathogen transmission.

Think Critically

Hepatitis A is spread through the oral-fecal route. In what ways could hepatitis A virus be spread in a restaurant if one of the employees is the reservoir?

PORTAL OF ENTRY

Pathogens can enter the body through the mucous membranes of the eyes, nose, mouth, trachea, or skin. Consuming food or water that is contaminated with disease-causing microorganisms is one example of how entrance can occur. Breathing in droplets containing pathogens and contracting a virus through broken skin or mucous membranes are other examples of portals of entry. Table 16.2 shows some of the pathogenic organisms that enter through various body portals.

Using only sterile and clean items when caring for patients reduces the entry of pathogens. Barrier precautions (gloves, masks, condoms), safe handling of food and water, good personal hygiene, avoidance of high-risk behaviors, and protection from insect bites and stings can prevent entry of microorganisms.

SUSCEPTIBLE HOST

A human **host** may be susceptible by virtue of age, state of health, or broken skin. Measures are used to prevent exposure to infectious agents and to improve a person's health by teaching good health and hygiene habits. Immunization to help protect against influenza or pneumococcal pneumonia is another means of decreasing susceptibility.

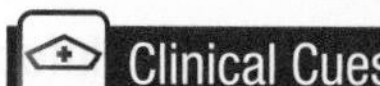

Influenza immunization is recommended yearly for all health care workers and anyone over 6 months of age.

Susceptible hosts can be protected by using aseptic techniques, barrier precautions, and protective isolation (see Chapter 17). Proper nutrition and a healthy lifestyle also increase resistance to infection. Table 16.3 lists factors that increase susceptibility to infection. Table 16.4 shows how the chain of infection can be broken at each link.

Susceptibility of the Older Adult

Many factors can place older adults at higher risk of infection. Poor nutrition, inadequate hygiene, impaired mobility, chronic illness, and physiologic changes all increase the risk of disease (Table 16.5). Older adults are hospitalized more frequently than younger people for problems caused by chronic illness or for treatment

Table 16.2 Portals of Entry for Selected Pathogenic Organisms

INFECTING ORGANISMS	RESULTANT DISEASES
Respiratory Tract	
Neisseria meningitides	Meningococcal pneumonia, meningococcal meningitis, meningococcemia
Cryptococcus neoformans	Cryptococcal meningitis, cryptococcal pneumonia
Mycobacterium tuberculosis	Tuberculosis
Influenza A virus	Influenza
Streptococcus pneumonia	Pneumococcal pneumonia
Measles virus (rubeola)	Measles
Legionella pneumophila	Legionnaires disease
Varicella-zoster virus	Chickenpox
Gastrointestinal Tract	
Salmonella enteritidis	Gastroenteritis
Salmonella typhi	Typhoid fever
Clostridium botulinum	Botulism
Poliovirus	Poliomyelitis
Hepatitis A virus	Hepatitis A
Escherichia coli O157:H7	Possibly, hemolytic uremic syndrome
Carbapenem resistant enterobacteriaceae (CRE)	Diarrhea (drug-resistant)
Genitourinary Tract	
Neisseria gonorrhoeae	Gonorrhea
Chlamydia trachomatis	Lymphogranuloma venereum, cervicitis, urethritis, endometritis
Enterobacteriaceae (*E. coli*, *Klebsiella* species, *Serratia* species, *Proteus* species)	Urinary tract infections
Intact Skin or Mucous Membranes	
Rhinovirus	Common cold
Respiratory syncytial virus	Pneumonia, bronchiolitis, tracheobronchitis
Schistosoma species	Schistosome dermatitis (swimmer disease)
Herpes simplex virus	Oral or genital herpes
Bloodstream	
Hepatitis B or C viruses	Hepatitis B or C
Plasmodium species	Malaria
Clostridium tetani	Tetanus
Human immunodeficiency virus (HIV)	Acquired immunodeficiency syndrome (AIDS)

From Ignatavicius DD, Workman ML. *Medical-Surgical Nursing: Patient-Centered Collaborative Care*. 5th ed. p. 509. Philadelphia: Elsevier Saunders; 2006.

Table 16.3 Factors That Increase Susceptibility to Infection

FACTOR	CONSEQUENCE
Age	Older adults and the very young are more susceptible to infection, likely because of the declining or immature immune function, respectively.
Malnutrition	Poor nutrition interferes with cell growth and replacement, which contributes to decreased immune function.
Excessive stress or fatigue	These states seem to interfere with the body's normal defense mechanisms.
Low leukocyte (WBC) count	Fewer white blood cells (WBCs) are available to fight infection.
Altered defense mechanisms	Body damage from trauma disrupts the natural defense mechanism of the skin and mucous membranes, allowing entry to microorganisms.
Alcoholism	This has an inhibiting effect on the immune system.
Chronic illness	Chronic illness upsets the homeostatic balance within the body, impairing the normal defense mechanisms. Serious illness taxes the immune system, causing greater susceptibility to other pathogens.
Indwelling tubes, devices, or equipment	Fracture pins, urinary catheters, intravenous (IV) cannulas, feeding tubes, prosthetic heart valves, and hip prostheses all provide either a portal of entry or a place for colonization of microorganisms.
Immunosuppressive treatment, chemotherapy, or corticosteroid treatment	Immunosuppressive treatment or chemotherapy depresses the immune system or harms the bone marrow, decreasing the number of leukocytes and macrophages. Corticosteroids depress the inflammatory response, inhibiting one of the body's defense mechanisms.

Table 16.4 Breaking the Chain of Infection

LINK	WAYS TO BREAK THE CHAIN	INTERVENTIONS
Reservoir		
Infected patient	Prevent transfer of microorganisms	Proper hand hygiene; use of gloves; Standard Precautions; Transmission-Based Precautions
Portal of Exit		
Secretions Feces Blood Urine Sputum	Prevent contamination	Thorough hand hygiene; Standard and Transmission-Based Precautions; not recapping needles; handling sharps correctly; containing contaminated materials; disinfection; following medical aseptic practices
Mode of Transfer		
Hands Contaminated food Contaminated supplies and other objects	Prevent contamination Eliminate vectors	Standard and Transmission-Based Precautions; proper hand hygiene; sterilization, proper cleaning, and refrigeration of foods; disinfection; proper disposal; surgical asepsis; pest control
Entrance		
Mouth Break in skin Mucous membranes	Put only clean things in mouth Protect skin Protect mucous membranes	Keeping objects out of mouth; good hygiene practices; good skin care; thorough cleansing of skin before an invasive procedure; covering skin breaks with occlusive dressing; Standard Precautions: goggles, face shield or mask, gloves, gown
Host		
Susceptible person	Protect natural body defenses by: • Good nutrition • Good hygiene • Adequate sleep • Decreased stress	Assessing degree of risk of infection; promoting natural body defenses; protective isolation; Standard and Transmission-Based Precautions; proper hand hygiene

Table 16.5 Increased Susceptibility of the Older Adult to Infection

Older adults are at higher risk of infection than younger adults. Any older adult with a chronic illness experiences increased stress on the body and a strain on the body's defense mechanisms from that disease; this makes the person more susceptible to other infections. The following factors also increase the risk of infection. You can institute certain interventions to try to decrease that risk.

AREA	FACTOR	NURSING INTERVENTION
Homeostasis	Older adults lose their homeostatic state more easily than younger adults as a result of loss of functioning cells in all body organs with aging.	Protect from exposure to pathogens. Promote good nutrition, exercise, and adequate rest to boost resistance to disease.
Immune function	Both immediate and delayed immune responses are decreased or altered.	Protect from exposure to pathogens. Immunize against influenza and pneumonia. Promote good nutrition to boost immune system.
Respiratory function	Impaired cough mechanism and impaired function of cilia decrease ability to expel foreign substances and mucus from the lungs, predisposing the person to respiratory tract infection.	Discourage smoking. Encourage deep breathing and intake of fluid to keep lung secretions thinned.
	Decreased macrophage activity in the lungs.	Encourage good oral hygiene to decrease potential for colonization of trachea and lungs with microorganisms.
	Less ability to expand the thorax predisposes older adults to atelectasis after surgery.	Help postoperative patients maintain a semiupright position (semi-Fowler) to aid lung expansion. Encourage use of incentive spirometer, deep breathing, and coughing. Ambulate as soon as possible.
Skin	Decreased elasticity, increased dryness, and decreased vascular supply make the skin susceptible to injury or breakdown and slower to repair. Breaks allow entry of microorganisms.	Instruct in appropriate skin care. Keep skin well moisturized. Prevent abrasions by using a lift sheet or a trapeze bar for positioning. Inspect skin at least once each shift for pressure areas.
Gastrointestinal system	Older adults have decreased secretion of gastric acid resulting in decreased destruction in the stomach of microorganisms ingested in food and drink.	Promote good oral hygiene to prevent swallowing pathogenic microorganisms.
	Pancreatic enzyme secretion is decreased, causing less destruction of microorganisms in the gastrointestinal (GI) tract.	Instruct in proper preparation and storage of food to prevent GI infection.
Urinary tract	Prostatic hypertrophy, cystocele, rectocele, and degeneration of nerves to bladder cause urine stasis in bladder as a result of incomplete emptying. Stasis predisposes to urinary tract infection.	Encourage intake of sufficient fluid to keep urine dilute. Encourage intake of cranberry juice and other foods that keep urine acidic, which will discourage the growth of microorganisms.

after a fall. This places them at higher risk for a **health care–associated infection (HAI)**—infection acquired by a patient after admission to a health care facility due to the transfer of microorganisms to the patient by contaminated hands or objects or infected people. Examples of HAIs include catheter-acquired urinary tract infection (CAUTI) and ventilator-acquired pneumonia (VAP) (see Chapter 17).

? Think Critically

Which organisms are you most frequently exposed to that could cause disease? How can you protect yourself against disease-causing microorganisms?

BODY DEFENSES AGAINST INFECTION

The body has many natural defenses against pathogen invasion. Intact skin serves as a **first line of defense** against harmful environmental agents. Skin functions as a protective barrier for the underlying tissues, helping maintain integrity. Sebaceous glands excrete sweat, lactic acid, and fatty acids to limit microbial growth.

Secretions from the mucous membranes lining the respiratory, gastrointestinal, and reproductive tracts contain an abundance of the enzyme **lysozyme,** which is bactericidal. Lysozyme is also found in tears and saliva. Cilia, which line the respiratory tract, trap microorganisms and **debris** (dead tissue or foreign matter) and propel them up and out of the body with a wavelike action. The bones protect the more delicate and vital organs from outside trauma. The bone marrow produces defensive blood cells.

The intestinal system is a major portal of entry for pathogens, and the liver is an essential part of the body's defense system. The Kupffer cells in the liver destroy bacteria that enter the portal liver circulation. Only about 1% of bacteria that enter the portal circulation from the intestines pass through the liver into the general circulation. The liver also detoxifies harmful chemicals by isolating various substances and facilitating their breakdown and excretion from the body.

Gastric secretions such as hydrochloric acid destroy ingested pathogens. Evacuation of feces flushes bacteria from the intestine, and the formation and elimination of urine flush the urinary system.

The body's **second line of defense** helps destroy pathogens that escape the first line of defense. This includes the mechanisms of fever, leukocytosis, phagocytosis, inflammation, and the action of **interferon** (biologic response modifier that affects cellular growth).

The body automatically raises its temperature in response to infection. A fever can slow the growth of many pathogens until other body defenses can be mobilized.

Clinical Cues

Fever is a natural defense mechanism. Therefore, a fever should not be treated right away unless it is dangerously high. In many instances, it is not desirable to lower the body temperature to normal. Rest and increased fluids are the correct treatment for the first few days.

Leukocytes, which are WBCs, are released in response to microorganisms, particularly bacteria, entering the body. This increased production or release of leukocytes is termed **leukocytosis.** They travel through the capillary walls out into the tissues to engulf the invader. Located in the lymphatic tissue, the alveoli of the lungs, the gastrointestinal system, the spleen, and the liver, **phagocytes** work to destroy or stop their invasion. The macrophages assist in body defense by removing cellular debris, engulfing and destroying bacteria and viruses, and removing metabolic waste products. Some phagocytes are called **tissue macrophages;** others, which are concerned with immunity, are the **lymphocytic cells.**

Phagocytosis is part of the inflammatory response, another defense mechanism of the body. When infection and leukocytosis occur, the WBC count is elevated. A large increase in the percentage of monocytes often indicates a bacterial infection. If the neutrophil count is decreased on the differential WBC count, while the monocyte count and lymphocyte counts are elevated, the cause of infection is probably viral. Increase in the percentage of basophils may indicate parasitic infection.

Interferons are produced in response to viral invasion of the cell. They stimulate antiviral proteins that prevent replication of viruses. Interferons can attack a wide variety of viruses, inhibiting or destroying them. Interferons stimulate the immune system, increase resistance to viral invasion, and interfere with viral replication.

INFLAMMATORY RESPONSE

The inflammatory response can be induced by any mechanical, chemical, or infectious disease-producing factor that injures cells of the body. Inflammation is an immediate response of the body to any kind of injury to its cells and tissues. The blood vessels dilate, bringing more blood to the damaged area, causing redness, warmth, and edema. **Inflammation is a localized protective response brought on by injury or destruction of tissues.** The basic purposes of the inflammatory response are to (1) neutralize and destroy harmful agents, (2) limit their spread to other tissues in the body, and (3) prepare the damaged tissues for repair. During inflammation, the chemicals **histamine** and **serotonin** are released. These chemicals act on the walls of the capillaries, causing them to be more permeable so that water, proteins, and defensive cells can pass out of the blood and into the fluid surrounding the damaged cells. This leakage of fluid is responsible for localized swelling, which in turn causes increased pressure and pain. Fibrinogen promotes clotting, blocking the lymphatic vessels. This results in a walling off of the area that delays spread of bacteria, toxins, and other harmful agents to other parts of the body (Concept Map 16.1). Purulent drainage, caused by the debris that sometimes results from the inflammation process, may accumulate at the site. Leukocytosis is then triggered and draws phagocytes to the damaged tissue to begin their work.

IMMUNE RESPONSE

The immune response is the **third line of defense** against pathogenic organisms. Microorganisms and other substances that do not belong in the body, such as pollen, are recognized as foreign invaders and trigger an **immune response** (the body's reaction to substances interpreted as nonself). For example, macrophages in the lungs engulf bacteria, dust particles, and any other foreign material that might threaten to damage the lung tissues. If the foreign particles are not expectorated, the leukocytes and later macrophages in the alveoli help wall them off, thereby preventing their spread to other tissues. An example of this process is the localizing of tubercle bacilli that have not been destroyed by the body's other defenses. *Mycobacterium tuberculosis* bacilli are walled off, preventing their dissemination to full-blown pulmonary tuberculosis.

The immune system response is specific to the type of invader. Unique antigens on the surface of individual cells aid the immune system in distinguishing self

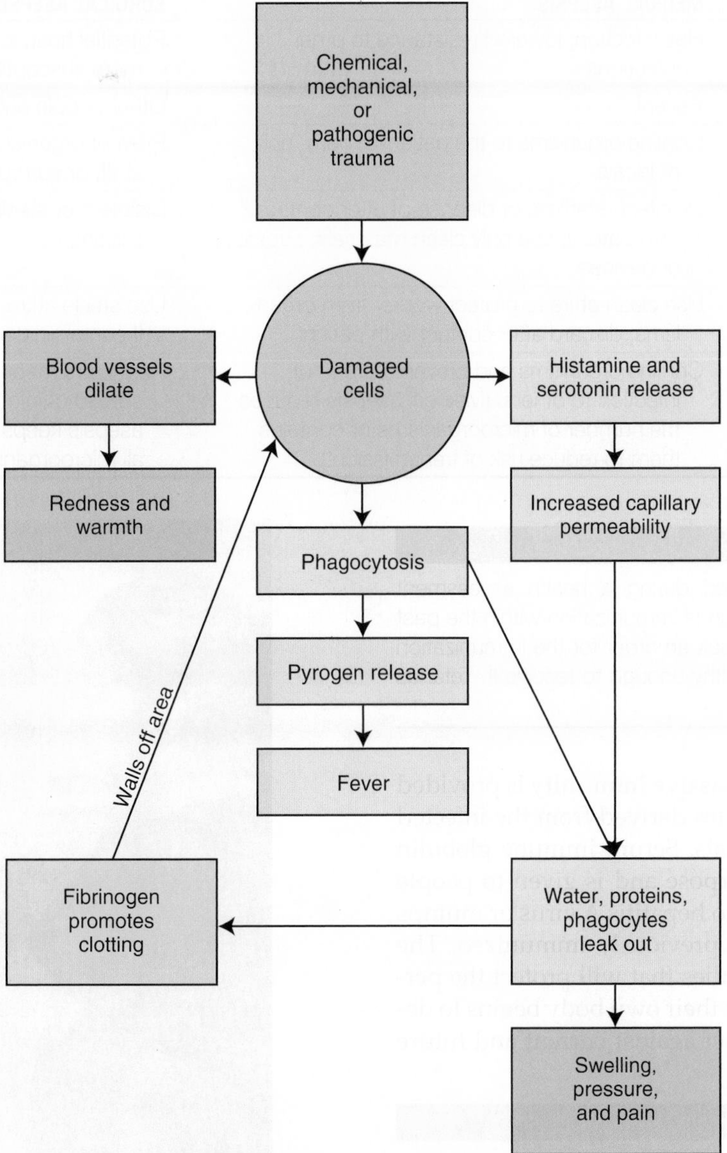

CONCEPT MAP 16.1 The inflammatory response.

from nonself (invaders) so it can destroy foreign material **(antigens).** Once exposed to a microorganism, the body produces **antibodies** against that invader. In this way, **naturally acquired immunity** occurs. Every antigen stimulates formation of a specific type of antibody. The next time that same microorganism invades the body, the antibodies respond and attempt to destroy it. Some types of naturally acquired immunity, such as with varicella (chickenpox), last a lifetime, but others, such as with influenza, last only a short time.

Passive acquired immunity occurs when a person is given an antitoxin or antiserum that contains antibodies or antitoxins that have been developed in another person. Tetanus antitoxin is an example of a substance that provides passive immunity. It protects a person from the current invasion of microorganisms but does not provide lasting immunity.

Naturally acquired passive immunity occurs when the fetus receives antibodies from the mother through placental blood before birth. This type of immunity is also acquired by the breastfeeding infant. It is temporary and typically lasts only until the infant's own immune system matures enough to function properly.

Artificially acquired immunity is achieved through injection of vaccines or immunizing substances that contain dead or inactive microorganisms or their toxins. The vaccine prompts the body to produce antibodies. Vaccinations against polio, measles, hepatitis B, influenza, tetanus, and diphtheria provide this type of immunity.

Table 16.6 Comparison of Medical Asepsis and Surgical Asepsis

FACTOR	MEDICAL ASEPSIS	SURGICAL ASEPSIS
Patient	Has infection, lowered resistance to other infections	Potential host; lowered resistance makes more susceptible
Reservoir of infection	Patient	Other people and the environment
Objective of barriers	Confine organisms to the patient's room, unit, or locale	Prevent organisms from reaching patient, staff, or surrounding area
Equipment and supplies	Disinfect, sterilize, or dispose of after contact with patient; use only clean materials, supplies, or devices	Disinfect or sterilize before contact with patient; use sterile materials
Nurse's protective attire: gown, mask, gloves	Use clean attire to protect worker from organisms; discard after contact with patient	Use sterile attire to protect patient; remedy if contaminated
Goal of nursing action	Confine organisms and prevent spread of infection to others. (Medical asepsis reduces the number of microorganisms or contains them to reduce risk of transmission.)	Reduce number of organisms and prevent spread of infection to patient. (Surgical asepsis keeps an area or objects free of all microorganisms for a period of time.)

Clinical Cues

All patients should be asked during a health assessment whether they have had a tetanus immunization within the past 10 years. If they have not, seek an order for the immunization as long as the patient is healthy enough to receive it. Tetanus can be deadly.

Artificially acquired passive immunity is provided by injection with antibodies derived from the infected blood of people or animals. Serum immune globulin is often used for this purpose and is given to people who have been exposed to hepatitis A virus or mumps and who have not been previously immunized. The injection provides antibodies that will protect the person for a short time while their own body begins to develop antibodies to protect against current and future exposure.

Think Critically

What alterations could you make in your lifestyle to make yourself less susceptible to infection?

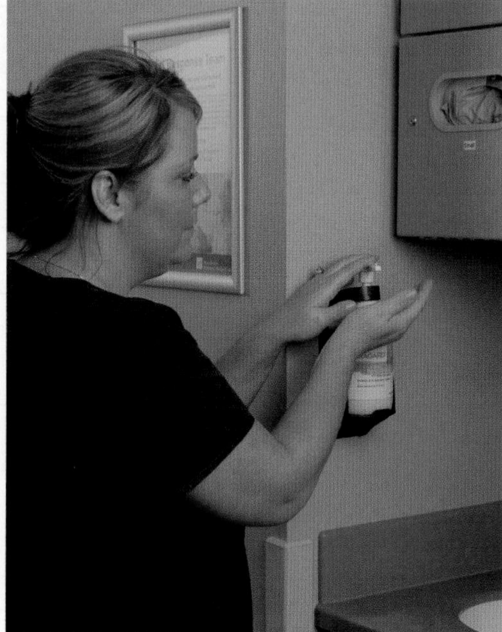

FIGURE 16.4 Nurse using an alcohol hand rub to cleanse the hands of microorganisms.

ASEPSIS AND CONTROL OF MICROORGANISMS

MEDICAL ASEPSIS AND SURGICAL ASEPSIS

Asepsis is the practice of making the environment and objects free of microorganisms. Two types of asepsis are practiced within health care agencies. The first, **medical asepsis**, is the practice of reducing the number of organisms present or reducing the risk for transmission of organisms. It prevents reinfection of the patient and the spread of infection from person to person. It involves cleanliness and is accomplished by protecting items in the environment from contamination and by disinfecting items that have been contaminated. Medical asepsis is referred to as **clean technique** because most, but not all, microorganisms are destroyed.

Surgical asepsis is the practice of preparing and handling materials in a way that prevents the patient's exposure to living microorganisms. Surgical asepsis is referred to as **sterile technique.** It involves sterilization of all instruments and inanimate equipment, as well as use of sterile supplies and sterile technique for procedures that invade the body and for wound care. Most microorganisms are destroyed. Timed hand scrubs may be used by people working in the operating room to reduce the number of microorganisms on the skin, or a hand rub with an alcohol-based product may be used instead. Barrier garments are used to prevent spread of microorganisms between the staff and the patient. The air in the operating room is filtered and exchanged at least 15 times an hour. The operating room must be thoroughly disinfected after each use. Table 16.6 compares medical and surgical asepsis. Techniques for surgical asepsis are covered in Chapters 17 and 37.

Box 16.2 Overview of the Current Centers for Disease Control and Prevention Hand Hygiene Guidelines

The Centers for Disease Control and Prevention recommendations for hand hygiene in health care settings should be followed by all health care agencies and workers. *Hand hygiene* is a term that applies to either handwashing with soap and water, use of an antiseptic alcohol-based hand rub, or surgical hand antisepsis (water and antiseptic agent).

QSEN Considerations: Evidence-Based Practice

Antiseptic Hand Rub

Evidence suggests that hand antisepsis—the cleansing of hands with an antiseptic hand rub—is more effective in reducing health care–associated infections than washing the hands with soap and water.

FOLLOW THESE GUIDELINES IN THE CARE OF ALL PATIENTS

- Continue to cleanse hands with either a non-antimicrobial soap and water or an antimicrobial soap and water (see Skill 16.1) whenever the hands are visibly soiled.
- Use an alcohol-based hand rub to routinely decontaminate the hands in the following clinical situations: (Note: If alcohol-based hand rubs are not available, the alternative is hand hygiene with soap and water.)
    - Before and after direct patient contact
    - After contact with a patient's intact skin (e.g., when taking a pulse or blood pressure or lifting and moving a patient)
    - Before donning sterile gloves when assisting in the insertion of central intravascular catheters
    - Before performing invasive procedures (e.g., urinary catheter insertion, nasotracheal suctioning) that do not require surgical asepsis
    - After contact with blood, body fluids, excretions, or other potentially infectious materials, mucous membranes, nonintact skin, and wound dressings
    - If hands will be moving from a contaminated body site to a clean body site during patient care
    - After contact with inanimate objects (including medical equipment) in the immediate vicinity of the patient
    - After removing gloves
- Before and after eating and after using a restroom, wash hands with a health care facility–approved alcohol-based hand rub or soap and water.
- Antimicrobial-impregnated wipes (i.e., towelettes) are not a substitute for using an alcohol-based hand rub or antimicrobial soap.
- If contact with spores (e.g., *Clostridium difficile, Candida albicans,* or *Bacillus anthracis*) is likely to have occurred, wash hands with soap and water. The physical action of washing and rinsing hands is recommended because alcohols, chlorhexidine products, iodophors, and other antiseptic agents have poor activity against spores.
- Do not wear artificial fingernails, extensions, tips, wraps, gels, or nail jewelry if you have direct contact with patients.

METHOD FOR DECONTAMINATING HANDS

When using an alcohol-based hand rub, apply product to palm of one hand and rub hands together, covering all surfaces of hands and fingers, until hands are dry. Follow the manufacturer's recommendations regarding the volume of product to use. Note how many applications of the product are permitted before handwashing with soap and water must be performed. Most products state no more than five applications before washing the hands with soap and water.

GUIDELINES FOR SURGICAL HAND ANTISEPSIS

- Surgical hand antisepsis reduces the resident microbial count on the hands to a minimum. See Skill 16.1 for the surgical hand scrub procedure.
- The CDC recommends using an antimicrobial soap and scrubbing hands and forearms up to the elbows for the length of time recommended by the manufacturer, usually 2 to 5 minutes. Refer to agency policy for time required.
- When using an alcohol-based surgical hand scrub product with persistent antimicrobial activity, follow the manufacturer's instructions. Before applying the alcohol solution, prewash hands and forearms with a non-antimicrobial soap, clean under the nails, and rinse and dry hands and forearms completely. After application of the alcohol-based product as recommended, allow hands and forearms to dry thoroughly before donning sterile gloves.

GENERAL RECOMMENDATIONS FOR HAND HYGIENE

- Use health care facility–approved hand lotions or creams to prevent irritant contact dermatitis associated with hand antisepsis or hand hygiene.
- Do not wear artificial fingernails or extenders when having direct contact with patients at high risk (e.g., those in intensive care units or operating rooms).
- Keep natural nails, with tips less than ¼-inch long.
- Wear gloves when contact with blood, body fluids, other potentially infectious materials, mucous membranes, or nonintact skin could occur.
- Remove gloves after caring for a patient (see Steps 16.1). Do not wear the same pair of gloves for the care of more than one patient, and do not wash gloves between uses with different patients.

HAND HYGIENE

Hand hygiene is one of the most effective ways to reduce the number of microorganisms on the hands, thereby preventing the transfer of microorganisms from one object to another or from person to person by the nurse. Any person may harbor microorganisms that are harmless to that person but may be potentially harmful to another person if they gain a portal of entry.

Gloves should be used to prevent contact with any blood or body fluids. **Health care workers must perform hand hygiene before and after giving care to a patient.** In 2002, the CDC concluded from research that alcohol-based hand rubs can be more effective than handwashing in ridding the hands of microorganisms (CDC, 2002). These guidelines were reinforced by the World Health Organization (WHO) (WHO, 2009) and remain the current guidelines at this time. Many hospitals and health care agencies provide alcohol-based hand rubs for personnel to use when hands **are not visibly contaminated** (Fig. 16.4). Box 16.2 provides an overview of the current CDC hand hygiene guidelines.

When hands are visibly soiled, the CDC recommends wetting the hands; adding soap; performing at least 15 seconds of vigorous rubbing (friction) to aid in spreading the soap over the hands, fingers, wrists, and thumbs; rinsing the hands under warm running water; and drying the hands thoroughly. Skill 16.1 provides the steps for correct hand hygiene. For a surgical scrub, the hands are washed with soap and water first and then scrubbed with a US Food and Drug Administration (FDA)–approved antimicrobial scrub agent or alcohol-based antiseptic hand rub agent. The procedure for surgical hand antisepsis is presented in Chapter 17.

Do not wear jewelry when you are providing patient care because microorganisms become lodged in the settings of stones, in the grooves of rings, and on the skin beneath the jewelry. The only exceptions are a plain wedding band and a watch with an expandable band that allows it to be pushed up above the wrist area for hand hygiene. Fingernails should be kept clean and short (no more than ¼ inch past

Skill 16.1 Hand Hygiene

 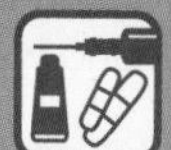 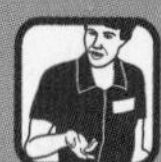  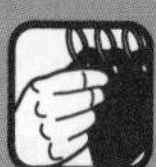 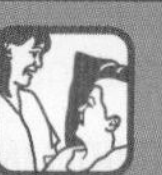 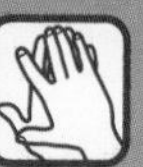 

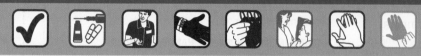

Perform hand hygiene at the beginning of the shift, before and after caring for each patient, before performing procedures, after toileting, before and after eating, before entering special care areas, and whenever the hands have become visibly soiled. Before beginning the shift, wash the hands vigorously for at least 15 seconds (30 seconds or longer if in specialty care areas), or according to agency policy. Thereafter, perform hand hygiene either by washing with soap and water or by use of a facility-approved alcohol-based hand rub product. The Centers for Disease Control and Prevention recommends that no artificial nails, extenders, gels, silk nail wraps, tips, or nail jewelry be worn and that natural nails should be kept no longer than ¼ inch past the fingertips.

Supplies

- Sink with warm running water
- Facility-approved liquid soap
- Disposable paper towels
- Trash can
- Facility-approved hand lotion
- Approved alcohol-based hand rub agent

Review and carry out the Standard Steps in Appendix A.

ACTION *(RATIONALE)*

Handy Hygiene With Soap and Water

1. Determine correct liquid soap agent to be used and length of time needed for handwashing according to task that was completed or degree of hand soiling that has occurred. *(The longer the washing with the approved agent, the more microorganisms are removed.)*

Planning

2. Check that soap and towels are nearby before beginning. *(Saves time.)*
3. Activate the towel dispenser so that towels are ready to tear off when needed before beginning. Push wristwatch and long sleeves (if present) up the arm. *(Activating the towel dispenser prevents contamination of clean, wet hands by the dispenser after washing. Two to four towels are necessary. Pushing the wristwatch and sleeves up the arm protects the watch and clothing from becoming soiled or wet.)*

Implementation

4. Turn on water and adjust to a comfortable temperature with medium water force. Keep body away from sink. *(Warm, continuously running water aids in the removal of microorganisms. Using medium water force to avoid splashing and not leaning against the sink help ensure your clothes are not contaminated.)*
5. Wet your hands with water, pointing your fingers toward the bottom of the sink. *(Water drains from the wrists to the fingertips, carrying organisms away.)*

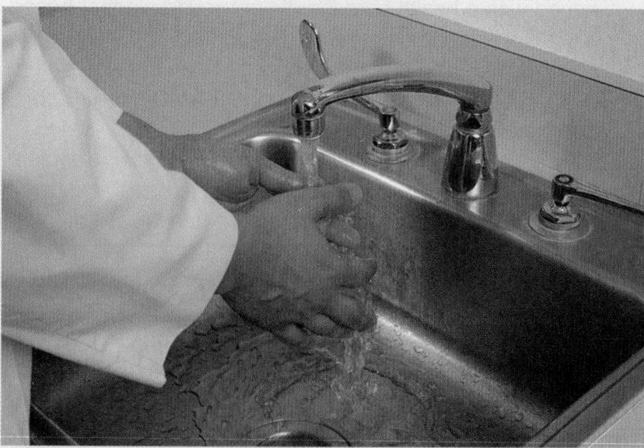

Step 5 **Wetting the hands.**

6. Apply a small amount of liquid soap (2 to 4 mL). *(Using liquid soap rather than a soap bar helps prevent transfer of microorganisms.)*

7. Wash your hands:
   a. Use 10 circular strokes for the palms while applying friction. *(Friction helps work up a lather and loosens or removes microorganisms.)*
   b. Wash the back of each hand with 10 circular motions. *(Vigorous rubbing removes organisms. Ten strokes should dislodge the organisms.)*
   c. Wash the fingers with 10 circular motions; rub the palms together, slide the back of one hand up the palm of the other while encircling the fingers with the opposite hand, and circle the thumb of opposite hand; run the hand over the back of other hand and around the wrist, alternating hands; and interlace the fingers of one hand with those of the other and, with friction, rub back and forth 10 times to clean the spaces between the fingers. Repeat as needed for the full length of the scrub. *(All surfaces of the fingers, hands, and wrists are washed.)*

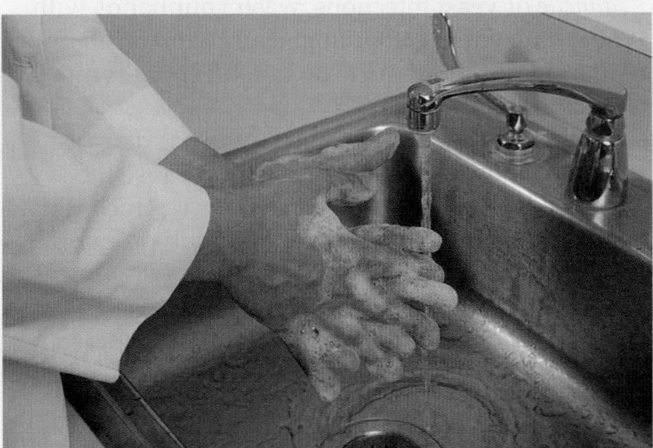

Step 7 **Scrubbing the hands.**

8. Begin rinsing at the wrists, then hands, and fingertips, keeping the fingers pointed downward. Avoid touching any part of the sink or faucet. *(Pointing hands and fingers toward the sink moves debris downward rather than upward onto cleaner areas. Touching the sink would contaminate the newly washed area of the hand or fingers.)*

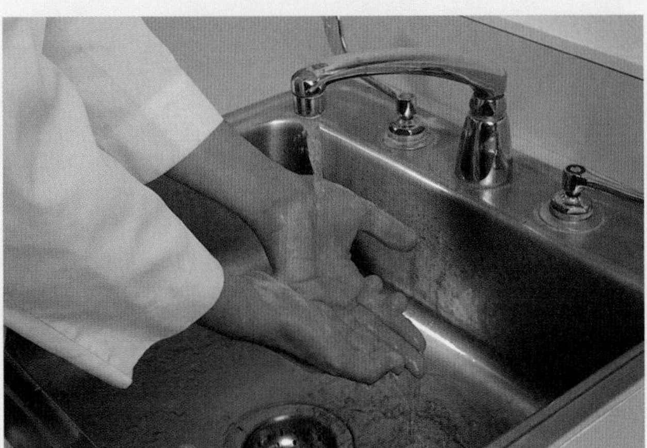

Step 8 **Rinsing the hands.**

9. Remove towels from the dispenser, and dry the hands and wrists thoroughly, beginning at the fingertips, working up the hand to the wrist. Pat hands and wrists dry rather than rub. *(Dry gently but thoroughly to prevent chapping of the skin. Use a clean towel for each combined wrist and hand.)*

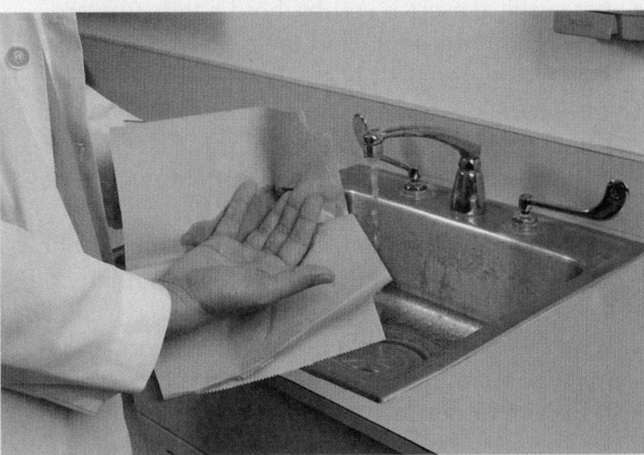

Step 9 **Drying the hands.**

10. With a dry paper towel, being careful not to touch the handles with the bare hand, turn off the water if hand controls are present. Discard towel in trash receptacle. *(Using a clean towel prevents recontamination of freshly washed hands.)*

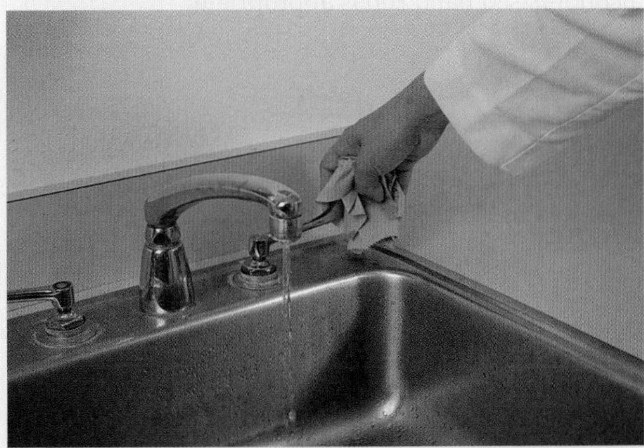

Step 10 **Turning off the water.**

11. Apply hand lotion if subject to chapping. *(Lubricates skin and keeps it soft; prevents cracking of the skin.)*

Evaluation

12. Check to see that hands are clean and dry and have been washed the proper length of time. Assess for breaks in the skin. *(Ensures hands are clean. Breaks in the skin provide a point of entry for microorganisms.)*

Documentation

None required. *(Hand hygiene does not ordinarily need to be documented.)*

Special Considerations

- Visibly soiled hands must be washed with soap and water.
- Wait until lotion has been absorbed before donning latex gloves to avoid increasing the risk of developing latex allergy.
- For surgical asepsis scrubs, hold hands upward throughout the scrub and the rinse. Sinks are used that accommodate this position. When possible, rinse hands with fingertips higher than the wrist.
- When working in a patient's home, a clean hand towel may be used in place of paper towels if no paper towels are available.
- Home care nurses should carry a container of liquid soap and alcohol-based hand rub in their bag.
- Caregivers and family members who have contact with the patient should be taught proper hand hygiene technique.
- If the rim or perimeter around the sink is wet, use a folded dry towel to dry it without contaminating your hands.
- If fingernails are dirty, clean with nail of other hand or with an orange stick.

Hand Hygiene With Approved Alcohol-Based Hand Rub Agent

If hands are not visibly soiled, then the use of an alcohol-based hand rub is appropriate.

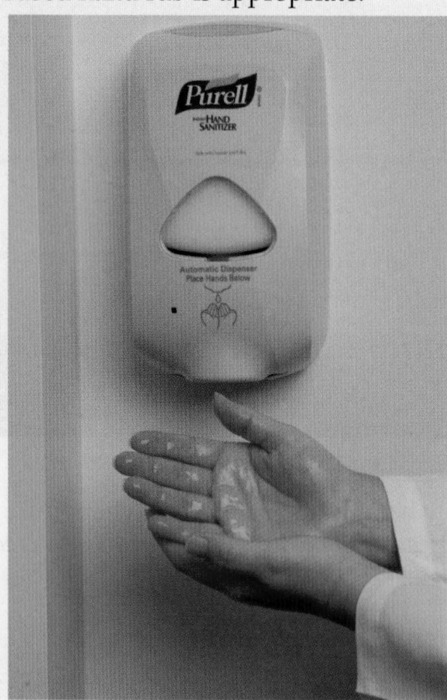

Step 2 **Using hand rub for hand hygiene.**

1. Dispense the required amount of hand rub into the palm of one hand. Using both hands, disperse the product over the entire surface of the hands and fingers to the wrists. *(Follow the manufacturer's written instructions regarding amount of hand rub to use and the number of times it may be used before handwashing with soap and water is required. Different products require different amounts to be used for hand hygiene. Often, after four or more uses of the hand rub, hands should be washed with soap and water. Product must make contact with all parts of the skin to eliminate microorganisms.)*
2. Continue to rub hands together over all surfaces of the wrists, hands, and fingers until all are completely dry. *(Contact with the skin until dry assists with elimination of microorganisms.)*

Special Considerations

- When working with a patient who has *Clostridium difficile* or yeast infections, wash your hands with soap and water rather than using a hand rub product. Hand rub products do not kill spore-forming microorganisms.
- When working with a patient who has diarrhea, wash hands with soap and water because the diarrhea may be caused by *C. difficile,* which is not eliminated by alcohol-based hand rub products.

Critical Thinking Questions

- When assigned to care for two patients, how long would you wash your hands when you have left the room of a patient with diarrhea before entering the room of a patient undergoing chemotherapy for metastatic cancer?
- If you just used an alcohol-based hand cleanser and you enter the room of a patient to perform a physical assessment and the patient states, "I didn't see you wash your hands," what would you do?

the fingertips), both for patient safety and for easier cleaning. Nail polish, if allowed, should not be chipped because it can harbor bacteria. No artificial nails, extenders, silk nail wraps or tips, gels, or nail jewelry should be worn. Proper hand care includes prevention of hangnails and skin abrasions, which provide a point of entry for bacteria.

Health Promotion/Health Promotion Points

Basics of Hand Hygiene

Perform hand hygiene before eating and after using the bathroom, bedpan, or commode. Wash hands thoroughly after handling raw meat. Use supermarket-provided sanitizing wipes to clean the grocery cart handle before using it. Perform hand hygiene after handling money.

Box 16.3 Centers for Disease Control and Prevention Standard Precaution Guidelines

Use Standard Precautions, or the equivalent, for the care of all patients. *Category IB*

A. HAND HYGIENE

1. Wash hands after touching blood, body fluids, secretions, excretions, and contaminated items, whether or not gloves are worn. Perform hand hygiene immediately after gloves are removed, between patient contacts, and when otherwise indicated to avoid transfer of microorganisms to other patients or the surrounding environment. It may be necessary to wash hands between tasks and procedures on the same patient to prevent cross-contamination of different body sites. *Category IB*
2. Use a plain (non-antimicrobial) soap for routine hand hygiene. *Category IB*
3. Use an antimicrobial agent or a waterless antiseptic agent for specific circumstances (e.g., control of outbreaks or hyperendemic infections), as defined by the infection prevention and control program. *Category IB*

B. GLOVES

Wear gloves (clean, nonsterile gloves are adequate) when touching blood, body fluids, secretions, excretions, and contaminated items. Put on clean gloves just before touching mucous membranes and nonintact skin. Change gloves between tasks and procedures on the same patient after contact with material that may contain a high concentration of microorganisms. Remove gloves promptly after use, before touching noncontaminated items and environmental surfaces, and before going to another patient, and wash hands immediately to avoid transfer of microorganisms to other patients or environments. *Category IB*

C. MASK, EYE PROTECTION, FACE SHIELD

Wear a mask and eye protection or a face shield to protect mucous membranes of the eyes, nose, and mouth during procedures and patient-care activities that are likely to generate splashes or sprays of blood, body fluids, secretions, and excretions. *Category IB*

D. GOWN

Wear a gown (a clean, nonsterile gown is adequate) to protect skin and to prevent soiling of clothing during procedures and patient-care activities that are likely to generate splashes or sprays of blood, body fluids, secretions, or excretions. Select a gown that is appropriate for the activity and amount of fluid likely to be encountered. Remove a soiled gown as promptly as possible, and wash hands to avoid transfer of microorganisms to other patients or environments. *Category IB*

E. PATIENT-CARE EQUIPMENT

Handle used patient-care equipment soiled with blood, body fluids, secretions, and excretions in a manner that prevents skin and mucous membrane exposures, contamination of clothing, and transfer of microorganisms to other patients and environments. Ensure that reusable equipment is not used for the care of another patient until it has been cleaned and reprocessed appropriately. Ensure that single-use items are discarded properly. *Category IB*

F. ENVIRONMENTAL CONTROL

Ensure that the health care facility has adequate procedures for the routine care, cleaning, and disinfection of environmental surfaces, beds, bed rails, bedside equipment, and other frequently touched surfaces, and ensure that these procedures are being followed. *Category IB*

G. LINEN

Handle, transport, and process used linen soiled with blood, body fluids, secretions, and excretions in a manner that prevents skin and mucous membrane exposures and contamination of clothing, and that avoids transfer of microorganisms to other patients and environments. *Category IB*

H. OCCUPATIONAL HEALTH AND BLOOD-BORNE PATHOGENS

1. Take care to prevent injuries when using needles, scalpels, and other sharp instruments or devices; when handling sharp instruments during and after procedures; when cleaning used instruments; and when disposing of used needles and other sharp devices. Never recap used needles, or otherwise manipulate them using both hands, or use any other technique that involves directing the point of a needle toward any part of the body; rather, use either a one-handed "scoop" technique or a mechanical device designed for holding the needle sheath. Do not remove used needles from disposable syringes by hand, and do not bend, break, or otherwise manipulate used needles by hand. Place used disposable syringes and needles, scalpel blades, and other sharp items in appropriate puncture-resistant containers, which are located as close as practical to the area in which the items were used, and place reusable syringes, needles, and other sharp devices in a puncture-resistant container for transport to the reprocessing area. *Category IB*
2. Use mouthpieces, resuscitation bags, or other ventilation devices as an alternative to mouth-to-mouth resuscitation methods in areas where the need for pulmonary resuscitation is predictable. *Category IB*

I. PATIENT PLACEMENT

Place a patient who contaminates the environment or who does not (or cannot be expected to) assist in maintaining appropriate hygiene or environmental control in a private room. If a private room is not available, consult with Infection Preventionist regarding patient placement or other alternatives. *Category IB*

STANDARD PRECAUTIONS

Infectious disease can be controlled by interrupting the chain of infection at any link, thus breaking the transmission cycle. The CDC has developed **Standard Precautions** to facilitate breaking the chain of infection. **These precautions protect both the nurse and the patient and are to be used for every patient contact; they include the use of hand hygiene and personal protective equipment (PPE)** (Box 16.3). PPE includes gloves, gowns, masks, protective eyewear, shoe coverings, and hair coverings. In addition, Transmission-Based Precautions may be implemented for patients with known or suspected specific diseases. This will be discussed in more detail in Chapter 17.

Gown

Wear a clean barrier gown that is impermeable to water and other fluids when there is a chance of being splashed with blood, body fluid, or other potentially infectious materials, or when these fluids may be aerosolized. Remove the gown after use, being careful not to contaminate the skin or clothing. Skill 16.2 explains how to put on and take off a barrier gown.

Mask

Apply a regular surgical face mask before entering the room if there is a chance that you will be in contact with airborne pathogens larger than 5 microns (e.g., influenza or meningitis) or splashed body fluids, such as when a patient is coughing or you are performing suctioning. Place the mask over the nose and mouth and secure it in place by an elastic band or ties

Skill 16.2 Using Personal Protective Equipment: Gown, Mask, Gloves, Eyewear

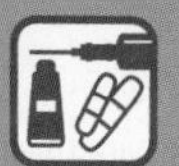
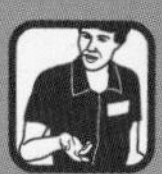

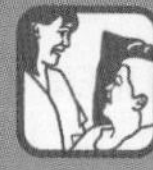
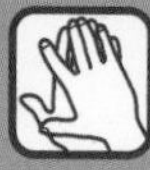

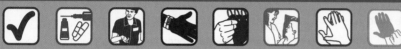

An isolation or barrier gown is most often an impermeable paper gown with long sleeves and cuffs, although a treated fabric gown may be provided. Use a gown whenever your clothing might be contaminated with body substances or airborne microorganisms from a patient who is undergoing isolation precautions. A mask is required when a patient is infected with an organism that can be transmitted by droplet or airborne particles. A mask is also necessary when entering a protective isolation unit to act as a barrier between you and the patient. It is helpful to speak to patients from the doorway and let the patients see your face before donning the mask. Use protective eyewear anytime there is a possibility of being splashed by blood, body fluids, or other potentially infectious materials. Carefully remove all PPE items after use to prevent transfer of microorganisms onto clothing or the environment.

Supplies

- Head cover
- Mask
- Eyewear
- Isolation gown
- Shoe covers
- Gloves

Review and carry out the Standard Steps in Appendix A.

ACTION *(RATIONALE)*

Assessment (Data Collection)

1. Determine PPE equipment necessary and assess cart or anteroom for available supplies. *(Ensures that items needed are present. [Assume that a gown, mask, gloves, and eyewear are needed.])*

Planning

2. Check supplies to see that sufficient numbers of each item are on the cart or in the anteroom for the entire shift. *(Prevents you from having to run to the supply room for an item when you or others are trying to provide care.)*

Implementation

3. Remove a head cover or surgical cap from the box. Place on head, ensuring all hair is covered. *(Minimizes the risk of hair falling onto patient during a procedure.)*
4. Remove a gown from the supply on the cart or in the anteroom of the isolation unit. Hold it by the neck area and allow it to unfold with the opening in the back toward you. *(Allows entry into the gown. A clean gown is used every time the patient's room is entered.)*

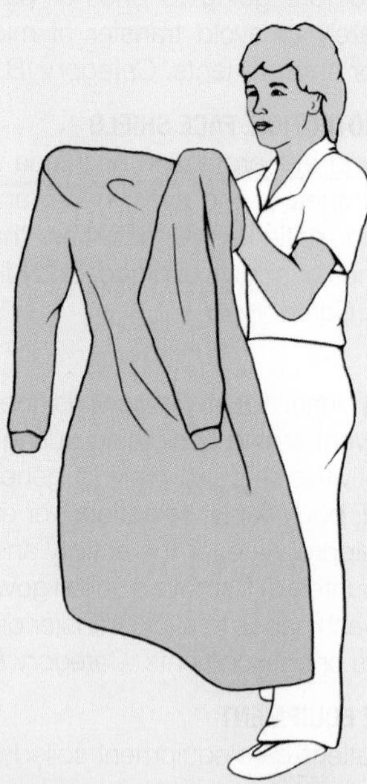

Step 4 **Donning a nonsterile gown.**

5. Slip arms into the sleeves and tie the ties at the back of the neck and the waist. *(The tied gown prevents contaminants from coming in contact with your clothing.)*

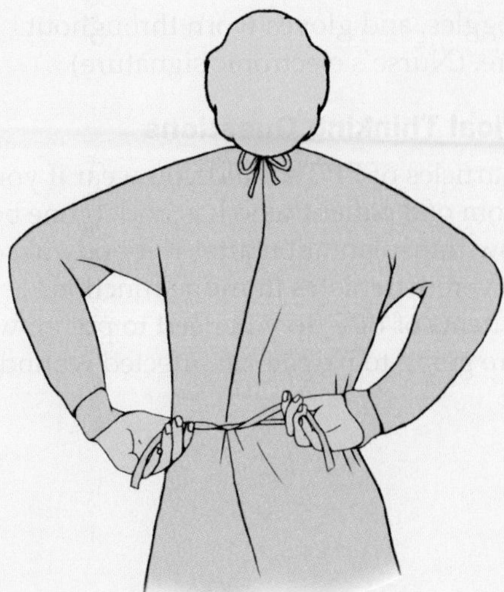

Step 5 **Tying the gown.**

6. Remove a mask from the cart or anteroom and place the mask with the metal band on the outside at the nose. Cover both the mouth and the nose. Secure the mask to the head with the elastic band, or tie the ties above the ears first. Adjust so that the bottom of the mask covers the mouth and chin, then tie it around the neck. *(A mask protects against airborne infection. The mask should fit close to the face without gaps. Accordion-type masks should cover the nose, mouth, and chin. Pinching the metal band so the mask conforms to the shape of your nose helps keep it from slipping. When a special respirator mask is needed, use only an N95 or higher respirator variety. These types of masks require specialized fit testing so that a tight seal is obtained and maintained each time the mask is worn. Regardless of the type, a mask must be replaced if it becomes moist.)*

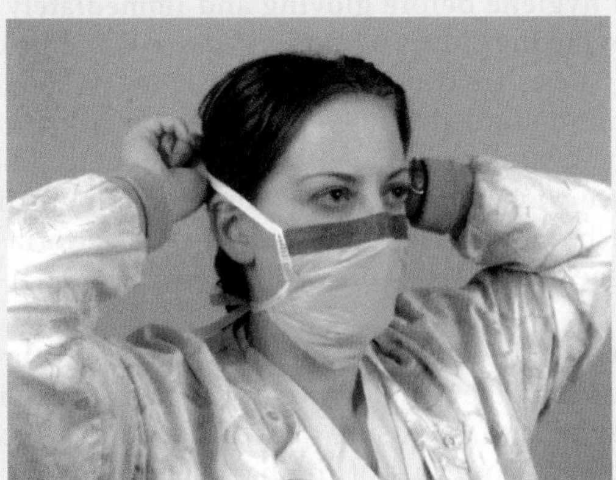

Step 6 **Putting on a mask.**

7. Wear shoe covers and a head cover if there is danger of contamination of the shoes and/or hair or for protective isolation. *(Disposable shoe covers and head cover protect the shoes and hair from contamination and from carrying microorganisms out of the isolation room.)*

8. Put on protective eyewear if such is not attached to the mask. *(Eyewear that has a full face shield that curves around the face, or top and side pieces to protect the eye area, keeps droplets and splashes from entering the mucosa of the eye.)*

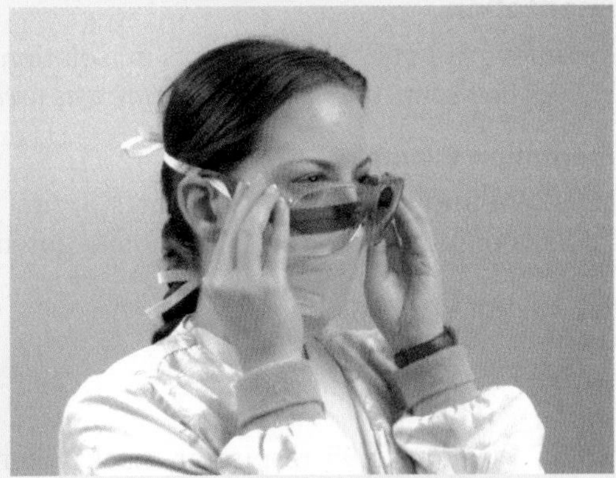

Step 8 **Putting on eyewear.**

9. Don gloves last. *(Glove cuffs are pulled up over the gown cuffs. This prevents any gap of unprotected skin at the wrists.)*

Removing Personal Protective Equipment

10. Remove the gloves without contaminating your hands (see Fig. 16.6 and Steps 16.1). *(If the skin of the hand touches the contaminated surface of the glove, microorganisms can be transferred.)*
11. Remove the protective eyewear without touching your face, and place disposable face covering in the trash. Place reusable eyewear in an impervious container so it can be disinfected. *(Careful handling of the contaminated eyewear prevents transfer of microorganisms.)*
12. If used, remove head cover carefully. *(Prevents possibility of contaminating self or environment.)*
13. Unfasten the waist tie on the gown, then the neck ties. Place your hands inside the neckline, and pull the gown down off the shoulders and over your upper arms. Slip your hands up inside each sleeve. Pull out your arms and hands and place the gown's outside surfaces together so it is turned inside out. Handle only the inside of the gown. Discard it in the proper receptacle. *(Prevents further contamination of the hands and clothing. Reduces transfer of microorganisms.)*
14. Remove the face mask by untying the lower strings first, then the upper ones; or remove it by the elastic band. Discard the used mask in the proper receptacle. *(Reduces transfer of microorganisms. A used face mask should never be allowed to dangle around the neck when not in use.)*
15. Perform hand hygiene. *(Removes microorganisms.)*

Evaluation

16. Ask yourself if the PPE was effective. Would you do anything differently the next time? *(Evaluates technique of garbing in PPE.)*

Documentation

17. Document use of PPE for patients in isolation. *(Verifies that correct protective procedure was used.)*

Documentation Example

10/12 2012 Wound irrigated with 10 mL NS; site clean, no s/s of infection or drainage noted; gown, mask, goggles, and gloves worn throughout procedure. (Nurse's electronic signature)

Critical Thinking Questions

1. What articles of PPE should you wear if you enter the room of a patient who has undergone bone marrow transplantation after full-body irradiation that severely depletes immune function?
2. What items of PPE do you need to put on when you are going to irrigate an infected wound?

PPE, Personal protective equipment.

(Fig. 16.5). Wear an N95 respirator mask when entering an area where airborne microorganisms less than 5 microns in size (e.g., *Mycobacterium tuberculosis* [TB]) are known to be present. N95 respirator masks must be approved by the National Institute for Occupational Safety and Health (NIOSH). They prevent passage of 95% of particulate matter. There are several styles of both regular and respirator masks. When removing masks, handle only the elastic band or ties and discard in a regular waste receptacle; do not leave them hanging around the neck or in a pocket. **Change the mask any time it becomes moist.**

Protective Eyewear

Wear protective eyewear to prevent fluid from entering the eye area and coming in contact with the mucosa or surface of the eye through splattering or aerosolization. Eyewear may be in the form of goggles, a face shield, or glasses with side and top pieces. Protective eyewear may be disposable or durable. If durable, the eyewear should be disinfected after each use. Wear eyewear for performing oral, nasotracheal, or endotracheal suctioning (unless a closed system is used); for performing wound irrigations; and for performing or assisting with procedures in which blood or other body fluids might splatter (e.g., the insertion of a central venous line).

Head Cover

Place a cap or head cover on the head if there is danger of contamination of the hair or if microorganisms resident in the hair might endanger the patient. After use, remove the cap by slipping the fingers beneath the elastic and handling only the inner surface of the head cover to prevent hand contamination. A head cover is also required in select locations such as the operating room because skin can shed into the operative site. This applies even to those who are baldheaded.

Shoe Covers

Cover skin around the ankles by appropriate protective covers whenever there is a chance of splashing body fluids during a procedure. **Shoes are covered so that pathogens are not carried out of the room; the covers are removed when exiting the room in the same manner as the head cover.** Many facilities no longer require staff to wear these; however, staff are encouraged to wear them in places like the delivery room or in the emergency department when dealing with trauma patients.

Gloves

Wear disposable gloves for Standard Precautions when there is a chance of contact with blood or body fluids, mucous membranes, nonintact skin, or secretions or excretions. Also use gloves for handling items contaminated with these substances. Put on gloves after the other pieces of PPE have been donned. When a gown is worn, pull gloves up over the cuffs of the gown. Gloves reduce the possibility of transmission of microorganisms between the nurse and the patient. **Perform hand hygiene before gloving and immediately after removing the gloves because no glove is 100% protective.** Gloves are contaminated once they are used and must be discarded before doing the next task or caring for the next patient. Steps 16.1 show how to properly remove contaminated gloves (Fig. 16.6). Immediately place the gloves in a trash receptacle and perform hand hygiene. **Never reuse or wash gloves.**

Latex allergy. Because of the greater exposure through glove use, more people have developed sensitivity or allergy to latex. Exposure may cause redness, local inflammation, pruritus of the hands, and anaphylaxis. People who have had multiple surgical procedures; who are allergic to bananas, kiwis, or avocados; or who have a history of reactions to other latex-containing products are at risk for developing this allergy. If a health care worker has a latex allergy, by law the employer must supply an alternative type of glove at no cost to the employee. Measures to help prevent latex sensitivity include using gloves in appropriate situations and not for routine tasks in which a blood, body fluid, or microorganism contact exposure is unlikely.

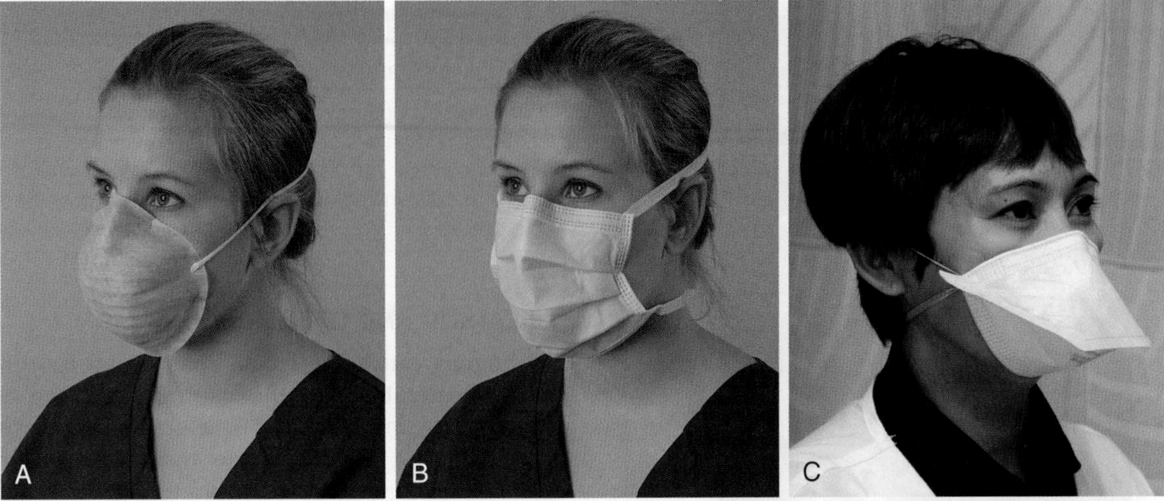

FIGURE 16.5 (A) Preformed mask. (B) Accordion mask with ties. (C) One type of N-95 (particulate filter) mask.

Steps 16.1 Removing Gloves

Use nonsterile gloves for Standard Precautions and most isolation procedures. After use, remove the contaminated gloves in a manner that prevents the spread of microorganisms.

ACTION (*RATIONALE*)

1. Grasp the cuff of the glove of one hand and slide the glove off the hand, folding the outside of the contaminated glove to the inside. *(Care must be taken not to touch the skin of the wrist or hand with the contaminated gloved hand, or microorganisms may be transferred.)*
2. Hold the glove removed in the palm of the other gloved hand, and slip the ungloved hand under the band of the second glove. Roll the glove off, turning it inside out over the first glove. *(Being careful not to touch the contaminated glove with the bare hand reduces transfer of microorganisms.)*
3. Touching only the inside surface of the rolled-up gloves, drop them in the trash. *(Rolling the contaminated gloves together with only the uncontaminated inner surface exposed helps prevent the transfer of microorganisms. Disposing of gloves properly helps reduce the spread of infection.)*

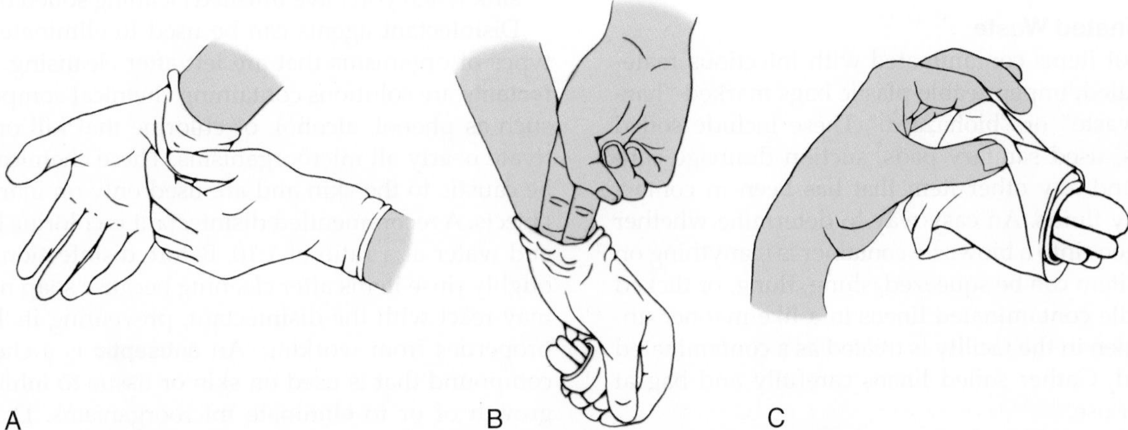

FIGURE 16.6 (A) Removal of the right glove. (B) Removal of the left glove. (C) Method of holding the removed gloves.

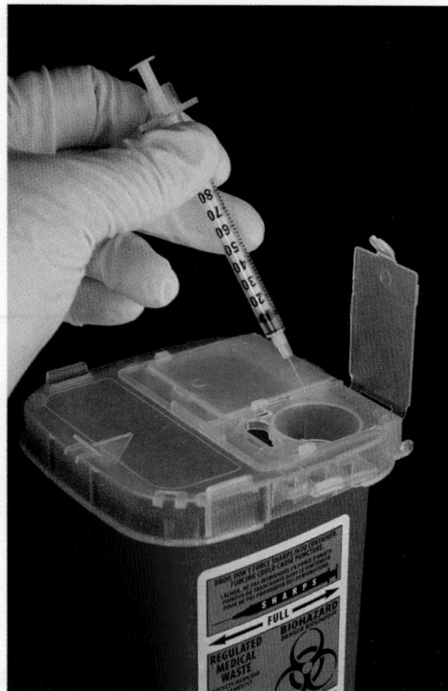

FIGURE 16.7 Deposit a used syringe and needle in a sharps container. (Photo copyright iStock.com.)

Gloves are removed directly over a trash receptacle without "snapping" them off. Do not use petroleum-based lotions under latex gloves because they attract latex proteins from the gloves, which can increase the risk of developing the allergy.

Disposal of Sharps

Disposable sharp instruments, referred to as "sharps," are placed directly into a special puncture-resistant sharps biohazard container immediately after use (Fig. 16.7). Place all needles, intravenous (IV) cannulas, and items that are sharp or might cause a skin break in the sharps container. Replace sharps containers when they are two-thirds full.

Contaminated Waste

Dispose of items contaminated with infectious material in sealed, impermeable plastic bags marked "hazardous waste" or "biohazard." These include soiled dressings, used sanitary pads, suction drainage containers, and any other item that has been in contact with body fluids. An easy way to determine whether an item goes into a biowaste container is if anything on or in the item can be squeezed, slung, flung, or flicked off. Handle contaminated linens in a like manner unless all linen in the facility is treated as a contaminated biohazard. Gather soiled linens carefully and bag at the site of use.

Clinical Cues

Keep used linens away from your uniform. Do not put them on the floor or chair because microorganisms from the patient can be spread this way. Place them directly into the linen hamper.

 **Safety Alert**

Disposing of Sharps

Drop used syringes and other sharps into the container designated for sharps disposal, and then activate the lever that drops the sharp into the container. Never allow your fingers to enter the container. Never recap needles that have been used on a patient.

CLEANING AND DISINFECTION

Pathogens can be killed or inactivated by disinfection, sterilization, or the use of sanitizing agents. Eliminating the reservoir is a good way to prevent transmission. Water, sewage treatment, and rodent control eliminate reservoirs for pathogens.

Appropriate cleaning removes and inhibits the growth of microorganisms. Always wear gloves when cleaning visibly soiled objects or performing wound care. Whether in the hospital, a long-term care facility, or a home setting, follow these steps to clean objects:

1. Rinse the object with cold water to remove organic material. Hot water coagulates the proteins contained in organic material, making them more adherent to the item being cleaned.
2. Once all visible organic material has been removed, wash the object in hot, soapy water. Soap's emulsifying action reduces surface tension and helps remove soil. (How the object is washed and the agent used depends on the object and the manufacturer's recommendation for cleansing and sanitizing.)
3. Use a stiff-bristled brush or abrasive to clean equipment with grooves and narrow spaces. Friction helps dislodge soil.
4. Rinse the object well with moderately hot water.
5. Dry the object; it is now considered clean, but not sterile.
6. Always disinfect the cleaning equipment and the sink when you have finished cleaning soiled objects.

Disinfectant agents can be used to eliminate some types of organisms that are left after cleansing. **Disinfectants** are solutions containing chemical compounds such as phenol, alcohol, or chlorine that kill or inactivate nearly all microorganisms. These chemicals can be caustic to the skin and are used only on inanimate objects. A recommended disinfectant is chlorine bleach and water at a ratio of 1:10. Before disinfection, thoroughly rinse items after cleaning because soap residue may react with the disinfectant, preventing its killing properties from working. An **antiseptic** is a chemical compound that is used on skin or tissue to inhibit the growth of or to eliminate microorganisms. Disinfectants and antiseptics have bactericidal or bacteriostatic properties. A **bactericidal** solution destroys bacteria; a **bacteriostatic** solution prevents the growth and reproduction of some bacteria. Povidone-iodine is an example of an antiseptic. Items that cannot be sterilized, such as skin, can be disinfected with antiseptic agents.

Wounds are cleansed using sterile normal saline or an antiseptic solution. Often a bacteriostatic cream or ointment is applied before the wound is dressed (Nursing Care Plans 16.1 and 16.2).

Sterilization

Sterilization is the best method of eliminating microorganisms from equipment and supplies. There are five methods of sterilization: steam under pressure (moist heat), dry heat, ethylene oxide, liquid chemicals, and hydrogen peroxide gas plasma.

Moist heat is most often used by applying steam under pressure in a device called an **autoclave.** Steam sterilization has four parameters: steam, pressure, temperature, and time. Since it is being applied under pressure, temperatures are higher than the boiling point. Under pressure, steam reaches temperatures of 250°F to 270°F (121°C to 132°C).

Ethylene oxide gas is effective against microorganisms and spores. It is used for heat-sensitive items and where good penetration is essential.

For cleansing items in the home, boiling in water is the easiest method. Items should be boiled for a minimum of 15 minutes. Items that cannot be boiled or disinfected by running them through the dishwasher's "sanitize" cycle can be exposed to direct sunlight for several hours. The heat and ultraviolet rays kill many exposed microorganisms.

Radiation. Ultraviolet light can be used for disinfection. Ionizing radiation is used to sterilize drugs, foods, and other items that would be damaged by heat. Irradiation is now being used on select fruits, vegetables, and meats as a way to ensure a safer food supply in the United States.

SEPSIS IN THE HOME ENVIRONMENT

Precautions are not as stringent in the home as in the hospital because the ordinary home does not contain the many pathogens found in a hospital environment. The number and degree of home precautions are based on whether there is an infected or immunocompromised person in residence and what microorganism is involved. Secure contaminated dressings and other disposable supplies in plastic zip-closure bags before disposal. Place linens contaminated with blood or body secretions in a sealed plastic bag until laundered. Rinse them in cold water as soon as possible, and then wash in hot, soapy water.

A 1:10 solution of chlorine bleach and water can be used to disinfect counters and bathrooms if they become soiled with body secretions. Running the dishwasher on the "sanitize" cycle or rinsing eating utensils with boiling water will reduce microorganisms.

Frequent "damp" dusting and vacuuming decrease the number of microorganisms in the environment. Exposing bedding and other items the patient uses that cannot be disinfected to 6 to 8 hours of sunshine may reduce the number of microorganisms on them. Tissues containing an infected patient's expectorated sputum or nasal secretions should be disposed of in a sealable plastic bag.

Forceps, scissors, and other small implements used for dressing changes can be washed with hot water and detergent, and then soaked in a bleach solution. They should be rinsed with hot water, drained, allowed to air dry, and then stored in a covered container. Drainage bags can be cleansed, disinfected, dried, and reused.

INFECTION CONTROL SURVEILLANCE

In most health care agencies, an infection prevention and control practitioner, known as an infection preventionist (IP), is responsible for ensuring that infection prevention and control measures are followed. When a patient is known to have an infection, the information is typically reported to the IP. This person works with the health care staff to ensure they understand which patient care and environmental cleaning measures are to be used. The IP also assesses the facility for spread of infection. All hospital patients are at risk for HAI, and each nurse must be vigilant in watching for signs of infection in each patient under his care.

Patients at high risk for infection are those who (1) are weakened by injury or severe illness; (2) have another chronic illness; (3) have a central venous catheter, IV cannula, indwelling drainage tube, or endotracheal tube for mechanical ventilation; (4) are very young or very old; (5) have an open wound; (6) have a surgical incision; or (7) have a compromised immune system from chemotherapy or immunosuppression. Whenever an infection is suspected, take additional precautions to prevent the possible spread of microorganisms, which if left untreated could lead to sepsis or even death.

Nursing Care Plan 16.1 Care of the Patient With Abrasions and Splenectomy

SCENARIO Terry Jackson, age 32, was admitted to the emergency department after a motorcycle accident in which he skidded and was thrown into a telephone pole. He has many abrasions on his legs and forehead and underwent a splenectomy for a ruptured spleen.

***PROBLEM*/NURSING DIAGNOSIS** *Incision*/Impaired skin integrity related to surgical incision and multiple abrasions.

Supporting Assessment Data *Subjective:* "These scrapes sting." *Objective:* Abdominal surgical incision covered with a dressing; abrasions on both legs and on forehead.

Goals/Expected Outcomes	Nursing Interventions	Selected Rationale	Evaluation
Surgical incision will heal within 2 weeks without signs of infection. Abrasions will heal within 2 weeks without signs of infection.	Change dressing as ordered using sterile technique.	Sterile technique will decrease likelihood of microorganisms entering the wound.	*Are incision and abrasions healing without signs of infection?* Yes, although the forehead abrasion is draining serous fluid.
	Inspect for signs of infection every shift.	Monitoring temperature, pulse, and WBCs, and inspecting wounds for redness, drainage, warmth, and pain help detect infection.	Temperature 99.0°F (37.2°C), pulse 78, WBCs 10,090. Incision clean and dry; abrasions beginning to scab. *Wound care performed?* Yes, ointment and fresh dressing applied daily.
	Cleanse wound site with prescribed method, then apply antiseptic ointment to abrasions.	Cleansing and then applying antiseptic ointment will decrease microorganisms at wound site.	
	Apply fresh dressing at least daily.	Dressing will prevent further microorganisms from entering the wound.	

PROBLEM*/NURSING DIAGNOSIS** *Surgical incisions*/Risk for infection related to abdominal surgery, splenectomy, and abrasions. **Supporting Assessment Data:** ***Objective: Spleen was removed after it was lacerated in motorcycle accident. Several abrasions sustained in accident.

Goals/Expected Outcomes	Nursing Interventions	Selected Rationale	Evaluation
Patient will not contract tetanus from introduction of microorganisms from road surface.	Administer 0.5 mL tetanus toxoid IM. Monitor for malaise or fever.	Tetanus toxoid vaccine increases antibody production to tetanus bacillus.	*Tetanus toxoid given?* Yes.
Patient will not contract HAI before discharge.	Discourage visitors who have an active infection.	Patients without a spleen are more susceptible to infection.	*Any signs of infection?* No.
	Maintain strict aseptic technique when handling IV lines and urinary catheter and when performing wound care.	Aseptic technique reduces the introduction of microorganisms to the patient.	*Aseptic technique maintained?* Yes. IV site clean, dry, and without redness. Urinary catheter draining clear urine without foul odor.
	Perform appropriate hand hygiene before touching patient, tubes, or dressings and on completion of any procedure.	Hand hygiene significantly reduces the spread of microorganisms to the patient and surrounding environment.	Hand hygiene performed rigorously.

Nursing Care Plan 16.1 Care of the Patient With Abrasions and Splenectomy—cont'd

Goals/Expected Outcomes	Nursing Interventions	Selected Rationale	Evaluation
	Assess for signs of surgical wound infection: chills, redness, swelling, increased pain in area, foul odor from wound, elevated WBC count, purulent drainage.	Serious infection may be averted if early signs of infection are noted.	*Any sign of surgical wound infection?* No, incision clean and dry without redness, swelling, or increased pain. WBC count 10,090. Continue plan.

CRITICAL THINKING QUESTIONS

1. What causes tetanus? Why is it a particular concern for Terry with this type of injury?
2. What other complications could occur if the surgical wound becomes infected?
3. Why are people who have lost their spleen more susceptible to infection?

IM, intramuscular; *IV*, intravenous; *WBC*, white blood cell; *HAI*, health care-associated infection.

Nursing Care Plan 16.2 Care of the Patient With a Foot Wound

SCENARIO Toby Jenkins, age 32, comes to the office after cutting his foot on a piece of glass in his backyard. He was playing barefooted with his dog. He has a ½-inch laceration on the bottom of the ball of his foot. It has been bleeding.

PROBLEM/NURSING DIAGNOSIS *Cut foot*/Impaired skin integrity related to laceration on bottom of foot.

Supporting Assessment Data *Subjective:* States cut foot on piece of glass in backyard; was barefooted. ***Objective:*** ½-inch bleeding laceration on ball of foot.

Goals/Expected Outcomes	Nursing Interventions	Selected Rationale	Evaluation
Laceration will heal within 10 days without signs of infection.	Soak foot in basin with antiseptic solution.	Antiseptic solution will decrease microorganisms in wound. Soaking allows solution to reach all portions of wound.	*Is laceration healing?* Not yet. Foot soaked bid.
	Irrigate laceration using small syringe and antiseptic solution.	Irrigation will reach areas of wound that soaking may not have reached. Pressure helps wash microorganisms from wound.	Laceration irrigated first 2 days.
	Apply antiseptic ointment to wound and dress.	Antiseptic ointment will decrease microorganisms at wound site. Dressing will prevent further microorganisms from entering the wound.	States has redressed wound daily.
	Instruct to stay off foot and keep it elevated as much as possible for 24 to 48 hours.	Elevation prevents pooling of blood and edema at wound site, allowing proper blood flow. Good blood flow allows macrophages to reach the area to help clean the wound.	Kept foot elevated as much as possible for 48 hours.
	Instruct to return in 2 days for reevaluation if redness, swelling, or increasing pain occurs.	Allows for visual assessment of wound for signs of infection.	Wound clean and dry. Progressing toward expected outcomes.

Continued

Nursing Care Plan 16.2 Care of the Patient With a Foot Wound—cont'd

PROBLEM/NURSING DIAGNOSIS *Contaminated wound*/Risk for infection related to laceration of foot with dirty piece of glass in yard.

Supporting Assessment Data *Subjective:* Piece of glass had been imbedded in the soil.

Goals/Expected Outcomes	Nursing Interventions	Selected Rationale	Evaluation
Patient will not contract tetanus from introduction of microorganisms from dirty piece of glass.	Administer 0.5-mL tetanus toxoid IM.	Tetanus toxoid vaccine provides antibodies to tetanus bacillus.	*Are there any signs of tetanus?*
	Instruct to report fever or general malaise.	Fever or malaise can indicate a complication from the vaccine or other infection.	Tetanus toxoid administered. Continue plan.

CRITICAL THINKING QUESTIONS

1. What causes tetanus? Why is it a particular concern for Mr. Jenkins with this injury?
2. What instructions would you give Mr. Jenkins regarding watching for infection and reporting signs and symptoms to the primary care provider?
3. How would you explain the rationale for keeping the foot elevated?

Get Ready for the NCLEX Examination!

Key Points

- Microorganisms are abundant in our environment, and many can cause infection if not controlled.
- Pathogens include bacteria, viruses, protozoa, rickettsia, fungi, prions, and helminths.
- The most effective way to destroy many kinds of microorganisms is to expose them to moist heat at a high temperature for 15 to 20 minutes.
- Standard Precautions are used for all patients to prevent the spread of microorganisms. Transmission-Based Precautions are used when a specific disease is known or suspected.
- The spread of infection is prevented by breaking any one of the six links of the infection chain (see Fig. 16.3).
- Older adults are typically more susceptible to infection due to the effects of natural aging on the body (see Table 16.5).
- Body defenses against infection are intact skin, the inflammatory process, and the immune response.
- The purposes of the inflammatory process are to neutralize and destroy harmful agents, limit their spread, and prepare damaged tissue for repair.
- There are five types of immunity: naturally acquired, passive acquired, naturally acquired passive, artificially acquired, and artificially acquired passive.
- Medical asepsis, or clean technique, reduces the number of microorganisms present and decreases the risk of transmission of microorganisms from one person to another.
- Surgical asepsis, or sterile technique, is a method of preparing and handling materials or equipment in such a way that microorganisms cannot be transferred from them to a person.
- Asepsis is not as stringent in the home environment as in a health care agency, but patients and families must be taught infection prevention and control techniques.
- Hand hygiene is the most effective way to prevent the transfer of microorganisms and is performed before and after caring for each patient.
- PPE is used to carry out Standard Precautions and includes items such as head cover, gowns, masks, protective eyewear, gloves, and sometimes shoe covers.
- Infection prevention and control are the responsibility of all health care workers.
- Pathogens can be killed or inactivated by disinfection, by sterilization, or by the use of antimicrobial agents.
- There are five methods of sterilization: steam/moist heat, dry heat/hot air, ethylene oxide, low-temperature gas plasma, and radiation.

Additional Learning Resources

SG Go to your Study Guide for additional learning activities to help you master this chapter content.

evolve Go to your Evolve website at http://evolve.elsevier.com/Williams/fundamental for additional online resources.

Review Questions for the NCLEX Examination

*Choose the **best** answer for each question.*

1. The most common method of microorganism transfer from one person to another in a hospital is prevented by:
   1. Disinfecting instruments in special solutions.
   2. Filtering the air in the hospital.
   3. Changing bed linens daily.
   4. Performing hand hygiene thoroughly and frequently.
2. The skin is the first line of defense and protects the body by: *(Select all that apply.)*
   1. Repelling microorganisms.
   2. Providing an intact physical barrier.
   3. Secreting bactericidal substances.
   4. Releasing macrophages.
   5. Shedding dead cells.

3. Means to decrease *susceptibility* of individuals to infection include: *(Select all that apply.)*
   1. Discouraging visitors who have an infectious illness.
   2. Using gloves and hand hygiene techniques properly.
   3. Giving antibiotics prophylactically at the time of surgery.
   4. Providing immunization as available.
   5. Promoting good nutrition and adequate rest.
4. Drug-resistant microorganisms are a problem within the community as well as within the hospital. Reasons for this include: *(Select all that apply.)*
   1. Overprescription of antimicrobial agents by health care providers.
   2. Lack of proper sanitation within communities.
   3. Discharging patients with infected wounds before treatment is complete.
   4. Patients who stop taking antimicrobial agents as prescribed.
   5. Overuse of inappropriate antimicrobials causing mutations in the microorganisms.
5. Malnutrition contributes to the susceptibility to infection because:
   1. There is little energy for healing.
   2. It decreases immune function.
   3. It prevents sufficient exercise.
   4. It upsets homeostatic balance in the body.
6. Medical asepsis differs from surgical asepsis in that surgical aseptic technique:
   1. Is only used in the operating room.
   2. Kills all microorganisms.
   3. Aims to prevent transmission of all microorganisms.
   4. Aims to prevent transmission of only disease-producing microorganisms.
7. Considering the chain of infection, a vector might be:
   1. An uninfected patient.
   2. *Staphylococcus* bacteria.
   3. A tick carrying Lyme disease.
   4. A contaminated water supply.

Critical Thinking Activities

Read each clinical scenario and discuss the questions with your classmates.

Scenario A

Discuss specific ways in which a person with a cold who goes to the movies can transmit the virus to others.

Scenario B

You are assigned to care for a patient who has viral pneumonia, a disease of the respiratory tract. What precautions would be necessary?

Scenario C

A parent asks you why her teenage son should be immunized against tetanus when he received the vaccine as a baby. How would you respond?

Scenario D

A neighbor who is an older adult keeps complaining about getting respiratory tract infections and small infected wounds. He asks you what he could do to prevent this. What would you tell him?

chapter

17 Infection Prevention and Control in the Hospital and Home

http://evolve.elsevier.com/Williams/fundamental

Objectives

Upon completing this chapter, you should be able to do the following:

Theory

1. Describe the four stages of infection.
2. List two common health care–associated infections (HAIs) and describe three ways to decrease the occurrence of each.
3. Explain how Transmission-Based Precautions are used with Standard Precautions.
4. Compare and contrast Airborne Precautions with Droplet Precautions.
5. Discuss the special requirements for Airborne Precautions when the patient has pulmonary tuberculosis.
6. Compare infection prevention and control procedures appropriate for the hospital with those used in the home.
7. List techniques for handling specimens; disposing of soiled linen, trash, and sharps; and cleaning equipment in the isolation setting.
8. Give three examples of how the nurse can provide psychosocial care of a patient in isolation.
9. State the four rules of surgical asepsis.

Clinical Practice

1. Use Standard Precautions when caring for patients.
2. Use Transmission-Based Precautions when caring for patients.
3. Properly bag and remove soiled linens and trash from an isolation room.
4. Teach a patient or family member how to properly dispose of soiled items at home.
5. Teach a patient or family member proper hand hygiene techniques.

Skills & Steps

Skill

Steps

Key Terms

airborne precautions (p. 245)
contact precautions (p. 245)
convalescent period (p. 243)
droplet precautions (p. 245)
health care–associated infections (HAIs) (p. 243)
human immunodeficiency virus (HIV) (ĭ-mū-nō-dĕ-FĬ-shŭn-sē, p. 244)
illness period (p. 243)
impervious (p. 246)
incubation period (ĭn-kū-BĀ-shŭn, p. 243)
infection prevention and control (p. 244)
isolation (ī-sō-LĀ-shŭn, p. 244)
leukocytosis (lĕw-kō-sī-TŌ-sĭs, p. 243)
malaise (mă-LĀZ, p. 243)
prodromal period (prō-DRŌ-măl PĔR-ē-ŏd, p. 243)
Standard Precautions (p. 245)
Transmission-based Precautions (p. 245)

Concepts Covered in This Chapter

- Infection
- Patient education
- Safety

INFECTION

STAGES OF INFECTION

Infection occurs when pathogenic microorganisms invade the body and multiply. The infectious process has four stages: the incubation period, the prodromal period, the illness period, and the convalescent period. The length of each period is influenced by many factors, including the organism itself, the host's overall health, and the environment in which infection has occurred.

The **incubation period** begins when the organism firsts enters the body and lasts until the onset of symptoms. During this period, the organism multiplies, and the duration of the period varies depending on the type of microorganism. In many viral diseases, the virus is transmitted during the incubation period.

The **prodromal period** is the short time from the onset of vague, nonspecific symptoms to the beginning of specific symptoms of infection. The patient may experience **malaise**, or a general feeling of discomfort or illness. They may also experience fatigue and elevated temperature. This period lasts a few hours to a few days. It is during this stage that patients are most contagious because microorganisms are most likely to be spread during this highly infectious stage. Typically, precautions against spreading the infection are not taken because people do not realize that they are ill until the more specific symptoms of infection appear.

During the **illness period**, localized and systemic signs and symptoms appear. The individual may have fever, headache, and malaise. Other specific signs of infection may be detected, such as rash, swollen lymph nodes, **leukocytosis** (increased white blood cells), purulent wound exudate, diarrhea, and vomiting. **The severity of the symptoms and the duration of the illness depend on the virulence of the pathogen and the person's susceptibility to the microorganism.** In this phase, people perceive that they are ill and may seek professional care.

The **convalescent** (recovery) **period** begins when the symptoms begin to subside, and it extends until the patient has returned to a normal state of health. This can take days to weeks, depending on the microorganism and the person's overall state of health. As the symptoms subside, patients may feel that they do not need to complete the prescribed medication regimen. Patient education by the nurse must emphasize the importance of finishing medication used to treat the infection, especially during this phase.

HEALTH CARE–ASSOCIATED INFECTIONS

Infections transmitted to a person while receiving health care services are called **health care–associated infections (HAIs)**. A health care worker can also contract an HAI (e.g., head cold, flu, and staphylococcal skin infection) if appropriate precautions are not used consistently. The Centers for Disease Control and Prevention (CDC) estimates that there were about 722,000 HAIs in acute care hospitals in 2011, with approximately 75,000 of these patients dying during their hospitalization (CDC, 2015).

Many invasive procedures predispose patients to infection either because the integrity of the skin or mucous membrane is altered or because an illness reduces the body's ability to defend itself against invading microorganisms. Device-associated infections include central line-associated bloodstream infections (CLABSI), catheter-associated urinary tract infections (CAUTI), and ventilator-associated pneumonia (VAP). If medical devices are not inserted using aseptic technique or appropriately maintained, the likelihood of a device-associated infection increases. Other patients at risk for HAIs include those with surgical incisions with or without drains, implanted prosthetic devices (such as heart valves, vascular grafts, or orthopedic joints, rods, and screws), patients requiring repeated injections or venipunctures for blood tests, and those with a compromised immune system from factors such as chemotherapy, human immunodeficiency virus (HIV) infection, or long-term steroid use.

The Institute for Healthcare Improvement (IHI) developed a VAP bundle based on research and Best Practices. According to the IHI (2012), health care providers can decrease the incidence of VAP by:

- Elevating the head of the patient's bed between 30 and 45 degrees, unless contraindicated.
- Daily "sedation vacation" (reducing sedation) for assessing the patient's ability to breathe independently, allowing mechanical ventilation to be discontinued as soon as possible.
- Prophylaxis (medication) for preventing peptic ulcer disease (PUD).
- Prophylaxis (medication) for preventing deep vein thrombosis (DVT).
- Daily oral care using chlorhexidine, an antimicrobial oral rinse.

The IHI (2015) suggests using the ventilator bundle checklist shown in Figure 17.1 to decrease the incidence of VAP in ICU patients. Although widely used, VAP guidelines are a source of clinical debate and may evolve or need to be changed based on the patient's condition. One area of controversy is the PUD prophylaxis recommendation. It has been shown that increasing gastric pH may promote bacterial growth in the GI tract (Munro & Ruggiero, 2014).

INFECTION PREVENTION AND CONTROL

Infection prevention and control involve:

- Observing patients for signs of infection.
- Recognizing individuals at high risk for infection and implementing appropriate precautions.
- Implementing procedures to contain microorganisms when an infection is suspected or confirmed.
- Monitoring diagnostic reports related to infection.
- Using approved sanitation methods.
- Properly handling and sterilizing or disposing of contaminated items and equipment.

The Infection Preventionist (IP) receives a report from the laboratory every time a culture is performed that is positive for a pathogenic microorganism. A report may also be sent to the IP from the nursing unit

VENTILATOR BUNDLE CHECKLIST
(Individual Patient)

Patient:______________________
Admit Date:______________________

ICU Day	**1**	**2**	**3**	**4**	**5**	**6**	**7**	**8**	**9**	**10**
1. Head of the Bed 30°	☐	☐	☐	☐	☐	☐	☐	☐	☐	☐
2. Daily sedative interruption and daily assessment of readiness to extubate	☐	☐	☐	☐	☐	☐	☐	☐	☐	☐
3. PUD Prophylaxis	☐	☐	☐	☐	☐	☐	☐	☐	☐	☐
4. DVT Prophylaxis	☐	☐	☐	☐	☐	☐	☐	☐	☐	☐
5. Daily Oral Care with Chlorhexidine	☐	☐	☐	☐	☐	☐	☐	☐	☐	☐

Adapted from:
Dominican Hospital
Santa Cruz, California, USA

FIGURE 17.1 Ventilator bundle checklist.

whenever a patient is identified as having an infectious disease or local infection. Appropriate precautions are then initiated for the type of organism present. The IP also investigates all HAIs, looking at possible causes, including breaks in the use of aseptic techniques or approved isolation precautions. The IP provides ongoing education regarding infection prevention and control methods for the health care staff.

Infection prevention and control techniques have undergone many changes over the past three decades. In the United States, current precautions are based on guidelines and regulations developed by the CDC and the Occupational Safety and Health Administration (OSHA). Initially, isolation techniques focused on hospitalized patients, but the evolution of **human immunodeficiency virus (HIV)**, hepatitis strains, Ebola, and a variety of drug-resistant bacteria has broadened the focus related to infectious diseases. Infection prevention and control practices are focused on protecting patients, health care workers, family members, and social contacts in all settings.

Health Promotion/Health Promotion Points

Specific Ways to Prevent Health Care–Associated Infections

- Perform hand hygiene before and after caring for the patient, before donning gloves and after their removal.
- Perform hand hygiene and change gloves between procedures that involve contact with mucous membranes, the perineal area, feces, wound drainage, or other contaminated matter.
- Help all patients on bed rest turn, deep breathe, and cough effectively at least every 2 hours.
- Use correct aseptic technique for cleansing the skin before performing an invasive procedure, such as intramuscular injections and catheter insertion.
- Assess intravenous line sites for signs of infection at least once per shift and each time you access the ports.
- Ensure that devices such as urinary catheters and intravenous are used only for appropriate reasons and remain in the patient only as long as needed.
- Keep the urinary catheter drainage bag below the level of the bladder at ALL times (even when transferring or transporting a patient).
- Clean residual urine off the catheter bag drainage tube after emptying the bag; do not let the tube touch the collection container or floor.
- Clean incontinent patients promptly. Carefully cleanse feces from the surface of indwelling catheters, the skin, and mucous membranes.
- Always cleanse from the urinary meatus toward the rectum (front to back).

Think Critically

What do you think are the most common types of health care–associated infections? Why do you think this?

Infection prevention and control rely on medical and surgical asepsis, Standard Precautions, and Transmission-Based Precautions to prevent or control the spread of microorganisms. The strict use of aseptic technique when performing all diagnostic and therapeutic procedures involving catheters, intravenous (IV) therapy, endotracheal and tracheostomy tubes, drainage tubes, and wound care reduces the incidence of HAIs. The current guidelines for infection precautions are delineated in Box 17.1. **Isolation** is a means of preventing contact between a patient and others to prevent the spread of infection. **Emphasis is placed on containing microorganisms and preventing their spread.**

Box 17.1 Transmission-Based Precautions Requirements

STANDARD PRECAUTIONS
Use for the care of all patients

AIRBORNE PRECAUTIONS
According to the Centers for Disease Control and Prevention, Airborne Precautions prevent transmission of infectious agents that remain infectious over long distances when suspended in the air. Use in addition to Standard Precautions for patients with known or suspected serious illnesses transmitted by airborne droplet nuclei. Examples of such diseases are:

- Measles (rubella).
- Varicella (including disseminated zoster).
- Pulmonary tuberculosis.

DROPLET PRECAUTIONS
Use in addition to Standard Precautions for patients with known or suspected serious illnesses transmitted by large-particle droplets. Examples of such illnesses are:

- Invasive *Haemophilus influenzae* type b disease, including meningitis, pneumonia, and epiglottitis.
- Invasive *Neisseria meningitidis* disease, including meningitis, pneumonia, and sepsis.
- Other serious bacterial respiratory tract infections spread by droplet transmission, including diphtheria (pharyngeal), *Mycoplasma* pneumonia, pertussis, and pneumonic plague.
- Streptococcal (group A) pharyngitis, pneumonia, or scarlet fever in infants and young children.
- Serious viral infections spread by droplet transmission, including adenovirus, influenza, mumps, parvovirus B19, and rubella (Nursing Care Plan 17.2).

CONTACT PRECAUTIONS
Use in addition to Standard Precautions for patients with known or suspected serious illnesses easily transmitted by direct patient contact or by contact with items in the patient's environment. Examples of such illnesses include:

- Gastrointestinal, respiratory, skin, or wound infections or colonization with multidrug-resistant organisms.
- Enteric infections with a low infectious dose or prolonged environmental survival, including *Clostridium difficile.*
- For diapered or incontinent patients, enterohemorrhagic *Escherichia coli* O157:H7, *Shigella*, hepatitis A, or rotavirus infection.
- Respiratory syncytial virus (RSV), parainfluenza virus, or enteroviral infections in infants and young children.
- Skin infections that are highly contagious or that may occur on dry skin, including diphtheria (cutaneous), herpes simplex virus (neonatal or mucocutaneous), impetigo, major (noncontained) abscesses, cellulitis, pressure injuries, pediculosis, scabies, staphylococcal furunculosis in infants and young children, and zoster (disseminated or in the immunocompromised host).
- Viral or hemorrhagic conjunctivitis.
- Viral or hemorrhagic infections (Ebola, Lassa, or Marburg virus).

Two premises underlie the current system of isolation. One is that infection may be present before the diagnosis is made. The second is that the greatest risk of transmitting infection for most microorganisms comes from direct contact by the caregiver's hands or equipment and supplies that have been soiled by blood, body fluids, and other potentially infectious materials. It is known that all body substances may harbor microorganisms and be infectious; therefore, contact with body substances must be avoided.

Current standards consist of two tiers developed by the Healthcare Infection Control Practices Advisory Committee (HICPAC) of the CDC. Tier 1 is Standard Precautions, and Tier 2 is Transmission-Based Precautions. **Standard Precautions** (see Chapter 16) delineate methods for avoiding direct contact with all body secretions except sweat, whether or not visible blood is present. This includes the mucous membranes and all nonintact skin. **Transmission-Based Precautions** (see Box 17.1) are based on interrupting the mode of transmission by identifying the specific secretions, body fluids, tissues, or excretions that might be infective. **Whether used singly or in combination, they are always used in addition to Standard Precautions.**

PERSONAL PROTECTIVE EQUIPMENT

CDC guidelines state that if full personal protective equipment (PPE) is required, it is donned in the following order: the gown, followed by the mask or respirator, and then the goggles or face shield, and finally the gloves. The sequence for removing PPE is gloves, followed by face shield or goggles, and then gown, and finally mask or respirator. Skill 16.2 shows the correct procedure for donning a gown and mask. Skill 17.4 shows the correct procedure for donning and removing sterile gloves. Always perform hand hygiene after removing gloves or any combination of PPE. A nurse who is coughing should wear a mask when in contact with patients.

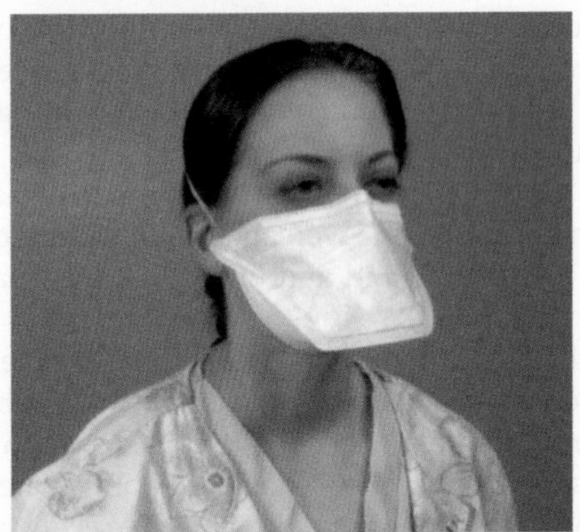

FIGURE 17.2 The N95 (particulate filter) mask.

When the patient has a known or suspected airborne infection such as pulmonary tuberculosis, you must wear a special particulate filter mask called an N95 (Fig. 17.2). Use the same type of mask when caring

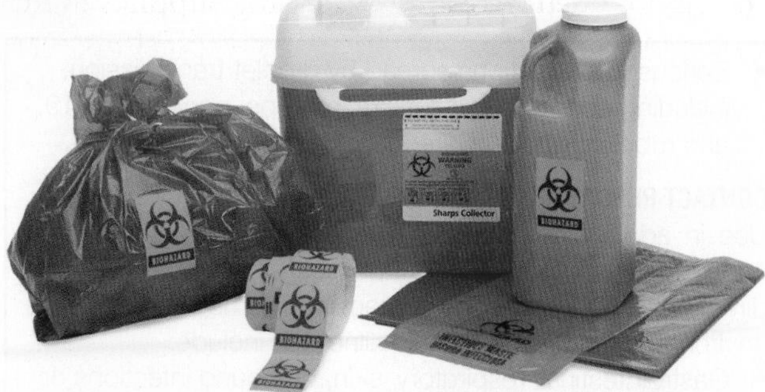

FIGURE 17.3 Biohazard waste bags and sharps containers. (Photo copyright istock.com)

for patients with known or suspected rubeola or varicella unless you are immune to these diseases.

Think Critically

Standard Precautions are to be used when there is possible or expected exposure to which body fluids?

Think Critically

Which Transmission-Based Precaution is used most often in a home care setting? Why?

Although Standard Precautions and Transmission-Based Precautions can seem overwhelming at first, the concepts are actually relatively simple. For example, never touch with bare hands anything that contains fluids from a body surface or cavity. Wear gloves for all contact with body fluids of any sort, including blood, saliva, urine, and feces. The only time gloves are not worn is for contact with intact skin or unsoiled articles. Perform hand hygiene well and often, paying close attention to areas around and under the fingernails and between the fingers.

Another precaution is to wear impermeable gowns when clothing may become soiled with body substances while providing patient care. Wear masks when contact with respiratory droplet secretions is anticipated, such as during oral suctioning. Add protective eyewear when there is the possibility of splashing body fluids. Dispose of all sharps in puncture-resistant containers located in the patient's room (Fig. 17.3), and activate the protective shield on the sharp item before disposal. Place trash and used linens in plastic bags. If items are visibly bloody or heavily soiled with blood or other infectious materials they must be placed in biohazard waste or **impervious** (moisture and particle proof) linen bags (Lillis, 2014).

NEEDLE STICK INJURIES

The CDC (2015) estimates that about 385,000 sharps-related injuries occur annually among health care workers in hospital; therefore, CDC and OSHA brought about guidelines for the development of needleless IV connection systems, syringes, and other devices that could cause a needle stick or puncture the skin with readily activated protective shields to cover needles or scalpel blades immediately after use. Use of these devices has significantly reduced the number of needle stick injuries, one of the major factors in health care worker exposure to pathogenic organisms.

QSEN Considerations: Safety

Decreasing the Spread of Infection

QSEN identifies as a competency that nurses "demonstrate effective use of strategies to reduce risk of harm to self or others" (QSEN, 2014). The nurse must adhere to the Transmission-Based Precautions and wear the appropriate PPE as indicated by mode of transmission. This is always done in conjunction with Standard Precautions.

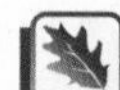

Life-Span Considerations

Older Adults

- Older adults are at greater risk for infection because their immune system is not as active as that of a younger person. The older the person the greater the infection risk.
- An older adult hospitalized for one infection has an increased risk of developing a second infection (a health care–associated infection) because the body's available defenses are already working to fight the first infection.
- Healing is slower in the older adult due to fewer immune cells available to fight infections.

❖ APPLICATION OF THE NURSING PROCESS

◆ ASSESSMENT (DATA COLLECTION)

At the first encounter with the patient, a baseline assessment should include assessing for signs of infection that may require Transmission-Based Precautions. Assess wounds each shift for signs of infection, and alert the primary care provider if an infection is suspected. The primary care provider will likely order a blood culture to confirm the presence of an infection and to determine the appropriate treatment. Admission laboratory studies may also indicate a possible infection (e.g., an increased white blood cell count). If the patient is frequently voiding small amounts of urine, experiencing pain on urination, or has a decrease in overall urine output, this may indicate an infection. A urinalysis will confirm if the patient has a urinary tract infection. If cultures were performed on any bodily fluids, check the reports to see if any microorganisms have been identified. Check the patient's temperature because a fever is usually indicative of an infection.

◆ NURSING DIAGNOSIS

The nursing diagnosis is risk for infection, related to surgical wound, open wound, invasive procedure, tube insertion, or weakened condition. The patient is no longer "At Risk" once the infection has been confirmed.

◆ PLANNING

Expected outcomes include "No HAI is evident." Standard Precautions are used until an infection is diagnosed. Adequate nutrition and hydration is necessary for healing. Patients with compromised immune status are often placed in protective isolation to reduce exposure to infectious organisms. People providing care for these individuals must wear gowns, gloves, and masks, and the patient needs to be in a private room. Specific guidelines vary with the facility and the degree of immunodeficiency. Know and follow your agency's policies and procedures.

If the outcome is not met and the patient contracts an HAI, the nurse must use Transmission-Based Precautions that require putting on PPE before each entry into the patient's room. Donning and doffing (removing) PPE can be time consuming so it is important for the nurse to plan. For example, will you need more linen? Are all the dressing supplies in the room? Does the patient need pain medication? Are routine medications due at this time? Is there drinking water in the room? Speaking to the patient in advance via the intercom can help ensure you will have everything necessary before donning PPE and entering the patient's room.

◆ IMPLEMENTATION

Teach a patient who is at risk for an infection about the disease process, modes of transmission, and precautions necessary to prevent spread of the infection (Nursing Care Plan 17.1). Explain Standard and Transmission-Based Precautions to any visitors.

Use Standard Precautions for each contact with every patient, regardless of whether infection is known to be present.

Nursing Care Plan 17.1 Care of the Patient Under Airborne Precautions

SCENARIO Doug Gamble, age 18, has pulmonary TB. He is in a private isolation room. It is his tenth day of hospitalization. He has just told the nurse he is feeling rejected because everybody wears a mask when they come in to see him.

PROBLEM/NURSING DIAGNOSIS *Does not understand infection precautions*/Deficient knowledge related to infection and mode of transmission.

Supporting Assessment Data *Subjective*: States he cannot understand why he has to stay in his room and why people have to wear masks to visit. *Objective*: Purified protein derivative (PPD) skin test positive. Sputum culture positive for acid-fast bacilli. Radiologic studies: Cavitations in apex of right lung. Medical diagnosis: Active pulmonary TB.

Goals/Expected Outcomes	Nursing Interventions	Selected Rationales	Evaluation
Patient will voice understanding of the pathogen and need for Transmission-Based Precautions.	Teach regarding pathogen that causes pulmonary TB, transmission of the organism, and need for masks and staying in room.	Understanding of disease transmission will help patient adhere to Transmission-Based Precautions.	*Does patient understand the need for precautions?* States he understands need for precautions.
	Teach specifics of good hand hygiene and respiratory etiquette, including covering the mouth when coughing and containment of used tissues and sputum.	Hand hygiene and proper respiratory etiquette will help prevent transmission of pathogen.	Attentive to hand hygiene, covers mouth when coughing, disposes of tissues appropriately: expected outcome being met.

PROBLEM/NURSING DIAGNOSIS *Under visitor precautions*/Impaired Social Interaction related to Transmission-Based Precautions

Supporting Assessment Data *Objective*: In private isolation room for Airborne Precautions. Visitors must wear an N95 mask when in the room. No visitors except parents since admission.

Goals/Expected Outcomes	Nursing Interventions	Selected Rationales	Evaluation
Patient will have visits with family or friends at least daily.	Speak with parents about the need for social interaction. Remind that people may visit if they wear the appropriate mask in the room.	Understanding may promote cooperation and obtain visitors for patient.	*Are visitors coming?* Parents verbalize understanding the need for social interaction.

Nursing Care Plan 17.1 Care of the Patient Under Airborne Precautions—cont'd

Goals/Expected Outcomes	Nursing Interventions	Selected Rationales	Evaluation
	Ask parents to call patient's friends and ask them to visit and arrange a visiting schedule.	A schedule for visiting will promote properly spaced visits that may increase social interaction without tiring the patient.	Mother is working on a visitor schedule. Continue plan.

PROBLEM/NURSING DIAGNOSIS *Feels rejected*/situational low self-esteem.

Supporting Assessment Data *Subjective*: States he feels rejected and dirty because people have to wear a mask whenever they are in his room. *Objective*: Transmission-Based Precautions call for an N95 mask whenever in the room.

Goals/Expected Outcomes	Nursing Interventions	Selected Rationales	Evaluation
Patient will adjust to Transmission-Based Precautions requirements by showing less anxious behavior when someone with a mask enters the room.	Remind patient of the route of transmission of TB. Assure him that the wearing of masks simply protects the visitors and caregivers.	Understanding the virulence of the organism and mode of transmission will help him understand the need for N95 masks and how they differ from surgical masks.	*Is patient less anxious?* Patient states he understands the danger of the organism and how it is transmitted.
	Ask that each health care person entering the room show her face at the door before donning a mask.	Showing the patient the face behind the mask makes the interaction more personal and friendly.	Each caregiver shows face and introduces self at the door.
	Show warm interest in the patient as a person. Include ordinary conversation during interactions so he knows he is seen as a person, not a disease.	Interest in the patient bolsters feelings of self-esteem.	Talking with patient about his interests appears to decrease feelings of isolation and help him cope. Progressing toward expected outcome.

CRITICAL THINKING QUESTIONS

1. How would you assess Doug's understanding of his illness?
2. Why is it important to schedule rest between activities for Doug?
3. Why is it important to keep Doug well nourished and hydrated?

TB, Tuberculosis.

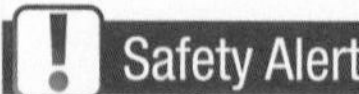

Safety Alert

Hand Hygiene

Hand hygiene is the most important action in preventing the transmission of infection (see Chapter 16). Perform hand hygiene before and after contact with a patient, wound care, or any invasive procedure. Perform hand hygiene before donning and after doffing gloves. Even tasks such as interviewing the patient requires that hand hygiene be performed before leaving the room, whether you touched the patient or not.

Always perform hand hygiene after touching the patient or anything in the patient's room. Methicillin-resistant *Staphylococcus aureus* (MRSA) and other pathologic organisms can survive for varying periods on almost any surface.

Think Critically

What personal protective equipment would you don to take the vital signs of someone under Airborne Precautions? How would this differ from someone on Droplet Precautions?

General Guidelines for Isolation Precautions

Specimen preparation and transportation. Before collecting body fluid or other potentially infectious material, verify the primary care provider's order and complete the correct laboratory requisition form. Next, label the specimen container with the patient's name and medical record number. Place the label on the container itself, not the lid because once the lid is removed in the laboratory, the specimen would be unlabeled. Don gloves and explain to the patient what is needed. Then collect the specimen without contaminating the outside of the container. Apply the lid, ensuring it is fully tightened. Clean or disinfect containers that are visibly contaminated before placing them in the laboratory transport bag. Place the secured laboratory specimen container in a plastic specimen bag and close the bag lock seal. Complete the laboratory requisition form and place it in the envelope pocket on the outside of the transport biohazard bag before leaving the patient's room. Both OSHA and the Clinical Laboratory Improvement Act (CLIA) require that specimens be transported to the laboratory in a plastic bag marked "biohazard." Remove gloves, perform hand hygiene, and then, following facility protocol, send the specimen to the clinical laboratory for processing.

Nursing Care Plan 17.2 Care of the Patient Under Droplet Precautions

SCENARIO Ricardo Hernandez, age 46, has streptococcal pneumonia. He is in a private isolation room. It is his third day of hospitalization. He is bored and has stated he feels upset because everyone has to wear a mask when close to him.

PROBLEM/NURSING DIAGNOSIS *Does not understand use of masks*/Deficient knowledge related to infection and mode of transmission.

Supporting Assessment Data *Subjective:* States that he cannot understand why he has to stay in his room and why people have to wear masks to visit. *Objective:* Sputum culture shows streptococci. X-ray diagnosis: pneumonia.

Goals/Expected Outcomes	Nursing Interventions	Selected Rationale	Evaluation
Patient will voice understanding of the pathogen and need for transmission precautions.	Teach regarding disease, pathogen that causes it, its transmission, and need for transmission precautions. Teach specifics of good hand hygiene and containment of tissues and sputum.	Understanding of disease, pathogen, and way it is transmitted helps patient adhere to transmission precautions. Hand hygiene decreases transmission of pathogens. Containment of tissues and sputum will help prevent transmission of pathogen.	*Does he express understanding of special precautions?* States that he understands need for precautions. Attentive to hand hygiene. Expected outcome being met.

PROBLEM/NURSING DIAGNOSIS *In isolation room*/Impaired social interaction related to transmission precautions.

Supporting Assessment Data *Objective:* In private isolation room for Droplet Precautions. Visitors must wear a mask if within 3 feet of the patient. Has had only two visitors in 3 days.

Goals/Expected Outcomes	Nursing Interventions	Selected Rationale	Evaluation
Patient will have visits of family or friends at least twice a day.	Speak with spouse about the need for social interaction. Remind that people do not need to wear a mask if they stay at least 3 feet away from the patient.	Understanding may promote cooperation and obtain visitors for patient.	*Are visitors coming twice a day?* Not yet. Spouse states she understands.
	Ask spouse to call friends, ask them to visit, and arrange a visiting schedule.	A schedule for visiting will promote properly spaced visits that may increase social interaction.	Spouse working on visiting schedule. Continue plan.

PROBLEM/NURSING DIAGNOSIS *Upset by Droplet Precautions*/Situational low self-esteem.

Supporting Assessment Data *Subjective:* States that he feels upset and dirty because people have to wear a mask when close to him. *Objective:* Droplet Precautions call for a mask when within 3 feet of the patient.

Nursing Care Plan 17.2 Care of the Patient Under Droplet Precautions—cont'd

Goals/Expected Outcomes	Nursing Interventions	Selected Rationale	Evaluation
Patient will adjust to transmission precautions requirements by showing less anxious behavior when someone with a mask enters the room.	Discuss the properties of the streptococcus organism. Discuss how streptococcal infection is transmitted. Assure patient that the wearing of masks simply protects the caregivers. Ask that each person entering the room show his or her face at the door before donning a mask. Show warm interest in the patient as a person. Praise patient for evidence of positive coping mechanisms.	Understanding the virulence of the organism and that it is transmitted by droplets will help him understand the need for masks to prevent transmission to caregivers. Showing the patient the face behind the mask makes the interaction more personal and friendly. Interest in the patient bolsters feelings of self-esteem. Positive reinforcement of good coping behaviors enhances self-esteem.	*Is patient less anxious when masked personnel are in the room?* Is less anxious. Patient states that he understands the danger of the organism and how it is transmitted. Each caregiver shows face and introduces self at the door. Talking with patient about his interests and occupation appears to decrease anxiety and help him cope. Progressing toward expected outcome.

CRITICAL THINKING QUESTIONS

1. How would you assess Mr. Hernandez to determine how to alleviate his boredom?
2. Why is it important to schedule rest between social or other activity for Mr. Hernandez?
3. Why is it important to keep Mr. Hernandez well hydrated?

Soiled linens. Soiled linen is handled as little as possible. Roll it up and place it inside the linen hamper in the patient's room. Never carry unbagged soiled linens in the hallway because it increases the risk of contaminating the surrounding environment. When the bag is two-thirds full, tie it closed and send it to the laundry according to agency policy. Double bagging is not necessary.

Trash and biohazard waste. Place disposable soiled equipment and supplies inside the plastic bag lining the waste receptacle in the patient's room. Red bags marked with a biohazard symbol are for biohazardous waste only. Ordinary trash is to be placed in standard trash bags and disposed of in the routine manner. Biohazardous waste requires special disposition that is very costly, and non-biohazardous trash should never be mixed in with it. To determine the type of trash receptacle to use, if an item were squeezed, slung, flung, or flicked, such as a soiled dressing, and it could release blood or body fluids, then it goes in the red biohazard bag. The biohazard bag is sealed when it is two-thirds full, removed, and sent to waste collection. The only time double bagging is necessary is if the plastic bag is soiled on the outside. In this instance, another nurse standing just outside the room's doorway holds open a second plastic bag, placing her gloved hands under the edge of the bag, which is folded outward to cover the nurse's hands. This further protects her hands from soiling. The nurse in the patient's room then places the first bag carefully inside the second one. The nurse outside the room ties the bag closed, being careful not to touch the inner first bag. Gloves are removed. The bag is taken to the soiled utility room for disposal. Then hand hygiene is performed.

Sharps. **Needles are not to be recapped before disposal.** Drop all used needles, scalpel blades, IV cannulas, suture needles, and other sharp items into a puncture-resistant sharps biohazard container. **Never put your fingers or hands inside the opening of the sharps container** (see **Chapter 35**). Shake the container gently to settle the contents and make more room if necessary. Replace sharps containers when they are two-thirds full. Seal the full sharps container and send it to the biohazard waste storage area for later removal. Federal policy and state laws require that sharps containers be secured in patient care areas, and that holding areas for biohazards must be accessible to staff only.

Other equipment. Clean reusable equipment if it is visibly soiled, and then send it to the central processing department to be disinfected. A disposable stethoscope and blood pressure cuff are issued to the isolation patient, and only these are to be used within the isolation room. When the patient is discharged, dispose of them in the regular trash. No special treatment is necessary for dishes. Some agencies use paper dishes, plastic utensils, and trays for a patient under Transmission-

Box 17.2 General Principles Regarding Isolation

- Floors are contaminated. Anything dropped on the floor is contaminated and must be discarded or cleaned carefully before reuse.
- Patients with communicable diseases should be grouped according to the epidemiology of transmission:
  - Contact through respiratory spread
  - Transmission by the gastrointestinal tract
  - Direct contact with wound or skin infection
- Minimize dust. Sweeping compounds or wet mops with disinfectants and damp dusting must be used for this purpose.
- Protect the patient from drafts.
- Establish contaminated and clean zones. The clean areas include those used by the health care worker. The patient should not use items outside the unit such as telephones. There should be a clean area in the isolation unit where no contaminated articles are permitted. Items not in the clean area are considered contaminated.
- Anything that is brought into the isolation area must not be removed except in proper containers, which are then placed in an outside container labeled "Hazardous Materials—Biohazard."
- Never rub your eyes or nose or put your hands near your mouth when taking care of a patient in an isolation unit.
- Never shake linen when removing it or placing it on the bed.
- Change gloves and perform hand hygiene after handling contaminated items.
- Provide a clean area for placement of supplies by putting a paper towel or square of paper on a dry surface.
- Keep a water pitcher and glass in the room. Ice and fresh water are brought to the door and transferred.
- Faucets should be turned on and off using a dry paper towel to protect the hands from recontamination.
- The same nursing procedures are carried out for these patients as for any patient, but you must use the appropriate barrier precautions.
- Use the room clock for taking the patient's pulse and respirations. If the room does not have a clock, your watch can be taken in by putting it in a clear plastic bag. When leaving the room, it can be emptied onto a clean paper towel.
- You should monitor your own level of resistance to infection and report to the unit director or charge nurse any skin lesion, sore throat, or other evidence of infection you may have. (You may be reassigned to protect yourself and the patient.)

Based Precautions, but this is not a CDC requirement. Box 17.2 presents other general principles.

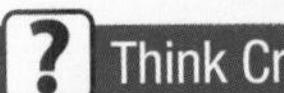

Think Critically

What types of trash would you place in a red biohazard bag? What type of procedure would require the nurse to use a red biohazard bag?

Natural defenses. Institute measures to protect and enhance the patient's natural body defenses (see Chapter 16). Protect intact skin and mucous membranes, promote a balanced diet and sufficient fluids, provide opportunity for adequate sleep and rest, and decrease stress as much as possible.

Patient placement. Place a patient in need of Transmission-Based Precautions in a private room. An exception can be made if another patient has the same type of infection: they can be roomed together. A patient with an airborne transmissible disease would be placed in an Airborne Infection Isolation Room (AIIR) and on Airborne Precautions. Keep the door to the room closed except when someone is entering or leaving. This helps ensure the organism remains contained and does not enter the rest of the unit. Box 17.3 presents isolation precautions recommended for hospitals.

Transporting the patient. Avoid transporting the isolation patient unless necessary. If transporting is unavoidable, give the patient a standard mask to wear while out of the room. For a patient under Droplet Precautions, take measures to prevent soiling of the environment. Notify the unit or department receiving the patient ahead of time that a patient under this particular type of Transmission-Based Precautions is coming to the area. Share information about any additional precautions required with those receiving the patient.

QSEN Considerations: Teamwork and Collaboration

Effective Communication

Follow communication practices that minimize risks associated with handoffs among providers and across transitions in care. It is vital that the nurse communicate to health care providers of other departments the type of Transmission-Based Precaution that the patient is on prior to transporting the patient. This will ensure all safety measures are implemented before the patient's arrival.

Infection Prevention and Control in the Home

The patient at home has less exposure to HAIs, but can still be at risk. Recent data indicate that around 3.5% of patients receiving home care develop an infection severe enough to require emergency treatment or hospitalization (Shang, Larson, Liu, & Stone, 2015). The emphasis in the home environment is on containing pathogens and preventing transmission to health care personnel, caregivers, and others in the household. The home health nurse must teach patients and families the importance of hand hygiene; how to dispose of contaminated medical supplies; and methods for cleaning the home environment, including how to dispose of dirty supplies safely (Box 17.4).

Box 17.3 Recommended Isolation Precautions in Hospitals: Transmission-Based Precautions (Tier 2)

AIRBORNE PRECAUTIONS

Use the Tier 1 precautions (Standard Precautions), as well as the following:

1. Place the patient in a private room that has negative air pressure: 6 to 12 air exchanges per hour and discharge of air to the outside or a filtration system for the room air.
2. If a private room is not available, place the patient with another patient who is infected with the same micro-organism. In select situations, approval from the local health department may be required (e.g., for a patient with pulmonary tuberculosis).
3. Wear a respiratory device (N95 respirator) when entering the room of a patient who is known to have or suspected of having primary tuberculosis.
4. Susceptible people should not enter the room of a patient who has rubella (measles) or varicella (chickenpox). If they must enter, they should wear an N95 respirator.
5. Limit movement of the patient outside the room to essential purposes. Place a surgical mask on the patient if possible.

DROPLET PRECAUTIONS

Use the Tier 1 precautions (Standard Precautions), as well as the following:

1. Place the patient in a private room.
2. If a private room is not available, place the patient with another patient who is infected with the same microorganism.
3. Wear a mask if working within 3 feet of the patient.
4. Transport the patient outside of the room only when necessary, and place a surgical mask on the patient if possible.

CONTACT PRECAUTIONS

Use the Tier 1 precautions (Standard Precautions), as well as the following:

1. Place the patient in a private room.
2. If a private room is not available, place the patient with another patient who is infected with the same microorganism.
3. Wear gloves as described in Standard Precautions.
   a. Change gloves after contact with infectious material.
   b. Remove gloves before leaving the patient's room.
   c. Cleanse hands immediately after removing gloves. Use an antimicrobial hand rub agent or soap and running water.
   d. After hand hygiene, do not touch possibly contaminated surfaces or items in the room.
4. Wear a gown when entering a room if there is a possibility of contact with infected surfaces or items, or if the patient is incontinent or has diarrhea, a colostomy, or wound drainage not contained by a dressing.
   a. Remove your gown in the patient's room.
   b. Make sure clothing does not contact possible contaminated surfaces.
5. Limit movement of the patient outside the room.
6. Dedicate the use of noncritical patient care equipment to a single patient or to patients with the same infecting microorganisms.

Box 17.4 Infection Prevention in the Home

1. Wash your hands often.
   - **When:** Before eating; before, during, and after handling or preparing food; before dressing a wound, giving medicine, or inserting contact lenses; after contact with body fluids or blood; after changing a diaper; after using the bathroom; after handling animals or their toys, leashes, or waste; after handling anything contaminated, such as trash, drainage, or soil.
   - **How:** Wet hands, apply soap, briskly rub hands together for 20 seconds, rinse thoroughly with warm water, and dry with a clean paper towel.
2. Routinely clean surfaces.
   - **In the kitchen:** Clean counters, cutting boards, and all other surfaces before, during, and after preparing food, especially meat and poultry. Use hot, soapy water and scrub cutting boards well.
   - **In the bathroom:** Clean and disinfect all surfaces routinely.
3. Handle and prepare food safely.
   - **Clean:** Clean hands and work surfaces often.
   - **Separate:** Do not cross-contaminate one food with another; use separate cutting boards for meat and fresh produce and keep food separate in the refrigerator.
   - **Cook:** Cook foods to proper temperatures; use a food thermometer. Find recommended food cooking temperatures at www.fightbac.org/cook or http://www.fsis.usda.gov/wps/portal/fsis/topics/food-safety-education/teach-others/fsis-educational-campaigns/is-it-done-yet.
   - **Chill:** Refrigerate foods promptly.
4. Get immunized.
   - Make certain you and your loved ones get the necessary shots suggested by your health care provider at the proper time, and maintain immunization records for the family. Ask your primary care provider about special programs that provide free shots for your child or older family members.
5. Use antimicrobials appropriately.
   - Take antimicrobials exactly as prescribed by your health care provider. Antimicrobials do not work against viruses such as colds or the flu.
6. Be careful with pets.
   - Follow the immunization schedule for your pets as recommended by the veterinarian.
   - Clean litter boxes daily.
   - Make certain your child does not put any object or hands in the mouth after touching animals.
   - Wash hands thoroughly after contact with animals, especially after visiting farms, petting zoos, and fairs.
   - Use flea and tick prevention treatment on cats and dogs.
7. Avoid contact with wild animals.
   - Do not leave food around, and keep garbage cans sealed around your home.
   - Clear brush, grass, and debris around your home.
   - Seal any entrance holes to animal dens, if any are found inside or outside of your home.
   - Use insect repellent to prevent ticks.

Home Care Considerations

Infection Prevention and Control Precautions for Patients in the Home Setting

- Teach patients, families, and caregivers the importance of hand hygiene. Stress that hands must be cleansed before caring for the patient and after care is finished. Gloves are needed in addition to hand hygiene for tasks such as tracheal suctioning and tracheostomy care, dressing changes and wound or drain care, tube feedings, and cleansing of personal areas of the body.
- Discard used dressings, tissues, wound-cleaning supplies, and any other item contaminated with body fluids into a plastic bag; seal the bag before placing it in the household trash for pickup.

When the patient has an infection, keep his towels, sheets, and clothes away from others until they can be washed. The patient's clothing and linens, in most cases, can be laundered with the household wash. Washing in warm water with standard laundry detergent is usually sufficient. Dry items thoroughly before use. Launder significantly contaminated clothing or linens separately from other household laundry.

Teach the patient to perform hand hygiene and to dispose of paper towels and facial tissues in an appropriate container. Instruct other family members to perform hand hygiene frequently. The bathroom should be cleaned daily with standard household cleaning agent or a 1:10 solution of chlorine bleach and water. Dishes should be washed on the hot (or sanitize) cycle of the dishwasher or soaked in scalding hot water after washing and allowed to air dry. Dispose of soiled dressings and wound care supplies in plain, unlabeled plastic bags that are tied up securely and stored in an appropriate trash receptacle for pickup with the rest of the household trash. Trash marked with the biohazard symbol, in accordance with state and federal laws, cannot be placed in the household trash receptacles. If these bags are found in the trash that is taken to a public dump site, the homeowner could be heavily fined for violating this law. Handling or transporting biohazard trash requires special permits.

A heavy plastic jug, such as an empty bleach bottle, with a secure top can be used to contain needles, syringes, and other sharp objects used in the patient's care. Placing a 1:10 solution of chlorine bleach and water in the container helps kill microorganisms. Disposal of the jug is subject to local regulations in the city, county, or province where the patient lives.

Use clean gloves for wound care unless there is an order for sterile dressing changes. Teach patients and family members to remove and dispose of contaminated gloves properly. Emphasize to wash hands before putting on gloves, and again after the gloves are discarded. Reinforce that gloves should never be reused.

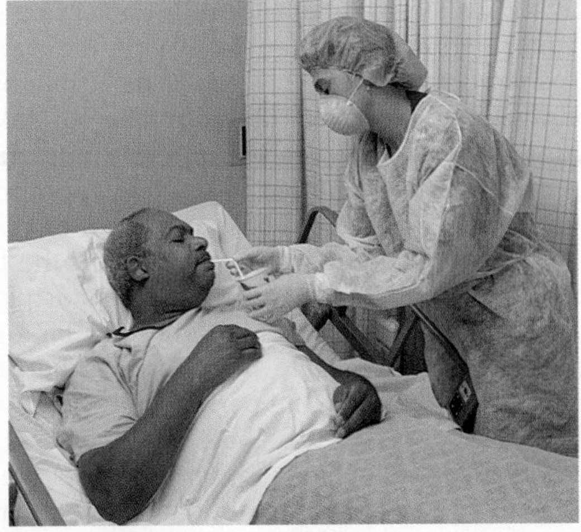

FIGURE 17.4 Nurse in personal protective equipment caring for a patient in a protective isolation room.

The patient's room should be cleaned frequently, with dust kept to a minimum. Allow fresh air to circulate in the room. Sunshine through the windows can elevate the patient's mood and decrease the presence of some microorganisms. Keep trash, newspapers, and clutter to a minimum to discourage transfer of microorganisms. Keep clean supplies in one area, well away from any contaminated items or trash.

Protective Environment

For a significantly immunocompromised patient, such as a bone marrow transplant recipient, it is important to protect him from exposure to potential pathogens. Place the patient in a special isolation room with its own ventilation system. Surfaces within the room are typically smooth to allow for thorough cleaning and disinfection. Do not allow anyone with an active infection, including health care workers, in the patient's room. In caring for this type of patient, all staff members require detailed education and training on protocols and procedures to ensure the patient's health and safety. Remain aware of your facility's policies and procedures regarding the care of a patient in protective environment isolation, and follow them at all times (Fig. 17.4).

Psychological Aspects of Isolation

The patient with Transmission-Based Precautions is at risk for both decreased self-esteem and sensory deprivation. This is particularly true for young children, who, under normal circumstances, are rarely alone and are often used to highly stimulating and entertaining environments. The elderly, too, can find isolation particularly trying, and it may lead to confusion secondary to the lack of normal stimulation and interaction. Assessment for sensory deprivation needs to be ongoing. The signs can include boredom, slowness of thought, disorganized thoughts, excessive sleeping during the day, anxiety, hallucinations, or panic attacks.

Having visitors can be helpful in preventing sensory deprivation. They can talk with the patient about shared interests. A visitor at mealtime often encourages improved nutritional intake by making mealtime more enjoyable. The nurse should learn about the patient's interests and provide appropriate activities such as games, books, puzzles, or crafts. The nurse can also suggest connecting to the hospital's Wi-Fi (if available) using their smartphone or tablet to listen to music or using their laptop to watch TV or a movie. However, avoid overtiring the patient by also allowing periods of rest between activities.

Sensory deprivation may occur if visitors are intimidated by the isolation precautions. There also may be decreased interaction with the health care team because of the need to put on PPE to enter the room. All of this can lead to a loss of self-esteem because the patient begins to feel that he is somehow unclean or unworthy of attention.

Listen to the patient's feelings. Make positive comments on grooming and activity efforts. Try to engage the patient in meaningful conversation by asking about interests or hobbies. Make visitors feel welcome, and help them understand that the patient benefits greatly from their presence. Addressing self-esteem needs is important for complete recovery, regardless of patient age.

Cultural Considerations

Cleanliness

The idea of being "contaminated," "soiled," or "dirty" can make the patient feel at fault or inferior. The patient may blame himself. The nurse can help overcome this with a warm, caring, and accepting attitude, and by avoiding displaying any irritation about the precautions or any evidence of distaste in dealing with the infection.

? Think Critically

How might you reassure a patient with pulmonary tuberculosis under Airborne Precautions who states that he feels everyone is avoiding him because he is "dirty"?

Infection Prevention and Control for the Nurse

OSHA regulations protect health care workers from occupational exposure to blood-borne pathogens in the workplace. In Canada, the Canadian Centre for Occupational Health and Safety addresses worker safety. These two agencies have determined that the three main modes of occupational exposure to blood-borne pathogens are as follows:

- Puncture wounds from contaminated needles or other sharps.
- Skin contact, allowing blood, body fluids, and other potentially infectious materials to enter through damaged or broken skin.
- Mucous membrane contact, allowing infectious materials to enter through the mucous membranes of the eyes, mouth, and nose.

Actions that decrease the nurse's risk for infection include frequent hand hygiene and other general medical aseptic techniques, wearing PPE, using needleless IV equipment and needles with guards, and avoiding carelessness in the clinical area.

It is also recommended that health care workers be immunized if they do not have an active immunity to certain diseases, including hepatitis B, influenza, mumps, measles, rubella, varicella (chickenpox), tetanus, diphtheria, pertussis, and meningococcal disease. In areas with high prevalence of pulmonary tuberculosis, yearly testing for tuberculosis is recommended for health care workers.

Surgical Asepsis

Surgical asepsis is another method used to prevent infection. Surgical asepsis is practiced in the operating room, obstetric areas, and special diagnostic areas and for procedures such as administering injections, changing wound dressings, performing urinary catheterization, and administering IV therapy. In the operating room, strict surgical asepsis is practiced, and head coverings, sterile gowns, masks, and gloves are worn. To perform a sterile dressing, change outside the operating room and use sterile gloves, a mask, and a sterile field. Talking during the dressing change is discouraged.

The four rules of surgical asepsis are:

1. Know what is sterile.
2. Know what is not sterile.
3. Separate sterile from unsterile.
4. Remedy contamination immediately.

The goal in surgical asepsis is to keep an area free of microorganisms. You must constantly be aware of which items and areas are sterile, clean, or contaminated to maintain surgical asepsis. The importance of maintaining sterility must become ingrained, and you must consistently maintain principles of surgical asepsis to protect patients (Box 17.5). By being constantly sensitive as to what is sterile, what is clean, and what becomes contaminated, you can catch and rectify breaks in sterile technique before microorganisms are transferred to the patient.

Surgical scrub. The surgical scrub (Skill 17.1) is more lengthy and vigorous compared with normal hand washing. Its purpose is to remove as many microorganisms as possible without damaging the skin of the hands. Water, a nail stick, an antiseptic agent, a scrub brush or sponge pad, and friction are used to cleanse the hands and forearms mechanically. The scrub begins at the tips of the fingers, working up the hands, and ends 2 inches above the elbows. All rinsing is done under warm, flowing water (Fig. 17.5). The timing

Box 17.5 Principles of Aseptic Technique

These principles form the basis of surgical asepsis:

1. A sterile surface touching a sterile surface remains sterile.
2. A sterile surface touching a nonsterile surface becomes contaminated.
3. Sterile materials must be kept dry; moisture transmits microorganisms and contaminates.
4. Only sterile items are used within the sterile field.
5. A sterile barrier must be considered contaminated after it has been penetrated.
6. The edges of a sterile package or container are considered contaminated after it is opened. An area of 1 inch surrounding the outer edge of the sterile field is considered unsterile.
7. When there is a doubt about the sterility of any item, it must be considered nonsterile.
8. Avoid reaching across or above a sterile field with bare hands or arms or with other nonsterile items.
9. Avoid coughing, sneezing, or unnecessary talking near or over a sterile field.
10. When wearing sterile gloves, keep hands in sight, away from all unsterile objects, and above waist level.
11. Gowns are considered sterile only in front, from the shoulder level to table level and the sleeves to 2 inches above the elbow.
12. Open the wrapper of a sterile pack away from the body, the distal flap first, the lateral flaps next, and the proximal flap toward the body last, thus making it unnecessary to reach over the sterile field.
13. Only the horizontal surface of a table is considered sterile.
14. The sterile field must be kept in sight at all times. Do not turn away from it or leave it. If this happens, you cannot be certain that it is still sterile.
15. The floor must be recognized as the most grossly contaminated area. Clean or sterile items that fall on to the floor should be discarded or decontaminated.

for the scrub does not include the rinsing time. Some agencies allow the use of the counted-stroke method of scrubbing rather than by-the-clock timing (Fig. 17.6). Current standards regarding the time for the traditional scrub are based on the recommendations of the antiseptic agent manufacturer, and, consequently, the recommended time varies from one agency to another, depending on the product used. A 2- to 4-minute scrub is average.

A newer brushless technique, which may be done with or without water, uses an antimicrobial agent that is at least 60% alcohol. This method was shown to be equally effective and "sustained efficacy" (hands remaining cleaner for longer) compared with a standard surgical scrub in a research study (Shen et al., 2015). For the brushless scrub technique, dispense 2 mL of antimicrobial agent into the palm of one hand. With the fingertips of the opposite hand, work some of the alcohol-based agent under the nails. Spread the remaining portion of the agent over all surfaces of the hand and arm to just above the elbow. Dispense another 2 mL of the antimicrobial agent into the palm of the other hand; repeat the procedure on the opposite hand and arm. Techniques vary depending on the product used. **Check the manufacturer's directions for the correct technique.** Allow the hands and arms to dry before gloving (Skill 17.2).

Opening sterile packs and packages and setting up a sterile field. Many sterile supplies are prepared commercially and are disposable or one-time use items. The package, set, or kit provides all the items commonly required in a variety of nursing procedures, such as catheterization, suture removal, dressing change, and irrigation. Individually wrapped items can be obtained to supplement the packs as needed.

Open packs and kits by removing the outer plastic or paper covering, take out the inner package, and aseptically unfold the wrapper to form a sterile field (Fig. 17.7). The principles of asepsis apply regardless of whether the package is disposable or a wrapped tray is prepared by the central supply department of the hospital. Skill 17.3 shows the steps for opening sterile packs and preparing a sterile field.

The principles to observe when opening sterile packages are:

- Perform hand hygiene.
- Open the sterile package away from the body.
- Touch only the outside of the wrapper.
- Do not reach across a sterile field; go around the sterile field if necessary to reach the other side.
- Always face the sterile field, even when moving to the other side.
- Allow sufficient space (at least 6 inches) between the body and the sterile field.

Most sterile items are available as individually wrapped or separate items, such as sterile packages of cotton-tipped applicators, tongue blades, 4 × 4 gauze dressings, abdominal (ABD) dressings, alcohol swabs, syringes, needles, Foley catheters, sterile gloves, and IV catheters. Instructions often appear on the outside of the package directing you where to open it, indicating the direction in which to tear, or showing where to peel at a certain point. Follow these instructions to avoid contaminating the contents.

When sterile supplies have been brought to the patient's bedside, never return them to the unit stock shelves. The outsides of these items are contaminated, and returning such supplies carries organisms from the patient's room back to the store of supplies for the unit. Do not stockpile supplies in the patient's room to avoid costly waste.

The procedure for pouring sterile liquids is listed in Steps 17.1.

Skill 17.1 Performing Surgical Hand Antisepsis: The Surgical Scrub

 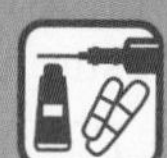 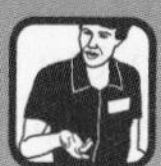 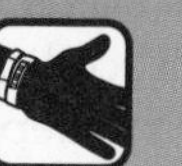 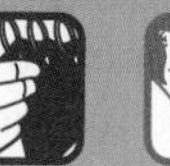 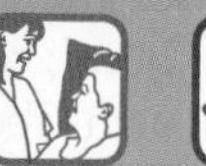 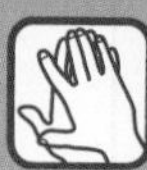 

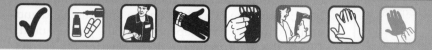

The purpose of the surgical hand scrub is to remove dirt, skin oil, and microorganisms from the hands and lower arms to reduce the microorganism count to as near zero as possible. The antiseptic residue remains on the skin to prevent the growth of microorganisms for several hours. A timed scrub is performed for the interval recommended by the manufacturer of the antiseptic agent used. Some agencies may allow a counted-stroke scrub.

A surgical scrub is performed before entering the operating room, the labor and delivery area, the newborn nursery, or the neonatal intensive care unit (NICU). The scrub is repeated before the next surgical procedure or delivery, or any time that the hands become visibly soiled or contaminated. A 5-minute scrub is presented here.

A brushless surgical scrub using an antimicrobial agent that is at least 60% alcohol may be substituted in some hospitals for the traditional surgical hand scrub (see Skill 17.2).

Supplies

- Sterile towels
- Foot faucet control
- Warm running water
- Antiseptic soap in a dispenser with foot control
- Scrub brush or sponge pad
- Nail stick

Review and carry out the Standard Steps in Appendix A.

ACTION *(RATIONALE)*

Assessment (Data Collection)

1. Determine whether all supplies needed are available before beginning. (*Missing supplies can mean interrupting the scrub to collect them and then having to start the scrub over.*)

Planning

2. Remove rings and watch. (*These items are unsterile and cannot be worn during a sterile procedure. Jewelry harbors microorganisms. No objects may be touched after beginning the surgical scrub.*)

Implementation

3. Adjust the water to a comfortable temperature using the foot control. (*The water remains running during the scrub and should be comfortably warm.*)

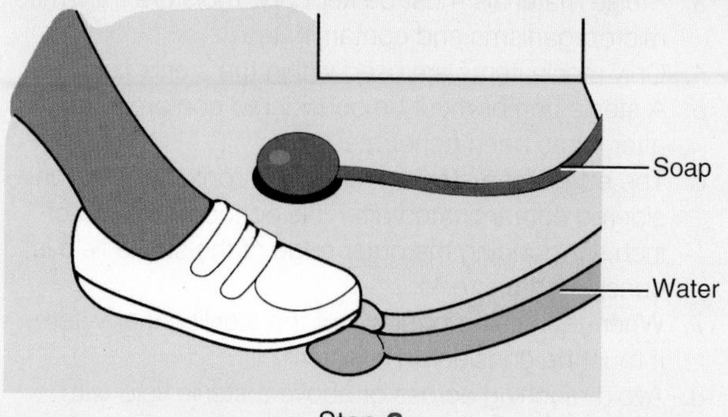

Step 3

4. Wet your hands and arms from above the elbows to the fingertips, with the hands kept higher than the elbows throughout the scrub. (*Moisture aids the formation of the cleansing lather. Keeping the hands higher than the elbows prevents microorganisms from draining over the cleansed hands.*)
5. Dispense the soaping agent onto the palms using the dispenser foot control, and rub hands together to work up a lather. Clean the fingernails with a nail stick. Wash the hands and forearms to a point at least 2 inches above the elbow. (*The soaping agent assists in cleaning dirt from under the nails and assists in removing microorganisms.*)
6. When using a prepackaged scrub brush or sponge pad, open the package, remove the nail cleaner, and clean the nails. Hold the nail stick until the nails have all been cleaned, and then discard it. Remove the brush or pad from the package and discard the package. Do not set down the brush or pad until the scrub is complete. If the brush or sponge pad is not impregnated with the cleansing agent, moisten the brush or pad and dispense the antiseptic agent onto it. (*Putting the brush or pad down during the scrub contaminates it. It must remain in the hands until the scrub is complete, and then be discarded*).

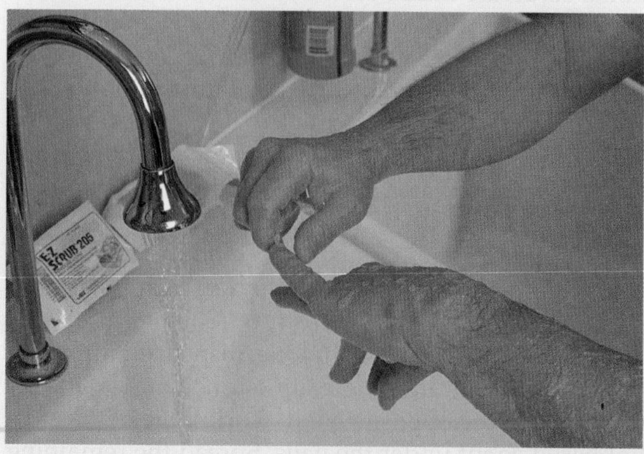

Step 6

7. Start at the fingertips and, with a circular motion, work around and between each finger, holding the scrub brush or sponge pad perpendicular to the fingers and nails. Use light to moderate friction. Scrub the back of the hand, the palm, and then the wrist with circular strokes. Scrub each hand and arm for 2½ minutes. Take care not to abrade the skin. *(Achieving the desired degree of skin asepsis requires an extended cleansing time. Excessive pressure can injure the skin and should be avoided.)*

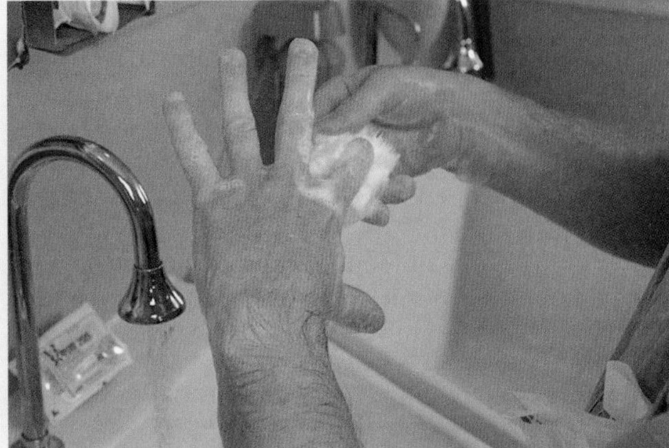

Step **7**

8. Continue up the arm to the elbow using circular scrub strokes on all surfaces, holding the brush or sponge pad parallel to the arm. *(Dirt and microorganisms need to be removed from portions of the arm that will be working in the surgical field even though these skin areas will be covered by a sterile gown and sterile gloves.)*
9. Rinse each hand and arm thoroughly, holding the hand above the level of the elbow and allowing the water to run from the fingertips down the hand to the wrist, the forearm, and off the elbow area. *(This maintains the hands as the cleanest area by not rinsing dirt from the arms over them.)*

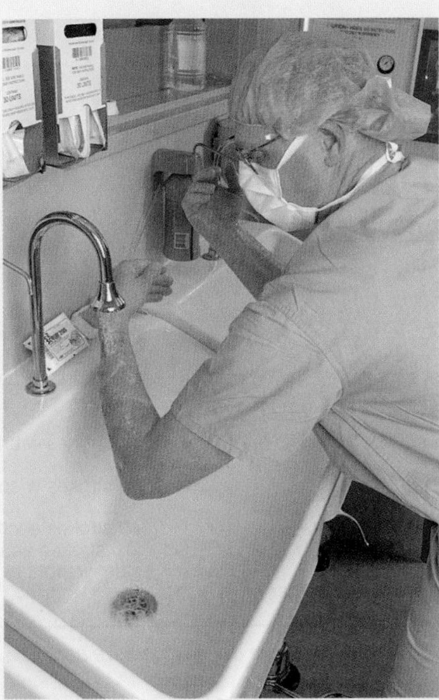

Step **9**

10. Turn off the faucet using the foot control. *(This prevents contamination of the hands from the faucet handle and maintains the sterility of the scrub.)*
11. Dry the hands with a sterile towel. Step away from the sterile field, lean slightly forward from the waist and unfold the towel, holding it by a corner and allowing it to unfold downward. Do not let the towel reach below waist level or come in contact with the body or any object in the room. *(When the towel is taken from a sterile field, it is lifted straight up and away from the sterile field, which keeps water from dripping on the sterile field. Maintaining the arms and hands above waist level and the hands above the elbows protects the scrubbed area. The hands are dried away from the sterile field. When working in the operating room or delivery room, the hands are dried on entering that room.)*
12. Keep the arms and hands above waist level and away from the body with the hands and fingers pointed up. Use the top half of the towel to blot the opposite fingers and hand dry, and move to the forearm. Use a rotary motion to move the towel from the forearm to the elbow. Do not go back over an area already dried. *(Starting with the fingers maintains the hands as the cleanest area. Moving back over an area previously dried contaminates it.)*
13. Grasp the lower end of the towel with the dried hand, and use the same procedure to dry the other hand and forearm. Discard the towel by dropping it into the proper receptacle when finished. Keep your hands and arms above waist level. *(Touching a damp part of the towel with the dried hand will contaminate that hand. Gowning and gloving are done next.)*

Evaluation

14. Ask yourself the following questions: Did the hands refrain from touching any part of the sink during the scrub? Were the hands higher than the elbows throughout the scrub? Was each hand and arm scrubbed for a full 2½ minutes? Were the hands dried without breaking technique? *(If the answer is yes to all of the questions, the scrub is complete. If contamination occurred, the scrub is repeated from the beginning.)*

Documentation

No documentation is required for this procedure.

? Critical Thinking Questions

1. Why should you avoid excessive pressure on the skin during the scrub?
2. If you are finished with the surgical scrub and are rinsing your hands and arms and accidentally touch the faucet spout, what would you do?

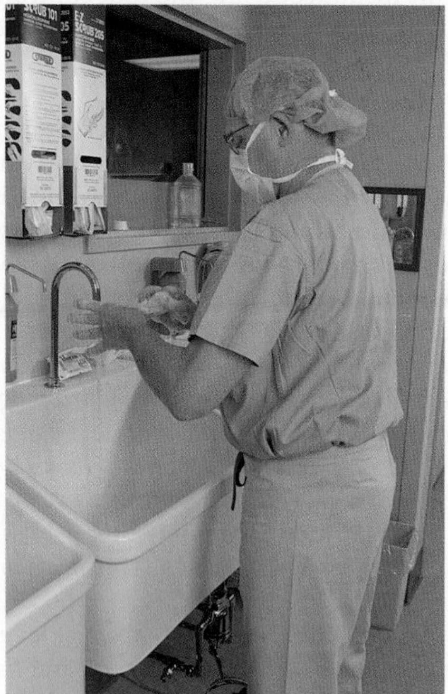

FIGURE 17.5 Nurse performing surgical scrub.

Sterile gloving. Sterile gloves must be used for sterile procedures. These gloves are made of various substances, including latex and nitrile, and are less permeable than the disposable plastic gloves. The method of donning and removing sterile gloves is presented in Skill 17.4.

Correcting breaks in asepsis. Whenever it becomes apparent that a break in surgical asepsis has occurred, you must rectify the error. A scrub is begun again if the hands touch the sink, which is always considered contaminated; sterile gloves are discarded and new gloves donned when any part of a glove touches a nonsterile area or item. Discard or put aside for resterilization any sterile supplies if they become contaminated, and open new packs or packages aseptically to replace them.

It is up to every nurse to point out breaks in sterile technique that occur when others seem unaware that they have contaminated themselves or the sterile field. Surgical asepsis is used in every aspect of nursing.

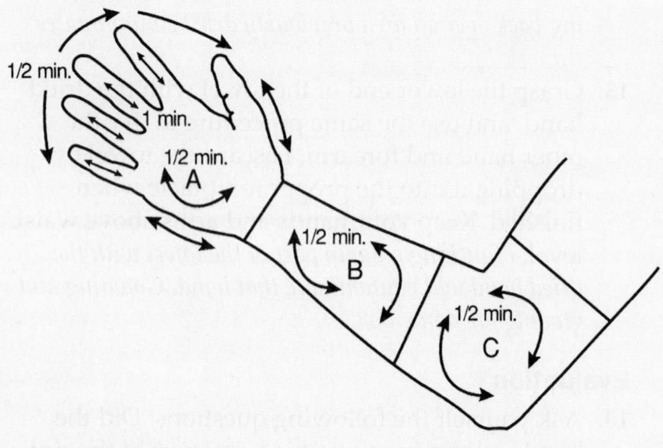

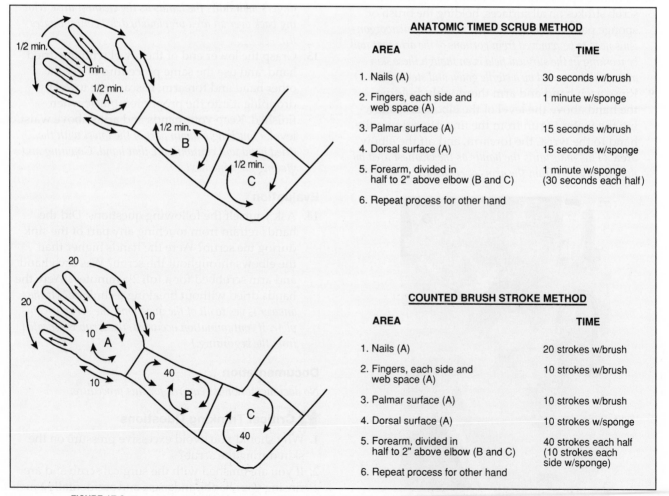

ANATOMIC TIMED SCRUB METHOD

AREA	TIME
1. Nails (A)	30 seconds w/brush
2. Fingers, each side and web space (A)	1 minute w/sponge
3. Palmar surface (A)	15 seconds w/brush
4. Dorsal surface (A)	15 seconds w/sponge
5. Forearm, divided in half to 2" above elbow (B and C)	1 minute w/sponge (30 seconds each half)
6. Repeat process for other hand	

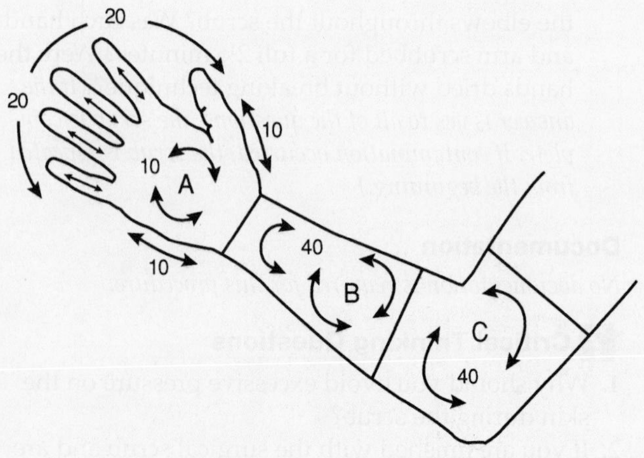

COUNTED BRUSH STROKE METHOD

AREA	TIME
1. Nails (A)	20 strokes w/brush
2. Fingers, each side and web space (A)	10 strokes w/brush
3. Palmar surface (A)	10 strokes w/brush
4. Dorsal surface (A)	10 strokes w/sponge
5. Forearm, divided in half to 2" above elbow (B and C)	40 strokes each half (10 strokes each side w/sponge)
6. Repeat process for other hand	

FIGURE 17.6 Surgical scrub techniques. (From Phippen, M.L., & Wells, M.P. [2000]. *Patient care during operative and invasive procedures.* Philadelphia, PA: Saunders.)

Skill 17.2 Performing Surgical Hand Antisepsis: The Surgical Hand Rub

 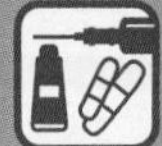 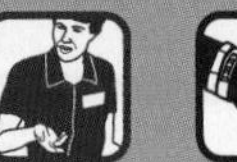 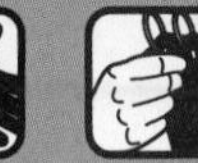 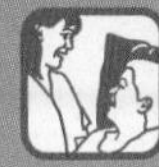 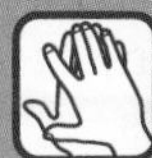 

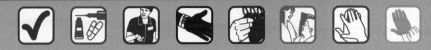

The surgical hand rub is an approved alternate method for removing dirt, skin oil, and microorganisms from the hands and lower arms and reducing the microorganism count to as near zero as possible. Antiseptic residue remains on the skin to prevent the growth of microorganisms for several hours.

A surgical hand rub is performed before entering the operating room, the labor and delivery area, the newborn nursery, or the neonatal intensive care unit. The rub is repeated before the next surgical procedure or delivery or any time that the hands become contaminated. It uses an antimicrobial agent that is at least 60% alcohol.

Supplies

- Sterile towels
- Foot faucet control
- Antiseptic soap
- Running water
- Antiseptic rub in a dispenser with foot control
- Scrub brush or sponge pad
- Nail stick

Review and carry out the Standard Steps in Appendix A.

ACTION *(RATIONALE)*

Assessment (Data Collection)

1. Determine whether all supplies needed are available before beginning. *(Missing supplies can mean interrupting the scrub to collect them and then having to start the scrub over.)*

Planning

2. Remove rings and watch. *(These items are unsterile and cannot be worn during a sterile procedure. Jewelry harbors microorganisms. No objects may be touched after beginning the surgical scrub.)*

Implementation

3. Adjust the water to a comfortable temperature using the foot control. *(The water remains running during the prewash and should be comfortably warm.)*
4. Wash hands and forearms thoroughly with antimicrobial soap and running water; cleanse under nails with nail stick. *(This removes surface soiling and dirt that might provide a barrier for microorganisms.)*
5. Rinse hands and arms under running water with hands held above the elbows. Dry thoroughly with paper towels. *(This removes soil loosened in the washing process without washing the soap down over the hands and possibly carrying microorganisms from the upper arms to the hands. Excess water on the skin may interfere with the action of the rub solution.)*
6. Dispense the antiseptic rub onto the palms using the dispenser foot control, and spread over hands and arms per manufacturer's instructions, which may vary depending on the product. Make certain that all surfaces are fully covered, paying particular attention to the thumbs, fingers, and space between each finger. Rub with the hands over all surfaces until they are dry. Begin rub at the fingers and end 2 inches above the elbows. Hold hands above the elbows and the arms away from the body. *(For the product to reduce microorganisms effectively, it must dry on the skin surfaces being disinfected. Working from the fingertips to the upper arms prevents carrying microorganisms or soil downward to the hands. Positioning the hands above the elbows and the arms away from the body prevents contamination from your body or the sink or countertop.)*
7. When the rub is dry, proceed immediately to the operating or procedure room to gown and glove. Keep the arms and hands above waist level and away from the body with the hands and fingers pointed up when moving from room to room. *(This keeps the hands and arms visible, preventing contamination by accidentally brushing against the body, doorway, or other personnel or surfaces.)*

Evaluation

8. Ask yourself the following questions: Did the hands refrain from touching any part of the sink or counter during the washing and rub? Were the hands higher than the elbows throughout the process? Was each hand and arm rubbed until the surface was fully dry? Were the hands and arms in full view and kept away from contact during the movement from the scrub area to the procedure or operating room? *(If the answer is yes to all of the questions, the rub is complete. If contamination occurred, the rub is repeated from the beginning.)*

Documentation

No documentation is required for this procedure.

? Critical Thinking Questions

1. Why should you pay particular attention to the fingers and thumbs during the procedure?
2. If you were finished with the surgical hand rub and accidentally brushed your elbow against the doorframe when moving into the procedure or operating room, what would you do?

◆ EVALUATION

If the patient is recovering without additional instances of infection from other organisms or infection of other body areas with a resident organism, goals are being met. Evaluation also includes assessing whether the patient's infection has been transmitted to any health care worker or any other patient on the unit or in the hospital. The IP monitors for this and, if it occurs, usually works in conjunction with the unit manager to ensure that staff members are correctly implementing infection prevention and control procedures.

Infection prevention and control are the responsibility of every nurse. The principles and techniques learned here will protect you and your patients from harmful microorganisms.

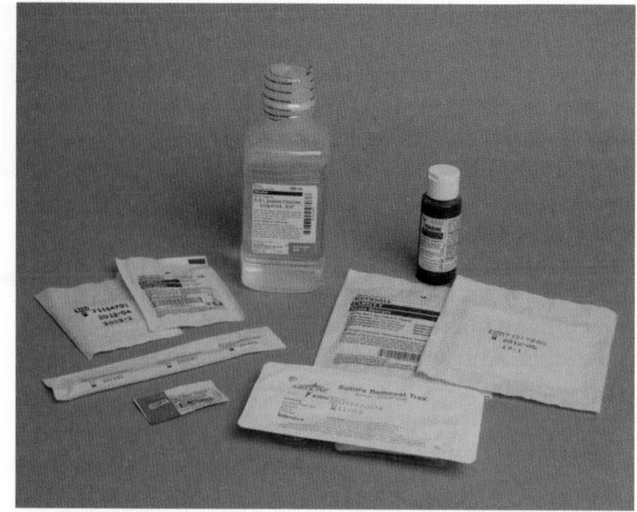

FIGURE 17.7 Know how to find the expiration date on a variety of supplies.

Skill 17.3 Opening Sterile Packs and Preparing a Sterile Field

 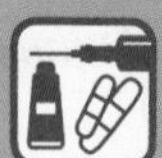 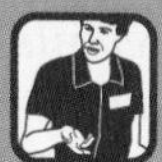  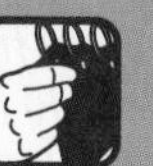 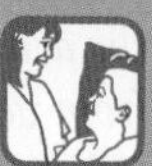 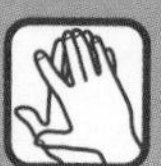 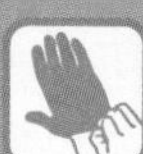

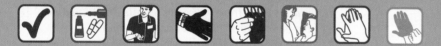

When sterile procedures are to be performed, sterile equipment and supplies are set up on a sterile field. Commercial disposable sterile sets of equipment and supplies are available for most standard procedures. Hospitals also wrap reusable equipment and cloth towels in packs that are sterilized before use. Hospital-prepared sterile packs are dated and are returned for resterilization if not used by the expiration date. Check the date before using a hospital-prepared sterile pack. Commercially prepared packs may also have expiration dates that need to be checked before use.

A sterile field is set up by using the inside of the wrapper on the sterile pack or by opening and draping a tabletop or instrument tray with sterile drapes and then placing the sterile items to be used on the field. The field is considered sterile to within 1 inch of its horizontal, or flat, border. The portion of the sterile drape that falls over the table or tray edge is always considered unsterile.

Supplies

- Sterile disposable equipment and supply tray
  or
- Hospital-prepared sterile pack and sterile drapes

Review and carry out the Standard Steps in Appendix A.

ACTION *(RATIONALE)*

Assessment (Data Collection)

1. Select a dry tabletop or instrument tray that is above waist level. *(Moisture can travel upward from the surface and contaminate the sterile field and supplies. Anything below waist level is considered contaminated according to principles of surgical asepsis.)*

Planning

2. Obtain the equipment tray and supplies to be used for the procedure, and explain the procedure to the patient if appropriate. *(This ensures that all needed equipment is on hand before scrubbing and gloving and that the patient is prepared for the procedure.)*

Implementation

3. Perform hand hygiene. *(This removes microorganisms.)*
4. Remove the plastic outer wrap, leaving the inner wrap in place. If a hospital-prepared pack does not have a plastic wrap, remove the tape holding it closed. When setting up a field at the bedside, you can use the plastic wrapper for discards. Place the pack so that the flap that opens to the back of the table is on top. *(The outside of the sterile pack is not considered sterile and can be touched. The first flap is to be opened away from the nurse's working area.)*
5. Facing the table, move to the far side and open the initial flap by lifting it upward away from the pack, and then outward and down over the edge of the table. If the pack is small enough, this can be done by reaching around the pack and opening the distal flap rather than moving to the other side of the field. *(Opening the distal flap first prevents contaminating the pack by reaching over the exposed sterile contents after the other flaps are opened.)*

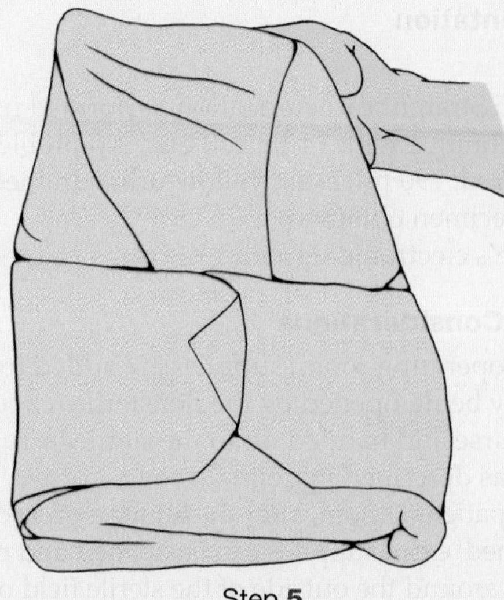
Step 5

6. With the left hand, move the flap on the left up and laterally away from the package. Pull the edge down over the edge of the table. Then open the right flap with the right hand in the same manner. Be careful to touch only the outside of the wrapper and not to reach across any area of exposed sterile supplies. *(This maintains the sterility of the inside of the pack and its equipment and supplies. Pulling the drape edges downward over table edges ensures that the wrap does not fall back over the field and contaminate it.)*

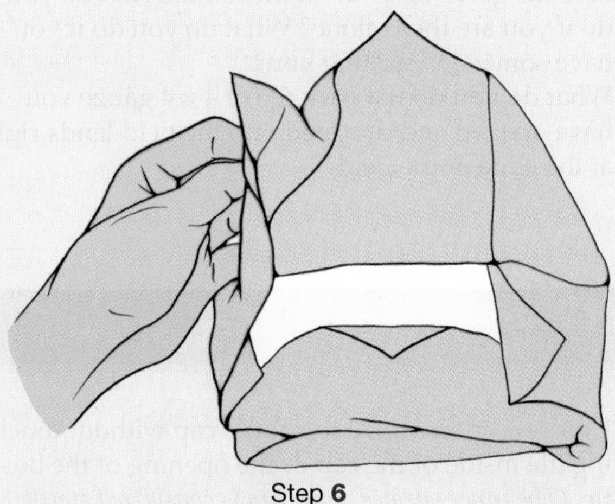
Step 6

7. Lift the front (proximal) flap up and toward you, handling only the outside of the wrapper or pull tabs. If the entire pack is to be handed off to someone in sterile gown and gloves, grasp the contents firmly in one hand from the underside, and pull each flap down over the hand that is grasping the contents of the package. Secure the flaps with your other hand when offering the pack contents to the sterile person who needs them. If the pack has an inner wrap, this is sterile and need not be opened before handing off the tray. *(This maintains the sterility of the pack contents. Holding back the flaps prevents them from falling forward and touching the gloved hands of the sterile person, or the hands of the nonsterile person from touching the sterile gloves.)*

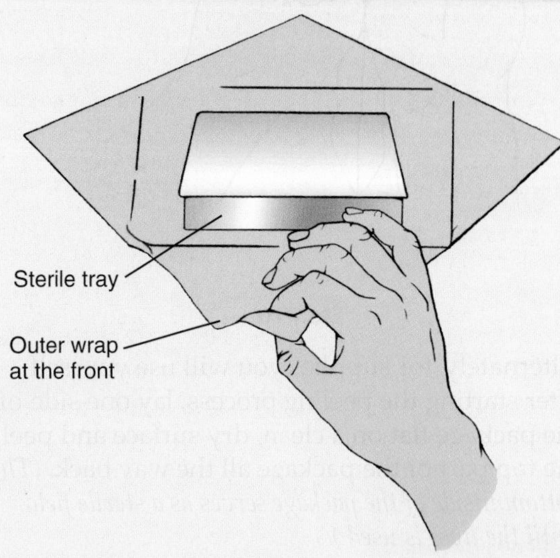

Step 7

8. The inside of the outer wrap is used as the sterile field. Using gloves and/or sterile forceps, arrange the equipment and supplies on the sterile field in the order in which they will be used. Keep all items at least 1 inch from the edge boundary. *(The inside of the wrapper that has not been touched is still sterile. Only sterile items may touch or move over the sterile field, or it will be contaminated. The outside 1-inch edge of the horizontal surface of the wrapper or field is considered contaminated because the edge is in contact with an unsterile surface or is hanging below waist level and subject to contact contamination. The entire field must remain dry to maintain sterility. You must continue to face the field. If your back is turned to the field or it is outside your line of vision, it is considered contaminated because it was not within your visual limits and something nonsterile could have fallen on it or touched it without your knowledge.)*

Adding Supplies or Equipment to the Sterile Field

9. Inspect the disposable package to see which edge is to be opened. Bring both hands together, and grasp the small flaps at the edge to be opened. *(This establishes the grip to open the package at the intended point.)*
10. Peel the two parts of the package apart by turning the hands outward to separate the sealed edges. *(Open the package, exposing the sterile contents. This allows the sterile person to extract the sterile contents of the package without being contaminated or it allows you to toss the supply item or piece of equipment gently onto your sterile field without contaminating it.)*

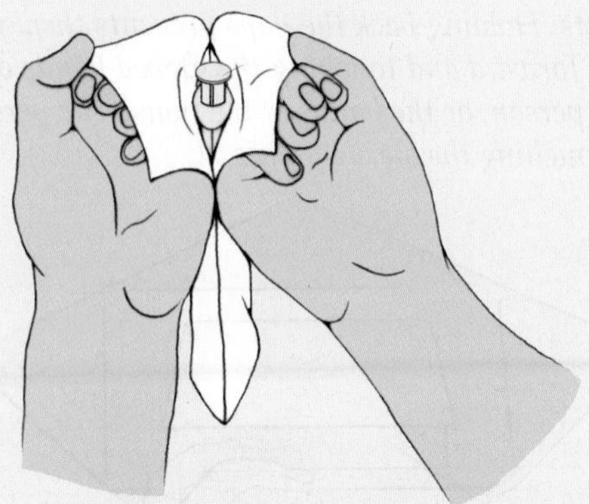

Step **10**

11. Alternately, for supplies you will use yourself, after starting the peeling process, lay one side of the package flat on a clean, dry surface and peel the top part of the package all the way back. *(The bottom inside of the package serves as a sterile field until the item is used.)*
12. Perform the sterile procedure, maintaining the principles of surgical asepsis (see Box 17.5). *(Any break in sterile technique contaminates the field, supplies, and equipment.)*

Evaluation

13. Ask yourself, Was the pack opened while maintaining sterile technique? Has the sterile field been within my line of vision during the whole procedure? Have I added supplies to the field in an aseptic manner? *(Answers will determine whether the field has been kept sterile.)*

Documentation

Example

9/17 1435 Straight catheterization performed using sterile technique with 14-Fr. catheter. No problems encountered; 190 mL clear, yellow urine drained; sterile specimen obtained.

(Nurse's electronic signature)

Special Considerations

- In the operating room, supplies are added to the field by being opened by the nonsterile (circulating) nurse and handed off to the sterile (scrub) nurse as described in point 7 above.
- In the patient's room, after the kit for a procedure is opened, extra supplies can be opened and positioned around the outside of the sterile field on their own wrappers, where they will be within reach.
- When offering a peeled package of supplies, keep the opened flaps over your hands so that the sterile person will not touch your nonsterile skin or the nonsterile flaps.

? Critical Thinking Questions

1. You have opened a sterile urinary catheter kit and are gloved. While cleansing the meatus (the hand touching the patient is now nonsterile, the hand with the swab is sterile), you accidentally contaminate the glove on your sterile hand. What do you do if you are there alone? What do you do if you have someone assisting you?
2. What do you do if a package of 4 × 4 gauze you have opened and dropped into the field lands right at the edge of the field?

Steps 17.1 Pouring Sterile Liquids

Sterile liquids are used during surgical procedures for wound irrigations and for cleansing during sterile procedures.

ACTION *(RATIONALE)*

1. Perform hand hygiene and, using sterile technique, set up the sterile field with a sterile container for the solution. Properly opened, the wrapper from a sterile kit such as an irrigation kit makes an appropriate sterile field at the bedside. *(This prepares an area where the sterile solution can be safely poured.)*
2. Check the solution label to verify that it is the ordered solution. Check the expiration date. *(This prevents using the wrong solution or an outdated solution. Sterile solutions are not considered sterile if the expiration date has passed.)*
3. Unscrew and remove the bottle cap without touching the inside of the cap or the opening of the bottle. *(The inner surface of the cap is considered sterile.)*
4. Place the cap with the inner surface facing up on the table outside the sterile field. *(This prevents contamination of the inside of the cap.)*
5. With sterile gloved hands or sterile transfer forceps, move the empty sterile container for the solution to 1 inch inside the edge of the sterile field. *(Positioning the container to 1 inch inside the edge of the sterile field allows you to pour the liquid without moving your arm or hand over the sterile field, while keeping the sterile container within the sterile field.)*
6. Hold the bottle about 6 inches above the empty sterile container and pour liquid into the container in a steady stream, preventing splashing of the liquid onto the sterile field. *(Pouring the*

liquid from this height and maintaining a steady stream prevents splashing. If splashing occurs, the field is contaminated, and a new sterile field must be prepared.)

7. When pouring is completed, pick up the cap by the outside and recap the bottle. Set it down outside the sterile field. *(In patient rooms and in the home setting, recapped solutions may be used if they have not become contaminated during recapping. In the operating room, remaining solution is discarded.)*
8. Write the date the solution was opened on the label and your initials. *(Solutions are considered unsterile after being open for a particular number of days, and some are single use only. Follow agency policy regarding discard dates for open solutions.)*
9. When pouring liquids from a previously opened bottle, pour a bit of solution over the lip of the bottle into a discard container, and then pour the solution into the sterile container. *(This washes the edge of the bottle and aids in preventing contamination of the solution being poured.)*

Skill 17.4 Sterile Gloving and Ungloving

 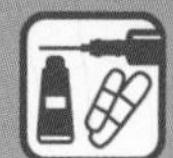 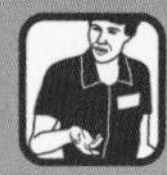   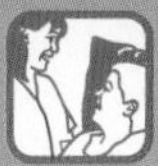 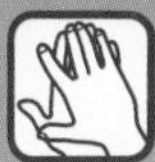 

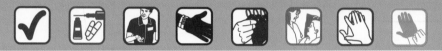

Sterile gloves are used for performing sterile procedures and handling sterile equipment and supplies. Sterile gloves are to be removed and replaced any time they become contaminated when performing a sterile procedure.

Supplies

- Package of sterile gloves in correct size

Review and carry out the Standard Steps in Appendix A.

ACTION *(RATIONALE)*

Assessment (Data Collection)

1. Determine what size gloves are needed. *(Gloves should fit snugly but not be so tight that they are extremely difficult to put on.)*

Planning

2. Select a clean, flat, dry surface above waist level on which to open the glove package. *(The glove package should remain stationary and easily accessible while putting on the gloves to decrease chance of contamination from contact with the surface of table. A wet surface will contaminate the gloves.)*

Implementation

Gloving

3. Place the package of correctly sized gloves on the flat surface. Perform hand hygiene. *(Hands must be clean and dry before gloving to reduce the transfer of microorganisms.)*
4. Peel open the outside wrapper, exposing the sterile glove package. *(The outer package keeps the inner pack sterile until opened.)*
5. Position the package so that the designation of right ("R") and left ("L") is visible right side up if this is indicated on the package. *(This places the gloves in correct association with the right and left hand, facilitating proper gloving. Some gloves can be used on either hand; those packages will not be marked R and L.)*
6. Use sterile technique, and open the glove package, handling only the outer wrapper. Handle the wrapper by the underneath part of the folded-back flaps. Pinch the corners of the flaps after pulling them open so that they remain open. *(Handling the outside of the wrapper only prevents contamination of the inner surface and the gloves. Allowing the wrapper to fall back on the gloves contaminates them.)*

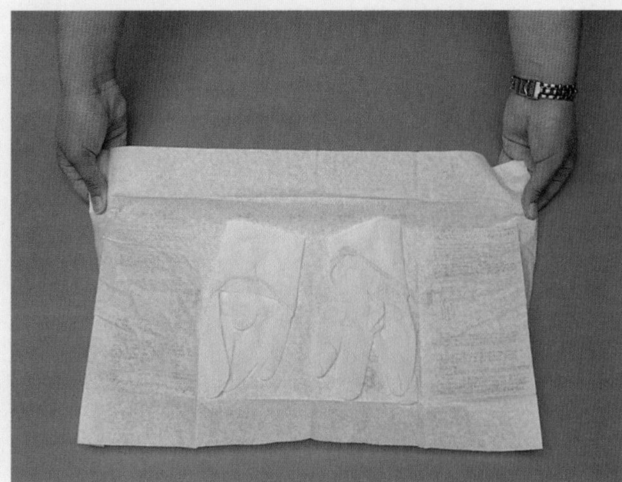

Step **6**

7. Pick up one glove by slipping the thumb into the opening and grasping the glove with the thumb

and fingertips at the folded-over cuff edge, and lift it up at least 12 inches off the wrapper, being careful not to touch the glove to yourself or any surrounding objects. *(Only the inside of the glove, which will be against the skin, is touched, leaving the outside sterile.)*

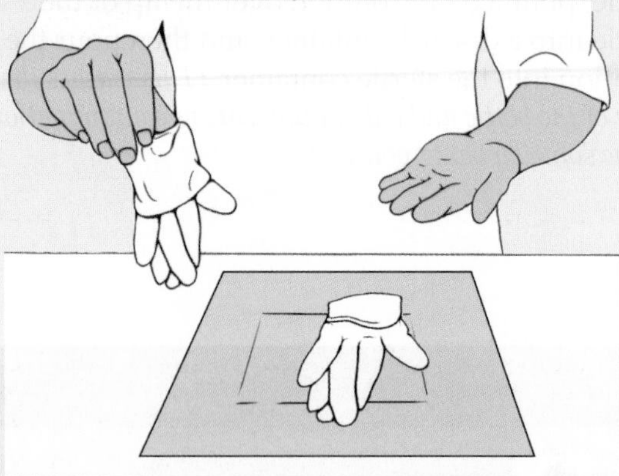

Step **7**

8. Insert the fingers of the other hand into the glove, and extend and hold the fingers slightly apart. Pull the cuff outward as you slip your hand into the glove. *(Touching only the inside surface of the glove prevents contaminating the outside sterile surface.)*
9. Pick up the second glove by placing the (sterile) gloved fingers under the cuff fold; slip the bare hand into the glove, being careful not to touch the outside of the glove or the other gloved hand with your bare skin. Once the hand is settled in the glove, slide the glove cuff up carefully over the wrist. *(Keeping the gloved fingers under the folded-over cuff of the second glove prevents the gloved hand from being contaminated by bare skin as the second glove is pulled on. Sliding up the cuff covers the exposed skin of the wrist.)*

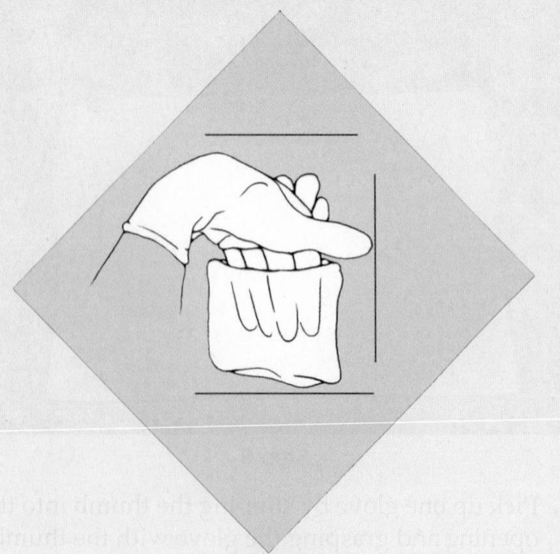

Step **9**

10. Adjust the fingers in the gloves as needed by pulling the glove fingers out with the opposite hand to straighten them and allow the proper finger to enter the space. *(Fingers must be situated correctly to permit hand dexterity while performing the procedure.)*

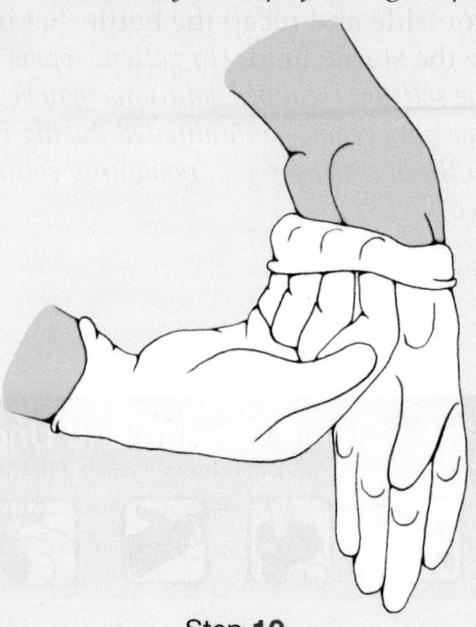

Step **10**

Ungloving

11. When finished with the sterile procedure, unglove by grasping the outside surface of one glove about 2 to 3 inches below the cuff edge with the opposite gloved hand. *(Grasping the glove in an area away from exposed skin prevents contaminating the skin with the now contaminated glove.)*
12. Pull the glove off the hand while turning it inside out and rolling it into the palm of your other gloved hand. *(This technique prevents organisms on the contaminated gloves from coming into contact with your skin.)*

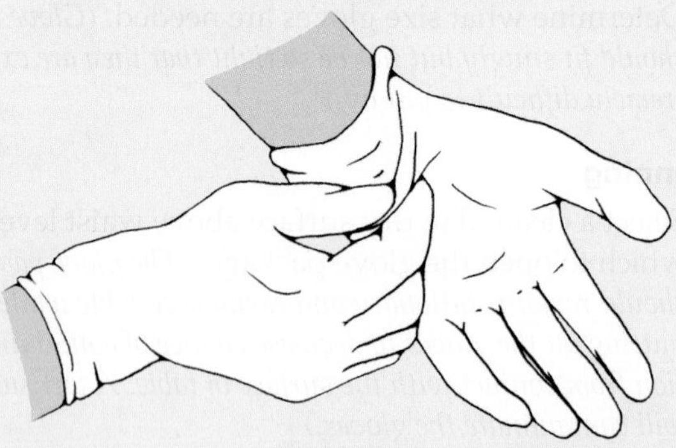

Step **12**

13. Still holding the first glove in the remaining gloved hand, place the fingers of your ungloved hand under the cuff of the remaining glove next to your skin. Slide the glove off, turning it inside out as you remove it. *(Touching only the skin of the hand with your bare hand prevents contaminating yourself with the outside of the now contaminated glove. The first glove's contaminated surface is now encased in the second.)*

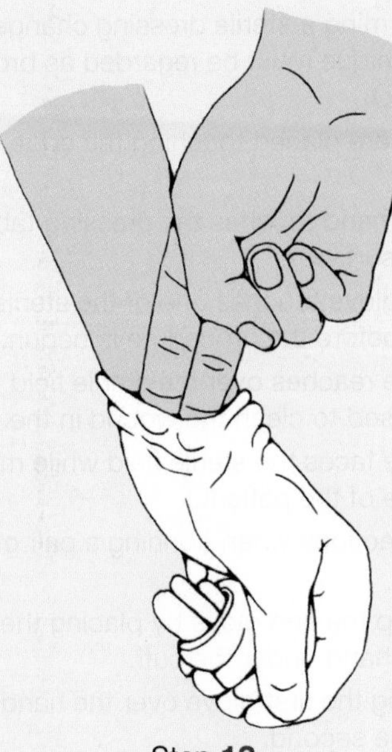

Step **13**

14. Dispose of the contaminated gloves in the proper receptacle. *(Because the contaminated surfaces of the gloves are on the inside of the gloves, they can be discarded in the trash.)*

15. Perform hand hygiene. *(This removes glove powder, if present, and removes any organisms that might have traveled through the gloves. Hand hygiene after removing gloves is required by Standard Precautions.)*

Evaluation

16. At all times during the wearing of sterile gloves, ask yourself, Have I touched a glove surface to an unsterile object? Have my gloved hands dropped below waist level? Do I need to reglove? *(If hands drop below waist level, they are considered contaminated because they are generally out of the field of vision.)*

Documentation

No documentation is required for this procedure.

Critical Thinking Questions

1. You are preparing to do a dressing change with the patient in bed, and set up the sterile field and supplies on the over-the-bed table. Where would you place the sterile glove pack to don the sterile gloves?
2. When donning sterile gloves, in what ways might the gloves become contaminated?

Get Ready for the NCLEX Examination!

Key Points

- Illness progresses through an incubation period, a prodromal period, an illness period, and a convalescent period.
- The present system of infection prevention and control consists of two tiers: Standard Precautions, to be used for all patients; and Transmission-Based Precautions, to be used for patients who have a transmissible organism.
- Transmission-Based Precautions are always used along with Standard Precautions.
- PPE is used to protect patients and health care workers. PPE includes head covering, protective eyewear, masks, gowns, gloves, and shoe covers. The mode of transmission of a microorganism determines which PPE is necessary.
- Hand hygiene is the best method of preventing HAIs.
- A special respirator (N95) mask is necessary to care for a patient under Airborne Precautions who has or may have pulmonary tuberculosis, varicella, rubeola, or severe acute respiratory syndrome (SARS). If the patient under Airborne Precautions must be transported, he must wear a mask.
- Laboratory specimens are labeled and bagged in a bag marked “biohazard” before removal from an isolation room.
- Linens and trash are deposited in specially marked biohazard bags before removal from an isolation room. Sharps are placed in a puncture-resistant container marked “biohazard.”
- Emphasis in the home environment is on preventing the transmission of microorganisms to others and containing pathogens.
- Protective isolation is used for severely immunocompromised patients. Full use of PPE is required for all people entering the patient’s room.
- The nurse should oversee appropriate activities and opportunities for contact with friends and family to prevent adverse psychological consequences for the isolation patient.
- Nurses must be knowledgeable about and strictly follow the principles of surgical asepsis and the use of sterile technique.

Additional Learning Resources

SG Go to your Study Guide for additional learning activities to help you master this chapter content.

evolve Go to your Evolve website at http://evolve.elsevier.com/Williams/fundamental for additional online resources.

Review Questions for the NCLEX Examination

*Choose the **best** answer for each question.*

1. The nurse is preparing to assist a patient with his bath. He has an infected, draining wound. What PPE would be required for these tasks? *(Select all that apply.)*
   1. Gown
   2. Mask
   3. Eyewear
   4. Gloves
   5. Face shield
2. Which step(s) are to be taken when preparing a sputum specimen to go to the laboratory? *(Select all that apply.)*
   1. Label the container.
   2. Collect the specimen and secure the lid.
   3. Place the container in a sealed plastic bag marked "biohazard."
   4. Place the biohazard bag in another plastic bag.
   5. Place the completed laboratory slip in the pocket on the bag.
   6. Put the container in the rack for the laboratory courier.
3. A nurse is working in a small hospital with a combined medical-surgical unit. The only beds available are in two-bed rooms, and each room already has one patient. The recovery room nurse is about to send up a 25-year-old woman who just had her tonsils removed. Who would be the most appropriate roommate?
   1. A 60-year-old woman newly diagnosed with bacterial pneumonia
   2. A 23-year-old woman with a draining wound
   3. A 15-year-old girl who had oral surgery yesterday
   4. A 50-year-old woman recovering from an alcohol overdose
4. A home care nurse has a patient with a wound infection who is also under Droplet Precautions. The patient's wife changes the dressing on the days that the nurse does not visit. The wound must be cleansed and then dressed. The nurse must teach the wife to: *(Select all that apply.)*
   1. Maintain strict surgical asepsis.
   2. Cleanse her hands and be careful to touch only the corners of the dressing with her bare hands.
   3. Store the used dressings and supplies in a sealed plastic bag before placing them in the trash.
   4. Wear a surgical mask as well as gloves when changing the dressing.
   5. Don clean gloves when removing the soiled dressings from the wound.
5. A patient under Contact Precautions wants to know if he may have visitors. The nurse tells him that:
   1. Visitors may come but they must wear a mask and gown.
   2. There are no special requirements for people visiting a patient under Contact Precautions.
   3. Visitors should check with the nurse to see whether they need to wear PPE.
   4. Visitors may come but should wash their hands before and after socially touching the patient.
6. When performing a sterile dressing change on a patient, correct technique must be regarded as broken if: *(Select all that apply.)*
   1. Supplies are placed touching the edge of the sterile field.
   2. A gloved hand touches the dressing table below the tabletop surface.
   3. A sterile glove touches one of the sterile dressings on the field before the procedure is begun.
   4. The nurse reaches over the sterile field when placing a swab used to clean the wound in the discard bag.
   5. The nurse faces the sterile field while moving to the other side of the patient.
7. The correct actions when donning a pair of sterile gloves include:
   1. Picking up the first glove by placing the fingers of the opposite hand under the cuff.
   2. Smoothing the first glove over the hand before putting on the second.
   3. Picking up the first glove by grasping it on the fold of the cuff.
   4. Adjusting the fingers of the first glove before donning the second glove.
8. A patient is taking medication for a respiratory infection. Which statement by the patient indicates the need for further patient education? *(Select all that apply.)*
   1. "I will take my medications until they are all gone."
   2. "Even if I feel better, I should finish this prescription."
   3. "I can stop taking these once my symptoms subside."
   4. "I will save the medication for when I start feeling sick again."
   5. "I will probably feel better before I finish the medication."

Critical Thinking Activities

Read each clinical scenario and discuss the questions with your classmates.

Scenario A

You are caring for a 43-year-old man who has an infected leg wound following a hiking accident. He is to keep his leg elevated and is under Contact Precautions. He has recently retired from the military and has just moved to the area. He is bored and restless. How would you help meet his psychosocial needs?

Scenario B

What would you do if you observed the physician's glove become contaminated during a sterile procedure and the physician appeared unaware that this had occurred? Be specific.

Scenario C

Your home care patient is an older man with a large abdominal wound that needs daily dressing changes. He lives with his wife, but she has severe arthritis in her hands and is unable to perform the procedure. You are scheduled for three visits per week. How would you solve the problem of getting his daily dressing change done on the days you are not scheduled to visit?

chapter

18

Safely Lifting, Moving, and Positioning Patients

http://evolve.elsevier.com/Williams/fundamental

Objectives

Upon completing this chapter, you should be able to do the following:

Theory

1. Describe the anatomy and function of the musculoskeletal system.
2. Explain the importance of proper body mechanics, alignment, and position change for both patient and nurse.
3. Discuss the principles of safe body movement and positioning, giving an appropriate example for each principle.
4. Identify ways to maintain the patient's correct body alignment in bed or in a chair.
5. Describe the proper method for transferring a patient between a wheelchair and a bed.

Clinical Practice

1. Correctly position a patient in the following positions: supine, prone, Fowler, and Sims.
2. Assist patients to sit up in bed.
3. Demonstrate complete passive range-of-motion (ROM) exercises for a patient.
4. Correctly transfer a patient from a wheelchair to a bed.
5. Transfer a patient from a bed to a stretcher.
6. Demonstrate the correct techniques for ambulating a patient and for breaking a fall while ambulating.

Skills

Key Terms

alignment (ă-LĪN-mĭnt, p. 269)
ambulate (ĂM-bŭ-lāt, p. 272)
bone (p. 268)
bursa (BŬR-să, p. 268)
cartilage (CĂR-tĭ-lĭj, p. 268)
contractures (kŏn-TRĂK-chŭrz, p. 271)
dangling (p. 284)
Fowler position (FŎW-lĕr, p. 272)
gait (p. 272)
gait belt (p. 288)
joint (p. 268)
kinesiology (kĭ-nē-sī-Ŏ-lō-jē, p. 269)
lateral position (LĂ-tĕr-ăl, p. 273)
ligaments (LĬG-ă-mĕntz, p. 268)
logrolling (LŎG-rō-lĭng, p. 280)
necrosis (nē-KRŌ-sĭs, p. 271)
pivot (PĬV-ŏt, p. 271)
pressure injuries (PRĔ-shŭr ŬL-sĕrz, p. 271)
prone position (PRŌN, p. 273)
semi-Fowler position (SĔ-mī FŎW-lĕr, p. 272)
shearing force (SHĒR-ĭng, p. 271)
side-lying (lateral) position (SĪD-lī-ĭng, p. 273)
Sims position (p. 273)
skeletal muscles (p. 268)
supine position (SOO-pīn, p. 272)
symmetry (SĬM-ĭ-trē, p. 271)
tendons (p. 268)
transfer belt (p. 288)

Concepts Covered in This Chapter

- Mobility
- Functional ability
- Safety

Lifting, moving, and positioning patients are integral parts of your workday. To provide the best patient care and prevent self-injury, you must know the principles of body mechanics. Coordinated movement involves using the bones, joints, and skeletal muscles properly. The Center for Disease Control (CDC) and the Occupational Safety and Health Administration (OSHA) have both published guidelines to assist nurses and employers with implementing policies to prevent injury to health care workers. Many institutions are moving toward a "no manual lifting" policy or to the use of a lift team to decrease health care worker back injuries from repetitive lifting, although lift teams alone are not a "magic bullet" and should be used in conjunction with appropriate equipment, staffing, and as part of a comprehensive safe patient handling program. Until comprehensive safe patient handling programs are in place in all health care institutions, there will be instances when a nurse must lift a patient without assistance or use of a mechanical device. The following principles and practices serve as guides to help prevent injury.

OVERVIEW OF THE STRUCTURE AND FUNCTION OF THE MUSCULOSKELETAL SYSTEM

WHICH STRUCTURES ARE INVOLVED IN POSITIONING AND MOVING PATIENTS?

- The musculoskeletal system contains skeletal muscles, ligaments, tendons, bones, joints, and cartilage.
- **Bone** is a dense, hard type of connective tissue. There are four basic types of bones—short, long, flat, and irregular—and they are made up of compact and spongy bone.
- A **joint** is the place of union of two or more bones in the body. Joints can be freely movable, slightly movable, or immovable.
- **Bursae** are small fluid-filled sacs that provide a cushion at friction points in freely movable joints.
- **Skeletal muscles** are striated muscles that are made of bundles of muscle fibers surrounded by a connective tissue sheath.
- **Tendons** are cords of fibrous connective tissue that connect a muscle to a bone to allow for joint movement.
- **Ligaments** connect bones or cartilage to provide support and strength.
- **Cartilage** is a fibrous connective tissue that acts as a cushion.

WHAT ARE THE FUNCTIONS OF BONES FOR POSITIONING AND MOVING PATIENTS?

- Bones provide the scaffolding or framework to the body (Fig. 18.1).
- The skeleton gives the body shape and supports the internal organs and skin.
- The bones provide places for the ligaments and tendons to attach, thereby allowing movement.
- The primary function of a joint is to provide movement and flexibility to the skeleton.

WHAT ARE THE FUNCTIONS OF MUSCLES FOR POSITIONING AND MOVING PATIENTS?

- Skeletal muscle contraction is accomplished through the stimulation of many muscle fibers.
- Contraction of skeletal muscles provides movement, stabilizes joints, produces body heat, and maintains posture.

WHAT CHANGES IN THE SYSTEM OCCUR WITH AGING?

- Bone strength and mass are lost because of mineral resorption. This may lead to osteoporosis, which

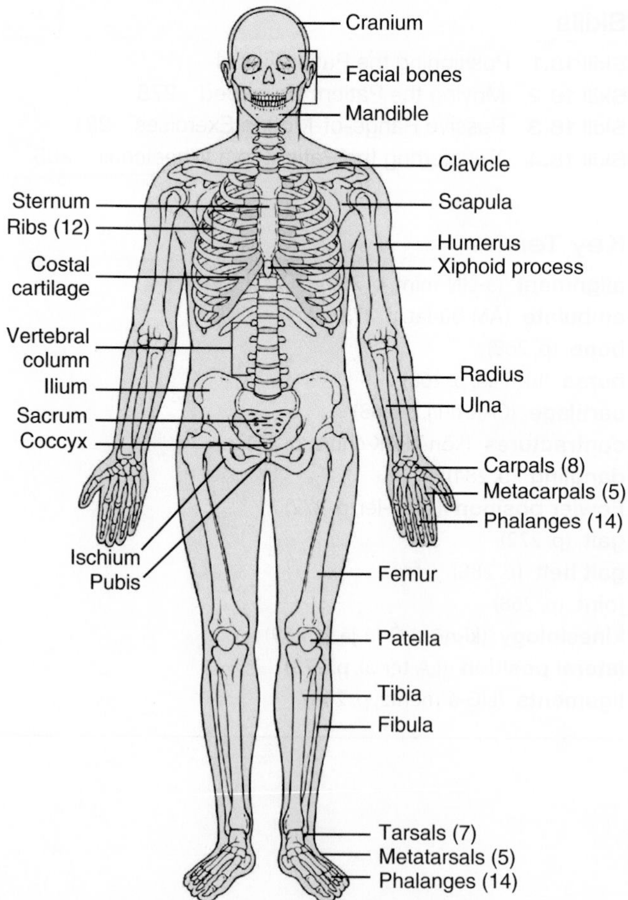

FIGURE 18.1 Anterior view of a normal skeletal system. (From Frazier, M. S., & Drzymkowski, J. W. [2009]. *Essentials of Human Disease and Conditions* [4th ed.]. St. Louis, MO: Saunders.)

is more common in women of Asian or Caucasian descent.

- The loss of bone density predisposes the older adult to fractures. The fractures do not heal quickly because of the decreased mineral uptake.
- Muscle cells are lost (sarcopenia) and replaced by fat. This leads to a loss of muscle strength and endurance.
- Muscle fiber elasticity is decreased or lost, causing decreased flexibility.
- Joint motion may decrease, limiting mobility, activity, and exercise.

 QSEN Considerations: Safety

Safety Concerns for the Older Adult

The older adult has an increased risk of falls related to sarcopenia and diminished balance. Decreased visual acuity, hearing loss, and decreased sensations create an increased risk for pressure injuries.

PRINCIPLES OF BODY MOVEMENT FOR NURSES

Kinesiology (also called body mechanics) is the study of the movement of body parts. The use of good body movement is important for the safety of both nurse and patient. The body functions best when it is in correct anatomic position or **alignment** (arrangement in a straight line, bringing a line into order). Correct body alignment is generally called "good posture" (Fig. 18.2). Correct, proper body movement is essential to prevent injuries. **One of the most common injuries for health care workers is lower back strain.** With proper use of body mechanics, many injuries can be avoided.

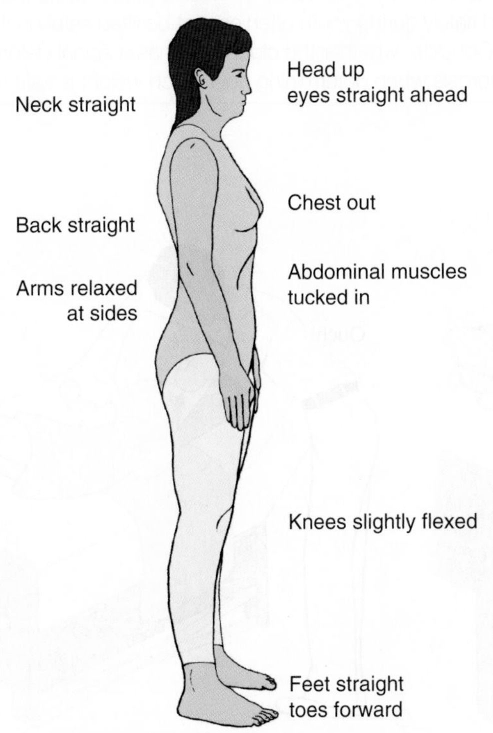

FIGURE 18.2 Correct standing body alignment.

 QSEN Considerations: Safety

Core Exercises

Core exercises can help keep your back healthy and strong. Core exercises train the muscles in your abdomen, pelvis, lower back, and hips to work together, leading to improved balance and stability.

In today's health care environment, more patients are being cared for at home. For these people and their caregivers to be safe, everyone must use correct lifting, moving, and positioning techniques (Box 18.1).

OBTAIN HELP WHENEVER POSSIBLE

It is always desirable to get help when moving patients. Combining the efforts of two or more health care workers to change a patient's position divides the work. Each worker has less weight or fewer parts of the body to move. Because of the increased acuity and overall increased workload of nurses, it is not always possible to find assistance to help with a move or lift; however, it is always better to wait for help than to risk injury. Encourage the patient to assist when transferring and moving if possible. Use devices such as mechanical lifts and slide boards where available. Properly used, these items decrease the workload and prevent injury.

USE YOUR LEG MUSCLES

In positioning and transferring, use the large muscles in legs as much as possible. Instead of bending over at the waist to pick up something from the floor, bend at the knees and lower slowly until you can pick up the item without straining the back (Fig. 18.3). Use the greatest number of muscles possible when lifting or moving an object. For instance, when turning a patient in bed, flex

Box 18.1 Guidelines for Moving and Lifting: Body Mechanics

- Obtain help whenever possible.
- Ask the patient to help if able.
- Bend or flex knees.
- Use the greatest number of muscles possible.
- Use thigh, arm, or leg muscles rather than back muscles.
- Use a wide base of support. Keep feet about shoulders' width apart.
- Use smooth coordinated movement; avoid jerking or sudden pulling motions.
- Keep elbows and work close to your body.
- Work at the same level or height as the object to be moved.
- If possible, pull objects toward you rather than pushing or lifting.
- Directly face the object or person to be moved.
- Keep your trunk straight; do not twist when lifting or pulling.
- Use your arms as levers when pulling the patient toward you. Lock the elbows and rock back on your heels, using the weight of your body to move the patient.

at the knees and use the muscles in the legs as well as arms. Without the power in the legs, the muscles in the arms will have to perform more work. It is far better to use thigh, arm, and leg muscles than back muscles.

PROVIDE STABILITY FOR MOVEMENT

Keep feet about shoulders' width apart. This establishes a wide base of support and provides stability for movement. It is easier to lose balance and move away from a center of gravity with feet placed close together. Keeping a wide base of support enables more even weight distribution and strength to carry heavier loads.

USE SMOOTH, COORDINATED MOVEMENTS

Use smooth, coordinated movements instead of jerking or sudden pulling motions. To coordinate effort, tell patients and other staff members to move, lift, or pull "on the count of 3." This will help to ensure that everyone is working at the same time to maximize the effort and decrease the individual load. This also provides good communication to minimize injury to other workers and promote overall team safety.

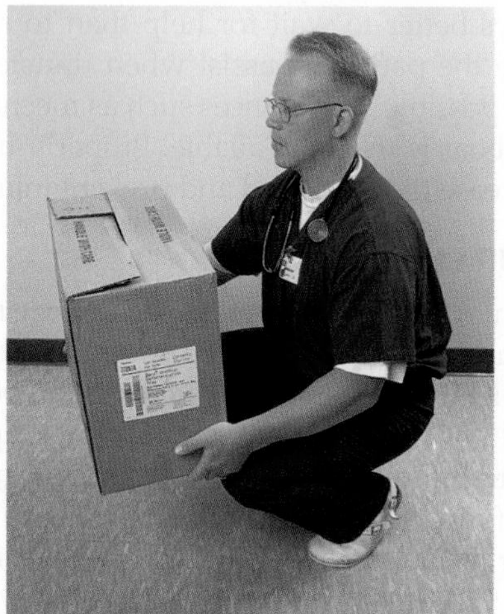

FIGURE 18.3 Using leg muscles to prevent back strain.

KEEP LOADS CLOSE TO THE BODY

Keep your elbows and work close to the body. This keeps the workload close to the waist and center of gravity.

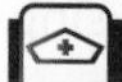

Clinical Cues

Nursing Tip

Pick up a large textbook and hold it close to your body. Although it is a heavy book, it is easily managed close to your center of gravity. Slowly extend your elbows forward. This moves the book farther from the center of gravity, and the book becomes increasingly heavy. Do not fully extend your elbows or you will put stress on your back muscles.

KEEP LOADS NEAR THE CENTER OF GRAVITY

Work at the same level or height as the object to be moved (Fig. 18.4). This keeps the workload near the worker's center of gravity. Changing bed linens is a good example of this principle. When changing linens or moving a patient, temporarily raise the bed to waist level to keep the work near the center of gravity. Injuries are more likely to occur the farther away the work is from the center of gravity.

Life-Span Considerations

Older Adults

Abilities, strength, and flexibility all change as we age. Older adults may need to be reeducated on how and what they may safely lift. As the body ages, there is a change in body posture (and center of gravity) and usually a decrease in muscle mass. Items that could be lifted safely during youth often cannot be lifted safely in the later years. Consider whether the older adult has a spinal deformity or osteoporosis when determining how much weight is safe to lift.

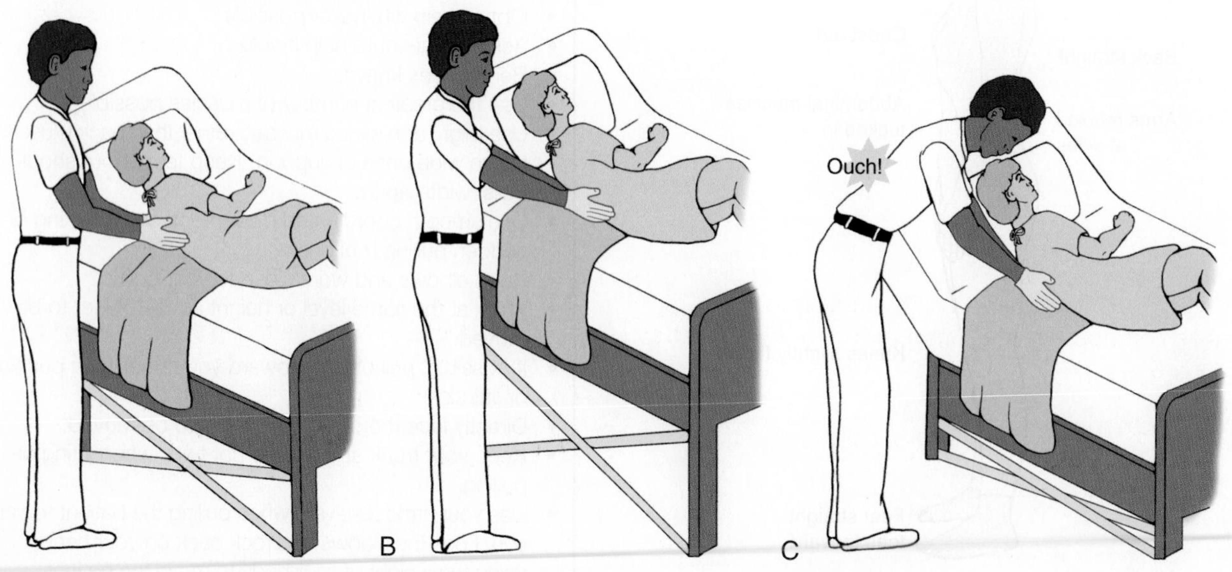

FIGURE 18.4 (A) Correct working height. (B) Work is too high. (C) Work is too low.

PULL AND PIVOT

Pulling actions require less effort compared with pushing or lifting. Whenever possible, use pulling motions. For example, when transferring a patient to a stretcher, two nurses should stand on the far side of the stretcher to pull the patient toward them onto the stretcher. This movement is easier than pushing because it brings the patient closer to each nurse's center of gravity.

Directly face the object or person to be moved. It is much easier to move an object if the nurse is facing in its direction.

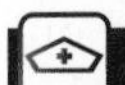 Clinical Cues

Nursing Tip

Place an object on the floor. Stoop down with the object in front of you and move the object forward. This is fairly easy. Now place the same object on the floor, stoop down, only this time with the object to the side. Moving the object forward is not as easy in this instance. To move the object at your side forward, you would need to twist to the side. To maintain proper body mechanics, keep your trunk straight when lifting or pulling. Avoid twisting. Instead, if turning is needed, **pivot** (turn or change direction with your feet while remaining in a fixed place). Pivoting prevents twisting, which can lead to back strain and injury

PRINCIPLES OF BODY MOVEMENT FOR PATIENTS

Body movement and alignment are also important for patients. Many patients are unable to change position or move in bed independently. There are two basic principles for patients:

- Maintain correct anatomic position.
- Change position frequently.

If these principles are not observed, the patient may experience complications or injury.

HAZARDS OF IMPROPER ALIGNMENT AND POSITIONING

Hazards of improper alignment and positioning include:

- Interference with circulation, which may lead to **pressure injuries** (tissue injuries that form from local interference with circulation).
- Muscle cramps and possible **contractures** (resistance to stretch in damaged muscle that pulls a joint into a fixed or "frozen" position).
- Muscle atrophy (decrease in muscle mass, flexibility, and strength).
- Fluid collection in the lungs.

Contractures, muscle cramps, and respiratory problems as complications of immobility are discussed in Chapter 39.

 Life-Span Considerations

Older Adults

Older adults have a greater risk for skin breakdown than younger patients do because they have decreased muscle mass, connective tissues, and elastin and collagen, as well as less moisture in their skin. This makes the skin more friable and prone to potential injuries such as shearing and pressure ulcers. Always handle older adults with care.

Pressure Injuries

Pressure injuries, formerly known as pressure ulcers, decubitus ulcers, or bedsores, occur from pressure on the skin. This pressure causes a local area of tissue **necrosis** (local death of tissue from disease or injury). Most often, the area of pressure occurs between a bony prominence and an external surface. Besides pressure, the other main factor in pressure injury development is **shearing force.** Shearing is an applied force that causes a downward and forward pressure on the tissues beneath the skin. Shearing forces occur when a patient slides down in a chair, bedclothes are pulled from beneath the patient, or the patient is slid up to the head of the bed without lifting the body. Pressure injuries are discussed in Chapters 19 and 38.

❖ APPLICATION OF THE NURSING PROCESS

◆ ASSESSMENT (DATA COLLECTION)

When assessing the **standing patient's** body alignment, begin by noting the head position in relation to the rest of the body (see Fig. 18.2). Is the head centered and erect? Are the shoulders and hips parallel? Are the knees and ankles slightly flexed and parallel to the hips and shoulders? Do the arms hang comfortably at the patient's side? Are the feet slightly apart to provide a base of support? During the assessment, also observe for any muscle weakness or paralysis, and check **symmetry** (equality in size, form, and arrangement of parts on the opposite sides of a plane; a mirror image) of extremities.

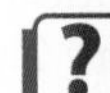 Think Critically

How would you describe your posture right now? Is your body in correct alignment?

When assessing the **sitting patient**, again observe for symmetry (Fig. 18.5). Determine whether the patient's head is erect and centered over the shoulders. Are the buttocks in the same plane as the shoulders, and are the thighs in line with the shoulders? The patient's weight should be distributed evenly over the buttocks and thighs. The knees should be flexed at about 90 degrees, with the feet resting comfortably on the floor. Provide a footstool if the feet do not reach the floor. The arms should lie comfortably in the lap or be supported by the chair armrests.

When assessing the **lying patient**, assess carefully for alignment and correct position. Patients often lie on their back when in bed. It is important to change this position frequently to prevent problems associated with immobility. Support the head with one pillow so the neck is not hyperflexed. The vertebral column should be centered and in alignment, without observable curves. The mattress should support the body in this position.

Finally, assess the patient's ability to **ambulate** (walk) and to change position independently. Observe the patient walking.

Concepts Covered in This Chapter

Professional Pointer

A primary care provider's activity order is needed for a patient to be out of bed.

Is the head centered over the vertebral column? Is the **gait** (style of walking) even and unlabored? Is the patient balanced? Is there any weakness or favoring of one side? This will determine the patient's ability to ambulate independently or determine the type of assistance needed.

◆ NURSING DIAGNOSIS

Nursing diagnoses commonly used for problems with body movement are:

- Risk for injury.
- Impaired physical mobility.
- Risk for impaired skin integrity.
- Impaired walking.

The patient's defining characteristics are added to the nursing diagnosis stem to individualize the care plan. Nursing diagnoses for patients with problems of immobility are covered more extensively in Chapter 39.

◆ PLANNING

The data collected during the assessment phase give information about how to best promote independence or assist the patient. If the patient is not able to move independently, change the patient's position at least every 2 hours to avoid complications. Your assessment will indicate whether you can move the patient independently or if you will need assistance. During planning, decide how to change the patient's position and whether you can delegate this task to unlicensed assistive personnel.

The home setting must also be considered when planning care for the patient. Will the family be able to turn or assist in turning the patient safely after discharge? Will the patient or family need any assistive devices, and do they know how to use them? Will extra pillows need to be purchased to assist with positioning? Will the patient be able to get around in and out of the home independently? Assessment and planning will answer these questions.

Expected outcomes are written for each nursing diagnosis. Examples related to the above mentioned nursing diagnoses are as follows:

- Patient will experience no musculoskeletal injury.
- Patient will return to former level of mobility within 6 months.
- Skin integrity will remain intact.
- Patient will not experience an injury while ambulating.

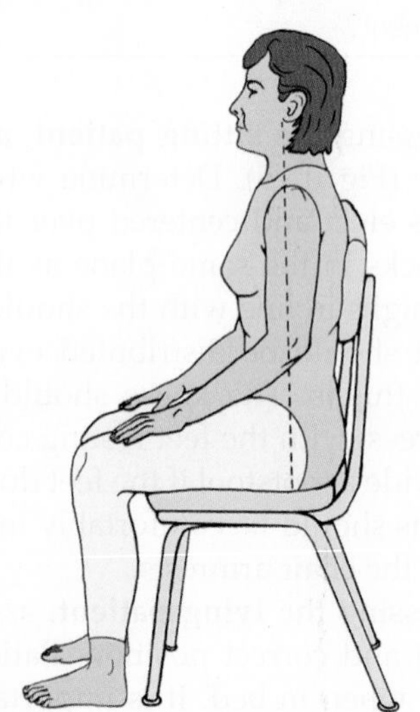

FIGURE 18.5 Correct sitting body alignment.

◆ IMPLEMENTATION

Positioning

Changing position accomplishes four things: (1) it provides comfort; (2) it relieves pressure on bony prominences and other parts; (3) it helps prevent contractures, deformities, and respiratory problems; and (4) it improves circulation. It is essential to know how to correctly support and position the patient while maintaining good body mechanics.

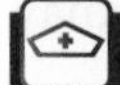

Clinical Cues

Maintain the patient's privacy through draping while changing positions. Many positions can leave a patient feeling vulnerable, and draping demonstrates respect for the patient and supports privacy.

Common Positions and Their Variations

While in bed, the patient can assume three basic positions: supine, side lying, and prone.

The **supine position** is appropriate for patients who are resting on their back. It is recommended after spinal surgery, cardiac catheterization, and after the administration of some types of spinal anesthetics. The supine position is similar to proper standing alignment except that the body is in the horizontal as opposed to the vertical plane.

Variations of the supine position are Fowler, semi-Fowler, and low Fowler positions. **Fowler position** is arranged by elevating the head of the bed 60 to 90 degrees. **Semi-Fowler position** is an elevation of 30 to 60 degrees, and low Fowler is an elevation of 15 to 30 degrees. Unless contraindicated, the knees can be raised 10 to 15 degrees in these positions. Alternatively, place a footboard at the bottom of the bed to brace the patient's feet in correct alignment. These positions improve cardiac output and respiration and promote urinary and bowel elimination. Do not place a patient who had abdominal surgery in a Fowler position unless ordered. Elevation of the knees above 15 degrees is contraindicated in older and postoperative patients because it is associated with decreased circulation of the lower extremities. Fowler position may help the patient who had a stroke and has paresis to swallow food and secretions.

Dorsal recumbent and **dorsal lithotomy positions** are other variations of the supine position. In the dorsal recumbent position, patients are on their back with knees flexed and soles of the feet flat on the bed (Fig. 18.6). This is used for a variety of procedures and examinations. The dorsal lithotomy position (Fig. 18.7) is used for examining the pelvic organs. It is like the dorsal recumbent position except the feet are usually placed in stirrups and the legs are spread farther apart and abducted. Patients with joint problems or arthritis may have difficulty assuming this position.

The **side-lying or lateral position** is achieved by having patients rest on their side. It alleviates pressure from bony prominences on the back. The major portion of the patients' weight is on the dependent shoulder and hip. Maintain the vertebral column in proper alignment as if they were standing. The oblique side-lying position removes pressure from the dependent shoulder and hip and is easier for patients to maintain.

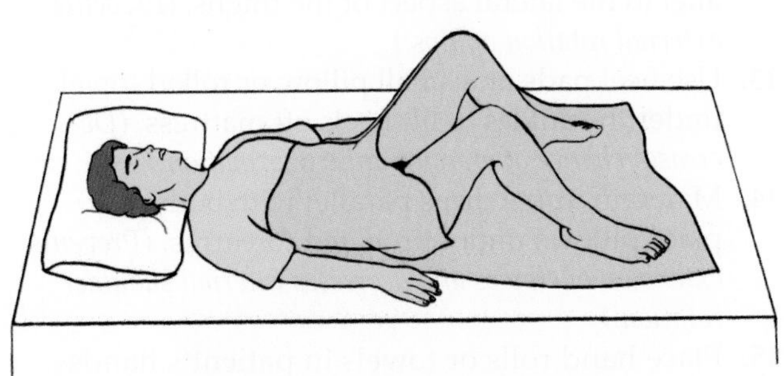

FIGURE 18.6 Dorsal recumbent position.

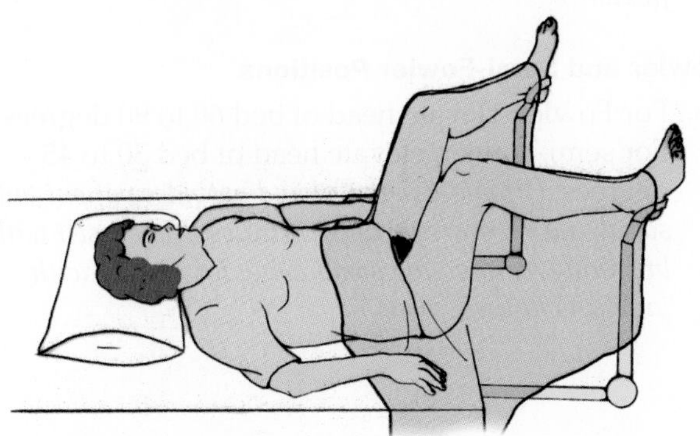

FIGURE 18.7 Lithotomy position.

Sims position is a variation of the side-lying position. It is used for rectal examinations, administering enemas, and inserting suppositories or for an unconscious patient. The distribution of weight is different from in the side-lying position because in the Sims position the weight is distributed over the anterior ileum, humerus, and clavicle. When positioning on the left side, place the patient's left arm behind her, and draw her right knee and thigh up above the left lower leg. Tilt the chest and abdomen forward so the patient is resting on them as well.

In the **prone position**, the patient is lying face down. It provides an alternative for patients on prolonged bed rest or who are immobilized. Spinal cord–injured patients sometimes use this position. The position is generally not well tolerated because it may be uncomfortable and deep breathing is difficult; it has been linked to sudden, unexpected death in patients with epilepsy (Liebenthal et al., 2015). One specific population subset, however, that may benefit from the prone position is critical care unit patients with severe acute respiratory distress syndrome (Drahnak & Custer, 2015). In the prone position, for patients who have not had a spinal cord injury, turn the head to one side or the other and support with a small pillow. If the head is not turned or the patient is not on a special bed with a removable piece at the head, the patient will not be able to breathe. It is often difficult for patients to access entertainment or to socialize in this position. Consider these factors when planning holistic care.

The **knee-chest position** is a variation of the prone position (Fig. 18.8). The patient is face down on the bed with the head turned to one side. The chest, elbows, and knees rest on the bed, and the thighs are perpendicular to the bed. The lower legs rest flat on the bed. This is used for rectal examinations and as a method to restore the uterus to a normal position. Do not leave the patient alone in the knee-chest position because the patient may become dizzy, faint, or fall. A patient with arthritis or joint abnormalities may not be able to assume this position.

Skill 18.1 describes how to place the patient in many of the above described positions.

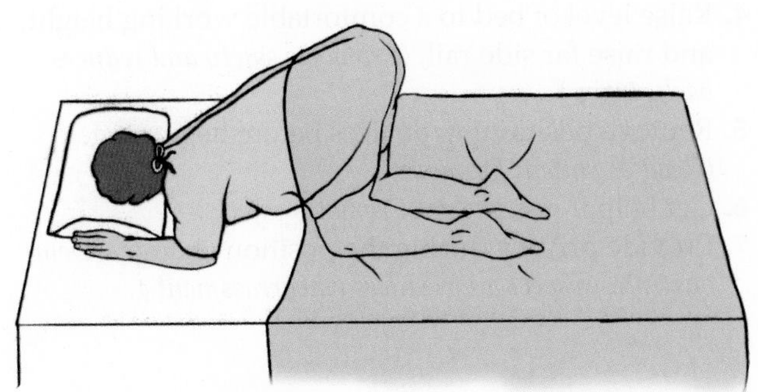

FIGURE 18.8 Knee–chest position.

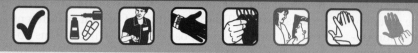

Skill 18.1 Positioning the Patient

 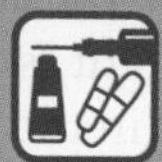 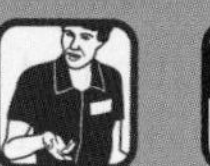 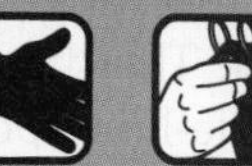 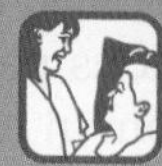 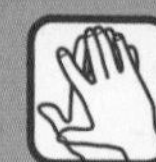 

Correct positioning of patients is essential for maintaining proper alignment. Many patients, because of injury, disease, helplessness, or therapeutic devices, need assistance with repositioning. Change the position of the patient in bed a minimum of every 2 hours. Obtain help to prevent injury to yourself and the patient. If rotating patients in the supine lying position, rotate between left side, right side, and back positions evenly. Consider keeping a chart to document the patient's position throughout the day.

Supplies

Positioning devices as needed for each position:

- Pillows
- Boots
- Trochanter rolls
- Hand rolls
- Trapeze bar
- Splints
- Side rails
- Sandbags
- Bed board
- Footboard or high-top sneakers

Review and carry out the Standard Steps in Appendix A.

ACTION *(RATIONALE)*

Assessment (Data Collection)

1. Assess for any restrictions to placing patient in particular positions. *(Provides baseline data and indicates positions that are contraindicated.)*

Planning

2. Gather positioning supplies. *(Provides easy access to equipment.)*
3. Explain what the patient is expected to do. *(Decreases fear and prepares patient to assist when possible.)*
4. Raise level of bed to a comfortable working height, and raise far side rail. *(Promotes safety and reduces back strain.)*
5. Remove positioning devices before beginning. *(Readies patient for move.)*
6. Get help if necessary. *(Promotes safety.)*
7. Provide privacy during the position change. *(Demonstrates respect and reduces embarrassment.)*

Implementation

8. Perform hand hygiene. *(Reduces transfer of microorganisms.)*
9. Move patient to head of bed (see Skill 18.2). *(Prepares patient to be repositioned properly in the bed.)*

Supine Position

10. Place patient on back with bed in flat position, if not contraindicated. *(Promotes working with gravity.)*
11. Place a pillow under patient's head, neck, and upper shoulders. *(Prevents flexion contractures of neck.)*

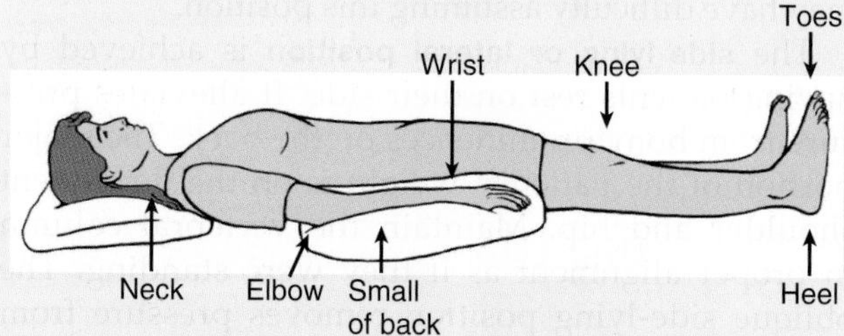

Step **11** **Body alignment**

12. If needed, place sandbags or trochanter rolls parallel to the lateral aspect of the thighs. *(Prevents external rotation of hips.)*
13. Use heel pads or a small pillow or rolled towel under the ankles to lift heels off mattress. *(Decreases chance of pressure injury formation.)*
14. Maintain upper arms parallel with body and place pillows under pronated forearms. *(Prevents extension of elbows and decreases internal shoulder rotation.)*
15. Place hand rolls or towels in patient's hands if needed to maintain correct slightly flexed position. *(Promotes thumb adduction and finger flexion.)*

Fowler and Semi-Fowler Positions

16. For Fowler, elevate head of bed 60 to 90 degrees. For semi-Fowler, elevate head of bed 30 to 45 degrees. *(Promotes comfort and provides patient with social and recreational opportunities. May assist with breathing, eating, and swallowing for patient with problems in these areas.)*

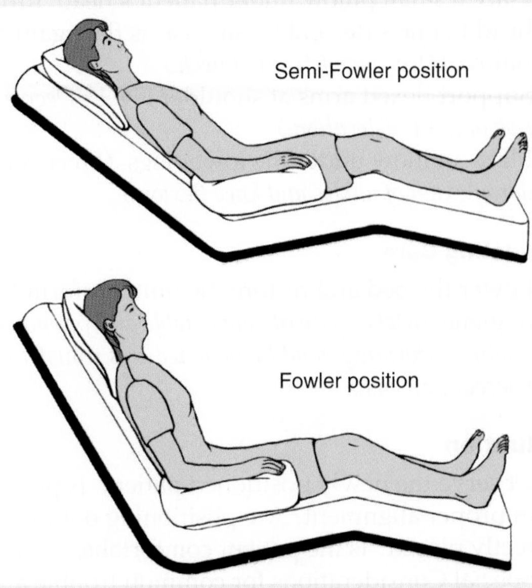

Step 16

17. Place patient's head and neck against small pillow on bed. *(Prevents cervical flexion.)*
18. Support patient's arms and hands with pillows if needed. *(Prevents flexion contracture of hands and wrists and shoulder dislocation from pull of arms and hands.)*
19. Place small pillow or towel roll under thighs. *(Provides comfort without hyperextension of knees or occlusion of popliteal artery.)*
20. Protect heels by using a small pillow, rolled towel, foam boots, or heel pads under patient's ankles. *(Decreases the chance of pressure injury formation.)*

Side-Lying Position

21. Place patient on back on flat bed, if not contraindicated, or with bed as low as patient can tolerate. Move patient slightly to far side of bed, starting with the head, torso, and then feet; align the body correctly. *(Promotes easy access and working with gravity. Body will be centered in the bed when in a new position.)*
22. Stand on side of bed to which you will turn the patient. *(Pulling requires less effort than pushing does.)*
23. Flex the patient's far knee across the near thigh. *(Supports and prevents injury to joints.)*
24. Ask patient to raise the near arm above the head. Place one hand on patient's far shoulder and the other hand on patient's far hip and roll patient toward you with a smooth motion, or use a lift sheet to turn patient smoothly onto the side. *(Supports and prevents injury to joints.)*

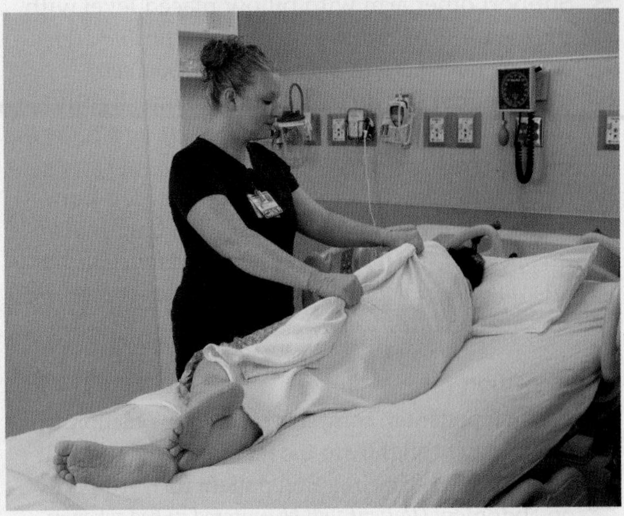
Step 24

25. Fold pillow lengthwise; tuck upper edge under the patient; roll the pillow against patient's back, rolling it toward the mattress. Place a lengthwise pillow between the flexed knees from knee to foot. *(Supports and promotes alignment. Prevents pressure injury formation. Prevents patient from rolling back to the prior position.)*

Side-Lying Oblique Position

26. Move patient's shoulder blade against the bed forward, toward you. *(Disperses weight so it is not centered on the shoulder.)*
27. Flex the arm next to the mattress; raise the hand so that it is even with the top of patient's head. *(Places less pressure on the shoulder and promotes comfort and flexibility of elbow.)*

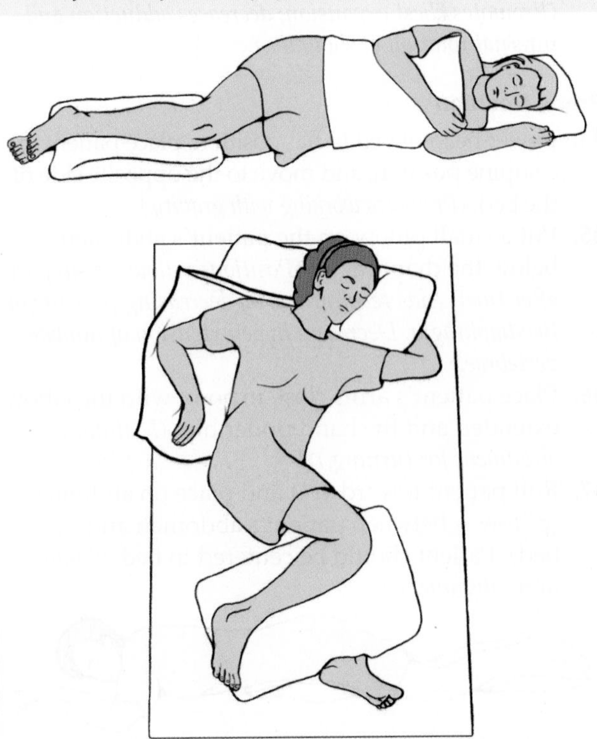
Step 27

28. Support other arm with pillow placed level with the shoulder. *(Promotes chest expansion and decreases adduction and internal rotation of shoulder.)*
29. Reach under hip area and pull the hip slightly forward. *(Decreases pressure on the hip by placing the body at an oblique angle.)*
30. Slightly flex knees and support upper leg from thigh to ankle with pillow(s) folded lengthwise. *(Supports the leg joints and decreases adduction and internal rotation of hip and thigh. Decreases pressure on bony prominences.)*

Sims Position

31. Position patient in complete side-lying position, but move patient slightly to the far side of the bed that patient's back is facing. Roll patient forward partly on abdomen. *(Patient will be centered in bed when repositioned. Rolling patient partly onto abdomen promotes even weight distribution.)*

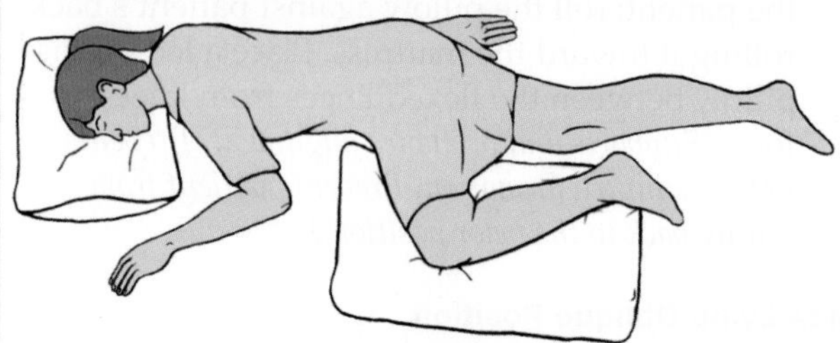

Step **31**

32. Slightly flex arm next to mattress behind patient. *(Prevents extension of elbow. Promotes comfort, and weight is not focused on shoulder joint.)*
33. Support flexed uppermost arm and leg with pillows so that the hand is level with the shoulder. *(Promotes chest expansion; decreases adduction and internal rotation of shoulder.)*

Prone Position

34. Lower head of bed to flat position, place patient in a supine position, and move to the opposite side of the bed. *(Promotes working with gravity.)*
35. Put a small pillow on the patient's abdomen, below the diaphragm. *(Positions pillow for support after turn. Aids respirations by decreasing pressure on the diaphragm. Decreases hyperextension of lumbar vertebrae.)*
36. Place patient's arms close to body with the elbow extended and the hand under hip. *(Maintains alignment for turning.)*
37. Roll patient toward you and place on abdomen (pillow is between patient's abdomen and the bed). Patient should be centered in bed. *(Maintains alignment.)*

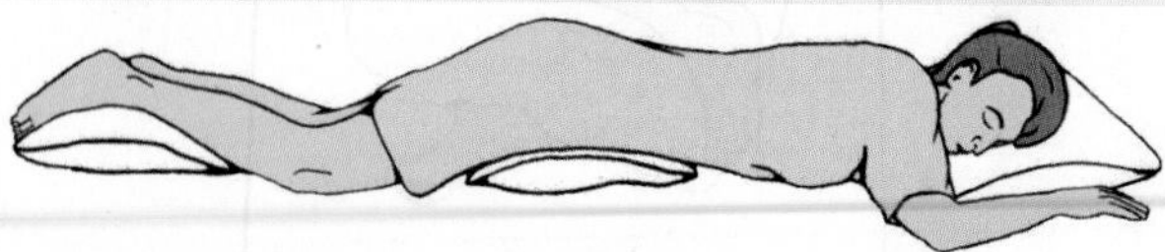

Step **37**

38. Place a small pillow under patient's head; turn head to one side, and be sure ear is flat against the pillow. *(Decreases flexion of neck.)*
39. Support flexed arms at shoulder level. *(Decreases risk of joint dislocation.)*
40. Place a pillow under the lower legs. *(Promotes dorsiflexion of ankles and knee flexion.)*

Completing Care

41. Lower the bed and restore the unit. Perform hand hygiene. *(Makes patient comfortable and promotes safety. Performing hand hygiene reduces transfer of microorganisms.)*

Evaluation

42. Observe the newly positioned patient. Is patient in proper alignment? Are positioning devices correctly placed? Is the patient comfortable? Check Special Considerations for common trouble areas with each position. *(Detects whether patient is in proper body alignment and position.)*

Documentation

43. Document in the medical record, depending on agency policy. Note date, time, position, and positioning devices used. *(Provides for consistency among personnel and validates actions provided.)*

Documentation Example

3/6 0800 Placed in supine position. Correct alignment maintained with pillows, hand rolls, and foot splints. (Nurse's electronic signature)

Special Considerations

- Wear gloves when moving or positioning a patient if you will be touching blood, body fluid, secretions, excretions, broken skin, mucous membranes, or contaminated items.
- For a patient who has edema or is dehydrated, turn and reposition more frequently than every 2 hours to avoid skin breakdown.

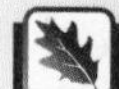 Life-Span Considerations

Older Adults

When repositioning an older adult, you must move slowly and carefully to avoid hurting the patient. Arthritis may cause the joints to be stiff and more difficult to move.

After positioning a patient, check the following areas to prevent possible problems.

Supine Position

- Feet: Maintain the feet in dorsiflexion; you may need to use a positioning device to decrease the chance of foot drop.
- Lower back: If the patient complains of lower back pain, place a small pillow or rolled towel under the patient's lumbar spine.

- Pressure points: Check for pressure on the occiput, lumbar vertebrae, elbows, and heels.

Fowler and Semi-Fowler Positions

- Circulation: Check to see that the lower extremities have palpable pulses, verifying that the popliteal artery is not occluded.
- Pressure points: Check for pressure on the scapula, sacrum, elbows, and heels.

Side-Lying Position

- Neck: Avoid lateral flexion.
- Pressure points: Check for pressure on the ankles, knees, trochanter, ileum, and ear.

Sims Position

- Hip and shoulder: Support properly to prevent internal rotation and adduction.
- Pressure points: Check for pressure on the clavicle, humerus, ileum, knees, and ankles.

Prone Position

- Feet: Position in dorsiflexion. Sustained extension with plantar flexion is undesirable.
- Pressure points: Check for pressure on the ear, chin, hips, and knees.

Critical Thinking Questions

1. If you use a pillow, you do not need to check for pressure points in that area. Is the statement true or false? Why?
2. What are some of the advantages of having a trapeze on a bed when the patient has a broken leg?

Positioning devices. Devices used for positioning include pillows, boots or splints, positioning wedges, footboards, cushioned boots or high-top sneakers, a trapeze bar (Fig. 18.9A), sandbags, hand rolls, trochanter rolls (see Fig. 18.9B), side rails, and bed boards. Use pillows to support the body or extremities and elevate body parts. Boots or splints help to maintain dorsiflexion of the feet and may help to prevent heel pressure. Footboards and high-top sneakers are alternative devices used to maintain foot dorsiflexion. Trochanter rolls prevent external rotation of the hips and legs when a patient is lying in a supine position. Sandbags immobilize an extremity, provide support, and maintain correct body alignment. Hand rolls and splints for the hands and wrists help to prevent contractures of the hands, promote thumb adduction, keep the fingers slightly flexed, and prevent dorsiflexion of the wrist. A trapeze bar allows a patient to adjust position by raising the trunk and buttocks off the bed. The patient may use it to move up in bed, transfer from bed to wheelchair, and strengthen upper extremities. Side rails assist the patient in changing position and turning in bed. Bed boards are boards that are placed under the home mattress to give more support to the mattress and thereby improve vertebral alignment. Similarly, blocks underneath the head of the bed may be used at home for elevation.

Moving Patients Up in Bed

Patients need different amounts of help moving in bed. After proper instruction, many are able to reposition and move themselves up in bed independently. Other patients are able to provide assistance after they are told what is expected of them. Dependent patients rely on the nursing staff for this procedure. Before moving a patient up in bed, one of the most important steps is to determine how much help will be needed. If lift equipment is available, use it. When manually lifting, if there is any doubt about whether a patient is too heavy or immobile to be moved by you, enlist at least one other person's help. Skill 18.2 describes how to move patients up in bed.

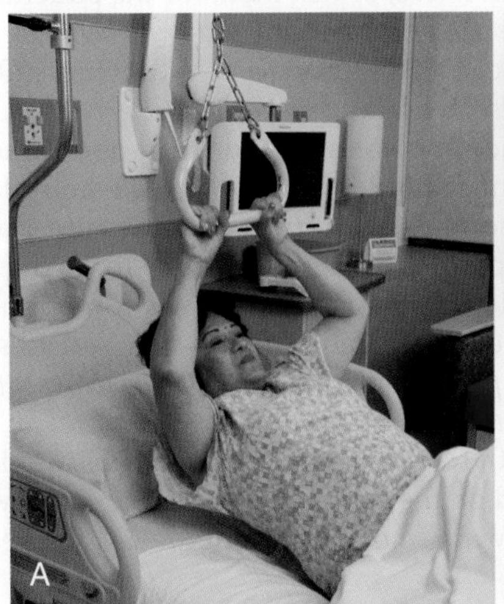

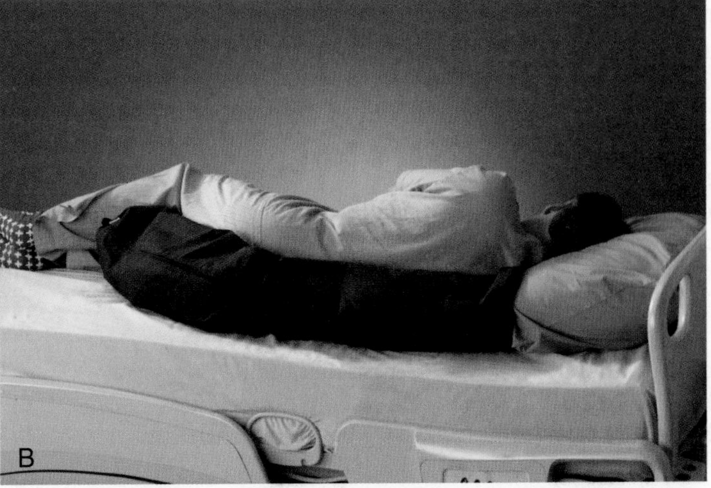

FIGURE 18.9 Positioning devices (A) Trapeze bar. (B) Trochanter roll. ([B] Courtesy Posey Co., Arcadia, California.)

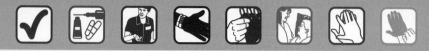

Skill 18.2 Moving the Patient Up in Bed

 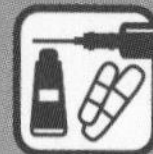 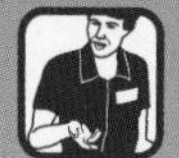   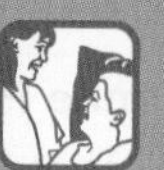 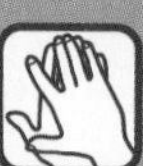 

Many healthy patients can reposition themselves in bed independently after proper instruction. Others, because of injury, disease, weakness, or therapeutic devices, may be able to help somewhat or will be totally dependent on you. It is always easier for two people to assist any patient in moving up in bed. If the patient is large or heavy, use lift equipment or a slide board (transfer board) or air-assisted transfer device if available instead of manually lifting. Check the agency policy.

Supplies

- Lift sheet or slide board for the patient who is dependent or requires assistance

Review and carry out the Standard Steps in Appendix A.

ACTION *(RATIONALE)*

Assessment (Data Collection)

1. Assess alignment, muscle strength, activity tolerance, and mobility. *(Indicates how much the patient can assist.)*

Planning

2. Gather positioning supplies and a lift sheet if needed. *(Promotes easy access to equipment.)*
3. Explain what you wish the patient to do. *(Prepares patient and decreases fear.)*
4. Raise level of bed to a comfortable working height. *(Promotes proper body mechanics and reduces back strain.)*
5. Remove positioning devices for patient's current position. *(Removes obstacles.)*
6. Get help if possible or needed. *(Promotes safety.)*
7. Provide privacy during the position change. *(Protects the right to privacy and reduces embarrassment.)*

Implementation

8. Perform hand hygiene. *(Reduces transfer of microorganisms.)*
9. Lock bed wheels and lower rail, if up, on the side closest to you. *(Prevents bed from rolling and provides access.)*
10. Place pillow upright against headboard. *(Prevents the patient from striking head against the headboard.)*

For the Patient Who Can Assist

11. Place the patient on back. Ask the patient to flex both knees, reach back with one or both arms, and grab the side rails (or hold trapeze bar if present), place chin on chest, then push down on the bed with both feet, lift the buttocks off the bed, and push upward. *(Allows the patient control while promoting exercise and independence. The chin on the chest prevents neck strain and decreases friction on the back of the head.)*

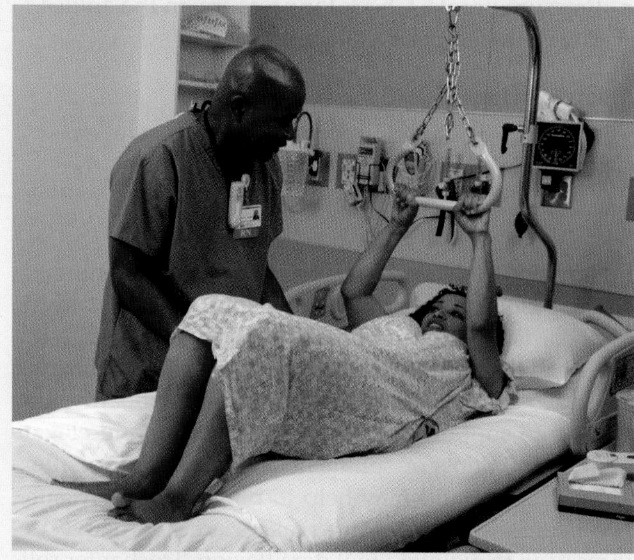

Step **11** Moving patient up in bed

For the Patient Who Needs Assistance (1 or 2 Nurses)

12.
    a. Place the patient on back. Face the head of the bed and, with a broad stance, place one foot in front of the other with the back foot closest to the bed. *(Prevents twisting and back strain. Provides a good base of support.)*
    b. Unless contraindicated, ask patient to flex both knees, or flex them for the patient. *(Decreases resistance of dragging legs.)*
    c. Place patient's arms across the chest. *(Decreases resistance of dragging arms.)*
    d. Place one hand and forearm under the patient's shoulder, support neck, and place the other hand and forearm under the patient's upper thighs. If you have help, each person holds the patient in this way on opposite sides of the bed. *(Supports the patient's heaviest parts. Having two people decreases effort needed.)*
    e. With rocking motion of your hips and legs, and on the count of 3, shift your body weight forward, moving patient toward the head of

the bed. Push with your arms as the patient lifts buttocks and pushes with both feet. *(Coordinates movement; helps to overcome forces of inertia.)*

For the Immobile Patient (1 Nurse)

13.
  a. Place patient supine. *(Promotes working with gravity.)*
  b. Stand diagonally next to the patient's legs in a broad stance with one foot in front of the other and the back foot closest to the bed; slide your arms under the legs. *(Prevents strain or twisting of back and provides a good base of support.)*
  c. Flex your knees and hips so your arms are level with patient's legs. Slide patient's legs diagonally toward head of bed. *(Allows a pulling motion, and legs are easier to move.)*
  d. Stand next to patient's hips; place one arm under patient's thighs and the other arm under patient's lower back. Slide the patient's hips diagonally toward head of bed. *(Maintains body alignment for you and aligns the patient's hips and feet.)*
  e. Place your arm nearest the head of the bed under patient's neck; support head and other shoulder. Place your other arm under patient's chest. Slide patient's trunk, shoulders, neck, and head toward head of bed. The patient is now in alignment on one side of the bed. *(Supports the patient's body weight during movement. Patient is aligned on one side of the bed.)*
  f. Raise side rail. Switch sides of the bed and repeat as necessary until patient reaches desired place in bed. *(Promotes safety and moves patient while maintaining alignment.)*
  g. Center patient in bed, moving the body in the three sections. *(Maintains alignment.)*

For the Immobile Patient (2 Nurses with a Lift Sheet)

14.
  a. Obtain a lift sheet. *(Less effort is needed to move patient on a sheet than to move with hands.)*
  b. With patient in a side-lying position, place lift sheet under patient by rolling up the edge of the sheet close to patient and placing it firmly against patient's back. *(Allows sheet to be pulled easily out from under the patient once turned. Supports the heaviest part of the patient.)*
  c. Roll patient back to the other side over the lift sheet. Pull sheet through. Place patient on back; with a nurse on each side of the bed, roll or fan-fold the sheet close to each side of the patient. *(Decreases risk of injury. If the patient is large, more than two nurses may be needed to transfer the patient safely.)*
  d. Each nurse places one foot slightly in front of the other, about shoulders' width apart, to form a broad base of support. *(Improves balance.)*
  e. With your hips and knees slightly flexed and your back straight, grasp the sides of the rolled or folded sheet as close as possible to patient. On the count of 3, lift patient to the head of the bed. *(Enables you to shift body weight in the direction of movement, decreasing the force needed to lift patient. Maintains proper body movement, decreasing chance of injury.)*

Completing Care

15. Smooth out lift sheet under patient. Position patient in desired position, raise side rails, lower bed, and replace call bell. *(Maintains alignment and promotes safety.)*
16. Restore the unit and perform hand hygiene. *(Promotes comfort and safety. Performing hand hygiene reduces transfer of microorganisms.)*

Evaluation

17. Observe patient's level of comfort, position, body alignment, and potential pressure points. *(Maintains support to body and decreases risk of injury.)*

Documentation

18. Repositioning for comfort and body alignment is documented in the medical record. Note the date, time, procedure, and position. *(Documents position changes and validates that they have been done.)*

Documentation Example

3/6 0900 Feet over end of mattress; moved to head of bed with assistance; repositioned supine for comfort; placed in proper alignment. Bed down, call bell within reach. (Nurse's electronic signature)

? Critical Thinking Questions

1. Explain how positioning yourself correctly when moving a patient up in bed aids the process.
2. Describe complications other than the development of a pressure injury that can occur from improper alignment and positioning.

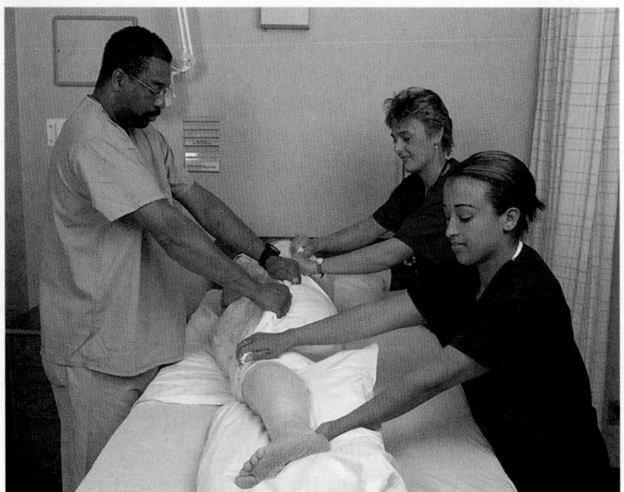

FIGURE 18.10 Logrolling a patient using a lift sheet.

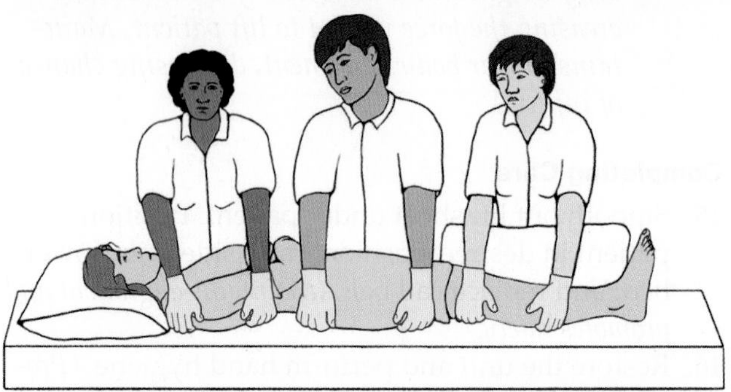

FIGURE 18.11 Logrolling a patient without a lift sheet.

One of the techniques to move patients in bed is called **logrolling**. Logrolling is turning the patient as a single unit while maintaining straight body alignment at all times. Logrolling is often used for patients with injuries or surgery to the spine and for those who must avoid twisting. The linens for an occupied bed are often changed by using the logrolling turn. Logrolling can be done either with or without a lift sheet. If a lift sheet is used, two or three people are needed to accomplish the move, depending on the patient's size (Fig. 18.10). It takes at least three people to logroll a patient safely without a lift sheet (Fig. 18.11).

When using a lift sheet, the nurse and preferably two assistants stand on opposite sides of a locked, flat bed at waist level. Leave a pillow under the patient's head and lower the side rails. Place pillows, if needed, between the patient's legs. All workers face the bed with one foot slightly in front of the other. Roll the lift sheet close to the patient's body and, on the count of 3, lift the patient to one side of the bed, keeping the patient's body in straight alignment. By lifting the patient to one side of the bed first, the patient should be centered in the bed after being logrolled. Position the tallest nurse on the far side of the bed, at the middle portion of the patient. The other two nurses are positioned one at the shoulders and neck and one at the legs and feet of the patient so that they can control movement of these parts. The nurse on the far side of the bed grasps the lift sheet. Again, hold the sheet as close to the patient's body as possible, and on the count of 3, roll the patient in one smooth, coordinated, even motion with the body in straight alignment. Rearrange the pillow under the patient's head and place any other positioning devices before lowering the bed and putting the call bell within the patient's reach.

Logrolling without a lift sheet is accomplished in a similar manner. Evenly space three nurses along one side of a locked, flat bed at waist level. One nurse supports, braces, and rolls the head, neck, and shoulder region as one unit; one supports and rolls the waist and hips; and the third supports and rolls the thighs and lower legs.

Box 18.2 Principles Guiding Range-of-Motion Exercise

- Move the body part to stretch the muscles and keep the joint flexible, but avoid movement to the point of discomfort.
- Perform ROM exercises of the joints of helpless or immobile patients at least twice a day, or more often if tolerated.
- Support the limb above and below the joint when performing passive exercises of arms and legs.
- Perform each movement a minimum of three to five times.
- Involve patients in planning their exercise program, and encourage active performance of the exercises if allowed and capability returns.

Therapeutic Exercise

Physical therapy is often ordered for the patient who is immobilized for an extended period. The primary care provider indicates the patient's problems, and the therapist performs an evaluation and then designs an exercise program to help the patient maintain or regain function and to prevent further musculoskeletal problems from occurring. If a physical therapist is not available, you must assist your patient in performing these exercises. The family or significant other can also be shown how to assist the patient with exercise.

Full range-of-motion (ROM) exercises should be performed either actively or passively several times a day. Active ROM exercises are used for the patient who independently performs activities of daily living but for some reason is immobilized or limited in activity or is unable to move one extremity because of injury or surgery. Passive ROM exercises are performed on the patient who cannot actively move. This patient cannot contract muscles, so muscle strengthening cannot be accomplished. All muscles over a joint are maximally stretched to achieve or maintain flexibility of the joint. This is accomplished by moving the muscles to the point of slight resistance but not beyond. To prevent joint injury in performing passive ROM exercises, support the limb to be exercised above and below the joint. Principles related to carrying out ROM exercises for patients are listed in Box 18.2. Skill 18.3 describes how to provide passive ROM exercises.

Skill 18.3 Passive Range-of-Motion Exercises

 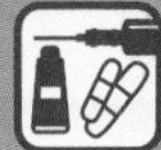 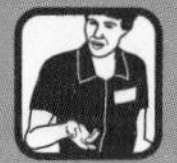   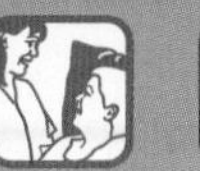 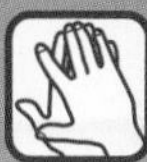 

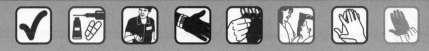

Many patients are paralyzed or have limited mobility of the extremities. To prevent joints from becoming rigid and immovable and to prevent contractures, it is necessary to provide motion to the joints on a regularly scheduled basis. Each exercise is repeated three to five times per session. The remainder of the patient is kept draped while one extremity is exercised.

Supplies

- Blanket or top sheet

Review and carry out the Standard Steps in Appendix A.

ACTION *(RATIONALE)*

Assessment (Data Collection)

1. Check the orders for any contraindication to performance of ROM. *(Avoids injuring the patient with ROM exercise.)*
2. Assess patient for areas of weakness or paralysis. *(Indicates which joints need passive ROM and which can be actively exercised.)*

Planning

3. Be certain wheels of bed are locked and bed is raised to working height. *(Prepares area for the procedure and prevents injury.)*

Implementation

4. Place patient in supine position, remove the pillow, and drape patient with sheet or blanket. *(Positions patient for the procedure. A drape provides privacy for the patient.)*
5. Perform passive ROM of the head and neck:
   - Support the head with your hands, and bring the head forward until the chin touches the chest.
   - Extend the neck by elevating the chin and having the patient look upward. Return the head to the neutral position.
   - Support the head with your hands, and turn it to face the right shoulder and then to the left shoulder. Pause in a neutral position.
   - Bend the head laterally to the right shoulder and then to the left shoulder. Return the pillow under the head. *(Exercises the neck and trapezius muscles. Promotes cervical spine mobility. Pillow makes patient more comfortable.)*

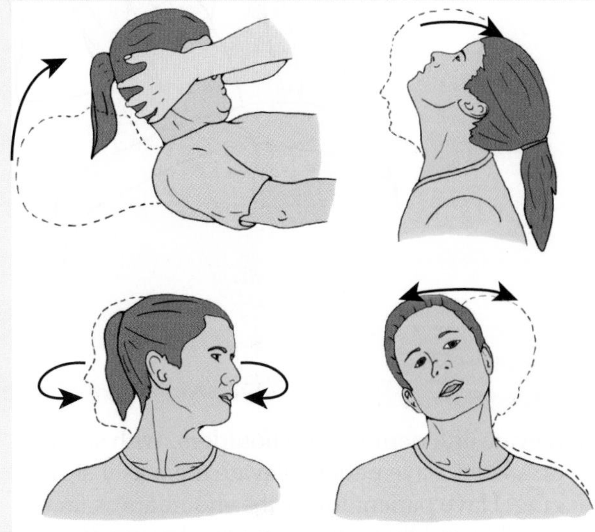

Step 5

6. Flex and extend the shoulder and elbow:
   - Supporting the patient's elbow with one hand, grasp her wrist with your other hand. Bring her arm straight up over the head, then lower it and bend the elbow. Return the arm to the patient's side.
   - Internally rotate the shoulder. Place one hand on the patient's arm above the elbow, and grasp the patient's hand with your other hand. Lift the arm and move it across the chest toward the other side. Return the arm to the original position.
   - Externally rotate the shoulder. Move the arm out from the patient's side in abduction. Flex the elbow, and move the forearm over the head. Return arm to the original position. *(Promotes joint movement and exercises the shoulder muscles.)*

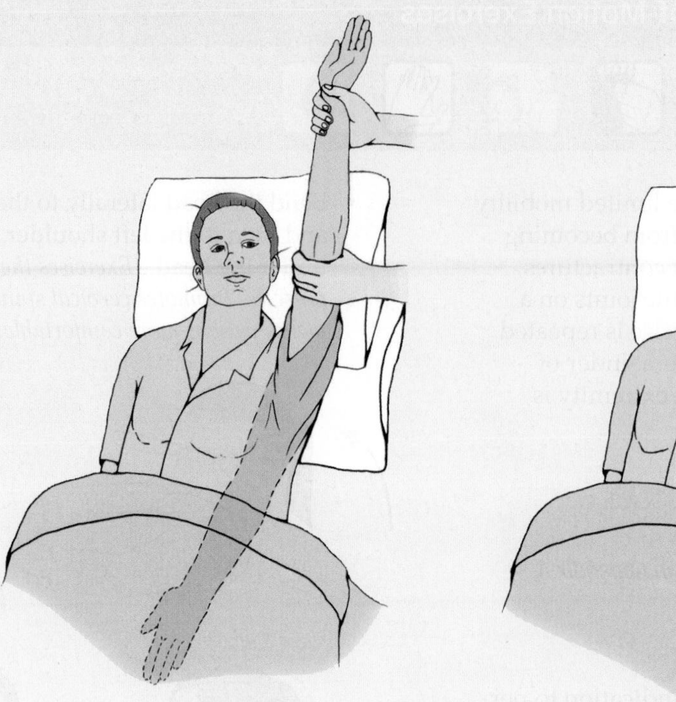

Step 6

7. Elevate and depress the shoulders. With shoulders level, have patient elevate them as if shrugging. Have patient lower the shoulders as far as possible and then return to a level plane. *(Loosens shoulder joints and promotes relaxation.)*
8. Flex the wrist:
   - Hold patient's wrist with one hand and the palm of the hand with your other hand, keeping patient's fingers straight. Hyperextend wrist by bending it backward. Extend the wrist by straightening.
   - Flex patient's wrist by bending the hand forward and closing the fingers to make a fist. Perform circumduction of the hand and wrist. Hold patient's wrist with one hand and the palm of patient's hand with your other hand, keeping the patient's fingers straight. Bend the wrist forward, and move it in a circular motion.
   - Rotate the wrist and hand. Grasp patient's wrist in both of your hands. Rotate wrist by turning the palm toward patient's face for supination and then toward the feet for pronation. *(Exercises the wrist. Circumduction promotes joint flexibility and prevents contractures. Rotation promotes joint flexibility and movement.)*

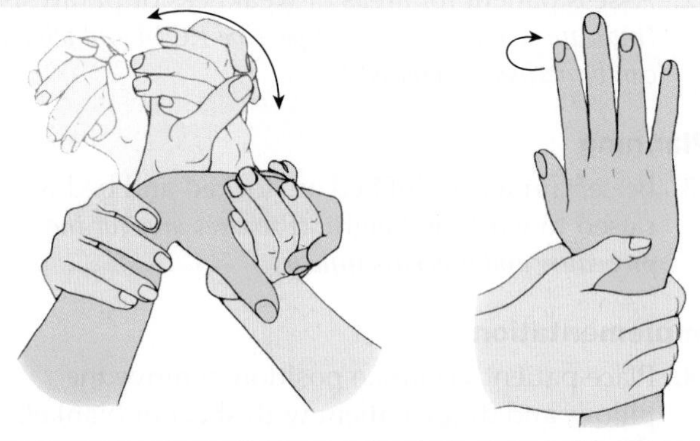

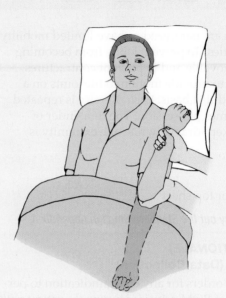

Step 8

9. Exercise the thumb and fingers:
   - Hold patient's hand with one hand and grasp patient's thumb with your other hand. Avoid pressing on the nail bed. Flex thumb and then fingers by bending them onto the palm.
   - Extend the fingers by returning them to their original position. Abduct the fingers by spreading them.
   - Adduct the fingers by returning them to a closed position. Circumduct the fingers and thumb by moving them in a circular motion.
   - Oppose the patient's thumb by touching it to each of her fingers in turn. *(Promotes opposition of thumb and grasp for other fingers needed to perform activities of daily living.)*

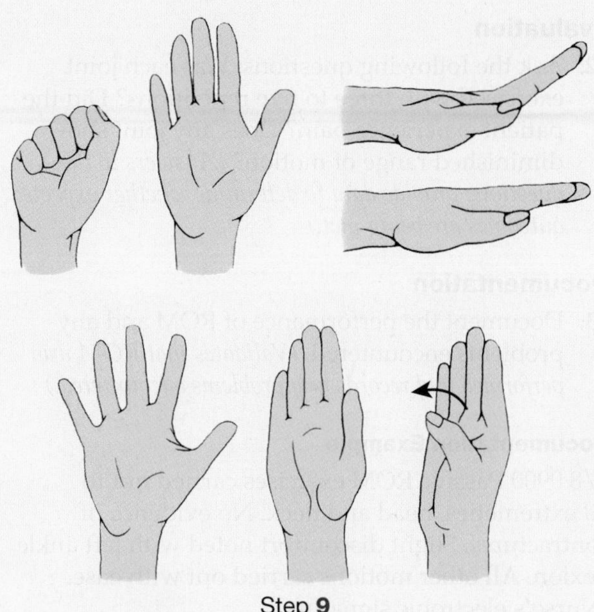

Step 9

10. Exercise the hip and knee:
    - Place one hand under patient's knee, and cup the heel in your other hand. Flex the leg by bending the knee and moving the leg toward the chest as far as it will go without causing pain. Extend the leg by lifting the foot upward and then lowering the leg to the bed.
    - Abduct the hip joint by keeping the leg straight and slowly moving the entire leg toward the edge of the bed. Adduct the hip joint by moving the leg back to the original position.
    - Rotate internally by keeping the leg flat on the bed, and roll the leg inward with toes pointed in toward the opposite foot. Rotate externally by keeping the leg flat on the bed; roll the leg outward with toes pointed away from opposite foot. *(Promotes successful mobility when the patient is able to resume ambulation and prevents hip contracture.)*

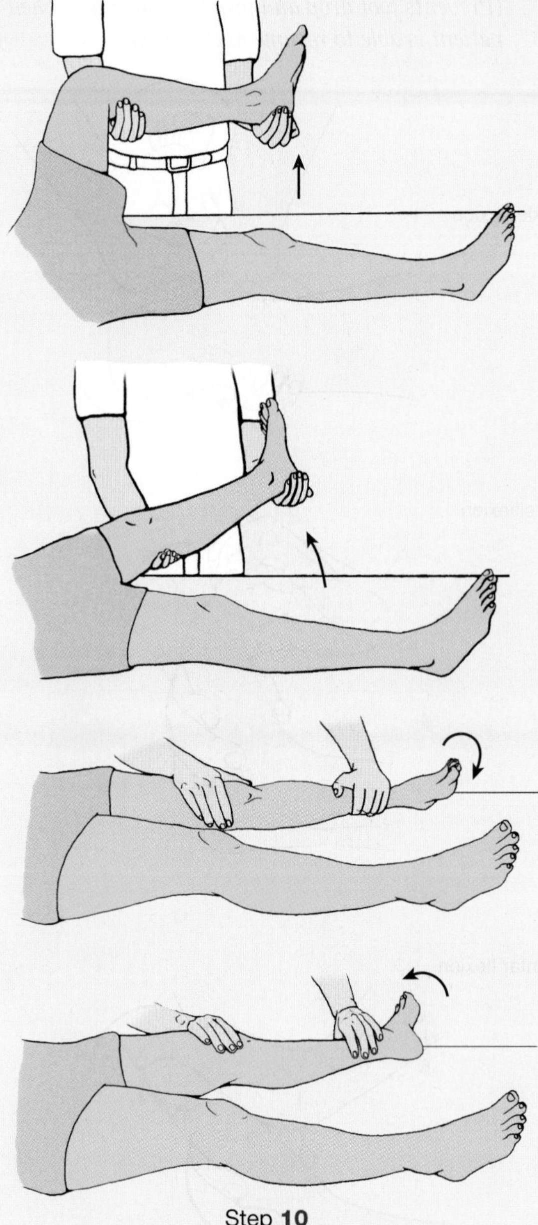

Step 10

11. Exercise the ankle and foot:
    - With the patient's leg on the bed, place one hand on the ball of the foot; then place the other hand just above the ankle.
    - Circumduct by holding the ankle with one hand and turning the whole foot outward and then inward in a circular motion. Perform ankle flexion, ankle extension, and toe circumduction as you did the fingers. Avoid holding the nail beds.
    - Perform dorsiflexion by pushing the foot forward toward the body and pushing down on the heel at the same time.
    - Perform plantar flexion by pushing the toes away from the body while pushing down on the heel.

(Prevents foot drop and promotes mobility when patient is able to resume ambulation.)

Ankle flexion

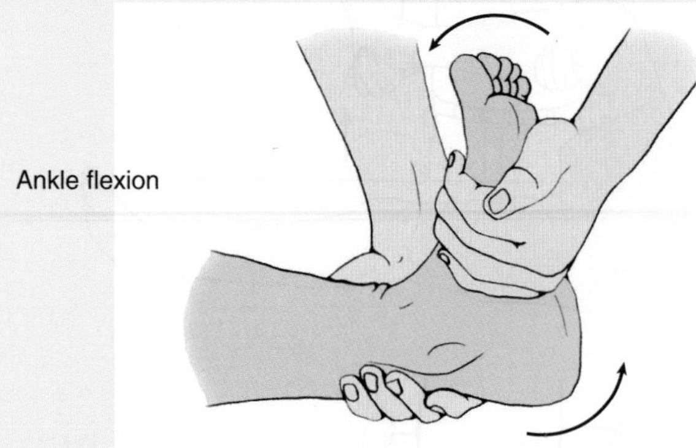

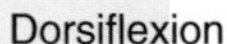

Dorsiflexion

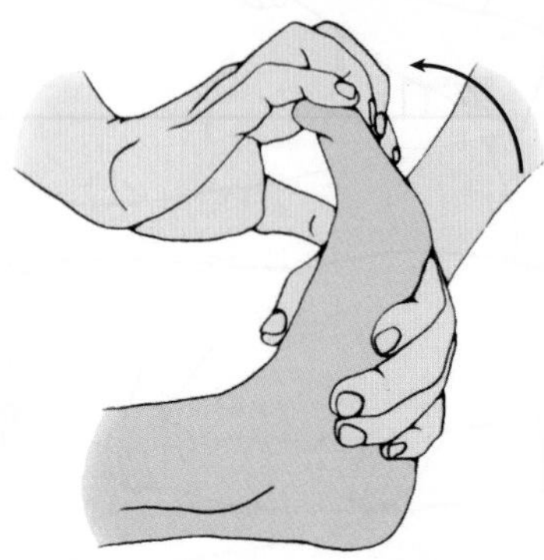

Plantar flexion

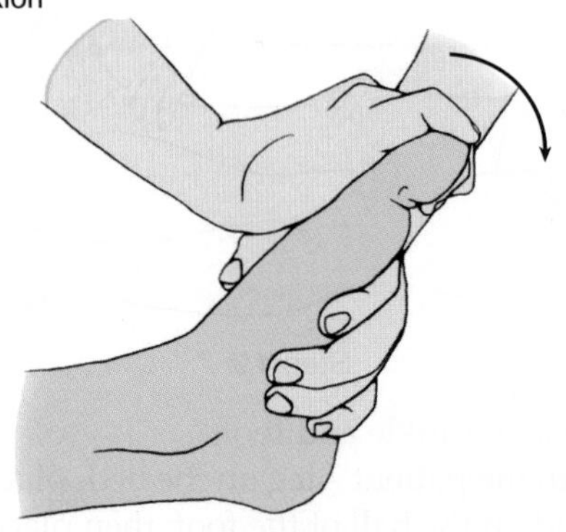

Step **11**

Evaluation

12. Ask the following questions: Was each joint exercised with three to five repetitions? Did the patient experience pain? Does any joint show diminished range of motion? *(Answers to these questions provide data to determine whether expected outcomes are being met.)*

Documentation

13. Document the performance of ROM and any problems encountered. *(Validates that ROM was performed and records any problems encountered.)*

Documentation Example

3/8 0900 Passive ROM exercises carried out to all extremeties, head and neck. No evidence of contractures. Slight discomfort noted with left ankle flexion. All other motions carried out with ease. (Nurse's electronic signature)

Special Considerations

- Encourage patients to perform active ROM on any joint they can safely move because this promotes muscle strength contraction and helps avoid muscle weakness and atrophy.
- If the patient becomes too tired with a full set of passive ROM exercises, divide the exercises into smaller sessions.

Life-Span Considerations

Older adults often have some arthritic joints. Ask the patient about this before beginning the exercises; medicate for pain as needed.

Home Care Considerations

Instruct the caregiver with the home patient on how to do the exercises. Leave a written schedule form for tracking performance.

Critical Thinking Questions

1. Your patient asks you why she needs to perform active ROM exercises. What would you tell her?
2. What benefits do you think will occur if you involve the patient in her exercise plan?

Clinical Cues

Watch the patient's face as you perform passive range-of-motion exercises so that you will know if you are causing pain. If the patient is expressing pain, you are moving the joint too far.

Lifting and Transferring

Lifting and transferring patients requires the use of proper body mechanics and positioning principles. Some patients may be independent or need minimal assistance to ambulate. Others may be completely dependent, needing to be transferred to a chair, wheelchair, or stretcher.

Before transferring a patient to a wheelchair, have her dangle her legs over the side of the bed first (Fig. 18.12). **Dangling** is the term used for the patient position of sitting on the side of the bed with the legs and feet over the side. **The feet either are on the floor or**

supported on a footstool. Dangling is often the first step before sitting in a chair or ambulating. The purpose of this is to accustom the body gradually to the position change. While the patient is dangling, assess the patient's balance, and monitor for orthostatic hypotension, dizziness, or nausea before getting the patient out of bed. If a patient has been on prolonged bed rest, she may only be strong enough to dangle for a few minutes and then will need to lie down again.

Wheelchairs are often used to transport an ambulatory patient to different areas for tests and procedures, or for the patient who is unable to walk or tolerate the fatigue associated with the effort. Either lift equipment or two nurses should transfer a patient to a wheelchair if the patient is unsteady, weak, or heavy (check agency policy) (Fig. 18.13). Transferring a patient to a wheelchair is described in Skill 18.4.

Stretchers may also be called litters, gurneys, or carts. They are used for transporting a patient who is unable to sit in a wheelchair or is having certain tests or procedures done: for example, surgery, CT scan, or MRI imaging. Stretchers have side rails and a safety belt that should be secured before moving the patient. Some hospitals require patients to be transferred with the head of the stretcher elevated to semi-Fowlers position to decrease potential for hospital-acquired pneumonia.

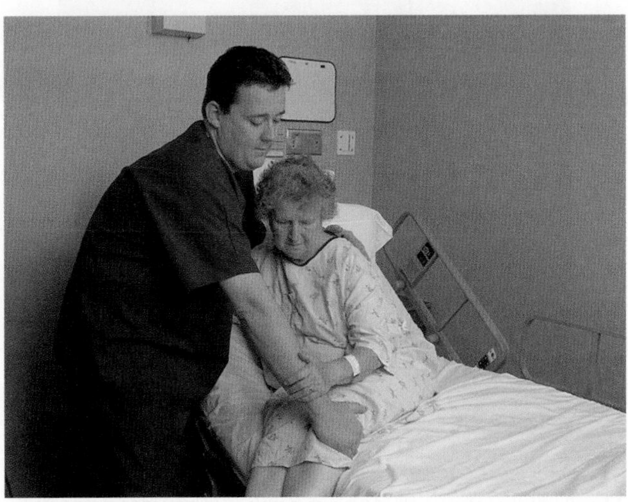
FIGURE 18.12 Assisting the patient to dangle at the side of the bed.

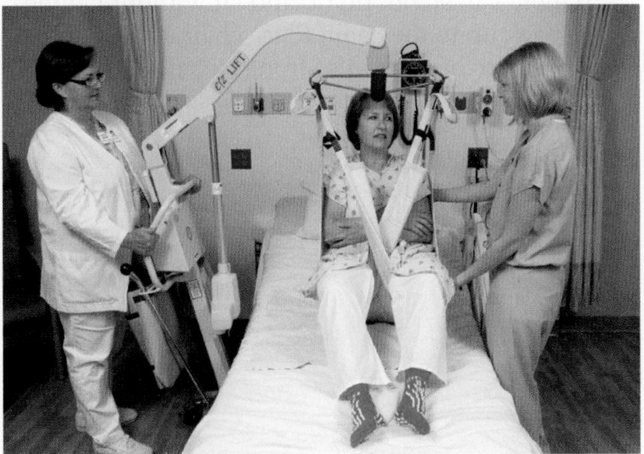

FIGURE 18.13 Mechanical lift system. (From Zerwekh, J., Garneau, A. *Nursing Today: Transition and Trends*, [8th ed.]. St. Louis, MO: Saunders.)

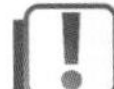 **Safety Alert**

LOCK THE WHEELS

For safety, always lock the wheels on the wheelchair and the bed or stretcher before attempting to transfer a patient into a wheelchair or stretcher or onto the bed. Otherwise, the wheelchair or stretcher could roll away, and the patient could be injured.

 **Think Critically**

Your 39-year-old patient has been on bed rest for 1 week. She has not been out of bed yet and needs to go to the x-ray department for a chest x-ray study. Do you use a wheelchair or a stretcher to send her? Why?

Moving a wheelchair or a stretcher is an exception to a principle of body mechanics discussed earlier in this chapter. Both devices are pushed rather than pulled. To pull a wheelchair or stretcher would cause back strain and twisting. Several manufacturers now make stretchers that have internal motors or require minimum amounts of pushing. These are designed with safe body mechanics in mind.

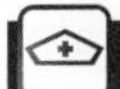 **Clinical Cues**

When transferring a patient into or out of a wheelchair, check positioning of the feet and arms to ensure they will not hit the chair or bed. Position the footrests where they will not interfere with the feet during transfer. Many skin injuries occur when transferring patients into or out of wheelchairs.

Transferring Devices

Devices that may be used in lifting and transferring patients include mechanical lifts, lift or pull sheets, air-assisted lateral transfer devices, slide boards, roller boards, and transfer (or gait) belts. Mechanical lifts are discussed in Chapter 39. Lift sheets are often used to move and transfer a patient. Low friction sheets may be used. Transferring a patient to a stretcher is discussed in Skill 18.5. Lift sheets may be used alone or with the following devices to help maintain the patient's alignment during a transfer.

A **slide board** (also called a transfer board) is a long semirigid polyurethane board, treated with an antistatic coating, to allow the patient to be transferred from bed to stretcher (or vice versa) smoothly and easily. To use a slide board to transfer a patient to a stretcher, turn the patient to one side, place the slide board, and lift sheet underneath the patient. Return the patient to

Skill 18.4 Transferring the Patient to a Wheelchair

 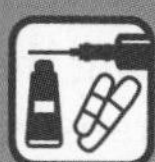 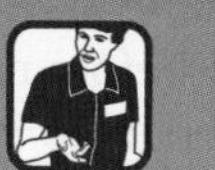 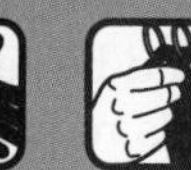 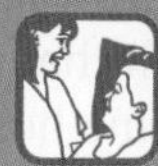 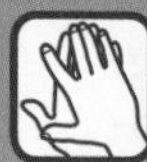 

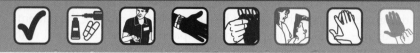

A patient is often transported to another area of the facility by wheelchair. Patients may be transferred to a wheelchair to provide greater independence. A similar procedure is used to transfer a patient to a chair. If the patient is large or heavy, use lift equipment for the transfer if available. Check agency policy.

Supplies

- Bed
- Wheelchair
- Safety jacket if patient is unstable when sitting
- Transfer belt if necessary
- Slippers or nonskid socks and robe

Review and carry out the Standard Steps in Appendix A.

ACTION *(RATIONALE)*

Assessment (Data Collection)

1. Assess patient's size, ability to assist in move, and ability to follow instructions. *(Provides baseline data; indicates what is needed for a safe transfer.)*

Planning

2. Gather wheelchair and transfer belt if needed. *(Provides easy access to equipment.)*
3. Maintain privacy by closing door and/or curtain. *(Protects right to privacy and reduces embarrassment.)*
4. Get help if needed. *(Promotes safety for you and patient.)*
5. Explain the procedure and what the patient is to do. *(Decreases fear of the unknown and prepares patient.)*

Implementation

6. Perform hand hygiene. *(Reduces transfer of microorganisms.)*
7. Place wheelchair parallel to the side of the bed. Lock wheelchair. *(Promotes easy reach and access. Locking wheelchair promotes safety.)*
8. Place transfer belt on patient if patient is weak or paralyzed on one side. *(Decreases the risk of a fall during transfer, and prevents pressure on patient's axillae.)*
9. Lower bed and side rail if elevated. Elevate the head of the bed to the highest level the patient can tolerate. *(Decreases the work for you and patient and promotes safety.)*
10. Help the patient turn onto side. Support the patient's shoulders with one arm and with the other arm at the patient's thighs, help the patient sit up and move the legs over the edge of the bed. Help patient move forward on bed until feet rest on the floor, and allow the legs to dangle. *(Maintains alignment and proper body mechanics; allows patient to adjust to being upright.)*

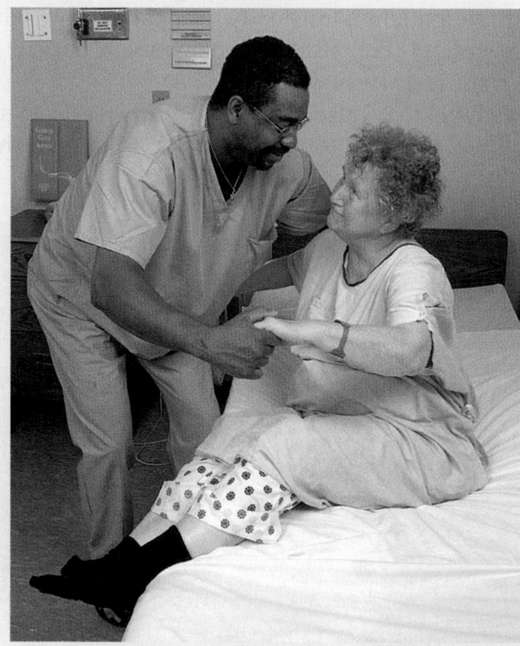

Step **10**

11. Assist patient in donning robe. *(Provides privacy.)*
12. Place slippers or nonskid socks on patient. *(Prevents patient's feet from slipping during transfer.)*
13. Reposition wheelchair closer if necessary so the patient can stand, pivot, and sit without having to back up to the chair. Place chair so that it is closest to the patient's strongest side. *(Reduces distance the patient must travel to sit safely in the chair.)*

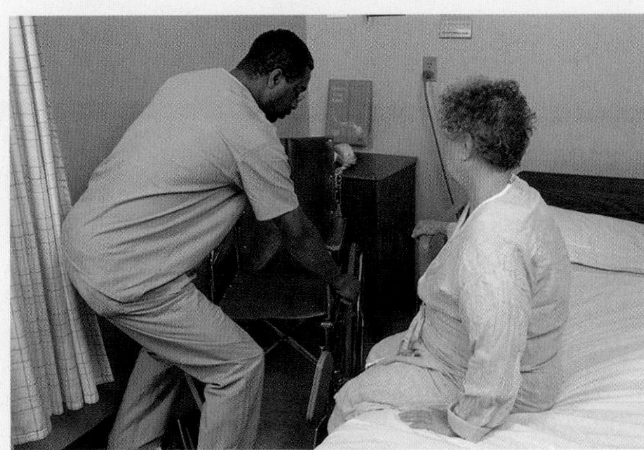
Step 13

14. Check that both wheels are still locked on wheelchair. *(Maintains safety because unlocked wheels allow chair to back away from patient as she sits. This can lead to patient's falling and possible injury for both parties.)*
15. Help patient stand by assuming a moderately wide stance in front of the patient; brace the patient's legs with your knees, which are slightly flexed. *(Provides base of support, maintains alignment, and prevents back injury.)*
16. Place your arms under the patient's axillae and your hands on the patient's scapula. If the patient is not able to push self off of the bed, have patient place arms around your shoulders (not your neck). If the patient is able to help push up from the bed, have patient place hands on the bed. *(Brings patient close to your center of gravity and provides a point of leverage for lifting.)*

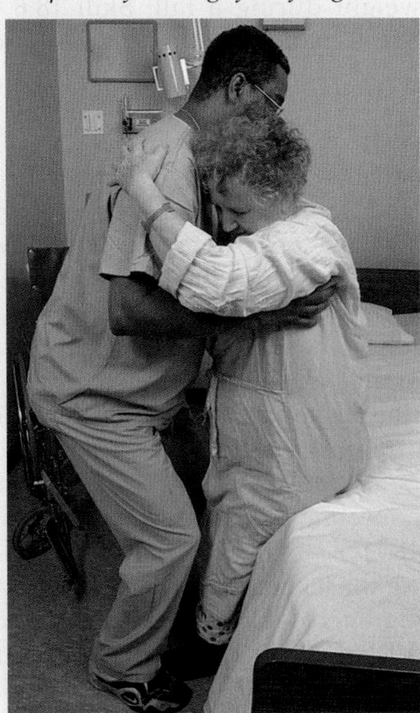
Step 16

17. On the count of 3, have the patient push on the bed, and lift patient upward while maintaining correct alignment in your back. Depending on your assessment of the patient's ability, a transfer belt or another nurse on the opposite side may be needed. *(Uses leverage to raise patient to a standing position. Assistance helps maintain safety.)*
18. Pivot 90 degrees so the patient's back is toward the seat of the chair. Have the patient reach back and grasp the arms of the chair, if able. Be certain patient's legs are against the seat of the chair, and lower patient into the chair. Flex your knees as patient lowers into the chair. *(Pivoting allows patient to sit down without twisting. Having legs against the seat places the patient's weight directly over the chair, providing safe support during sitting. Flexing your knees prevents self-injury.)*

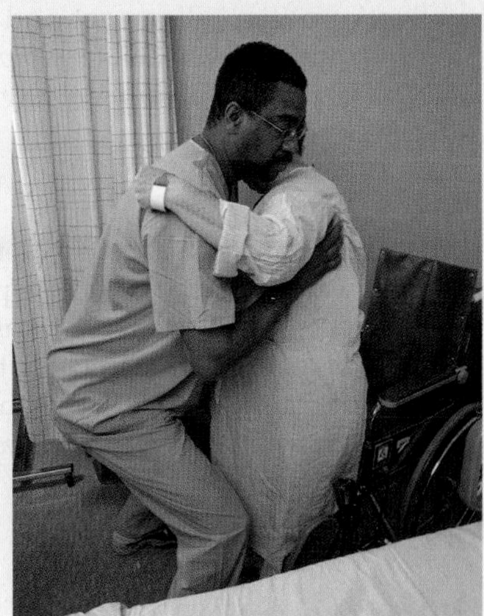
Step 18

19. Assist the patient in placing the feet on the footrests. Avoid striking the patient's ankles while fixing the footrest. Apply a protective device if ordered. Position patient in the chair in correct alignment—hips should be back in the chair. If necessary, help patient to reposition farther back in the chair. Provide support for weak or paralyzed extremities. *(Maintains alignment and prevents injury.)*

Transferring the Patient Back to the Bed (a Reversal of the Procedure)

20. Check to ensure the brakes are locked on the wheelchair. Have patient grasp both arms of the chair and push up and out of the chair to a standing position. Assist patient by placing one arm under the axilla and the other under the elbow. *(Maintains safety. Patient assists with lifting. Hands under the axilla and elbow stabilize the patient.)*

21. Help the patient pivot 90 degrees so patient's back is next to the bed. When the patient is able to stand unassisted, remove the robe. Have patient place hands on bed and lower self to sit on bed. *(Pivoting allows patient to sit without twisting. Having patient stand aids in removal of robe because patient is not sitting on robe.)*
22. Remove slippers. Have patient lean against the elevated head of the bed, and assist in swinging legs up into bed, maintaining good body mechanics. *(Positions patient at head of bed so patient will not need to be moved up in bed.)*
23. Cover the patient, raise side rail if necessary, and place call bell within reach. *(Maintains privacy and institutes safety measures.)*

Evaluation

24. Assess patient's position, alignment, and comfort level. Modify as necessary. *(Maintains support of body and decreases chance of injury resulting from poor positioning or movement.)*

Documentation

25. Document, noting date, time, position, length of time patient was out of bed, and how patient tolerated the procedure. If the patient was transported to another area for a test, include this information. Note number of personnel needed to complete the transfer. *(Validates effectiveness of nursing care and activity of patient and provides data for transferring patient.)*

Documentation Example

3/8 1000 Assisted out of bed to wheelchair by standing and pivoting, with assistance of one nurse. No weakness or difficulty noted during transfer. Returned to bed after 30 minutes. (Nurse's electronic signature)

Special Considerations

- When transferring a patient to a wheelchair, you may need to help the weak patient readjust position in the wheelchair. To do this, stand behind the wheelchair with your knees flexed. Place your arms under patient's axillae and lift the patient up and back by using your leg muscles. Reposition and place the call bell within patient's reach.

? Critical Thinking Questions

1. Dangling the legs at the side of the bed is important, especially for the patient who has not been out of bed. Why?
2. Your patient had a right stroke with left-sided paresis. In transferring the patient to the wheelchair, which side of the patient should be closest to the chair? Why?

a supine position and place the stretcher against the bed with the side rail down. Lock the stretcher wheels. One or more nurses are on the far side of the bed, and you and another nurse are on the far side of the stretcher. Hold the lift sheet as close to the patient as possible. On the count of 3, pull the patient across the transfer board. The nurse(s) on the far side of the bed support the patient's head and feet and help guide the patient to the stretcher.

A less commonly used piece of equipment, the **roller board,** works similarly to a slide board except that it contains several roller bars between fixed end bars and it rolls the patient in a "conveyor belt" sort of way.

A **transfer belt** or **gait belt** should be used to ambulate or transfer the weak or unsteady patient. It is made of a tightly webbed canvas material and is very sturdy. Place and buckle the belt around the patient's waist before having the patient stand. Tighten it just enough to allow space for your hand to grasp it from the rear. **Insert your hand into the belt from the bottom so that, if the patient falls, you will be able to support the weight.** If you hold the belt from the top, it could slip out of your hand from the patient's weight during a fall. Skill 18.6 discusses how to assist a patient in ambulation and how to break a fall.

◆ EVALUATION

During evaluation, determine whether the expected outcomes and goals from the planning phase have been met. Evaluate your use of proper body mechanics. Obtain feedback from the patient and other personnel regarding positioning and transfers. Did you position the patient safely and correctly? Was the patient comfortable when you finished, or did you need to readjust the position? Did pressure areas develop on the skin? If the plan needs to be changed, document the changes for other personnel. Record the progress achieved in meeting the goals and outcomes (Nursing Care Plan 18.1).

Practicing the techniques of proper body mechanics and alignment will increase your confidence in being able to safely move and position any patient. Using your muscles and these techniques correctly will help protect your back. Preventing back injuries is a major concern for all health care professionals.

Skill 18.5 Transferring the Patient to a Stretcher

 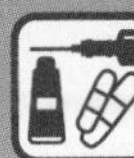 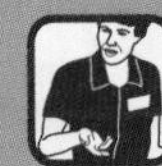 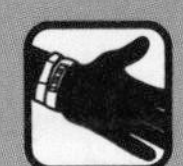 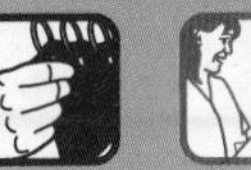 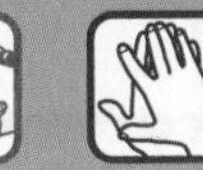 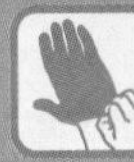

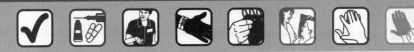

Patients are transferred to a stretcher to be moved from place to place in the hospital for diagnostic tests or surgery. Care must be taken to prevent injury to the patient and yourself during this task. As with any skill, it is important to have the correct number of staff members to transfer the patient safely. Observe proper body movement and alignment to prevent injury. Three staff members or more are needed, depending on patient size. Use a slide board or air-assisted transfer device if available.

Supplies

- Bed
- Stretcher
- Bath blanket or sheet
- Second bath blanket or sheet
- Slide board or air-assisted transfer device

Review and carry out the Standard Steps in Appendix A.

ACTION *(RATIONALE)*

Assessment (Data Collection)

1. Assess patient's size and ability to assist in move (e.g., folding arms on chest). *(Provides baseline data and indicates the number of additional staff needed for transfer.)*

Planning

2. Gather stretcher and other supplies needed for the transfer. *(Promotes access to equipment for safe transfer.)*
3. Maintain patient's privacy by closing door and/or curtain. *(Protects the patient's right to privacy and reduces embarrassment.)*
4. Get other staff members needed to help with transfer. *(Provides for a safe transfer.)*
5. Explain the procedure to the patient. *(Decreases fear of the unknown and prepares patient for what will occur.)*

Implementation

6. Perform hand hygiene. *(Reduces transfer of microorganisms.)*
7. Lock the wheels of the bed and raise it level with the height of the stretcher. *(Prevents the patient from falling between bed and stretcher. Level surfaces allow maintenance of proper body movement and alignment.)*
8. Fold the top covers to the foot of the bed, making certain feet are uncovered. Remove any positioning devices from bed. Cover patient with bath blanket or sheet. *(Moving covers prevents feet from becoming tangled in bed linen during transfer. Removing positioning devices prevents obstruction during transfer. Covering the patient provides privacy during transfer.)*
9. Check for any tubes (e.g., intravenous [IV], nasogastric, urinary catheter, or chest tube), and position them so they will not be pulled out or dislodged during transfer. *(Prevents patient injury and loss of access, as with an IV.)*
10. Lower the bed's side rail on the side where the transfer will occur, and have one nurse remain at the bedside to protect the patient from falling. *(Improves access to patient and provides for safety.)*
11. Place the lift sheet and/or slide board and/or special sheet needed for the air-assisted device under the patient as described in Skill 18.2. The slide board is placed beneath the lift sheet. Air-device sheets are used instead of lift sheets. *(Lift sheet minimizes shearing forces. The slide board makes transfer much easier.)*
12. Place patient on back; have both nurses grasp the edge of the sheet, and on the count of 3, move patient to the open edge of the bed. *(Decreases the risk of injury by using more people. If the patient is large, more than three nurses may be needed to transfer the patient safely. If air-assisted device is used, fewer staff may be needed.)*
13. Place the stretcher firmly against the open side of the bed and lock its wheels. *(Maintains safety and prevents patient from falling.)*
14. Two nurses stand with a correct stance on the far side of the stretcher. The third nurse stands or kneels on the other side of the bed to assist in guiding the patient from the bed to the stretcher. On the count of 3, the two nurses pull and the third nurse lifts and guides the patient to the stretcher. *(Pulling is easier than pushing, and it promotes a smooth transfer.)*

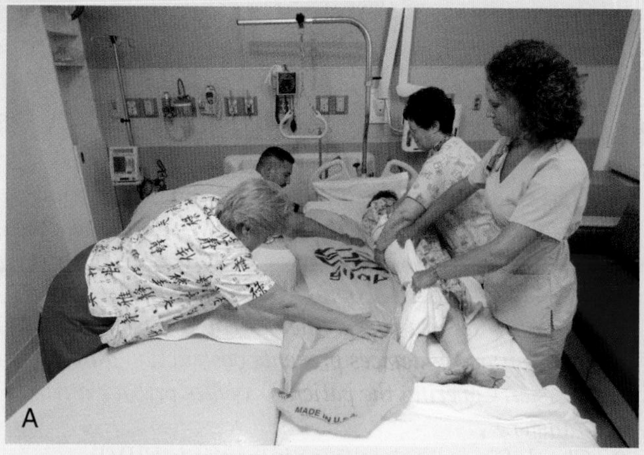

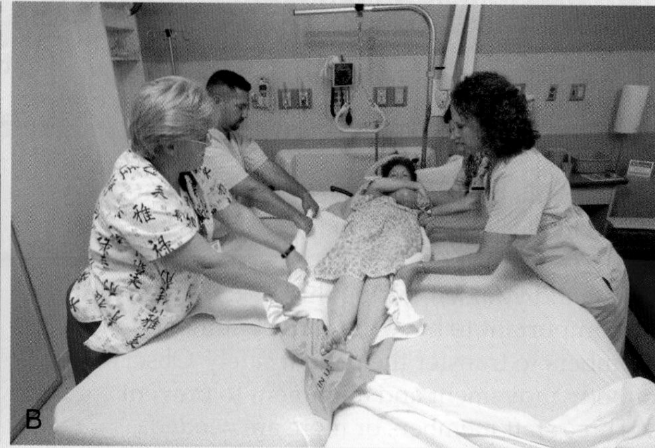

Step **14**

15. Smooth out the lift sheet under the patient. Check and straighten the patient's body alignment. Fasten the safety belt securely over the patient, and raise the side rail of the stretcher. *(Provides safety.)*
16. Cover the patient for more warmth if needed, and put a pillow under the patient's head. *(Provides comfort.)*
17. Unlock the wheels, move the stretcher away from the bed, and raise the opposite stretcher rail. *(Allows patient to be moved to the test or procedure site.)*
18. Remake or straighten the patient's bed in preparation for patient's return. *(Conserves time because bed is ready for patient on return.)*

Evaluation

19. Assess patient's position, alignment, and comfort level. Modify as necessary. *(Maintains support of body and decreases chance of injury resulting from poor positioning or mechanics.)*

Documentation

20. Document the transfer: date, time, type of transfer, number of personnel necessary, and how patient tolerated the procedure. If patient was transported to another area for a test, include this information. *(Notes that patient was transferred off unit.)*

Documentation Example

3/18 1330 To x-ray. Transferred from bed to stretcher by three staff members using a pull sheet without incident. Safety belt applied. (Nurse's electronic signature)

? Critical Thinking Questions

1. Why are two nurses placed on the side to which the patient is being moved onto the stretcher?
2. What purpose does a slide board serve in transferring your patient to the stretcher?

Skill 18.6 Ambulating the Patient and Breaking a Fall

 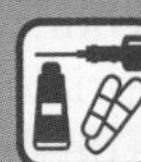 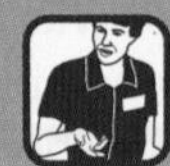  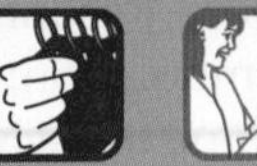 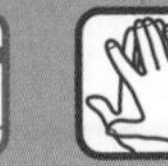 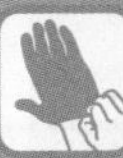

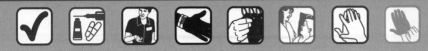

A patient may need assistance with ambulation because of unsteadiness from illness or trauma, weakness from prolonged bed rest, or a need to manage therapeutic equipment such as drains or intravenous (IV) lines. Sometimes during ambulation, a patient may begin to fall unexpectedly. It is important to know how to properly ambulate the patient and break a patient's fall to prevent injury to both the patient and yourself. The patient must be able to stand unassisted before attempting to ambulate.

Supplies

- Robe
- Socks
- Slippers or shoes
- Transfer or gait belt (if necessary)

Review and carry out the Standard Steps in Appendix A.

ACTION *(RATIONALE)*

Assessment (Data Collection)

1. Check the patient's written activity order. *(A written order is required to get the patient out of bed.)*
2. Assess patient's comfort level, coordination, activity tolerance, strength, and balance. *(Provides baseline data and informs you if more than one staff member will be needed.)*

Planning

3. Gather patient items and transfer belt if necessary. *(Provides easy access.)*
4. Get additional help if necessary. *(Promotes safety.)*
5. Explain the procedure to the patient. *(Decreases fear of the unknown and prepares the patient for what will occur.)*

Implementation

Ambulating the Patient

6. With the patient seated on the side of the bed with robe, socks, and slippers on, place patient's feet firmly on the floor. Position yourself in front of the patient with your feet apart and outside of the patient's feet. Place your arms under the axillae and hands over both scapulae, and assist the patient to a standing position. (Alternative: For the weak patient, use a transfer or gait belt. Hold belt behind the patient with one hand from underneath.) Support the patient's arm/elbow on the side closest to you. Check and secure all tubes. *(Forms a support base for you and the patient and provides leverage for lifting. Maintains patient's center of gravity at midline. Transfer or gait belt enables you to support the patient's weight. Tubes must not be pulled on or trip the patient.)*
7. Move to the patient's side, and provide support as the patient balances before walking. Allow patient to stand for a couple of minutes. Check patient's posture, and encourage patient to walk with head up and eyes open, looking forward. *(Promotes balance.)*

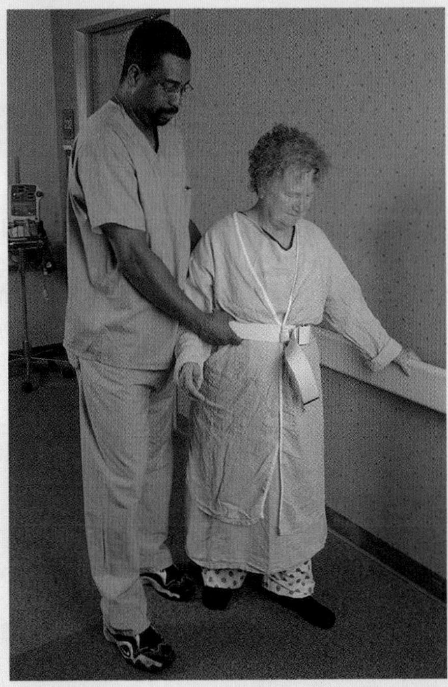

Step 7

8. Walk at the patient's side. Match your gait with the patient's. The patient may hold your elbow or hand for stabilization. *(Conveys caring and provides stability, thus encouraging the patient to achieve greater mobility. Support prevents loss of balance and falling.)*

Breaking a Patient's Fall

During ambulation, a patient may unexpectedly stumble or begin to fall.

9. If the patient begins to fall, stand with your feet apart slightly behind the patient and grasp the patient's body firmly at the waist or under the axilla. *(Provides a broad base of support.)*

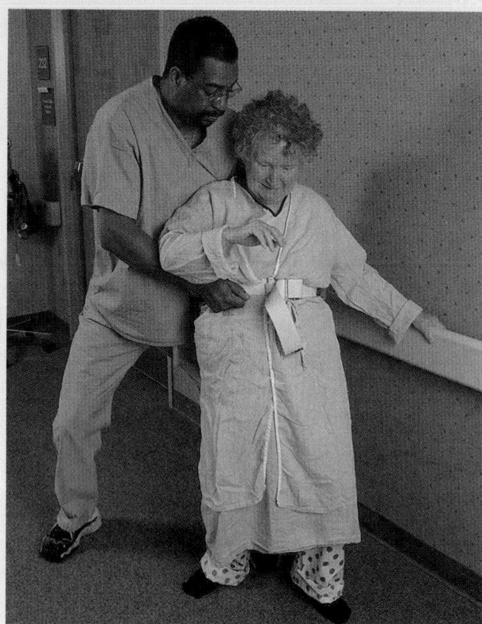

Step 9

10. Extend your near leg against the patient's leg, and slowly slide the patient down your leg to the floor, keeping your body in straight alignment. *(Slows the rate of descent, decreasing the risk of injury. Straight alignment keeps your line of gravity within your base of support.)*

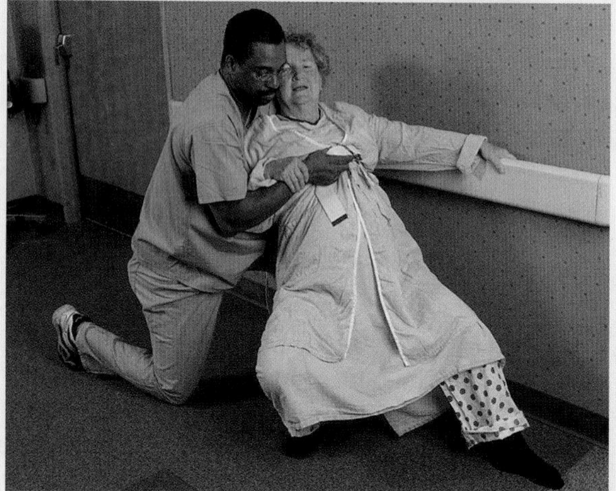

Step 10

11. As the patient slides, bend your knees to lower your body while continuing to support the patient. *(Maintains weight within your center of gravity.)*
12. Call for additional help, check the vital signs, and examine patient for any injuries incurred because of the fall before allowing the patient to rise. *(Prevents any further injury or discomfort to the patient.)*

Assisting the Patient Back to Bed After Ambulating

13. Walk to the side of the bed and have patient turn with the buttocks facing the bed. Patient reaches back for the mattress with both hands for support. Reconnect tubing that was disconnected for ambulation; secure all tubing appropriately. Continue to assist patient back to bed as described in Skill 18.4. *(Mattress provides support and security. Alignment is maintained. IV tubing, urinary catheter, drainage tubes, and suction must be resecured and checked for patency.)*

Evaluation

14. For ambulating, note patient's posture during ambulation, effort, tolerance, comfort level, and the distance ambulated. *(Provides data for comparison and modification if necessary.)*
15. For breaking a fall, note the difficulty encountered, whether injury occurred, and whether primary care provider was notified. Did patient stumble or feel dizzy? Was patient hypotensive? *(Provides data for prevention of falls and highlights necessary modifications.)*

Documentation

16. For ambulating, record distance ambulated, patient's tolerance of procedure, and any assistive devices or personnel necessary. *(Records effectiveness of nursing care and provides for consistency of care among personnel.)*

Documentation Example

3/18 1430 Assisted to ambulate the length of the hall. Walked slowly with minimal assistance. No complaint of weakness or dizziness. Back to bed, placed in a semi-Fowler position for comfort. Bed down, call bell in reach. (Nurse's electronic signature)

17. For breaking a fall, document the fall and its consequences per institutional policy. Note any perceived or patient-stated cause of fall, any injury sustained, and measures taken. *(Documents incident; presents assessment findings and care provided.)*

Documentation Example

3/18 1030 While ambulating in hallway, patient stated became dizzy and began to fall. Fall broken and patient gradually supported in slide to the floor. Checked for injuries. No cuts, bruises, or abrasions noted. BP, 110/76; pulse, 92; respirations, 24. Complains of no discomfort, only weakness. Assisted to wheelchair and back to bed. Bed down, call bell in reach. Primary care provider and charge nurse notified. (Nurse's electronic signature)

Special Considerations

- Assess for signs and symptoms of orthostatic hypotension when the patient is dangling at the side of the bed.

- If the patient is weak or partially paralyzed on one side, support the patient on the opposite, unaffected side, so that the assistive device (such as a cane) can be used on the affected side. Otherwise, support the patient on the affected, weaker side.
- Only suction tubing and oxygen cannula should be disconnected when ambulating the patient out of the room. The IV line needs to be checked for the correct drip rate after the patient is returned to bed. All tubes should be checked for kinks and to determine patency.
- Do not overtire the patient when ambulating.
- Support the patient's head when breaking a fall.
- For minimal support, hold the patient's arm with your hand.
- For moderate support, encircle the patient's waist with your near arm and use the other arm to support the patient's near arm and hand.
- For maximal support, have another person help you so that support can be provided on each side of the patient.

Critical Thinking Questions

1. What steps would you take to avoid having a patient fall during ambulation?
2. On which side do you support a patient who has left-sided weakness? Why?

Nursing Care Plan 18.1 Care of the Patient at Risk for Injury

SCENARIO Darla Porter, age 74, a patient on your orthopedic unit, sustained a proximal fracture of the right tibia during a motor vehicle accident. Mrs. Porter has a long leg cast and a history of arthritis in her hands. You implement this plan of care.

Problem/Nursing Diagnosis *Leg in cast*/Risk for injury related to inability to change position independently.

Supporting Assessment Data *Subjective:* States since car accident is unable to move in bed without help. ***Objective:*** Arthritis in her hands makes using a trapeze bar difficult. She is not able to shift her position independently.

Goals/Expected Outcomes	Nursing Interventions	Selected Rationales	Evaluation
Patient will remain free of injury until able to move independently.	Inspect skin for signs and symptoms of impaired integrity q 2 hour.	Patient at risk for development of pressure injury because of inability to move independently.	*Has any injury occurred?* No redness, blanching, or pallor noted on skin pressure points.
	Encourage patient to perform ROM exercises twice a day; assist PRN	ROM exercises help to maintain joint mobility.	ROM performed 1 time this shift.
	Inspect musculoskeletal system for joint contractures q day.	Early detection is key for intervention, thus avoiding contractures.	No contractures noted.
	Reposition patient at least q 2 hours using appropriate devices such as pillows and footboard to maintain anatomic alignment.	Adjusting position at least every 2 hours helps to prevent skin breakdown. Positioning devices help maintain anatomic alignment and therefore decrease chance of injury.	Correct anatomic alignment maintained.
	Encourage patient to cough and deep breathe q hour.	Coughing and deep breathing help prevent collection of fluid in the lungs.	Expected outcome is being met.
	Teach patient and family correct transfer techniques.	Correct transfer techniques protect patient and family member from injury.	

CRITICAL THINKING QUESTIONS

1. What are some other possible nursing diagnoses this patient might have? Construct a care plan for one or two of those diagnoses using some of the above mentioned information.
2. Describe the benefits of using positioning devices.

ROM, Range-of-motion. *PRN*, as needed; *q*, every

Get Ready for the NCLEX Examination!

Key Points

- The musculoskeletal system is involved in positioning and moving patients.
- Observing proper body alignment and mechanics helps prevent injuries. Lower back strain is one of the most common injuries for health care workers.
- Get help when necessary before moving or positioning a patient.
- Observing these principles helps to prevent the hazards of improper positioning: pressure injuries, muscle contractures, and fluid collection in the lungs.
- Pressure and shearing force are the main factors in developing pressure injuries.
- There are three basic positions: supine, side lying, and prone. Other positions include Fowler, semi-Fowler, low Fowler, and Sims.
- Common positioning devices include pillows, boots, splints, high-top sneakers, trochanter rolls, sandbags, trapeze bars, side rails, and bed boards.
- Logrolling is a technique in which the patient is turned as a single unit.
- A lift sheet supports a patient from the shoulders to below the buttocks, and it facilitates transfers.
- While the patient is dangling, monitor for orthostatic hypotension, dizziness, or nausea before getting the patient out of bed.
- Lock the wheels on stretchers and wheelchairs before transferring patients.
- Transferring devices include mechanical lifts, air-assisted transfer devices, slide boards, lift or pull sheets, low friction sheets, and transfer (or gait) belts.
- Pulling motions are better than pushing motions, except that wheelchairs and stretchers are pushed to maintain alignment.

Additional Learning Resources

SG Go to your Study Guide for additional learning activities to help you master this chapter content.

evolve Go to your Evolve website at http://evolve.elsevier.com/Williams/fundamental for additional online resources.

Review Questions for the NCLEX Examination

*Choose the **best** answer for each question.*

1. An older adult may need to be reeducated on how to lift safely because: *(Select all that apply.)*
   1. Muscles and bones lose strength as one ages.
   2. Bone density is decreased.
   3. Muscle mass is decreased and posture has changed.
   4. Memory decreases with age.
2. Forgetting to reposition a patient in a wheelchair for more than 1 hour may lead to:
   1. The beginning of a pressure injury.
   2. Muscle atrophy.
   3. Pooling of lung secretions.
   4. Skin abrasions from shearing forces.
3. When preparing to move a patient who can assist up in the bed, you would *first:*
   1. Pull the bed covers down to the foot of the bed.
   2. Raise the bed to a good working height.
   3. Ask the patient to grab the upper guardrails.
   4. Ask the patient to bend the knees and plant the feet on the mattress.
4. You have assisted your patient to the prone position. Which intervention is most important?
   1. Ask if he has any neck discomfort.
   2. Count his respirations.
   3. Offer him a magazine.
   4. Place the call bell within reach.
5. When changing the patient's position, it is most important to:
   1. Use only those muscles necessary.
   2. Stand with feet close together for greater strength.
   3. Work at the same level or height as the patient.
   4. Push rather than pull, as your weight helps.
6. You are dangling your patient in preparation for getting her out of bed. Your plan is to dangle her for 2 minutes and then transfer her to the chair. After 1 minute, she complains of nausea and states that she sees "stars." What should you do?
   1. Reassure her that this will pass.
   2. Get the blood pressure (BP) cuff from across the room.
   3. Gently lie her back down.
   4. Wait 2 more minutes and then check her BP.
7. When a patient falls, you document in the nurse's notes:
   1. Your best guess about what happened.
   2. A statement concerning how you believe the hospital was negligent.
   3. Any patient-stated cause of fall.
   4. As little as possible to avoid liability.

Critical Thinking Activities

Read each clinical scenario and discuss the questions with your classmates.

Scenario A

You are to get a patient who has left-sided paresis out of bed and into a chair for the first time. The patient has been in this country only a short time. How would you go about doing this? Would you need assistance?

Scenario B

You and three other nurses are logrolling a patient. You are 5 feet, 6 inches tall, and the other nurses are all at least 3 inches taller. How high do you position the bed to logroll the patient?

Scenario C

Your patient became weak while walking and you broke her fall and assisted her to the floor. What would you do next? What procedures would need to be followed?

chapter 19

Assisting With Hygiene, Personal Care, Skin Care, and the Prevention of Pressure Injuries

http://evolve.elsevier.com/Williams/fundamental

Objectives

Upon completing this chapter, you should be able to do the following:

Theory

1. Describe the structure and function of the integumentary system.
2. Describe factors that influence personal hygiene practices.
3. List the skin areas most susceptible to pressure injuries.
4. Discuss risk factors for impaired skin integrity.
5. Discuss the purposes of bathing.
6. Describe how hygienic care for the younger and the older patient differs.

Clinical Practice

1. Describe how to prevent and stage a pressure injury.
2. Perform a complete bed bath and back rub.
3. Provide oral care for an unconscious patient.
4. Prepare to provide personal care for a patient, including nail care, mouth care, perineal care, and shaving.
5. Assist a patient with the care of contact lenses.
6. Instruct a patient in ways to prevent buildup of cerumen in the ears.

Skills & Steps

Key Terms

blanch (p. 297)
caries (KĀ-rēz, p. 310)
cerumen (sĕ-RŪ-mĕn, p. 296)
dermis (DĔR-mĭs, p. 296)
diaphoresis (dī-ă-fō-RĒ-sĭs, p. 297)
epidermis (p. 296)
eschar (ĔS-kăr, p. 299)
exacerbation (ĕg-zăs-ĕr-BĀ-shŭn, p. 308)
halitosis (hăl-ē-TŌ-sĭs, p. 310)
hygiene (HĪ-jēn, p. 297)
induration (ĭn-dū-RĀ-shŭn, p. 299)
integumentary (ĭn-tĕ-gū-MĔN-tăr-ē, p. 296)
maceration (mă-sĕr-Ā-shŭn, p. 297)
melanin (MĔL-ăw-nĭn, p. 296)
reactive hyperemia (rē-ĂK-tĭv hī-pĕr-Ē-mē-ă, p. 297)
sebaceous (sē-BĀ-shŭs, p. 296)
sebum (SĒ-bŭm, p. 296)
syncope (SĬN-kō-pē, p. 307)

Concepts Covered in This Chapter

- Culture
- Infection
- Inflammation
- Mobility
- Nutrition
- Pain
- Patient education
- Perfusion
- Safety
- Sensory perception
- Tissue integrity

The skin is the largest organ of the body, and it must be kept clean to prevent skin disorders and pressure injuries. Hygiene is the proper care of the skin, hair, teeth, and nails to promote good health by protecting the body from infection and disease and to provide a sense of well-being. You are responsible for maintaining safety, privacy, and warmth when providing or assisting patients in hygiene practices. You must also encourage patients to function at their highest level of independence.

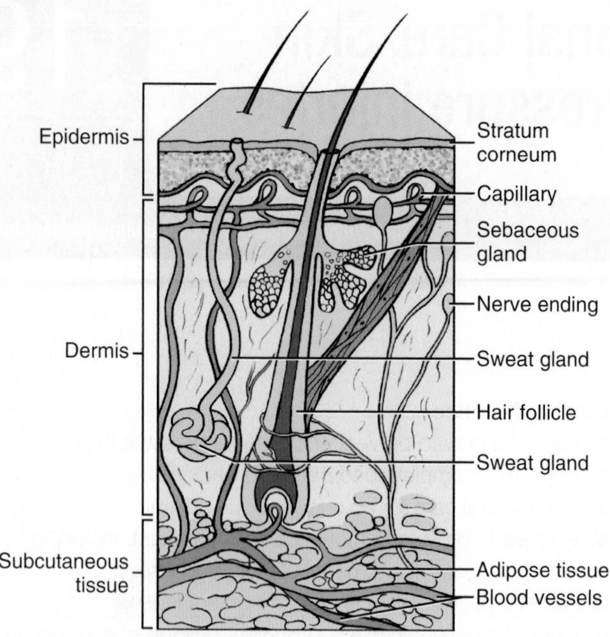

FIGURE 19.1 Cross section of the skin.

OVERVIEW OF THE STRUCTURE AND FUNCTION OF THE INTEGUMENTARY SYSTEM

WHAT IS THE STRUCTURE OF THE SKIN?

The **integumentary** system contains the skin, hair, nails, and sweat and sebaceous glands. The skin, the largest organ in the body, has two main layers: the epidermis and the dermis (Fig. 19.1).

- The **epidermis** (outer, thicker layer) consists of stratified squamous epithelial tissue and does not contain blood vessels. It receives its nutrition by diffusion from vessels in underlying tissues. It is also called the **stratum corneum.**
- The bottom layer of the epidermis contains melanocytes that secrete **melanin**, the main determinant of skin color.
- The **dermis** (inner, thinner layer) is made of dense connective tissue that gives the skin strength and elasticity. It is also called the **corium.**
- The dermis contains blood vessels, nerves, fibroblasts, the base of hair follicles, and glands; the nails are derived from the epidermis. Fibroblasts produce new cells to heal skin after injury.
- Hair and nails are made of keratin and have no nerve endings or blood supply.
- **Sebaceous** glands secrete an oily substance called **sebum.** Sweat glands secrete sweat, and ceruminous glands (modified sweat glands) secrete a waxy substance called **cerumen.**
- Mucous membranes line the cavities or passageways of the body that open to the outside, such as the mouth and digestive, respiratory, and genitourinary tracts. Like skin, they are made of a surface layer of epithelial tissue over a deeper layer of connective tissue.

WHAT ARE THE FUNCTIONS OF THE SKIN AND ITS STRUCTURES?

- The skin has four main functions: protection, sensation, temperature regulation, and excretion and secretion.
- The skin is the first line of defense in protecting the body from bacteria and other invading organisms. It protects tissues from thermal, chemical, and mechanical injury.
- The sebaceous glands produce sebum, which helps make the skin waterproof by preventing water loss from underlying tissues and too much water absorption during bathing and swimming.
- Melanin absorbs light and protects against ultraviolet rays. When exposed to ultraviolet light, the skin makes vitamin D, which is needed for absorbing phosphorus and calcium.
- The skin has sensory organs for touch, pain, heat, cold, and pressure.
- The skin regulates temperature by dilating and constricting blood vessels and activating or inactivating sweat glands.
- Sweat glands assist in maintenance of homeostasis of fluid and electrolytes. They serve as excretory organs because sweat contains nitrogenous wastes. As sweat evaporates, it produces a cooling effect. Sweat glands in the axillae and external genitalia also secrete fatty acids and proteins.
- Sebum lubricates the skin and hair, keeping these structures softer and more pliable. It also decreases the amount of heat lost and bacterial growth.
- Mucous membranes protect against bacterial invasion, secrete mucus, and absorb fluid and electrolytes.

WHAT CHANGES IN THE SYSTEM OCCUR WITH AGING?

- Loss of elastic fibers and adipose tissue in the dermis and subcutaneous layers causes skin to be thinner and more transparent, with wrinkling and sagging.
- Loss of collagen fibers in the dermis makes the skin more fragile and slower to heal.
- Decreased sebaceous gland activity causes dry and itchy skin.
- Temperature control is altered by the decreased sebaceous gland activity and the loss of skin density. This results in cold intolerance and puts the person at risk for heat exhaustion.
- Hair becomes thin and grows more slowly because of a decrease in the number of hair follicles. Hair loses its color from the loss of melanocytes at the hair follicles.
- Nail growth decreases and the nails thicken.

❖ APPLICATION OF THE NURSING PROCESS

◆ ASSESSMENT (DATA COLLECTION)

The bath provides an excellent opportunity for assessment of the patient. Assess the individual factors affecting the patient's hygiene and his ability to perform self-care. During a bath, assess the condition of the patient's skin and his overall physical appearance, emotional and mental status, and learning needs.

Factors Affecting Hygiene

Hygiene practice is affected by many variables such as economics, ability to perform self-care, and personal preference. One of the most basic factors is a patient's sociocultural background. **Different cultures have different views on hygiene practices.** In some cultures, people do not use deodorant products or bathe daily. Other cultures consider the use of deodorant products and a daily bath essential. The patient's economic status may affect his hygiene because the money for supplies may or may not be available. The patient may lack knowledge of a particular aspect of hygiene. The ability to perform self-care may be affected by the patient's mental or physical condition, which may be altered because of illness or injury.

QSEN Considerations: Patient-Centered Care

Bathing Preference

One important factor affecting hygiene practice is personal preference. One patient may prefer to bathe at night, whereas another may prefer to bathe every 2 days.

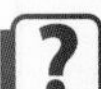
Think Critically

Your patient is an older adult and complains of being cold.

What safety concern would you have with him preparing his own bathwater?

QSEN Considerations: Patient-Centered Care

Self-Care Abilities

Assess your patient's ability to provide self-care by assessing cognitive and physical function. Do any factors such as poor vision, decreased sense of touch, or limited range of motion interfere with self-care? Are coordination, muscle strength, and balance adequate? A patient with limitations in these areas may need additional, if not total, help with hygiene.

Skin and Pressure Injuries

A pressure injury is an injury that forms from a local interference with circulation (see Chapter 18) and may involve either intact or ulcerated skin. The interference with circulation causes the skin to **blanch** (turn white or, in darker skin, become pale). If the pressure is relieved at this point, the skin will become red or a darker color because of vasodilation. **Reactive hyperemia** is the process in which the blood rushes to a place where there was a decrease in circulation.

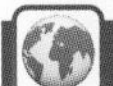
Cultural Considerations

Dark Skin Assessment

When assessing for stage I pressure injuries in patients with darkly pigmented skin, use natural light or a halogen lamp to look for skin color changes. Pressure areas may have purple hues. Compare the skin around bony prominences with skin over the prominences. Damaged skin may be boggy or stiff, or warmer or cooler. Moistening the skin can assist in identifying changes in color.

Risk factors for pressure injuries. There are many risk factors in the development of pressure injuries; the most common ones can be found in Box 19.1.

The first two risk factors listed deal with a patient's mobility. If a patient is confined to a bed or chair, the same areas of the body sustain pressure. This also happens if a patient cannot change position independently (e.g., a patient who is paralyzed or unconscious.

Moisture can lead to pressure injuries in a patient who is **incontinent** (has lost bowel or bladder control). Skin that is frequently wet leads to **maceration** (softening of tissue that increases the chance of trauma or infection). **Diaphoresis** (perspiration), not drying a patient properly after a bath, and the use of incontinence briefs also place a patient at risk because of moisture.

A balanced diet is necessary to prevent injury development. Without proper calories, protein, fluids, vitamins, and minerals, the body's cells, capillaries, and tissues are easily damaged. Altered sensory perception places a person at risk for pressure injuries because he may not receive the body's signals of discomfort reminding him to change position. Lowered mental awareness is another factor because patients who have lost the concept of time may not realize they have been in the same position for a prolonged period. Lowered mental awareness may be caused by medication, anesthesia, or health problems.

Think Critically

Why do you think an obese patient might be more prone to problems of tissue integrity?

Skin assessment for pressure injuries. Perform a skin assessment for pressure injury risk on admission. The Braden Scale for Predicting Pressure Sore Risk is commonly used (Fig. 19.2). After the initial assessment, reassess every 24 hours. This may be done while you are bathing your patient. Pay attention to the skin over bony prominences (Fig. 19.3). Check pressure areas when turning and repositioning your patient.

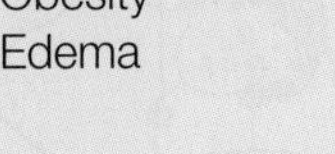

Box 19.1 Pressure Injury Risk Factors

MAJOR FACTORS
- Immobility
- Inactivity
- Moisture
- Malnutrition
- Advanced age
- Altered sensory perception
- Lowered mental awareness
- Friction and shear

CONTRIBUTING FACTORS
- Dehydration
- Obesity
- Edema

Braden Scale

FOR PREDICTING PRESSURE SORE RISK

Patient's Name________________ Evaluator's Name ________________

					Date of Assessment			
SENSORY PERCEPTION Ability to respond meaning fully to pressure-related discomfort	**1. Completely Limited:** Unresponsive (does not moan, flinch, or grasp) to painful stimuli, due to diminished level of consciousness or sedation. OR limited ability to feel pain over most of body surface.	**2. Very Limited:** Responds only to painful stimuli. Cannot communicate discomfort except by moaning or restlessness. OR has a sensory impairment which limits the ability to feel pain or discomfort over 1/2 of body.	**3. Slightly Limited:** Responds to verbal commands, but cannot always communicate discomfort or need to be turned. OR has some sensory impairment which limits ability to feel pain or discomfort in 1 or 2 extremities.	**4. No Impairment:** Responds to verbal commands. Has no sensory deficit which would limit ability to feel or voice pain or discomfort.				
MOISTURE Degree to which skin is exposed to moisture	**1. Constantly Moist:** Skin is kept moist almost constantly by perspiration, urine, etc. Dampness is detected every time patient is moved or turned.	**2. Very Moist:** Skin is often, but not always moist. Linen must be changed at least once a shift.	**3. Occasionally Moist:** Skin is occasionally moist, requiring an extra linen change approximately once a day.	**4. Rarely Moist:** Skin is usually dry, linen only requires changing at routine intervals.				
ACTIVITY Degree of physical activity	**1. Bedfast:** Confined to bed	**2. Chairfast:** Ability to walk severely limited or non-existent. Cannot bear own weight and/or must be assisted into chair or wheelchair.	**3. Walks Occasionally:** Walks occasionally during day, but for very short distances, with or without assistance. Spends majority of each shift in bed or chair.	**4. Walks Frequently:** walks outside the room at least twice a day and inside room at least once every 2 hours during waking hours.				
MOBILITY Ability to change and control body position	**1. Completely Immobile:** Does not make even slight changes in body or extremity position without assistance.	**2. Very Limited:** Makes occasional slight changes in body or extremity position but unable to make frequent or significant changes independently.	**3. Slightly Limited:** Makes frequent though slight changes in body or extremity position independently.	**4. No Limitations:** Makes major and frequent changes in position without assistance.				
NUTRITION <u>Usual</u> food intake pattern	**1. Very Poor:** Never eats a complete meal. Rarely eats more than 1/3 of any food offered. Eats 2 servings or less of protein (meat or dairy products) per day. Takes fluids poorly. Does not take a liquid dietary supplement. OR is NPO and/or maintained on clear liquids or IV's for more than 5 days.	**2. Probably Inadequate:** Rarely eats a complete meal and generally eats only about 1/2 of any food offered. Protein intake includes only 3 servings of meat or dairy products per day. Occasionally will take a dietary supplement. OR receives less than optimum amount of liquid diet or tube feeding.	**3. Adequate:** Eats over half of most meals. Eats a total of 4 servings of protein (meat, dairy products) each day. Occasionally will refuse a meal, but will usually take a supplement if offered. OR is on a tube feeding or TPN regimen that probably meets most of nutritional needs.	**4. Excellent:** Eats most of every meal. Never refuses a meal. Usually eats a total of 4 or more servings of meat and dairy products. Occasionally eats between meals. Does not require supplementation.				
FRICTION AND SHEAR	**1. Problem:** Requires moderate to maximum assistance in moving. Complete lifting without sliding against sheets is impossible. Frequently slides down in bed or chair, requiring frequent repositioning with maximum assistance. Spasticity, contractures or agitation leads to almost constant friction.	**2. Potential Problem:** Moves feebly or requires minimum assistance. During a move skin probably slides to some extent against sheets, chair, restraints, or other devices. Maintains relatively good position in chair or bed most of the time but occasionally slides down.	**3. No Apparent Problem:** Moves in bed and in chair independently and has sufficient muscle strength to lift up completely during move. Maintains good position in bed or chair at all times.					
Key: at risk, 15-18; Moderate risk, 13-14; High risk, 10-12; Severe risk, 9.				Total Score				

FIGURE 19.2 Braden scale for predicting pressure sore risk. *IV*, Intravenous; *NPO*, nothing by mouth; *TPN,* total parenteral nutrition. (Copyright 1998 by Barbara Braden and Nancy Bergstrom. Reprinted with permission.)

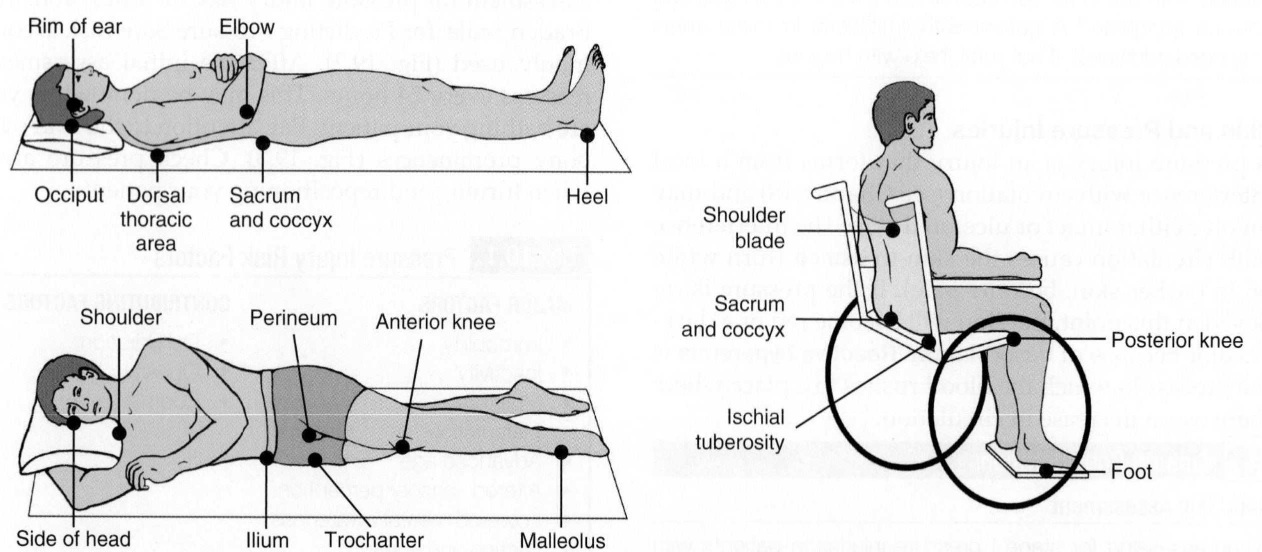

FIGURE 19.3 Pressure points where pressure injuries often occur.

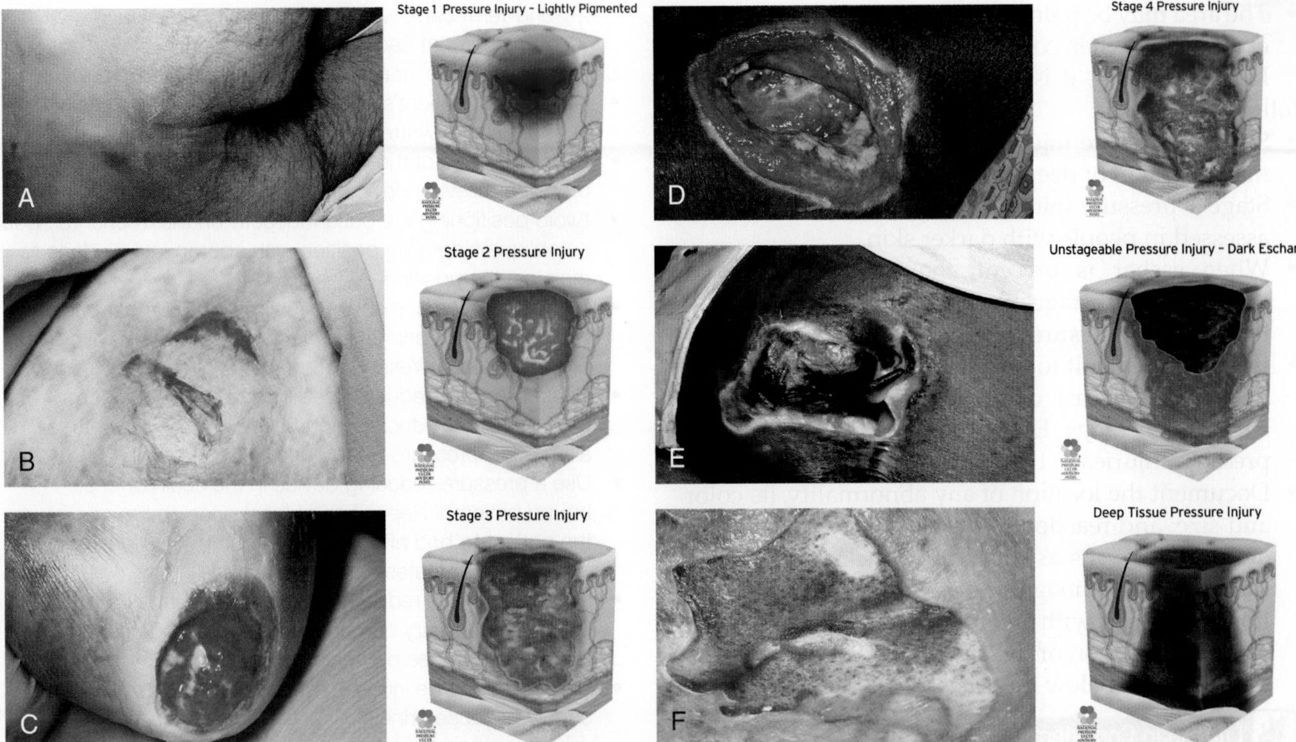

FIGURE 19.4 (A to D) Four stages of pressure injuries. (E) Unstageable Pressure Injury. (F) Deep Tissue Pressure Injury. (Used with permission of the National Pressure Ulcer Advisory Panel, 2016).

Clinical Cues

Medicare will not reimburse health care facilities for "reasonably preventable" pressure injuries. Pressure injuries present on admission must be documented thoroughly and accurately. Treatment for stage 3 or 4 pressure injuries will be reimbursed at a higher rate if they are documented in the medical record within 2 days of inpatient admission (Waters et al., 2015).

Redness can normally be expected to be present for one-half to three-fourths as long as the pressure prevented blood flow. If the redness subsides during this time or the area blanches from fingertip pressure, then damage to the tissues is not expected. For example, your patient has been in a supine position for an hour and is now turned to a right side-lying position. You notice a 1-inch diameter area of redness on the sacrum. If there has not been damage, then you expect the redness to subside in 30 to 45 minutes. If the redness persists after that time, then the pressure has damaged the skin and the underlying tissues because they have not received an adequate supply of blood, oxygen, and nutrients. Unrelieved, the damage eventually will lead to tissue necrosis and a pressure injury.

If you note a reddened area when repositioning a patient, reassess later to see whether reactive hyperemia is present. If the redness remains and the skin does not blanch to fingertip pressure, then the patient has a stage 1 pressure injury.

The National Pressure Ulcer Advisory Panel (2016) has issued an international staging system for pressure injuries (Fig. 19.4):

- **Stage 1 Pressure Injury:** An area of intact skin that is red, deep pink, or mottled skin that does not blanch with fingertip pressure. In people with darker skin, there may be discoloration of the surrounding skin. Warmth, edema, and **induration** (an area that feels hard) in comparison to surrounding tissue may be signs of a stage I pressure injury.
- **Stage 2 Pressure Injury:** Partial-thickness skin loss with exposed dermis. The wound bed is pink or red and moist, and may appear as an intact or ruptured blister.
- **Stage 3 Pressure Injury:** Full-thickness skin loss that looks like a deep crater and may extend to the fascia. Subcutaneous tissue is damaged or necrotic; fat is visible. Undermining and tunneling may be present. There may be damage to the surrounding tissue.
- **Stage 4 Pressure Injury:** Full-thickness skin loss with extensive tissue necrosis or damage to muscle, bone, or supporting structures; sinus tracts may be present. Infection is usually widespread. The injury may appear dry and black, with a buildup of tough, necrotic tissue **(eschar),** or it can appear wet and oozing.
- **Unstageable Pressure Injury:** Loss of full thickness of tissue. The base of the injury is covered by eschar (tan, brown, or black) in the wound bed, or the base of the injury contains slough (yellow, tan, gray, green, or brown).
- **Deep Tissue Pressure Injury:** Localized discolored intact skin that is maroon or purple or a blood-filled blister resulting from damage to underlying soft tissue from pressure or shearing.

- The area may be painful, firm, mushy, boggy, warmer, or cooler when compared to adjacent tissue.

During staging, it is important to be aware of the following:

- Stage 1 pressure injuries may be just superficial or may be a sign of deeper tissue damage.
- Stage 1 pressure injuries are not always accurately assessed in people with darker skin.
- When eschar is present, the pressure injury is described as unstageable. **Eschar must be removed to stage the pressure injury properly.**
- It may be difficult to assess pressure injuries if your patient has a cast or other orthopedic device or support stockings. Extra care is necessary to assess pressure injuries in these instances.
- Document the location of any abnormality, its color and size, and reaction to the blanch test. Add other descriptive terms as they apply, including induration, blisters, drainage, odor, or eschar. Some institutions use forms with an outline of a body so you can draw the location of the area(s) involved. A Braden score of 18 or below indicates pressure injury risk.

 Life-Span Considerations

Older Adult

- Older adults have an increased risk of developing impaired skin integrity from normal aging changes. They have thinner skin, decreased subcutaneous fat, decreased sebaceous gland activity, and decreased elasticity in their skin. This makes them less able to tolerate pressure, shearing, and friction forces.

Healing pressure injuries are not "reverse staged." For example, a stage 4 is not called a stage 3 pressure injury as it improves. This pressure injury would be called a "healing stage 4 pressure injury." Document the pressure injury by objective description and measurement.

Prevention of pressure injuries. **Excellent nursing care is the main factor in the prevention of pressure injuries.** It is your responsibility to be aware of any risk factors your patient may have and attempt to lessen them. New wireless, wearable patient sensors that track individual patients and alert staff when patients are due to be turned are being used in some hospitals. A comprehensive pressure injury prevention program that includes staff education and proactive measures and skin care protocols can reduce hospital-acquired pressure injuries (Swafford et al, 2016). **Prevention is less time-consuming and less costly than pressure injury treatment is.**

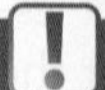 Safety Alert

Prevention of Pressure Injuries

- National Pressure Ulcer Advisory Panel (2016) recommends using a structured risk assessment such as the Braden Scale as soon as possible after admission (but within 8 hours), followed by re-assessment at the following intervals:
    1. acute care: every shift
    2. long-term care: weekly for 4 weeks, then quarterly
    3. home care: at each nurse visit

Skin that is red, blue, or mottled indicates impaired circulation.

- Change the patient's position at least every 2 hours when in bed, using a written schedule.
- Keep the heels of the immobile patient off the bed. Use pressure-relieving devices on the bed.
- Avoid positioning the patient directly on the trochanter. Use an oblique side-lying position with appropriate wedges to maintain the position.
- Minimize friction and shear forces by using proper positioning, transferring, and turning techniques. The use of creams, protective films, dressings, and padding reduces friction.
- Use a pressure-reducing bed device such as a foam pad, pressure-reducing mattress, low friction sheets, or alternating-pressure pad.
- Use a pressure-reducing device in the chair for chair-bound patients. Reposition at least once an hour or return the patient to bed after 1 hour. Encourage self-weight shifting every 15 minutes.
- Do not massage reddened skin because it has already suffered temporary damage. Do not massage directly over bony prominences because this is harmful.
- Wash and dry the incontinent patient promptly and thoroughly because urine and feces irritate the skin. Avoid using incontinence briefs unless the patient has severe diarrhea or is leaving the unit for a procedure.
- Avoid mechanical or physical injury from improperly fitting splints, braces, casts, and prostheses. Place a thin dressing (foam or breathable material) underneath medical devices.
- Avoid burns caused by excessively hot or cold applications such as hot water bottles, ice bags, heating pads, and heat lamps.
- Provide adequate nutrition and fluid intake.

Treatment and care for pressure injuries. The team approach is the most effective method of pressure injury treatment. The team should include the patient, the family or caregivers, and health care providers. Some units have developed specialized skin care teams. Treatment options should be explained, and the patient should be encouraged to be an active participant. The plan should be consistent with the individual patient and family preferences, goals, and abilities. Include education on development and prevention of pressure injuries.

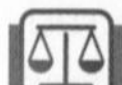 Legal and Ethical Considerations

Document Preventive Measures

Document all measures taken to prevent pressure injuries to show that all possible measures were instituted in case the patient develops a pressure injury in spite of your care. This can protect you from charges of negligence if the pressure injury does not heal and the patient brings a lawsuit against you.

The initial care of a pressure injury involves debridement, wound cleansing, and the application of dressings. In many cases, the pressure injury is infected and antibiotic therapy is used. Surgery is needed to repair some pressure injuries. Wound care is discussed in more depth in Chapter 38.

Box 19.2 Nursing Diagnoses for Hygiene and Skin Integrity Problems

- Acute pain
- Chronic low self-esteem
- Chronic pain
- Dressing self-care deficit
- Imbalanced nutrition: less than body requirements
- Impaired physical mobility
- Impaired skin integrity
- Ineffective peripheral tissue perfusion
- Risk for impaired skin integrity

◆ NURSING DIAGNOSIS

Nursing diagnoses for a patient with potential hygiene and skin integrity problems are listed in Box 19.2. To individualize the care plan, add the defining characteristics to the nursing diagnosis stem based on the information you obtained regarding your patient.

◆ PLANNING

The data collected during the assessment will enable you to plan hygiene care. Include the patient's ability to perform the hygiene tasks and any personal preferences or habits. Efforts should be made to help the patient maintain a positive body image. Educational needs and the home environment must also be considered.

Nursing goals for hygiene might include:

- Patient's skin integrity will be maintained.
- Patient's hair is clean and neatly styled each day.
- Patient's mouth is intact and free from odor.

Planning must include the times during the day that care will be needed. See Box 19.3 for examples.

◆ IMPLEMENTATION

Bathing

Bathing has four basic purposes: (1) cleanse the skin, (2) promote comfort, (3) stimulate circulation, and (4) remove waste products secreted through the skin.

Water should be warm but should not burn the patient (approximately 105°F [40.6°C], or according to agency policy). When water cools, replace it. Bed rails must be up when you are away from that side of the bed because the bed is raised to working height. Fully draw curtains around the bed to maintain privacy. Do not leave any gaps that could expose the patient to others in the room. Place a sign on the outside of the door to indicate that a bath is in progress. Close the patient's door and windows to decrease drafts. Appropriately drape the patient for warmth and comfort. Only the part of the body being bathed should be exposed at any one time. Encourage independence, but offer assistance as needed. Depending on the patient's ability and activity level, you may need to give either a partial or a complete bath.

Box 19.3 Scheduling Hygiene Care

Each patient has different needs and abilities, but, in general, care is provided on the following basis. Individual needs are always addressed while encouraging the patient to perform to an optimal level of functioning.

EARLY-MORNING CARE

- Offer a bedpan or urinal or provide help to the bathroom or bedside commode.
- Wash the hands and face.
- Clean and clear the over-the-bed table.
- Provide oral care.
- Prepare for tests or surgery (e.g., enemas, shaves, or other pre-procedure requirements).

AM CARE OR MORNING CARE

Generally occurs after breakfast and is the main hygiene care.

- Offer a bedpan or urinal.
- Provide oral care.
- Bathe (complete or partial bed bath, shower, or tub bath).
- Give a back rub.
- Shave and provide hair care.
- Care for nails.
- Dress.
- Straighten the patient unit.

AFTERNOON CARE

- Provide care after any diagnostic or special test as needed; for example, electroencephalography (EEG) may leave electrode paste in the patient's hair.
- Offer a bedpan or urinal.
- Provide oral care.

HOUR-OF-SLEEP CARE (BEDTIME)

- Offer a bedpan or urinal.
- Wash the hands and face.
- Provide oral care.
- Change to a gown if needed.
- Give a back rub.
- Adjust or help the patient adjust position in bed.
- Straighten the patient unit.

Linens are straightened or changed as needed throughout the day.

Types of baths. A bath may be cleansing or therapeutic, and complete or partial. With a complete bath, all areas of the patient's body are washed.

 **Assignment Considerations**

Baths

When assigning baths to the unlicensed assistive personnel (UAP), be explicit about which type of bath or shower the patient requires. Ask the UAP to inspect the skin and report any lesions or problems to you. Remind the UAP to abide by the patient's cultural practices and to explain to the patient what will be done. Ask that the patient be allowed to perform as much self-care as possible, but not to the point of becoming excessively tired.

The term *partial bath* has two different meanings depending on your institution. In one case, it means that only certain parts of the body are bathed, such as the face, hands, axillae, back, and perineal area. In the other case, a *partial bath* means that a complete bath is done—partially by the patient (the areas that can be reached) and partially by you (all other areas).

Life-Span Considerations

Older Adult

- Because of decreased sweat and sebaceous gland activity, a full bath is not needed every day. Personal preference must be considered.
- Because of thinner skin and decreased subcutaneous fat, chilling is more likely during the bath. Prevent this by prewarming the bath area and providing adequate draping.
- Older adults have less subcutaneous fat, and their skin is more fragile and drier. Use warm (not hot) water and minimal amounts of mild soap, rinse thoroughly, and thoroughly pat dry to minimize skin irritation. Bath oils may be used, but special care needs to be taken to prevent slips and falls.

QSEN Considerations: Evidence-Based Practices

Bathing Cloths

- While in the hospital, chlorhexidine-impregnated cloths may be used instead of soap to reduce the risk of hospital-acquired infection (Powers & Fortney, 2014).
- Moisturize the skin immediately after the bath with lotion or cream. Apply this while the skin is still damp to trap additional moisture.
- Evaluate the home environment for safety aids such as nonskid tub or shower mats, safety bars, and shower or bench chairs if appropriate.

Cleansing baths. The most common type of bath is a cleansing bath. It is generally provided in a bed, tub, or shower. Bed baths are given to patients who are unable to use a tub or shower. Skill 19.1 details how to administer a bed bath.

Skill 19.1 Administering a Bed Bath and Perineal Care

 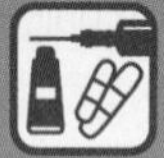 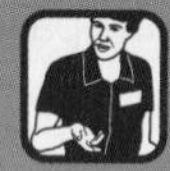 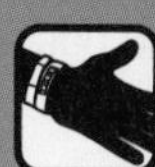  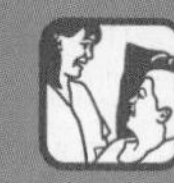 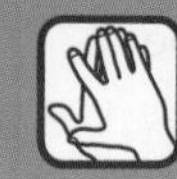 

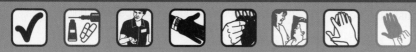

A complete bed bath is given when the patient is dependent and unable to provide hygiene self-care. Examples of such instances are patients with severe pain, injuries, or diseases that limit movement, or when the primary care provider has ordered that the patient not expend the energy to self-bathe. In some instances, special perineal care is ordered.

Supplies

- Basin of warm water
- Soap
- Towels and washcloths
- Bath blanket
- Clean linen for bed
- Clean gown
- Body lotion
- Toilet articles
- Hamper or bag for soiled linen
- Bedpan or urinal, toilet paper

For Perineal Care

- Underpad
- Gauze pads or washcloths
- Pitcher and water or ordered solution

Review and carry out the Standard Steps in Appendix A.

ACTION *(RATIONALE)*

Assessment (Data Collection)

1. Assess patient's preferences, including cultural factors. *(Demonstrates respect for patient preference and encourages participation in care.)*

Planning

2. Gather supplies. *(Provides easy access to equipment needed for hygiene and personal care bathing.)*
3. Explain the procedure to the patient. *(Decreases fear of the unknown and prepares patient.)*
4. Prepare environment for bathing: close doors and windows, adjust room temperature if necessary, pull curtains around bed, and place a sign ("Bath in progress") on the door. *(Promotes comfort by warming room and decreasing chance of drafts. Placing sign on door provides privacy.)*
5. Offer bedpan or urinal. *(Provides comfort and decreases chance of interruption during bath.)*

Implementation

6. Perform hand hygiene. Wear gloves if you or patient has any broken skin. Gloves must be worn while cleansing perineal area. *(Reduces transfer of microorganisms.)*

7. Raise the side rails and raise the level of bed to a comfortable working height. Lower rail on side closest to you and position patient in a comfortable position close to you. *(Promotes proper body alignment because work is at your center of gravity. Provides comfort for patient.)*
8. If a bath blanket is available, fan-fold the blanket horizontally and place it across patient's chest. Ask the patient to hold the top edge of the bath blanket. Pull the blanket and the covers to the foot of the bed. Remove the top covers out from underneath the bath blanket. Use the top sheet if a bath blanket is not available for a drape. *(Drapes patient, protecting privacy.)*

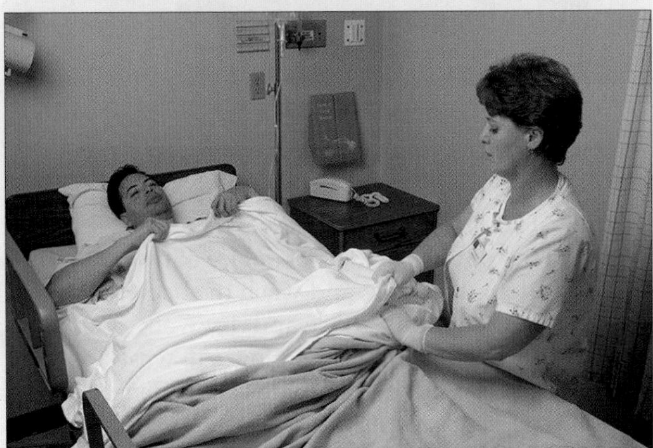

Step **8**

9. Remove linens as directed in Skill 20.2. *(Prepares linens to be replaced on bed.)*
10. Remove patient's gown, being careful to keep patient draped. If the patient has an intravenous (IV) line in place, remove the gown by gently pulling the gown off the patient's arm over the IV line without pulling on the line or disturbing the IV cannula. Lift the IV bag and tubing and thread them through the sleeve from the outside toward the inside of the gown to free the gown. If patient has a weak or paralyzed side, undress the unaffected side first. *(Prepares patient for bathing. Careful removal of gown protects the IV site.)*

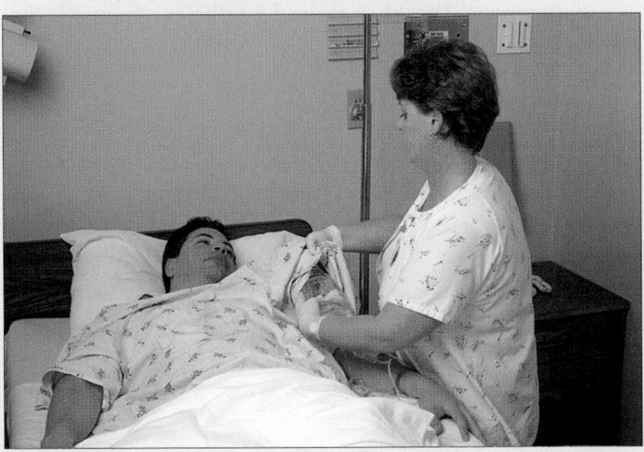

Step **10**

11. Raise the side rail while preparing the bathwater. Water should be warm and checked with either a bath thermometer or the inside of your wrist. Do not leave the soap in the water. Change water when it cools or becomes soiled or when a soap film develops. *(Provides for safety. Warm water is soothing, and maintaining warm, clean water is comforting.)*
12. Lower rail and remove the pillow under the patient's head or place a towel over the pillow. Make a bath mitt by grasping the washcloth at an edge and folding one-third of it over your fingers. Bring the opposite edge across your fingers and hold it with your thumb. Bring the top end of the cloth down to your palm and tuck that end under the lower edge. *(Provides better control of the washcloth; loose ends do not drag across patient. Loose ends cool quickly and chill the patient.)*

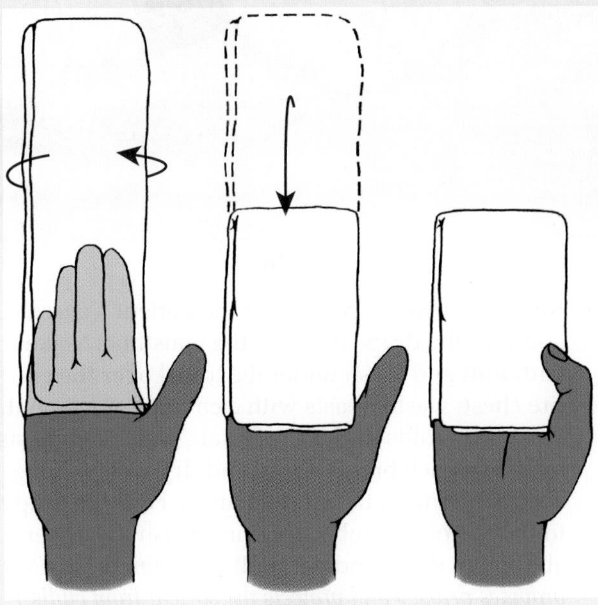

Step **12**

13. Fold drape to expose only the area being cleaned. Spread a towel across the patient's chest. *(Protects patient privacy and prevents chills.)*
14. Ask the patient about preference of using soap on the face. Moisten the bath mitt with water and wash one eye area from the nose to the outer edge near the ear; use a separate part of the mitt to wash the other eye area. Do not use soap near eyes. Wash patient's face and neck. Dry well. Rinse cloth and wash forehead from the center to each side; wash the rest of face, using a circular motion around the mouth. Rinse and dry the face well. Wash, rinse, and dry each ear and the neck. Patient may wash own face if able. *(Using different parts of the cloth to wash eye area prevents moving bacteria from one eye to the other. Rinsing well prevents the soap from drying the skin.)*

15. Place a towel under the far arm, make a bath mitt, use soap, and wash the entire arm with long, sweeping strokes from distal to proximal (toward the axilla). Give special care to the axilla with extra soaping. Rinse and pat dry well. Wash the hands and fingers, rinse, and dry. Move the towel, and wash and dry the near arm and hand in the same manner. *(Towel protects the mattress from getting wet and is available for drying. Washing distal to proximal promotes circulation. Bacteria collect in the sweat gland areas, and extra cleansing of axilla is needed to remove secretions and decrease body odor.)*

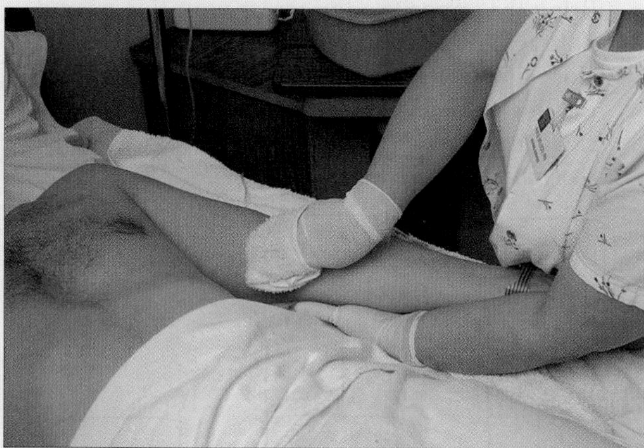

Step **15**

16. Keep the towel in place over the patient's chest, and pull the drape down to the waistline. Make a bath mitt and wash under the towel over the entire chest; wash breasts with a circular movement. Wash skin folds under the female patient's breasts by lifting each breast. Rinse and dry well, paying special attention to skin fold areas. Fold the drape to the top of the pubic bone and wash the lower abdomen. Rinse and dry well. *(Washing in sections provides privacy and protects the patient from chills.)*
17. Expose the far leg, and tuck the bath blanket around the patient to prevent chilling. Flex the leg and place a towel lengthwise on the bed. Wash from the foot to the knee with long, sweeping strokes and then from the knee to the hip in the same manner. Rinse and dry the leg well. Place the bath basin on the towel and lift the foot, placing your hand under the heel, and place it into the water. Wash the foot and dry it. Dry each toe separately, and place the leg and foot under the drape. Wash the near leg in the same manner. *(Tucking bath blanket around patient keeps the patient warm. Stroking from distal to proximal encourages venous return. Placing the foot into warm water is soothing and comforting to the patient.)*

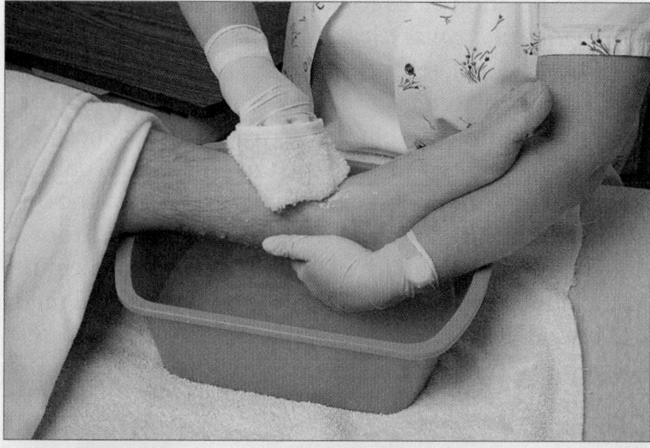

Step **17**

18. Change the bathwater after washing the legs and feet. *(Prevents using water that has been used on the feet on other parts of the body.)*
19. Turn the patient to the side, place a towel lengthwise along the back, and wash the back with long, sweeping motions. Rinse and dry well. Offer a back rub at this time. Don gloves to wash the folds of the buttocks and anus well. *(Towel protects mattress from moisture.)*
20. Change water and washcloth. Provide privacy for the patient to wash the genital area. If patient is unable, don gloves if not done in Step 6; place an underpad beneath the perineum to protect the mattress and wash the area thoroughly, rinse well, and pat dry carefully. For the female patient, wash from the front to the back. For the uncircumcised male patient, retract the foreskin and clean the head of the penis, rinse, and reposition the foreskin. Lift the scrotum and clean the area well. If a catheter is in place, carefully wash around it with soap and water, and rinse the area. Dry the penis and scrotum. Remove the underpad. *(Promotes privacy because many patients wish to wash their own perineum. Cleanses areas patient cannot manage. Washing around a catheter removes body secretions.)*

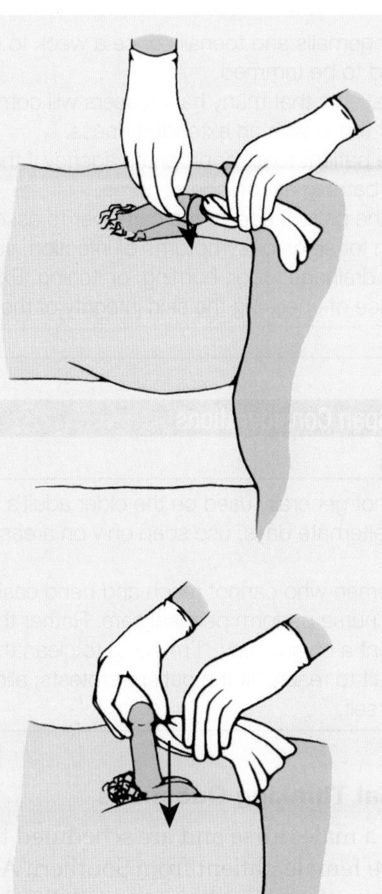

Step 20

For Specially Ordered Female Perineal Care

21. Place patient in the dorsal recumbent position in bed. Drape with a bath blanket diagonally (it should look like a diamond resting on the patient). Take the point of the bath blanket by the patient's feet and fold it up to the pubic area. Place the outer sides of the bath blanket over patient's knees and wrap the corners around each foot. *(Provides privacy and prevents chills.)*
22. With gloves in place, remove any peripad or dressings and observe characteristics of the drainage. Discard soiled items in a sealable plastic bag. *(Standard Precautions must be used when handling items soiled with body substances.)*
23. Slip an underpad under the patient's hips and position patient on the bedpan as described in Chapter 29. Raise the head of the bed slightly or use pillows to support the patient's head. *(Underpad prevents soiling the linens and mattress. Positioning the patient prevents back strain by supporting the head and shoulders.)*
24. Carefully pour warm water or the prescribed solution over the perineal area to rinse off urine, feces, or vaginal drainage. *(Cleanses outer perineum.)*
25. Use the nondominant hand to separate the labia majora, and, with downward strokes from the pubic area to the rectum, cleanse the skin folds with cotton balls, gauze pads, or a washcloth. Use only one downward stroke with each gauze pad, cotton ball, or portion of the washcloth. Rinse and pat the area dry with clean towel or fresh gauze pads. Remove the underpad and replace peripad or redress as needed. *(Cleaning with downward strokes prevents carrying bacteria from the dirty rectal area up to the vaginal area and urinary meatus. Peripad or dressing provides for collection of secretions.)*

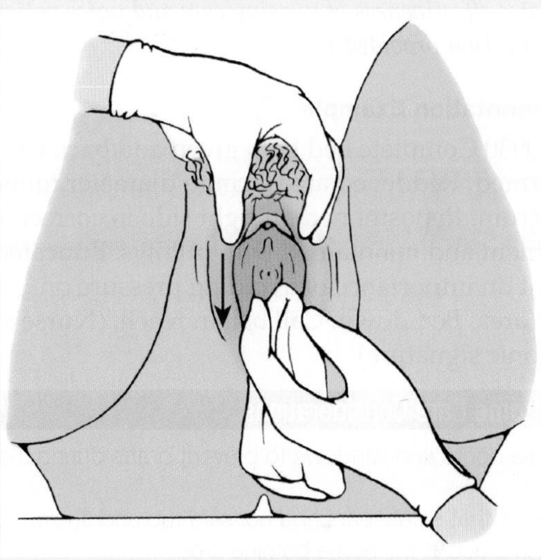

Step 25

Completing Care

26. Put a clean gown on the patient. If the patient has an IV in place, lift the IV bag and line and put it through the sleeve of the gown from the inside of the gown to the outside, *just as the arm will go through the sleeve.* Then carefully place the patient's arm through the sleeve of the gown. If a patient has a weak or paralyzed side, dress this extremity first. *(Maintains IV site and prevents the IV cannula and tubing from coming apart. Dressing is more comfortable and easier for the patient and you.)*
27. Complete personal care by combing the patient's hair, caring for fingernails and toenails, and permitting the male patient to either shave himself or be shaved (see Steps 19.2). *(Increases patient's sense of well-being and self-esteem.)*
28. Lower the bed, lower unneeded side rails, and restore the unit. Empty, rinse, and wipe out the basin before returning to storage. *(Makes patient comfortable and safe. Cleaning basin prepares it for the next use; wiping removes soap scum that rinsing alone leaves behind.)*

29. Make the occupied bed if needed (see Skill 20.2). *(The patient who needs a bed bath may not be able to get out of bed.)*

Evaluation

30. Observe the newly bathed patient. Is the patient comfortable? Did the bath tire the patient? Are there any modifications you would make in providing future hygiene care for this patient? *(Determines if any changes are needed.)*

Documentation

31. Document on the flow sheet or in the nurse's notes depending on agency policy. Note the type of bath performed or given, the patient's tolerance of the procedure, any patient education done, and any abnormalities found during the bath. *(Validates effectiveness of nursing care and notes patient education provided.)*

Documentation Example

6/25 0930 Complete bed bath given and back rub performed. Reddened area 2 cm in diameter found on sacrum. Repositioned on right side in correct body alignment and maintained with pillows. Educated patient on importance of avoiding pressure on the sacral area. Bed down. Call bell in reach. (Nurse's electronic signature)

Home Care Considerations

- Close doors and windows to prevent drafts during the bath.
- Ensure that safety bars and nonskid tub and shower pads are in place in the home bathing area.
- Caution patients to always check the water temperature before entering the bathtub or shower.
- Trim nails after bathing while the nails are soft.
- Check fingernails and toenails once a week to decide if they need to be trimmed.
- Inform patients that many hairdressers will come to the home for those with an extended illness.
- Refer the patient to an appropriate agency if there is a need for bathing assistance at home.
- Instruct the patient and/or the caregiver to assess the perineum for signs or symptoms of infection, such as redness, drainage, odor, burning, or itching. Explain the importance of checking the skin integrity of the perineal area.

Life-Span Considerations

Older Adults

- Soap is not generally used on the older adult's skin every day. On alternate days, use soap only on areas visibly soiled.
- Older women who cannot reach and bend easily need to have the nurse perform perineal care. Rather than giving this patient a choice, say, "I'm going to clean the areas that are difficult to reach." If the patient protests, allow her to wash herself.

Critical Thinking Questions

1. You are a male nurse and are scheduled to care for a mature female patient from Southern Asia. Does your patient's culture have any implications for her care? Why or why not?
2. The patient in your assignment is the same age as you but of the opposite sex. You will need to provide special perineal care to this patient. What is the best approach in completing this task?
3. Describe three things you would do to promote your patient's comfort during a complete bed bath.

Steps 19.1 Providing a Tub Bath or Shower

When inpatients can safely bathe by themselves, the bathing area is prepared, and then patients are readied for the bath or shower. Patients must be checked on frequently while in the tub or shower.

ACTION (*RATIONALE*)

1. Schedule use of tub or shower room. Clean according to institution's policy. Place towel on floor outside of tub or shower and nonskid mat in tub or shower. *(Scheduling ensures area is available when patient is ready. Cleaning prevents spread of microorganisms. Towel provides a dry, warm area for the patient to step on, and the mat decreases chance of falls.)*
2. Gather supplies and assist patient to area. Completely drape patient or have robe and slippers. *(Assisting the patient promotes safety. Draping or robing decreases chance of chills and provides privacy.)*
3. Place "occupied" sign on door; demonstrate use of call bell system. *(Maintains privacy and promotes safety.)*
4. Fill tub halfway with warm water; check the temperature per policy and adjust as needed. If using the shower, turn on water and adjust temperature as needed. A handheld sprayer allows you or the patient to control water flow and prevents you from becoming soaked. Place toiletry articles within patient's reach. Assist patient as needed. *(Checking*

water temperature prevents burns. Placing toiletry articles within reach decreases chance of falls. Assistance promotes hygiene by helping patient with hard-to-reach areas.)

5. Instruct patient not to stay in the tub or shower longer than 20 minutes. Check on the patient every 5 minutes; knock on the door before entering. Remain within calling distance if the patient has a history of **syncope** (fainting), light-headedness, or dizziness, or is taking a shower or bath for the first time after surgery or illness. *(Time limit decreases chance of light-headedness or dizziness resulting from vasodilation from the warm water. Checking on patient and remaining within calling distance provide privacy and promote safety.)*
6. Assist patient out of tub or shower. Encourage the use of safety bars during transfer. Assist with drying and dressing. Transport back to room. *(Promotes safety. Drying and dressing patient maintain warmth by preventing chills.)*
7. Clean tub or shower per institution's policy. *(Prevents transfer of microorganisms.)*
8. Document type of bath taken, tolerance of procedure, condition of skin, and amount of assistance needed by patient. *(Promotes continuity of care.)*

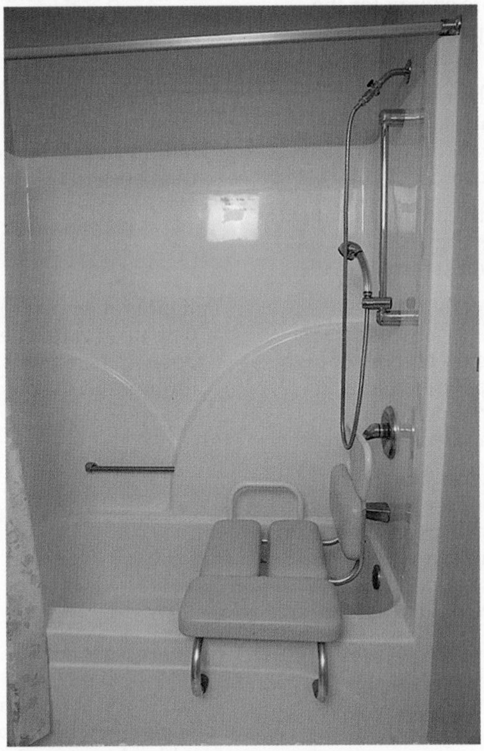

FIGURE 19.5 Shower bench and grab bar assist the weak patient.

Steps 19.1 explain the procedures for providing a tub bath or shower. Offer the use of the toilet before running the bathwater or placing the patient in the tub or shower. A shower chair or bath bench and grab bars are used for the patient who is weak or not ambulatory (Fig. 19.5). If the patient does not have balance problems, assist the patient into a tub that is half filled with warm water. Once the patient is in the tub or shower, add warmer water as desired. Place a call bell within easy reach of the independent patient. Check on the patient every 5 minutes, and inform the patient that the bath should not exceed 15 to 20 minutes.

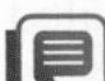 Communication

Assisting the Weak Patient

Bob Rodriguez is 59 years old and was admitted to the hospital yesterday for a right-sided stroke. He has some left upper extremity weakness but no other deficits. Mr. Rodriguez has just pushed his tray onto the floor. His nurse enters his room after hearing the crash.

Nurse: "Mr. Rodriguez, I heard your tray fall to the floor. Are you all right?"

Mr. Rodriguez: "No! I am not sure if I will ever be all right again."

Nurse: "You're not sure if you'll be all right . . . what do you mean?"

Mr. Rodriguez: "I am left-handed and got disgusted trying to feed myself."

Nurse: "Using your right hand to feed yourself breakfast was very frustrating for you, wasn't it?"

Mr. Rodriguez: "Yes! I just don't know how I will ever be able to take care of myself."

Nurse: "You're worried, and I understand your concern. It is still too early to tell how much weakness will remain on your left side. The therapists from physical and occupational therapy and I will work with you to teach you how to care for yourself while you are here in the hospital."

Mr. Rodriguez: "Do you really think that I will be able to feed and bathe myself at home?"

Nurse: "Yes. There are many techniques and devices available to help people care for themselves independently. Would you like something else to eat? I could call the kitchen for another tray."

Mr. Rodriguez: "Thank you, but I don't really want anything right now."

Nurse: "Would you like to start your bath? I could begin teaching you some of the techniques now, if you are ready for me to help you with your bath. What do you think?"

Mr. Rodriguez: "Yes, I would like to learn. Thank you."

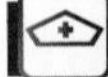 Clinical Cues

If the patient is weak, provide assistance with the bath and do not leave the bathroom.

Provide a towel for the patient to drape the genital area while in the tub for privacy. Nursing Care Plan 19.1 presents one plan for hygienic care.

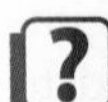 Think Critically

Your patient does not want a bath now, but your instructor expects the bath to be done by 10 am. What do you do?

Nursing Care Plan 19.1 Care of the Patient With a Self-Care Deficit

SCENARIO Herman Gray, age 67, has a diagnosis of **exacerbation** (an increase in the severity or symptoms of a disease) of chronic obstructive pulmonary disease. Mr. Gray is widowed. He lives alone. He was admitted to your unit this morning, and you devised the following plan for hygiene care.

PROBLEM/NURSING DIAGNOSIS *Fatigue*/Bathing self-care deficit related to intolerance to activity.

Supporting Assessment Data *Subjective:* States, "I get too tired standing at the sink to wash myself." *Objective:* Visibly tired with minimal activity. Becomes short of breath with exertion.

Goals/Expected Outcomes	Nursing Interventions	Selected Rationales	Evaluation
Patient will participate in hygiene care each day.	Gather supplies for patient.	Patient participation in self-care will maintain or increase self-esteem.	*Participating in hygiene care?* Washed face and hands. Bathing after morning rest period.
	Plan hygiene care when the patient is well rested.	Provides more energy for the patient to perform the self-care.	
Patient completes hygiene care without fatigue by discharge.	Provide a chair for the patient to sit by the sink for bathing.	Sitting in a chair takes less energy than standing does; it allows patient to complete more self-care.	*Experiencing fatigue with hygiene care?* Some fatigue noted, but less than yesterday.
	Assist with hygiene when patient becomes tired.	Assisting with care helps patient conserve energy for self-care he deems most important.	
	Suggest scheduling hygiene activities throughout the day to minimize fatigue. If patient has a PRN oxygen order, have patient use oxygen during bath.	Breaking up care conserves patient energy and allows patient to complete more of own care in smaller increments. The ability to perform self-care enhances self-esteem.	Patient is able to participate in care when done in increments throughout the day. Outcome met.
	Advise patient of assistive devices available for bathing, such as long-handled sponge and shower chair or bench.	Assistive devices may help conserve energy by making hard-to-reach areas easier to clean and minimizing exertion. Chairs or benches also help ensure patient safety.	
Patient makes decisions about obtaining hygiene care at home before discharge.	Refer to visiting nurses association or home health agency for home care if needed.	Provides for care after discharge.	*Have decisions been made?* No referral necessary at this time. The patient has applicable phone numbers and contacts.

CRITICAL THINKING QUESTIONS

1. When you consider Mr. Gray's ability to care for himself at home, what other self-care activities might be a problem based on his statement?
2. On discharge, it is noted that Mr. Gray is able to perform his own hygiene activities. What devices do you think he should have at home to perform these tasks?

PRN, As needed.

Therapeutic Baths. *Therapeutic* means having healing or medicinal qualities. Therapeutic baths are performed to achieve a desired effect. There are several types of therapeutic baths. A whirlpool bath is done in a bathtub or special whirlpool tub that has a device that agitates the water. The heat of the water and agitation gently massage the skin. Whirlpools are used to cleanse, stimulate peripheral circulation, and provide comfort. Starch or oatmeal baths, using plain instant oatmeal, are used for patients with dermatitis. Commercial products are also available and are added according to package directions. The skin is patted dry after the bath so the nerve endings are not stimulated by rubbing.

Sitz baths are used to apply moist heat and clean the perineal or anal area (Fig. 19.6). The bath promotes

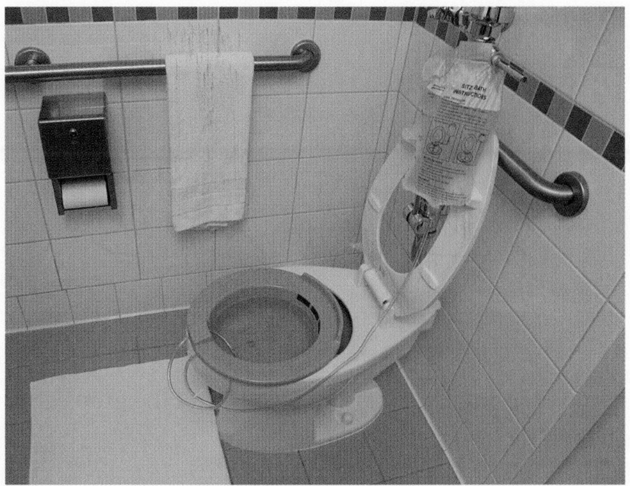
FIGURE 19.6 Sitz bath.

healing and relieves pain and discomfort. It is commonly used after birth and vaginal or rectal surgery. Body soaks are usually indicated to cleanse open wounds or apply medicated solutions to an area. Feet and arms are the parts of the body most often soaked. Cooling sponge baths are also known as tepid sponge baths. An order is usually needed before this type of bath can be used to bring down a fever. A cooling sponge bath can be soothing but also may be uncomfortable if the patient's fever is high.

Variations of the Bed Bath. A bag bath is a variation of the bed bath. Instead of using a basin, which has been found to be a potential reservoir of bacteria (Powers & Fortney, 2014), a self-contained bag is used. This self-contained bag contains several premoistened disposable cloths. The cloths are moistened with a cleansing agent that does not need rinsing. They may be heated or used directly from the bag. The bag contains many cloths, so a different cloth may be used for different body parts. The major disadvantage to this system is that it is more costly.

Clinical Cues

Keep in mind these key points when bathing a patient:
- Maintain safety.
- Provide privacy.
- Prevent chills.
- Encourage independence.

Back Massage

A back massage is an important part of hygiene care, and it involves the sense of touch. Benefits of the back rub include:
- Communicates caring
- Fosters trust in the nurse–patient relationship
- Provides an opportunity to assess the skin on the back
- Stimulates circulation of blood to the area
- Reduces tension and promotes relaxation

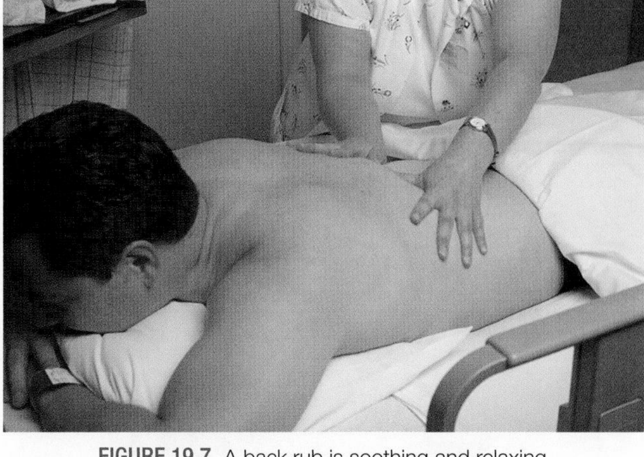
FIGURE 19.7 A back rub is soothing and relaxing.

Box 19.3 notes to perform a back rub with morning care and at bedtime. It is essential to provide one to patients confined to bed. Use oils or lotions according to patient preference and the skin's condition. Avoid open wounds and areas of pressure injury while performing a back rub.

Use more pressure on upward strokes toward the head and less pressure on downward strokes. The pressure should be firm but should not cause tensing or discomfort for the patient. After a few minutes, rub in any remaining lotion using short circular strokes, paying particular attention to the shoulders and neck. During the back rub, remember the following safety and comfort issues:
- Move the patient close to you to maintain proper body mechanics to prevent self-injury.
- Raise the bed to an appropriate height, and lower the rail only on the side where you are standing during the back rub.
- Make certain your hands are warm and relaxed before beginning. Warm any lotion or oils in your hands before placing them on the patient. Cool hands and cold lotions cause the patient to tense and pull away.

An effective back rub should last approximately 3 to 5 minutes (Fig. 19.7).

Perineal Care

Usually a patient will accept your assistance with perineal care, although a few try to avoid it because they feel embarrassed. Proper draping helps promote comfort with the procedure (Fig. 19.8). You can reduce your feelings of embarrassment by remembering your purpose is to assist the patient. Explain the procedure to reassure the patient and gain cooperation. Maintain a matter-of-fact attitude and be objective; avoid any sexually suggestive conversation or actions. A professional and dignified attitude can help reduce embarrassment.

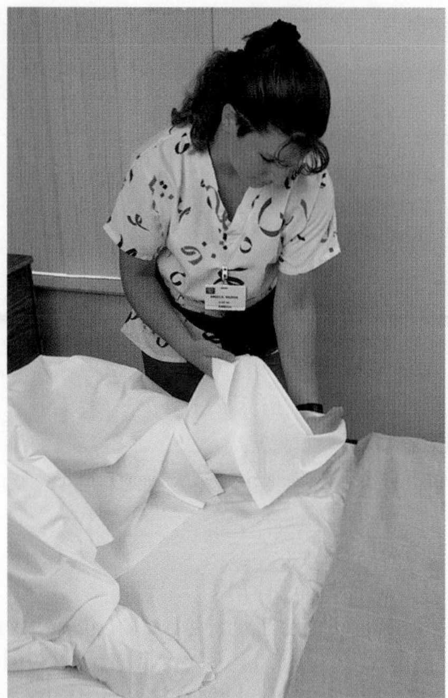

FIGURE 19.8 Draping the female patient in the lithotomy position for perineal care.

Mouth Care

Mouth care removes food particles and secretions, which prevents **halitosis** (bad breath), feelings of uncleanliness, and dental **caries** (cavities). Oral hygiene promotes a better appetite and maintains the healthy state of the mouth, gums, teeth, and lips. Fluoride-containing toothpaste, soft or powered toothbrush, and flossing have been shown conclusively to promote oral health. Lack of oral hygiene can have serious consequences, including increased risk of stroke, heart disease, and pneumonia (Heavey, 2014). Provide oral care on a regular basis, ideally, four times a day (see Box 19.3).

Mouth care for the conscious patient. To assist a patient with mouth care, raise the head of the bed 45 to 90 degrees. Wear gloves when providing or assisting with mouth care. If the patient is unable to sit up, turn the patient to the side facing you. Place a towel under the chin. Moisten the toothbrush with water and apply toothpaste. Brush from the gum line to the edge of the teeth. All surfaces of each tooth should be brushed (Fig. 19.9). Have the patient rinse the mouth and spit the solution into the emesis basin. Repeat as desired or necessary. Provide the patient with a cloth or tissue to wipe the mouth when finished.

To assist the patient in flossing the teeth, obtain 12 to 15 inches of floss. Loosely wrap the ends of the floss around the index finger on each hand and work the floss between each tooth. Slide the floss gently down to the gum line, pulling the floss back and forth. If tooth brushing is performed before flossing, then the fluoride can come into direct contact with the tooth surfaces to prevent dental caries. Rinse and wipe the mouth again. Report any excessive bleeding of the gums after flossing.

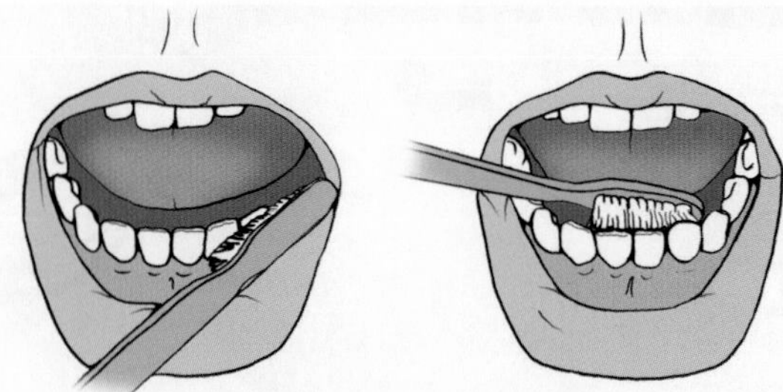

FIGURE 19.9 Brushing the teeth.

Mouth care for the unconscious patient. **Provide full mouth care to an unconscious patient at least once every 4 hours.** If the patient is mouth breathing, perform care every 4 hours. Mouth breathing causes the tongue to dry and become crusty. Remove any dry secretions because they cause halitosis and may obstruct airflow. Perform moist swabbing of the mouth every 2 hours or as needed to maintain the integrity of the oral cavity. Mouth care of the unconscious patient is described in Skill 19.2.

Denture care. Patients with dentures who are confined to bed, are comatose, are weak, or have trouble with hand and finger dexterity may need assistance to care for their dentures. Dentures should be cleaned to prevent irritation to the gums and infection. A patient may use an adhesive for a better fit. Usually, a patient who uses adhesive does not like to remove the dentures during the day. Care should then be provided in the morning and at bedtime. Do not place dentures on a meal tray because they are often lost when the trays are removed. Dentures should be removed for at least 6 hours daily to relieve pressure on mouth tissues and to allow saliva to cleanse the tissues. **When not in the mouth, dentures are kept in a labeled denture container filled with water or normal saline.** Skill 19.3 details how to clean dentures.

! Safety Alert

Use Denture Adhesive Safely

Caution patients that denture adhesives are safe when used as directed but can be harmful if overused because of the zinc they contain. Some adverse reactions including myelopathy have been reported to the Food and Drug Administration when patients have used much greater amount (e.g., a tube of adhesive lasting 4 days instead of 7 weeks).

Hair Care

Provide hair care regularly during illness, during or after the morning bath. Hair care consists of brushing and combing, shampooing, shaving, and mustache and beard care. Morale and body image are improved

Skill 19.2 Administering Oral Care to the Unconscious Patient

 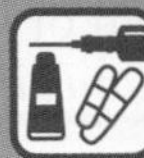 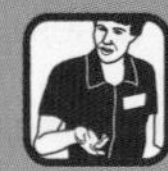   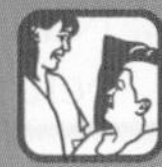 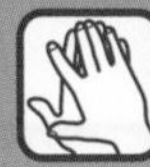 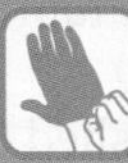

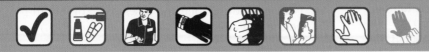

Unconscious patients require frequent mouth care. Cleansing is especially important for these patients because they often breathe through their mouths, which leads to dryness and crusting of the area.

Supplies

- Toothbrush and toothpaste
- Mouthwash
- Mouth suction device
- Gloves
- Water-soluble lubricant
- Water
- Paper towels
- Tongue blade and 4 × 4 gauze pads
- Towel or toothettes
- Emesis basin
- Irrigation syringe

Review and carry out the Standard Steps in Appendix A.

ACTION *(RATIONALE)*

Assessment (Data Collection)

1. Assess for gag reflex. *(Identifies risk of aspiration.)*

Planning

2. Gather supplies and place on paper towels on the over-the-bed table. *(Provides easy access to equipment. Paper towels keep table clean.)*
3. Explain the procedure to the patient. *(Provides stimulation because unconscious patients may be able to hear.)*
4. Close door or pull curtain. *(Provides privacy.)*

Implementation

5. Raise bed level to a comfortable working height. Turn patient laterally on side of bed nearest you. Lower side rail. *(Promotes good body mechanics; work is at your center of gravity.)*
6. Turn on the suction and place the suction device under the corner of the pillow near you. Put a towel under the patient's head and the emesis basin beneath patient's mouth and chin. *(Readying suction device provides for immediate use of suction in case patient gags. Towel and basin keep gown and linens clean.)*
7. Wear gloves. Use toothettes or toothbrush and toothpaste to cleanse the teeth and mouth. Use mouthwash or water to clean the interior of the cheeks, roof of the mouth, teeth, and tongue. A 4 × 4 gauze pad may be wrapped around an index finger or tongue blade to remove crusts. Repeat as necessary. *(Observes Standard Precautions. Mouthwash and water are good cleansing agents. Removing crusting and debris maintains a healthy mouth.)*
8. Floss by holding a 12- to 15-inch piece of floss with the ends wrapped around the middle finger of each hand. Using index fingers and thumbs, gently work floss between each tooth, moving down to gum line and back up to tooth edge. *(Removes tartar and plaque.)*

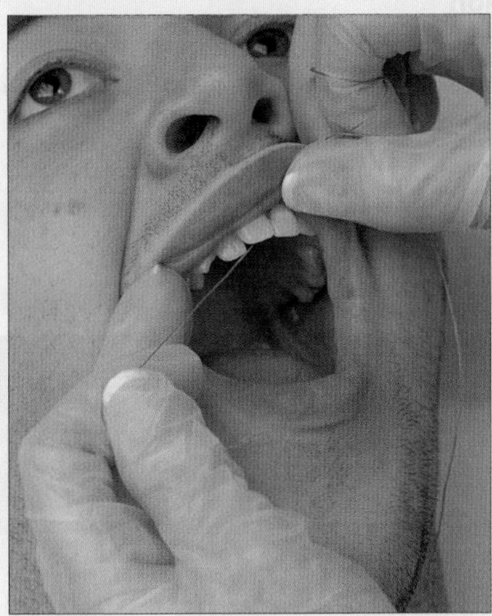

Step 8

9. With patient's head turned to the side, intermittently rinse the mouth by gently squirting water in with the syringe; use the suction device to remove water and debris. *(Using small amounts of water and turning the head to the side promote drainage and reduce risk of aspiration.)*

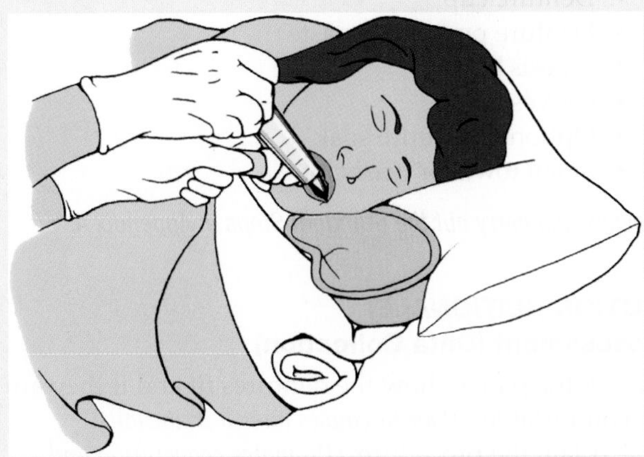

Step 9

10. Wipe patient's mouth and lubricate the lips and corners of the mouth with water-soluble lubricant. *(Prevents drying and cracking of lips.)*
11. Explain to the patient that you have finished the procedure. *(Provides stimulation because the unconscious patient may be able to hear.)*
12. Remove gloves and dispose of them properly. Reposition patient, raise side rail, and lower bed. *(Proper removal and disposal of gloves prevents spread of microorganisms. Repositioning patient and restoring unit promote safety and comfort.)*
13. Clean supplies and tidy unit. *(Readies equipment for next use and straightens patient's environment.)*

Evaluation

14. Put on gloves and inspect mouth to check effectiveness of procedure. *(Determines if other actions are needed.)*

Documentation

15. Note procedure done and assessment of mouth before and after care. *(Notes any abnormalities.)*

Documentation Example

7/28 0800 Mouth heavily crusted. Cleansed with mouthwash. Teeth brushed. No signs of aspiration during procedure. No bleeding or areas of inflammation noted. (Nurse's electronic signature)

Critical Thinking Questions

1. Complete oral care is necessary for the patient who is comatose. What precautions will you take to ensure this patient's safety and your own?
2. Every 8 hours, complete oral care is needed for the comatose or unconscious patient. Will you perform any other actions between the full care? If so, what?
3. What purpose does talking to the patient during the procedure serve?

Skill 19.3 Providing Denture Care

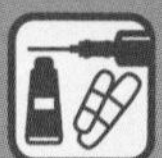
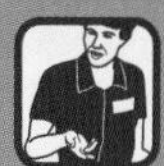
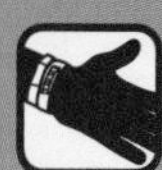
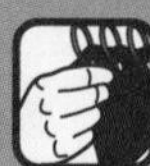
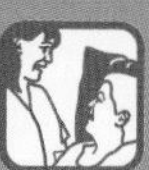

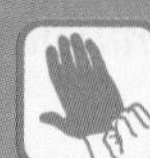

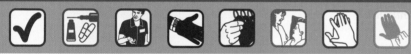

Dentures must be cleaned at least twice a day to maintain oral hygiene and promote oral health. If the patient is unable to perform this task independently, then you must provide assistance or clean the dentures yourself.

Supplies

- Denture brush or toothbrush
- Denture adhesive
- Denture cup
- Denture powder or paste
- Emesis basin
- Gloves
- Optional: denture soak
- Small towel or washcloth

Review and carry out the Standard Steps in Appendix A.

ACTION *(RATIONALE)*

Assessment (Data Collection)

1. Ask the patient how the dentures fit and if they are comfortable. *(Poor fit causes mouth irritation.)*
2. Explain the procedure. *(Promotes cooperation and understanding; decreases any anxiety over procedure.)*

Planning

3. Arrange supplies on over-the-bed table or near sink. *(Provides access to equipment.)*
4. Pull curtain and close door. *(Provides privacy. Many patients are reluctant to be seen without their dentures in place.)*
5. Ask patient to remove dentures. If he is unable, put on gloves and remove upper denture by grasping the front teeth with the thumb and index finger. Move denture up and down slightly to break the vacuum seal. Turn slightly and slip it out of the mouth. Place in the emesis basin. Grasp the lower denture with thumb and index finger and pick it up; turn slightly and carefully remove it from the mouth without stretching lips. Place in the emesis basin. *(Allows full access to mouth. Protects dentures until cleaned.)*
6. Assess the mouth and gums. *(Detects any irritation, redness, or swelling.)*

Implementation

7. Take emesis basin to the sink and place a washcloth or small towel in the sink. Fill sink with tepid water to about 1 inch in depth. *(Placing*

towel in sink decreases chance of breakage if dentures are accidentally dropped. Tepid, rather than hot, water prevents the dentures from becoming softened or deformed.)

8. Brush all surfaces with brush and paste or powder. Dentures may be soaked first in a commercial cleansing soak. *(Prevents accumulation of food and bacteria, thereby reducing odor and stains.)*

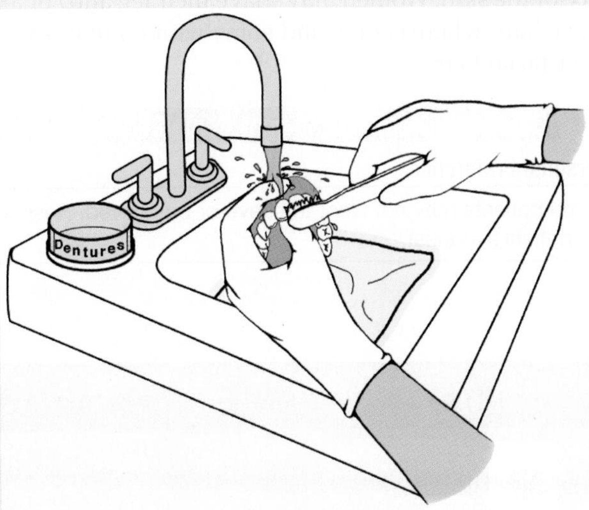

Step 8

9. Rinse well in tepid water and place in denture cup or emesis basin that is half filled with cool water. *(Rinsing removes toothpaste or powder, bacteria, and food. Placing dentures in cup keeps dentures safe until needed.)*
10. Clean the patient's mouth (gums, palate, and tongue) with a soft brush and toothpaste. *(Promotes oral hygiene by removing debris and stimulating circulation.)*
11. Assist the patient in replacing moistened dentures or replace them yourself. Use a dental adhesive if requested or needed. Insert the top denture first by reversing removal procedure (tilt slightly and push up onto gum), and press into place. Insert lower denture. *(Wetting dentures aids insertion and provides comfort. Adhesive promotes a better seal and increases comfort for some patients. Upper denture is easier to place first because it is larger. Pressing into place creates a seal against the roof of the mouth.)*
12. Store dentures in a labeled denture cup in cool water if they are not being replaced immediately in the mouth. *(Prevents loss because cup is labeled. Most patients do not sleep with their dentures in place.)*
13. Clean equipment and tidy unit. *(Readies supplies for next use and straightens the patient's environment.)*

Evaluation

14. Ask patient if the dentures are comfortable. *(Determines if the dentures were inserted correctly or if there is any irritation.)*

Documentation

15. Document on flow sheet or nurse's notes per policy. Note any areas of irritation or abnormality and action taken. *(Validates care and promotes continuity. Indicates if there are any problems or abnormalities.)*

Documentation Example

7/28 2200 Dentures cleaned; c/o small area of irritation on front gum line of lower denture; 1-cm diameter area of redness noted. Mouth swished with mouthwash. Dentures left in labeled denture cup on bedside stand; reassess area in A.M. (Nurse's electronic signature)

? Critical Thinking Questions

1. Many people feel self-conscious when they remove their dentures. What can you do to make the patient more comfortable during this task?
2. What is the purpose of placing a washcloth or small towel in the sink before cleaning dentures?
3. After removing your patient's dentures, you note an area of irritation on the right lower gum. What do you do?

when the patient is comfortable with his appearance. Brushing and combing the hair stimulates circulation, which helps to promote hair growth, prevent hair loss, distribute oil along hair shafts, and bring nutrients to the roots.

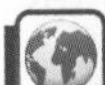 Cultural Considerations

Caring for African American Hair

The hair of African Americans tends to be fragile and may be easily injured or damaged. It should be washed every 7 to 14 days. It can be rinsed daily. This type of hair breaks easily, and a wide-toothed "pick" comb should be used to comb out tangles. The hair should be combed while wet. A leave-in type of conditioner should be used daily. Do not use heat for drying the hair. A satin pillowcase, scarf, or cap may be desired for sleep to decrease tangling. Alternatively, the hair may be plaited or tied back for sleep, making sure it is not too tight. Style is a matter of individual preference.

Brushing and combing. Use a clean brush or comb to brush from the scalp toward the hair ends to decrease pulling. Separate the hair into three sections; then each of those sections may be split into smaller sections. It is easier and more comfortable for the patient to brush or comb small sections of hair at a time. Be gentle when providing hair care.

A patient may have tangled or matted hair. To decrease pain, hold the hair between the scalp and the area you are brushing or combing. Braiding the hair helps to reduce tangles. Ask permission from the patient before braiding. Alcohol, astringents, or water may be used to loosen hair strands that are tangled or matted. Do not cut the hair to remove tangles. **A written, informed consent is necessary to cut a patient's hair.**

Shampooing. Shampooing removes dirt, soil, blood, or solutions from the hair, and it stimulates circulation of the scalp and eases brushing and combing. A patient who is able to shower or bathe may be shampooed without difficulty. If the patient is able to be out of bed in a chair, you may shampoo the hair in front of the sink. You must do the shampooing in bed if the patient is bedridden (Skill 19.4). Dry or rinseless shampoo that does not require water is available for cleaning the hair. It is usually sprayed into the hair. Another option is a shampoo cap such as the ReadyBath shampoo cap. Brushing removes the dirt and oils.

Shaving. Shaving is the removal of hair from the surface of the skin. Women may shave their leg and/or axillary hair, whereas men and some women may shave their facial hair.

QSEN Considerations: Patient-Centered Care

Personal Preference

Some patients may not want to shave or be shaved. Respect the patient's request.

Skill 19.4 Shampooing Hair

 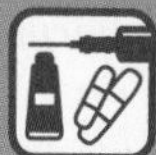 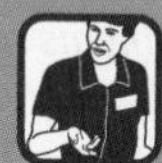  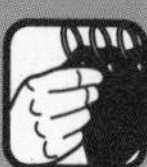 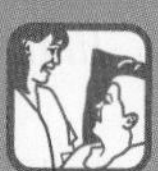 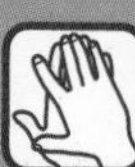 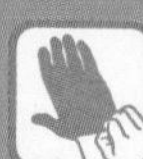

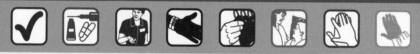

Assistance is given for shampooing the hair when the patient is unable to perform this procedure and the hair needs to be shampooed.

Supplies

- Shampoo
- Comb and brush
- Hair dryer
- Pitcher
- Waterproof pad
- Basin or pail for waste water
- Rinse or conditioner (optional)
- Shampoo tray or plastic trough
- Washcloth
- Bath blanket
- Bath towels (2 to 4)

Review and carry out the Standard Steps in Appendix A.

ACTION *(RATIONALE)*

Assessment (Data Collection)

1. Assess need for shampoo. Assess for contraindications to performing hair wash. *(Prevents injury to patient.)*
2. Check written order to see if a special shampoo is ordered. *(Medicated shampoos may be ordered in cases of dandruff, head lice, or other conditions.)*

Planning

3. Gather supplies. *(Provides easy access to equipment.)*
4. Explain the procedure to patient. *(Decreases fears and anxiety over procedure.)*

Implementation

5. Wear gloves if patient's scalp has lesions, cuts, or infestation or there is dried blood in the hair. *(Prevents spread of microorganisms.)*
6. Raise the bed, lower the near side rail, remove the pillow, and move the patient to the near side of the bed. Place a waterproof pad under the patient's shoulders and head. Drape patient with a bath blanket. Place a towel around patient's shoulders. *(Promotes proper body alignment and mechanics. Waterproof pad keeps linens dry. Drape prevents chills, and the towel helps to keep patient dry.)*
7. Brush or comb patient's hair. *(Removes tangles.)*
8. Place basin or pail on chair at the head of the bed to collect the waste water. Place the shampoo tray under the patient's head. Lower bed and obtain warm water. *(Shampoo tray keeps runoff water in basin or pail and protects bed from moisture. Using warm water promotes comfort.)*
9. Raise bed and lower near rail. Offer patient a folded washcloth to cover the eyes. Pour a small amount of water through patient's hair, starting at the front hairline and moving to the back of the head; wet entire hair surface completely. Apply shampoo and lather. Use your fingertips to massage all parts of the scalp. Again, start from the front and work to the back. Lift the head slightly to massage fully and wash the back of the head. Add water as needed to maintain lather. *(Promotes proper body alignment. Washcloth protects the*

eyes from soap and water. Friction aids in making the lather, which will cleanse the hair.)

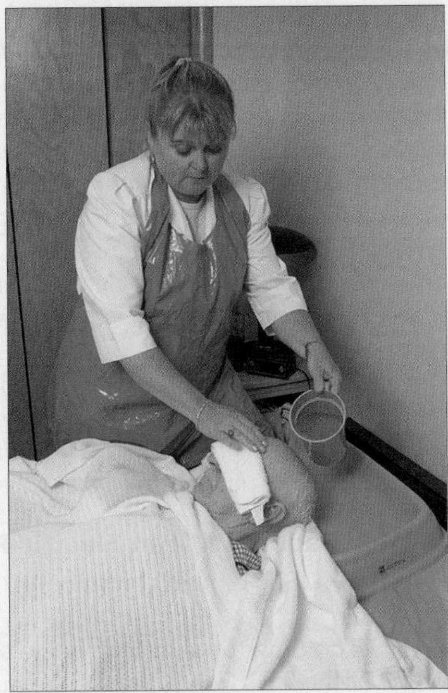

Step 9

10. Rinse thoroughly by pouring warm water through the hair. Rinse until the soap is completely out of the hair. Repeat washing and rinsing hair if needed (if the patient can tolerate the procedure again). *(Hair should be adequately cleaned.)*
11. Apply a cream rinse or conditioner if requested or ordered. Rinse thoroughly. *(Decreases tangles and adds moisture.)*
12. Wrap head in towel; dry face and shoulders. Remove shampoo tray and basin. *(Towel decreases chills. Removing tray and basin prevents spills.)*
13. Towel dry hair and scalp, using more towels if needed. Comb hair; use a hair dryer if needed. *(Towel drying promotes quicker drying of the hair. Combing removes tangles and styles the hair.)*
14. Position patient for comfort and finish arranging the hair as desired by patient. *(Promotes comfort and demonstrates respect for patient's wishes.)*
15. Clean equipment and restore the unit, lowering the bed and raising the side rail. *(Cleaning readies equipment for next use. Restoring unit promotes safety.)*

Evaluation

16. Assess condition of hair and scalp. How does patient feel now? *(Promotes a sense of well-being and cleanliness as hair is left clean and groomed.)*

Documentation

17. Document the patient response and tolerance of the procedure. Note any abnormalities of the hair or scalp found during the procedure. *(Validates effectiveness and provides for consistency among personnel.)*

Documentation Example

8/2 1030 Bed shampoo given. Complained of being tired and weak. Stated it felt "very good to have clean hair again." No abnormalities of hair or scalp noted. Bed down and call bell within reach. (Nurse's electronic signature)

Critical Thinking Questions

1. What needs to be done before determining how to give your patient a shampoo in bed?
2. People, especially the women, in some cultures cover their hair. What would you do if your patient is Muslim and a medicated hair shampoo is ordered?

Shaving may be done before, during, or after the bath. Many patients confined to bed can shave themselves if you set up the equipment. A weak or otherwise debilitated person will need your assistance with shaving. Either a safety razor or an electric razor may be used. Check an electric razor before use for any possible electrical hazard. Any razor should be used on only one patient to provide for infection control. Be gentle and use short strokes with the safety razor (Fig. 19.10). Check the patient's medical record to see whether the patient has any bleeding tendencies or is receiving medication that would contraindicate the use of a safety razor. A safety razor should not be used when a patient has a low platelet count, is receiving an anticoagulant, is undergoing chemotherapy, or is on aspirin therapy. Steps 19.2 describe how to shave a male patient.

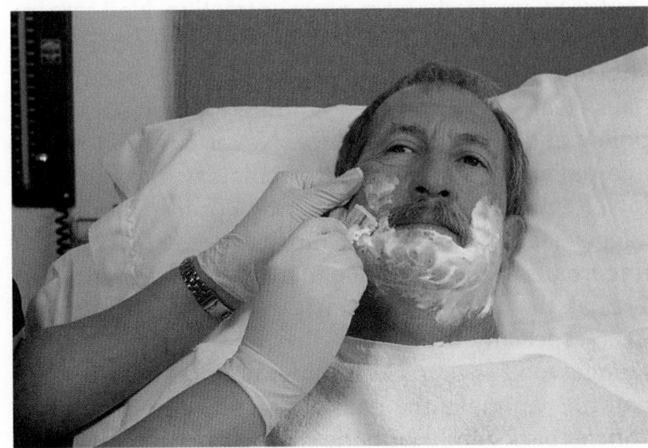

FIGURE 19.10 Shaving in the direction of hair growth.

Steps 19.2 Shaving a Male Patient

Shaving can improve a man's appearance and give him a sense of well-being. Unless he has his own electric razor, you must use a safety razor. Practicing by shaving a family member or friend will increase your confidence in the procedure.

ACTION (*RATIONALE*)

Shaving a Male Patient With a Safety Razor

1. Clean the face and neck with warm water. Place a warm washcloth on the patient's face for several minutes. Drape the patient and protect the bed linens from water. *(Cleaning reduces the surface bacteria should a cut occur. Application of warm washcloth reduces the chance of cuts because warm water softens the skin. Draping patient keeps linens dry and promotes patient comfort.)*
2. Apply shaving cream to face and neck or use lathered soap as a substitute. *(Lubricates skin so the razor glides more easily.)*
3. Hold a safety razor at a 30- to 45-degree angle in your dominant hand. Carefully pull patient's skin taut with your other hand. Use firm, short motions in the direction of hair growth to shave the area. *(Decreases the chance of cutting or nicking the skin. Prevents pulling of the skin. Many patients, if able, will instruct the nurse on personal preference regarding shaving technique.)*
4. Rinse the razor every two or three strokes, changing the water as needed. *(Cleans razor of hair and ensures a closer, even shave. Clean water prevents contamination.)*
5. Short downward strokes are used for the upper lip area. *(Decreases chance of cuts or nicks.)*
6. Rinse area with a washcloth and clean, warm water. Dry area. *(Promotes comfort, removes shaved hair, and decreases surface bacteria.)*
7. Assess area for cuts, nicks, or hair. Apply lotion or aftershave if desired by patient. *(Lotion promotes comfort by moisturizing the skin. Aftershave closes the pores opened by the moist heat through astringent action.)*

Shaving a Male Patient With an Electric Razor

1. Apply preshave lotion or skin conditioner. *(Softens beard and skin.)*
2. Turn on razor; holding the skin taut, begin shaving one side of the face. Gently stroke the razor downward in the direction of hair growth. *(Prevents pulling of the facial hairs and skin abrasion.)*
3. Offer lotion or aftershave when finished. *(Provides comfort.)*

Mustache and Beard Care. A patient with a mustache and/or beard needs daily care to these areas. Keep the facial hair clean and free of food particles. Cleanse mustaches and beards with a warm, damp washcloth or wash with soap or shampoo. **You may not shave off a beard or mustache without a written, informed consent.**

Nail Care

Most patients can perform nail care for themselves as part of their daily hygiene routine. You may need to provide care for those who are unconscious, blind, confused, unsteady, or in a cast or traction. Nail care includes regular trimming, cleaning under the nails, and cuticle care, and is usually done with the bath. Keep nails clean and trimmed according to the institution's policy and patient preference. Never cut the toenails of a patient with diabetes or circulatory disease of the lower extremities without a written order. Check your agency's policy to see if an order is needed to trim the fingernails of the diabetic patient.

Soak the nails in warm soapy water for 5 to 10 minutes, especially if they are dirty or thickened. Use an orangewood stick to clean under nails because a metal nail file can make the nails rough and trap dirt. Push cuticles back gently with the stick to prevent hangnails, which are pieces of skin that are partially detached at the base of the fingernail. Hangnails are painful and a possible source of infection.

Use nail clippers to cut the toenails straight across to prevent them from growing into the skin along the sides (Fig. 19.11). This can cause pain or infection and leads to a condition called ingrown toenails. Ingrown toenails often require a surgical procedure to correct.

Observe the color of the nail beds to monitor circulation in the extremities. Examples of when such monitoring is needed are after surgery, during traction, when the patient is in a cast, or when there is a risk of failure in the general systemic circulation. Nail polish needs to be removed in these instances to allow monitoring.

Patient Education

Hygiene and Skin Care

Good hygiene practices and appropriate skin care techniques can be taught to patients during bath time. The following points should be covered:

- Hygiene care is important in maintaining health.
- Use warm, not hot, water and a mild soap when bathing.
- For patients who spend time outdoors, use sunscreen year round with a minimum sun protection factor (SPF) of 15 on all exposed areas; reapply every 2 hours.
- Check skin for any changes such as redness and rashes, changes in moles, or skin growths.
- Address safety concerns, such as water temperature and prevention of falls in the shower and tub.

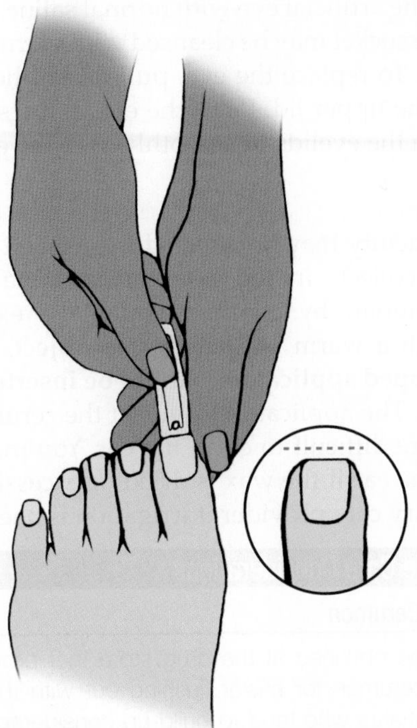

FIGURE 19.11 Cut toenails straight across and then smooth the corners.

- Prevent dry skin by avoiding cold or dry air and using creams or oils on the skin.
- Eat a balanced diet.
- Remove moisture on the skin from urine, stool, perspiration, or wound drainage.
- Clip toenails or file straight across; smooth any sharp edges.

Eye Care

Assess your patient's eyes for drainage, crusting, or redness. Notify the primary care provider if any abnormalities are found. Routine eye care is described in Skill 19.1. If crusting is noted, soak the eyelid with a warm, damp washcloth for 2 to 3 minutes to soften the crust and ease its removal. Use a different part of the cloth for each eyelid. Perform more frequent eye care for unconscious patients; administer lubricating drops as ordered. Older adults will have the nursing diagnosis: Risk for dry eye.

Health Promotion Points

Eye Recommendations for Older Adults

- Have glaucoma screening done every 2 to 3 years after age 40. Glaucoma is one of the leading causes of blindness.
- Be regularly checked for cataracts and macular degeneration.
- Use an Amsler grid at home to detect signs of macular degeneration.
- Wear a brimmed hat and dark glasses when outdoors to help prevent cataracts.
- Use artificial tears if you experience dry eyes to help prevent infection.

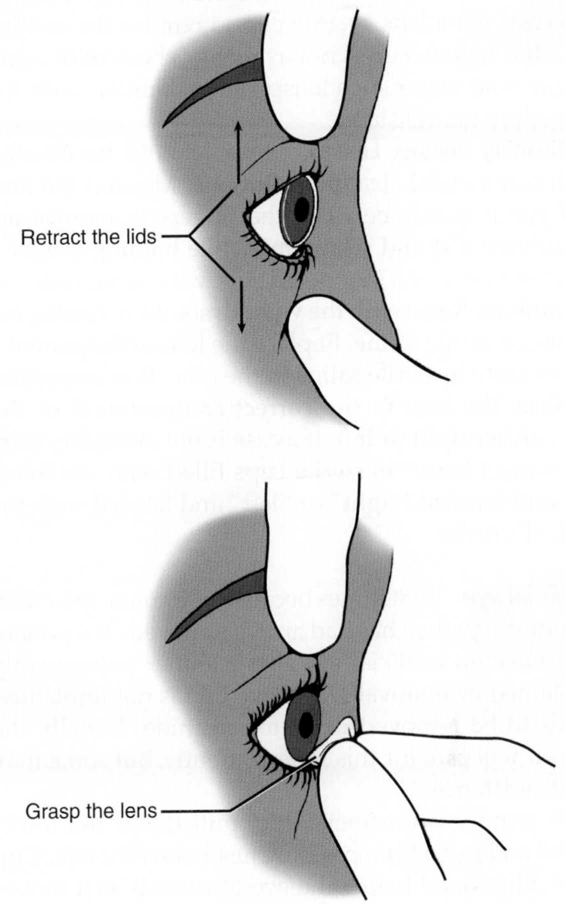

FIGURE 19.12 Removal of a soft contact lens.

Glasses and contacts. Store glasses in a case when not in use. Most glasses today have plastic lenses that are easier to scratch than glass. To clean either type of lens, use clean warm water and a soft cloth to wipe dry. Do not use a paper towel on plastic lenses because it may scratch them.

Contact lenses are classified as to whether they are hard or soft. Hard lenses feel like a firm plastic disk, whereas soft lenses have the consistency of a thick plastic food wrap. Many contact lenses may be worn for an extended period.

Removal of Contact Lenses. To remove a hard lens, perform hand hygiene and don clean gloves. Cup your nondominant hand below the patient's eye. Move the lens directly over the cornea. Pull the upper eyelid up above the edge of the lens; pull the lower lid down to the lower edge of the lens. Press slightly on the lower lid at the edge of the lens; the lens should slide out between the eyelids.

To remove a soft lens, perform hand hygiene and don clean gloves. Place a drop of wetting solution or sterile saline in the eyes to moisten the contact surface. Using your nondominant hand, open the eye with your middle finger and thumb. Use the index finger of your dominant hand and place it gently on the lower edge of the lens. Slide the lens down toward the lower lid. Gently pinch the lens between your index finger and thumb, and lift the lens out (Fig. 19.12).

Sometimes the techniques described do not work. In this case, get a lens suction cup to remove the contact lens. If a suction cup is not available, check with a colleague who wears such lenses and is familiar with the procedure for assistance.

Cleaning Contact Lenses. Lenses should be cleaned with commercial cleaning solutions. Moisten the lens and rub it gently between the fingers to remove accumulated dirt and secretions while holding it over a basin of water or a stoppered sink with some water in the bottom. Rinse with the wetting solution, rinsing solution, or sterile saline. Replace the lens in the patient's eye or store in sterile saline in the case. **It is important to place the lens in the correct compartment of the case, either right or left.** If a case is not available, store the contact lenses in sterile cups filled with sterile saline and marked "right" or "left" and labeled with the patient's name.

Artificial eye. Sometimes because of trauma, infection, or tumor, a patient has had an eye removed. The patient may have an artificial eye that is either permanently implanted or removable. An eye that is not implanted needs to be removed daily for cleaning. Usually the patient will care for this independently, but some may need assistance.

To remove an artificial eye, pull down the lower eyelid and put a little pressure just below the eye. Cup your other hand below the eye to catch it as it moves out of the socket. Assess the socket for any signs of infection. Report any redness or drainage immediately. Cleanse the artificial eye with normal saline. The edges of the eye socket may be cleansed with warm tap water or saline. To replace the eye, pull down the lower lid and lift the upper lid. Place the eye in the socket, and be certain the eyelids fit smoothly over the eye.

Ear Care

Hearing acuity may be affected if cerumen or foreign material collects in the external ear canal. Remove these materials by gently washing the external ear canal with a warm washcloth. **No object, including cotton-tipped applicators, should be inserted into the ear canal.** The applicators compact the cerumen, making it more difficult to clean the ear. You may need to irrigate the ear if the wax is dried or excessive. Notify the primary care provider if irrigation is needed.

Home Care Considerations

Removing Cerumen

A kit can be obtained at the drug store that provides drops to soften cerumen for easier flushing out with the small ear syringe. Patients who tend to build up considerable cerumen should be encouraged to use the kit periodically.

Hearing aids. Hearing aids amplify sound and must be cleaned daily (Fig. 19.13). There are five types of hearing aids: (1) behind the ear, (2) "mini" behind the ear, (3) in the ear, (4) in the ear canal, and (5) completely in canal. Do not drop or bump hearing aids because this can cause damage. Store the aid in its case to pre-

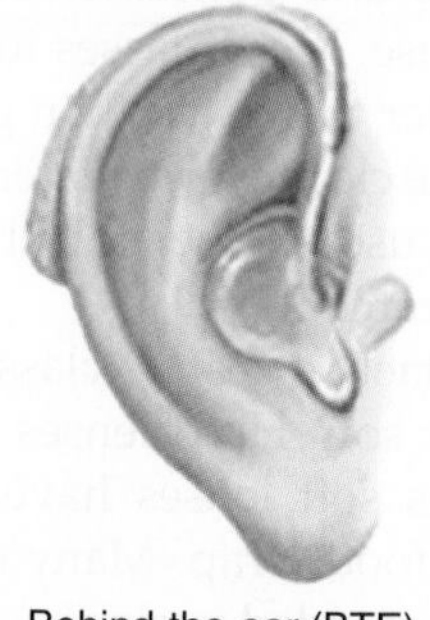

Behind-the-ear (BTE)

"Mini" (BTE)

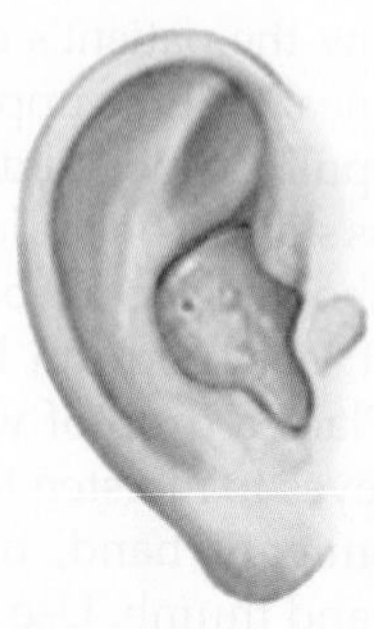

In-the-ear (ITE)

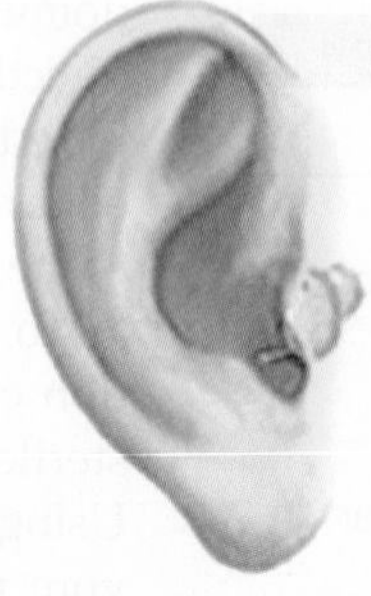

In-the-canal (ITC)

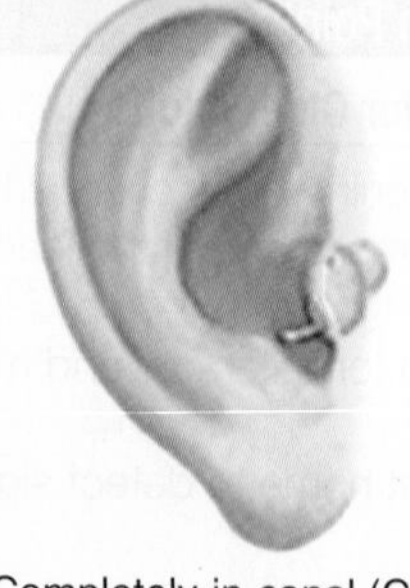

Completely-in-canal (CIC)

FIGURE 19.13 Hearing aids.

vent damage and to avoid an accumulation of dust and dirt when not in use. Clean the hearing aids as directed to decrease buildup of wax and drainage, which can damage the hearing aids. Do not submerge the hearing aid in water. If the hearing aid is not working, check to make certain that the unit is turned on, the battery is installed correctly (it may need to be replaced), and there are no cracks or breaks in the plastic housing or tubing. Replace dead batteries immediately.

Clinical Cues

When the hearing aid is out of the ear and in its case, the battery cover should be opened so that the battery disengages.

◆ EVALUATION

During evaluation, you determine whether the expected outcomes set during the planning stage of the nursing process have been met. Evaluation statements indicating the expected outcomes for hygiene have been met are as follows.

- Patient has no evidence of redness, irritation, or breaks in skin integrity; skin integrity is maintained.
- Hair is clean and neatly styled each day per patient preference.
- The mucous membranes are pink and moist, without signs or symptoms of irritation or odor.

Feedback from the patient and other personnel should be obtained during evaluation. Self-evaluation is important too. Did you encourage the patient to function independently? Did you use good body alignment when providing care? Were active measures taken to prevent pressure injuries? The information gathered will indicate if any changes need to be made in the plan. If so, document the progress made and the changes for other staff.

Get Ready for the NCLEX Examination!

Key Points

- The skin is the largest organ of the body. The main functions of the skin are to protect, sense, regulate temperature, excrete, and secrete.
- Changes from aging may cause the skin to (1) wrinkle and sag, (2) become dry and itchy, (3) have altered temperature control, and (4) be more fragile and slower to heal.
- Hygiene is the practice of cleanliness that helps to preserve health. To determine self-care abilities, assess the patient's physical and cognitive ability.
- A pressure injury forms from local interference with circulation. Pressure injuries are graded according to four stages plus the categories "unstageable" and "deep pressure tissue injury." Pressure injury staging may be inhibited in dark-skinned patients, when eschar is present or in patients with orthopedic devices.
- Pay particular attention to assessing areas over bony prominences.
- The purposes of bathing are to cleanse the skin, promote comfort, stimulate circulation, and remove waste products from the skin.
- When providing perineal care for a female, wipe from front to back to prevent infection. When providing perineal care for an uncircumcised male, reposition the foreskin after cleansing.
- Maintaining oral hygiene prevents halitosis, feelings of uncleanliness, and dental caries.
- Hair care improves morale and body image. Hair and beards may not be cut without a written, informed consent.
- Shaving with a safety razor is contraindicated in patients who are on anticoagulants, chemotherapy, or aspirin or who are immunocompromised.
- Trim toenails straight across. An order is needed to trim the toenails of patients with diabetes or peripheral vascular disease.
- To provide eye care, wipe from the inner to the outer part of the eye using a different portion of the washcloth for each eye.

Additional Learning Resources

SG Go to your Study Guide for additional learning activities to help you master this chapter content.

evolve Go to your Evolve website at http://evolve.elsevier.com/Williams/fundamental for additional online resources.

- Animations
- Answer Guidelines for Think Critically boxes and Critical Thinking Questions and Activities
- Answers and Rationales for Review Questions for the NCLEX Examination
- Glossary with pronunciations in English and Spanish
- Interactive Review Questions for the NCLEX Examination and more!

Review Questions for the NCLEX Examination

*Choose the **best** answer for each question.*

1. Which patient is at greatest risk for developing a pressure injury?
   1. A 40-year-old paraplegic man who is obese and uses a self-propelling wheelchair
   2. An 80-year-old woman with Alzheimer disease, peripheral neuropathy, and urinary incontinence
   3. A 55-year-old man who had surgery this afternoon and is difficult to arouse
   4. A 75-year-old woman who is postoperative day 2 for hip replacement surgery

2. A factor in skin problems common to older adults is: *(Select all that apply.)*
   1. Skin tends to be dry because of increased gland activity.
   2. Hair becomes thicker and grows more slowly.
   3. Nails become thin and more brittle.
   4. Fewer nutrients are available from the reduced diet.
   5. Skin is less elastic and more fragile.
3. Your patient has an area at the left trochanter that is reddened with slightly abraded skin. You would stage this as a __________ pressure injury.
   1. Stage 1 Pressure Injury
   2. Stage 2 Pressure Injury
   3. Stage 3 Pressure Injury
   4. Unstageable Pressure Injury
4. The extremities are washed from distal to proximal because this:
   1. Promotes safety.
   2. Cleanses the skin better than proximal to distal does.
   3. Supplies vital skin oils.
   4. Promotes venous return to the heart.
5. The primary reason some hospitals prefer a bag bath to a traditional bed bath is:
   1. Cost savings.
   2. Time savings.
   3. Infection control.
   4. Less mess.
6. When providing foot care for the diabetic patient, you must remember to:
   1. Cut the cuticles to prevent hangnails.
   2. Never soak the feet.
   3. Check for an order before trimming the nails straight across.
   4. Check for an order before trimming the nails in a curved manner so there are not any sharp points to irritate the skin.
7. Prevention of pressure injuries is promoted by: *(Select all that apply.)*
   1. Changing the patient's position every 2 hours.
   2. Directly massaging reddened areas.
   3. Keeping the heels of the immobile patient off the bed.
   4. Using lift devices such as a trapeze bar to move patients.

Critical Thinking Activities

Read each clinical scenario and discuss the questions with your classmates.

Scenario A

While assisting a female patient during her bath, you notice that she cleanses herself by wiping from the rectum to the pubic area. You remember that she has a history of having recurrent vaginal infections. What will you do? How will you explain perineal care and proper toileting techniques to her?

Scenario B

Your postoperative patient has a history of a stroke with weakness on his left side. In the hospital, he has performed most of his hygiene care independently and states that he "likes doing things for himself." What would you tell the family of your patient when they say they always do their father's complete bath at home so that he does not get tired?

chapter 20

Patient Environment and Safety

http://evolve.elsevier.com/Williams/fundamental

Objectives

Upon completing this chapter, you should be able to do the following:

Theory

1. Discuss nursing responsibilities for environmental management.
2. Identify common noises in health care facilities and ways to minimize their effects on patients.
3. Explain the importance of neatness and order in the patient's environment.
4. Describe methods to prevent mechanical and thermal accidents and injury in health care facilities and the home.
5. Discuss the various forms of bioterrorism, safety measures to be taken, signs and symptoms of agents used, and measures to treat or contain the threat.
6. Discuss the principles for using protective devices.
7. Demonstrate knowledge of the legal implications of using protective devices.

Clinical Practice

1. Discuss how the health care facility's environment affects your patient.
2. Using correct technique, make an unoccupied and an occupied bed.
3. Explain, according to your facility's procedures, how to clean up a biohazard spill.
4. Discuss your clinical facility's response plan to a bioterrorism threat.
5. Given an emergency scenario, practice triaging the victims.
6. Correctly apply an extremity immobilizer.

Skills

Key Terms

acute radiation sickness (ARS) (p. 333)
alarm fatigue (p. 330)
biohazard (bī-ō-hă-zărd, p. 332)
bioterrorism (p. 333)
environment (ĕn-VĪ-rŏn-mĕnt, p. 321)
humidity (hū-MĬ-dĭ-tē, p. 322)
poison (p. 335)
ventilation (p. 322)

Concepts Covered in This Chapter

- Communication
- Infection
- Pain
- Patient education
- Safety
- Sensory perception
- Thermoregulation

The **environment** is the total of all elements and conditions that surround us and influence our development. Caring for the patient's environment is important in providing holistic care. The goal is to ensure safety while making the patient as comfortable as possible. This chapter presents information on the factors that are controllable by the nurse in keeping a patient's environment safe. Additionally this chapter demonstrates nursing skills such as proper bed making, and when and how to apply a protective device.

FACTORS AFFECTING THE ENVIRONMENT

The same environmental factors Florence Nightingale wrote about more than a century and a half ago are still important today. Temperature, ventilation, humidity, lighting, odor, and noise all are factors that must be controlled.

TEMPERATURE

Infants and older adults may need their rooms warmer than other patients do because of their poor thermoregulation. Keep room temperature between 68°F and 74°F (20°C and 23°C). Operating rooms and critical care areas are kept slightly cooler to reduce the patient's metabolic demands.

VENTILATION

Ventilation is the process or act of supplying a building or room continuously with fresh air. Most health care facilities have central air-conditioning units that regulate temperature, humidity, and air exchange. Most hospital windows cannot be opened for safety reasons and are not a source of ventilation. Fans are discouraged because air currents spread microorganisms. A table fan may be ordered if the patient has a respiratory condition because the patient may find it easier to breathe when air movement is felt; however, the nurse should be vigilant of ensuring the fan has an appropriate blade protection screen. At home, windows may be opened at the top and bottom to encourage air circulation. For some patients (those with transmittable respiratory diseases or burns), a negative-airflow room (maintaining airflow into the room) might be indicated; for other patients a positive-airflow room (maintaining airflow out of the room) might be needed.

HUMIDITY

Humidity is the amount of moisture in the air. A range from 30% to 50% is normally comfortable. Very low humidity dries skin and respiratory passages. Most hospitals maintain a low humidity setting to discourage the growth of microorganisms. Vaporizers or humidifiers may be ordered for a patient with a respiratory condition who requires more humidity.

LIGHTING

A sunny, cheerful room can improve a patient's spirits. Areas must have adequate lighting for tasks and to prevent accidents and injury. The light should be bright enough to see without glare and to avoid eyestrain, and be soft and diffuse to prevent sharp shadows. Ideally, your patient will be able to control the lights independently. Appropriate interior and exterior lighting in the home helps protect against crime.

Clinical Cues

At night when the patient is sleeping, use a flashlight to provide low diffuse light to check the patient without disturbing her. Use a flashlight to check fluid levels in drainage containers, the amount of intravenous fluid remaining, and other data.

ODOR CONTROL

Illness changes sensory perceptions. Odors that ordinarily are pleasant may make the patient feel nauseated. Health care facilities may have unpleasant odors from bedpans, urinals, wounds, and other sources. Good ventilation and cleanliness will effectively control odors. Box 20.1 lists odor control measures.

NOISE CONTROL

Noise is inevitable in health care facilities. The hospital should be a place for rest and quiet, yet a patient may experience sensory overload from all of the noise. Noise disturbs patient sleep, may increase blood pressure, and interfere with healing. Noise is the top complaint in patient satisfaction surveys, and Medicare bases reimbursement partially on patient satisfaction survey results (Landro, 2013).

Clinical Cues

If not contraindicated, the patient who is disturbed by noise during sleep might try using foam earplugs to mask the noise. They will not prevent a patient from hearing a fire alarm and can be helpful for a restful night's sleep.

Equipment being moved in the halls, visitors, and health care personnel all combine to raise the sound level. Sound-absorbing flooring and ceiling materials, carpeting, and plastic equipment are used to reduce noise. The main cause of noise is people. To reduce noise, avoid long conversations on the intercom by going to the patient's room to talk. Encourage staff to limit conversations in the hallway and to speak in lowered voices. Tact is important when dealing with patients, their visitors, and colleagues. Soft, pleasant background music may be played to mask other sounds and promote relaxation. Some hospitals employ professional musicians, often harpists, to play soft music and promote a calm environment.

Box 20.1 Odor Control

- Reduce offensive odors by emptying and rinsing the bedpan, bedside commode, urinal, and emesis basin promptly. Change soiled linens as soon as possible.
- Dispose of used dressings, catheters, urine bags, tubing, intravenous bags, and other disposable equipment by placing in a closed plastic bag according to Standard Precautions guidelines and facility procedure. Dispose of them in the dirty or soiled utility room. **Do not dispose of anything that could become odorous in the patient's unit trash can.**
- Avoid being the source of odors yourself. Odors that linger include cigarette smoke; strong foods, such as onions, garlic, or curry; and perspiration or body odors. Eliminate these by bathing, using unscented deodorant, wearing clean clothes, and performing oral hygiene after food or coffee breaks. **Perfumes, scented lotions, or scented cosmetics should not be worn in a patient care setting.**
- Remove old, disintegrating flowers and stagnant water promptly.
- Consult with your patient before using a room deodorizer or spray. These items can help control lingering odors, but your patient may be allergic or sensitive to the deodorizer itself. You might offend the patient if you spray a deodorizer throughout the room without asking permission first.

Think Critically

Your patient's roommate has the television on very loud and your patient is unable to get any rest. What would you do to help your patient?

INTERIOR DESIGN

Patients' rooms and public areas often look more like a hotel now as opposed to the stark white of the past (Fig. 20.1). Rooms are tastefully decorated. The goal is to provide a homelike environment for the patient.

NEATNESS

It is important to provide a neat, tidy atmosphere for your patient. Keep the unit in enough order to be safe, but not so rigid that the patient may not have possessions from home. **Straighten the patient unit after making the bed. Remove old dishes and unused equipment promptly.** Clear and wipe the over-the-bed table before serving meals. Obtain the patient's permission before disposing of newspapers or magazines. Check and straighten the unit each time you enter and as time permits. Be mindful of area rugs and inform patients of this potential fall hazard.

PRIVACY

Privacy is essential for a patient's well-being. Always knock gently and identify yourself before entering the room. In multiple-patient rooms, close the curtain around the patient for personal tasks such as using a bedpan and bathing. Post a sign on the door informing others of such tasks to discourage them from entering the room.

PATIENT UNIT

Each acute care patient unit contains a bed, bedside cabinet, over-the-bed table, chair, call light, and closet. The unit usually has an over-the-bed light and a television and/or radio. Newer patient rooms may have Internet access or movies on demand. Long-term care units are more homelike with dressers, photographs, and mementos.

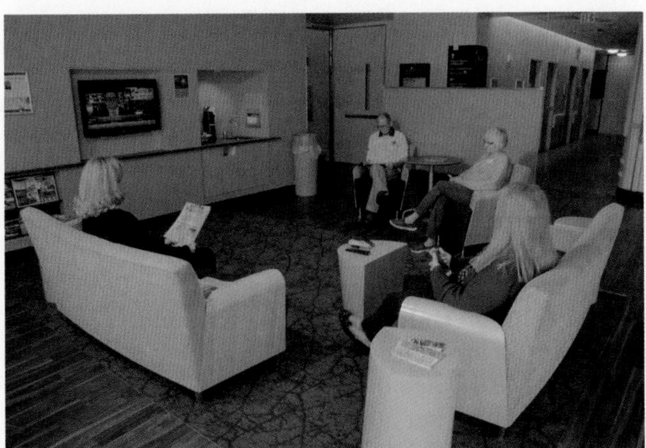

FIGURE 20.1 Common areas in the hospital environment often resemble a hotel lobby.

BEDS

A health care facility mattress is usually firm and has a covering that can be cleansed easily between patients. An overlay (air or gel filled) may be used with a mattress to reduce the risk of pressure injuries, but newer mattresses are designed to reduce pressure areas. Beds used for health care are usually on wheels and equipped with side rails. The patient may use the rails to change position or to get out of bed. Specialty beds such as low bed frames (closer to the floor) may be used for someone who is at risk for falling.

 QSEN Considerations: Safety

Memory Jogger

Side rails can be a safety hazard and are considered restraints by the Health Care Financing Administration because they restrict movement (US Food and Drug Administration, 2014).

You need to make certain that the mattress fits snugly to the rails and that the rails are close enough together so that the patient's head is not able to fit through them. **Always check to be certain the bed wheels are locked, unless you are moving the bed.**

BED POSITIONS

Most hospitals have electric beds, with controls on the side rails for changing the position. Other facilities use manual beds, with a crank for changing the position. The bed is usually kept in the "low position" (i.e., close to the floor). The bed can be placed in various positions (Fig. 20.2).

 Home Care Considerations

Home Bed Safety Rail

A small-handle side rail or transfer rail may be purchased for a regular bed at home. This rail is attached to a large board that is placed under the mattress. The weight of the patient and mattress secures the rail, which the patient uses to adjust position or get in or out of bed.

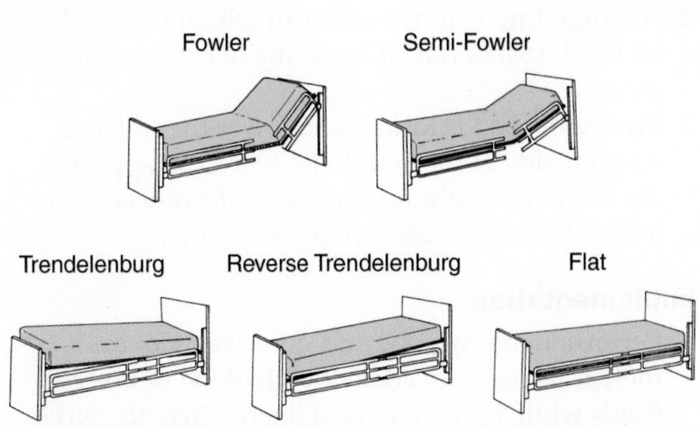

FIGURE 20.2 Hospital beds can be adjusted to different positions. (From Potter, P.A., Perry, G.A. [2009]. *Fundamentals of Nursing* [7th ed.]. St. Louis: Mosby.)

BED MAKING

Bed rest may be an important part of the treatment for your patient. Most patients may be out of bed for short periods as they recover. An unoccupied bed is made when the patient is out of bed in the chair or out of the room for a diagnostic procedure or therapy. **An occupied bed is made only if the patient absolutely cannot be out of bed.** For example, a patient whose activity order is bed rest with bathroom privileges would have the bed made while using the bathroom. Skills 20.1 and 20.2 describe how to make an unoccupied and an occupied bed, respectively. Bed linens should be neat, orderly, and wrinkle-free. Linens that are rumpled may interfere with movement, place pressure on vulnerable skin areas, or cause the patient to fall when getting out of bed. Some important guidelines for making any bed are listed in Box 20.2.

Skill 20.1 Making an Unoccupied Bed

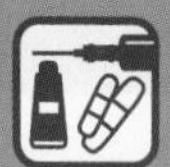
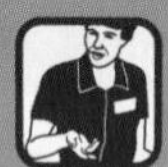

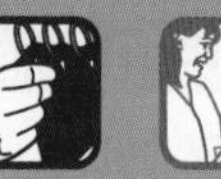
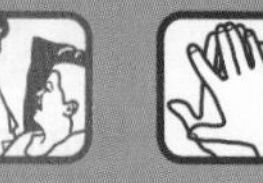

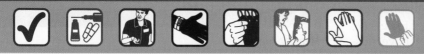

Most beds are made when they are unoccupied. Many patients may be out of bed for the length of time it takes to make the bed. If the patient is allowed out of bed, make the bed at that time to reduce the work for both you and the patient.

Supplies

- Straight or fitted bottom sheet
- Waterproof underpad (if needed)
- Drawsheet or lift sheet (if needed)
- Top sheet
- Pillows (one or more)
- Linen bag or hamper
- Bedspread and/or blanket
- Pillowcases (one or more)

Review and carry out the Standard Steps in Appendix A.

ACTION *(RATIONALE)*

Assessment (Data Collection)

1. Check patient's orders and ability to be out of bed. Obtain help if necessary. *(Promotes safety for you and patient.)*

Planning

2. Arrange linens in the order in which they will be used. *(Saves time if linens are in correct order for use.)*
3. Ensure the bed is locked and lower the side rail on your side of the bed. Raise bed to an appropriate working height for you. *(Provides easy access to materials. Prevents back strain and injury.)*

Implementation

4. Perform hand hygiene and don clean gloves if there is a chance of contact with blood or body fluids while removing used linen. *(Prevents spread of microorganisms.)*
5. Loosen all linens on one side of the bed. Go to other side, lower that rail, and loosen the linens from the head to the foot of the bed. Fold bedspread if not soiled; place over the back of patient's chair. Remove sheets and pillowcases, removing each separately. Place pillows on a clean surface, roll linens together, and put them in the pillowcase, linen hamper, or bag. Avoid shaking or fanning the linens. Do not place sheets on the floor. *(Loosening permits linens to be removed easily; bedspread and pillows are ready to be replaced. If no linen hamper or bag is available, place the soiled linen in the pillowcase. Place on the foot of the bed or over-the-bed table to prevent spread of microorganisms.)*

Make the Bed on One Side

6. Check the mattress. Clean if soiled. Move mattress to the head of the bed if needed by grasping it in the center and at the bottom edge while facing the head of the bed, and slide it up. *(Mattress is cleaned before making the bed. Mattresses tend to move to the foot of the bed when the head of the bed is raised.)*
7. Make the bed on one side at a time. Place all center folds in the linens at the center of the bed. *(Decreases the number of steps for the nurse. Centering linens puts the same amount of sheet on both sides of the bed.)*
8. Place and center the bottom sheet on the mattress. Unfold the sheet right side out so that the wide hem end is at the top of the mattress and the narrow hem end is at the foot of the bed. Tuck about 12 inches of the sheet smoothly over the top of the mattress. If a fitted sheet is used, fit the top and bottom corners of the mattress into it on your side. *(Secures sheet snugly to the head of the bed and evenly distributes linens.)*
9. Miter the corner at the head of the bed by picking up the side edge of the sheet so that it forms

a triangle with the head of the bed, with the side edge perpendicular to the bed. Using the palm of your hand, hold the sheet against the side of the mattress and tuck excess under mattress. Drop the sheet over your hand; then withdraw your hand and tuck the flap of the sheet under the mattress. *(Holds the corners in place.)*

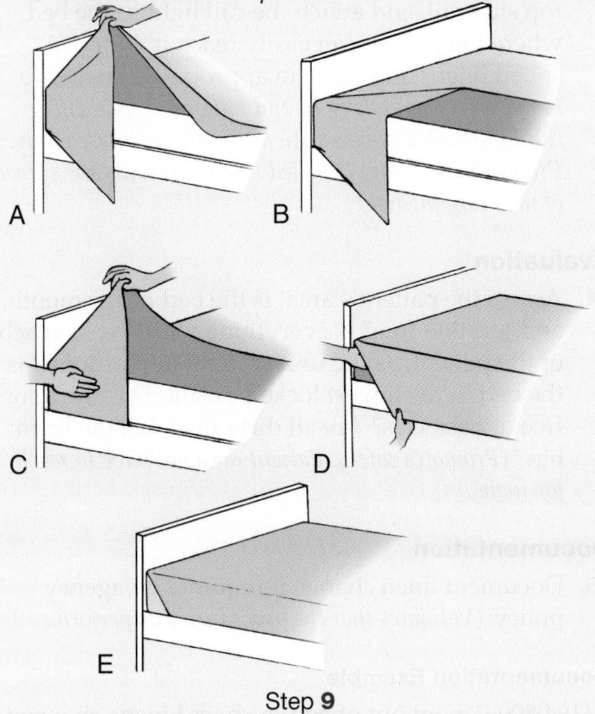

Step **9**

10. Position the drawsheet or lift sheet (if used) over the middle of the bed. Unfold and tuck both sheets in, on this side, from head to foot. If a lift sheet is used, do not tuck it under the mattress. *(Protects the bottom linens from soiling by placing the drawsheet from the patient's shoulders to below the hips. A lift sheet aids in repositioning the patient.)*
11. Place upper edge of the top sheet at the top of the mattress, seam (bottom) side up, and unfold it toward the foot of the bed. *(Placing top sheet seam side up avoids irritation from the seam when a cuff is formed over the bedspread.)*
12. Position the blanket or bedspread 4 inches from the top of the mattress and unfold it toward the foot. Repeat for extra blankets. *(Allows sheet to be cuffed over top covers.)*
13. Tuck the sheet, blankets, and bedspread under the bottom of the mattress as one unit if a toe pleat is not needed. Miter the corner by lifting the top linens away from the mattress and up onto the bed about 18 inches from the bottom of the bed. A triangle should be formed. Tuck excess linens hanging below mattress level under it, bring down the upper portion of the linens, and smooth them into a neat diagonal line. *(Secures linens under the mattress. Top covers are not tucked under down the sides of the mattress to allow the patient to get in and out of bed easily.)*

Make the Bed on the Other Side

14. Fanfold the top linen back toward the center of the bed while tucking in the bottom sheet and drawsheet. Miter the corner. *(Folding top linen back allows you to see any wrinkles and remedy them. Mitering holds the bottom sheet in place.)*
15. Grasp the edges of the bottom sheet tightly in both hands with the knuckles on top. Pull tightly down over the side; tuck under the mattress along the side, working down the side from head to foot. Pull sheet diagonally at the bottom corner of the mattress to remove wrinkles. *(Provides a smooth bottom sheet without wrinkles that may cause pressure areas.)*

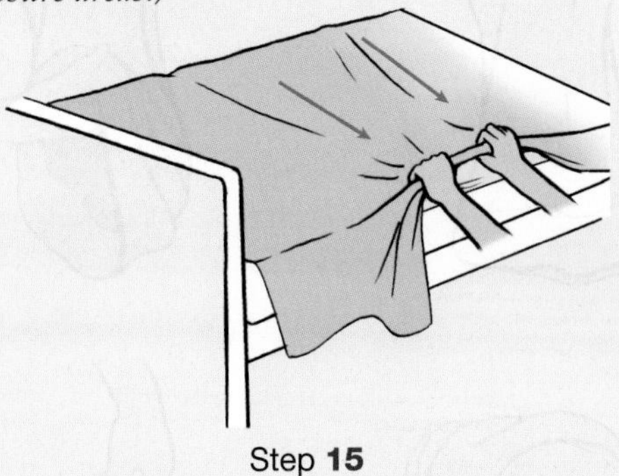

Step **15**

16. Grasp the drawsheet (if used); pull tightly and tuck it in over the side of the mattress. If this is to be used as a lift sheet, do not tuck it under the mattress. *(Saves time because a lift sheet is used often.)*
17. Smooth top linens from the head to the foot of the bed if a toe pleat is not needed. Fold sheet, blanket, and bedspread under the mattress at the foot of the bed as one unit. Miter the corner of the top linens. *(Provides patient with a wrinkle-free bed.)*
18. Make toe pleats as indicated. The following are two examples of toe pleats:
    a. At the center of the top linens, at the foot of the bed, make a 6-inch lengthwise pleat in the top linens before tucking the covers under the mattress.
    b. Fold a 2-inch horizontal pleat, 6 to 8 inches from the foot of the bed, across the top linens before tucking the covers under the mattress. *(Allows room for the patient's feet to move and prevents formation of pressure injuries from the weight of the linens on the toes.)*
19. Move to the head of the bed and fold back the top sheet, forming a cuff 4 to 6 inches over the edge of the blanket and bedspread. *(Provides a smooth edge under patient's chin and prevents soiling of blanket and bedspread.)*

20. Apply the pillowcase by grasping the closed end of the pillowcase and, with the other hand, gathering one side of the open pillowcase up over the hand at the closed end. Grasp the pillow at the center of one end through the pillowcase while holding the pillow away from your body. With the other hand, grasp the open edge of the pillowcase and pull it down over the pillow. Do this until the pillow is completely covered. Adjust the pillow inside the case, keeping it from being contaminated by contact with your uniform. *(Places pillow smoothly in the case without contaminating it.)*

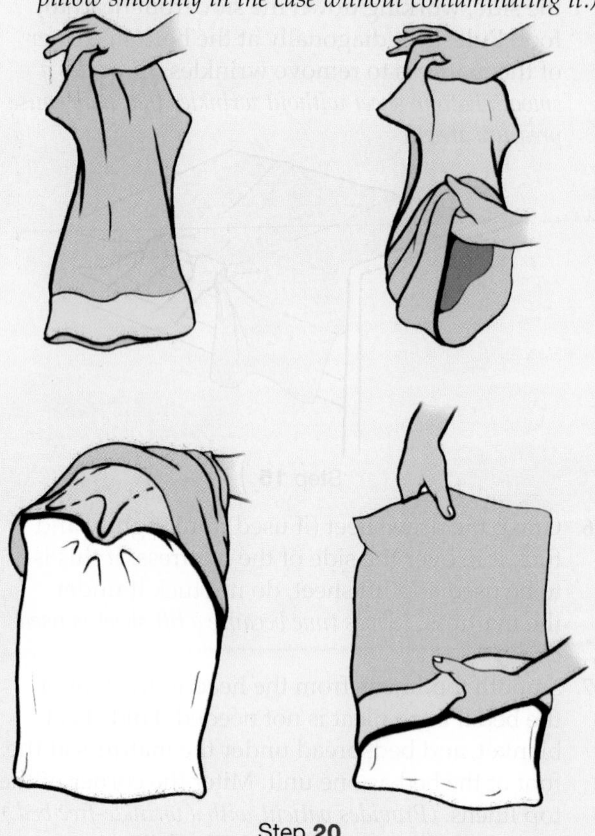

Step 20

21. Place the pillow(s) at the head of the bed with the open ends away from the door. *(Fitting the pillowcase evenly over the pillow with the corners at the correct locations provides a neater appearance.)*
22. Follow agency policy, or open the bed by folding the top linens back. *(Allows patient to enter the bed easily.)*
23. Place the bed in its lowest position, raise the far, top side rail, and attach the call light to the bed where the patient can easily reach it. Remove soiled linens and place in appropriate area. *(Promotes safety in getting in and out of bed. Attaching call light to bed allows patient to call the nurse easily. Promptly disposing of soiled linens prevents the spread of microorganisms.)*

Evaluation

24. Assess the patient's area. Is the bed neat, smooth, and wrinkle-free? Is everything within easy reach of the patient? Is the unit straight and orderly? Is the bed in the lowest locked position? Is the floor free of obstacles? Are all dirty linens in the linen bin? *(Promotes safety. Patient does not have to reach for items.)*

Documentation

25. Document linen change if required by agency policy. *(Validates that the procedure was performed.)*

Documentation Example

4/19 0800 Patient out of bed in chair. Linens changed, bed locked and in low position, call light within reach. (Nurse's electronic signature)

? Critical Thinking Questions

1. Why is it inadvisable to gather and deliver linen needed for two or three rooms at the beginning of the shift?
2. Why is it a good idea to pull the old linens apart and separate them if they are bunched up, before rolling them together to take off the bed and put into the linen hamper?

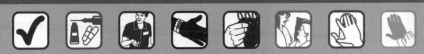

Skill 20.2 Making an Occupied Bed

 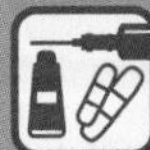 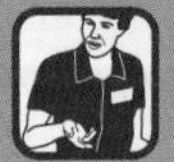 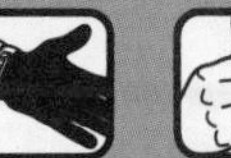 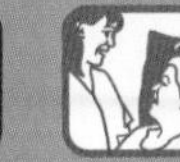 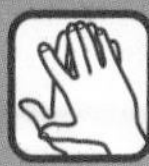 

Linens are changed with the patient in bed if bed rest has been ordered. The procedure is easier and quicker when carried out by two people. Nursing research has shown that many patients experience greater benefit from getting out of bed than remaining on total bed rest. Hence, fewer beds are now made as occupied beds.

Supplies

- Bath blanket
- Bath supplies (if combining with a bed bath)
- Linens (as listed in Skill 20.1)

Review and carry out the Standard Steps in Appendix A.

ACTION *(RATIONALE)*

Assessment (Data Collection)

1. Check patient's orders to ensure patient is not allowed out of bed. Obtain help if necessary. *(Ensures medical plan will be followed. Promotes safety.)*

Planning

2. Arrange linens in the order in which they will be used. *(Saves time.)*
3. Ensure bed is locked and lower the side rail on your side. The other rail should be raised. Raise bed to an appropriate working height. *(Prevents back strain and injury.)*

Implementation

4. Perform hand hygiene and don clean gloves if there is a chance of contact with blood or body fluids during procedure. *(Prevents spread of microorganisms.)*
5. Loosen the blanket and bedspread from the foot of the bed and remove each piece separately. If unsoiled, fold and place item over the back of patient's chair. Place any soiled linens in the soiled linen or hamper bag. *(Placing unsoiled items over the chair back saves time by readying linens to be replaced.)*
6. Place a bath blanket over the patient and the top sheet, unfold it, and ask the patient to hold the top or tuck under the patient's shoulders. Remove the top sheet from beneath the bath blanket, and place in linen hamper or bag. *(Provides warmth and privacy.)*
7. Move the mattress to the head of the bed. Patient may help by grasping the headboard and pulling if able, or have another staff member help you. *(Allows more room for the feet at the end of the bed.)*
8. Move patient into a side-lying position at the far side of the bed, facing away from you. Assist patient into proper alignment. Place a pillow under the head and at the patient's back to keep patient in place if necessary. *(Provides safety. Allows near side of bed to be made.)*
9. Loosen the bottom linens from the top and side of the bed; roll each piece of linen as close to the patient as possible.
   a. Smooth the mattress cover (if present), and put the bottom sheet on the bed with the center fold at the center of the mattress. Fanfold the portion of the sheet that is for the other side of the bed with the centerfold at the center of the mattress.
   b. Push the folded linen under the rolled, soiled bottom sheets that are being removed. Tuck the near side of the bottom sheet under the head of the mattress, and miter the corner. Tuck the sheet under the mattress from the head to the foot of the bed. *(Allows soiled linens to be removed and clean linens to be placed when patient rolls to the other side of the bed.)*

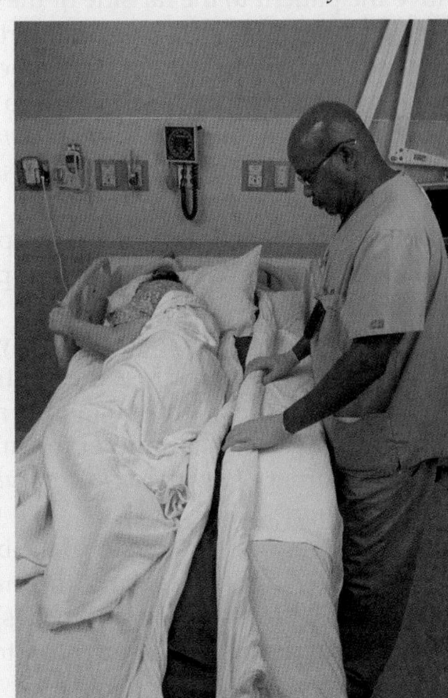

Step 9a

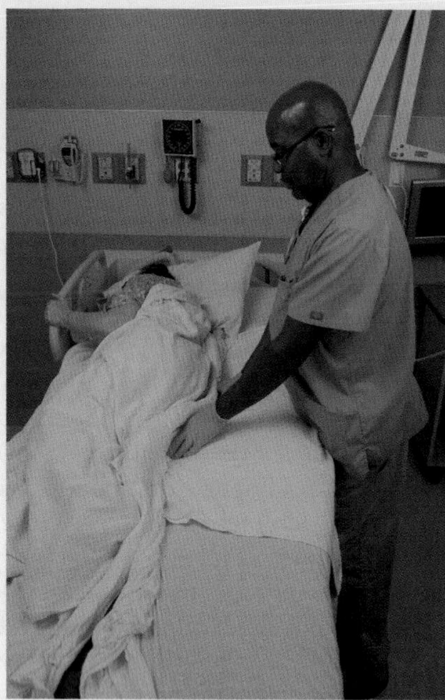
Step 9b

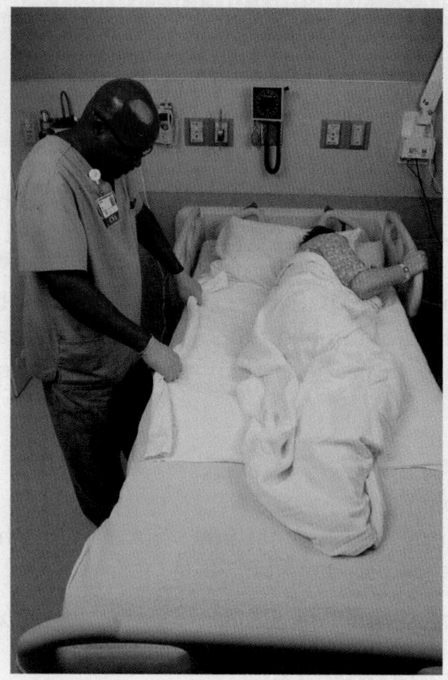
Step 14

10. Place drawsheet on the bed (optional), centering it on the mattress so that it reaches from the patient's shoulders to below the hips. Fanfold the far side of the sheet, and push it under the rolled bottom sheets. Tuck the near side under the mattress. Raise the side rail. *(Allows removal of a soiled drawsheet when the patient is turned.)*
11. Go to the other side of the bed, lower that rail, and move the patient to the far side of the bed. If the patient can turn easily, ask patient to roll to the opposite side. Adjust patient's alignment, and reposition the bath blanket. Ask patient to grab the raised side rail for support. *(Allows removal of soiled linens and placement of clean linens. Raised rail provides safety.)*
12. Loosen the bottom linens and roll them up. Place in the linen hamper or bag or in the used pillowcase. *(Prevents spread of microorganisms.)*
13. If a mattress cover is used, smooth out any wrinkles. Pull the bottom sheet across the mattress, fold over the top of the mattress, smooth, and tighten. Tuck the excess sheet under the mattress and miter the corner. *(Prevents wrinkles that may cause pressure injuries.)*
14. Pull the drawsheet from the center of the bed; to pull tightly, place your knee against the mattress while pulling. Tighten, smooth, and tuck sheets under the side of the mattress from head to foot. *(Protects the bottom sheet from soiling.)*
15. Allow the patient to roll onto back. Place the top sheet over the patient and the bath blanket with the top edge folded down a few inches beneath the chin. Have the patient hold the top of the sheet and remove the bath blanket. Position the blanket (if used) and bedspread in the same manner. Smooth top linens and tuck the excess at the foot under the bottom of the mattress if a toe pleat is not needed. Miter the corner on the near side and then miter the far side. Fold the top edge of the sheet over the blanket, and bedspread to form a cuff. *(Keeps the patient warm and protects privacy while the top linens are placed.)*
16. Make a toe pleat in the top sheet and blanket if desired as described in Skill 20.1, Step 18. *(Provides extra room for the feet.)*
17. Remove the used pillowcase and place in the linen hamper or bag. Apply the clean pillowcase by grasping the closed end of the case in one hand and gathering one side from the open end up over the other hand. Grasp the pillow at the center of one end through the pillowcase while holding the pillow away from your body. Smooth the pillowcase down over the pillow. Place beneath the patient's head with the open end away from the door. *(Places the pillow in the case without contaminating it. Fitting the pillowcase evenly over the pillow with the corners at the correct locations provides a neater appearance.)*
18. Lower the bed, replace call light, and restore the unit. Remove the linen hamper or bag and place in appropriate area. *(Provides safety for patient and a method to call the nurse. Promptly disposing of soiled linens helps prevent spread of microorganisms.)*

Evaluation

19. Assess patient's area. Are the linens neat, smooth, and wrinkle-free? Is the unit restored? *(Restoring the unit promotes safety because the patient does not have to reach for items and it includes ensuring the area is the free of obstacles and all dirty linens are in the linen bin.)*

Documentation

20. Document linen change on the flow sheet or in the nurse's notes, depending on agency policy. *(Validates completion of the procedure.)*

Documentation Example

10/15 0900 Linens changed on occupied bed, which is in locked, low position. (Nurse's electronic signature)

Special Considerations

- If the patient is in traction, the bed may have to be made from the top to the bottom (head of bed to foot of bed), instead of side to side. The same principles are applied from top to bottom. The patient may use the trapeze bar if able to help lift as you work the sheets down the bed.
- Linens should be smoothed, with wrinkles removed, whenever the patient is turned.

Home Care Considerations

- For the home care patient, a large plastic bag can be used crosswise under the hip area to protect the mattress from soiling. It is placed beneath the mattress pad to prevent any discomfort to the patient.

Critical Thinking Questions

1. For work efficiency, is it better to work with a colleague, helping him make occupied beds and then having him help you, or to make your occupied beds on your own?
2. When a patient is to be on bed rest, how can you sometimes make the bed when she is not in it?

Box 20.2 Guidelines for Bed Making

- Use good body alignment, a wide base of support, and a proper working height when making the bed. Face the direction of movement and bend at the knees, not the waist.
- Complete the linen change on one side before moving to the other side to save time and conserve energy.
- Avoid contaminating clean linen. Once linens enter a unit, they are exposed to that patient's microorganisms and must not be returned to the clean supply or used elsewhere.
- Unfold linens onto the bed. Do not flip or fan linens, to avoid stirring up air currents. Microorganisms travel on air currents and could be carried out of the unit.
- Remove linens one piece at a time to avoid wrapping dentures, eyeglasses, religious objects, or other patient belongings in soiled linens.
- Do not place used or soiled linen from one patient on the bed, table, or chairs belonging to another patient's unit.
- Carry used or soiled linens away from the body and place them in closed linen hampers or bags. Use a pillowcase if a linen bag is not available, and transport it to the linen hamper or chute. **Do not place soiled linens on the floor.**

QSEN Considerations: Safety

Memory Jogger

Safety is a primary concern when caring for your patients. Safety is needed to prevent accidents and possible injuries to patients, visitors, and health care personnel.

SAFETY

Methods of meeting the following 2016 National Patient Safety Goals from The Joint Commission are presented in the appropriate chapters of this text.

Acute care:

- Identify patients correctly.
- Improve staff communication.
- Use medicines safely.
- Use alarms safely.
- Prevent infections.
- Identify patient safety risks.
- Prevent mistakes in surgery.

Long-term care:

- Identify residents correctly.
- Use medicines safely.
- Prevent infection.
- Prevent residents from falling.
- Prevent bed sores.

The most common accidents among patients are falls, burns, cuts, and bruises. Fights with others, loss of personal possessions, choking, and electrical shock may also occur. Home safety is another issue you need to discuss with your patients. You must be aware of possible safety hazards and correct them to prevent accidents. Box 20.3 describes nursing actions to promote patient safety.

HAZARDS

Falls

Falls are a safety hazard. The three most common factors that predispose a person to falls are impaired physical mobility, altered mental status, and sensory and/or motor deficits. All patients and their

Box 20.3 Nursing Actions to Promote Patient Safety

IN A HEALTH CARE FACILITY

- Orient the patient and family when admitted to the room with regard to hospital procedures and operation of the call bell system, bed, restroom, television, and radio. Verify that the patient can operate the controls.
- On admission, assess the patient's gait and risk for falling. If the patient is considered to be at risk for falls, implement your facility's fall risk prevention program.
- Evaluate the patient's drug regimen for side effects that may increase the risk of falling (e.g., those that affect the central nervous system or cause orthostatic hypotension, dizziness, or drowsiness).
- Keep the bed in the low position if not giving direct care.
- Put the mattress onto the floor or a low platform if there is a high risk for a fall and the patient does not ask for help when getting out of bed.
- **Toilet the patient on a regular schedule to decrease the chance that the patient will try to get out of bed unassisted.**
- Lock the bed wheels to prevent the bed from rolling when the patient attempts to get in or out.
- Provide a night-light to aid patients in going to the bathroom at night, to decrease disorientation, and to prevent bumping into furniture.
- Encourage the use of firm, nonskid slippers to prevent slipping while walking.
- Answer call lights quickly so that the patient learns to trust you and does not feel the need to get up without help.
- Tell the patient when you will next check in, and be prompt.
- Be certain the patient is comfortable and all desired items including the call bell are in easy reach before you leave the room.
- Encourage use of grab bars for the toilet, tub, and shower.
- Place the high-risk or restless patient in a room close to the nurses' station so you can check on the patient often.
- Stay with the patient who is confused, agitated, or unsteady whenever the patient is up.
- Restrict fluids after 6 pm if a patient is up at night frequently to empty the bladder and has a history of injury when out of bed.
- Provide appropriate diversionary and social activities for confused and restless patients. Seating patients confined to a wheelchair close to the nurses' station often provides enough stimulation to occupy their thoughts and reduce their need to wander.
- Be certain wheelchair brakes are locked before transferring a patient into or out of it.
- Perform change-of-shift safety checks of the unit.

IN THE HOME

- Place a nonskid bath mat in the tub and shower.
- Use night-lights for moving from the bedroom to the bathroom at night.
- Suggest the installation of grab bars for the bathroom by both the toilet and bathtub or shower.
- Install door buzzers or bed alarms that sound when the patient leaves the bed or opens an outside door.
- Keep the furniture arrangement and position of personal items constant to decrease confusion and eliminate the need to search for items.
- Maintain sufficient activity during the day to prevent too much napping, which can lead to nighttime wandering.
- Encourage removal of extension cords as they may cause a fall.
- Caution the patient that items on the floor and animals may cause falls. Removing a companion animal from the home because of the risk of a fall must be carefully weighed against the social and emotional importance of a pet's companionship.
- Inform the patient and the family that hospital beds may be obtained or rented for home use. Provide appropriate community resources as indicated.

environment must be assessed and periodically reassessed for the risk for falling. An evaluation of the patient's medications should be included in this assessment as they are correlated with an increased risk for falls. Patient's rooms should be clear of floor clutter including spills, clutter, and area rugs. Action must be taken to mitigate identified risks. An example of a fall risk assessment tool is presented in Fig. 20.3. Chapter 40 provides safety tips to prevent the older adult from falling in the home. In most facilities, a patient at risk for falls is given a color-coded wrist or leg band to alert the staff of this increased risk. Assistive devices, hip protectors (Fig. 20.4), and personal alarms have been shown to decrease fall risk. Personal alarms sense a change in position or pressure and sound an alarm to alert caregivers that patients are attempting to get out of bed or a chair (Fig. 20.5).

These bed and chair alarms along with cardiac and oxygen sensor alarms are among the alarms specified in the 2016 National Patient Safety Goal of improving the safety of medical alarms. All medical equipment alarms need to be closely monitored and checked for functionality and volume at the start of the shift and frequently throughout the shift. Steps need to be taken to prevent the catastrophic outcomes of **alarm fatigue** (Box 20.4). Alarm fatigue occurs when nurses become desensitized to patient care alarms and then miss or delay response to an alarm. These absent or delayed responses have resulted in adverse patient outcomes (Sendelback & Funk, 2013).

Life-Span Considerations

Older Adult

Falls are the most frequent cause of injury for the older adult in an acute care facility.

Fall Risk Assessment

Place a check mark in front of the items that apply to the patient.

General Information
____ Age over 70
____ History of falls*
____ Confusion at times
____ Confused most of the time*
____ Impaired memory or judgment
____ Unable to follow directions*
____ Needs assistance with elimination
____ Visual impairment
____ Feels physically weak*

Medications
____ Receiving central nervous system suppressants (narcotic, sedative, tranquilizer, hypnotic, antidepressant, psychotropic, anticonvulsant)
____ Receiving medication that causes orthostatic hypotension (antihypertensive, diuretic)*
____ Medication that may cause diarrhea (cathartic)
____ Medication that may alter blood glucose levels (insulin, hypoglycemics)

Gait and Balance
____ Poor balance when standing*
____ Balance problems when walking*
____ Swaying, lurching, or slapping gait*
____ Unstable when making turns*
____ Needs assistive device (walker, cane, holds on to furniture)*

Note: A check mark on any starred item indicates a risk for falls. A combination of four or more of the unstarred items indicates a risk for falls.

FIGURE 20.3 Fall risk assessment tool.

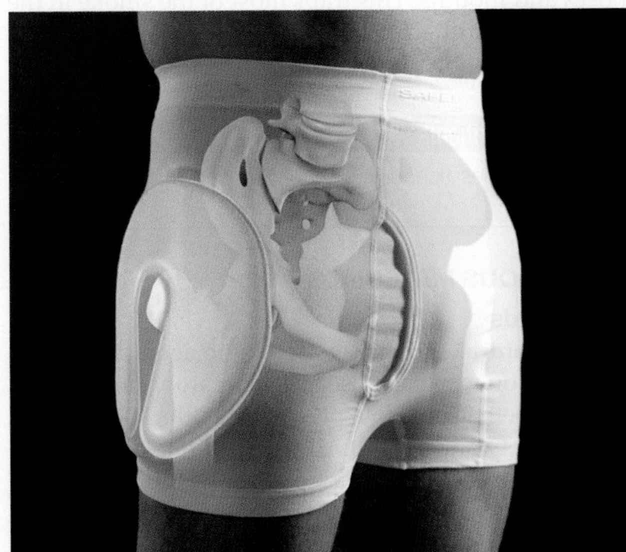

FIGURE 20.4 Hip protectors disperse the force of a fall to soft tissues, decreasing the risk of hip fracture. (Courtesy HIProtector, www.HipProtector.com)

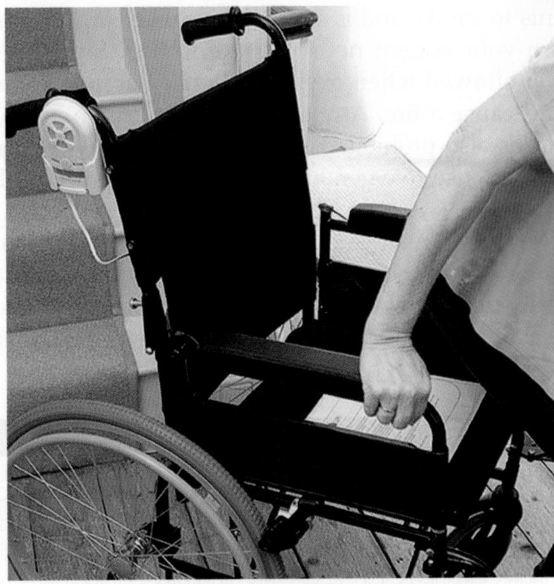

FIGURE 20.5 Wheelchair alarm.

Box 20.4 Bed or Chair Alarm Safety Guidelines

- Educate staff regarding the effects of delayed response to alarms.
- Check on patients regularly and implement bedside handoffs.
- Educate the patient and family regarding the purpose of the alarm and use of call light.
- Reevaluate the need for a bed alarm every shift.
- Attach a bed alarm to the call light system.
- Use alarms that turn off automatically when the patient stops attempting to get out of bed.

Data from Daniels, K. (2014). Fighting bed alarm fatigue in orthopedic units. *Nursing*, 44(9), 66-67.

Burns

Burn prevention includes protecting the patient from accidental thermal injury and the threat of fire. Thermal injuries may be caused by either hot or cold materials. A person who has diabetes, impaired circulation, or paralysis or who is taking medications that alter mental awareness is more easily burned than a healthy person is. To prevent these injuries, use a barrier between the patient's skin and the thermal application. Check the temperature of oral liquids before giving them to the patient. Warn the patient if a food or drink is hot. Caution the patient to avoid lying on, or sleeping with, heating pads or ice packs. Inspect electrical cords for frayed or broken areas that may cause sparks or fires. The engineering staff must check all electrical appliances brought from home into the hospital before use to ensure safety.

Smoking

Smoking is banned in most health care facilities; however, some long-term care agencies allow smoking in designated areas. Carefully supervise the patient who wants to smoke and is sedated, confused, or irrational. Warn your patient not to smoke in bed. **Smoking is never allowed when oxygen is in use because a spark could cause a fire.** Any equipment that might cause a spark is also prohibited near oxygen. Inform your patient who uses oxygen at home, and the family, of this risk.

We must create social and physical environments that promote good health for all. Environmental air quality free of smoke is one such environment. Encourage your patients not to smoke (Centers for Disease Control and Prevention, 2015a).

Health Promotion/Health Promotion Points

Smoking Cessation

Patients and residents of long-term care facilities who smoke should be given information on how to quit smoking. Smoking damages the lungs, blood vessels, and other vital organs and decreases the oxygen-carrying capacity of the blood. Positive reinforcement for efforts to quit smoking is very important. Many patients want to quit and would accept suggestions from nursing. Clear, consistent advice; individual or group therapy; nicotine replacement therapy; and frequent telephone contact have been shown to increase a smoking cessation program's effectiveness.

Fire

Fire is a possibility in any setting. **You must know and be familiar with your institution's fire regulations.** This includes knowing the location of the fire extinguishers, fire alarms, and escape routes, as well as notifying the telephone operator of a fire in your area.

There are three basic types of fire extinguishers: A, B, and C. Type A is a water-under-pressure extinguisher that is used for paper, wood, or cloth fires. Type B contains carbon dioxide and is used for gasoline, oil, paint, fat, and flammable liquid fires. Type C also contains carbon dioxide but is used for electrical fires. The most commonly seen extinguisher is an ABC combination extinguisher that can be used on any kind of fire.

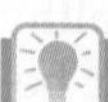

QSEN Considerations: Safety

Using a Fire Extinguisher

The acronym PASS serves as a reminder for using a fire extinguisher correctly:
Pull the pin
Aim at the base of the fire
Squeeze the trigger
Sweep side to side

Most agencies use the *RACE* acronym to respond to a fire because it is easy to remember. Should a fire occur, you must:

- **R**escue any patients in immediate danger by removing them from the area.
- **A**ctivate the fire alarm system.
- **C**ontain the fire by closing all doors and any open windows.
- **E**xtinguish the flames with an appropriate extinguisher or **E**vacuate.

Use proper body mechanics to evacuate patients to prevent injury. Protect against possible smoke inhalation by placing wet towels across the bottom of closed doors, and have people hold wet washcloths over their noses and mouths. This traps most of the smoke in the washcloth during breathing. Box 20.5 lists home fire safety precautions.

Box 20.5 Fire Safety in the Home

- Make certain that each room has two clear exits and everyone knows and has practiced using the escape routes.
- Install smoke detectors on each level of your home.
- Never smoke in bed. Use sturdy, nonspill ashtrays. Check furniture for any smoldering cigarette butts after parties.
- Identify your house with large, easily seen address numbers for the fire department.
- Keep matches, lighters, and flammable liquids out of the reach of children. Store paints, thinners, and other flammable liquids in their original containers, away from heat, sparks, or flame. **Never store gasoline or propane inside the home.**
- Never leave cooking food unattended. Keep cooking areas clear of combustible materials.
- Keep your attic free from combustibles such as magazines and newspapers.
- Have chimneys and central heating systems inspected at least once per year and cleaned if necessary.
- Never overload electrical circuits or bypass fuses or circuit breakers. Do not run extension cords under furniture or carpets or across doorways.
- Use portable space heaters with care.
- Do not allow smoking in a home where oxygen is in use.

Think Critically

Why do facilities schedule announced and unannounced fire drills?

HAZARDOUS MATERIALS

Biohazards

A **biohazard** is defined as a biologic agent, chemical, or condition (such as unsecure laboratory procedures) that can be harmful to a person's health. The Occupational Safety and Health Administration (OSHA) classifies materials in the work environment according to the degree of hazard to health that they impose. OSHA publishes specific guidelines for labeling, handling, cleaning spills, and disposing of these materials. Mercury is an example of a biohazard, as are blood and

Table 20.1 Common Diseases Spread Through Bioterrorism

BIOLOGIC AGENTS USED AS WEAPONS	SYMPTOMS	TYPICAL INCUBATION PERIOD (DAYS)
Anthrax	Fever, malaise, fatigue, dry cough, chest discomfort progressing to severe respiratory distress, and shock. Death typically 24–36 hours after onset of severe symptoms.	1–6
Botulism	Difficulty speaking and swallowing, ptosis (drooping eyelids), blurred or double vision; respiratory distress, descending muscular paralysis leading to respiratory arrest.	1–3
Ebola virus *(Filovirus)*	Abrupt onset of fever, severe headache, muscle pain, swollen lymph nodes, nausea, vomiting, diarrhea, maculopapular rash on the trunk, weakness, and progressive bleeding.	2–21
Lassa fever (arenavirus)	Fever, weakness, malaise, headache, sore throat, shock, facial swelling, profuse bleeding, chest pain, tremor, and hearing loss.	6–21
Plague	High fever, headache, chills, mucopurulent sputum, chest pain, hemoptysis, and purpura.	1–6
Ricin (cytotoxin from castor beans)	Fever, chest tightness, cough, dyspnea, nausea, and arthralgias present first. Pulmonary edema occurs within 18-24 hours. Death occurs in 36-72 hours.	4–8 hours
Smallpox	Initially, malaise, fever, vomiting, headache, and backache; 2-3 days later, chickenpox-like lesions starting on the face and extremities, with progression from macules to papules to pustular vesicles.	12
Tularemia	Fever, chills, headache, swollen lymph nodes, and nonproductive cough.	3–6

Data from U. S. Army Medical Research Institute of Infectious Diseases (2012), CDC Ebola (Ebola Virus Disease) (2015b), and World Health Organization (2015).

most body fluids. A material safety data sheet (MSDS) should be available for each biohazard substance stored or used on the nursing unit. These sheets, often available electronically on the unit, are consulted for recommended methods of storage, labeling, handling spills, and disposal. Everyone must comply with these guidelines.

Bioterrorism and Other Terrorism Agents

Terrorist activities are designed to cause panic, fear, and chaos and disrupt an area's rescue and medical systems. **Bioterrorism** is the release of pathogenic microorganisms into a community to achieve political and/or military goals. Common diseases, symptoms, and incubation periods for agents used in bioterrorism are listed in Table 20.1. It is important to know the early signs and symptoms of these agents because many of them initially manifest with vague or flulike symptoms.

Chemical terrorism is the use of certain compounds to cause destruction to achieve political and/or military goals. Health care agencies and institutions have developed plans and methods to handle these threats to safety. Chemical agents come in liquid, gas, and solid forms. Temperature and pressure can affect the form of the chemical agents. There are several types of chemical threats, including pulmonary agents, cyanide agents, nerve agents, vesicants, and incapacitating agents. Table 20.2 lists the agents used in the different kinds of chemical threats and the symptoms associated with each type.

Radiation is a form of energy that can come from manufactured sources as well as the sun and outer space. Some elements that release radiation, such as uranium, exist naturally in the soil. Plutonium, which is used in nuclear power plants, is also used to make nuclear bombs. Terrorists may use radioactive substances attached to an explosive device (a "dirty bomb") to disperse radiation. The body can be protected from radiation in three basic ways: time (decrease the amount of time near a source), distance (increase your distance from a source), and shielding (use a barrier or shield between you and the source). **Acute radiation sickness (ARS)** develops when most or all of the body is exposed to a high dose of radiation, usually over a short period. The initial symptoms of ARS are nausea, vomiting, and diarrhea. Loss of appetite, fatigue, fever, skin damage, hair loss, and potentially seizures, coma, and death are possible later effects.

You must be familiar with your institution's policies and procedures for handling victims of a terrorist attack. Knowing how to respond to terrorist attacks with various agents will help prepare you should a crisis happen in your area. Being prepared will help alleviate your anxiety and increase your confidence in dealing with such unpredictable events. In turn, this will help you manage your patients' fears and give care that is more effective.

Decontamination. When a terrorist attack has occurred, such as the one with Sarin gas in a Tokyo subway in 1995, a portable decontamination

Table 20.2 Types, Symptoms, and Effects of Chemical Weapons

TYPE	EXAMPLES	SYMPTOMS	EFFECTS
Pulmonary agents	Phosgene (CG) Diphosgene (DP) Chloropicrin (PS) Chlorine (CL)	Irritation of the eyes and tracheobronchial tree. Tears, coughing, and chest discomfort. May appear minor at first but gets worse to include dyspnea and tachypnea.	Damages alveolar-capillary membranes during inhalation. Can result in pulmonary edema.
Blood agents	Hydrogen cyanide (AC) Cyanogen chloride (CK)	Odor of bitter almonds on the breath is a classic sign but may not be detected. Severe respiratory distress in an acyanotic person. Skin coloring may be cherry red, cyanotic, or normal. Irritation of eyes, nose, and airways.	Work by being absorbed into the blood. Cyanide prevents intracellular oxygenation. Exposure to high concentrations can lead to death in 6–8 minutes. Severe exposure may result in asystole.
Nerve agents	Tabun (GA)Sarin (GB)Soman (GD)VX	Pupil constriction, red eyes, reduced vision, airway constriction, uncontrolled rhinorrhea, salivation, tearing, and sweating. Uncontrolled secretions in the gastrointestinal and respiratory tracts as well. May lead to convulsions, paralysis, and death.	Prevent the nervous system from working properly. Most toxic of the known chemical agents. Major effects seen in skeletal and smooth muscles.
Vesicants/blister agents	Sulfur mustard (H, HD) Lewisite (L) Phosgene oxime (CX)	Irritate exposed skin and membranes. Mustard is the only one that does not cause immediate symptoms, but it can cause tissue damage within several minutes without burning or redness. Typical onset for all agents is 4–8 hours.	Cause blisters or vesicles in the eyes, respiratory tract, and skin, which is how this type gets its name. Some can be deadlier than pulmonary agents or cyanide because of their immediate action and lack of effective antidotes.
Incapacitating agents	3-Quinuclidinyl Benzilate (BZ)	Range of usual onset is 30 minutes–4 hours. May see paranoia to full-blown delirium and periods of deep sleep with clawing or climbing movements. Person at risk of hyperthermia and injury from own random movements.	Designed to impair, not kill, victims through hallucinations, illusions, and nausea and vomiting. In most cases, do not cause death.

unit with a specially trained staff is set up outside the emergency department (ED). The staff must wear masks and protective clothing that are impervious to chemicals and cover *all* skin surfaces (Fig. 20.6). Military mission-oriented protective posture (MOPP) suits may be used that have a hooded pullover top, drawstring trousers, rubber boots, and gloves. A chemical mask with filtered respirator must be worn with the suit. An emergency protocol from the local health department's disaster response plan is followed to decontaminate victims before they enter the hospital building. Thorough scrubbing of all of the person's skin is often part of the protocol.

Triage and treatment. Patients are triaged as they enter the ED. The word "triage" comes from the French word *trier* ("to sort"), as French physicians in the battlefields of World War I devised a plan to sort patients according to who would be likely to survive. Patients

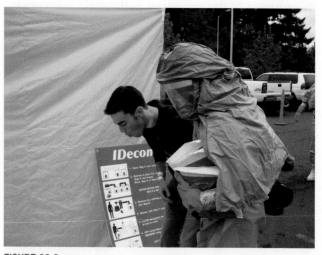

FIGURE 20.6 Biohazard suits worn by personnel assisting victims (drill at PeaceHealth Southwestern Medical Center, Vancouver, Washington.)

are assessed and labeled according to the priority of care: immediate, delayed, minimal, or expectant. Patients who require lifesaving care are labeled "immediate"; care for those in need of major or prolonged care can be "delayed" briefly; those with minor injuries to be attended to are labeled "minimal"; and "expectant" indicates those with severe life-threatening injuries who probably will not survive even with medical care. Triage priorities are based on the premise that limited medical resources should be used on those patients who will most likely live if they receive treatment.

Treatment is based on the type of agent to which the patient was exposed and the degree of exposure. Antibiotics are used for some of the biologic agents, and antidotes may be used for some chemicals and poisonous gases. Otherwise, treatment is directed at supporting organ function while the body tries to recover. If needed, life support measures including medications, ventilators, and dialysis are used.

Poison

A **poison** is a substance that, when ingested, inhaled, absorbed, applied, injected, or developed within the body, may cause functional or structural disturbances. This is possible even if only a small amount of the poison is encountered. Agents used in chemical terrorism fit into this category. Treatments and antidotes for poisoning can be obtained from a poison control center or are listed on some containers. **Some poisons do not have antidotes or treatments.** When reporting a known or suspected poisoning, have the label handy. Report the following:

- Name of the product.
- Patient's age.
- Amount of product involved.
- Any symptoms and/or complaints.

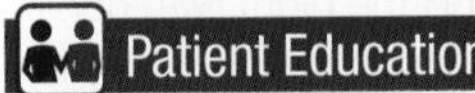

Patient Education

Poison Prevention

All patients should be taught these safety precautions:

- Never call medicine "candy." Store all medicines in child-proof containers and above a child's reach.
- Keep toxic substances in a locked cabinet or closet out of the reach of children and older adults with knowledge deficit and limited memory recall. Label with poison stickers. Remember herbal remedies including vitamins should be included.
- Always keep toxic substances in their original labeled container. Never put toxic substances in beverage or food containers.
- Obtain the poison control center number from your local operator. Keep it near the telephone so you do not need to search for it in an emergency.
- Never induce vomiting unless instructed by a professional. Depending on the type of poison (e.g., lye, gasoline, grease, or some cleaning and petroleum products), inducing vomiting may cause further damage.
- Older adults may obtain prescription medications and herbal remedies in bottles that are not childproof. If young grandchildren visit, these items should be kept in a locked cabinet.

PROTECTIVE DEVICES

Protective devices, formerly called *restraints*, were overused in the past and may not be allowed (depending on state law) in long-term care facilities. If they are allowed in a setting, strict rules apply regarding length of order and frequency of patient assessment. Restricting movement on a long-term basis causes problems such as muscle weakness, atrophy, loss of bone mass, joint contractures, constipation, incontinence, pressure injuries, depression, and cognitive impairment. The patient's self-concept and mood are negatively affected, and both the patient and family can be emotionally affected. In the past, some staff used these devices as a way to punish or discipline a patient. **This is an illegal, unethical, and unacceptable practice that constitutes malpractice.**

Restraints are used in two types of situations: for behavioral or nonbehavioral indications. A protective device is used for a behavioral health reason if the patient is in a psychiatric setting or has demonstrated a sudden change in mental status or behavior. Nonbehavioral usage is for the continuation of medical treatments. An example of a nonbehavioral use would be an older adult with a history of dementia who needs to have her intravenous (IV) site protected from attempts to dislodge the catheter. Health care workers must check patients in a behavioral health protective device more frequently. The array and use of physical and chemical protective devices (i.e., medication) in psychiatric or behavioral health settings are not covered in this text. **It is your responsibility to be aware of and follow the regulations in your facility and area.**

LEGAL IMPLICATIONS OF USING PROTECTIVE DEVICES

Federal and local laws protect the patient from physical and mental abuse and from physical and chemical restraints except those that are authorized by a physician, in writing, for a specified and limited time, or that are needed in an emergency. The devices must be applied by licensed, qualified personnel.

The Joint Commission supports the use of protective devices if clinically necessary, but only as a last resort. This text has described the use of the bed's side rails as a way to increase a patient's independence in changing position or getting in or out of bed. However, in some situations and facilities, full side rails are considered restraints because they limit a patient's ability to move, whereas half-rails do not, and are not considered restraints. The evidence demonstrates that using bed rails as a restraint can be harmful.

ALTERNATIVES TO PROTECTIVE DEVICES

The standard of practice is to consider alternatives to restraints before using them. Many of the actions described in Box 20.3 involve frequent observations of the patient, which help prevent patient injury and decrease the use of the devices.

Box 20.6 Principles Related to the Use of Protective Devices

- The use of protective devices must help the patient or be needed for the continuation of medical therapy.
- Use the least amount of immobilization needed for the situation.
- Obtain a written order for all devices that limit movement or immobilize the patient. Notify the primary care provider as soon as the device is no longer needed.
- Apply the device snugly but not so tightly as to interfere with blood circulation or nerve function.
- Remove the device and change the patient's position at least every 2 hours. Perform active or passive exercises for immobilized joints and muscles.

 QSEN Considerations: Safety

Sitting With the Patient

Encourage the family and friends of a patient who is confused to sit with the patient to promote safety.

PRINCIPLES RELATED TO THE USE OF PROTECTIVE DEVICES

Box 20.6 lists five principles related to the use of protective devices. In general, the device must directly benefit the patient.

 Life-Span Considerations

Older Adults

Older adults often become more confused in unfamiliar surroundings such as an acute care facility. Having familiar items from home, such as photographs or mementos, will help older adults orient to the facility and feel more comfortable. Reorient the older adult frequently to reduce the need for a protective device.

For example, a patient who is confused may try to pull out a nasogastric tube, IV line(s), or any other medical device. To continue medical treatment, the patient's hand may be placed in a mitten. If after additional assessments and reorientations this does not prevent the patient from pulling out the medical device(s), then a wrist or extremity device may be ordered.

If an assessment shows cause, the order must be obtained and in effect before applying a device. In an emergency, some agencies permit a device to be applied without an order, but one must be obtained as soon as possible. When the protective device is no longer needed, obtain an order to discontinue it. The order usually specifies the type of device and how long it may be used (usually no more than 24 hours, depending on the patient's age).

 Communication

Explaining the Need for a Protective Device

The situation below shows how a caregiver can explain the need for using a protective device to a family member.

Helen Klein is a 68-year-old patient in your unit. She was admitted for a right total hip replacement and has a history of Alzheimer disease. Mrs. Klein returned to the postoperative unit 2 hours ago. Because of her diagnosis of Alzheimer disease, you have placed her in a room near the nurses' station. Mrs. Klein is very confused and only oriented to person. Shortly after she returned to the unit, her family went to dinner. You have tried repeatedly to orient her while her family is at dinner. You are now exiting the room after finding that Mrs. Klein was trying to get out of bed and has removed her dressing, drain, and IV line. You see her daughter coming down the hall. The daughter asks you, "How is my mother? Is she resting?"

Nurse: Your mother is fine, she is awake. May I talk with you for a minute?

Ms. Klein: Sure.

(You should find a quiet, private place, out of Mrs. Klein's hearing, to talk with the daughter.)

Nurse: Ms. Klein, although your mother is stable, being in the hospital and changing her routine has added to your mother's confusion. While you were at dinner, she removed her dressing, drain, and IV line and was trying to get out of bed. We already have her in a room close to the nurses' station so that we can check on her more frequently. Is it possible for you or another family member to spend the night with her?

Ms. Klein: Why would you want me to do that? I did not think family members could stay with patients.

Nurse: For some patients, it is safer and they rest better if someone they are familiar with stays with them. This helps keep the patient oriented and calm. If this is not possible, we may need to use an extremity immobilizer for your mother so that she does not pull out her lines again.

Ms. Klein: You mean tie her hands? That is cruel.

Nurse: Extremity immobilizers are secured to the bed. This is not meant to be cruel. It is a protective measure. The purpose is to keep your mother safe while she is receiving treatment(s). I do not want her to pull out her tubes and drains. That would endanger her safety.

Ms. Klein: I see what you mean. I'll talk with my brothers and sisters and see if one of us can spend the night with her. If we are with her, will she need to be tied down?

Nurse: It has been my experience that when a family member stays, the patient rests and remains in bed, so no, we would use extremity immobilizers only if necessary to protect your mother.

When applying the protective device, make certain that the patient's movements will not impair circulation or nerve function. Padding the device with a soft washcloth or gauze pads will prevent skin irritation. The device should fit snugly when applied, but should not compromise the patient's neurovascular status. **You should be able to fit your index and middle fingers between the patient and the device easily.** A device that is secured too tightly may cause injury. Skill 20.3 describes how to apply different protective devices.

Secure the ties of a protective device to an immovable part of the bed frame. Do not tie it to the side rails because lowering the rails may cause the device to be pulled too tightly around the patient or cause strain on a joint of an immobilized extremity. Place the ties under the armrests of a chair and secure at the back. This

Skill 20.3 Applying a Protective Device

 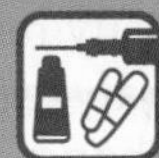 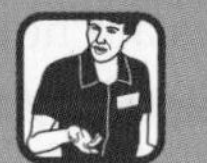 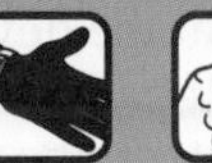 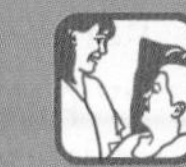 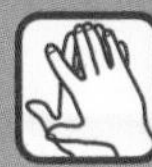 

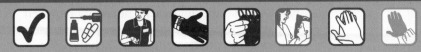

A protective device is used only after all alternative methods have been tried. Each type of device has its own purpose or main uses. A security or safety belt is used for the patient who is at a high risk for falls or to secure a patient to a stretcher. An extremity immobilizer is used to prevent disruption to dressings, skin grafts, intravenous (IV) lines, urinary catheters, nasogastric tubes, and so forth. A mitten or hand mitt is used to keep the patient from scratching, grasping tubes and catheters, or pulling the ties on a limb immobilizer.

Supplies

- Protective devices
- Belt
- Extremity immobilizer
- Mitten or hand mitt
- Soap, washcloth, towel, and lotion

Review and carry out the Standard Steps in Appendix A.

ACTION *(RATIONALE)*

Assessment (Data Collection)

1. Assess whether all other possible measures have been used to resolve the safety problem and whether they have been effective. *(Confirms that all possible methods of ensuring patient safety have been tried before using a protective device.)*
2. Check to see whether there is an order for a protective device; if not, obtain one. *(Use of a protective device requires a written order.)*
3. Review your agency's policy and procedure for use. *(Keeps your practice within legal parameters.)*
4. Assess the skin and circulation in the area where the device will be applied. *(Provides baseline data before application of the device.)*

Planning

5. Review manufacturer's instructions about the application of the device and obtain help if necessary. *(Promotes correct usage and safety for you and patient.)*

Implementation

6. Explain the purpose and need for the device to the patient and family. *(Decreases anxiety of patient and family.)*
7. Lock brakes on wheelchair or bed before proceeding. *(Promotes safe application.)*
8. Apply the device and tie with a half-bow knot. *(A half-bow knot fastens the device, yet can be untied easily and quickly by you in an emergency.)*

For the Security or Safety Belt

9. With patient sitting in a wheelchair, place the security belt around the waist or upper legs and slip one end of the tie through the slit on the opposite side. *(Secures belt to patient before it is attached to chair.)*

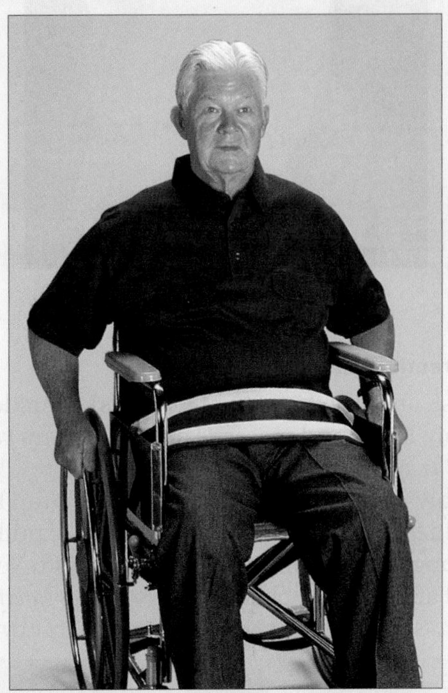

Step 9

10. Bring both ends under the armrests and behind the chair (one on each side) and tie to the frame or fasten the buckle, if present. *(Prevents patient from untying the protective device.)*

For a Chair With a Tabletop

11. Ensure the patient is awake and sitting fully upright in the chair. *(Prevents patient from sliding down.)*
12. Carefully slide the table top into a secure and locked position, ensuring that fingers are not near the latch mechanism. *(Prevents injury while the table top is being secured.)*
13. Place patient near high traffic area of the unit, such as the nurses' station. *(Prevents unsupervised use of chair with tabletop.)*

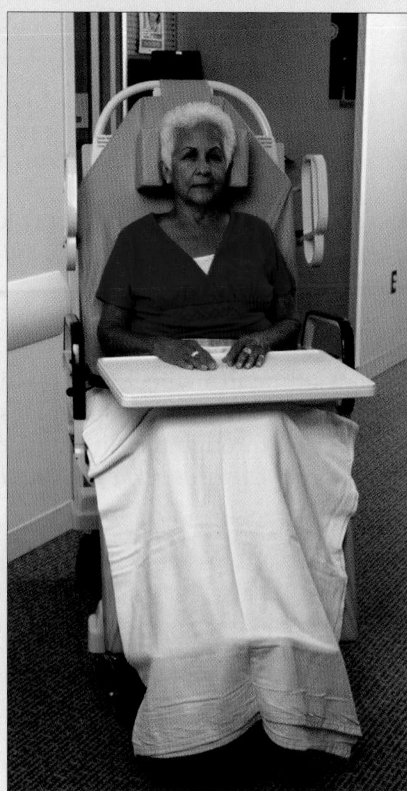
Step **13**

For Extremity Immobilizers

14. Wash and dry the patient's wrist(s) or ankle(s); apply lotion and massage areas. *(Prepares patient for the application.)*
15. Apply immobilizer to the extremity. Wrap the padded end around the wrist or ankle; pull the tie through the slit or buckle, or fasten with Velcro and attach to the bed frame. *(Promotes safety and decreases chance of impeding circulation of extremity.)*

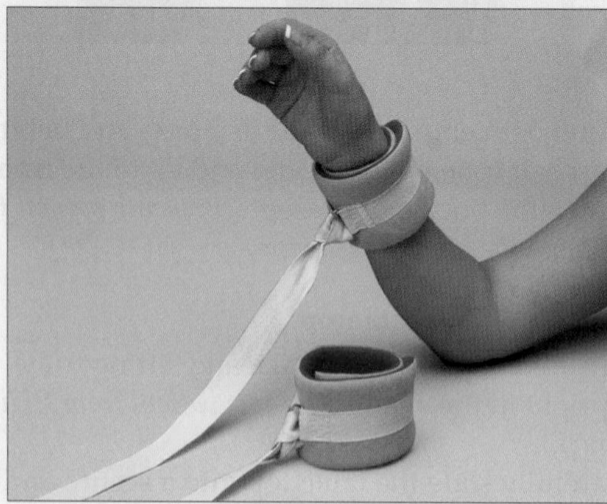
Step **15**

For a Mitten or Hand Mitt

16. Wash and dry the patient's hand thoroughly; apply lotion and massage hands. *(Prepares patient for the application.)*
17. Slip hand into mitt, and slip tie around wrist and secure. It is usually better to apply mitts to both hands so that the devices are not easily removed by patient. If patient is partially paralyzed, use only one mitt on the nonparalyzed hand. *(Promotes safety and prevents using fingers to pull out tubes and IV lines.)*

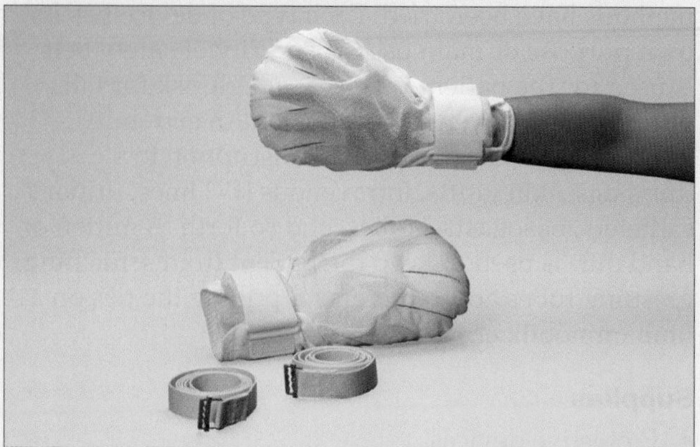
Step **17**

Evaluation

18. Check on the patient at least every 15 to 30 minutes or as directed by your agency and observe neurovascular function and patient's position and needs. *(Monitors patient for problems with the device and positioning and prevents patient's needs from going unmet.)*
19. At least every 2 hours (or according to agency policy), release the ties, change the patient's position, supervise active or provide passive range-of-motion (ROM) exercise, and assess the condition of the skin under the device. Remove only one device at a time. *(Provides safety while preventing joint stiffness and muscle aches; minimizes risk of pressure injuries.)*
20. Provide access to a call bell or other method to summon the nurse. *(Provides safety and makes patient feel less isolated.)*
21. Assess for the continued need for the device. *(Prevents patient from being in a device longer than necessary.)*

Documentation

22. Note the patient's behavior, alternative methods tried, explanation to patient and family, and condition of skin before applying the device. Ongoing documentation includes periodic reevaluation of need for device, skin condition, pulses, patient's tolerance of device, times restraints were removed and then reapplied, and time when device was removed and discontinued. *(Validates the need for the use of a device and that the device is being used correctly.)*

Documentation Examples

10/15 1400 Oriented to person only, thrashing in bed, and unable to understand directions to prevent removal of IV line. Primary care provider notified, order obtained for right wrist protective device, and device applied. Skin intact; fingers warm, dry, and with quick capillary refill. Call bell within reach. (Nurse's electronic signature)

10/15 1600 Right wrist immobilizer removed and reapplied. Skin remains intact; passive ROM to R arm, wrist, and fingers. Sensation intact; no evidence of circulation impairment. (Nurse's electronic signature)

Home Care Considerations

You must consider the family or caregivers when:

- Assessing their ability to stay with the patient attentively in an effort to avoid the use of protective devices.
- Instructing them on interventions to try before using protective devices.
- Developing a written schedule for removal of device, skin care, and exercise.
- Providing a documentation tool to track actual removal of the device and the care given.
- Informing them whom to notify should any abnormality be found.

Critical Thinking Questions

1. What would you do if your patient has extremity immobilizers ordered and there is an IV in the right wrist area?
2. What can happen if a restraint is too tight and circulation is impaired in an extremity?

also prevents the patient from sliding the tie up and off the back of the chair.

Use a half-bow knot to secure the device to the bed frame or chair. The half-bow knot is a secure knot that will not slip, even if tugged upon, yet can easily be undone by health care workers. It is similar to that used when tying shoes except only one loop is made (Fig. 20.7).

Remove the device at least every 2 hours and offer food and toileting. Perform active or passive range-of-motion exercises for immobilized joints and muscles to prevent complications. Use supportive pillows and pads for positioning. Check circulation and pulses distal to the device every 15 to 30 minutes. Signs that the circulation or nerve function has been impaired include skin coolness, change in color (particularly pallor or a bluish hue), numbness, pain, edema, and loss of sensation or movement. Remove the device immediately and contact the primary care provider if any of these signs occurs.

Think Critically

Your confused patient keeps getting out of her wheelchair. What could you do to try to keep her in the chair? If that does not work, what safety device do you think you would use?

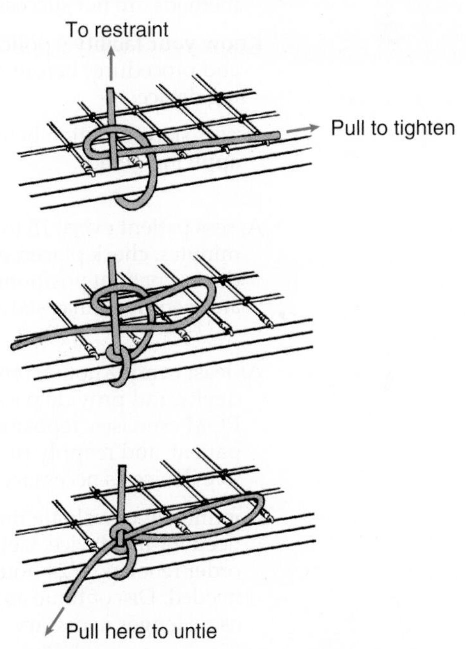

FIGURE 20.7 Tying a half-bow or safety knot.

DOCUMENTATION OF THE USE OF PROTECTIVE DEVICES

Describe the objective behaviors you observed (the reason) that led you to believe there was a risk for injury. Document every alternative action and method that was tried, and their effectiveness, before placing the device. Document the time and from whom the order for the device was obtained, the type of device applied, the time of application, the name of the person applying the device, and the location of the device on the patient's body. Include the patient and family education performed before placement of the device. Obtain an informed consent as necessary. Document the periodic observations you make of the patient, including sensation, circulation (skin color, distal pulses, and capillary refill), and movement. Lastly, record the time when the device was discontinued and your name or the name of the person discontinuing the device. Nursing Care Plan 20.1 describes the care of a patient needing a protective device.

Nursing Care Plan 20.1 Care of the Patient Wearing a Protective Device

SCENARIO Hirosha Kumoto has Alzheimer disease. She is in a room by the nurses' station. While her family was at dinner, you checked on her every 15 minutes. You tried to orient Ms. Kumoto to her surroundings. She is oriented ×1 only. Because Ms. Kumoto's family was not able to spend the night with her, it was decided to apply extremity immobilizers.

PROBLEM/NURSING DIAGNOSIS Patient is pulling out tubes and trying to get out of bed/Risk for injury related to confusion and disorientation.

SUPPORTING ASSESSMENT DATA *Subjective:* Asks repeatedly, "Where am I? Why am I here?" *Objective:* Observed patient trying to get out of bed and climb over the side rails. Patient removed postop dressing, drain, and IV.

Goals/Expected Outcomes	Nursing Interventions	Selected Rationales	Evaluation
Patient will experience injury during recovery period.	Assess patient's ability to follow the medical regimen.	Assessment provides current information and data on patient condition.	*Has any injury been sustained?* No evidence of injury at this time.
	Try all alternative methods first, such as orienting patient, placing patient in room by the nurses' station, asking family to sit with patient PRN.	Protective devices are used only if alternative methods fail and are documented as failing.	Family member is with the patient intermittently.
	Obtain an order to apply protective device if above methods are not successful.	An order is required for any application of a protective device that restrains movements.	PRN order obtained from primary care provider.
	Know your facility's policies and procedures before placing device.	Facilities differ on policies and procedures. You must follow your institution's rules.	
	Assess skin condition before applying device.	Assessing skin condition prevents placing item over irritated uncovered area.	Skin intact without redness.
	Assess patient every 15 to 30 minutes: check placement of device, patient positioning, and neurovascular status.	Frequent checks ensure patient has not untied device and that device is in proper position with adequate neurovascular status.	Patient checked q 15 minutes. No problems noted.
	At least every 2 hours, remove device and provide passive ROM exercises, reposition patient, and reapply protective device as necessary.	Allows joint movement, helps prevent contractures, prevents skin breakdown, and is refreshing for patient.	Repositioned and ROM provided q 2 hours.
	Continually reevaluate the need for the device. Get the order renewed q 24 hours as needed. Discontinue as soon as no longer necessary.	Devices are discontinued as soon as possible.	No fall or injury sustained. Meeting expected outcome.
Patient's family will verbalize understanding of the need for use of protective devices.	Explain to family the reasons for protective devices. Explain monitoring for safety.	When family understands that the goal is to keep family member safe, they are more likely to agree with use.	Does the family understand? Family verbalizes the need for using protective device when they are not present.
	Explain that all alternatives will be tried before placing protective device.	Communication helps prevent misunderstanding.	Full explanation given to family.
	Explain that device will be removed as soon as is possible.	Reassures family that the patient will not always be restrained.	Expected outcome being met.

Nursing Care Plan 20.1 Care of the Patient Wearing a Protective Device—cont'd

Goals/Expected Outcomes	Nursing Interventions	Selected Rationales	Evaluation
Medically necessary devices will remain in place.	Use least restrictive protective device to ensure outcomes.	Reassures family that the patient will not always be restrained.	Intravenous line and dressing remained in place. Expected outcome being met. Continue plan.

CRITICAL THINKING QUESTIONS

1. The extremity immobilizers help prevent accidental removal of tubes and drains. Would you use any other type of device for Ms. Kumoto? Why or why not? If so, what device would you consider using?
2. Does your facility offer any other alternatives to restraint use? Which policy do you feel is best? Why?

PRN, As needed; *ROM*, range of motion.

Get Ready for the NCLEX Examination!

Key Points

- Many factors can be controlled in the patient's environment.
- Bright lighting is needed for performing procedures.
- Adequate night lighting is needed to prevent injury when going to the bathroom.
- The most common cause of noise pollution in a health care agency is people.
- Keep rooms neat and clean, while allowing patients to have personal items close to them.
- Privacy is important to a patient's well-being.
- A bed should be neat, clean, dry, and free from wrinkles.
- Bed making should be done, if possible, while the patient is out of bed.
- Safety is a primary concern when caring for patients.
- Falls are the most frequent cause of injury for the older adult patient in an acute care facility.
- *RACE* is the acronym for how to proceed in case of a fire.
- Know your agency's policy for cleaning up a biohazardous spill and handling bioterrorism or chemical terrorism occurrences.
- Triage involves assessing and labeling patients according to the priority of care.
- Protective devices are used only as a last resort.
- Use the least restrictive immobilizing device for the situation and monitor the patient frequently.
- A protective device should be applied snugly but should not impair neurovascular status.

Additional Learning Resources

SG Go to your Study Guide for additional learning activities to help you master this chapter content.

evolve Go to your Evolve website at http://evolve.elsevier.com/Williams/fundamental for the following FREE learning resources:

- Animations.
- Answer Guidelines for Think Critically boxes and Critical Thinking Questions and Activities.
- Answers and Rationales for Review Questions for the NCLEX Examination.
- A glossary with pronunciations in English and Spanish.
- Interactive Review Questions for the NCLEX Examination and more!

Review Questions for the NCLEX Examination

*Choose the **best** answer for each question.*

1. In making a bed, it is important to remember: *(Select all that apply.)*
   1. To place soiled linens on the floor to avoid contaminating the bed.
   2. To unfold linens on the bed to avoid stirring up air currents.
   3. To return unused linens to the floor's clean linen area to prevent waste.
   4. To raise the bed during the linen change to prevent back strain.
2. Which patient might be most likely to suffer a burn if left to bathe in a tub alone?
   1. An adult female who is to have abdominal surgery tomorrow
   2. An adult male who has been having back pain after a cystoscopy
   3. A patient taking drugs that alter mental awareness
   4. An alert older adult patient who prefers tub bathing
3. Which action would help prevent the most frequent cause of injury to the older adult patient?
   1. Keeping pathways clear of papers and objects
   2. Grounding all electrical apparatuses in use
   3. Checking temperatures of fluids before serving them
   4. Reviewing the dose and frequency for all ordered medications with the patient

4. If a biohazard spill occurs in the dirty utility room on your unit and you are unfamiliar with the product involved, you would first:
   1. Dilute the spill with water.
   2. Find the MSDS.
   3. Don gloves.
   4. Call a housekeeper.
5. The correct sequence of action in a fire is:
   1. Call for help, activate the alarm, rescue a patient in danger, and extinguish the fire.
   2. Rescue a patient in danger, activate the alarm, contain the fire, and extinguish the fire.
   3. Call the hospital operator, race to close the fire doors, activate the alarm, and evacuate all patients.
   4. Race to close the fire doors, activate the alarm, call the hospital operator, and evacuate all patients.
6. What is the most appropriate triage classification for an alert, oriented, and mobile patient with an obvious broken arm?
   1. Immediate
   2. Delayed
   3. Minimal
   4. Expectant
7. You are considering applying a protective device to your patient. What needs to be done **first**?
   1. Obtain an order from the primary care provider.
   2. Discuss your intentions with the patient.
   3. Discuss your intentions with the family.
   4. Determine that all other safety measures have been attempted to try to resolve the safety issue.

Critical Thinking Activities

Read each clinical scenario and discuss the questions with your classmates.

Scenario A

Two of your friends and fellow nursing students are talking and laughing loudly at the nursing station. What would you do?

Scenario B

While giving a bath to your bedridden patient, you notice smoke coming from the bathroom. What is your first action? After that, how would you proceed?

Scenario C

During a home care visit, you find several safety hazards in the patient's home. How would you handle the situation?

Scenario D

You notice a foul odor in your patient's room. How would you proceed?

chapter 21

Measuring Vital Signs

http://evolve.elsevier.com/Williams/fundamental

Objectives

Upon completing this chapter, you should be able to do the following:

Theory

1. List the anatomic structures involved in the regulation of the vital signs and describe their functions.
2. Identify the physiologic mechanisms that regulate temperature, heart rate, blood pressure, and respiration.
3. List the factors that affect body temperature.
4. Discuss normal and abnormal characteristics of the pulse.
5. Describe the respiratory patterns considered to be normal and abnormal.
6. Explain the relationship of Korotkoff sounds to systolic and diastolic blood pressure.
7. State why pain is considered the fifth vital sign.

Clinical Practice

1. Demonstrate measuring and recording the body temperature of an adult and a child at the oral, rectal, axillary, and tympanic (eardrum) sites using electronic or tympanic thermometer.
2. Demonstrate measuring and recording an apical pulse and a radial pulse.
3. Demonstrate counting and recording respirations.
4. Demonstrate measuring and recording blood pressure.
5. Demonstrate using an automatic vital signs machine to monitor pulse and blood pressure.
6. Recognize deviations from normal vital sign patterns.
7. Determine factors that might be adversely affecting the patient's temperature, pulse, respiration, or blood pressure.

Skills

Key Terms

apex (p. 357)
apnea (ĂP-nē-ă, p. 363)
arrhythmia (ă-RĬTH-mē-ă, p. 360)
auscultation (ăw-skŭl-TĀ-shŭn, p. 364)
auscultatory gap (ăw-SKŬL-tă-tō-rē GĂP, p. 369)
axillary (ĂX-ĭ-lă-rē, p. 348)
basal metabolic rate (BMR) (BĀ-sĭl mĕ-tă-BŎ-lĭk RĂT, p. 344)
Biot respirations (bē-ŌT rĕs-pĭ-RĀ-shŭns, p. 363)
bradycardia (brăd-ē-KĂR-dē-ă, p. 358)
bradypnea (brăd-ē-PNĒ-ă, p. 363)
cardiac output (p. 345)
Cheyne-Stokes respirations (chān stōks rĕs-pĭ-RĀ-shŭns, p. 363)
chills (p. 349)
core temperature (p. 348)
crackles (KRĂK-ŭlz, p. 363)
crisis (p. 349)
cyanosis (sī-ă-NŌ-sĭs, p. 362)
defervescence (dĕ-fĕr-VĔ-sĕns, p. 349)
diastolic pressure (dī-ă-STŎ-lĭk, p. 347)
dyspnea (DĬSP-nē-ă, p. 363)
eupnea (YĔWP-nē-ă, p. 362)
febrile (FĒB-rĭl, p. 349)
fever (p. 344)
hypertension (hī-pŭr-TĔN-shŭn, p. 369)
hyperthermia (hī-pŭr-THĔR-mē-ă, p. 349)
hyperventilation (p. 363)
hypotension (hī-pō-TĔN-shŭn, p. 370)
hypothermia (hī-pō-THĔR-mē-ă, p. 350)
hypoxemia (hī-PŎK-sē mē-ă p. 363)
hypoxia (hī-PŎK-sē-ă, p. 345)
Korotkoff sounds (kō-RŎT-kŏf SŎWNDS, p. 369)
Kussmaul respirations (KŪS-măl rĕs-pĭ-RĀ-shŭnz, p. 363)
lysis (LĪ-sĭs, p. 349)
metabolism (mĕ-TĂ-bō-lĭsm, p. 344)
orthostatic hypotension (ŏr-thō-STĂT-ĭk hī-pō-TĔN-shŭn, p. 370)
overhydration (ō-vĕr-hī-DRĀ-shŭn, p. 347)
oximeter (ŏk-SĬM-ĕ-tĕr, p.364)
oximetry (ŏk-SĬM-ĕ-trē p. 364)
palpate (p. 357)
pulse deficit (p. 358)
pulse pressure (p. 364)
pyrexia (pī-RĔX-ē-ă, p. 345)
pyrogens (PĪ-rō-jĕnz, p. 344)

Key Terms—cont'd

respiration (p. 345)
rhonchi (RŎNG-kī, p. 363)
shock (p. 370)
sphygmomanometer (sfĭg-mō-mă-NŎM-ĕ-tĕr, p. 365)
stertor (STĔR-tŏr, p. 363)
stethoscope (STĔTH-ō-skōp, p. 358)
stridor (STRĪ-dŏr, p. 363)
stroke volume (p. 345)
systolic pressure (sĭs-TŎL-ĭk, p. 347)
tachycardia (tăk-ĕ-KĂR-dē-ă, p. 358)
tachypnea (tăk-ĭp-NĒ-ă, p. 363)
tympanic membrane (tĭm-PĂN-ĭk, p. 348)
vital signs (p. 344)
wheeze (p. 364)

 **Concepts Covered in This Chapter**

- Acid-base balance
- Cellular regulation
- Infection
- Pain
- Stress
- Safety
- Thermoregulation

The **vital signs**—temperature, pulse, respiration, blood pressure, and pain level, plus oxygen saturation level—give some indication of a person's state of health. They represent interrelated physiologic systems of the body. Learning to measure vital signs is the beginning step in gathering assessment data for patients. Evaluation of vital sign data requires several readings so that a patient's true status can be determined.

 **QSEN Considerations: Teamwork and Collaboration**

Assigning Vital Signs

If another health care worker is assigned to take vital signs on your assigned patients, check the measurements to see how they fit with your assessment and in the overall picture of the patient's health.

It is important to understand the physiologic mechanisms that regulate vital signs and the factors that can affect each one.

OVERVIEW OF STRUCTURE AND FUNCTION RELATED TO THE REGULATION OF VITAL SIGNS

HOW IS BODY HEAT PRODUCED?

- Heat production is a by-product of **metabolism** (cellular chemical reactions in the body).
- When metabolism increases, more heat is produced. This is what causes **fever** (elevated temperature). When pathogens invade the body and the body attempts to destroy them, the increased activity (metabolism) causes fever. **Pyrogens** (agents that cause fever) produced by some pathogens act on the body's thermostat and raise the body temperature.
- **Basal metabolic rate (BMR)** is the rate at which heat is produced when the body is at rest. The average BMR depends on the person's body surface area.

WHAT FACTORS AFFECT BODY HEAT PRODUCTION?

- BMR is affected by thyroid hormone. Excessive amounts of thyroid hormone cause an increase in the metabolic rate and the person feels warm and their body temperature rises; insufficient thyroid hormone results in a decreased metabolic rate and the person's body temperature falls.
- Other hormones that affect metabolic rate are epinephrine, norepinephrine, and testosterone. Because of their levels of testosterone, men have a higher BMR than women.
- Voluntary muscle movement of exercise increases the BMR and heat production.
- The involuntary muscle action of shivering can increase heat production up to five times normal. (This is why you shiver when you are cold.)

HOW IS BODY TEMPERATURE REGULATED?

- The hypothalamus, located between the cerebral hemispheres, acts as a thermostat and controls body temperature by a feedback mechanism (Fig. 21.1).
- The chemical reactions that occur in the body as it fights a pathogen cause the thermostat to reset to a higher level (a new set point).
- When the body heat rises above normal, the hypothalamus sends out a signal through the nervous system that causes vasodilation, sweating, and inhibition of heat production.
- If the body temperature drops below normal range, the hypothalamus sends messages for vasoconstriction of surface blood vessels to conserve heat and messages to induce shivering to increase heat production.
- Heat loss occurs through the skin's exposure to the environment. It occurs through (1) radiation, (2) conduction, (3) convection, and (4) evaporation.
- Blood flow from the internal organs carries heat to the skin. The heat is radiated to cooler objects in the person's vicinity.
- When objects in the surroundings are warmer than the body, heat is radiated to the body and absorbed.
- When warm skin touches a cool object, heat is lost to the object by conduction. Ice bags applied to the skin increase conductive heat loss.

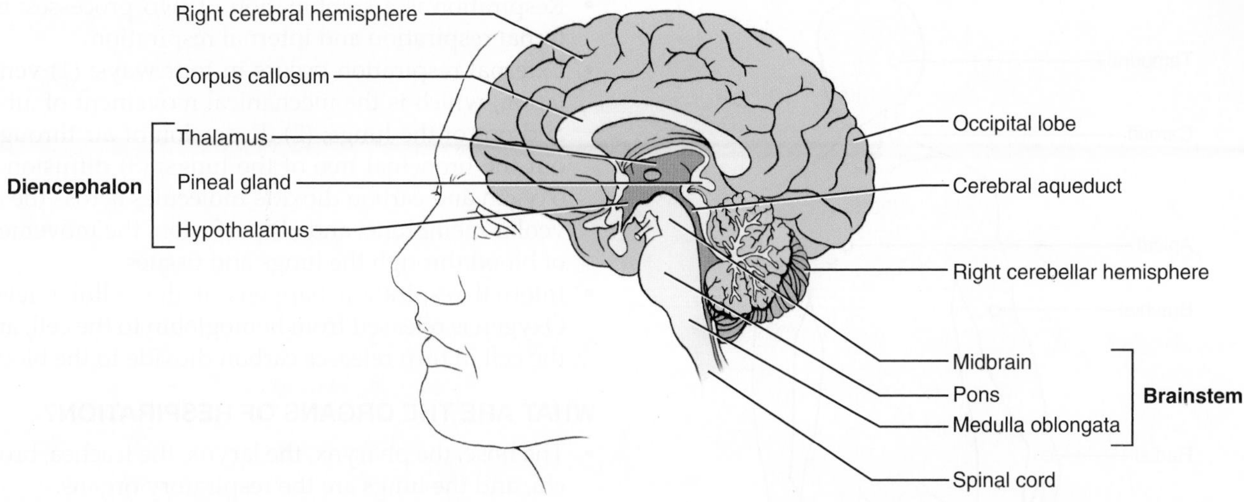

FIGURE 21.1 The hypothalamus acts as the body's thermostat.

- Air movement causes heat to be transferred from the skin to the air molecules by convection. Fast-moving air from an electric fan cools by convection. Heat loss increases when the skin is moistened and evaporation occurs.
- Sweat glands contribute to evaporative loss by secreting sweat in response to a message from the hypothalamus when the body temperature rises too high.
- As water evaporates from the skin, heat is transferred to the air. Heat is continuously lost from the body by evaporation, resulting in a daily loss of 800 mL of water from the skin and lungs.

HOW DOES FEVER OCCUR, AND WHAT ARE ITS PHYSIOLOGIC EFFECTS?

- **Pyrexia** (fever) occurs when normal mechanisms of the body cannot keep up with excessive heat production and body temperature rises. Pyrexia occurs when the body temperature rises above 100.2°F (37.9°C).
- When **pyrogens** (substances that cause fever) such as bacteria cause an immune response in the body, the hypothalamus is stimulated to raise the body's temperature set point.
- Altering the body's internal environment and allowing it to become hotter before triggering natural cooling mechanisms permits the body to become more hostile to the bacteria, and the immune system can more effectively destroy them. Fever also stimulates the immune system to produce substances to fight viruses.
- If the temperature rises above the new set point, the skin becomes flushed and moist.
- **Diaphoresis** is excessive sweat production, which attempts to cool the body by evaporation.
- When the metabolic rate rises and there is a greater demand for oxygen at the cellular level, fever occurs.
- Heart and respiratory rates rise to help the body meet the increased metabolic demand. If the oxygen demand cannot be met, cellular **hypoxia** (state of insufficient oxygen) occurs. Cerebral hypoxia (insufficient oxygen to the brain) may cause confusion in the individual.

WHAT PHYSIOLOGIC MECHANISMS CONTROL THE PULSE?

- Cardiac contractions produce the pulse. The surge of blood into the aorta causes a pressure wave that can be felt over a peripheral artery. Figure 21.2 shows the points on the body where the pulse may be felt.
- Cardiac contractions are normally initiated by the electrical impulse emerging from the sinoatrial (SA) node within the right atrium of the heart. Any problem with electrical conduction in the heart affects the pulse rate.
- When the heart contracts, an average of 60 to 70 mL of blood is propelled into the aorta. **Stroke volume** is the volume of blood pushed into the aorta with each heartbeat. Stroke volume affects the character of the pulse. A weak pulse may indicate a fall in stroke volume.
- The amount of the blood circulating in the vascular system and the degree of vasodilation or vasoconstriction of the blood vessels can also affect stroke volume and the pulse.
- The pulse rate multiplied by the stroke volume equals the **cardiac output**. Cardiac output is the amount of blood pumped by the left ventricle in 1 minute. Average cardiac output in the adult is about 5 L of blood per minute.

WHAT IS RESPIRATION?

- **Respiration** is the exchange of oxygen and carbon dioxide in the lungs and tissues and is initiated by the act of breathing.

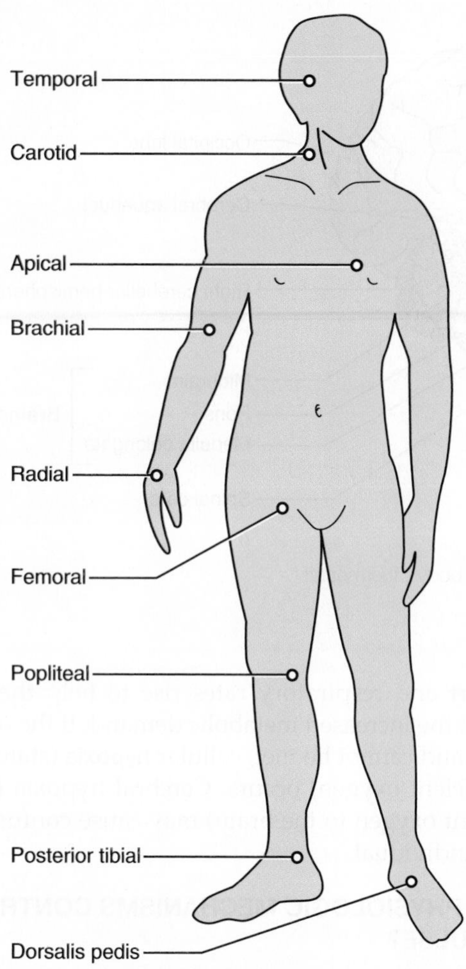

FIGURE 21.2 Pulse points.

- Respiration is a combination of two processes: external respiration and internal respiration.
- External respiration occurs in four ways: (1) ventilation, which is the mechanical movement of air in and out of the lungs; (2) dispersion of air throughout the bronchial tree of the lungs; (3) diffusion of oxygen and carbon dioxide molecules across the alveolar membrane; and (4) perfusion, the movement of blood through the lungs and tissues.
- Internal respiration happens at the cellular level. Oxygen is released from hemoglobin to the cell, and the cell in turn releases carbon dioxide to the blood.

WHAT ARE THE ORGANS OF RESPIRATION?

- The nose, the pharynx, the larynx, the trachea, bronchi, and the lungs are the respiratory organs.
- There are three lobes in the right lung and two lobes in the left lung.
- The bronchial tree, consisting of the bronchi and the bronchioles, carries oxygen to the various parts of the lungs (Fig. 21.3).
- Movement of the diaphragm controls inhalation and exhalation. The slight negative pressure created in the chest during inspiration draws air into the lungs.
- Gas exchange with the blood occurs in the alveoli, tiny thin-walled sacs.
- Surfactant secreted by cells in the walls of the alveoli is necessary for alveoli to remain open; it reduces surface tension on the alveolar wall, allowing expansion.

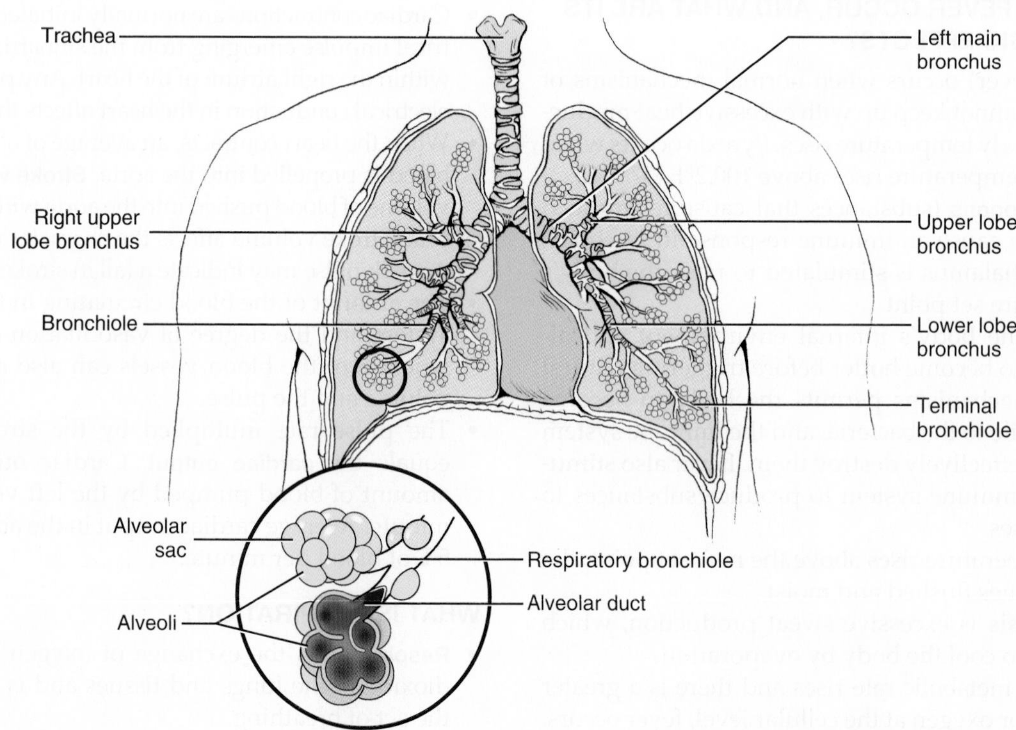

FIGURE 21.3 Respiratory structures.

HOW IS RESPIRATION CONTROLLED?

- Breathing is an involuntary, automatic function controlled by the respiratory center located in the pons and medulla of the brainstem (see Fig. 21.1).
- The respiratory center works together with feedback mechanisms. The carotid body receptors in the common carotid arteries and the aortic body receptors lying adjacent to the aortic arch signal the respiratory centers to alter the rate or depth of respiration in response to decreased oxygen levels in the blood.
- Increasing levels of carbon dioxide and increasing hydrogen ion (H^+) concentration in the blood can also activate these receptors.
- Messages are sent from the respiratory center to the respiratory muscles controlling the diaphragm and the intercostal muscles, thereby altering the respiratory rate or depth.
- The pumping action of the heart brings blood through the lung capillaries, where diffusion of oxygen and carbon dioxide can take place across the alveolar membrane.
- Carbon dioxide is mainly carried as bicarbonate ion (HCO_3-) in the blood until it reaches the lung. Carbon dioxide diffused into the lungs is released with exhalation.

WHAT IS BLOOD PRESSURE?

- Blood pressure is the pressure exerted on the arterial wall. The pressure changes depending on whether the heart is pumping or resting.
- **Systolic pressure** is the maximum pressure exerted on the artery during left ventricular contraction (systole).
- **Diastolic pressure** is the lower pressure exerted on the artery when the heart is at rest between contractions (diastole).

WHAT PHYSIOLOGIC FACTORS DIRECTLY AFFECT THE BLOOD PRESSURE?

- The amount of cardiac output (stroke volume × heart rate) affects the blood pressure. Blood pressure increases as stroke volume increases.
- If cardiac output falls, blood pressure falls.
- When vasoconstriction causes peripheral vascular resistance to rise, the pressure within the arterial system increases to push the blood along.
- When vasodilation occurs, vascular resistance drops and the pressure within the arterial system decreases.
- If blood volume increases, as in **overhydration** (excess fluid volume), blood pressure increases because of the greater volume of blood in the same space (the vascular system).
- If blood volume decreases, as with bleeding or dehydration, blood pressure decreases.
- If the blood becomes thicker, as when excessive blood cells are manufactured, blood pressure increases because more pressure is needed to push the thicker fluid through the vascular system.
- When the vascular walls lose elasticity, as happens with arteriosclerosis (hardening of the arteries) and aging, blood pressure increases to push the blood through more rigid pathways.

WHAT CHANGES OCCUR IN VITAL SIGNS WITH AGING?

- Temperature is a less reliable indicator of health in the older adult. Fever is less likely to develop, but heat loss occurs more readily and can lead to hypothermia. Older adults often have a lower normal temperature than the average adult. This may be due to a lower metabolic rate.
- The normal range for the heart rate does not change in the healthy older adult, but the rhythm may be slightly irregular.
- Respiratory rate may rise slightly as decreases in vital capacity and respiratory reserve occur.
- The systolic blood pressure rises slightly because the aorta and major arteries tend to harden with age. In many older adults, the diastolic pressure rises also.

MEASURING BODY TEMPERATURE

Normal body temperature ranges from 97.5°F to 99.5°F (36.4°C to 37.5°C) and varies considerably among individuals. Two scales are used to measure temperature: Fahrenheit and Celsius. Table 21.1 presents temperature correlations between the two scales. The temperature in a healthy young adult averages 98.6°F (37°C). It varies within the normal range as the body adjusts to changes in the amount of heat produced or the amount of heat lost. Some people run a low-normal or a high-normal temperature consistently; this represents the normal body temperature for them. It is important to

Table 21.1 Comparison of Temperature Scales[a]

FAHRENHEIT	CELSIUS (CENTIGRADE)
95.0°	35.0°
95.9°	35.5°
96.8°	36.0°
97.7°	36.5°
98.6°	37.0°
99.5°	37.5°
100.4°	38.0°
101.3°	38.5°
102.2°	39.0°
103.1°	39.5°
104.0°	40.0°
104.9°	40.5°

[a]To change Celsius to Fahrenheit, multiply by 9/5 and add 32. To change Fahrenheit to Celsius, subtract 32 and multiply by 5/9.

know the patient's usual temperature and then compare changes with that measurement.

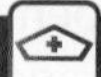 Clinical Cues

The patient's temperature usually does not indicate a fever unless it is over 100.2°F (37.9°C). Sometimes the temperature elevation is a body reaction to surgery or injury, rather than an indication of fever, and is expected to occur.

FACTORS INFLUENCING TEMPERATURE READINGS

The temperature reading obtained varies according to the site used. Measurement sites are the mouth, rectum, axilla (armpit), ear, and skin. Most temperatures are measured orally, rectally, via the **tympanic membrane** (eardrum), or via the temporal artery. Rectal temperatures are usually about 1°F (0.5°C) higher and axillary temperatures are about 1°F lower than those measured orally. The **axillary** temperature is the temperature taken in the armpit. The electronic thermometer is switched to the rectal setting and attached to a different probe before taking a rectal temperature (the rectal probe is usually red), and the reading should be recorded as a rectal temperature. The rectal temperature is usually taken with the patient in the left Sims position so that the rectum is positioned to accept the thermometer probe.

Sometimes the primary care provider indicates the site of temperature to be taken; when it is not indicated, follow agency protocol.

The temporal artery thermometer is the most accurate noninvasive way to measure body temperature. It is passed over the temporal artery in the forehead. It captures the naturally emitted heat from the skin over the temporal artery, taking 1000 readings per second and selecting the highest reading. It provides an accurate arterial temperature. The probe is gently stroked across the forehead to the far side (Fig. 21.4). Arterial temperature is close to rectal temperature but almost 1°F (0.5°C) higher than oral temperature. Ideally the temporal artery thermometer should be slid across the forehead above the brow ridges in a relatively straight line. Temporal artery temperature is unaffected by eating, drinking, smoking, or mouth breathing. If the person has been side-lying with part of the forehead into the pillow, allow the skin to cool to room temperature before using the thermometer.

Measuring tympanic temperature involves inserting the thermometer probe into the auditory canal. The probe must be pointed at the tympanic membrane for the reading to be accurate. This is another easy and quick method of measuring temperature. The graduated size of the probe prevents injury to the tympanic membrane. Tympanic membrane temperature is a good indicator of core body temperature. **Core temperature** is the temperature of the deep tissues of the body. The thermometer measures heat radiated as infrared energy from the tympanic membrane. The same blood vessels serve the hypothalamus and the membrane, so the temperature is close to core temperature at the hypothalamus. Temperatures taken with a tympanic thermometer are not subject to variations caused by eating hot or cold foods or liquids, smoking, or chewing gum. They can be affected, though, by an ear infection, excessive wax blocking the canal, or someone with a small, curved ear canal, such as a child.

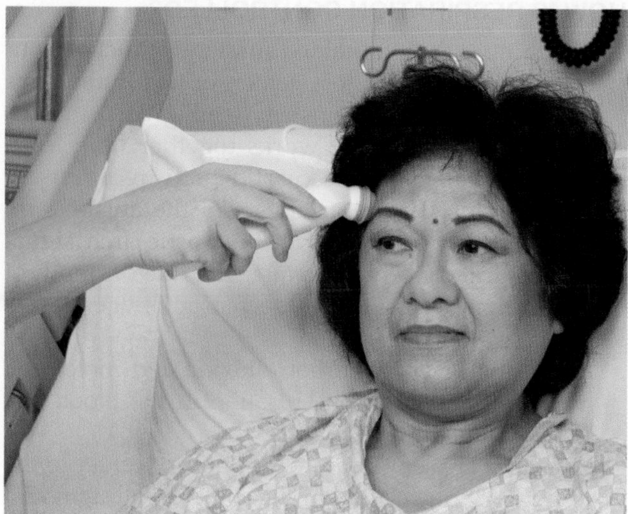

FIGURE 21.4 Slide the temporal artery thermometer across the forehead.

? Think Critically

Can you name three advantages of a tympanic thermometer over an oral thermometer? What is the advantage of a temporal artery thermometer?

Tympanic and temporal artery thermometers are more expensive than home electronic thermometers and are not universally used at home. Oral temperatures are convenient for older children and adults. The glass clinical thermometer is falling out of favor due to the length of time they take and their risk of breaking. The newer types of electronic, chemical, and infrared thermometers register in much less time and are in common use today. If the patient has recently swallowed hot or cold foods or liquids or has been smoking or chewing gum, wait 15 to 30 minutes for these effects to pass for a more accurate measurement of oral temperature. **A glass thermometer is never used orally if the patient is uncooperative or at risk for biting on the thermometer.**

Rectal temperatures are taken when an accurate temperature cannot be obtained orally and a tympanic or temporal artery thermometer is not available. The rectal route may be used when the patient has nasal congestion, has undergone nasal or oral surgery, is unable to keep the mouth closed, or is at risk for seizures. Rectal temperatures should not be used for cardiac

Box 21.1 Factors That Affect Body Temperature

- **Time of day (circadian rhythm):** The body temperature on awakening is generally in the low-normal range because of inactivity of the muscles. Conversely, the afternoon body temperature may be high-normal owing to the body's metabolic processes, the patient's activity, and the temperature of the atmosphere.
- **Environmental temperature:** As might be expected, the body temperature is lower in cold weather and higher in hot weather.
- **Patient's age:** At birth, heat-regulating mechanisms are generally not fully developed, so the infant may have marked ups and downs in body temperature during the first year of life.
- **Physical exercise:** Physical exercise uses large muscles, which create body heat by burning up the glucose and fat in the tissues. Muscle action generates heat, and core temperature rises.
- **Menstrual cycle and pregnancy:** Body temperature drops slightly just before female **ovulation** (the normal monthly ripening and release of the ovum) and then may rise 1°F above normal during ovulation. Within a day or two preceding the onset of the next menstrual period, the temperature drops again. During pregnancy, the body temperature may consistently stay at high-normal because of an increase in the patient's metabolic rate.
- **Emotional stress:** Highly emotional states cause an elevation in body temperature. The emotions increase hormone secretion, and the body activities required for this increase heat production.
- **Disease conditions:** Bacteria, viruses, and toxins from some infective agents and the chemical reactions of the inflammatory response may produce fever. Fever is a protective defense mechanism that the body uses to fight pathogens and their toxins.
- **Drugs:** Certain drugs may cause temperature elevation because of the chemical action they have in the body.

patients or patients who have had rectal surgery and is generally the choice of last resort.

Axillary temperatures are taken when oral temperatures are contraindicated and a tympanic or temporal artery thermometer is not available. They are a less reliable measure. Factors that may affect body temperature are listed in Box 21.1.

? Think Critically

Can you explain the physiologic process that causes a pregnant woman's temperature to be higher than that of the nonpregnant woman?

PROBLEMS OF TEMPERATURE REGULATION

Hyperthermia

A condition in which the patient's temperature is above the normal range (100.2°F [37.9°C]) is called a fever, a febrile state, or pyrexia. However, fever is often not considered significant until the temperature reaches 101.3°F (38.5°C). A fever is usually a common symptom of infection, in which the heightened temperature helps destroy invading bacteria. Very high fevers, such as those greater than 105.8°F (41°C), cause damage to body cells, particularly those of the central nervous system. **Hyperthermia** (above-normal body temperature) may also occur after brain injury.

Life-Span Considerations

Older Adults

Patients older than 75 tend to have a lower base body temperature. A frail older adult individual often may have a base temperature of 97.2°F (36.2°C) (Williams, 2016). If an elevation of 2°F (1.1°C) occurs, fever is present.

In fever the physiologic thermostat is reset at a higher level than normal and the body's heat-producing mechanisms elevate the body temperature to the new setting. Because of chemical reactions in the body, **chills** (sensations of cold and shaking of the body) may occur. The metabolic rate increases by about 7% for each degree Fahrenheit (10% for each degree Celsius) rise in temperature.

The course of a fever can be observed on the recorded graph in the patient's medical record. Fever occurs in three distinct stages: onset, febrile, and **defervescence** (abatement of fever). Onset may occur gradually or suddenly. The body responds to a pyrogen by trying to conserve and manufacture heat to raise the set point for core temperature. The person feels cold and adds clothes or covers, curls up in a ball, and turns up the heat to feel warm. Chills, increased respiratory rate, and increased pulse rate mark this stage. During the **febrile** stage, the body temperature rises to the new set point established by the hypothalamus and remains there until the cause of the fever resolves. **If the fever is very high or if it lasts for an extended period, dehydration, delirium, and convulsions may occur.** Dehydration occurs as fluid is lost with perspiration and more rapid breathing. Delirium and convulsions may occur because neurologic function is affected when the temperature in the brain rises. The stage of defervescence brings lowering of the body temperature to normal. The person feels warm and the skin may be moist.

A **crisis** (abrupt decline in fever) may occur when the body controls the infection, or a **lysis** (gradual return to a normal temperature, when applied to fever) may mark the decline of the fever. Fevers are classified as constant, intermittent, remittent, or relapsing (Box 21.2).

Life-Span Considerations

Older Adults

The temperature in the older adult may not reflect the seriousness of the illness because temperature may not rise significantly.

Box 21.2 Fever Patterns

- **Constant:** The temperature is continuously elevated with less than 1°F of variation within a 24-hour period.
- **Intermittent:** The temperature alternates rising and falling (e.g., low in the morning and high in the afternoon, or low for 2 to 3 days followed by a high temperature for 2 to 3 days).
- **Remittent:** A high temperature falls, usually in the morning, and again rises later in the day. The temperature never falls to normal in this type of fever until recovery occurs.
- **Relapsing:** The temperature falls to normal and then rises again in a repeating pattern.

Hypothermia

Hypothermia (subnormal body temperature) refers to a lowering of the temperature of the entire body, not just a portion of it. The thermal regulating center in the hypothalamus is greatly impaired when the temperature of the body falls below 95°F (35°C). At this level, the activity of the cells is reduced, less heat is produced, and sleepiness and coma are likely to develop. Those at risk for hypothermia include postoperative patients who have been cooled during surgery, newborn infants whose skin is exposed to cool room temperatures, older adults or debilitated patients, the chronically ill, patients taking certain medications, and those exposed to cold temperatures for prolonged periods, such as homeless persons.

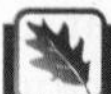 **Life-Span Considerations**

Older Adults

- Older adults, like infants, lose considerable body heat through the scalp. Wearing a hat, even indoors, helps prevent heat loss in cold weather.
- The older adult with inadequate home heating is at risk for hypothermia during cold weather.

People exposed to extremely cold weather often suffer frostbite of the ears, nose, fingers, and toes, where exposed tissue and feet and hands freeze. If the frozen part is thawed immediately, there is little effect on tissues. If frostbite is prolonged, it causes death of cells and loss of the frozen area.

Nursing activities for treating the patient with a below-normal body temperature should focus on reducing heat loss and supplying additional warmth: (1) provide additional clothing or blankets for warmth (many hospitals use "blanket warmers" to provide warm blankets); (2) give warm fluids, if permitted; (3) adjust the temperature of the room to 72°F (22.2°C) or higher; (4) eliminate drafts; (5) increase the patient's muscle activity; and (6) submerge frostbitten areas in a warm bath, with water temperature no warmer than 107°F (41.7°C).

 **Safety Alert**

Electric blankets should be avoided due to risk of electric shock via wires being accidentally pinched by hospital beds.

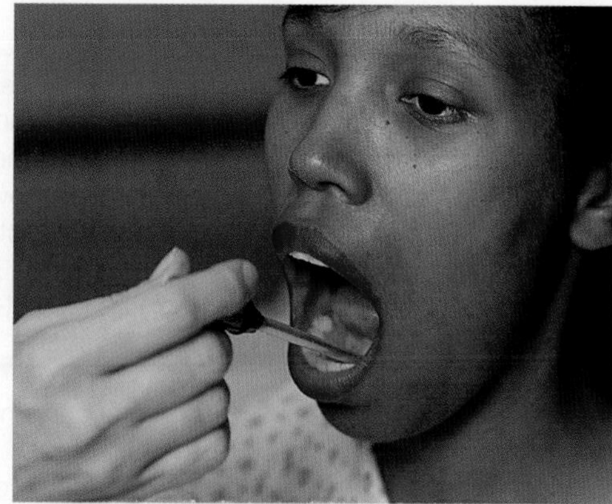

FIGURE 21.5 Measuring oral temperature. Place the tip of the thermometer under the tongue in the sublingual pocket. (From Potter, P.A., Perry, A.G., & Ostendorf, W. [2016]. *Nursing Interventions & Clinical Skills* [6th ed.]. St. Louis, MO: Mosby.)

MEASURING BODY TEMPERATURE

Clinical thermometers are used to measure the body temperature, and a growing number of different types are on the market. Thermometers made of glass with mercury-filled bulbs are not used anymore because if they are broken, they release mercury and its vapor, which are toxic. Glass thermometers are now filled with nonmercury material. Health facilities often use electronic digital thermometers; tympanic thermometers; temporal artery thermometers; and disposable, single-use thermometers.

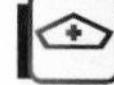 **Clinical Cues**

Before taking an oral temperature, be certain the patient has not eaten, drank fluids, or smoked within the previous 15 minutes, since this will cause an erroneous reading. A glass thermometer must remain in the sublingual pocket for 3 to 5 minutes to accurately reflect the body temperature.

Taking an Oral Temperature

The tip of the thermometer or probe with a plastic sleeve or probe cover should be placed in the sublingual pocket (Fig. 21.5). The patient should keep the tongue down, close the mouth, and keep the lips closed. Remove the cover before reading a glass thermometer.

Taking a Rectal Temperature

Provide privacy and ask the patient to turn to the side, facing away from you with the knees slightly flexed; drape the patient to reveal only the anal area. Don gloves and lubricate the tip of the rectal thermometer or probe; lift the upper buttock slightly so that the anus can be clearly seen. Insert the lubricated bulb into the rectum, directed toward the umbilicus, about 0.5 to 1.5 inches. Hold the thermometer in place for 3 to 5 minutes or until the correct temperature is indicated. Wipe the thermometer or probe from the stem toward the bulb or probe tip. Wipe the buttocks to remove lubricant or stool. Correctly dispose of tissues and gloves and perform hand hygiene.

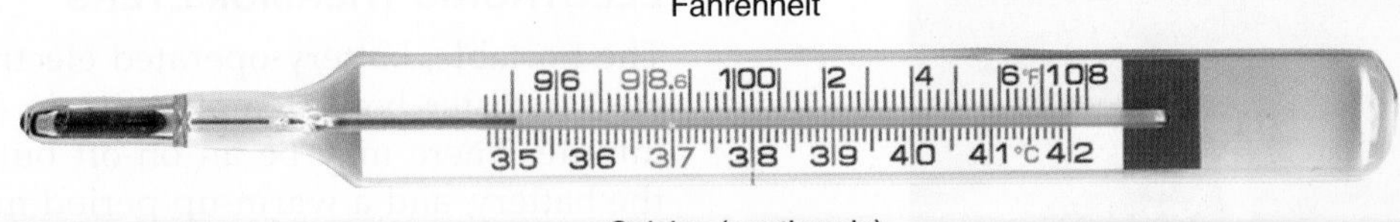

FIGURE 21.6 Nonmercury Geratherm glass thermometer. (Courtesy R.G. Medical Diagnostics, Southfield, Michigan.)

Taking an Axillary Temperature

Place the thermometer in the center of the patient's dry axilla (armpit). A wet axilla will produce a false reading. Ask the patient to hold the arm tightly against the chest. The arm may rest on the chest. Leave the thermometer in place for 3 to 8 minutes or until the thermometer indicates the reading is complete. Remove and wipe the thermometer clean from the stem to the tip.

GLASS THERMOMETERS

The glass thermometer has a bulb containing an alloy of elements called galinstan and a stem in which the substance can rise (Fig. 21.6). On the stem is a graduated scale representing degrees of temperature from 94°F to 106.8°F. (The range on a Celsius thermometer scale is 34°C to 43°C.) The alloy in the bulb expands when the bulb is in contact with body heat and registers on the scale in the stem. The bulb may be long and slender or blunt like the short, fat bulb used for rectal thermometers. Rectal thermometers often have a red tip or color on the stem to signify that they are for rectal use only and should not be used orally. Oral thermometers may be used to take axillary temperatures. All glass thermometers must have an alloy below the normal range before being used; this is accomplished by shaking down the alloy—that is, by holding the thermometer firmly by the distal glass end and flicking the wrist in a quick motion several times to bring the alloy down to the bulb. Glass style thermometers are being used less commonly than previously due to the risk of them breaking and the length of time it takes to use them.

Safety Alert

Glass Thermometers

A glass thermometer should not be used orally if the patient is unconscious, subject to seizures, confused, or agitated, because it might break if the patient bites on it. This thermometer should not be used orally on an infant or toddler who cannot hold it in the mouth properly or who might bite down on it. Rectal and oral thermometers must be kept separated so they are not confused. Glass thermometers are slippery when soapy; be especially careful when washing the thermometer. Glass thermometers may still be used in homes, since not all households will have other types of thermometers. Nurses should be able to teach parents how to read a glass thermometer (Fig. 21.7).

Reading the Glass Thermometer

Hold the thermometer horizontally at eye level and rotate it toward you until you can clearly see the column of alloy. Note where the end of the alloy is

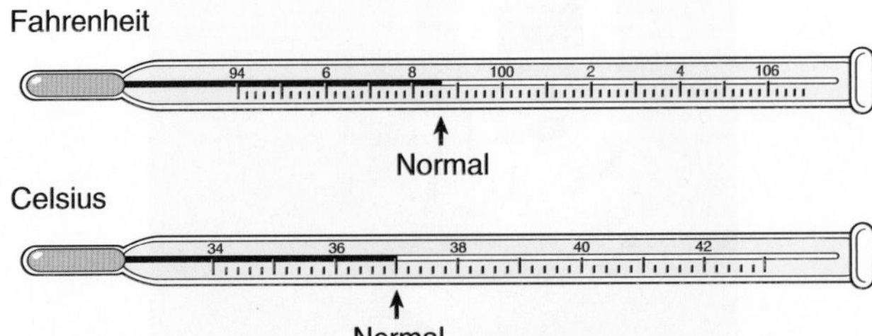

FIGURE 21.7 Reading the thermometer in Fahrenheit and Celsius.

on the lined scale. The stem of the galinstan alloy–in-glass thermometer contains the scale for measuring the temperature. The scale may be calibrated in either Fahrenheit or Celsius degrees, or it may have both scales. The Celsius scale has long lines indicating the degree and short lines for each one-tenth of a degree. In contrast, the Fahrenheit scale has an arrow marking the normal temperature of 98.6°F. Long lines on the scale represent each degree, but only the even-numbered degrees are written as 96°, 98°, 100°, and so on. Short lines between the degree lines represent two-tenths of a degree. All temperatures are recorded as ending in an even number when using this thermometer because it does not measure odd tenths of a degree. For example, one would read and record 99.2°F or 99.8°F but never 99.3°F or 99.7°F. To convert temperature from one scale to another, use these formulas:

$$\text{Fahrenheit to Celsius: } (\text{Fahrenheit} - 32) \times 5/9 = \text{Celsius}$$

$$\text{Celsius to Fahrenheit: } (\text{Celsius} \times 9/5) + 32 = \text{Fahrenheit}$$

Use lukewarm water to wash a glass thermometer, and rinse it with cold water. Oral and rectal thermometers should be stored separately to avoid confusing them.

Home Care Considerations

Taking the Temperature at Home

- Teach the home care patient or family to cleanse the thermometer by using a clean tissue and wiping with a twisting motion from the tip toward the bulb, and then washing it in warm, soapy water and rinsing with cold water.
- The thermometer should be disinfected in 70% to 90% isopropyl alcohol or a 1:10 solution of household bleach and water.
- The thermometer should be rinsed after disinfection, dried, and stored in a dry container.

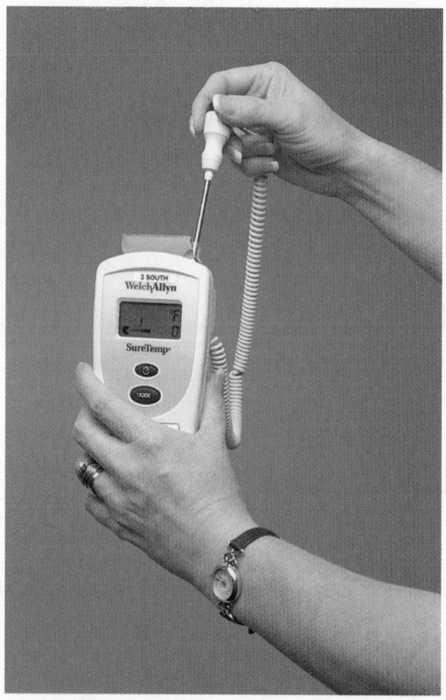

FIGURE 21.8 An electronic thermometer.

ELECTRONIC THERMOMETERS

The portable, battery-operated electronic thermometers register body temperature in 5 seconds to 1 minute. There may be an on-off button to activate the battery, and a warm-up period may be required (Fig. 21.8). The oral probe is placed in a plastic cover or sheath that is used one time and then discarded. The correct disposable probe cover and the correct setting should be used for the electronic thermometer when taking an oral or rectal temperature. The temperature is displayed digitally on a small screen on the handheld unit. The reading is in tenths of a degree, so temperatures taken with this unit may end in odd numbers, such as 99.5°F (37.5°C). Skill 21.1 describes the use of an electronic thermometer.

Tympanic Thermometers

These portable, battery-operated electronic thermometers register temperatures in 1 to 2 seconds. A switch on many units may be set for infant and toddler or for child and adult. The auditory canal

Skill 21.1 Measuring Temperature With an Electronic Thermometer

 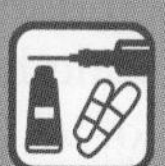 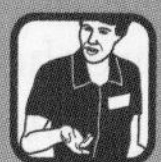  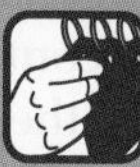 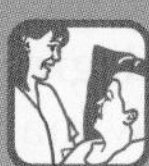 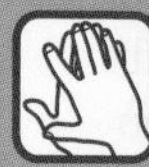 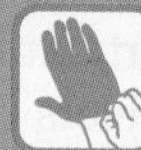

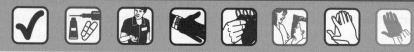

An electronic thermometer may be used to measure temperature, without worry about injury, for patients who are at risk for seizure disorders. If a rectal temperature is desired, a special rectal probe is used along with a rectal probe cover.

Supplies

- Electronic thermometer
- Probe covers
- Pencil and paper

Review and carry out the Standard Steps in Appendix A.

ACTION *(RATIONALE)*

Assessment (Data Collection)

1. Perform hand hygiene, identify the patient, and explain the procedure. Ask whether the patient has had anything to eat or drink in the past 15 minutes. *(Reduces transfer of microorganisms, ensures that correct patient is undergoing the procedure, and puts patient at ease. Eating, drinking, or smoking alters the temperature of the oral cavity.)*

Planning

2. Check to be certain there are probe covers in the container. Check the low battery light to ensure proper functioning of the thermometer. *(Probe must not be used without a cover. A low battery must be recharged or replaced to obtain an accurate temperature measurement.)*

Implementation

3. Remove probe from the unit, and push it down into a probe cover until a slight click is heard. *(The probe cover must be firmly in place for the unit to operate correctly.)*

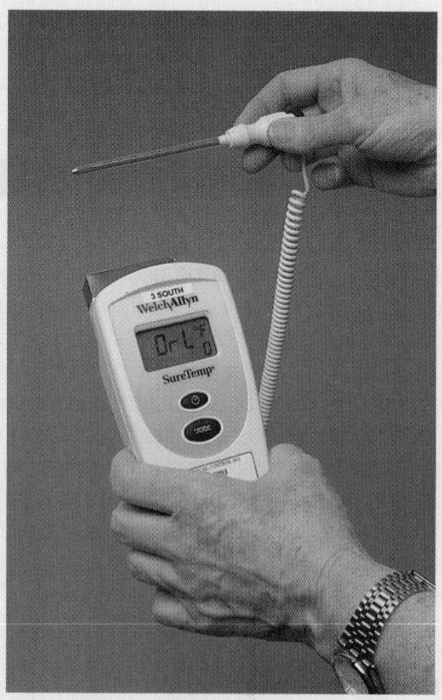

Step 3

4. Place probe under patient's tongue in the side sublingual pocket. Ask patient to close the lips

and keep them closed. *(The probe must be in contact with tissue rich in blood supply to obtain an accurate temperature.)*

5. Hold the unit steady, or allow the patient to hold it, and read the temperature on the screen when the light stops flashing or the unit beeps. *(Many units beep when the correct temperature is recorded. If probe is not positioned correctly, the unit will not beep or will refuse to register a temperature.)*

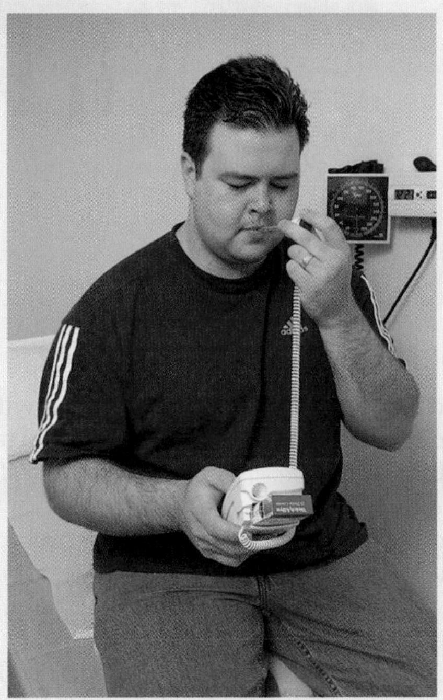

Step 5

6. Remove probe from the mouth, and discard the probe cover into the waste container by pressing the ejector button. *(Ejecting probe cover directly into the waste can prevent handling its contaminated surface. Probe covers are never reused. Be careful not to accidentally leave a probe cover in the bed.)*
7. Note the temperature, and clear the register by returning the probe to its holder. *(Returning the probe to its holder turns off thermometer and saves the battery.)*
8. Record patient's temperature on your worksheet. *(Noting the time and temperature on your worksheet makes it readily available when documenting.)*

Evaluation

9. Ask yourself: Is the temperature elevated? Is it higher or lower than the last reading? *(Provides data to determine trend of the temperature.)*

Documentation

10. Record the time and temperature on the graphic sheet or computer flow sheet. Record measures taken if the temperature was elevated in the nurse's notes. *(Verifies temperature was taken and makes measurement data available.)*

Documentation Example

6/18 1200 T 99.8°F.

Special Considerations

- If thermometer does not function, the probe cover may be loose. Remove the cover, insert the probe back into its storage location to reset, pull it out, and replace the cover, being certain it is snapped into place.
- A rectal probe attachment and probe cover may be used to take a rectal temperature if this probe is available.

Critical Thinking Questions

1. If the temperature reading obtained does not fit with the clinical symptoms and history, what would you do?
2. Many care providers think that using an electronic thermometer is more accurate than using a tympanic thermometer for an ill adult. What do you think is the reasoning behind this?

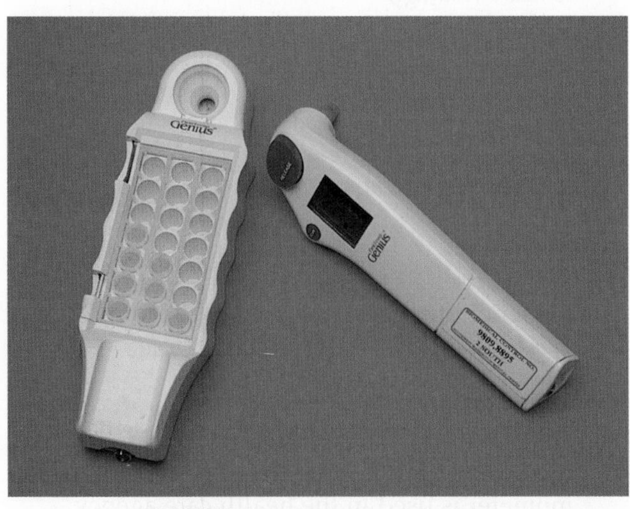

FIGURE 21.9 A tympanic thermometer.

probe is placed in a plastic cover that is used one time and then discarded. The temperature is displayed digitally on a small screen on the hand-held unit. The reading is in tenths of a degree and can be displayed in degrees Fahrenheit or Celsius (Fig. 21.9). Using a tympanic thermometer is explained in Skill 21.2.

Temporal Artery Skin Thermometer

The temporal artery thermometer is moved over the skin of the forehead over the temporal artery. It is an electronic thermometer that is fast and accurate. It is less invasive than the tympanic thermometer and more reliable when used correctly (see Fig. 21.4).

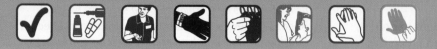

Skill 21.2 Measuring Temperature With a Tympanic or Temporal Artery Thermometer

 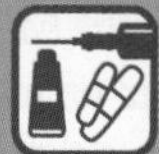 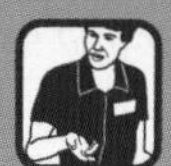 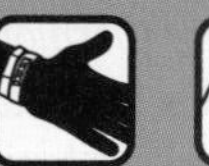 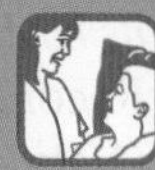 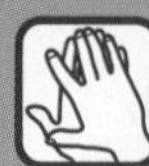 

When placed into the auditory canal, a tympanic thermometer produces a reading of core temperature. It is especially useful for measuring temperature in children. A temporal artery thermometer provides a more accurate reading, since positioning and wax in the ear canal may alter the tympanic reading.

Supplies

- Tympanic or temporal artery thermometer
- Probe covers
- Pencil and paper

Review and carry out the Standard Steps in Appendix A.

ACTION *(RATIONALE)*

For a Tympanic Thermometer

Assessment (Data Collection)

1. Determine reason for measuring the tympanic temperature. *(Tells whether measurement is routine or infection is suspected.)*

Planning

2. Check the low battery light. Set unit for the desired mode: infant-toddler or child-adult. *(If battery is low, the unit will not function. An inaccurate reading will be obtained if the wrong mode is used.)*
3. Check to see that there are probe covers in the container before going to the patient. *(Prevents an unnecessary trip to obtain the covers.)*

Implementation

4. Perform hand hygiene. *(Reduces transfer of microorganisms.)*
5. Remove probe from the unit and attach a probe cover. *(The probe cover must be securely in place to obtain a reading. A disposable cover prevents transmission of microorganisms from one patient to another.)*
6. Gently place probe in the ear canal until it seals the opening. Grasp the top of the pinna and gently pull up and back to straighten the ear canal of the adult if needed. Pull the lobe of the ear down or back to straighten the canal of a child under age 2 years if needed. Point probe slightly toward the face. *(Probe must be pointed at the tympanic membrane and be sealed in the canal for an accurate measurement. The auditory canal should be inspected for redness, swelling, discharge, or presence of cerumen [earwax] or a foreign body before insertion of probe.)*

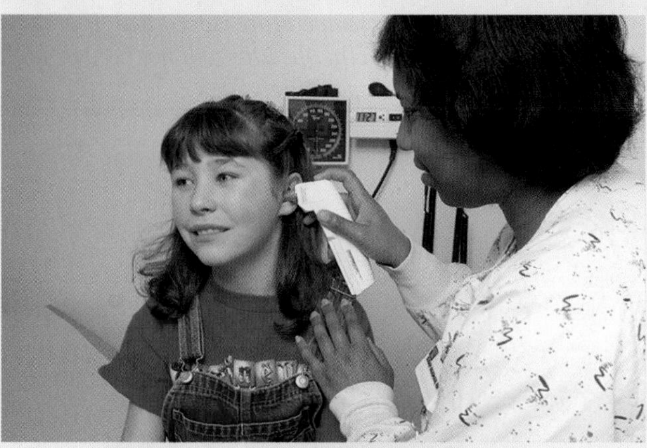

Step 6

7. Hold the unit steady. Steady the head with one hand if needed, and press the button to take the reading. *(Head movement will break the seal of the probe in the canal.)*
8. Read the temperature and remove probe. Praise a child for cooperating, if appropriate. *(Temperature will be displayed on the small screen on the unit when it has been obtained.)*
9. Discard probe cover in waste receptacle. *(Probe covers are contaminated and not designed to be reused.)*
10. Return thermometer to the base unit for recharge. *(Prepares for the next use.)*
11. Perform hand hygiene. *(Reduces transfer of microorganisms.)*

For a Temporal Artery Thermometer

12. Remove cover and place probe in the center of the forehead. Press the button to turn on thermometer. *(Positions thermometer properly and turns it on to take a reading.)*
13. Lightly slide probe across the forehead into the hairline. If perspiration is present, lift probe and touch on the neck just behind the ear. *(Perspiration may interfere with the reading.)*
14. Release the button; read the temperature. *(Measures the arterial temperature.)*

Evaluation

15. Ask yourself: Is the temperature elevated? Is it higher or lower than the previous reading? *(Provides data to determine temperature trend.)*

Documentation

16. Document the time and temperature on the medical record. If more than one type of thermometer is used in the health care agency,

designation of an aural temperature should be made. *(Notes that temperature was taken and makes measurement data available.)*

Documentation Example

6/18 1200 T 100.3°F.

Special Considerations

- A tympanic thermometer should not be used if the patient has an inflammatory condition of the auditory canal or if there is discharge from the ear.
- Moving the probe laterally back and forth with small movements assists in positioning the probe so that it seals the canal.

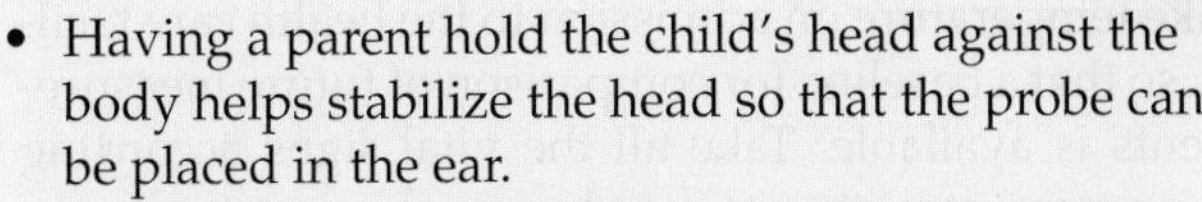

- Having a parent hold the child's head against the body helps stabilize the head so that the probe can be placed in the ear.
- Approaching the small child or very older adult patient with a slow, smooth movement after explaining what you are going to do decreases reflex "ducking."

Critical Thinking Questions

1. Will wax in an ear interfere with a tympanic thermometer reading? Why or why not?
2. If a 2-year-old child keeps turning his head away and squirming when you try to take a tympanic temperature, what would you do?

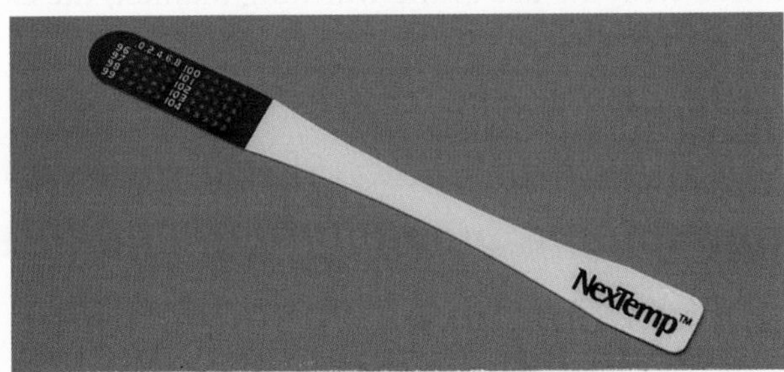

FIGURE 21.10 A disposable thermometer.

DISPOSABLE THERMOMETERS

Various types of single-use, disposable thermometers are available; among them are temperature-sensitive tapes that are placed on the forehead or abdomen to record the heat of the body. These are often used in newborn nurseries. Another type is the NexTemp thermometer (Fig. 21.10). The sensor end of the shaft contains a series of dots arranged so that each one changes color at a different temperature. Directions on the package explain how to use these thermometers. Most disposable thermometers register the temperature within 2 minutes.

❖ APPLICATION OF THE NURSING PROCESS

◆ ASSESSMENT (DATA COLLECTION)

Choose the appropriate site for temperature measurement based on the patient's age and condition and the type of thermometer available. Determine whether any factors might alter the temperature reading. The axillary or rectal method may be used when a tympanic or temporal artery thermometer is not available for patients who have wired jaws, who have a nasogastric tube in place and cannot breathe easily with the mouth closed, or who may have seizures.

Check the electronic thermometer battery before measuring the patient's temperature. A low battery may make the measurement inaccurate.

Choose the right mode (infant-toddler or child-adult) on the tympanic thermometer before measuring the patient's temperature. An inaccurate reading will result if the thermometer is not set properly.

Health Promotion/Health Promotion Points

Promoting Home Use of a Thermometer

When working with patients outside of the hospital setting, be certain that they own a thermometer and know how to use it. Many people do not own a thermometer. Teach the patient and family how to care for the thermometer.

◆ NURSING DIAGNOSIS

Nursing diagnoses for patients with alterations of normal temperature might be:

- Hyperthermia related to infection or excessive heat exposure.
- Hypothermia related to prolonged exposure to cold.
- Ineffective thermoregulation related to neurologic injury.

Abnormalities found on assessment of the other vital signs (pulse, respiration, blood pressure) may indicate problems in various body systems. When such findings remain abnormal, nursing diagnoses would be written that address those problems.

◆ PLANNING

Expected outcomes are written for each nursing diagnosis. For example,

- Patient's temperature will return to normal after 3 days of antibiotic therapy.
- Normal body temperature will be regained within 6 hours.
- Temperature will be maintained below 102.5°F with use of hypothermia blanket.

Further expected outcomes are written for nursing diagnoses, established by abnormalities in other vital signs.

◆ IMPLEMENTATION

Take temperature on admission to the health care facility so that a baseline for comparison of future measurements is available. Take all the vital signs according to primary care provider orders or agency standards. Other times the temperature should be taken are

- Every 4 hours when a known infection is present.
- Every 2 to 4 hours when a fever is present.
- When the patient is "not feeling right."
- When the patient is receiving drugs that may affect the temperature.
- Before surgery or an invasive procedure, then at regular intervals afterward as prescribed by hospital protocol.

Measures to reduce fever are presented in Box 21.3. Other interventions are presented in Nursing Care Plan 21.1.

Box 21.3 Nursing Interventions to Reduce Fever

- Encourage large fluid intake unless contraindicated.
- Lower the room temperature by adjusting the thermostat or opening doors or windows.
- Increase the rate of circulating air with a fan.
- Remove items of clothing or bed covers.
- Control or reduce the amount of body activity.
- Carry out the primary care provider's orders for cooling measures and supportive treatment: tepid sponge bath, cooling blanket, high-calorie diet and fluids, or medication to lower temperature and combat the disease.

◆ EVALUATION

To evaluate the plan's success, determine whether expected outcomes have been met. Evaluate measures to keep temperature within normal range by analyzing the trend of the temperature on the graphic record. A fever that is decreasing when the patient is receiving antibiotics for an infection is one indication that the antibiotic therapy is effective. For the hypothermic patient, if the temperature returns to normal with the use of the warming blanket, the expected outcomes are met.

Nursing Care Plan 21.1 Care of the Patient With Elevated Body Temperature

SCENARIO Mr. Hubert, age 76, came to the clinic with flu symptoms, malaise, and temperature elevation. He has been ill for several days.

PROBLEM/NURSING DIAGNOSIS *Temperature 102.2°F (39°C), chills*/Hyperthermia related to infectious process.

Supporting Assessment Data *Subjective:* "I feel terrible and I'm really weak." *Objective:* Temperature 102.2°F (39°C), flushed skin, skin warm to touch; pulse 98, BP 132/84, respiratory rate 26.

Goals/Expected Outcomes	Nursing Interventions	Selected Rationale	Evaluation
Patient's temperature will decrease 1°F within 8 hours.	Instruct to keep clothing and linen dry and to use only light clothing or linens.	Allows heat loss through conduction and convection.	*Is body covering kept to the minimum needed to prevent chilling?* Patient acknowledges instructions.
Patient's temperature will return to patient's baseline within 48 hours.	Advise to monitor temperature at home and to administer acetaminophen q 6 hours as ordered for temperature over 102.2°F (39°C).	Tracks temperature trend; antipyretic will reduce temperature.	*Does patient have a thermometer at home, and does he know how to use it?* States he will monitor his temperature with his thermometer.
	Instruct to limit activities and to increase frequency and length of rest periods until temperature is normal.	Activity increases metabolic rate, contributing to heat production.	*Does patient agree to limit his activities?* States he wants to go to church tomorrow but will stay home and rest.
	Instruct to increase oral fluid intake to at least 2000 mL/day with desired fluids.	Fluids will be insensibly lost and need to be replaced to lower temperature.	*Is patient willing to increase fluid intake?* States he has juice, tea, water, and soft drinks at home and will increase his intake.

CRITICAL THINKING QUESTIONS

1. If the patient's temperature continues to rise, what interventions would you suggest?
2. How does using only light bed covers and sleepwear or light clothing assist specifically in lowering the body temperature?

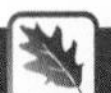 Life-Span Considerations

Older Adults

- The average temperature in the older adult is 96.5°F to 97.5°F (35.8°C to 36.4°C).
- Body temperature in the very older adult tends to be low in the morning on awakening, because of decreased metabolic rate and activity during sleep.
- The lack of subcutaneous fat allows the older adult's body to cool more readily than bodies of younger people.

Evaluation to determine whether expected outcomes have been met for nursing diagnoses related to abnormalities in the other vital signs includes measurements indicating that those vital signs are now within normal limits.

MEASURING THE PULSE

Each time the heart contracts to force blood into an already full aorta (artery leading from the heart), the arterial walls in the vascular system must expand to accept the increase in pressure. The pressure wave causing this expansion is called the pulse. By counting each pulsation of the arterial wall, you can determine the pulse rate.

COMMON PULSE POINTS

The pulse can be felt wherever a superficial artery can be held against firm tissue, such as a bone (see Fig. 21.2). The pulse is felt most strongly over the following areas:

- Radial artery in the wrist at the base of the thumb
- Temporal artery just in front of the ear
- Carotid artery on the front side of the neck
- Femoral artery in the groin
- Apical pulse over the **apex**, the pointed end of the heart
- Popliteal pulse behind the knee
- Pedal pulse of the posterior tibial artery on the inside of the ankle behind the malleolus, in the groove between the malleolus and Achilles tendon and dorsalis pedis on the anterior aspect (top) of the foot (see Fig. 21.12)

The radial artery in the wrist is most often chosen to **palpate** (feel) the pulse when taking vital signs. It is best found by placing the flat part of the first two fingers against the tendon, or cord, on the thumb side of the inner wrist and then rolling the fingers slightly outward into the little trough on the thumb side of the wrist. Skill 21.3 describes measurement of the radial pulse. When it is difficult to find or to count the radial pulse, the apical beat of the heart is counted for a full minute with the use of

Skill 21.3 Measuring the Radial Pulse

 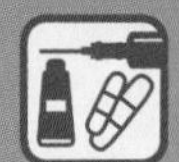 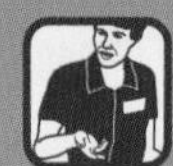  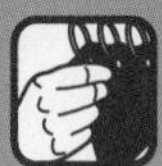 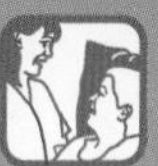 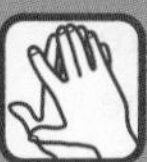 

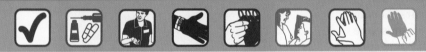

The radial pulse is measured whenever vital signs are taken. The pulse quality and character should be noted while the pulse is being counted. When the radial pulse is irregular, the apical pulse should also be taken.

Supplies

- Digital watch or watch with second hand
- Pen and paper

Review and carry out the Standard Steps in Appendix A.

ACTION *(RATIONALE)*

Assessment (Data Collection)

1. Identify the patient. *(Ensures pulse will be recorded for the correct person.)*

Planning

2. Explain the procedure. *(Puts patient at ease.)*

Implementation

3. Perform hand hygiene. *(Reduces transfer of microorganisms.)*
4. Place the pads of two or three fingers lightly over radial artery with patient's hand palm down. *(Fingers are used rather than the thumb because your thumb has a strong pulse that could be confused with that of the patient.)*

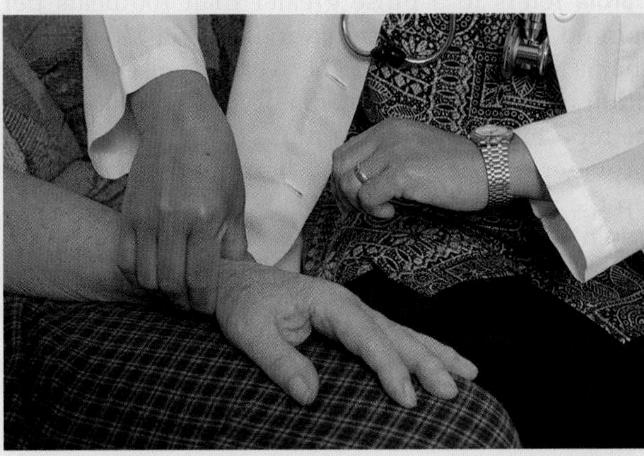

Step **4**

5. Begin with a beat, and count the next beat as "1." Count the pulsations for 30 seconds and multiply by 2 to obtain the rate per minute. Note regularity, strength, and character of the pulse. Whenever pulse is irregular, very rapid, or very slow, count for a full minute. *(If the first beat is counted "1," the total count will be inaccurate because you should count only each full cardiac cycle. Counting for 30 seconds rather than 15 provides a more accurate measurement of the pulse. Count for a full minute if there is an irregular heart rate.)*
6. Jot down the count. *(Prevents forgetting the result.)*
7. Perform hand hygiene. *(Reduces transfer of microorganisms.)*

Evaluation

8. Ask yourself: Is the result within normal range for the patient? Is the pulse slower or faster than previous readings? Has the patient ever had a pulse irregularity? *(Provide data regarding any alteration from normal for the patient.)*

Documentation

9. Record the time and pulse rate on the medical record. Note any abnormalities in quality or rhythm in the nurse's notes. Report abnormalities as appropriate. *(Notes pulse measurement and any abnormality.)*

Documentation Example

6/18 1200 P 92; irregular.

Special Considerations

- If the pulse is difficult to palpate, use lighter pressure. Change to the other wrist if there is still difficulty.

Critical Thinking Questions

1. If a radial pulse is difficult to feel or thready, how would you count the pulse?
2. If an adult patient's pulse rate is 105 bpm, what questions should you ask before assuming that this the patient has a heart problem?

a **stethoscope**. Count the apical pulse when it is important to have an accurate measure of the heart rate and when ordered by the care provider for patients with heart conditions. Routinely take an apical pulse before administering digitalis and beta blocker medication. The apical, rather than the radial, pulse is also taken on children younger than 2 years. Locate the apical heart sound by placing the stethoscope on a point midway between the imaginary line running from the middle of the left clavicle through the left nipple in the fifth intercostal space (Fig. 21.11; Skill 21.4).

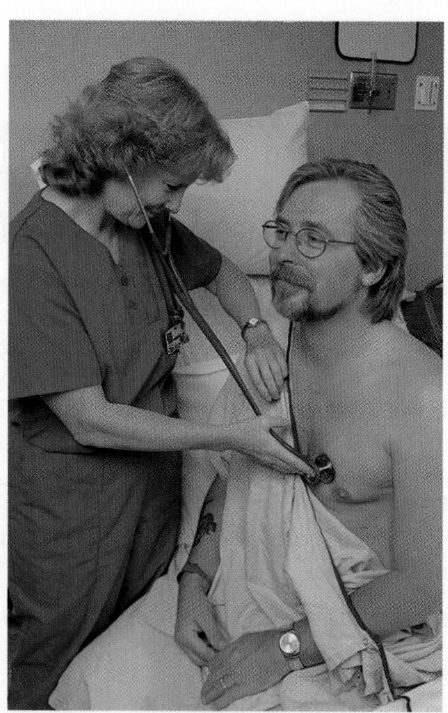

FIGURE 21.11 Counting the apical pulse.

PULSE RATE

The pulse rate varies widely and is influenced by a large number of factors (Table 21.2). The term **tachycardia** refers to a pulse greater than 100 beats per minute (bpm); **bradycardia** indicates a slow pulse that is less than 60 bpm. The average pulse rate in an adult is 72 bpm. Tachycardia or bradycardia should be reported to the charge nurse or the primary care provider. Medications may be prescribed to speed up the pulse when it is too slow or to slow it down when it is too fast. Table 21.3 shows average pulse rate by age.

Occasionally, you may need to take both a radial pulse and an apical pulse when the radial pulse is irregular, skips beats, or is difficult to count. This requires two people to count the radial and apical pulses at the same time to determine whether there is a **pulse deficit** (difference between the apical and radial pulse). The nurses use one watch visible to both when counting the apical-radial pulse and begin and end counting at the same time. One nurse counts the radial pulse and the other counts the apical pulse. The radial pulse subtracted from the apical pulse equals the pulse deficit.

As the blood travels farther away from the heart, the distinct wave of the pulse begins to fade, but the pulse can be palpated at the ankle or top of the foot.

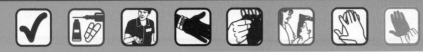

Skill 21.4 Measuring the Apical Pulse

 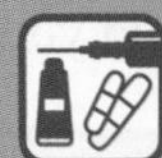 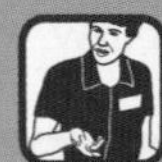 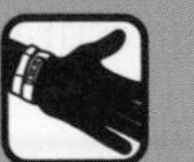  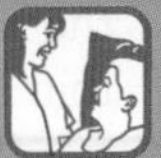 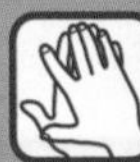 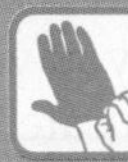

The apical pulse is measured during a physical examination; whenever the radial pulse is irregular; or when the patient has heart failure, has an arrhythmia, has had heart surgery, or is recovering from a myocardial infarction. An apical pulse measurement is required before the patient is given digitalis or beta blocker–type heart medication.

Supplies

- Stethoscope
- Digital watch or watch with second hand
- Pen and paper

Review and carry out the Standard Steps in Appendix A.

ACTION *(RATIONALE)*

Assessment (Data Collection)

1. Determine whether the patient has a known heart arrhythmia. *(Provides a baseline against which to compare the apical pulse.)*

Planning

2. Perform hand hygiene. Provide privacy; explain the procedure. Eliminate extraneous noise. *(Reduces transfer of microorganisms, protects patient's right to privacy, and puts patient at ease. Turning off TV and closing door provides a quieter environment.)*

Implementation

3. Expose left side of the chest. Warm the diaphragm of stethoscope in the palm of your hand for a minute or two. *(Sounds are transmitted through the stethoscope best if it is placed on bare skin. A cold stethoscope is unpleasant for the patient.)*

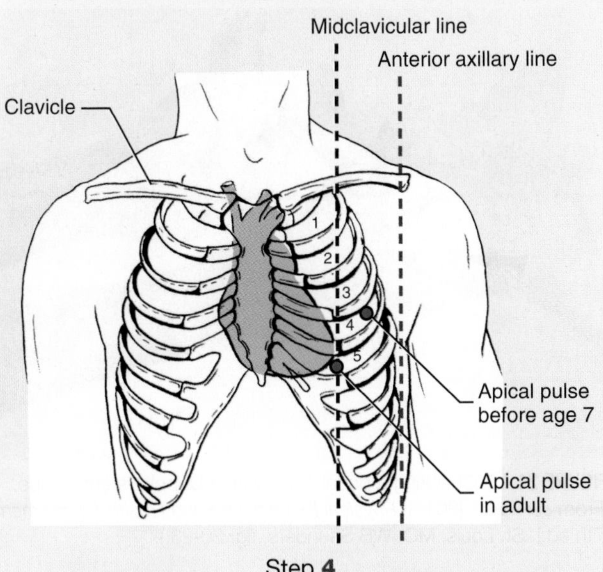

Step 4

4. Locate apex of the heart by palpating for the fifth intercostal space at the midclavicular line. *(The apex of the healthy heart is located at the fifth intercostal space, midclavicular line.)*
5. Listen to heart sounds with the diaphragm of the stethoscope. *(High-pitched heart sounds are heard best with the diaphragm. If sounds are not heard clearly, move stethoscope around slightly until sound is heard.)*
6. Count the number of beats for 1 minute. *(While counting, note rhythm and the strength of the beat.)*
7. Jot down the apical pulse. Cover the chest, make the patient comfortable, and restore the unit. *(Prevents chilling and protects privacy. Restore patient's personal belongings to their former places, place the call light at hand, and raise side rails if needed to provide for safety.)*
8. Perform hand hygiene. *(Reduces transfer of microorganisms.)*

Evaluation

9. Ask yourself: Was the apical pulse irregular? Has it been irregular before? Is this the same type of irregularity? *(Answers to questions provide further data regarding the patient's heart status.)*

Documentation

10. Note on the graphic record that the pulse was taken apically. If the apical pulse was irregular, note the finding in the nurse's notes. *(Identify the method by which the pulse was taken. Any abnormality should be documented in the nurse's notes.)*

Special Considerations

- An apical pulse is the preferred method of measuring the pulse in children under 2 years of age.
- Care should be taken not to frighten a patient if the radial pulse is irregular and you then take the apical pulse. Explain to the patient that you could not obtain an accurate count radially and wish to listen to the heart directly.
- Do not start counting the apical pulse until you can hear it clearly. This sometimes takes a few beats to tune the ear to the soft beat.
- If the sound is difficult to hear, ask the patient to lean forward to bring the heart closer to the chest wall.

Critical Thinking Questions

1. If your patient has a very thick chest and it is difficult to hear the apical pulse, how would you verify the heart rate you measured as being accurate?
2. When a patient's vital signs are being taken by an electronic vital signs monitor, can you be certain the heart rate is accurate? How would you verify that it is?

Table 21.2 Factors Affecting Pulse Rate

FACTOR	EFFECT
Age	The pulse rate gradually diminishes from birth to adulthood.
Body build and size	Tall, slender people may have a slower pulse rate than short, stout people.
Blood pressure	When the blood pressure rises, it causes a decrease in the pulse rate. When the blood pressure is lower, the pulse rate increases because the heart is attempting to increase the output of blood.
Drugs	Stimulants increase the pulse rate. Depressants decrease the pulse rate.
Emotions	Acute anxiety stimulates the sympathetic nervous system, increasing the heart rate.
Blood loss	Excessive blood loss, as with hemorrhage, increases the heart rate as the body tries to meet the tissue oxygen demands.
Exercise	Exercise increases the pulse rate because the heart pumps faster to meet circulatory needs.
Increased body temperature	The pulse rate increases at the rate of 7–10 beats for each degree of temperature increase.
Pain	Pain increases the pulse rate.

Table 21.3 Average Pulse Rates

AGE GROUP	AVERAGE PULSE RATE AT REST (BPM)
Normal pulse range	60–100
Some athletes	45–60
Adult male	72
Adult female	76–80
Child (age 5 years)	95
Child (age 1 years)	110
Newborn	120–160

Pedal pulses are checked to determine whether there is any blockage in the circulation in the artery up to that point, especially in patients who have had cardiac catheterization using the femoral artery for the insertion of the catheter or those who have had surgery on the leg. Mark an X on the skin over the spot where the pedal pulse is felt so that all staff can use the same location. When the pedal pulse is difficult to locate, a Doppler ultrasound stethoscope must be used (Fig. 21.12).

PULSE CHARACTERISTICS

When counting the pulse, note the rate, the rhythm, and the volume. **Begin timing with a beat that is not counted; the next beat is "1."** An **arrhythmia** (irregular pulse) has a period of normal rhythm broken by periods of irregularity or skipped beats. This can occur as a temporary condition from emotional stress or fright. A continuing arrhythmia may be indicative of heart disease or a medication's side effects and should be reported to the charge nurse or the primary care provider and recorded. Figure 21.13 shows various pulse rates and rhythms.

Health Promotion/Health Promotion Points

Monitoring of the Pulse by a Patient With a Heart Condition

If the patient has a known heart condition, teach him to take his own pulse correctly and to assess the pulse characteristics. Ask him to keep a log of his pulse rates. Inquire if he knows when or what he should report to the primary care provider.

The volume, or strength, of the pulse is just as important as the rate. With moderate pressure of the first two or three fingers on the vessel, a strong pulse will

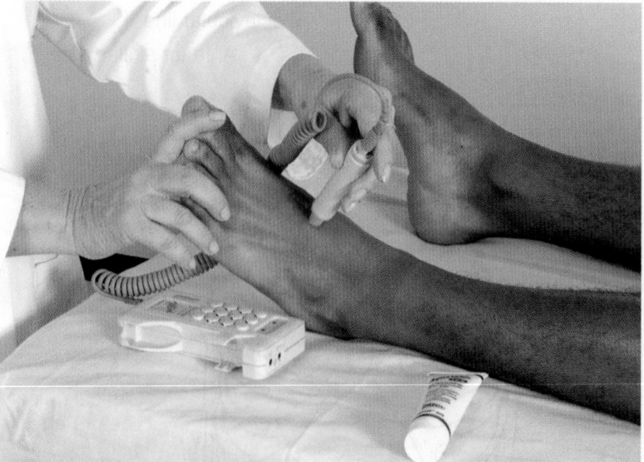

FIGURE 21.12 Checking a pedal pulse with a Doppler stethoscope. (From Jarvis, C. [2016]. *Physical Examination and Health Assessment* [7th ed.]. St. Louis, MO: WB Saunders, fig. 20-23.)

be felt regularly and with good force. Some of the most common terms to describe the strength of a pulse are:

- Weak and regular (even beats with poor force), or 1+
- Strong and regular (even beats with moderate force), or 2+
- Full and bounding (even beats with strong force), or 3+
- Feeble (barely palpable)
- Irregular (both strong and weak beats occurring within 1 minute)
- Thready (generally indicates that it is weak and may be irregular)
- Absent (no pulse palpable or heard on auscultation)

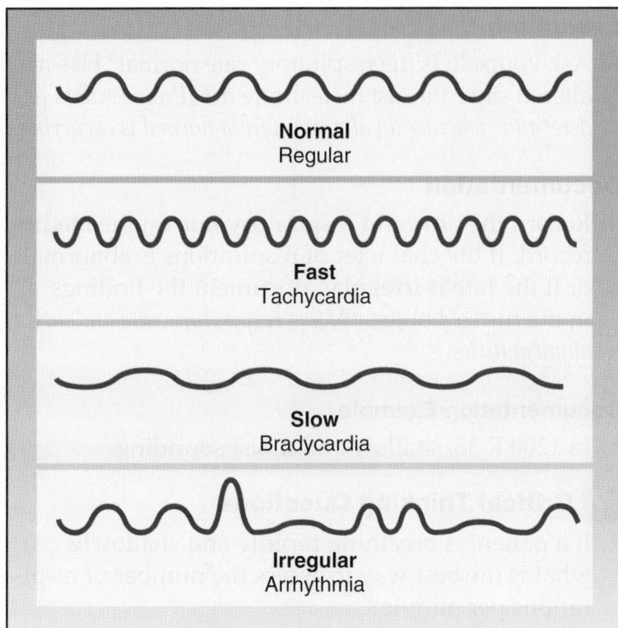

FIGURE 21.13 Pulse rhythms.

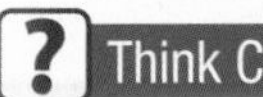

Think Critically

If an older adult patient who is receiving intravenous therapy had a pulse of 78 bpm, strong and regular, at 8 am and at noon the pulse is 84 bpm, full, and bounding, what might account for the change?

❖ APPLICATION OF THE NURSING PROCESS

Pulse rate and characteristics are assessment factors used to help determine cardiovascular health. Pulse abnormalities are defining characteristics for a variety of nursing diagnoses and are considered together with other assessment data. Changes in pulse rate are used for evaluation of the patient's response to different types of interventions, such as ambulation, bathing, dressing, or exercising.

MEASURING RESPIRATIONS

Respirations are measured each time a full set of vital signs is taken. **A change in respiratory rate may indicate a change in a patient's condition but is always considered along with the other vital signs and assessment data.** Count the respirations for 30 seconds and multiply by 2. In someone who is known to be very ill or who has irregular respirations, count for a full minute (Skill 21.5).

Skill 21.5 Five Measuring Respirations

 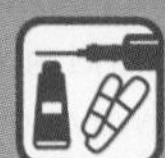 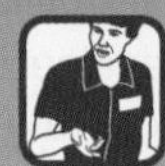 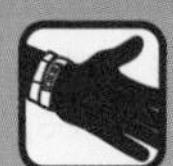  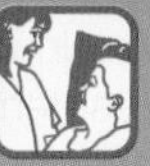 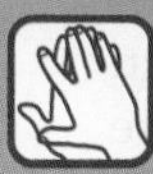 

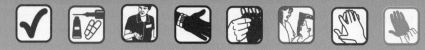

Respirations are measured each time vital signs are obtained. The depth and character of respirations, as well as the number of breaths per minute, should be noted. The most accurate measurement is obtained when the patient is unaware that you are counting respirations.

Supplies

- Digital watch or watch with second hand
- Pencil and paper

Review and carry out the Standard Steps in Appendix A.

ACTION (*RATIONALE*)

Assessment (Data Collection)

1. Look for a way to distract the patient while you count respirations. *(Respiration measurement is more accurate when obtained with the patient unaware of the procedure.)*

Planning

2. Plan to count the respirations after measuring the radial pulse as if you were still counting the pulse. *(May make the patient unaware that you are counting respirations.)*

Implementation

3. Perform hand hygiene, and tell the patient you are going to take the vital signs. *(Reduces transfer of microorganisms. Puts patient at ease.)*
4. After taking the radial pulse with the wrist lying on the chest, continue holding wrist while counting respirations or position your hand on the chest. Position the watch so that you can see both its dial and the rise and fall of the chest. *(Doing this makes it appear as if you are counting the pulse while you are watching the chest rise and fall. This strategy helps distract the patient from his breathing. Alternately, having*

your hand on the patient's chest allows you to feel the rise and fall of the chest so you can count the respirations.)

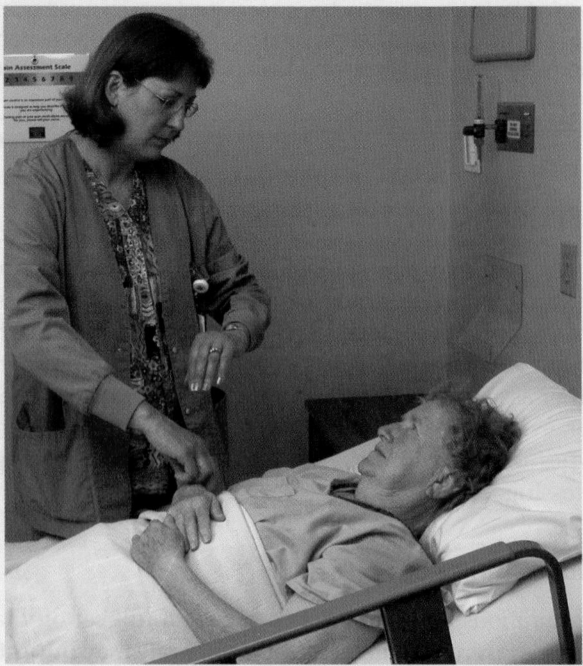

Step 4

5. Count the respirations, noting rate, depth, pattern, and sounds. Count for 30 seconds by the watch and multiply by 2 to get the rate for 1 minute. If respirations are irregular, count for a full minute. *(Recall that a respiration includes both inspiration and expiration. Thirty seconds is sufficient for an accurate count if respirations are regular.)*
6. Jot down the measurement along with the pulse rate. *(Prevents forgetting the count.)*
7. Perform hand hygiene. *(Reduces transfer of microorganisms.)*

Evaluation

8. Ask yourself: Is the respiratory rate normal? Has it altered since the last measurement? *(Provides data to determine whether an alteration from normal is occurring.)*

Documentation

9. Record the time and respiratory rate on the medical record. If the character of respirations is abnormal or if the rate is irregular, document the findings in the nurse's notes. *(Notes respiratory rate and any abnormalities.)*

Documentation Example

6/18 1200 R 36, shallow and moist sounding.

? Critical Thinking Questions

1. If a patient is breathing rapidly and shallowly, what is the best way to assess the number of respirations per minute?
2. What do you think is a better measure of a patient's respiratory status than counting respirations?

Many of the factors that affect the pulse rate also affect the respiratory rate because the heart and lungs are closely connected in providing oxygen to sustain life. Although the rate and depth of respirations are controlled by the respiratory center in the brain, they are easily influenced by emotions, pain, the degree of activity, age, fever, drugs, and disease conditions. The respiratory center is sensitive to changes in the carbon dioxide level in the blood and, to a lesser degree, in the oxygen level. Individuals can voluntarily control the rate and depth of respirations somewhat, as may happen when patients are aware that their respirations are being counted.

Respiratory rates vary according to age. Table 21.4 shows the normal range. The ratio of respirations to heartbeats is fairly constant at approximately 1 respiration to 4 heartbeats. In addition, the rate of respirations increases during fever as the body attempts to remove excess heat. Increased levels of carbon dioxide or lower levels of oxygen in the blood cause an increase in the respiratory rate to restore the chemical balance and expel the carbon dioxide. Head injury or any increased intracranial pressure depresses the respiratory center and results in shallow or slow breathing.

! Safety Alert

Certain drugs, such as narcotic analgesics and some sedatives, tend to depress the respiratory rate. Always monitor the patient's respiratory quality and rate when you administer narcotic analgesics and/or sedatives.

If an adult does not breathe at a minimal rate of 12 respirations per minute and in sufficient depth, some of the following symptoms of hypoxia may be noted as a result of low oxygen supply in the blood:

- Apprehension and restlessness
- Confusion, dizziness, and change in the level of consciousness
- **Cyanosis** (bluish discoloration) or skin color changes, particularly around the mouth and in the nail beds

RESPIRATORY PATTERNS

As respirations are being counted, observe for variations in the pattern of breathing (Fig. 21.14). **Eupnea** (a normal, relaxed breathing pattern) is effortless, evenly spaced, regular, and automatic. The inspiratory phase is a bit shorter than the expiratory phase. Changes from this normal pattern are described in a variety of ways.

Table 21.4 Normal Range of Respirations

AGE GROUP	RESPIRATIONS PER MINUTE
Older adult	16–20
Healthy adult	12–20
Adolescent	16–20
Child (age 3 years)	20–30
Infant (age 1 year)	20–40
Newborn	30–80

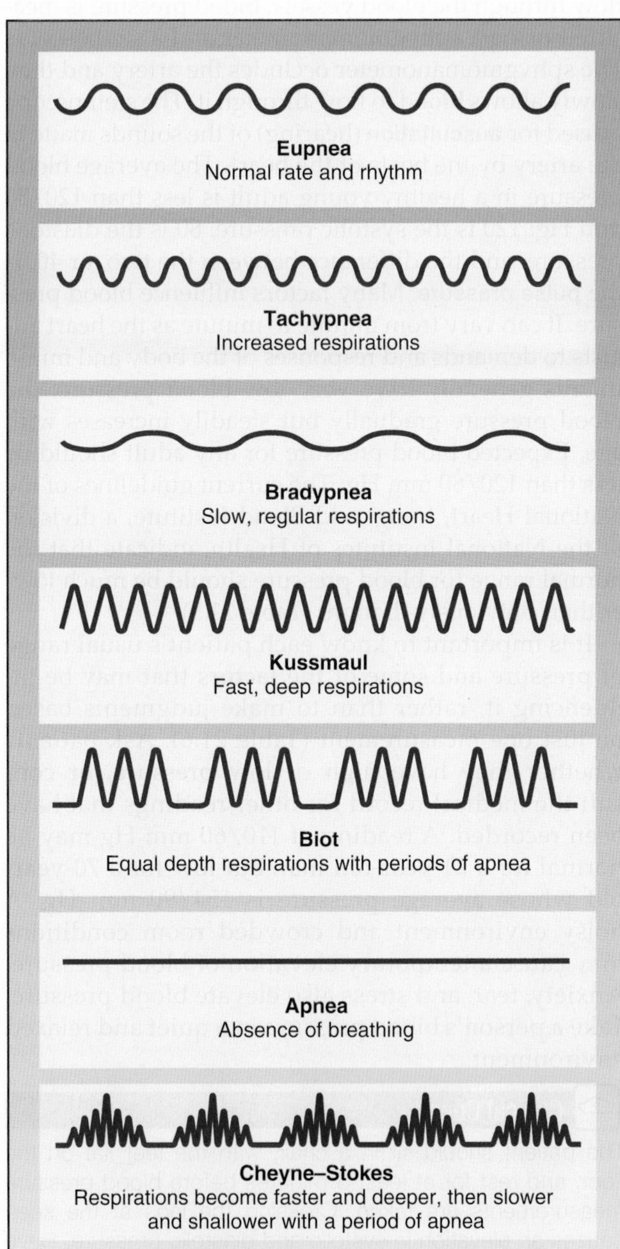

FIGURE 21.14 Respiratory patterns.

Dyspnea (difficult and labored breathing) is often accompanied by flared nostrils, anxious appearance, and statements such as "I can't get enough air." It is important to know how much activity causes the dyspnea: Does it occur when walking down the hall, trying to eat a meal, or even when trying to talk?

Tachypnea (increased or rapid breathing) results from the presence of fever and a number of diseases. Breathing rate increases about four breaths for each 1°F (0.5°C) increase in temperature.

Bradypnea (slow and shallow breathing) results when a limited amount of air is exchanged and less oxygen is taken in. This type of breathing often leads to **hypoxemia** (decreased levels of oxygen in the blood). It is often seen in patients who are under medical sedation, who are recovering from anesthesia or abdominal surgery, or who are in a weak or debilitated condition.

Hyperventilation is a pattern of breathing in which there is an increase in the rate and the depth of breaths and carbon dioxide is expelled, causing the blood level of carbon dioxide to fall. The condition is seen after severe exertion, during high levels of anxiety or fear, and with fever and conditions such as diabetic acidosis.

Kussmaul respirations have an increased rate and depth with panting and long, grunting exhalation. Kussmaul respirations are seen in patients with diabetic acidosis and renal failure.

Biot respirations are four to five breaths of equal depth alternating with irregular periods of **apnea** (absence of breathing). These respirations occur in patients with increased intracranial pressure. Such changes from the normal respiratory pattern of breathing should be reported to the charge nurse or the primary care provider so that appropriate treatment can be initiated.

Cheyne-Stokes respirations consist of a pattern of dyspnea followed by a short period of apnea. Respirations are faster and deeper, then slower, and are followed by a period of no breathing, with continuation of this cycle. This is seen in critically ill patients with brain conditions, in patients with heart or kidney failure, and in cases of drug overdose.

Some of the terms used to describe adventitious breath sounds (abnormal lung sounds) are:

- **Crackles**: Abnormal, nonmusical sound heard on auscultation of the lungs during inspiration; formerly called rales (sound like hair rubbed between the fingers next to the ear).
- **Rhonchi**: Continuous dry, rattling sounds heard on auscultation of the lungs caused by partial obstruction.
- **Stertor**: Snoring sound produced when patients are unable to cough up secretions from the trachea or bronchi.
- **Stridor**: Crowing sound on inspiration caused by obstruction of the upper air passages, as occurs in croup or laryngitis.

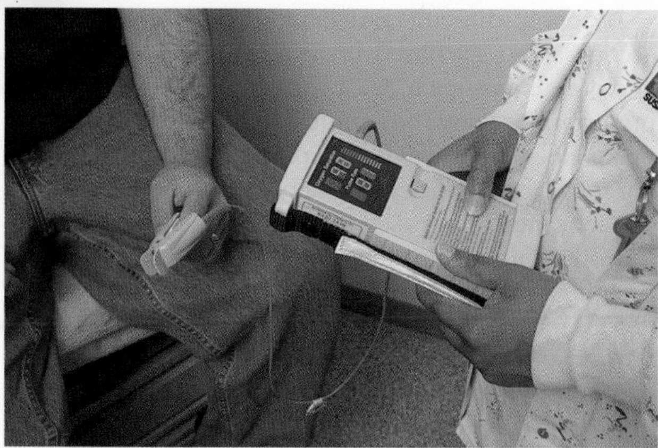

FIGURE 21.15 Measuring oxygen saturation with a portable pulse oximeter.

- **Wheeze**: Whistling sound of air forced past a partial obstruction, as found in asthma or emphysema.

Abnormal patterns of respiration are covered more fully in Chapter 28.

The respiratory rate and pattern must be analyzed together with other data such as breath sounds and arterial oxygen saturation to determine a patient's specific problem. Measurement of respirations may be performed to evaluate a patient's response to activity.

MEASURING OXYGEN SATURATION OF THE BLOOD

Another method of monitoring function of the respiratory system is pulse **oximetry** (measurement of oxygen). With a pulse **oximeter** (machine that measures oxygen in the blood), changes in arterial oxygen saturation can be tracked. Oxygen saturation may be spot-checked or continuously monitored (Fig. 21.15). The device measures oxygen saturation by determining the percentage of hemoglobin that is bound with oxygen. A sensor or probe is attached to an area of the patient through which infrared and red light can reach the capillary bed. Oxyhemoglobin absorbs more infrared than red light. A microprocessor in the monitor receives the information from the sensor probe, computes the saturation value, and displays it on the monitor screen. A finger or toe clip-on probe is most commonly used, but adhesive sensors can be applied to the nose or the forehead. A clip-on probe is available for use on an earlobe or an infant's foot.

Many agencies use a combination vital signs monitor and oximeter for scheduled vital sign measurements. The oxygen saturation is documented with the vital signs. Further information about pulse oximetry is found in Chapter 28.

MEASURING THE BLOOD PRESSURE

By measuring the blood pressure (BP), you obtain information about the effectiveness of the heart contractions, the adequacy of the blood volume in the system, and the presence of any obstruction or interference to flow through the blood vessels. Blood pressure is measured using a sphygmomanometer and a stethoscope. The sphygmomanometer occludes the artery and then slowly allows blood to flow through it. The stethoscope is used for **auscultation** (hearing) of the sounds made in the artery by the beats of the heart. The average blood pressure in a healthy young adult is less than 120/80 mm Hg: 120 is the systolic pressure, 80 is the diastolic pressure, and the difference between the two, or 40, is the **pulse pressure**. Many factors influence blood pressure. It can vary from minute to minute as the heart adjusts to demands and responses of the body and mind. Infants generally have very low blood pressure; the blood pressure gradually but steadily increases with age. Expected blood pressure for any adult should be less than 120/80 mm Hg. The current guidelines of the National Heart, Lung, and Blood Institute, a division of the National Institutes of Health, indicate that the normal range for blood pressure should be much lower than previously thought (Table 21.5).

It is important to know each patient's usual range of pressure and some of the factors that may be influencing it, rather than to make judgments based on just one measurement (Table 21.6). Ask patients whether they have high or low pressure, or consult the medical record for other readings that have been recorded. A reading of 110/60 mm Hg may be normal for a 21-year-old man but low for a 70-year-old whose average pressure is 154/90 mm Hg. A noisy environment and crowded room conditions may cause a temporary elevation of blood pressure. Anxiety, fear, and stress also elevate blood pressure. Take a person's blood pressure in a quiet and relaxed environment.

Table 21.5 Classification of Blood Pressure

CLASSIFICATION	SYSTOLIC BLOOD PRESSURE (MM HG)	DIASTOLIC BLOOD PRESSURE (MM HG)
Normal	<120	and <80
Prehypertension	120–139	or 80–89
Stage 1 hypertension	140–159	or 90–99
Stage 2 hypertension	≥160	or ≥100

Clinical Cues

The patient should sit in a chair, with the feet flat on the floor, and rest for at least 5 minutes before blood pressure measurements are taken. Crossing the legs at the knee causes an elevation in systolic and diastolic pressure. Have the patient rest supine for at least 1 minute before a supine measurement is taken. In either position, the arm should be elevated so that the brachial artery site for the reading is at the level of the right atrium. Prop the arm on a pillow when using the supine position.

Table 21.6 Factors That Influence Blood Pressure

FACTOR	INFLUENCE
Age	Newborns and infants have the lowest blood pressure, ranging from 75/50 to 100/70. Blood pressure increases with age. It is highest in older adults because of a decrease in the elasticity of vessels. However, a blood pressure reading above 140/90 mm Hg is not considered normal.
Stress and emotions	Stress, pain, and strong emotions raise blood pressure by releasing hormones and stimulating the sympathetic nervous system, leading to vasoconstriction and an increased heart rate. Regular exercise can lower stress levels.
Medication	Medications from several categories can be given to lower blood pressure, including diuretics, calcium channel blockers, ACE inhibitors, and many more. Other medications that lower blood pressure as a side effect include narcotics, tranquilizers, hypnotics, diuretics, antihypertensives, and certain cardiac medications. Medications that raise blood pressure include nonsteroidal anti-inflammatory medications (NSAIDs), antihistamines, migraine medications, weight loss drugs, and hormone therapy (estrogen and corticosteroids).
Diurnal variation	Blood pressure is typically lowest at night with sleep, gradually rises during the day with increased activity, and peaks midafternoon.
Sex	Starting at puberty, men tend to have higher blood pressure than women. After menopause, women tend to have higher blood pressure than men.
Exercise	Blood pressure increases with activity and exercise (especially weight training) as the sympathetic nervous system responds to an increased need for oxygen.
Body position	Blood pressure is lowest with lying down. It is slightly higher with standing because of sympathetic nervous system stimulation and baroreceptor activity.
Right vs. left arm	About one quarter of the population has a difference of 10 (±5) mm Hg between the right and left arms. A difference less than 10 mm Hg is not considered significant.
Vasodilation	Parasympathetic nervous system stimulation increases blood vessel lumen diameter, thereby lowering blood pressure. This may happen in response to warm temperatures, fever, and relaxation.
Vasoconstriction	Sympathetic nervous system stimulation decreases blood vessel lumen diameter, thereby raising blood pressure. This may happen in response to cold temperatures.
Head injury	Injuries to the head and increased intracranial pressure result in increased blood pressure and pulse pressure.
Reduced blood volume	Blood pressure decreases in response to inadequate blood volume, as from decreased cardiac output, hemorrhage, or shock.
Increased blood volume	Excessive fluid volume in the cardiovascular system increases blood pressure.

Sources: American Heart Association (2016). Types of blood pressure medications. <www.heart.org/HEARTORG/Conditions/HighBloodPressure/PreventionTreatmentofHighBloodPressure/Types-of-Blood-Pressure-Medications_UCM_303247_Article.jsp#.VpfBcVLm6eB; Charbek, E. (2015). Normal vital signs. http://emedicine.medscape.com/article/2172054-overview

Mayo Clinic Staff (2015). High blood pressure (hypertension). www.mayoclinic.org/diseases-conditions/high-blood-pressure/basics/definition/con-20019580; Shaw, B.H., & Protheroe, C.L. (2012). Sex, drugs and blood pressure control: The impact of age and gender on sympathetic regulation of arterial pressure. J Physiol, 590(12), 2841-2843.

EQUIPMENT USED FOR MEASURING BLOOD PRESSURE

Although direct measurement of blood pressure with an arterial catheter is the best method, the **sphygmomanometer** (device used to indirectly measure blood pressure) with an occlusive cuff and the stethoscope are commonly used pieces of equipment for measuring blood pressure (Fig. 21.16). Two types of manometers were traditionally used in clinical settings: the mercury gauge, when greater accuracy is needed, and the aneroid gauge, which is a smaller unit and easy to carry but less accurate. Many hospitals in the past had manometers attached to the wall in each patient's room. Mercury has been designated as a biohazard, and its use in medical equipment is being phased out. The aneroid type is prone to mechanical alterations that affect the accurate calibration of the device. Aneroid sphygmomanometers should be recalibrated every 6 to 12 months.

Electronic vital sign monitors are replacing both the aneroid type and mercury manometers in hospitals. An electronic sphygmomanometer takes the blood pressure almost automatically. The cuff is placed on the arm or wrist and pumped up. As the air is released, the systolic and diastolic pressures are displayed on a screen in the unit. This model does not require the use of a stethoscope for listening to pressure sounds, but it is much more expensive than the traditional manometer. The traditional manometer consists of a gauge for measuring the blood pressure;

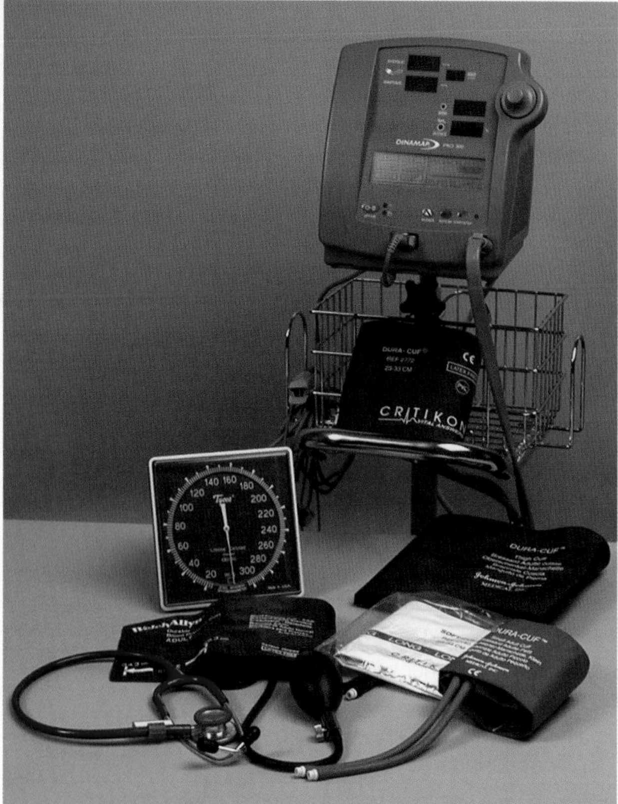

FIGURE 21.16 Equipment for measuring blood pressure. *Left,* Aneroid sphygmomanometer. *Right,* Electronic sphygmomanometer. *Front,* Stethoscope.

tubing running from the gauge to a cuff, which is wrapped around the arm or leg; and a control bulb that inflates and deflates the cuff. This sphygmomanometer is particularly useful for home monitoring. Many nurses are becoming reliant on the electronic sphygmomanometer, but it will not give nurses the opportunity to hear the pulse and identify an arrhythmia or other abnormality, as they could if using manual manometers.

The cuff must be the correct size to obtain an accurate blood pressure reading. A narrow cuff is used for small children, and a wider cuff is needed for muscular or obese people. Using the wrong size produces errors as great as 25 mm Hg. The proper width is 21% larger than the diameter of the arm, and the inflatable bladder should go around at least three-fourths of the arm. A standard acoustic stethoscope with Y tubing, soft ear tips, and a diaphragm head is satisfactory for taking vital signs (Skill 21.6).

Clinical Cues

Always use the markings on the cuff to measure the arm-to-cuff width to verify that the cuff is the correct size. If in doubt, use a larger cuff, since cuffs that are only slightly too large will not alter the readings. If the sounds are very faint, try using the other arm, or use a Doppler stethoscope to amplify the sounds so that accurate readings occur.

Skill 21.6 Measuring Blood Pressure

 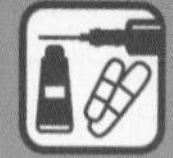 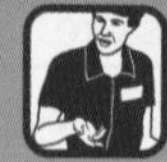  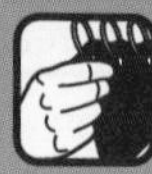 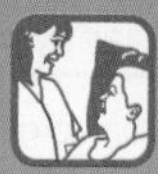  

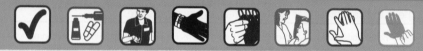

Blood pressure is measured each time vital signs are taken. Trends in blood pressure are monitored to detect early signs of complications from surgery, illness, or trauma.

Supplies

- Stethoscope
- Sphygmomanometer with correct size cuff
- Pencil and paper

Review and carry out the Standard Steps in Appendix A.

ACTION *(RATIONALE)*

Assessment (Data Collection)

1. Identify the patient. Check to see the patient's typical blood pressure. *(Ensures that blood pressure is recorded for the correct person. Knowing the usual pressure assists in knowing how high to inflate the cuff.)*
2. Assess the size of patient's arm to determine cuff size needed. *(The bladder of the cuff should cover two-thirds of the upper arm circumference.)*
3. Assess whether there is a contraindication to taking the blood pressure on either arm. *(If a patient has had a mastectomy, a serious injury, or a lymph node dissection, or has an intravenous line or a dialysis shunt on one arm, use the arm on the other side. If both arms are contraindicated, use a thigh cuff on a leg.)*

Planning

4. Provide privacy and reduce environmental noise. Explain the procedure and perform hand hygiene. *(A quieter environment allows you to hear blood pressure sounds more accurately. Explaining procedure puts patient at ease. Hand hygiene reduces transfer of microorganisms.)*
5. Place patient in a comfortable position, sitting down with feet on the floor or lying down, and allow blood pressure to stabilize for 5 minutes before measuring it. *(Position changes alter hemodynamics within the body; blood pressure stabilizes within 5 minutes.)*

Implementation

6. Apply cuff smoothly to patient's arm, positioning the center of the bladder over the brachial artery and placing cuff 1 to 2 inches above the antecubital space. Wrap cuff firmly and smoothly around the arm and fasten it. Alternatively, position cuff over the popliteal artery on the underside of the thigh. *(Center of the cuff's bladder must be over the brachial or popliteal artery for an accurate measurement.)*

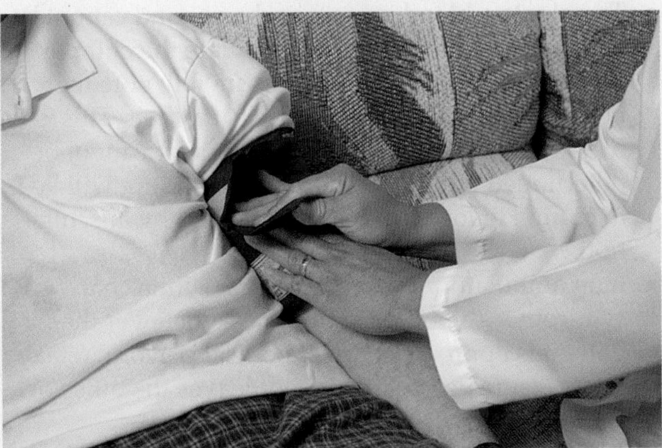

Step 6

7. Position gauge so it can be easily visualized. *(Straining to see lines on the gauge may cause an inaccurate reading.)*
8. Position and support patient's arm or leg at heart level. *(An arm or leg positioned above or below heart level may cause an inaccurate reading.)*
9. Close the valve of the air pump by turning the screw valve clockwise until closed, but not so tightly that it cannot be easily released. *(Closing the valve directs airflow into the cuff when the bulb is squeezed.)*

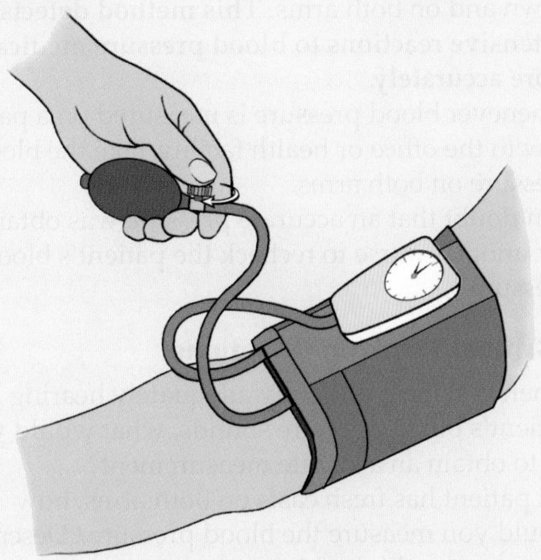

Step 9

10. Palpate the brachial or popliteal artery for the strongest pulse area. Pump up the cuff until the artery is occluded, then release the valve and let the air out of the cuff. Radial artery may be palpated instead of brachial. *(Locating the pulse before pumping up the cuff is essential to determine the approximate level of the systolic pressure. Locating where pulse is strongest over brachial artery allows placement of stethoscope to best hear the sounds.)*

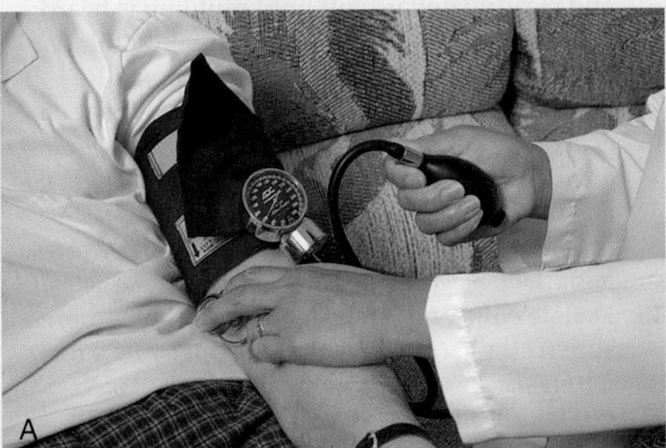

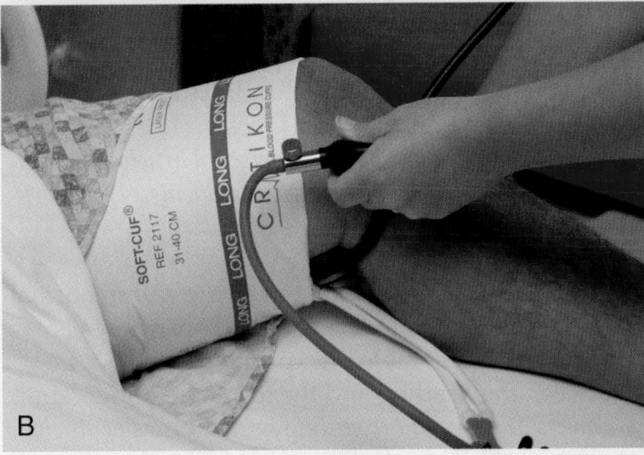

Step 10

11. Direct earpieces of the stethoscope slightly forward, and place them in your ears. Place diaphragm or bell of the stethoscope over the brachial or popliteal pulse. *(The bell is smaller and fits more closely over the skin than the diaphragm. When the bell is used, it should be only lightly applied to the skin. The diaphragm must be held firmly in contact with the skin to hear sounds clearly.)*
12. When 30 seconds have passed, reinflate the cuff quickly, while watching the gauge, to at least 30 points higher than the point at which you can no longer feel the pulse. *(Ensures cuff is inflated to a point above the patient's systolic blood pressure and prevents missing an auscultatory gap [period where sound disappears]. Keeping the mercury column at eye level gives a more accurate reading. The aneroid gauge should be read with the eyes directly over or in line with it.)*

13. Deflate cuff at a constant rate of 2 mm Hg/second by unscrewing the valve on the bulb pump counterclockwise. *(Deflating too rapidly or too slowly gives false readings. Avoiding contact of the stethoscope tubing with the clothing, cuff, or tubing of the sphygmomanometer decreases the possibility of extraneous noise.)*
14. Listen for the first Korotkoff sound, and note this as the systolic blood pressure. Continue to listen and steadily deflate cuff until muffling is heard; note this point. Continue deflating until the last Korotkoff sound is heard; note this point. Replace the patient's clothing if needed. *(The point of muffling of Korotkoff sounds is considered the most accurate measurement of blood pressure in children; the point at which the last Korotkoff sound is heard is considered most accurate for adults. If sleeve was pushed up, replacing it shows courtesy to the patient.)*
15. Deflate cuff completely. Jot down the blood pressure reading. *(Deflating prepares cuff for next use. Jotting the measurement on your worksheet makes it readily available when recording in the medical record.)*
16. Perform hand hygiene. *(Reduces transfer of microorganisms.)*
17. If you turned off the TV or radio, turn it back on. Restore the unit as it was. *(Shows courtesy and caring to the patient. Replacing personal articles and call light within reach helps prevent accidents.)*

Evaluation

18. Ask yourself: Is the blood pressure within normal range? Is it elevated? Is it dangerously low? Is there a considerable unexplained difference between this reading and the former reading? *(Answers provide data regarding further assessments that may need to be made. Excessively high or low pressure should be reported to primary health care provider.)*

Documentation

19. Document the time and pressure on the graphic sheet; record any new abnormality in the nurse's notes with your assessment. Blood pressure is recorded with the systolic pressure as the top number of a fraction and the diastolic pressure as the bottom number. *(Demonstrates blood pressure trend and communicates any abnormality.)*

Documentation Example

6/18 1200 BP 136/84. (If muffling occurs, record as 136/92/84. If thigh cuff is used, note that it is a thigh blood pressure.)

Special Considerations

- Use appropriate cuff size with the bladder of the cuff covering two-thirds of the arm circumference. Three sizes should be available: pediatric, adult, and large adult. A poorly fitting cuff provides an inaccurate measurement.
- When using a thigh cuff, wrap the cuff about 2 inches above the knee. Place the stethoscope over the popliteal artery. Turn the patient onto the abdomen, if possible.
- To palpate a blood pressure when sound cannot be heard, locate the radial pulse, inflate the cuff per usual routine, and let the pressure fall; note the point at which the radial pulse is first felt. This is the systolic pressure; diastolic pressure cannot be determined by this method. This measure will be 2 to 5 mm Hg lower than that obtained by auscultation.
- If an ambulatory care patient has "white coat syndrome" (blood pressure rises whenever the patient is approached by a medical person), retake the pressure before the patient leaves the office or clinic.
- Teach hypertensive patients the importance of monitoring their blood pressure frequently.
- Encourage the purchase of a home blood pressure unit.
- If a wrist blood pressure monitor is used, advise that the wrist must be positioned at the level of the heart for accuracy. An arm monitor is preferred, since it is more accurate.
- Digital blood pressure monitoring systems with large number readouts are available for older adults with poor vision.
- An older adult with hypertension should regularly be checked with the patient standing and lying down and on both arms. **This method detects hypotensive reactions to blood pressure medication more accurately.**
- Whenever blood pressure is measured on a patient new to the office or health facility, take the blood pressure on both arms.
- If in doubt that an accurate pressure was obtained, ask another nurse to recheck the patient's blood pressure.

? Critical Thinking Questions

1. When you have difficulty adequately hearing a patient's blood pressure sounds, what would you do to obtain an accurate measurement?
2. If a patient has fresh casts on both arms, how would you measure the blood pressure? Describe how you would do this.

Box 21.4 Guidelines for Measuring Blood Pressure

To obtain an accurate reading and to avoid problems that lead to errors, use the following guidelines when measuring blood pressure:

- Have the patient lie down or sit and rest for 5 minutes. If sitting, the patient should keep the feet flat on the floor.
- Use the brachial artery in the elbow joint of either arm. The arm should be supported on a surface at the level of the heart.
- Check the condition of the equipment, and position the manometer gauge so it can be seen at eye level from a distance of 1 to 3 feet. The gauge indicator should be at zero when the cuff is deflated. Use the correct cuff size.
- Bare the arm, and place the cuff and stethoscope directly on the skin. Bunched or wrinkled clothing prevents the correct cuff placement.
- Palpate the brachial or radial artery before taking the blood pressure when the patient is new to you. Inflate the cuff while palpating the artery and note the level at which the pulse disappears. Deflate the cuff. Wait 30 to 60 seconds before reinflating for the auscultated readings. (For repeated measurements on familiar patients, you may forgo the palpated pressure, but inflate to 10 to 20 points above the person's usual systolic reading.)
- Make certain the diaphragm of the stethoscope is placed firmly but lightly over the artery or the bell is placed lightly. All surface edges of the diaphragm should be in contact with the skin. Do not place the thumb over the bell or top of the stethoscope to hold it in place; use your index finger and ring finger on the base of the diaphragm.
- Inflate the cuff to 30 mm Hg above where the pulse disappeared on palpation with inflation to prevent missing an auscultatory gap (period when no sound is heard).
- Allow the cuff to deflate very slowly at 2 mm Hg/second. Any faster causes erroneous readings of both systolic and diastolic pressure.
- Once the cuff is starting to deflate, continue to deflate slowly all the way to zero. Do not stop midway and begin to inflate again, since this gives a false reading.
- Listen for the different sounds while steadily deflating the cuff, and identify the systolic and diastolic pressures. The phase I sound is the systolic pressure; the disappearance, or phase V, sound is the diastolic pressure. If the sound persists down to zero, then indicate the point at which the phase IV sound occurred and record all three numbers, as in this example: 130/62/0 (see Skill 21.6).

KOROTKOFF SOUNDS

While measuring blood pressure, you may hear certain sounds that relate to the effect of the blood pressure cuff on the arterial wall. These sounds, called **Korotkoff sounds**, were identified by a Russian surgeon and are numbered as follows:

Phase I: Tapping—Systolic pressure indicated by faint, clear tapping sounds that gradually grow louder

Auscultatory gap: No sound—Silence as cuff deflates for 30 to 40 mm Hg; common with hypertension

Phase II: Swishing—Murmur or swishing sounds that increase as the cuff is deflated

Phase III: Knocking—Louder knocking sound that occurs with each heartbeat

Phase IV: Muffling—A sudden change or muffling of the sound (indicates diastolic pressure in children and some adults)

Phase V: Silence—Disappearance of sound (marks diastolic pressure in adults)

It is important to continue to listen until the cuff is deflated so that you do not mistake an auscultatory gap for the last Korotkoff sound. Follow the guidelines in Box 21.4 when measuring the blood pressure.

When the blood pressure cannot be determined by auscultation, the palpation method is used to estimate systolic pressure. Diastolic pressure cannot be measured this way. With the blood pressure cuff in place on the upper arm, palpate the radial artery. Inflate the blood pressure cuff 30 mm Hg above the point at which the radial pulse disappears. Release the valve and allow mercury to fall 2 mm Hg/second, noting the point on the manometer when the radial pulse is again felt.

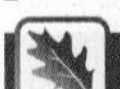 **Life-Span Considerations**

Older Adults

- It is wise to always first palpate the artery to detect at what level on the manometer no pulse is felt before taking the blood pressure of an older adult.
- Many older adults with hypertension have an auscultatory gap in their Korotkoff sounds. If you simply pump up the cuff until you do not hear any sound and then let air out of the cuff, you may miss the upper point of the systolic blood pressure.

HYPERTENSION

Pressure consistently elevated above 140 systolic and/or 90 diastolic is called **hypertension**. Hypertension is more common in African Americans, who get it earlier and more frequently than Caucasian or Hispanic Americans. Other risk factors include older age, obesity, unhealthy lifestyles, and long-lasting stress. Men and women are equally affected; however, before age 45 men get hypertension more frequently, whereas after age 65, women are affected to a greater degree (National Heart, Lung, and Blood Institute, 2012). Some people may have hypertension without any risk factors. **Prolonged hypertension can cause permanent damage to the brain, the kidneys, the heart, and the retina of the eye. It is the cause of many strokes.**

Life-Span Considerations

Older Adults

- The pulse pressure of the older adult person is often widened because systolic pressure tends to rise with age more quickly than diastolic pressure.
- The older adult often experiences **orthostatic hypotension** (drop in blood pressure when arising to a standing position) because the elasticity of the blood vessels decreases with old age. This predisposes them to pooling of blood in the lower extremities on standing and may cause dizziness. These patients are at risk for falls. Placing special elastic stockings on the lower extremities may lessen the problem.

A systolic pressure 140 mm Hg or higher and a diastolic pressure 90 mm Hg or higher are regarded as being outside of the normal range (hypertension). Prehypertension is a systolic pressure above 120 mm Hg and a diastolic pressure above 80 mm Hg. A large study was recently stopped early because it demonstrated that lowering systolic blood pressure to 120 instead of the recommended 140 reduced rates of heart attacks and strokes by 30% and deaths by 25% in people over age 50 (AJN, 2015). Blood pressures consistently higher than these should be reported to the charge nurse or the primary care provider if the patient usually has normal blood pressure.

Health Promotion/Health Promotion Points

Promoting Home Blood Pressure Monitoring

If the patient has been diagnosed with hypertension, encourage home monitoring of his blood pressure. Have him obtain a sphygmomanometer that is reliable, and teach him to use it properly. Readings should be documented and tracked for changes.

The Healthy People 2020 overarching goal (Chapter 2) to attain high quality, longer lives free of preventable disease, disability, injury, and premature death includes the following objectives concerning elevated blood pressure:

- Increase the proportion of adults with hypertension in clinical health systems whose blood pressure is under control.
- Increase the proportion of adults who have had their blood pressure measured within the preceding 2 years and can state whether their blood pressure was normal or high.
- Reduce the proportion of persons in the population with hypertension.
- Increase the proportion of adults with prehypertension or hypertension who meet the recommended guidelines for body mass index, saturated fat consumption, sodium intake, physical activity, and moderate alcohol consumption.
- Increase the proportion of adults with hypertension who are taking the prescribed medications to lower their blood pressure.

 Think Critically

Why are several blood pressure readings required before a diagnosis of hypertension can be made?

HYPOTENSION

Low blood pressure is called **hypotension**. Some people have blood pressure that is normally below 90/60 mm Hg, and they are healthy with no other symptoms. However, hypotension with symptoms of **shock** (circulatory collapse) is a dangerous condition that can rapidly progress to death unless treated. Shock is caused by hemorrhage, vomiting, diarrhea, burns, and myocardial infarction, among other conditions.

Signs and symptoms of shock include a decrease in blood pressure, an increase in pulse rate, cold and clammy skin, dizziness, blurred vision, and apprehension. Report such signs and symptoms to the charge nurse or the primary care provider without delay, and assist in treating the shock. See Chapter 37 for information about shock and its treatment.

Some patients experience postural or orthostatic hypotension (drop in blood pressure occurring with change from supine to standing or from sitting to standing position) from drug therapy, a neurologic problem, or dehydration. Blood pressure should be taken in both the standing and sitting positions for these patients. A drop of 15 to 20 mm Hg from the patient's normal baseline pressure combined with symptoms of faintness, blurred vision, dizziness, or syncope signifies orthostatic hypotension. It is caused by a failure of vasomotor compensatory mechanisms in response to position changes or to baroreceptor reflex impairment (Box 21.5).

❖ APPLICATION OF THE NURSING PROCESS

Blood pressure measurements are considered along with the pulse rate in evaluating the general health of the cardiovascular system. Abnormalities such as hypotension, hypertension, and narrow or wide pulse pressure are defining characteristics for various nursing diagnoses and are considered along with other assessment data when choosing an appropriate diagnosis. Blood pressure is often assessed to determine how the patient is responding to a procedure or to drug treatment. This measurement is used to evaluate the patient's response to medication for hypertension. It is an important measurement in evaluating cardiovascular disease and in monitoring for shock.

Box 21.5 Technique for Determining Orthostatic Hypotension

When the patient is experiencing fatigue, light-headedness, falls, visual blurring, or syncope, check for orthostatic hypotension.

- Measure the pulse rate. Then, with the patient supine and the brachial artery at the level of the heart, measure the blood pressure. While measuring, support patient's arm and back; patient should have legs uncrossed. Record the measurements.
- Assist the patient to a standing position. Immediately measure the pulse. Again with the brachial artery at the level of the heart, measure the blood pressure at 1 minute and 3 minutes after standing.
- Determine the difference between the supine and standing systolic blood pressures and the difference between the supine and standing diastolic blood pressures.

If there is a 20 mm Hg decrease in the systolic blood pressure or a 10 mm Hg decrease in the diastolic blood pressure when standing, the patient has orthostatic hypotension. Variations in heart rate are helpful in determining the cause of the orthostatic hypotension. A tachycardic response (increase in heart rate over 20 beats per minute) indicates dehydration or volume depletion. If the patient has both a decrease in blood pressure of 20 mm Hg and an increase in heart rate of 20 beats per minute it is "doubly" significant (KeithRN, 2016) - **the patient could be in serious trouble!**

PAIN, THE FIFTH VITAL SIGN

The Joint Commission's standards have included pain as the "fifth" vital sign since they developed a Pain Management Standard in 2001.

 **QSEN Considerations: Patient-Centered Care**

Pain

The identification and management of pain is an important component of patient-centered care (The Joint Commission, 2014).

For this reason, pain is assessed and findings are often recorded along with the other vital signs in the medical record. The assessment must include pain location, intensity, character, frequency, and duration. The same version of a standardized pain scale should be used at each assessment. Follow up on the assessment findings and treatment of pain are done according to agency policy. Chapter 31 presents further information on the assessment and treatment of pain.

AUTOMATED VITAL SIGN MONITORS

Lightweight, portable, automated units are available that measure blood pressure and heart rate simultaneously (Fig. 21.17). Measurements can be obtained in 21 to 45 seconds. It is also possible to program most units to measure these vital signs at specified intervals. The vital signs are displayed digitally and may be retrieved using the unit's stored data capability. If a blood pressure reading is considerably different from the patient's normal blood pressure, check the pressure with a manual sphygmomanometer. The machine may be malfunctioning or may need calibration.

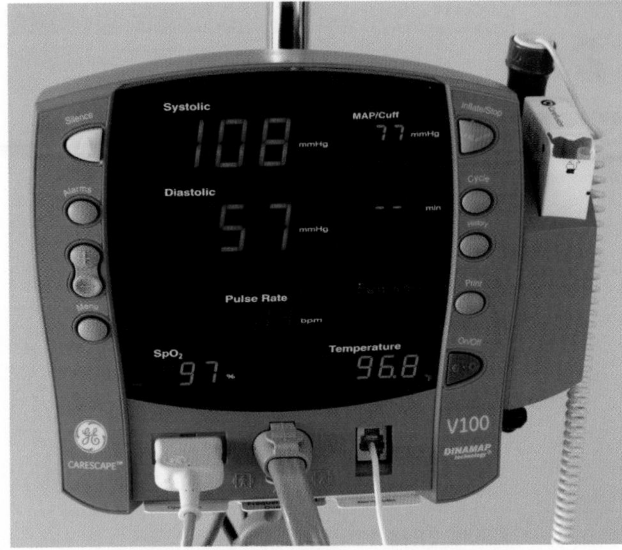

FIGURE 21.17 Automated vital signs monitor.

DOCUMENTING VITAL SIGNS

Carry a small pad and pen with you and write vital signs down as soon as the measurements are obtained. It is easy to make errors or to forget the readings, especially when measuring vital signs for more than one patient. If computer entry is used, enter the vital signs before going to the next patient. Some nursing units record the vital signs on a jot board or worksheet used as a quick reference by nurses and physicians. For paper-based systems, the vital signs are recorded on the patient's medical record by the unit secretary or the nurse. In addition, any unusual or abnormal findings may be written in the nurse's notes because of their importance to the patient's condition. In electronic health records, vital signs are documented within the correct screen on the computer for each patient (Fig. 21.18).

RECORDING TEMPERATURE MEASUREMENTS

For manual graphing, note that the range of degrees for temperature is 96°F to 105°F. Guidelines for documenting on the graphic record are as follows:

- Record in even numbers. The graphic sheet is scored so that each line equals two tenths of a degree. Do not use odd numbers unless an electronic thermometer was used with measurements accurate to one tenth of a degree.
- Place a dot on the center of the appropriate line; the dot should be at the intersection of the appropriate hour and temperature reading.
- Connect the dots with a straight, accurate line.
- If the temperature is rectal, write ® above the dot.

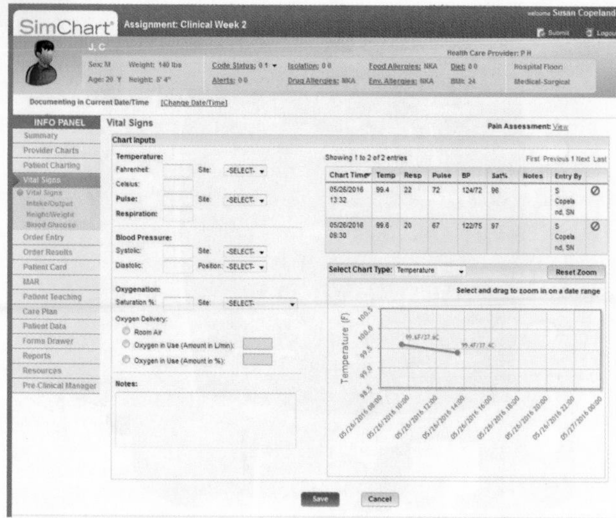

FIGURE 21.18 Vital signs electronic screen.

- If the temperature is axillary, write @ above the dot.
- With computerized documentation, the graphing is done automatically when the numbers are entered.

RECORDING PULSE MEASUREMENTS

The pulse is documented on the same page as the temperature in a table or on a graph. On a graph, each line between the bold lines represents 10 pulse beats.

Record the pulse on a graph in even numbers, such as 80, 86, and 102. Connect the dots with a straight, accurate line when a hard copy graph is used. For electronic entry, simply enter the pulse measurement in the correct place on the vital signs screen.

RECORDING RESPIRATION MEASUREMENTS

The lower portion of a hard copy graphic sheet is sometimes used for recording the respiratory rate on a graph or in a table. When the respiratory rate to be recorded on a graph is one of the numbers indicated on the sheet (such as 20 or 40), place the dot in the center of the appropriate line. Otherwise, the dot is centered at the correct vertical distance between two lines. Record on a graph in even numbers, such as 22 and 46. Connect the dots with a straight, accurate line. Enter the respiration measurement in the correct spot on the vital signs screen for electronic documentation.

RECORDING BLOOD PRESSURE MEASUREMENTS

Hard copy graphic sheets contain a section labeled "blood pressure" and provide space for recording the readings. Write the systolic pressure above the slanted line and the diastolic pressure below the line. For electronic documentation, enter the blood pressure measurement in the correct location on the vital signs screen.

EVALUATING VITAL SIGN TRENDS

When vital signs are outside the expected norms, reflect a gradual trend, or have changed significantly compared with the previous vital signs, nursing actions may be indicated. The nursing actions may be independent of the primary care provider's orders or dependent and based on a written order. Because a change in vital signs is an early indication of physiologic change in the patient, the primary care provider should be notified of any significant change. After notification of the care provider and implementation of nursing actions, monitor the effectiveness of the actions by measuring the vital signs repeatedly until they return to acceptable limits.

When vital signs merit notification of the health care provider or implementation of nursing actions, make a narrative entry in the patient's medical record. The narrative entry should include the time at which the vital signs were measured, subjective and objective observations, the actions implemented, and the result of the actions. Document contact with the primary care provider or office personnel, including the name of the person to whom the message was given.

Many hospitals use a separate frequent vital sign sheet for patients whose condition requires repeated vital sign measurement. Frequent measuring of vital signs may be ordered for a patient who has had an invasive procedure, who is taking specific cardiac medications, or whose condition is unstable.

Get Ready for the NCLEX Examination!

Key Points

Temperature

- Normal body temperature ranges from 97.5°F to 99.5°F (36.4°C to 37.5°C). Average temperature of a healthy adult is 98.6°F (37°C).
- Temperature alterations should be compared with the patient's normal temperature.
- Rectal temperatures are about 1°F higher, and axillary temperatures are about 1°F lower, than oral temperatures.
- Measurement by tympanic thermometer comes closest to core body temperature.
- Temperature is affected by time of day, environment, age, exercise, hormones, emotional stress, disease conditions, and certain drugs.
- A temperature over 100.2°F (37.9°C) is abnormal and is termed *pyrexia* or *fever.* A temperature of 105.8°F (41°C) or higher may cause damage to body cells.
- Hypothermia occurs when the temperature falls below normal range.
- The oral route is never used for temperature measurement for the unconscious or uncooperative patient or one who may have a seizure.

Pulse

- The pulse is initiated by contractions of the heart sending blood out into the arteries.
- The pulse is normally assessed at the radial artery in the wrist or at the apex of the heart.
- Normal pulse rate in the adult ranges from 60 to 100 bpm, with the average being 72 bpm.
- A pulse rate greater than 100 bpm is called tachycardia.
- A pulse rate lower than 60 bpm is called bradycardia.
- When counting a pulse, begin counting with "0"; the next beat is "1."
- Pulse measurement includes noting the pulse's rhythm, volume, and rate.
- Besides being a measure of cardiovascular status, pulse rates are used to evaluate response to treatment and activity.

Respiration

- Respiratory rate is always considered in conjunction with other assessment data because many factors can affect it.
- The normal range of respirations for the healthy adult is 12 to 20 per minute.
- Symptoms of hypoxia include restlessness, confusion, change in level of consciousness, and cyanosis.
- Abnormal breathing patterns are dyspnea, tachypnea, bradypnea, and hyperventilation; Cheyne-Stokes, Kussmaul, and Biot respirations.
- Respiratory rate is considered along with other data such as breath sounds and arterial oxygen saturation for assessment of the respiratory system.
- Measurement of arterial oxygen saturation may be done with a pulse oximeter.

Blood Pressure

- A sphygmomanometer and stethoscope are used to measure blood pressure. An electronic sphygmomanometer or vital sign monitor may also be used.
- The cuff must be the appropriate size for the patient for blood pressure measurement to be accurate.
- Errors in technique of blood pressure measurement may cause inaccurate readings.
- The phase IV Korotkoff sound (muffling) is used to determine diastolic pressure in children and in some older adults. Generally, the disappearance of sound (silence, phase V) marks the diastolic pressure.
- Optimal blood pressure in the healthy adult is less than 120/80 mm Hg; pressure over 140/90 mm Hg or below 90/60 mm Hg is considered abnormal.
- A blood pressure consistently over 140/90 mm Hg constitutes hypertension. A symptomatic blood pressure below 90/60 mm Hg is called hypotension.
- Signs and symptoms such as cold clammy skin, apprehension, dizziness, blurred vision, and an increase in pulse rate may accompany hypotension and indicate shock.
- Vital signs are recorded on the graphic record or the electronic medical record. Abnormalities of vital signs are noted in the nurse's notes along with further assessment data.
- Abnormal blood pressures should be reported to the charge nurse or the primary care provider.

Additional Learning Resources

SG Go to your Study Guide for additional learning activities to help you master this chapter content.

evolve Go to your Evolve website at http://evolve.elsevier.com/Williams/fundamental for additional online resources.

Review Questions for the NCLEX Examination

*Choose the **best** answer for each question.*

1. The nursing assistant reports to the nurse that the temperature of a patient who is first day postoperative is 100.2°F. Which action should the nurse take **first**?
   1. Notify the surgeon of the temperature elevation.
   2. Check the preoperative temperature reading.
   3. Tell the nursing assistant to take the temperature again in 2 hours.
   4. Prepare to administer an acetaminophen PRN-ordered suppository.

2. Temperature greater than 105.8°F (41°C) should be treated promptly to reduce the fever to prevent which health risk?
    1. Chemical reactions to oxygen in the bloodstream
    2. Potential damage to the cells of the central nervous system
    3. Heavy perspiration causing dehydration
    4. The increased workload of the heart
3. Pulse oximetry readings should be correlated with which other assessment or findings?
    1. The respiratory assessment
    2. The vital signs
    3. The hemoglobin level of the blood
    4. Changes in blood pressure
4. Which health condition or intervention may put a patient at risk of developing orthostatic hypotension? (*Select all that apply.*)
    1. Receiving 3 L of IV fluid in 24 hours
    2. The patient has had diarrhea and vomiting for 3 days.
    3. Taking medication for hypertension
    4. The patient has been somewhat nauseous for 48 hours.
    5. The patient has a sinus infection and fever with a temperature of 101.4°F.
5. Which are the signs and symptoms of shock that may be seen with hypotension? (*Select all that apply.*)
    1. Tachypnea
    2. Apprehension
    3. Tachycardia
    4. Cool, clammy skin
    5. Increased blood pressure
6. When assigning vital sign measurement to the nursing assistant, the nurse says to take the apical pulse for the full 60 seconds. For which patient would this instruction be *most* important?
    1. A patient who is bradycardic
    2. A patient whose usual heart rate is 76 bpm
    3. A patient who is tachycardic
    4. A patient whose heart rate is irregular
7. A patient is receiving an opiate-based medication to help manage pain. Which assessment has the highest **priority** when monitoring his condition?
    1. Temperature
    2. Pulse
    3. Respirations
    4. Blood pressure

Critical Thinking Activities

Read each clinical scenario and discuss the questions with your classmates.

Scenario A

A mother brings her toddler into the clinic because he has been pulling at his ear and seems feverish. The child cried most of the night and is upset now.

1. How would you obtain accurate vital signs on this child?
2. Will a heart rate or respiratory rate be accurate if taken when a child is crying?

Scenario B

Robert Jaisal comes to the clinic for the first time because he has a sore throat. You find that his blood pressure measurement is 176/104 mm Hg.

1. Do you think this is an accurate measurement?
2. What would you do next?
3. What factors might be affecting Mr. Jaisal's blood pressure at this time?
4. What are the guidelines for determining whether a patient has hypertension?

Scenario C

Theresa Hernandez comes to the clinic after pulling a back muscle. She is experiencing considerable pain. Her vital signs are usually BP 124/82, pulse 76, respirations 14, and temperature 97.8°F. What would you expect to find when you take her vital signs during this visit to the clinic?

chapter 22

Assessing Health Status

http://evolve.elsevier.com/Williams/fundamental

Objectives

Upon completing this chapter, you should be able to do the following:

Theory

1. Discuss the types of assessment used in various situations.
2. Demonstrate the techniques used during physical examination.
3. Describe how to gather information for a comprehensive database for a patient.

Clinical Practice

1. Assess the patient's psychosocial and physical functioning by gathering information in an organized way.
2. Perform a basic physical examination on a patient.
3. Perform a visual acuity test on a patient.
4. Carry out focused physical assessments of the cardiovascular, respiratory, gastrointestinal, and neurologic systems.
5. Teach patients the assessment techniques for the early detection of cancer.
6. Educate patients about the recommendations for periodic diagnostic testing.
7. Assist with a medical examination by positioning and draping the patient and organizing the equipment.

Skills & Steps

Key Terms

adventitious sounds (ăd-vĕn-TĬ-shŭs, p. 384)
auscultation (ăw-skŭl-TĀ-shŭn, p. 380)
bronchovesicular sounds (brŏn-cō-vĕ-SĬ-kū-lăr, p. 384)
dual-energy x-ray absorptiometry (DXA) (p. 394)
edema (ĕ-DĒ-mă, p. 379)
kyphosis (kĭ-FŌ-sĭs, p. 383)
lesions (p. 378)
lordosis (lŏr-DŌ-sĭs, p. 383)
nystagmus (p. 395)
olfaction (ōl-FĂK-shŭn, p. 380)
palpation (păl-PĀ-shŭn, p. 379)
percussion (pĕr-KŬ-shŭn, p. 380)
quadrant (KWĂ-drănt, p. 387)
scoliosis (skō-lē-Ō-sĭs, p. 383)
tremors (p. 380)
turgor (TŬR-gŏr, p. 379)
vesicular sounds (vĕ-SĬ-kū-lŏr, p. 384)

Concepts Covered in This Chapter

- Culture
- Patient education

DATA COLLECTION AND ASSESSMENT

Assessment is a vitally important nursing function. It is a continual process for determining the patients' condition and progress. You are expected to assess lung sounds properly, identify abnormal heart sounds, determine when something might be wrong in the abdomen, monitor circulatory status, detect neurologic changes, note skin problems, and recognize signs and symptoms of problems in any body system. When an illness occurs, it is likely to affect more than one body system. Although a staff nurse rarely has time to do a thorough physical examination of each patient assigned, a quick focused assessment and a survey of all body systems are performed for each patient at the beginning of each shift. Nurses are with patients more than other health care providers are, and they must monitor for subtle changes in condition. Strong assessment skills can quickly identify new signs and symptoms that indicate complications of an illness or adverse side effects of medical therapy. This is especially important when working with home care or long-term care patients because the nurse is often the only health professional who sees the patient at regular intervals. The licensed practical nurse/licensed vocational nurse (LPN/LVN) charge nurse in the long-term care facility acts as the "eyes and ears" of the primary care provider, as does the home care nurse.

Most people have had a physical examination at some time in their lives. Physical examinations are usually required for entry into schools, for the issuance of insurance policies, for employment, for particular types of driver's licenses, and for induction into military service. A complete physical examination is performed on patients who seek primary preventive care every 1 to 5 years, depending on age and health condition. A nurse often assists with the primary care provider's examination of the patient.

Think Critically

Can you describe your last physical examination? What was done? What questions were you asked?

APPLICATION OF THE NURSING PROCESS

ASSESSMENT (DATA COLLECTION)

When a patient is admitted to the hospital, long-term care facility, home care service, or other agency, an initial assessment is performed. This assessment usually includes gathering a history and demographic data and performing a brief physical examination. This type of assessment is covered in Chapter 5, along with interviewing (see Boxes 5.2 and 5.3).

Data Collection

In addition to the physical examination, you are also expected to obtain some historical data concerning the patient's past and present state of health. The type of information required for the admission history form is covered in Chapters 5 and 23. Students are often required to complete a history form to turn in with a nursing care plan or concept care map. The health history and psychosocial data provide pertinent information about the patient to assist in administering daily care. Certainly, knowledge of the current health problems is essential, and you should review the medical record for these data or obtain them from the patient if the data are not yet in the record.

Psychosocial and Cultural Assessment

To care for the whole patient rather than just tend to an area of physical need, you must be aware of how the illness is affecting the patient's life. Exploration of concerns regarding not only health but also all other areas of the patient's life is appropriate. If a mother is worried about the care of her small children at home, her energy will be focused on them rather than on healing.

Assess for cultural preferences and health beliefs so that an individualized plan of care can be formulated. Cultural assessment includes asking the patient and family about preferences for food, bathing, and personal care; what they think about their illness and treatment; and who should be consulted about decisions. Phrase questions in a positive, nonthreatening way. Do not assume that just because a patient is a member of a certain ethnic group, she has beliefs and practices common to that group. Box 22.1 provides a patient interview guide. Specific questions regarding potential physical, sexual, and alcohol abuse are presented in Box 22.2. Further information on cultural assessment is presented in Chapter 14.

Life-Span Considerations

Older Adult

If the older adult has difficulty with memory, data may be gathered from a family member or significant other.

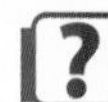
Think Critically

What specific areas would you include in an overall assessment of a patient?

Physical Assessment

When patients are first encountered, observe their behavior and appearance to begin to form an opinion about their health status. Some of these data may lead to the conclusion that a person is ill, has an elevated temperature, or is malnourished. Detecting possible signs of abuse should be included in the assessment (Box 22.3). In addition to observations, it is essential to ask the right questions and measure various body functions. The assessment thus provides a complete picture of physiologic functioning. When combined with the health and psychosocial history, it forms a health database for the individual. The information gathered from the physical assessment can be used for a variety of purposes, including:

- Determining the patient's level of health and physiologic functioning
- Arriving at a preliminary nursing diagnosis of a health problem
- Confirming a diagnosis of dysfunction, disease, or inability to carry out activities of daily living (ADLs)
- Indicating specific body areas or systems for additional testing or examination
- Evaluating the effectiveness of prescribed treatment and therapy and observing for adverse side effects
- Monitoring for changes in body function
- Determining whether there are any signs of abuse

Box 22.1 Patient Interview Guide

SOCIAL DATA

- What is your marital status? Who is a significant person in your life?
- Do you have health insurance?
- What is [was] your occupation?
- How has your admission affected things at home?
- Do you have any visual or hearing deficits?
- Do you wear dentures?
- Do you have any prostheses, such as an artificial limb or joint?
- Are you an active member of any organization?
- Do you belong to a religious group or participate in spiritual practices?
- Are there cultural practices we should know about to care for you properly?
- Are you allergic to any medications? What happens when you take them?
- What prescription drugs do you take and how often? What over-the-counter medications do you take regularly or occasionally? Do you take any herbal products or supplements?
- Do you have any food allergies? Any allergies to any other substances? What happens when you eat or come into contact with any of these things?
- What do you like to eat? Are you currently on a special diet? Any special favorite foods? Do you have any food dislikes or intolerances?
- Do you or have you ever smoked? How much? For how long? When did you quit?
- Do you drink wine or other alcohol? When and about how much do you drink?
- Do you need assistance with your activities or with your personal care?
- Have you had previous surgeries or serious injuries?
- What health problems do you have?
- Do you routinely see other care providers? For what?
- What brought about your admission here?

PHYSICAL DATA: REVIEW OF SYSTEMS

Head and Neck

- Do you have frequent headaches or dizziness?
- Do you have problems with your ears? Are you hard of hearing? Do you have ringing in your ears or use a hearing aid?
- Do you have visual problems, or wear contact lenses or glasses? Have you ever been told you have glaucoma, cataracts, or any problems with your eyes in general? When was your last eye examination?
- Do you have frequent colds or nasal allergies, sinus infections, sore throats, hoarseness, trouble swallowing, or swollen glands?
- When was your last dental examination? Any problem with gum disease or mouth sores?
- Do you have difficulty sleeping at night? Do you often take naps?

Chest

- Do you have a frequent cough? Is it a dry cough, or do you bring up sputum? Can you describe the sputum for me?
- Do you have a history of lung problems such as pneumonia, asthma, wheezing, bronchitis, or emphysema?
- Have you had or ever been exposed to tuberculosis?
- Have you had any occupational exposure to any respiratory hazards?
- Have you ever had angina, chest pain, heart attack, or irregular heartbeats? Any palpitations, murmurs, or shortness of breath?
- Do you experience leg pains or cramps after walking a short distance?
- Do you have a pacemaker? Automatic defibrillator?
- Have you ever been told you have high blood pressure (hypertension)?
- Female: When was your last mammogram? Do you have any discharge from your nipples or any breast lumps?

Abdomen

- Do you have frequent indigestion, gas, bloating, heartburn, nausea, or vomiting?
- Do you experience excessive thirst or hunger?
- Do you have frequent bowel movements, a change in your bowel routine, or a change in the appearance of your bowel movements? Frequent diarrhea or constipation?
- Have you ever had rectal bleeding or black or tar colored stools? Do you have excessive gas?
- Have you ever had hemorrhoids?
- Have you ever had problems with your gallbladder or liver?

Genitourinary

- Have you had problems urinating? Do you regularly have to get up during the night to urinate? If so, how many times during the night?
- Have you experienced urgency or frequency on a regular basis? Do you get the urge to urinate and then cannot void?
- Do you have problems with dribbling of urine or unexpectedly urinating when you laugh or cough?
- Have you ever had a urinary tract infection? Do you have them often?
- Any history of kidney stones?
- Female: Are you sexually active? Any vaginal problems or problems in the genital area? Any problems with your menstrual cycle? When was your last menstrual period? Any bleeding between periods or after menopause? When was your last Pap smear? Have you had any unusual vaginal discharge? Any history of herpes or other sexually transmitted infections?
- Male: Are you sexually active? Any genital problems or penile discharge? Any history of herpes or other sexually transmitted infections? Any prostate problems?

Extremities and Musculoskeletal

- Do you have any joint pain or stiffness?
- Any muscle pain or back problems?
- Are you able to move your body in a full range of motion?
- Do you have any problems with circulation in your legs or arms?
- Do you bruise easily or have any skin lesions?
- Any history of phlebitis, thrombophlebitis, gout, or arthritis?
- Any fractures or injuries?
- Any artificial joints?
- Any sign of abuse?

Endocrine

- Have you ever been diagnosed with thyroid problems? Hyperthyroid or hypothyroid?
- Have you ever been told you have diabetes? Type 1 or type 2? How long ago were you diagnosed? Do you take insulin or an oral agent to control your blood glucose?

Box 22.2 Questions to Detect Potential Physical, Sexual, or Alcohol Abuse in the Adult

- Does your spouse or partner ever physically hurt or threaten you?
- Are you restricted by your partner or spouse from seeing other people?
- Has your partner or spouse forced you to perform activities that you refused to do or that made you uncomfortable?
- Is there an adult close to you of whom you are afraid?

POTENTIAL ALCOHOL ABUSE

Ask these questions:

- Have you thought that you should decrease the amount you drink?
- Have you ever become irritated when people comment on your drinking?
- Have you ever felt remorseful about your drinking?
- Have you ever had a drink in the morning to feel better?

When the patient is seen with a new illness or complaint, obtain a history of that illness or complaint with the questions in Box 22.4.

The physical assessment can be performed in a variety of settings, such as hospitals, health centers, clinics, schools, long-term care facilities, and primary care providers' or nurse practitioners' offices.

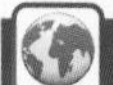

Cultural Considerations

Ask Before Touching

Many cultures, including those of India, China, and the Arab countries, do not permit a male outside of the family to touch a female. Male nurses should seek permission from the female patient before touching her and should understand that it is not a personal issue if she requests a female nurse or primary care provider.

The examination can be performed by a physician, nurse, physician assistant, nurse practitioner, clinical nurse specialist, or other clinician, depending on the type of assessment, its purpose, and the policies of the particular agency. The assessment of physiologic functioning ranges from a comprehensive, in-depth examination that includes all systems of the body to a brief, scanning type of examination confined to a specific body part or system. Vocabulary specific to physical assessment is provided in Box 22.5.

Physical Examination Techniques

Because assessment is also a tool for nurses to use in planning nursing care, attention must be focused on methods of gathering information. In addition to using interviewing and communication skills, information is obtained by using the senses: sight, hearing, smell, and touch. The most helpful of these senses is sight, closely followed by touch.

Box 22.3 Signs and Symptoms of Possible Abuse

FOR CHILDREN

- Evidence of physical injuries or neglect, including old bruising or fractures, poor hygiene, dirty clothes, malnourishment.
- Explanations about injury that are conflicting from child and parents.
- Injuries that are inconsistent with the explanation of how they happened.
- Child's inappropriate response to examination and questions such as pulling away from touch or looking at the caregiver before answering a question.
- Frequent visits to the primary care provider or ER for injury or illness.
- Being overly affectionate or sexually knowledgeable for age.
- Fear of someone well known to the child.
- Resistance to having clothing removed for examination.
- Chronic genital itching, pain, or evidence of sexually transmitted infection.

FOR AN OLDER ADULT

- Dehydration or malnutrition without an underlying illness.
- Evidence of burns or neglected pressure ulcers.
- Bruises on the upper arms and trunk, both older and newer.
- Inadequate clothing or shoes for the weather.
- Verbalization of a lack of food, medicine, or care.
- Fear of the caregiver.
- Poor hygiene with body odor and soiled clothing.
- Verbalizes that someone has taken control of finances or life without consent.

FOR SPOUSE OR PARTNER

- Frequent injuries that are referred to as from an "accident."
- Dressing in clothing designed to hide bruises or scars (long sleeves in hot weather, sunglasses worn indoors).
- Rarely go out without the partner or spouse.
- Have limited access to money or family car.
- Considerable anxiety or depression.
- Are afraid of the spouse or partner or seem extremely anxious to please that person.
- Talk about their partner or spouse's temper or possessiveness.

Inspection and observation. Through the sense of sight, you are able to inspect the various parts of the body and observe the patient's behavioral responses. When assessing the patient's physiologic condition, use inspection to make observations about the patient's general appearance, contours of the body, skin tone and color, rashes, scars and **lesions** (tissue damage or abnormality), deformities or extremity weakness, characteristics of movements, and respirations.

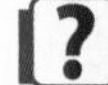

Think Critically

Can you think of other signs you might observe during physical examination?

Box 22.4 Taking a History of a New Illness or Problem

When a patient is seen with a new problem or illness, ask:

- What is the problem?
- When did it start? How did it start?
- Are the symptoms getting worse or remaining the same?
- Did anything seem to precipitate this illness or problem?
- How is it affecting you? Does it interfere with your usual activities?
- How often do the symptoms occur? Under what circumstances? Is there a relationship to meals? Is this a seasonal problem for you?
- If there is pain, where is it? Can you describe it? How would you rate it on a scale of 0 to 10?
- What, if anything, seems to relieve your symptoms?

Palpation. The sense of touch can be used to obtain a great deal of clinical information about patients. **Palpation** involves using the hands to feel various parts of the body. Palpation can be used to detect the size, shape, and position of parts of the body and the texture, temperature, and moisture of the skin. Palpation is used to ascertain:

- Muscle spasm or rigidity
- Pain, swelling, or a growth
- Any restriction in movement of a body part
- Skin temperature, **turgor** (elasticity), and **edema** (fluid in the tissues)

Skillful palpation is based on knowing how to use the fingers and hands effectively. The backs of the hands

Box 22.5 Vocabulary Specific to Physical Assessment

ADLs: Activities of daily living: for example, bathing, dressing, grooming, cleansing teeth, shaving, and toileting.
Ascites: Abnormal accumulation of serous fluid within the peritoneal cavity.
Bruit: Abnormal sound heard on auscultation; a kind of swishing sound.
Cognitive: Relating to the mental process of knowing, remembering, and relating; connected thinking.
Cyanosis: A bluish tinge to the skin, nail beds, or mucous membranes, indicating a significant decrease in oxygenation.
Ecchymosis: Blue or purplish patch on the skin or mucous membrane that is not elevated; bruising.
Erythema: Redness of the skin caused by congestion of the capillaries in the lower layers of the skin that occurs with any skin injury, infection, or inflammation.
Extension posture: Arms stiffly extended, adducted, and hyperpronated with hyperextension of the legs and plantar flexion of the feet; indicates disruption of the motor fibers in the midbrain and brainstem; formerly called *decerebrate posture.*
Fissure: A narrow slit.
Flexion posture: Internal rotation and adduction of the arms with flexion of the elbows, wrists, and fingers, resulting from neurologic injury and interruption of voluntary motor tracts; extension of the legs may also be seen; formerly called *decorticate posture.*
Guaiac: A test for blood in the stool.
Gurgles: Also known as low-pitched wheezes. Wet sounds heard when auscultating the lungs; newer term for rhonchi; gurgle sounds also occur in the bowel.
Inspection: Visual examination for detection of abnormal signs or qualities.
Integument: The skin covering the body.
Jaundice: Yellowness of the skin, sclera, mucous membranes, and excretions resulting from hyperbilirubinemia and deposition of bile pigments; also called *icterus.*
Jugular venous distention (JVD): Visible protrusion of the jugular veins when the patient is positioned sitting in bed at a 15- to 35-degree angle; assessed as a sign of heart failure or overhydration.
Lethargy: Abnormal drowsiness or stupor.
Murmur: A periodic sound of short duration of cardiac or vascular origin.
Ophthalmoscope: Lighted instrument used for viewing the interior of the eye.
Orientation: Awareness of one's environment with reference to person, place, time, and event.
Otoscope: Lighted instrument used to visualize the tympanic membrane and interior of the ear canal.
Pallor: Paleness of the skin.
Papanicolaou (Pap) smear: A microscopic laboratory examination used to determine the presence of malignant cells from body secretions (respiratory, genitourinary, or digestive tract).
Patent: Freely open (e.g., a patent drain).
Petechiae: Pinpoint, round, purplish red spots that are not raised, caused by intradermal or submucosal hemorrhage; a significant sign for various diseases.
Pigmentation: The deposition of coloring matter in the skin.
Proctoscopic examination: Examination of the rectum with a lighted instrument.
Rinne test: A test to compare bone and air conduction of sound, performed with a tuning fork.
Sanguineous: Bloody.
Scar: A mark remaining after the healing of a wound.
Serosanguineous: Composed of serum and blood.
Sigmoidoscopy: An examination of the sigmoid colon using a lighted instrument.
Sign: Any objective evidence of disease or dysfunction.
Sore: A term for a painful lesion of the skin or mucous membrane.
Speculum: A short, funnel-like tube for examining canals, such as the nasal canal and the vaginal canal.
Sputum: Mucous secretions of the lungs ejected through the mouth.
Symptom: Any indication of disease perceived by the patient; subjective information.
Tinnitus: A noise in the ears such as ringing, buzzing, or roaring.
Tuning fork: A forked metal instrument used to test hearing and the sense of vibration.
Vertigo: A sensation of rotation or whirling movement; dizziness.
Weber test: A test of bone conduction of sound performed with a tuning fork placed in the center of the forehead.
Wheeze: A high-pitched respiratory sound that often indicates narrowed airways; it is common in patients with asthma.
Wound: Bodily injury caused by physical means with disruption of the skin or other structure.

and fingers are used to investigate differences in skin temperature over an inflamed joint or a foot with poor circulation. The skin is thinner on the back of the hand and more sensitive to changes in temperature. The pads of the fingers are used to palpate the size, position, and consistency of various structures, such as the lymph nodes and breast tissue. The palm of the hand is used to detect vibrations or **tremors** (involuntary fine movement of the body or limbs), and the thumb and index finger are used to check skin turgor, joint position, and the firmness of muscles and other tissues.

Palpate the abdomen lightly to identify painful or tender areas or to locate masses or abnormal collections of fluid. The pads of the fingers are used in light palpation, and pressure is exerted to indent the skin about 1 to 2 cm (½ to ¾ inch) (Fig. 22.1). Deep palpation depresses the skin 4 to 5 cm (1½ to 2 inches) and can be done using one or both hands. When palpating, watch the patient's face for signs of discomfort and discontinue if pain occurs.

Percussion. **Percussion** supplies other information about structures of the body. It involves light, quick tapping on the body surface to produce sounds. Variations in the sounds reflect the characteristics of the organs or structures below the surface. Percussion is used primarily over the chest and abdomen to determine the size, location, and density of organs that lie within. The most common type of percussion consists of striking the middle finger of one hand with the index or middle finger of the other hand. When tapping, do not move the forearm; all the force is generated by a quick snap of the wrist (Fig. 22.2). The tapping finger makes a quick contact with the other hand, and after two or three taps in one location, the hands are moved to another area. Different sounds are emitted as the examiner moves from one resonant area to a less or more resonant one. The sounds vary in their intensity, pitch, and duration, depending on the presence of underlying air, fluid, or a solid organ.

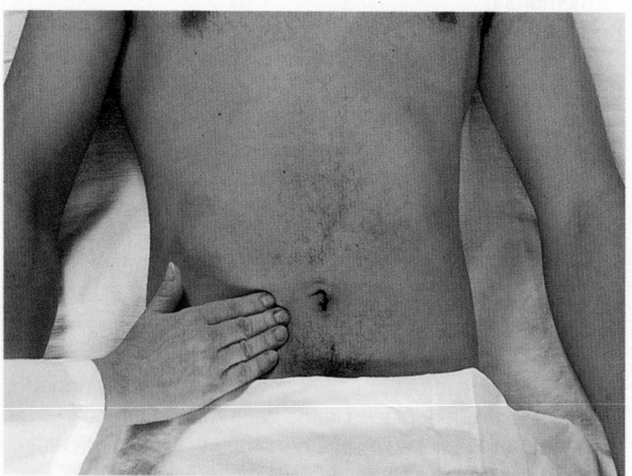

FIGURE 22.1 Palpate the Abdomen for Areas of Tenderness. (From Potter, P. A., Perry, A. G., Stocjert, P., & Hall, A. [2014]. *Fundamentals of nursing* [8th ed.]. St. Louis, MO: Mosby; fig. 30.64.)

Auscultation. **Auscultation** is the process of listening with the aid of the stethoscope to sounds produced in the body. It is particularly valuable in hearing sounds produced in the heart, lungs, and abdomen. Use the stethoscope to take blood pressure readings, to listen to the lungs, to assess heart sounds, and to check for the presence of bowel sounds. When listening to the lungs, use the diaphragm of the stethoscope; heart valve sounds are best assessed through the bell of the stethoscope placed lightly on the chest wall. To use a stethoscope properly, place the earpieces in your ears so that they point forward toward your nose. The diaphragm is used to detect high-pitched sounds: breath, bowel, and normal heart sounds. The diaphragm (larger, flat surface) is held firmly against the skin, and it may leave a ring on the skin when lifted. The bell piece (smaller, cupped piece) is used to detect low-pitched sounds such as abnormal heart sounds made by the valves. It is held lightly against the skin; pressing harder obliterates the low-pitched sounds.

Clinical Cues

Do not place your thumb over the bell of the stethoscope when holding the diaphragm against the skin. If you do, you may only hear your own pulse transmitted via your thumb.

Olfaction. **Olfaction** is the sense of smell. The nose is used to identify characteristic smells associated with specific problems. A fruity odor to the breath can indicate diabetic acidosis; alcohol on the breath can provide a clue to the patient's lethargy or irrationality. Foul mouth odor may indicate periodontal disease or poor oral hygiene. A foul or sweet odor coming from under a cast or a wound indicates infection. A foul odor in the female genital area may indicate a vaginal infection.

Basic Physical Examination

The basics of physical examination are the foundation on which you begin to build expertise. As you study medical-surgical conditions, pediatrics, and obstetric care, you will learn more specialized assessment skills.

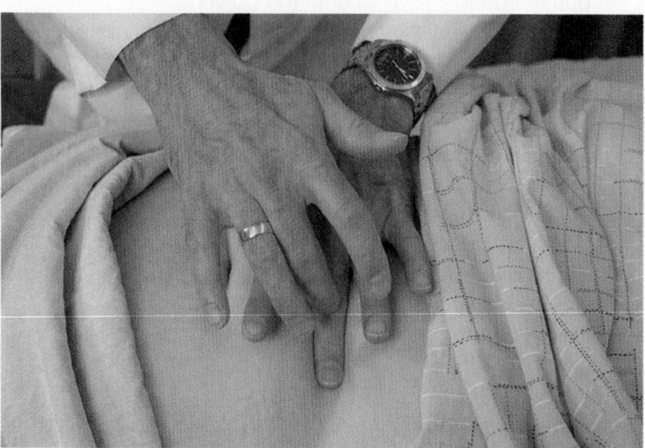

FIGURE 22.2 Technique for Percussion.

Height and weight. A basic nursing function is to weigh and measure the patient. Adult weight is most frequently measured on the standing scale (Fig. 22.3). Weight can also be measured by using a built-in scale in a bed or a chair scale. Weight is measured consistently with or without shoes, depending on the practice setting. Steps 22.1 provide the procedure for weighing the adult. Infants are weighed on an infant scale (Fig. 22.4). The infant is placed on a clean paper cover or the scale is cleansed after each weighing. The infant is weighed with one hand hovering closely to prevent a fall while adjusting the scale weights. **Never leave an infant unattended on the scale.**

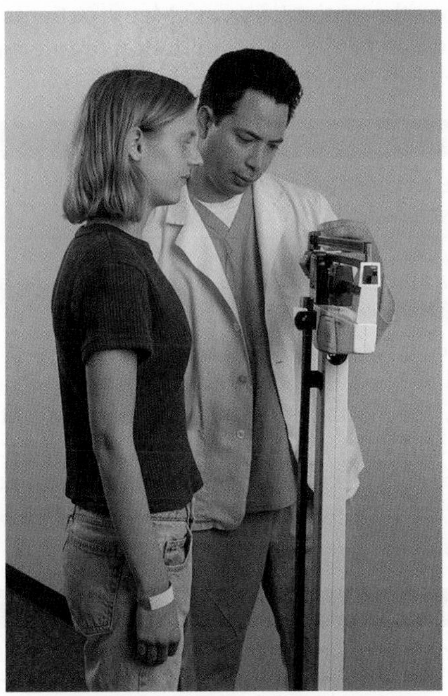

FIGURE 22.3 Weighing the Adult.

Height is measured from the sole of the foot to the crown of the head. A vertical measuring rod is generally used with the patient standing erect and looking straight ahead. Shoes should not be worn when the patient is measured. The most common device used to measure adults and older children is the height rod attached to a standing scale. Raise the rod to a height greater than the person to be measured, and raise the extension bar. The person stands with the feet together centered under the rod with the back to the rod and looks straight ahead. Lower the extension rod while keeping it at a 90-degree angle until it rests level on the patient's head.

Infants and children younger than 3 years of age are measured in the supine position with the legs fully extended. In the primary care provider's office, when an infant measurement board is not available, the length can be closely approximated by placing the infant on the paper covering an examining table, marking at the top of the head with the head in good alignment and the infant looking up, and then making another mark at the base of the heel with the leg fully extended. Measure the distance between the marks with a measuring tape. A second person is usually needed to help position the infant or toddler. Most measuring devices are marked in inches and in centimeters, with fractions of these units to ensure an exact measurement.

Historically, height and weight charts were used to determine if the patient's weight is within normal limits, but these have been replaced by body mass index charts (see Table 26.8 in Chapter 26). For children, standard growth charts can help the primary care provider determine if growth is within the expected range (Fig. 22.5).

Children are weighed and measured frequently to track growth and determine whether there is expected progression. Older adult patients should be measured

Steps 22.1 Weighing the Adult With a Standing Balance Scale

The adult is weighed on admission to the health care facility and periodically during clinic or office visits.

ACTION *(RATIONALE)*

1. Check that the scale is properly calibrated and balanced by moving both weights to zero. The bar should rest in the middle of the space. *(Ensures that patient's weight measurement will be accurate.)*
2. Place a clean paper cover on the footplate of the scale. *(Prevents transfer of microorganisms.)*
3. Assist patient onto the scale, without shoes. Be certain that both feet are totally on the scale. *(Shoes add to normal body weight. If a part of the foot is off the scale, the scale will not weigh accurately.)*
4. Move the large weight indicator on the lower part of the scale to the general range of the patient's weight (e.g., 50, 100, 150, 200, 250, or 300 lb). *(Prepares the scale by approximating patient's weight.)* Ask the patient to remain still, while adjusting the weights. Slide the other weight along upper portion of the scale along the weight beam until the balance bar rests in the middle of the space. *(If patient moves, the scale balance beam will swing wildly.)*
5. Record weight. *(Recording the number immediately helps to prevent forgetting the exact number.)*
6. Assist patient off the scale and allow her to put shoes on. *(Assisting the patient prevents falls when getting off scale.)*

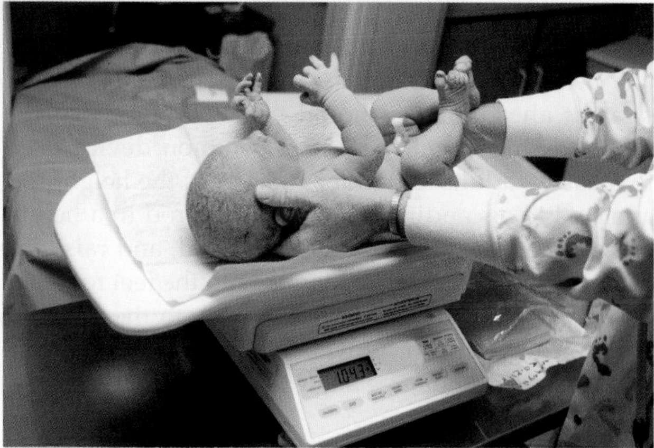

FIGURE 22.4 **Weighing the Infant.** (Photo copyright istock.com.)

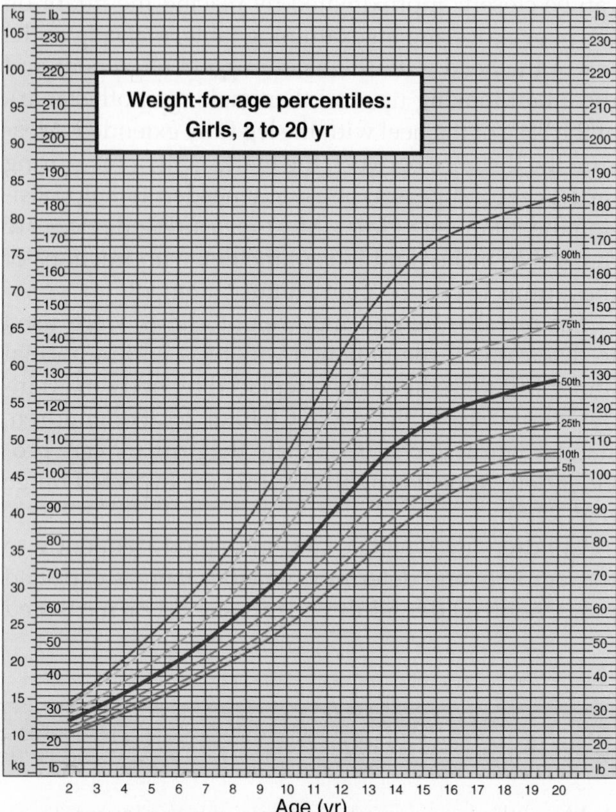

FIGURE 22.5 **Growth Chart Showing Percentile Curves for Weight by Age for Girls.** (From Dorland. [2012]. *Dorland's illustrated medical dictionary* [32nd ed.]. Philadelphia, PA: Saunders. VitalBook file.)

yearly to track decreases in height that might indicate alterations in the spine such as those caused by osteoporosis.

Vital signs measurement. Vital signs should be measured at the time of the physical examination. If previous measurements are available, the present ones are compared with them. Blood pressure should be measured on both arms after the patient has been quietly sitting or lying down for at least 5 minutes.

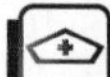 **Clinical Cues**

The blood pressure reading will be more accurate if the patient's feet are flat on the floor, the brachial artery is at the level of the right atrium, and neither you nor the patient talks during the procedure. (See Chapter 21 for guidelines for measuring blood pressure.)

If blood pressure is abnormal, it should be measured on both arms and with the patient in a standing position as well. Never take the blood pressure on the arm containing a dialysis shunt or intravenous site or on the side where a mastectomy and lymph node dissection have occurred. If blood pressure is elevated during an office or clinic visit, take the pressure again just before the patient leaves. Many patients become anxious when facing an examination or interview with a primary care provider.

 **Think Critically**

If you take a patient's blood pressure and it measures 148/94 mm Hg, what would you do?

The radial pulse is assessed and, if it is irregular, the apical pulse is counted. Respirations are also assessed, as is the temperature. Techniques for measuring vital signs are presented in Chapter 21. In office practice, the temperature is taken if the patient has a complaint that might alter the body temperature. Respirations are counted if there is a problem in the respiratory system. **In the hospital, the full set of vital signs is assessed.**

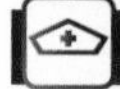 **Clinical Cues**

Whenever an illness affecting the respiratory system is present, count the respirations for a full minute. Note the character and depth of the respirations, as well as the rate.

Review of Body Systems

Head and neck. Assess the patient's general appearance, the color and tone of the skin and its condition, the appearance of the eyes, and the condition of the hair. Does the nose seem stuffy? Is there drainage? Do the teeth appear clean? Does the patient seem to have difficulty hearing? Are the pupils equal in size? Do the eyes move in unison? Are there any extra movements of the eyes or lids? Are the corneas and lens clear, or is there an opacity? When was the last eye examination? Is the patient alert and oriented? Does thinking seem logical? Does the neck appear normal? Are there complaints about swollen lymph nodes? Is the neck positioned midline to the head? Does neck movement seem normal and without stiffness? Perform a visual acuity examination as described in Steps 22.2 (Fig. 22.6). Hearing can be tested quickly and easily using the audioscope (Fig. 22.7). Directions for testing are included with the unit. Each ear is tested with four frequencies.

Steps 22.2 Testing Visual Acuity

The Snellen eye chart is used to test visual acuity. The test is performed by the nurse during a physical examination at an office or clinic and when there is a question of a problem with vision. Sometimes testing is done first without glasses and then with glasses.

ACTION *(RATIONALE)*

1. Position the patient 20 feet from the Snellen chart (see Fig. 22.6). *(Accuracy of the test depends on maintaining correct distance from the chart.)*
2. Ask patient to leave on corrective lenses (except reading glasses) and cover one eye with an opaque card. *(Vision of each eye is tested individually.)*
3. Instruct patient to read the chart to the smallest line in print possible, reading from left to right. *(Identifies the person's visual acuity in that eye.)*
4. Record the fraction at the end of the last line read, and indicate the number of missed letters and whether corrective lenses were worn (e.g., 20/30, –2 with contact lenses). *(The number beside the smallest print read is the visual acuity score; other designations indicate how the test was performed.)*
5. Test the other eye and record the visual acuity. *(Vision must be tested in both eyes individually.)*
6. Perform the test with both eyes uncovered. Record the score. *(Tests acuity in both eyes together.)*
7. If patient cannot read the top number even with glasses, position her closer to the chart. *(The score distance is altered according to how far patient is from the chart.)*
8. Record the scores. *(Documents results of test.)*

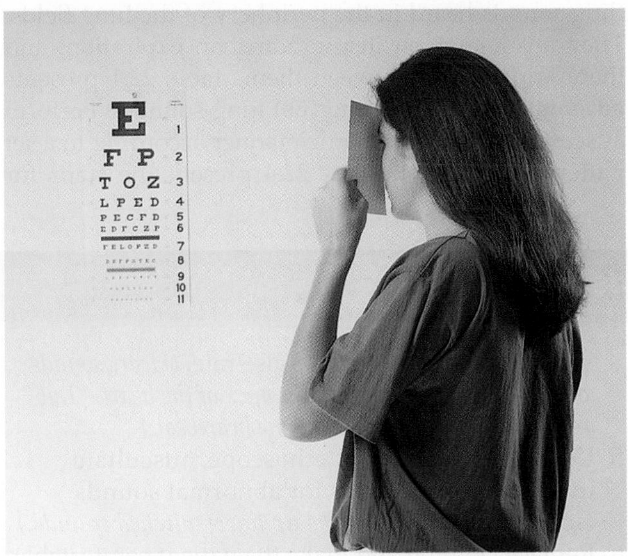

FIGURE 22.6 Testing Visual Acuity. (From Jarvis, C. [2008]. *Physical examination and health assessment* [5th ed.]. Philadelphia, PA: Saunders.)

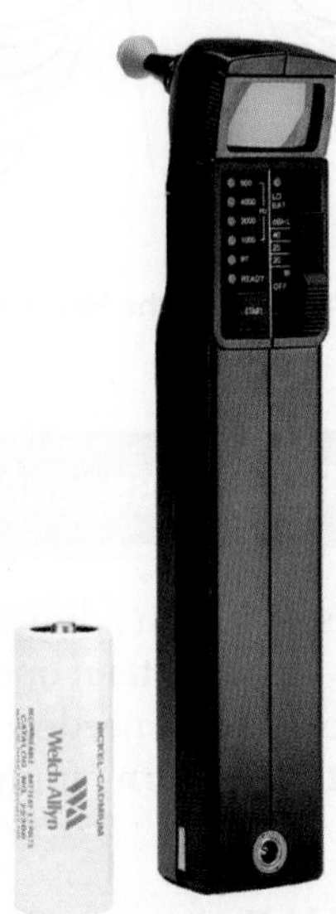

FIGURE 22.7 Audioscope Instrument for Testing Hearing. (Courtesy Welch Allyn, Skaneateles Falls, New York.)

Chest, heart, and lungs. The chest should rise and fall with respiration symmetrically on both sides of the body. By placing the thumbs over the posterior vertebrae at the level of the tenth rib and noting whether the movement of each thumb is the same on inspiration, you can observe chest excursion. Inspect the spine from the rear and the side. It should be in midline with gentle concave and convex curves when viewed laterally. The shoulders should appear to be at equal height. Note whether **lordosis** (exaggerated lumbar curve), **kyphosis** (increased curve in the thoracic area), or **scoliosis** (pronounced lateral curvature of the spine) is present.

Inspect the anterior chest to see if there is a noticeable point of maximal impulse (PMI) of the heart. It will be located at or close to the fifth intercostal space at the left midclavicular line. Place the diaphragm of the stethoscope over this area and listen for the heart sounds S_1 and S_2. S_1 is the "lub" sound, and S_2 is the "dub" sound. S_1 is loudest at the apex of the heart in the mitral area. S2 is softer at this location and can be heard more loudly over the aortic area (Fig. 22.8). The sounds are heard best if the stethoscope is placed against the skin rather than the cloth of the gown or shirt. Count the apical pulse and note whether it is regular. Determine whether any sounds present aside from the two normal heart sounds, such as the swish of a murmur (Steps 22.3). After mastering basic heart sounds, you can practice listening to the valve sounds with the bell of the stethoscope placed lightly on the skin.

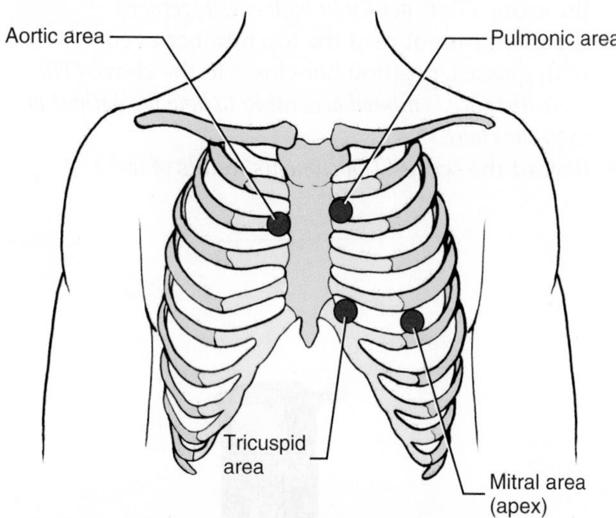

FIGURE 22.8 **Auscultate the Heart in Each Area.**

The locations for listening to the valves are shown in Figure 22.8. It takes considerable practice to hear all but the loudest heart murmurs and to determine the type. You will learn more about abnormal heart sound assessment and further techniques for assessing each body system in your medical-surgical nursing courses.

Lung sounds are auscultated using the diaphragm of the stethoscope. The sounds are created by air moving through passageways of varying diameter and length. The sounds vary in pitch and duration depending on the area of auscultation (Fig. 22.9).

Sounds over the trachea are loud and coarse. They are equal in length for inspiration and expiration and have a slight pause between them. When auscultation is done over the upper area of the chest over the bronchi, the sounds are harsh and loud and are shorter on inspiration than expiration. There is a pause between the two sounds. The **bronchovesicular sounds** are those heard over the central chest or back. Normally they are equal in length during inspiration and expiration and have no pause between them. They are medium in tonality and loudness. **Vesicular sounds** are the soft, rustling sounds heard in the periphery of the lung fields. They are longer on inspiration than expiration, and there is no pause between them. Table 22.1 presents **adventitious sounds** (abnormal lung sounds). Perform auscultation in a systematic manner according to a set pattern (Fig. 22.10). Steps 22.4 present the steps for

Steps 22.3 Basic Assessment of Heart Sounds

Heart sounds are assessed on admission to the health facility or agency's care and then once each shift in the hospital. A quiet room is needed to assess heart sounds; ask the patient to turn off music or the television.

ACTION *(RATIONALE)*

1. Perform hand hygiene and explain the procedure. Provide privacy by closing the door or curtains. *(Reduces transfer of microorganisms; explaining the procedure places patient more at ease. Closing the door or curtains protects patient's right to privacy and prevents embarrassment.)*
2. Have patient sit upright or elevate head of bed 45 to 90 degrees if not contraindicated. *(Sitting position brings the heart closer to anterior chest wall.)*
3. Loosen or remove clothing. *(Allows anatomic landmarks to be identified and the stethoscope to be placed on the skin.)*
4. Place the diaphragm of the stethoscope at the apex of the heart (fifth intercostal space, left midclavicular line) and identify S_1 and S_2, the "lub" and "dub" sounds. Count the apical pulse rate. *(Heart sounds are normally the loudest at the apex of the heart. "Lub" and "dub" together make up one heartbeat.)*
5. Using the bell of the stethoscope, auscultate in the four valve areas for abnormal sounds (see Fig. 22.8). *(Bell picks up lower-pitched sounds.)*
6. Replace clothing and make the patient comfortable. Lower the bed and raise the side rails if they were moved. Assist patient with music or TV when finished. *(Prevents chilling, protects privacy, and shows consideration and caring.)*
7. Report murmurs or any sound that is different from an S_1 or S_2 *(Abnormal sounds may indicate a change in condition.)*
8. Record the apical heart rate and presence of normal or abnormal sounds. *(Notes rate and any abnormal sounds: for example, "Apical rate 74, regular with normal S_1S_2.")*

performing lung auscultation. Perform auscultation on initial assessment and once per shift for all patients who are on bed rest, who have a respiratory problem, or who are at risk for a respiratory problem.

Skin and extremities. The skin is inspected for any rash or lesions (Table 22.2), and the assessment frequently includes the Braden Scale for Predicting Pressure Sores. There should be no flaking or excessive dryness. Check turgor by gently pinching up a bit of skin on the arm or over the sternum. If the skin is slow to return to a flat position, the patient is most likely dehydrated. If the skin returns to the original position in less than 3 seconds, the turgor is "brisk." Ask about any changes in moles or other lesions. Check the nails for discoloration or abnormal appearance. Nail fungus may cause such changes. Abnormally shaped fingertips may indicate a cardiopulmonary problem.

Check capillary refill time by observing the color of the nail bed and then compressing the nail bed with the thumbnail or the distal end of a capped pen. Release the pressure and note how quickly the color returns to the nail bed. If the color returns slowly, check again and count the seconds ("one-one thousand, two-one thousand," etc.) to estimate the number of seconds it takes for the color to return. **Normal refill time is less than 3 seconds.** This is not a comprehensive assessment of circulation, but it can be useful.

Compare peripheral pulses bilaterally. It is most important to check the dorsalis pedis pulse because it is an indication of the quality of circulation in the lower extremities.

Assess for generalized edema by checking for weight gain over a short time. Ask about shoe and ring tightness and sock patterns left on the ankles when socks are removed. Look for eye and hand puffiness and abdominal fullness. To check for dependent edema, press the fingers into the tissue over the tibia just above the ankle. If an indentation remains, **pitting edema** is present (Fig. 22.11). To describe edema, you can use the terms *taut, tight, puffy, indented,* or *pitting*. If pitting is present, it is classified according to its depth.

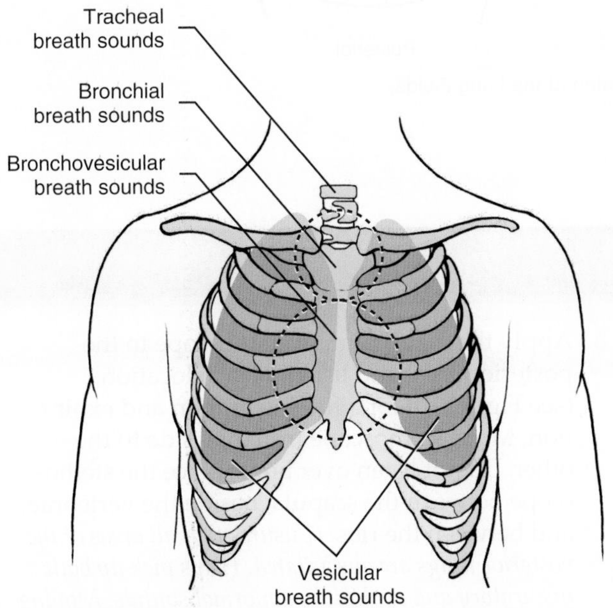

FIGURE 22.9 Locations of Normal Lung Sounds.

Table 22.1 Abnormal Lung Sounds

SOUND	DESCRIPTION
Wheeze	Whistling, musical, high-pitched sound produced by air being forced through a narrowed or partially obstructed airway.
Gurgle or low-pitched wheeze	Coarse, low-pitched, sonorous, rattling sounds caused by secretions in the larger air passages; sometimes called rhonchi.
Crackles	Fine or coarse nonmusical sounds. Fine crackles are high in pitch. Coarse crackles are louder and low in pitch. Crackles are similar to the sound produced by rubbing hairs between the fingers close to the ear.
Stertor	Snoring sound produced by inability to cough up secretions from the trachea or bronchi.
Stridor	Croaking or crowing sound heard when there is partial obstruction of the upper air passages.
Pleural friction rub	Grating or scratchy sound similar to creaking shoe leather or opening a squeaky door, caused when irritated pleural membranes rub over each other.

Life-Span Considerations

Older Adult

- The skin of the older adult is less elastic and drier than that of the younger person. Skin begins to sag. Skin turgor is not an accurate measure of hydration in the older adult. Checking the mucous membranes is a better assessment technique.
- Older adults are prone to develop lesions related to aging, such as brown spots **(lentigines)** and **actinic keratoses** (reddened, flaky areas that are precancerous).

Inquire about any abnormal sensations in the skin. Is there any tingling or twitching? Can the patient feel the difference between warmth and cold? Inquire about any change in muscle strength. Does the patient ambulate normally? Is there weakness or paralysis of any extremity? Inquire about fatigue level. Does the patient have any difficulty bending and moving, as when getting in and out of a chair or a car?

The abdomen. Assess bowel sounds on admission and once per shift for all patients. Bowel sounds are produced by the contractions of the small and large intestine. They are wavelike clicks and gurgles that 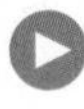 occur from 5 to 30 times a minute. They are particularly active after eating; between meals, it is normal to hear only a few sounds. Bowel sounds are

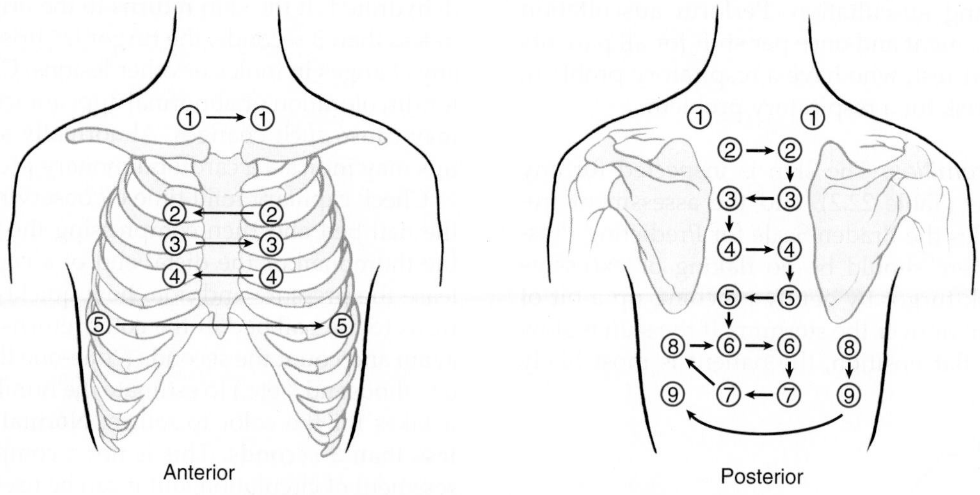

FIGURE 22.10 Sites for Auscultation of the Lung Fields.

Steps 22.4 Auscultating the Lungs

ACTION *(RATIONALE)*

1. Perform hand hygiene and explain what you are going to do. *(Prevents spread of microorganisms. Prepares patient for the procedure.)*
2. Eliminate extraneous noise from the area: ask patient to turn off music or the TV, close the door as needed, and ask patient not to talk. *(Lung sounds are heard more clearly without noise interference.)*
3. Provide privacy by drawing curtain around the bed or closing the door to the room; adjust blinds if the window faces a walkway or if others can see in easily. *(Protects patient's privacy; displays care and courtesy.)*
4. Help patient assume a sitting position with the back away from the bed or chair. Raise bed to working height. *(It is easier to auscultate the posterior of the lungs with patient in a sitting position. If a sitting position is not possible, patient can be turned to the side to auscultate over the back. Raising the bed makes it easier to auscultate without straining back muscles.)*
5. Remove or loosen clothing so that stethoscope can be applied to the skin in the correct locations. *(It is easier to visualize anatomic landmarks if clothing is removed or loosened. Sounds are heard more clearly when stethoscope is placed on the skin rather than on fabric.)*
6. Warm the diaphragm of stethoscope with your hand. *(Reduces discomfort for patient.)*
7. Ask patient to breathe in and out slowly and deeply through an open mouth. *(Reduces air turbulence noise and helps prevent hyperventilation.)*
8. Apply the diaphragm of stethoscope to the posterior chest and listen in each location (see Fig. 22.10) for a full inspiration and expiration. Move stethoscope from one side to the other. Do not listen over bone; place the stethoscope between the scapula, beside the vertebrae, and between the ribs. *(Ensures that all areas of the posterior lungs are auscultated. Helps pick up both inspiratory and expiratory abnormal sounds. Moving from side to side helps to compare sounds heard.)*
9. Move around to the front of the patient and auscultate the anterior and lateral areas of the lungs in a methodical side-to-side fashion. *(Provides a comprehensive assessment.)*
10. If noise from hair on the chest is heard, press the diaphragm more firmly onto chest. *(Hair noise obscures lung sounds.)*
11. If gurgles or low-pitched wheezes or crackles are heard, ask the patient to take a couple of deep breaths and to turn the head away and cough. *(Deep breathing and coughing may clear the passages.)*
12. Compare sounds heard on the right with those on the left for each area. *(Aids in the detection of abnormal sounds.)*
13. Rearrange the patient's clothing and help the patient turn music or the TV back on. Lower the bed if it was raised, and make the patient comfortable. *(Restoring the unit protects privacy and promotes comfort and safety.)*
14. Perform hand hygiene. *(Reduces transfer of microorganisms.)*
15. Document findings. *(Provides data for future comparison.)*

Table 22.2 **Types of Primary Skin Lesions**

LESION	DESCRIPTION	LESION	DESCRIPTION
Macule	Circumscribed, flat area with a change in skin color; smaller than 0.5 cm in diameter; if lesion larger than 0.5 cm, it is a patch *Examples:* freckles, petechiae, measles, flat mole (nevus), café-au-lait spots, vitiligo (complete depigmentation)	**Plaque**	Circumscribed, elevated, superficial, solid lesion; larger than 0.5 cm in diameter *Examples:* psoriasis and seborrheic and actinic keratoses
Papule	Elevated, solid lesion; smaller than 0.5 cm in diameter, if the lesion is larger than 0.5 cm in diameter, it is a nodule *Examples:* wart (verruca), elevated moles, lipoma, and basal cell carcinoma	**Wheal**	Firm, edematous, irregularly shaped area; diameter variable *Examples:* insect bite and urticaria
Vesicle	Circumscribed, superficial collection of serous fluid; smaller than 0.5 cm in diameter *Examples:* varicella (chickenpox), herpes zoster (shingles), and second-degree burn	**Pustule**	Elevated, superficial lesion filled with purulent fluid *Examples:* acne and impetigo

From Lewis, S. L., Dirksen, S. R., Heitkemper, M. M., Bucher, L., & Camera, I. (2014). *Medical-surgical nursing: Assessment and management of clinical problems* (9th ed.). St. Louis, MO: Elsevier Mosby.

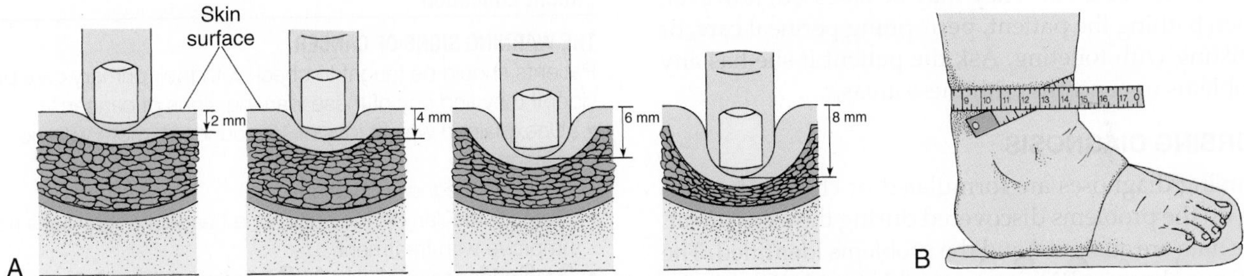

FIGURE 22.11 (A) Measuring pitting edema. (B) Measuring pedal edema. (From deWit, S. C. [2017]. *Medical-surgical nursing: Concepts and practice* [3rd ed.]. Philadelphia, PA: Saunders.)

described as **hyperactive** if they are very frequent, **hypoactive** if there are long periods of silence, and **absent** if no sound is heard for 2 to 5 minutes in any of the four quadrants. With the patient in a supine position, lightly place the stethoscope over a **quadrant** (quarter) of the abdomen and listen; if no sound is heard, progress through the other quadrants until sounds are heard or listen for at least 2 minutes (Fig. 22.12).

Clinical Cues

If you press when you palpate the abdomen before auscultating or press too hard with the stethoscope, you may cause bowel sounds to occur that would not have normally been there.

Next, if the patient has a gastrointestinal problem, percuss over each quadrant of the abdomen (see Fig. 22.2). The sound will be dull over solid tissue and resonant over air-filled areas. If several resonant areas are present, a large amount of gas is in the bowel.

Life-Span Considerations

Older Adult

- Skin sensation and sensory function tend to diminish with aging.
- Muscle strength and joint flexibility may be decreased in the older adult.

After auscultating and percussing, gently palpate each quadrant of the abdomen looking for areas of

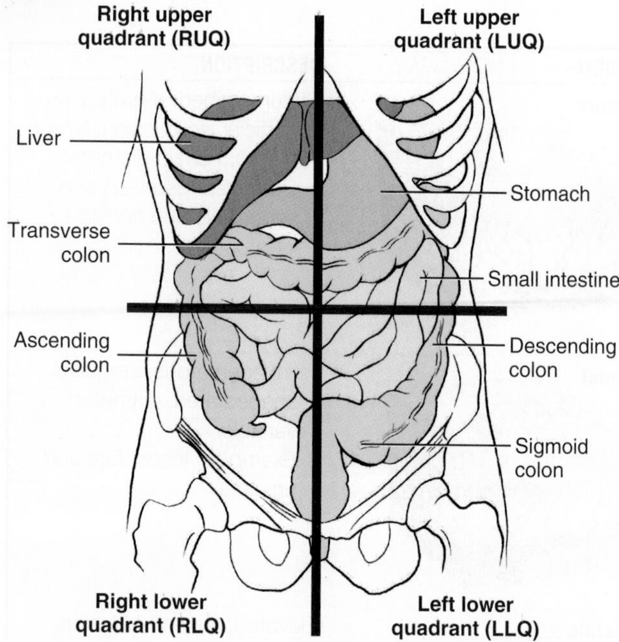

FIGURE 22.12 Auscultation of bowel sounds; listen in each quadrant. *LLQ,* Left lower quadrant; *LUQ,* left upper quadrant; *RLQ,* right lower quadrant; *RUQ,* right upper quadrant.

tenderness, pain, and abnormal masses. When documenting the findings, note the size of the abdomen to establish a baseline for future comparison.

Genitalia, anus, and rectum. Unless the patient has a specific complaint in these areas, the nurse does not visually assess them. They may be assessed, however, when bathing the patient, performing perineal care, or assisting with toileting. Ask the patient if she has any problems or concerns with these areas.

◆ NURSING DIAGNOSIS

Nursing diagnoses are formulated or chosen depending on the problems discovered during the assessment. The data are analyzed and the problems identified. The registered nurse (RN) is responsible for identifying the nursing diagnoses; however, the LPN/LVN may need to choose the appropriate diagnoses from the North American Nursing Diagnosis Association–International (NANDA-I) list if no RN is present during the shift.

◆ PLANNING

Appropriate goals or expected outcomes are written for each nursing diagnosis identified. Set priorities of care based on the most urgent needs of each assigned patient. Make a work organization plan incorporating all of the tasks and assessments that need to be made during the shift.

◆ IMPLEMENTATION

Assessment of patients involves interviewing and gathering a history, performing the physical examination, or assisting the primary care provider while the physical examination is performed.

In many instances, a nursing assessment of the areas of basic need is more appropriate than a total physical assessment is. A systematic way to perform such an assessment is to use the acronym RNS HOPE. The acronym stands for:

- **R**est and activity
- **N**utrition, fluids, and electrolytes
- **S**afety and security
- **H**ygiene and grooming
- **O**xygenation and circulation needs
- **P**sychosocial and learning
- **E**limination

The data to be covered for this assessment of psychosocial and physiologic functioning are listed in Box 22.6. Information gathered from this assessment is then analyzed, and a nursing care plan is prepared using the nursing process. After the initial assessment and development of the care plan, gather additional information in pertinent areas to update the plan and evaluate progress. Skill 22.1 describes the systematic performance of a physical examination.

Each patient should also be assessed at the beginning of each shift or shortly thereafter. This is a quick head-to-toe assessment to enable the nurse to establish priorities of care and organize the work for the shift (Box 22.7).

Patient Education

Patient Education

THE WARNING SIGNS OF CANCER

Patients should be taught to check with their primary care provider if they find any of these warning signs of cancer:

- Unexplained weight loss of 10 pounds or more with no reason.
- Extreme tiredness or fatigue.
- Pain, particularly in the back, or a headache that does not improve with treatment.
- Skin changes: Any wart, mole, or freckle that changes appearance; other skin changes such as color change, pruritus, and excessive hair growth.
- Lesions that do not heal (e.g., on the mouth, skin, or genitals).
- Change in bowel or bladder habits: Long-term constipation, diarrhea, a change in the size of the stool, pain when passing urine, blood in the urine, or a change in bladder function (such as needing to go more or less often than usual).
- White patches inside the mouth or on the tongue: could be precancerous lesions.
- Unusual bleeding or discharge: from the stool, vagina, urine, nipple, or coughing up blood.
- Lump (or red/thickened skin): breast, testicle, lymph nodes (glands), and the soft tissues (but can happen anywhere).
- Persistent indigestion or trouble swallowing.
- Persistent nagging cough or hoarseness.

Source: American Cancer Association (2015). American Cancer Society releases new breast cancer guideline. <www.cancer.org/cancer/news/news/american-cancer-society-releases-new-breast-cancer-guidelines>.

Box 22.6 Basic Needs Assessment

REST AND ACTIVITY NEEDS
- Body proportion and appearance
- Range of motion in joints
- Muscular strength
- Balance and equilibrium
- Ability to perform activities of daily living (e.g., bathing, dressing, grooming, feeding, elimination, and ambulation)
- Sleep pattern, including interruptions and quality
- Hours of bed rest per day
- Pain

NUTRITIONAL, FLUID, AND ELECTROLYTE NEEDS
- Height and usual weight
- Unusual weight gain or loss
- Caloric needs for level of activity
- Amount and type of food ingested daily
- Vitality level and amount of appetite
- Compliance with prescribed diet
- General body appearance
- Fluid intake and output during past 24 hours, even if intake and output records have not been kept (Question patient and family to arrive at an estimated amount.)
- Abnormal loss of body fluid through suctioning, vomiting, diarrhea, hemorrhage, wound drainage, burns, and so forth
- Tubes used to instill or drain fluids (e.g., intravenous therapy, catheters, food supplements, and total parenteral nutrition)
- Fluid volume; edema; weight change
- Normal filling of neck veins
- Turgor of skin and moistness of mucous membranes
- Laboratory values of blood factors (e.g., hemoglobin, hematocrit, and electrolyte levels)

SAFETY AND SECURITY
- Risks for injury: skin condition, pressure areas, falls
- Sensory deficits (e.g., deafness, blindness, or aphasia)
- Muscular weakness (e.g., paresis or paralysis)
- Language spoken at home
- Understanding of written and spoken English
- Any indication of physical or emotional abuse
- Need for prosthetic, security, or safety devices

HYGIENE AND GROOMING
- Ability to bathe, dress, and groom self
- Amount of assistance needed
- Preferred routines

OXYGENATION AND CIRCULATION NEEDS
- Rate, depth, and pattern of breathing
- Breath sounds, upper and lower air passages, auscultated front and back
- Cough and sputum production
- Level of consciousness
- Orientation to reality
- Blood pressure
- Heart sounds
- Pulse rate and characteristics
- JVD
- Peripheral pulses
- Skin color and temperature
- Laboratory values (e.g., CBC, arterial blood gases) (if available)
- Tolerance for usual ADLs

PSYCHOSOCIAL AND LEARNING NEEDS
- Desire for spiritual assistance
- Support system
- Mental outlook
- Usual coping mechanisms
- Need for social service consult
- Financial worries
- Fears and concerns
- Knowledge deficits and learning needs

ELIMINATION
- Characteristics and amount of urinary output
- Characteristics and regularity of bowel movements
- Control of urinary and anal sphincters
- Alterations in elimination (e.g., use of laxatives or presence of catheter or ostomy)
- Bowel sounds and abdominal characteristics
- Presence of pain, burning, or other discomfort
- Signs of dehydration and temperature control

Skill 22.1 Performing a Physical Examination

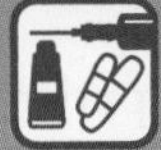
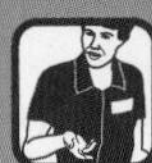
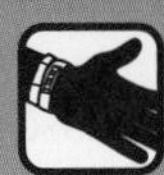

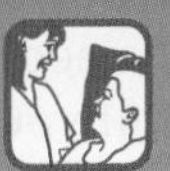
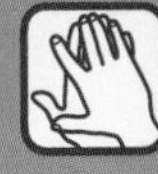

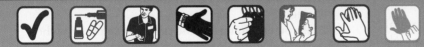

Nursing physical assessments are of various types and depth, depending on the situation and the need. The assessment guide presented here is for a basic nursing physical examination. Further assessment would be indicated for areas where abnormalities are detected. With experience, you will add other assessment techniques to this basic examination.

Supplies
- Stethoscope
- Sphygmomanometer
- Thermometer
- Scale with measuring rod
- Patient gown

Review and carry out the Standard Steps in Appendix A.

ACTION *(RATIONALE)*

1. Interview the patient and obtain a thorough history. *(Provides data regarding past medical problems, current complaints, and risk factors for various disorders.)*
2. Ask the patient to put on a patient gown. *(Provides easy access to various parts of the body for examination.)*
3. Weigh and measure patient. Record the measurements. *(Establishes baseline height and weight.)*
4. With patient seated, examine the head and neck. *(Allows the blood pressure to stabilize while performing another part of the examination.)*
5. Examine the skin and joints of the extremities. Check and compare the peripheral pulses bilaterally. *(Provides data about possible joint problems, skin lesions, and circulatory problems; detects the presence and quality of peripheral pulses.)*
6. Measure the blood pressure, pulse, respirations, and temperature. *(Supplies information about vital functions of the body.)*
7. Auscultate the heart, listen in valve areas, and count the apical heart rate. *(Determines abnormalities of heart rate and rhythm and the presence of abnormal sounds.)*

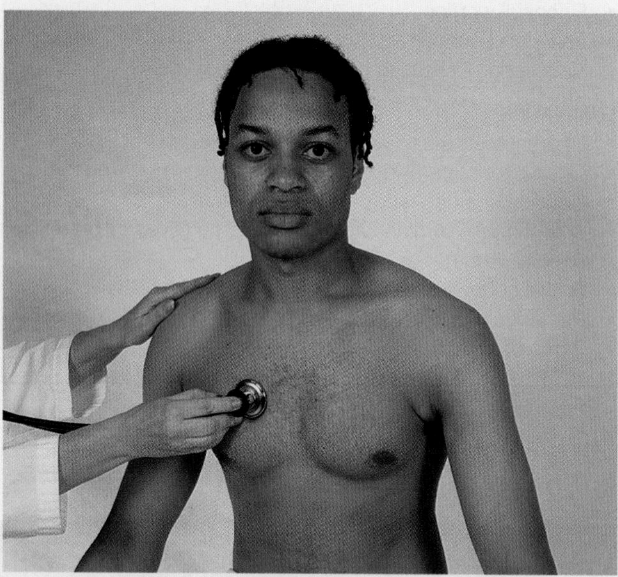

Step 7

8. Auscultate the lungs and check for bilateral equal chest movement with respiration. *(Noting rate, rhythm, and depth of respiration and comparing sounds from one side with the other help determine whether lung abnormalities are present.)*
9. Have the patient recline to a supine position on the examining table or bed and assess the abdomen. Auscultate for bowel sounds, percuss for areas of excessive gas, and palpate gently for tenderness. *(Determines whether bowel sounds are present and normal, whether excess air is in the colon, and whether tenderness is present.)*
10. Obtain any needed specimens. *(Provides specimens for ordered diagnostic tests.)*
11. Direct further attention to any area in which a problem was discovered or in which patient has a complaint. *(Gathers data to be brought to the attention of the physician, nurse practitioner, or physician's assistant.)*
12. If an eye examination is indicated, check visual acuity. *(Determines whether further eye examination is needed for visual correction.)*
13. If need indicates, check hearing using an audioscope. *(Screens for hearing abnormalities requiring referral for further testing.)*
14. Document findings of the physical examination. *(Provides a written record of the findings. Provides baseline data for comparison with future assessment.)*
15. Allow patient to dress and ask if there are any questions. *(Shows courtesy and care.)*

SPECIAL CONSIDERATIONS

- Review the physical changes of aging before deciding that a finding is "abnormal" in the older adult.
- Allow the older adult patient time to adjust to position changes, and assist with ambulation, if needed.
- If any neurologic abnormality is noted, perform a neurologic check (see Skill 22.2).
- During the assessment, question the patient about the most recent dental and eye examinations. Inquire as to the status of diagnostic tests recommended periodically for preventive health care and cancer detection.

? Critical Thinking Questions

1. If you have a patient who cannot communicate verbally with you and who seems confused, how would you obtain the assessment data you need?
2. If you are doing an assessment on a patient who came in with a respiratory problem and you notice a suspicious-looking mole on the lower leg, how would you get the primary care provider to pay attention to that finding?

Provide patient education about the purpose of diagnostic tests ordered and explain what they will experience when undergoing them. Every patient should inquire about recommended diagnostic tests: checking stool for occult blood, sigmoidoscopy or colonoscopy, mammography and conventional (Papanicolaou [Pap] smear) or liquid-based cytology (women), blood glucose level, complete blood count (CBC) and metabolic panel of laboratory tests, urinalysis, full eye examination, and hearing test.

Patient Education

Topics for Patient Education

A good time to provide patient education about preventive health care is while you are assessing the patient. Topics can include:

- The need for regular physical examinations
- Recommended periodic diagnostic tests
- The need for immunizations
- The necessity of regular dental examinations
- The warning signs of cancer
- When to notify their primary care provider

Cultural Considerations

Modesty

Some cultures are modest when it comes to touch and may be uncomfortable touching their own bodies. It is essential to understand this reluctance when patient education involves self-examination. Stressing the benefits of the procedure may help overcome the problem.

Assisting With a Physical Examination

You may be asked to do the initial screening of the patient before the patient is seen by the examiner. Obtain a brief history of any complaints, measure vital signs, and prepare the patient for the examination. You should explain the examination procedure to the patient, answer any questions the patient has, and generally try to put the patient at ease. The examiner will explore each part of the body in considerable depth.

Positioning and draping. You will prepare the patient for the particular type of examination the examiner is

Box 22.7 Shift Head-to-Toe Assessment

INITIAL OBSERVATION
- Skin color
- Appearance
- Affect
- Ease of respiration
- How the patient is feeling

HEAD
- Ability to respond to questions
- Appearance of eyes
- Ability to communicate
- Level of consciousness
- Presence of confusion
- Presence of JVD

VITAL SIGNS
- Temperature
- Pulse rate, rhythm, and quality
- Respiration rate, depth, and pattern
- Blood pressure; compare with previous readings
- Oxygen saturation of the blood

PAIN
- Level of pain
- Frequency of use of medication
- Present status; need for medication
- Patient-controlled analgesia (PCA) pump functioning; medication left

CHEST: GENERAL HEART AND LUNG ASSESSMENT
- Auscultate lung fields
- Listen to heart rate at apex
- Inspect for equal bilateral movement of chest wall

ABDOMEN
- Appetite
- Shape
- Soft or hard
- Bowel sounds
- Time of last bowel movement
- Voiding status

EXTREMITIES
- Normal movement bilaterally
- Skin turgor and temperature
- Skin lesions or pressure areas
- Sensation
- Presence of edema
- Peripheral pulses; compare bilaterally
- Signs of possible abuse

TUBES AND EQUIPMENT
- Intravenous catheter: condition of site, fluid infusing, rate, additives; time next bag is to be started
- Nasogastric tube: suction setting; amount and description of drainage; patency of tube, security of tube
- Urinary catheter: description and quantity of drainage; tube not under patient
- Dressings: location, drains in place; wound suction devices; amount and description of wound drainage
- Oxygen cannula or mask: flow rate in liters; tracheostomy site; ventilator settings
- Pulse oximeter: intact probe and readings
- Traction: correct weight and body alignment; weights hanging free
- Other equipment: applied properly and functioning as ordered

ASSESSMENT OF NEEDS
- Call bell in reach
- Tissues and waste container in reach
- TV control in reach
- Water and personal items positioned conveniently
- Room temperature suitable
- Room neat and tidy
- Determine what supplies will be needed in the room for the remainder of the shift

going to perform. Most examinations begin with the patient in a gown, seated on the end of the examination table with a drape over the lap and legs. The patient then assumes a supine position, and the drape is pulled up over the upper body to expose the chest and/or abdomen. For the lithotomy position used to examine the female genitalia and for the pelvic examination, stirrups hold the patient's feet in an elevated position. To drape for the lithotomy position, provide a draping sheet or a bath blanket turned so that one corner forms a triangle that falls between the legs. The pillow can be brought down from the head of the table to cushion the patient's head while in this position. The patient's buttocks should be right at the end of the table.

Life-Span Considerations

Older Adult

- An older adult will become chilled quickly because less subcutaneous tissue is present. Be certain draping is sufficient to prevent chilling.
- An older adult may become stiff when in a particular position on the examining table and should be slowly helped to a seated position for a few minutes and then assisted from the table to stand.

The knee-chest position is sometimes used for a rectal examination. A lateral or Sims position is used for a flexible sigmoidoscopy examination of the lower colon. A prone position may be needed for an examination of (or to remove lesions on) the back or the back of the legs (Fig. 22.13).

The primary purpose of draping the patient is to prevent unnecessary exposure of the body during the examination. **A patient who feels exposed and embarrassed will be tense, restless, and less able to cooperate.** Proper draping contributes to the patient's feeling of being cared for, and it promotes relaxation. The drapes also provide some warmth and prevent chilling.

The drapes may be of cloth or paper. The examining gown is also used for draping, since it can be arranged to expose and cover different parts of the body as needed.

Elements of the physical examination. Before a pelvic examination, the patient should empty the bladder. If a urine specimen is required, it is obtained before the patient undresses for the examination. Provide the patient a labeled container and directions for specimen collection.

Ask the patient to disrobe and don the examination gown. Prepare the examination table with a fresh paper cover, provide a drape, and prepare the necessary equipment for the physical examination (Box 22.8). Explain to the patient how to don the gown and how to place the drape. If a pelvic examination and Pap smear (either conventional or liquid-based cytology) are to be performed, place a vaginal speculum, gloves, and lubricating jelly in a convenient location. Place fixative for the slide within reach; open the ThinPrep jar if needed. Place large cotton-tipped swabs within reach. Open and label the kit for the smear, and place the patient's name and the date on the end of the slide, in pencil. Affix the label to the ThinPrep jar if used. Fill in the laboratory requisition slip. Position the examination light so that the examiner can adjust it.

A female nurse may be requested to be present in the room when a male health care provider performs a pelvic or breast examination of a patient. When the

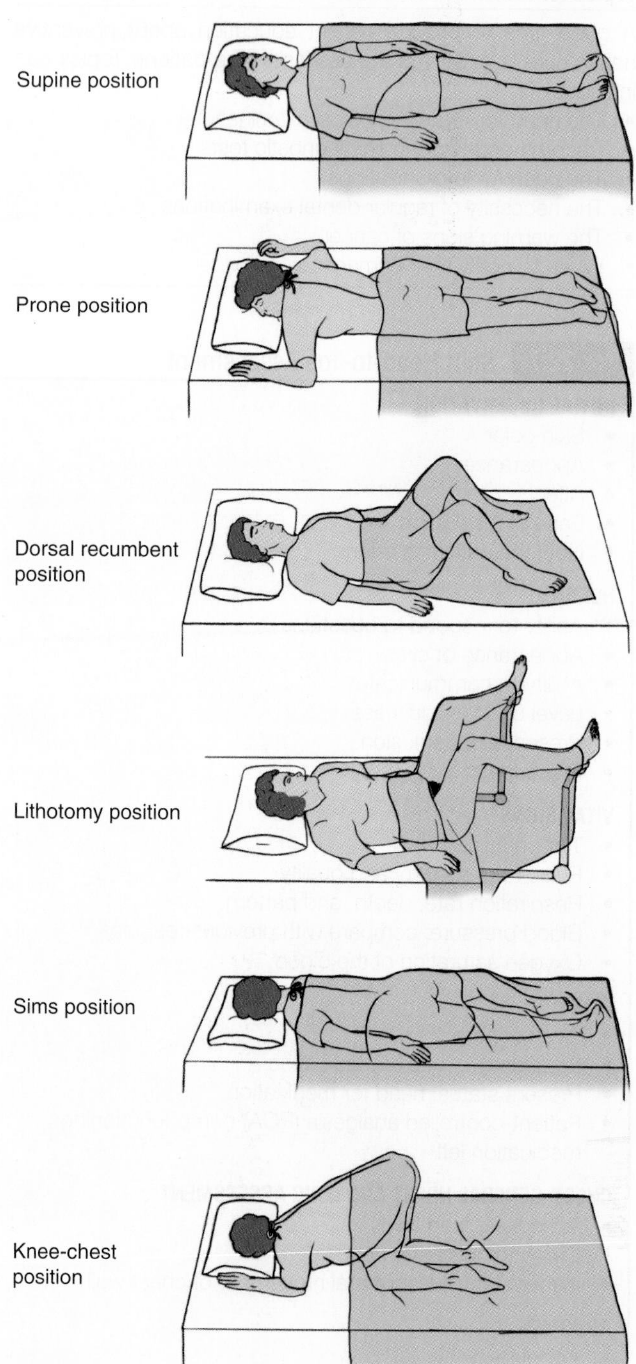

FIGURE 22.13 Positions for Physical Examination and Procedures.

examiner is ready, pull out the stirrups on the examination table and help the patient assume a lithotomy position. Keep the drape over the lower half of the patient's body during positioning. The examiner obtains specimens for the Pap smear and then performs the pelvic examination.

For the male patient, a glove, lubricant, and a test card for occult blood in the stool are placed adjacent to the examination table.

Other common procedures that you may be asked to perform are a urine dip, a hemoglobin measurement, a random blood glucose measurement, an electrocardiogram, and possibly a spirometry reading. Blood may need to be drawn for blood chemistry tests and a CBC. These procedures are described in Chapter 24.

After the patient has been prepared, the examiner systematically assesses every body system. The ophthalmoscope is used to check the interior of the eye (Fig. 22.14). The light in the room is dimmed for this procedure. Pupil response is tested by shining the light into first one eye and then the other and watching the pupils constrict. Ocular pressure is tested for glaucoma in specialized offices, surgery centers, or eye clinics.

The ears are examined with an otoscope after the outer ear is palpated for tenderness or nodules. With this instrument, the health care provider can visualize the ear canal and the tympanic membrane (Fig. 22.15). It is normal for cerumen to be in the ear. If there is excessive cerumen, the ear may need to be lavaged.

Clinical Cues

If the ear is to be lavaged, it is helpful to instill a wax dissolver into the ear and to let it sit for 10 to 30 minutes before lavaging. This makes the lavage procedure shorter and more comfortable for the patient.

Hearing may be initially tested with the Weber test, which is performed by striking a tuning fork and placing it in the middle of the patient's forehead or the skull. The patient says whether the sound is heard equally in both ears. The Rinne test compares air versus bone conduction of sound; sound is normally heard longer by air conduction. The tuning fork is struck and placed beside the ear. It is then struck and placed on the bone behind the ear. The patient says which sound lasted longer.

After the head and neck, chest, lungs, and heart have been examined, the patient is asked to lie down on the examination table. The abdomen is assessed with the patient in this supine position.

Box 22.8 Equipment and Supplies for the Physical Examination

The examiner should have the following items available to perform a physical examination:

- Examination gown
- Drape(s)
- Stethoscope
- Thermometer
- Sphygmomanometer
- Scale with height rod
- Tape measure
- Otoscope
- Ophthalmoscope
- Percussion hammer
- Tuning fork
- Tongue blades
- Cotton-tipped applicators
- Laboratory and x-ray request forms
- Examination lamp
- Flashlight
- Nasal speculum
- Vaginal speculum
- Rectal speculum
- Lubricant
- Snellen eye chart
- Tonometer
- Eye occluder or card
- Audioscope or ticking watch
- Papanicolaou smear supplies
- Test card for occult blood

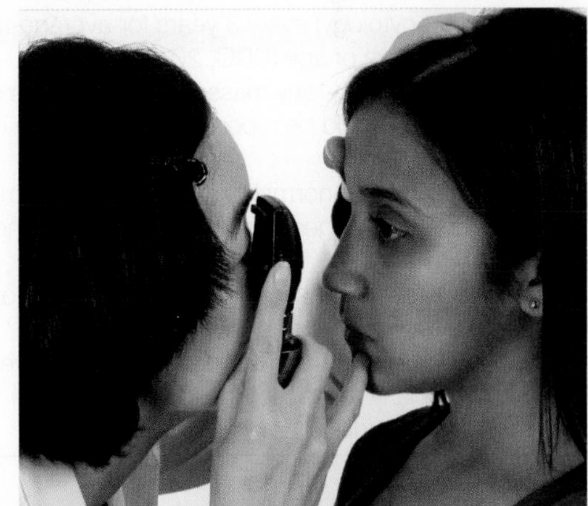

FIGURE 22.14 Checking the Eye With an Ophthalmoscope. (From Jarvis, C. [2016]. *Physical examination and health assessment* [7th ed.]. Philadelphia, PA: Saunders.)

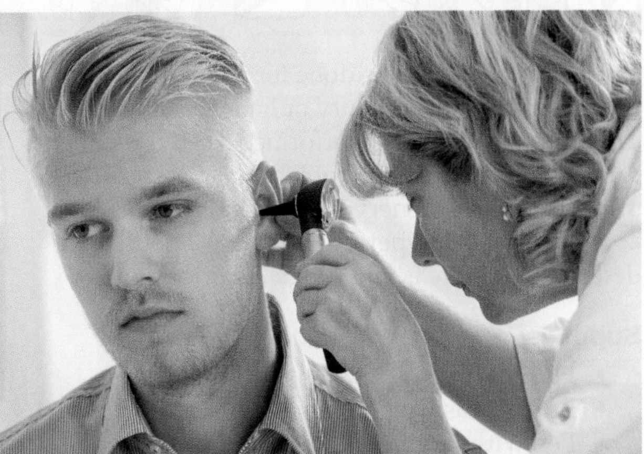

FIGURE 22.15 Checking the Ear With an Otoscope. (Photo copyright istock.com.)

 Health Promotion

Recommended Periodic Diagnostic Tests

Patients should be taught that the following diagnostic tests should be performed periodically to prevent health problems or detect cancer:

- **Blood pressure**—annual measurement; more frequently if elevated above 140/90 mm Hg.
- **Cholesterol**—measurement every 1 to 3 years; more frequently if above 200 mg/dL.
- **Blood glucose**—measurement every 1 to 3 years; more frequently if above 100 mg/dL.
- **Bone density**—screening for osteoporosis with a **dual-energy x-ray absorptiometry** (DXA) of the hip and lumbar spine for women aged 65 years and older.
- **Breast**—mammogram beginning at age 45 and then every 2 years after age 55, continuing as long as a woman is in good health (American Cancer Society, 2015). Women may begin screening at age 40 if desired, and may continue with annual mammography at age 55. They should determine these choices in collaboration with their primary care provider.
- **Colon-rectum**—fecal occult blood testing, sigmoidoscopy or colonoscopy, performed at age 50 and continuing until age 75 years (CDC, 2014b).
- **Cervix and uterus**—if the cervix and uterus are present, pelvic examination every year, and Pap smear (conventional or liquid-based cytology) every 3 years for average-risk women 21 to 65 years of age (CDC, 2014a).
- **Testicles and prostate**—any masses in the testicles or difficulties urinating should be reported to the primary care provider.
- **Skin**—any moles with abnormal pigmentation, asymmetry, irregular borders, or changes should be reported to the primary care provider.
- **Oral**—yearly dental examination; inspect sides and bottom of the tongue every few months.
- **Eye**—examination every 3 to 5 years; after age 40 every 2 to 3 years, particularly testing for glaucoma; more frequently for those with diabetes or eye disease.

Further assessment of the extremities may be performed. When the examination is complete, the patient is often asked to dress, and then the findings are discussed.

Special Focused Examinations

At times, you will need to perform a neurologic check, which is a brief form of a neurologic examination. The neurologic check is performed at regular intervals on patients who have experienced a head injury or who have had brain surgery. **It is done for any patient at risk of increasing intracranial pressure.** A decrease in level of consciousness is an indicator of neurologic deterioration. Skill 22.2 presents the steps of the neurologic check.

The pupil size is measured under normal light conditions. Pupils are normally round and equal in size. A flashlight is used to make the pupils constrict. They should constrict briskly when stimulated by the light. Both pupils should get smaller when either eye is stimulated by the light; this is called the **consensual reflex.** Pupils also constrict when looking at a near object and then dilate when viewing a far object; this is called **accommodation.** Normal findings are often documented using the acronym PERRLA, meaning *P*upils *E*qual, *R*ound, and *R*eactive to *L*ight and *A*ccommodation. Eye muscles are tested by checking extraocular movements (EOMs). Ask the patient to track your finger or an object as it is moved to six different positions. The eyes normally move in a coordinated manner. Absence of movement or irregular movement may indicate cranial nerve damage or a neurologic problem.

The Glasgow Coma Scale is used in most hospitals to score the neurologic examination for patients with decreased level of consciousness (Table 22.3). It provides a baseline against which changes can be evaluated.

Skill 22.2 Performing a Neurologic Check

 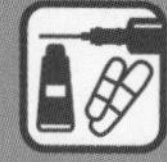 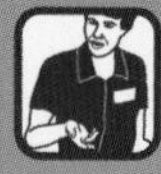  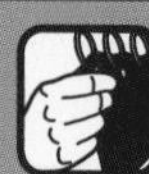 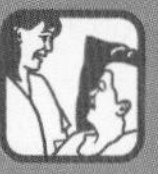 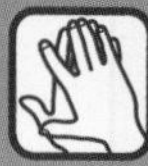 

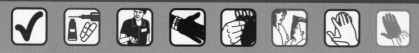

The neurologic check is done for any patient who has sustained a head injury or had cranial surgery. This assessment is also performed for those patients who have a neurologic problem such as seizures or a suspected central nervous system infection. This assessment is often performed every 2 hours to determine if there is neurologic deterioration.

Supplies

- Flashlight
- Pupil measuring guide
- Pen with the cap on

Review and carry out the Standard Steps in Appendix A.

ACTION *(RATIONALE)*

1. Ask the patient questions to test orientation to person, place, time, and event. Ask if the patient remembers where she is, what month it is, who is president, when she was born, or other relevant questions. Do not ask the same questions each time the neurologic check is performed. *(Checks degree of mental orientation.)*
2. With room lights subdued, but not dim, examine the size of the pupils and determine whether they are equal in size. Measure the size. *(Increasing intracranial pressure, when extreme, causes one or both pupils to dilate.)*

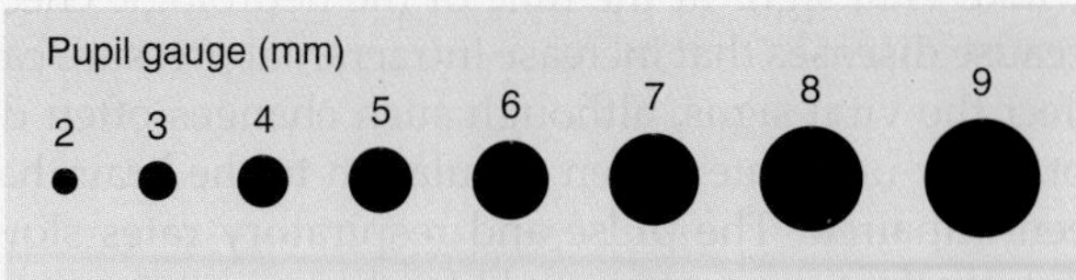

Step **2**

3. Turn the flashlight on and position it lateral to the eye on the same plane. Slowly bring it over to shine directly on the pupil of the eye on that side and watch to see whether the pupil constricts. Quickly move the light back away to the side of the head. Briefly shine the light directly onto the pupil again and watch the other eye for pupil constriction, indicating a consensual reflex. *(The pupil of that eye should constrict briskly and return to its former size after the light is averted. The pupil of the eye that did not have light shone in it should also constrict, demonstrating consensual reflex)*
4. Perform the same maneuver for the other eye. Briefly shine the light directly onto the pupil and watch for the pupillary reaction. Briefly shine the light directly onto the pupil again and watch the other eye for pupil constriction, indicating a consensual reflex. *(If the pupil reacts sluggishly, it indicates that intracranial pressure is rising. Report this to the primary care provider immediately.)*
5. Ask the patient to follow your finger, pen, or pencil with her eyes as you move it to the cardinal (primary) points. Test on one side and then the other. *(Watch the patient's eyes to see whether the patient tracks your finger without* **nystagmus** *[jerky movements]. Checking these eye movements provides information about cranial nerves III, IV, and VI.)*

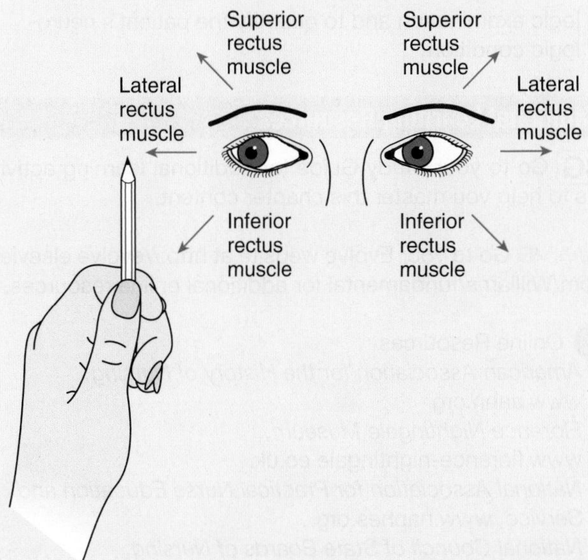

Step 5 (Adapted from Ignatavicius, D. D., & Workman, M. L. [2002]. *Medical-surgical nursing: Critical thinking for collaborative care* [4th ed.]. Philadelphia, PA: Saunders.)

6. Ask the patient to follow your commands. Ask the patient to do specific things, such as rotate the left foot at the ankle or touch the nose with the right index finger. *(The ability to follow commands indicates intact cognition and motor pathways.)*
7. Test extremity muscle strength by having the patient push against your hands with the sole of one foot and then with the other. Then cross your middle and index fingers on both hands, and have the patient grasp each set of fingers with the hand opposite it. Check for the degree of strength and equality of strength on both sides. *(Decreases in muscle strength can indicate pressure on certain areas within the brain or a problem within the spinal cord or muscles themselves. When weakness occurs on one side only, it can indicate a problem on the opposite side of the brain. Crossing the fingers prevents excessive pain.)*

For the Comatose Patient

8. Check the patient's response to a stimulus by pressing on the area near the base of a fingernail with a hard object or by applying pressure with two fingers in a grasp position on the trapezius muscle. *(Note whether the patient grimaces, withdraws from the stimulus, displays flexion posture, or displays extension posture. The Glasgow Coma Scale may be used to rank the patient's condition [see Table 22.3].)*
9. Make the patient comfortable. Document the findings, precisely describing any abnormalities found. *(Making the patient comfortable shows care and concern. Documentation notes result of the examination and provides data for future comparison.)*

Critical Thinking Questions

1. Can you explain why pupils might react sluggishly when intracranial pressure is rising?
2. What other questions could you ask the patient besides Where are you? What day is it? and Who is president? that would give you a good indication of the patient's orientation?

Table 22.3 Glasgow Coma Scale[a]

EYE OPENING	POINTS
Spontaneous	4
To sound	3
To pain	2
Never	1
Motor Response	
Obeys commands	6
Localizes pain	5
Normal flexion (withdrawal)	4
Abnormal flexion posturing	3
Extension posturing	2
None	1
Verbal Response	
Oriented	5
Confused conversation	4
Inappropriate words	3
Incomprehensible sounds	2
None	1

[a]The highest possible score is 15. A score of 7 or less indicates coma.

Take vital signs at the time of the neurologic check because diseases that increase intracranial pressure can affect the vital signs, although such changes often do not occur until late, when circulation to the brain has been impaired. The pulse and respiratory rates slow, whereas the temperature and blood pressure rise.

◆ EVALUATION

Evaluating the techniques of physical assessment and the thoroughness of data collection is an individual responsibility. Questions to ask are:

- Were all areas assessed adequately?
- Were any pieces of data missing from the assessment form?
- Was the patient comfortable during the assessment?
- Did the interaction remain focused on the assessment?
- Was all equipment available for the examination?
- Was the patient positioned and draped appropriately?
- Were procedures and their purpose explained to the patient?

A thorough, efficient assessment takes considerable practice. Assessment skills will improve with practice over time.

Get Ready for the NCLEX Examination!

Key Points

- Nurses are expected to perform a basic physical assessment.
- Time and practice will improve assessment skills.
- One of the most important nursing roles is assessing ill patients for signs of complications.
- Assessment of the home care patient is especially important because you are acting as the primary care provider's "eyes and ears" for the patient who cannot go to the office.
- Data collection is a vital part of a physical assessment, and it requires a comprehensive interview.
- A holistic assessment requires psychosocial, spiritual, and cultural data.
- Auscultation, percussion, palpation, and olfaction are used as methods of assessment.
- Auscultation of the lungs and heart must be done carefully and thoroughly.
- The physical assessment provides an excellent patient education opportunity about preventive health care.
- You will assist the examiner with various types of physical examinations by positioning and draping the patient and setting up the required equipment.
- You must be able to assist the patient in assuming the supine, lithotomy, prone, Sims, and lateral positions.
- Draping protects the patient's privacy and modesty and helps prevent chilling.
- Laboratory requisitions must be filled out for all specimens to be sent for analysis.
- A neurologic check is often performed by nurses every few hours on patients at risk of increasing intracranial pressure.
- The Glasgow Coma Scale is used to score the neurologic examination and to quantify the patient's neurologic condition.

Additional Learning Resources

SG Go to your Study Guide for additional learning activities to help you master this chapter content.

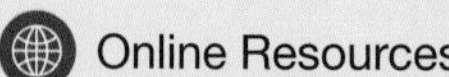 Go to your Evolve website at http://evolve.elsevier.com/Williams/fundamental for additional online resources.

Online Resources

- *American Association for the History of Nursing*, www.aahn.org
- *Florence Nightingale Museum*, www.florence-nightingale.co.uk
- *National Association for Practical Nurse Education and Service*, www.napnes.org
- *National Council of State Boards of Nursing*, www.ncsbn.org
- *National Federation of Licensed Practical Nurses*, www.nflpn.org
- *American Nurses Association*, www.nursingworld.org

Review Questions for the NCLEX Examination

*Choose the **best** answer for each question.*

1. A holistic nursing assessment of a patient is necessary to:
   1. Formulate an effective nursing care plan.
   2. Establish patient trust in the nurse.
   3. Determine the patient's physical problems.
   4. Detect adverse effects of treatment.
2. When performing an auscultation for heart rate and rhythm (S_1 and S_2), it is most important to listen:
   1. At the base of the heart with the bell.
   2. To an area above the left nipple with the bell.
   3. Two inches below the right nipple with the diaphragm.
   4. At the fifth intercostal space, left midclavicular line, with the diaphragm.
3. When auscultating lung sounds, you should: *(Select all that apply.)*
   1. Use the bell of the stethoscope.
   2. Turn off music or the TV.
   3. Use the diaphragm of the stethoscope.
   4. Listen in two or three places.
   5. Follow a systematic pattern of stethoscope placement.
4. Neurologic checks are performed for the patient who has experienced an intracranial injury to determine: *(Select all that apply.)*
   1. State of cognition.
   2. An increase in intracranial pressure.
   3. A lack of coordination.
   4. Pupil reactions.
   5. Decrease in consciousness.
5. When preparing a patient for a pelvic examination, you would first position her on the table in the ____________ position until the examiner is ready to perform the examination.
   1. Supine
   2. Sims
   3. Knee-chest
   4. Lithotomy
6. When planning care for a patient with a respiratory complaint, which pieces of information are most important to consider? *(Select all that apply.)*
   1. Back and joint pain
   2. Decreased appetite
   3. Abnormal breath sounds
   4. Feelings of dyspnea
   5. Decreased activity tolerance
7. When performing an initial assessment on a patient, which piece of information is of highest priority?
   1. Where the patient is living
   2. Any allergies to medications
   3. Treatment for previous illnesses
   4. Date of previous diagnostic tests
8. When checking blood pressure with an automated machine, if the reading is considerably outside the previous reading for the patient, the nurse should first:
   1. Check the BP in the other arm.
   2. Take the BP with the patient supine.
   3. Wait 20 minutes and take another reading.
   4. Measure the BP with a manual sphygmomanometer.

Critical Thinking Activities

Read each clinical scenario and discuss the questions with your classmates.

Scenario A
How could you obtain needed information for your initial assessment from a patient who is deaf?

Scenario B
If you were not certain that the blood pressure measurement you obtained is accurate, what would you do?

Scenario C
How would you handle the situation if your patient refuses to answer the questions you ask during your assessment interview?

Scenario D
What would you do if you are to assess a patient of the opposite sex and the person does not want you to do the assessment?

chapter 23

Admitting, Transferring, and Discharging Patients

http://evolve.elsevier.com/Williams/fundamental

Objectives

Upon completing this chapter, you should be able to do the following:

Theory

1. Differentiate between routine and emergency admissions.
2. Describe the role of the admitting department.
3. Identify the elements included in a patient's orientation to the nursing unit.
4. Discuss five types of information that must be included in the discharge form sent with a patient going to another facility.
5. Delineate the necessary information to include on a patient's discharge instructions when the patient is going directly home.
6. Explain the procedure for pronouncing and recording a patient's death.

Clinical Practice

1. Orient a patient to the patient unit and the hospital.
2. Assist with the performance of an admission assessment.
3. Assist with the transfer of a patient to another unit.
4. Use correct communication techniques to ensure safe handoff of a patient to another nurse, department, or facility.
5. Interact with the social worker regarding the discharge needs of an assigned patient.
6. Demonstrate appropriate interaction with the family of a patient who has died.

Key Terms

autopsy (ăw-tŏp-sē, p. 405)
co-pays (cō–pāz, p. 399)
coroner (cŏ-rŏ-nĕr, p. 405)
deductibles (dē-dŭc-tĭ-blz, p. 399)
discharge planner (p. 403)
do not resuscitate (DNR) (p. 404)
emergency admissions (ē-mĕr-gĕn-cē ăd-mĭsh-ŭnz, p. 399)
health maintenance organizations (HMOs) (p. 399)
managed care plans (p. 399)
Medicaid (mĕd-ĭ-cād, p. 399)
medical social worker (MSW) (p. 404)
Medicare (mĕd-ĭ-cār, p. 399)
routine admissions (rū-tēn, p. 398)

 Concepts Covered in This Chapter

- Anxiety
- Collaboration
- Communication
- Culture
- Mobility pain
- Patient education

TYPES OF ADMISSIONS

Each day thousands of people are admitted to acute care facilities. This is part of the daily routine for the nurse, but for the patient, it is a major event. Do not lose sight of the admission's impact on the patient. Illness, injury, and the need for surgery are highly stressful, particularly if associated with loss of function, chronic health problems, a change in body appearance, or a terminal diagnosis. The financial impact can be devastating because of both the cost of care and the loss of income. These stressors extend to include the family and often close friends and associates as well.

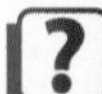 Think Critically

If you learned you needed to be admitted to the hospital today, how would it affect or alter your life right now?

ROUTINE ADMISSIONS

Routine admissions are those that are scheduled in advance. The primary care provider and patient have agreed to the admission as the most appropriate way to address the medical need, and the patient has had at least a short time to make plans and arrangements for this interruption in the usual routine.

 QSEN Considerations: Patient-Centered Care

Family Care

In some cultures, family members are expected to go with the patient and stay with him in the hospital. It is up to the nurse to ensure that the family is allowed to spend time with their loved one without causing disruptions for the other patients. Providing a family room or a secluded corner and allowing one or two visitors at a time can help to meet this need.

Many facilities have specific units that provide same-day surgeries. Patients arrive a few hours before their procedure and, after a short recovery period in the day-surgery unit, they are discharged home. Although considered outpatients, same-day surgery patients must meet the routine admissions criteria. If their condition is such that they cannot go home the same day, they are admitted to an inpatient nursing unit.

EMERGENCY ADMISSIONS

Emergency admissions are those for which there was no prior planning. These occur when sudden illness, injury, or abrupt worsening of an existing condition requires immediate admission for treatment. Such admissions tend to be particularly stressful for both the patient and close family and friends. In addition to worry and fear about the medical problem, the patient may have prior commitments that now cannot be met or children who need care. These concerns can have a direct effect on the patient's response to treatment.

ADMISSION PROCESS

PREADMISSION PROCEDURES AND REQUIREMENTS

Routine admissions often take place the day of a scheduled procedure. For this reason, most facilities require that the patient come in a day or two before admission to complete the administrative paperwork and have any admitting laboratory work or other diagnostic tests completed.

Insurance companies and health care regulatory organizations mandate that specific criteria be met when an individual is admitted to the hospital. For routine admissions, these are completed in advance. In an emergency, however, they take place as the patient is being stabilized in the emergency department and prepared for admission.

Authorization for Admission

Most third-party payers require prior authorization for hospital admission. There are a variety of third-party payers including private or employer-provided coverage through major insurance companies, **managed care plans** (health care plans in which all medical care except emergency care is managed and must be preauthorized by the insuring group), and **health maintenance organizations (HMOs)** (organizations that provide most outpatient care at organization clinics, may provide inpatient care at organization hospitals, and must authorize usage of outside services). Government plans include **Medicaid** (state medical care coverage for low-income individuals and families), **Medicare** (medical care coverage provided through the Social Security Administration, primarily for people age 65 and over), and TRICARE (coverage in civilian facilities for military staff, family, and retirees).

In most cases, the primary care provider's office is responsible for obtaining authorization for hospital admission. If authorization is denied, it means that the patient's insurance carrier has refused to accept liability for payment. All payment programs and plans have criteria that define the services covered. For example, most plans do not cover procedures that are regarded as purely cosmetic, such as a facelift or breast augmentation, but these same plans may cover cosmetic procedures if they are to repair the effects of an injury or a necessary surgical procedure such as a mastectomy.

Admitting Department Function

The admitting department is responsible for making sure that all admission criteria are met. They collect the personal and insurance information and verify the authorization for admission. In many facilities, the admitting department is part of the business office, and is responsible for making payment arrangements on insurance **deductibles** and **co-pays** (the amounts the insurance carrier may require the patient to pay for care). They may also collect deposits and make payment arrangements for noncovered services.

For an emergency admission, this process may become the responsibility of the emergency department clerical staff.

Laboratory Work and X-Ray Examinations

Laboratory work and examinations related to the planned course of treatment are commonly done before a routine admission. This includes procedures such as x-ray examinations, computed tomography (CT) scans, and magnetic resonance imaging (MRI).

DAY OF ADMISSION

Patients arrive at the hospital 1 or 2 hours before the scheduled procedure. For early procedures, this often means that they arrive near the end of the night shift rather than on the day shift. Day-surgery units typically begin the day shift early, at 5 or 6 am, to accommodate the early arrivals.

Patient Orientation to the Nursing Unit

Newly admitted patients, particularly those who have never been hospitalized before, may be nervous and unsure of what to expect. You can do a great deal to alleviate their anxiety during the initial contact by orienting them to the nursing unit.

You should smile, make eye contact, and call the patient by name. A good example of the initial contact would be, "Hello, Mr. Jones. My name is Sandra Smith. I'm an LPN, and I'll be one of your nurses today." It is important that the patient be given the names of all caregivers and their specific roles. **Never assume that a patient wishes to be called by his or her first name.** Address patients in the manner that is most comfortable for them.

Proceed to orient the patient to the unit. Show the location of the call bell and demonstrate its use. Show the location of the bathroom and use of the emergency call bell next to the toilet. In addition, show the patient how to operate the bed, lights, television, and telephone and explain information on the status board if used (Fig. 23.1). Explain the daily routine including meal times, times of shift change, and visiting hours. If possible, give the patient a printed orientation handout with this information. If the patient is to receive nothing by mouth (NPO), explain or reinforce this information. If the patient is not NPO and has no ordered fluid restriction, obtain a diet order and then fill the water pitcher and place it within the patient's reach.

Although this initial contact is frequently brief and may immediately precede hurried preparations for surgery or other procedures, the patient must be made to feel welcome and valued. **The patient must also be given many opportunities to have questions answered and procedures explained.** If the patient is too ill at the time of admission for a full orientation, it should be done as soon as the patient's condition permits.

 **Life-Span Considerations**

Older Adult

Age and failing health can decrease an older person's ability to cope with and understand change. These patients often need extra time and support in adjusting to a hospital stay.

Care of patient belongings. Hospitals provide little space for personal belongings, but patients may find great comfort in wearing their own bathrobe or having a special picture on the bedside table or shelf. Help your patients put belongings in the closet and encourage them to send home anything that they will not need during their stay. Valuables such as credit cards, money, or jewelry should be sent home with a family member. If this is not possible, obtain a valuables envelope and arrange for safe storage of these items following your facility's protocol. Document all other items such as dentures, hearing aids, or walkers on the patient belongings list and label items with the patient's name when appropriate. Items that plug into electrical outlets need to be checked by the maintenance department to ensure that they are properly grounded. During the patient's stay, update the list to indicate things sent home or new items brought in for the patient's use.

Some patients bring in their medications from home. Each facility has a specific protocol regarding these medications. The medication reconciliation process should be used, comparing the patient's medication orders to all of the medications that the patient has been taking. Most facilities ask that any medications

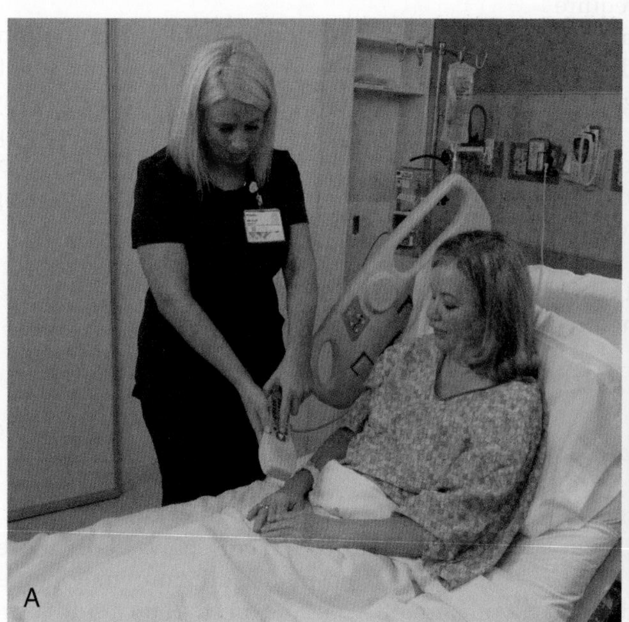

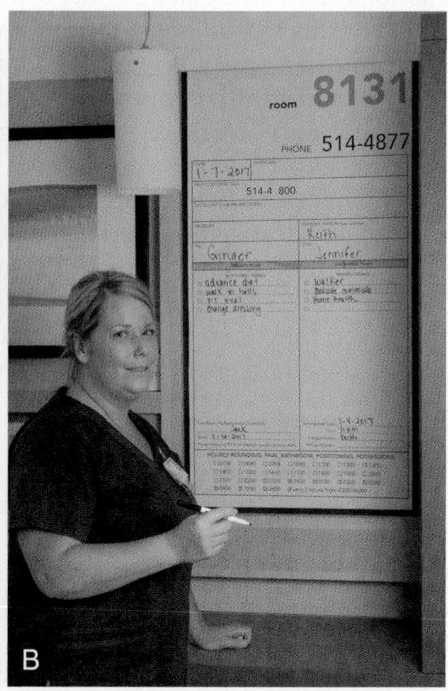

FIGURE 23.1 The Nurse Orienting the Patient to the Unit. (A) Orienting the patient to call bell; (B) orienting the patient to the status board.

brought in be sent home. **It is important to notify the primary care provider of any medications the patient has been taking at home that are not included in the present orders.** Know the proper procedure for your facility and follow it at all times.

Initial Nursing Assessment (Data Collection)

The nursing assessment in an acute care facility is performed and documented by the registered nurse (RN), but the licensed practical nurse/licensed vocational nurse (LPN/LVN) can greatly assist in this process by gathering data during the initial contact. Vital signs, lists of medications (including all over-the-counter medications, supplements, and herbals taken by the patient), and information about allergies, previous hospital stays, illnesses, and surgeries can all be obtained by the LPN/LVN and given to the RN. In some facilities, the nursing assessment is done during a preadmission interview, which significantly reduces the tasks that must be accomplished before patients are sent for scheduled procedures.

LPN/LVNs are frequently charge nurses in skilled nursing facilities and are responsible for completing the written assessment and beginning the care plan. When documenting an assessment, it is important to describe your findings accurately. Most facilities use a check-off system, but a narrative description is still required. Table 23.1 shows the items to be assessed and gives examples of descriptive terms.

Chapter 5 gives specific information on assessment data collection and use of nursing diagnoses. Chapters 5 and 6 discuss the formulation of care plans.

Initiating the Medical Record

In an acute care facility, the patient will have an electronic medical record. In a skilled nursing facility, the charge nurse usually transcribes orders and prepares the paper medical record, laboratory slips, x-ray requests, and consent forms. It is the charge nurse's responsibility to check that everything has been accurately transcribed. The nurse must be able to set up a chart and do the transcription if the charge nurse is not available. Regardless of who does the actual transcription of orders and completion of request forms and consents, the nurse who checks and signs the orders is directly responsible for their accuracy. In most acute care facilities, the RN verifies orders, but in some acute facilities, and in most skilled nursing facilities, this duty is performed by the LPN/LVN.

Admission orders are often long and complex. For safety, the individual transcribing the orders should make a check mark by each order as it is processed. The nurse who reviews the orders must verify that each order has been processed and that the transcription is accurate. **This means the nurse must read every laboratory slip, procedure request, and consent form, correcting as necessary.** If an error has been made on a document to be signed, any changes must be clear and must be initialed. Any deletions are crossed out with a single line, with the nurse's initials, date, and reason for the error written above the line. If a consent form has been transcribed inaccurately, or if the primary care provider orders a change in the wording, it should be destroyed and a new consent written for the patient's signature.

TABLE 23.1 Admission Assessment Data Gathering

ASSESSMENT CATEGORY	EXAMPLES OF DATA
Level of consciousness	Alert, lethargic, drowsy, difficult to arouse, unresponsive to unpleasant stimuli, comatose
Vital signs	Temperature (include how taken [e.g., oral, tympanic, temporal artery, rectal, or axillary], and whether Fahrenheit or Celsius). Pulse rate and quality (e.g., bounding, thready, regular, or irregular). Respiratory rate and quality (e.g., labored, shallow). Respiratory status (e.g., unlabored, labored, wheezing, cough [productive or nonproductive], shortness of breath, use of accessory muscles, or abnormal breath sounds on auscultation [name or describe abnormal sounds]). Blood pressure (systolic and diastolic). Height and weight (the patient should be weighed and measured rather than accepting the stated height and weight unless the medical condition prevents this)
Ability to communicate	Language spoken, any speech impediment or impairment, or decreased ability to understand verbal communication
Vision and hearing	Visual impairment including type and degree; hearing impairment including degree; ability to read Braille, use sign language, or read lips
Condition of skin	Skin breaks or tears, bruises, abrasions, pressure areas, excessive dryness, birthmarks, rashes, surgical incisions, wounds
Prosthetic and assistive devices	Hearing aid, glasses, contact lenses, dentures, braces, walker, wheelchair, cane, artificial limbs, and wigs
Other health problems and concerns	Pain or discomfort, loss of function or loss of normal control of function, restricted movement, alteration in sensation, additional diagnoses other than that for which admission is occurring (e.g., diabetes mellitus or heart disease)

Once transcription of the orders has been verified, the orders are signed. A line is drawn along the left margin of the orders being verified, and then the nurse signs with the date and time immediately below the last order and the care provider's signature. The facility may require that this be done in red ink or have some other specific protocol. Know and follow your facility's policy.

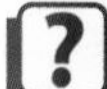

Clinical Cues

Avoid conversing with co-workers while signing off orders to help ensure that mistakes are not made because of interruption and distraction.

Hospitals and other facilities have specific policies for noting allergies. In most institutions, they are written on the plan of care and displayed prominently in the medical record. In addition, patients wear a colored wristband with the allergies clearly listed.

REACTIONS TO ADMISSION

Patients may have various reactions to admission. They may experience anxiety over what will happen to them, concern over being away from home or work duties, financial concerns, fear of a possible diagnosis, fear of loss of privacy, or concerns about comfort and quality of care. Feelings of loneliness or loss of identity may occur. Discover how the patient feels about admission and ask about any fears or concerns.

Think Critically

What would you do if your patient being admitted tells you that she has no one at home to care for her children and that she was supposed to pick them up from school?

PLAN OF CARE

QSEN Considerations: Teamwork and Collaboration

Memory Jogger

Preparation of the care plan is part of the assessment, and it is done by the nurse in collaboration with all health team members.

The basis of the plan of care is the nursing process and nursing diagnosis, both of which are covered in detail in Chapters 4 to 6.

PATIENT TRANSFER TO ANOTHER HOSPITAL UNIT

Changes in condition may require that a patient be transferred from one nursing unit to another. As patients in the intensive care unit (ICU) or cardiac care unit (CCU) become stable, they are often transferred to a step-down unit SDU or to the medical-surgical unit. A patient who was originally admitted to the medical or surgical unit may become less stable and be transferred to the SDU, ICU, or CCU.

Before a patient is transferred, the patient's primary care provider must be notified and approve the transfer. If the patient's condition suddenly deteriorates, he may be moved immediately per established hospital protocols, but in general, transfers from one nursing area to another require a specific order by the attending physician. The admissions office, or in some facilities the business office, must be notified of any transfers.

It is also important that the patient's family or significant other be notified, preferably before the actual transfer. In emergencies, notification should be made as soon as possible.

Each facility has specific guidelines on documentation, but the transfer must always be recorded in the nursing notes by both the nurse transferring the patient and the nurse receiving the patient. The care plan must be reviewed and revised and a full report given to the receiving nurse when the patient arrives on the new unit. The ISBAR-R (Introduction, Situation, Background, Assessment, Recommendations, and Read back) format should be used while giving report (see Chapter 8).

Failure to pass on necessary information in the process of transferring a patient has been cited as a major factor in patient care errors. The major accrediting body in the United States, The Joint Commission, has included "improve staff communication" in its patient safety goals. Its guidelines state that every facility is to have procedures in place that provide for accurate communication of patient information at the time of any transfer, whether to another nursing unit, to an ancillary department for tests or procedures, or to another facility. This information includes a complete listing of the patient's current medications. The Joint Commission further states that the procedures should include the opportunity for the person receiving the patient to ask questions regarding the patient and the plan of treatment.

Loss of patient belongings is most likely to happen during a transfer from one unit to another. This is particularly true of durable medical equipment such as walkers, canes, and wheelchairs because they are often overlooked on the assumption that they belong to the facility rather than the patient. **For this reason, all equipment brought to the hospital by the patient should be clearly labeled, usually with a wide piece of tape on which the patient's name is written in large letters.**

Glasses, dentures, hearing aids, and jewelry are the other most frequently lost items, and replacement can be expensive for the facility. Check the drawers, shelves, patient bathroom, and bed linens carefully to ensure that such things are not accidentally thrown away or sent to the laundry.

DISCHARGING THE PATIENT

Discharge planning begins at admission, particularly when the diagnosis indicates the patient will need rehabilitation or long-term assistance. Members of the health care team must document needs to be addressed so the patient can be discharged from acute care. The **discharge planner** (an RN who organizes and implements the plan for patient discharge) uses this information, along with information gathered from the patient, the family, and the primary care provider, to make appropriate discharge arrangements for the patient. Necessary durable medical equipment and home care agency assistance, if needed, should be arranged before discharge.

The actual discharge orders are written by the primary care provider. When discharge orders are received, you should assist as needed with notifying the family or significant other, collecting patient belongings, and preparing the patient for the ride home or to a new facility. Just before discharge, retrieve any valuables stored in the hospital safe and have the patient sign for them in accordance with hospital protocol. The business office must be notified of the impending discharge. The medication reconciliation sheet must be completed and a copy given to the patient. When the patient leaves, housekeeping must be notified so that they can do the terminal cleaning of the patient unit.

DISCHARGE TO AN EXTENDED-CARE OR REHABILITATION FACILITY

Acute hospital stays are often short, and patients may not be well enough to go directly home at the time of discharge. A growing number of patients are being discharged to rehabilitation or extended-care facilities.

To ensure that information regarding necessary treatments, medications, and special needs is clearly communicated, the RN completes a detailed patient information sheet for the receiving facility. Information recorded includes primary and secondary diagnoses; current orders; medications (including over-the-counter medications, dietary supplements, and any herbals the patient takes), noting dosage, route, frequency, and time of last dose given; care provider names and telephone numbers; and a brief synopsis of the hospital stay. It is preferable but not always possible for the discharging nurse to call the admitting nurse at the new facility and give a verbal report before sending the patient.

If the patient is to be transferred by ambulance, the hospital discharge planner arranges for this service. If the patient is able to go by private car and the primary care provider agrees, the patient is usually taken to the car via wheelchair by a staff member.

Any records to be transferred with the patient must be ready in an envelope before the transporting vehicle arrives. Often a copy of the discharge summary and instructions is also faxed to the receiving facility to allow them to make advance arrangements for the patient's arrival.

Assist the patient with packing personal belongings before discharge. You should also help the patient as necessary to dress in a manner appropriate to the mode of transport and the weather conditions.

Life-Span Considerations

Older Adults

The need to be transferred from the hospital to a rehabilitation or long-term care facility can be confusing and frightening for older adult patients. Whenever possible, have a family member or a close friend either travel with patients or meet them when they arrive at the new facility to smooth this transition.

DISCHARGE HOME

Patients being discharged directly home require essentially the same preparations as those discussed above. Most patients discharged directly home travel by private car, but special transport may be needed for patients with severe mobility restrictions. It is the nurse's responsibility to verify that necessary arrangements have been made so the discharge goes smoothly for the patient and the family.

Written discharge instructions are prepared by the nurse and reviewed with the patient and often family members (Box 23.1). Both the patient and the nurse sign the form, a copy is given to the patient, and one is placed in the medical record. The discharge form lists medications, activity restrictions, special diet instructions, and ordered follow-up appointments. The primary care provider's name and phone number are also listed. This is particularly important if the patient is being cared for by a new provider. For example, an accident victim may have been assigned an orthopedic surgeon during admission through the emergency department and will need to know how to contact this physician for care following discharge.

Box 23.1 Checklist for Discharge Patient Education

Cover these topics:

- Telephone number of primary care provider; date and time of follow-up appointment
- Diet instructions
- Activity restrictions and exercise instructions
- Medications and schedule for administration
- Over-the-counter medications not to take while on current prescriptions
- Instructions about bathing and hygiene
- Dressing-change instructions
- Instructions for any new prosthesis or brace
- Signs and symptoms to report to the primary care provider
- Any requirements for follow-up laboratory work

Discharge patient education is performed, preferably in an unhurried environment that permits time for questions. It is desirable for a family member or significant other to be present for the patient education session. Written instructions are sent home with the patient. Documentation of what was covered is entered into the nurse's notes.

Home Health Care

Many patients, particularly the older adults, receive home health care following discharge. Home health services may include skilled nursing such as wound care, diabetic care, and patient education, and intravenous medication administration. Physical, occupational, or speech therapy; respiratory care; and personal care performed by a home health aide are also often part of home care services. Counseling and information regarding long-term planning, financial assistance, and community services can be provided by a **medical social worker (MSW)**. Many services that were once available only to hospital patients are now routinely provided in the home setting.

Home health care has many advantages including reduced cost, decreased exposure to potentially serious infections, and, most important, provision of care in a familiar, comfortable environment. Medicare, Medicaid, and some insurance and managed care plans provide for payment of portions or all of these services for a period of time when ordered by a primary care provider.

Discharge Against Medical Advice

Occasionally a patient insists on leaving the hospital against the primary care provider's advice. The patient has the right to make this choice. It is the responsibility of the health care team to help patients understand how the decision to leave the hospital may affect their health. Listen to what the patient has to say, answer questions, and offer to ask the primary care provider or the supervising nurse to talk with the patient.

If the patient ultimately decides to leave, notify the primary care provider immediately. If the primary care provider thinks it is inappropriate for a discharge order to be written, the patient is asked to sign a form stating that he is leaving against medical advice (AMA). Sometimes a patient refuses to sign. You must document this, and then date and sign the form in the space provided. Additionally, document the names of any witnesses to the refusal to sign. The patient's stated reasons for leaving are written in the nursing notes.

When patients choose to leave AMA, they must be informed of additional potential consequences. These include that they will not receive prescriptions for medications or treatment, and that if insurance carriers refuse to pay the hospital bill, they would become liable for monies owed. Document that you relayed this information in the medical record.

DEATH OF A PATIENT

Despite a growing trend toward remaining at home to die, most deaths still occur in the hospital, long-term care, or hospice facilities. It is often a difficult time for family and friends, and at times, even for the hospital staff. Death after a long, good life or at the end of lingering illness or pain may be seen as a kind and welcome release. Death of a vigorous active adult or a child, however, is often viewed as unfair and even unthinkable. Death may also greatly disrupt family life, especially if the individual was the primary wage earner or provider of care for the family children. See Chapter 15 for more about care of the dying patient.

PROVIDING SUPPORT FOR SIGNIFICANT OTHERS

Often the most important gift you can give the bereaved is just being there. Simply sit and listen while they talk of their loss and the fears about the changes it will bring. People need to grieve; it is an important step in healing.

Many people derive significant comfort from spiritual or religious beliefs and practices. Offer to call their priest, minister, rabbi, or spiritual advisor. If death is anticipated, doing this while the patient is still alive can be particularly helpful, especially if the religious beliefs include specific pre-death rituals.

You can also offer to make telephone calls or arrangements for someone to come and take the significant other home if this seems appropriate. An older widow or widower alone at the bedside of the just-deceased spouse, for example, may have difficulty making a decision to leave without some guidance or assistance.

Allow the family and friends adequate time at the bedside to say their good-byes. Crying, touching their loved one, and hugging each other are all part of a necessary human process in dealing with grief.

It is important to note that you must deal with your own feelings about death before you can be a good support person for someone else. Young nurses should not feel personally rejected if the family looks to older staff members for comfort and assistance. Older individuals have usually had more opportunity to experience loss through death, and family members frequently think they will have a deeper understanding of the effect.

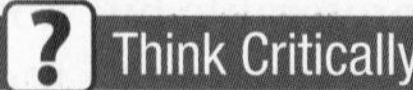

Think Critically

How do you feel about caring for a patient who is dying?

PRONOUNCEMENT OF DEATH

Most states require a physician to pronounce death unless the patient has a **do not resuscitate (DNR)** order. In these cases, many states permit RNs to pronounce death. You must be familiar with the policy and procedure for your facility and adhere to it. The time life signs ceased, the time death was pronounced, and the name of the person making the official pronouncement must be documented in the nursing notes.

AUTOPSIES

Most deaths are not followed by an **autopsy** (examination of the remains by a pathologist to determine cause of death). An autopsy is usually performed when a death is sudden or unexpected, the result of injury or suspicious circumstances (such as suspected homicide), or had not been seen within a specific period by a physician. In such cases, the death becomes a coroner's case, and the **coroner** (city or county medical officer responsible for investigating unexplained death) orders and authorizes the autopsy. The laws governing autopsy in these instances vary, and facility policies will follow local state law.

An autopsy may also be performed when it is believed that information valuable to medical research may be obtained, or when the family has questions about the cause of death. In such cases, the next of kin must authorize the autopsy. If an autopsy is requested by the family, they may have to incur the costs.

ORGAN DONATION

The need for donor organs grows continually. Thousands of people each year owe their opportunity for a longer, healthier life to an organ donation. Unfortunately, the gap between people needing organ transplantation and donors for organs keeps widening each year. Requests to the family for organ donation are usually done by a physician, a specially trained nurse, or an organ donation organization representative. When handled in a sensitive, caring manner, requests for organ donation can be an opportunity for the family to allow something good to come out of a personal tragedy.

Get Ready for the NCLEX Examination!

Key Points

- An admission may be planned or it may occur in response to a medical emergency, but it is always a stressful event for the patient.
- Many procedures including surgery are now done as outpatient services, with the patient being cared for in a day-surgery unit.
- The majority of health care payment plans require that authorization be obtained by the primary care provider's office before a routine or elective admission.
- The admission department is responsible for determining that all admission criteria have been met and payment arrangements have been made.
- Because patients are often admitted only 1 or 2 hours before a procedure, laboratory work and x-ray studies are frequently done a day or two before admission.
- You must make patients feel welcome and orient them to the unit and hospital routine.
- Patients should be asked to send all valuables, unnecessary items, and medicines home if possible.
- Patient belongings, particularly those that are necessary for their care such as wheelchairs, walkers, and canes, should be clearly labeled with the patient's name.
- In an acute care facility, the admission assessment and care plan are developed by an RN with the LPN/LVN providing data for this purpose.
- LPN/LVNs may be charge nurses in some skilled nursing facilities, and they assume full responsibility for the initial assessment and initiating the care plan. The RN reviews the plan and makes alterations if necessary.
- Transfer of a patient from one unit to another requires an order from a primary care provider, and care must be taken that the family is notified and all patient belongings are moved with the patient.
- The RN discharge planner begins discharge plans at the time of admission to ensure that patient needs will be adequately met after leaving the facility.
- Written discharge instructions, complete with medications, treatments, and copies of necessary medical records must accompany the patient being transferred to another facility.
- Patients discharged to their homes must be provided with written instructions regarding medications, treatments, and follow-up care.
- Home health care may be ordered before discharge, particularly for older adult patients. This may include skilled nursing, personal care assistance, therapy, and assessment by a social worker.
- If a patient chooses to leave the hospital AMA, the nurse must notify the primary care provider and ask the patient to sign a form acknowledging that the primary care provider advises against leaving.
- Death is usually pronounced by the physician and must be accurately noted in the medical record, including the time life signs ceased and the time death was officially pronounced and by whom.
- Autopsy is performed only for specific reasons and must be ordered by the coroner or authorized by the next of kin.

Additional Learning Resources

SG Go to your Study Guide for additional learning activities to help you master this chapter content.

evolve Go to your Evolve website at http://evolve.elsevier.com/Williams/fundamental for additional online resources.

Review Questions for the NCLEX Examination

*Choose the **best** answer for each question.*

1. When instructing a patient scheduled for same-day surgery, you tell him to: *(Select all that apply.)*
   1. Bring his medications with him.
   2. Bring only essential items to the hospital.
   3. Have someone available to take him home after the procedure.
   4. Report to the same-day surgery unit 1 to 2 hours before the scheduled procedure.
   5. Bring a robe and slippers and any overnight supplies such as a denture care kit.
2. In an acute care facility the person responsible for the initial nursing assessment is:
   1. The admissions staff.
   2. The RN.
   3. The RN or LVN.
   4. The primary care provider.
3. Orders are verified and signed off by:
   1. The unit secretary.
   2. The licensed nurse.
   3. The physician.
   4. The nursing supervisor.
4. If a patient brings credit cards, cell phone, and jewelry to the hospital, you can provide for their security by: *(Select all that apply.)*
   1. Sending items home with the family.
   2. Storing the items in the bedside drawer.
   3. Placing the contents in a valuables envelope to be stored in a safe.
   4. Making a list of all the items on a "belongings list" and placing it in the medical record.
   5. Hiding the valuables in the closet.
5. When transferring a patient to another facility, copies of pertinent medical records:
   1. Are the responsibility of the family to deliver.
   2. Must be faxed to the facility or must accompany the patient.
   3. Are mailed at the time of transfer.
   4. Must be delivered by hospital messenger because they are confidential.
6. What information should be included in a discharge summary? *(Select all that apply.)*
   1. Patient's present condition
   2. Activity restrictions
   3. Medications administered in the hospital
   4. Topics covered in discharge patient education
   5. Diet to be followed
7. If a patient wants to leave AMA, the nurse:
   1. Detains him until the primary care provider can speak with him.
   2. Explains that insurance may not pay his bill if he leaves.
   3. Immediately calls the nursing supervisor to speak to the patient.
   4. States that security people will prevent his leaving.
8. An autopsy may be required when: *(Select all that apply.)*
   1. A patient dies after a 4-day hospitalization.
   2. A patient dies at the hands of another.
   3. A patient dies without being under a primary care provider's care outside the hospital.
   4. The cause of death is unknown.
   5. The patient dies because of an accident.

Critical Thinking Activities

Read each clinical scenario and discuss the questions with your classmates.

Scenario A

What might you say to make a nervous patient and family feel more relaxed during the admission process?

Scenario B

What would you do if a family wanted to discuss organ donation?

chapter 24

Diagnostic Tests and Specimen Collection

http://evolve.elsevier.com/Williams/fundamental

Objectives

Upon completing this chapter, you should be able to do the following:

Theory

1. Discuss appropriate psychosocial care and education for patients undergoing diagnostic tests or procedures.
2. Prepare to perform a capillary glucose test, a venipuncture, a throat culture, an electrocardiogram, a urine dipstick test, and a stool for occult blood test.
3. Describe each of the categories of tests that are commonly performed.
4. Explain factors to be considered when an older adult is to undergo diagnostic testing.

Clinical Practice

1. Provide pretest and posttest nursing care, including appropriate education, for patients undergoing diagnostic tests and procedures.
2. Attend to psychosocial concerns of patients undergoing various diagnostic tests.
3. Perform a random blood glucose test using capillary blood and a glucometer.
4. Perform patient education for magnetic resonance imaging (MRI).
5. Describe how to prepare a patient for and assist with aspiration procedures such as lumbar puncture, thoracentesis, paracentesis, bone marrow aspiration, and liver biopsy.
6. Correctly use Standard Precautions whenever obtaining or handling specimens for diagnostic tests.
7. List the steps for assisting with a pelvic examination and Pap test.
8. Correctly fill out laboratory and test requisition forms.

Skills & Steps

Skills

Steps

Key Terms

anemias (ă-nē-mē-ăz, p. 409)
aspiration (ăs-pĕr-ā-shŭn, p. 416)
biopsy (bī-ŏp-sē, p. 416)
colonoscopy (KŌ-lŏn-Ŏ-skō-pē, p. 426)
culture (cŭl-chŭr, p. 408)
cystoscopy (sĭst-Ŏ-skō-pē, p. 427)
electroencephalogram (EEG) (ē-LĔK-trō-ĕn-SĔ-fă-lō-grăm, p. 428)
endoscope (ĔN-dō-skōp, p. 425)
gastroscopy (găs-TRŎ-skō-pē, p. 425)
hematoma (hē-mă-TŌ-mă, p. 425)
jaundice (JĂWN-dĭs, p. 427)
panel (p. 411)
polyps (PŎL-ĭps, p. 426)
smears (p. 430)
transducer (trăns-DŪ-sĕr, p. 416)
venipuncture (VĔN-ĭ-pŭnk-chŭr, p. 411)

Concepts Covered in This Chapter

- Anxiety
- Fluid and electrolyte balance
- Glucose regulation
- Infection
- Inflammation
- Patient education
- Perfusion
- Safety

DIAGNOSTIC TESTS AND PROCEDURES

Diagnostic tests and procedures provide important information about complex chemical reactions that affect the body's function. Laboratory examinations of blood, urine, and other body fluids and tissues provide accurate information about the function of various organs and physiologic mechanisms. The information is helpful in making or confirming a diagnosis or in evaluating the effectiveness of a treatment. It is necessary to check the instructions from the particular department of the facility in which the test is to be performed for the specifics of patient preparation because this may vary somewhat from facility to facility. Box 24.1 provides terms with definitions specific to diagnostic testing.

❖ APPLICATION OF THE NURSING PROCESS

◆ ASSESSMENT (DATA COLLECTION)

When a diagnostic test or procedure is ordered, determine what the patient knows about the test to establish what patient education is needed. Inquire about concerns the patient may have about the test. Determine if any special nursing measures are needed to protect the patient's safety. Inspect wounds each shift for signs of infection so that the primary care provider can be alerted to the need for a **culture** (the growing of microorganisms in or on a medium designed for their growth). Assess the patient for allergies to medication and to iodine and other procedure skin-prep solutions used for diagnostic testing.

◆ NURSING DIAGNOSIS

Nursing diagnoses are those pertinent to the problems for which a diagnostic test or procedure is ordered. "Deficient knowledge" related to the type of diagnostic test is appropriate if the patient is unfamiliar with the test. A few examples of nursing diagnoses for which diagnostic tests might be part of the treatment plan include:

- Impaired urinary elimination related to dysuria and foul-smelling urine.
- Acute pain related to raw, sore throat.
- Acute pain related to inflammation and swelling at wound site.

◆ PLANNING

Check to see that pretest medications and supplies are available on the unit 1 to 2 hours before the scheduled test time. Plan when to do any patient education about the test or procedure. Include the pretest and posttest care in your work schedule. A test involving the colon requires the administration of enemas, which can be time consuming. Many diagnostic tests require frequent vital sign measurement when the patient returns to the nursing unit. Expected outcomes are written for the particular nursing diagnosis associated with the problem for which the test is being performed.

Assignment Considerations

Posttest Assessments

Carefully consider before assigning vital sign measurements to the unlicensed personnel (UAPs) after invasive diagnostic tests. Vital signs are not the only parameters that are usually needed to assess a patient. The patient may need to be monitored for bleeding, neurologic abnormalities, decreases in sensation or function, increasing pain, and general changes in condition. The licensed nurse's assessment should encompass all considerations for the patient.

◆ IMPLEMENTATION

Make certain that the patient has received adequate education about the test or procedure to be performed and that their concerns have been addressed. Carry out the pretest and posttest actions for the particular test or procedure, including the signed consent for any invasive procedure requiring one. Remind the patient that test results often are not available the same day and often take up to a week or more to be reported.

Patient Education

Patient Education

DIAGNOSTIC TESTS

You should also consider the instructions for the preparation for the specific test available from the department performing the test. Teach the patient:

- The purpose of the test.
- What will be experienced during the test.
- Whether it is necessary to refrain from eating or drinking before the test and for how many hours.
- Whether the test requires special preparation (medications, special diet, laxatives, enemas, or the need to drink a lot of water).
- Whether routine medications may be taken before the test.
- When the result will probably be available.
- Any posttest measures such as drinking more water, taking a laxative, or remaining on bed rest for a certain number of hours.
- Whether it is necessary to arrange for someone to drive the patient home after the test.
- About how long the test usually takes.
- Any after effects of the test or procedure.

Box 24.1 Terminology for Diagnostic Testing

Angiography: A method of injecting a dye into an artery and obtaining an x-ray study of blood vessels, tumors, and lesions.

Arteriography: Radiography of an artery or arterial system after injection of a contrast medium into the bloodstream.

Bronchoscopy: Inspection of the interior of the tracheobronchial tree through a bronchoscope.

Cardiac catheterization: Introduction of a catheter into the heart chambers to confirm a diagnosis or to evaluate the extent of the disease process.

Colposcopy: A gynecologic examination that uses the colposcope to examine the walls of the vagina and the cervix.

Complete blood count (CBC): Includes type and number of red blood cells, white blood cells, platelets, and hemoglobin.

Computed tomography (CT) scan: Through use of a computer, cathode ray tubes emit radiation at different depths to show the density of tissues and organs, indicating malformations, tumors, or other irregularities; also called *computed axial tomography (CAT) scan.*

Conization: Coring or removal of the mucous lining of the cervical canal and its glands by means of cutting with a high-frequency current; performed when a Pap smear indicates abnormal cells.

Cytology: The study of the structure, function, and pathology of cells.

Endoscopic retrograde cholangiopancreatography (ERCP): Examination of the biliary system done through a flexible endoscope and instillation of contrast medium into the ampulla of Vater of the pancreas.

Esophagogastroduodenoscopy (EGD): Endoscopic examination of the esophagus, stomach, and duodenum.

Fluoroscopy: Examination by means of fluoroscope using x-ray studies displayed on a fluorescent screen.

Glucometer: A small machine used to measure glucose content of capillary blood.

Hematology: The study of blood and its components.

Histology: The branch of anatomy dealing with the structure, composition, and function of tissues.

Intravenous pyelography (IVP): Injection of a dye into a vein to show urine flow through the renal pelvis, ureters, and bladder on x-ray examination.

KUB x-ray: X-ray study of the kidneys, ureters, and bladder.

Liquid-based cytology (LBC): This type of Pap smear performed in approximately 90% of Pap smears in the United States. In contrast to the traditional Pap, it produces a sample that has improved clarity and quality. Instead of cells being directly placed onto a microscope slide, they are deposited into a small bottle of preservative liquid.

Lumbar puncture: Insertion of a hollow needle into the subarachnoid space between the third and fourth lumbar vertebrae to withdraw samples of cerebrospinal fluid for analysis and to measure the pressure; also called *spinal puncture* and *spinal tap.*

Magnetic resonance imaging (MRI): A noninvasive method, based on magnetic fields, of visualizing soft tissue without the use of contrast media or ionizing radiation.

Papanicolaou (Pap) smear: A laboratory test to detect cancer, especially cervical, vaginal, or uterine cancer; use began in the 1950s. Later the test was improved by use of LBC.

Paracentesis: A needle puncture of the abdomen to remove ascites fluid, to perform a lavage, or to initiate peritoneal dialysis.

Proctosigmoidoscopy: Examination of the rectum and sigmoid colon with a sigmoidoscope.

Radiography: The making of film records of internal structures of the body by exposure of film sensitized to x-rays.

Radioimmunoassay (RIA): Use of radionuclides, following principles of immunology, to measure materials present in blood in minute amounts.

Radionuclides: Radioactive substances that disintegrate with the emission of electromagnetic radiation.

Radiopharmaceutical: A radioactive pharmaceutical substance used for diagnostic or therapeutic purposes.

Sequential multiple assay (SMA): A series of assay tests for a variety of chemical substances performed one after another on one blood or serum sample by a chemical analyzer.

Thoracentesis: Insertion of a needle through the chest wall to the pleural space to drain fluid or air or to instill medication.

Treadmill stress test: A test that measures heart rate and blood pressure response to clinically controlled active exercise on a treadmill (a machine with a moving belt on which one walks while staying in one place).

Ultrasonography: A technique in which deep structures of the body are visualized by recording the reflections (echoes) of ultrasonic waves directed into the tissues.

Laboratory Tests

Tests can be performed on body fluid or tissue to detect changes from the normal state. Because blood bathes and nourishes all body tissues and collects waste products for elimination, chemical changes in the blood can be signs of disease. Analysis of urine also provides a rich source of information about cellular activity.

Hematology tests. **Hematology** is the study of blood and its components. The complete blood count (CBC) provides information about the state of health or presence of illness (Table 24.1). Changes in the number, size, or appearance of red blood cells (erythrocytes) occur in diseases associated with types of anemia. The **hematocrit** refers to the separation of blood and is the amount of blood cells in relation to the amount of plasma. It is decreased in severe **anemias** (low red blood cell count) and massive blood losses but is higher than normal in dehydration and shock.

During infections, the type and number of white blood cells **(leukocytes)** increase **(leukocytosis).** The

Table 24.1 Example of a Complete Blood Count (Adult)

COMPONENT	TEST VALUE	NORMAL RANGE
WBC	6.8 k/µL	5.0-10.0/mm^3
RBC	4.59 M/µL	4.2-6.1/mm^3
Hgb	14.0 g/dL	12.0-18.0 g/dL
HCT	40.8 mL/dL	37.0-52.0 mL/dL
MCV	89.0 fL	80.0-95.0 fL
MCH	30.6 pg/cell	27.0-31.0 pg/cell
RDW	11.3%	11.6-14.6%
PLT	252,000/mm^3	150,000-400, 000/mm^3
Segmented neutrophils	50%	54%-62%
Lymphocyte	36%	28%-33%
Monocyte	12%	3%-7%
Eosinophil	2%	1%-3%
Basophil	0%	0%-1%
RBC morphology	Normal	Normal

Hgb, Hemoglobin; *HCT*, hematocrit; *MCH*, mean corpuscular hemoglobin; *MCV*, mean corpuscular volume; *PLT*, platelet; *RBC*, red blood cell; *RDW*, red cell distribution width; *WBC*, white blood cell.

neutrophil count, in particular, can be significant. When infection is severe, the bone marrow releases more granulocytes as a compensatory measure; many young, immature polymorphonuclear neutrophils called "bands" are released into the bloodstream.

Clinical Cues

Most laboratories report the cells on the differential white blood cell (WBC) count by order of maturity, with the less mature cell forms being on the left side of the report. Therefore, a "shift to the left" in the number of cells, or an increase in bands, may indicate infection.

Life-Span Considerations

Older Adults

Because of normal changes with aging, older adults may not be able to mount a significant leukocytosis; therefore, even a moderate rise in WBCs can indicate infection.

Certain drugs may cause a sharp fall in leukocytes **(leukopenia),** making the individual less able to fight off infection. Hemoglobin testing shows the blood's capacity to transport oxygen from the lungs to the tissues. Hemoglobin levels drop when there is bleeding within the body.

In addition to the CBC, tests of bleeding and clotting time of the blood may be done. Knowledge about the length of bleeding time is essential before most surgeries or extensive dental extractions are performed. Common tests for clotting time are the prothrombin time (PT) and activated partial thromboplastin time (APTT). PT is prolonged in certain

Table 24.2 Blood Chemistry Tests and Their Purpose

TEST	ORGAN CHECKED OR PURPOSE
Glucose	Diabetes or hypoglycemia
Bilirubin, ALT, ALP, and albumin	Liver
AST	Liver or coronary artery disease
BUN and creatinine	Kidney
LDH, CK, and troponins	Heart
Calcium	Parathyroid and calcium metabolism
Cholesterol	Potential for atherosclerotic heart disease
Phosphate	Renal failure, bone metastasis, and hypercalcemia
Total protein	Malnutrition, liver disease
Uric acid	Gout

ALT, Alanine aminotransferase; *ALP*, alkaline phosphatase; *AST*, aspartate aminotransferase; *BUN*, blood urea nitrogen; *CK*, creatine kinase; *LDH*, lactate dehydrogenase.

diseases of the liver and in certain blood disorders. **PT is widely used to adjust dosages of anticoagulant drugs such as sodium warfarin (Coumadin).** This test is reported using International Normalized Ratio (INR) numbers. The partial thromboplastin time is used for monitoring clotting time during heparin therapy.

! Safety Alert

Bleeding Danger

A normal platelet count is 150 to 400/mm^3 of blood. Platelet activity is essential to blood clotting.

Spontaneous bleeding is a serious danger when the platelet count falls below 20,000/mm^3 of blood. Observe for bleeding gums, blood in the urine, and oozing from needle sticks.

The erythrocyte sedimentation rate (ESR or "sed rate") measures the rate at which the red blood cells settle out of unclotted blood in 1 hour. Inflammatory conditions cause the cells to settle more rapidly: the more rapid the settling, the higher the ESR.

? Think Critically

The patient's hemoglobin level when she was admitted was 13.8 g/dL. Two days later, the level is 13.2 g/dL. Is this significant? What could it mean?

Blood chemistry tests. Blood chemistries are commonly obtained to detect changes in biochemical reactions in the body and to determine a diagnosis. They provide information about the electrolyte balance, the body's ability to metabolize nutrients, the function of organs, and the presence or accumulation of toxic substances (Table 24.2). Most laboratory reports list the normal values (reference range) for each test with the results of the test.

Food and drink are usually withheld for 8 to 12 hours before blood chemistry tests. The blood specimen for a CBC, chemistry, or serology test is obtained by **venipuncture** (puncture of the vein with a needle). Wear gloves and implement Standard Precautions; take steps to prevent continued bleeding from the puncture site. The blood specimens are collected in tubes with color-coded stoppers, which indicate the type of anticoagulant or preservative, if any, the tubes contain (Skill 24.1).

Blood glucose tests are essential in the diagnosis and control of diabetes. They are also commonly ordered when a patient is receiving total parenteral nutrition (TPN, described in Chapter 27). Testing the amount of blood glucose can be done outside the laboratory using capillary blood from a finger stick, test strips, and a machine called a glucometer (Skill 24.2).

Other tests are used to determine toxic levels of substances such as barbiturates, lead, arsenic, and medications. **Most laboratories are equipped with automated and computerized instruments that carry out multiple tests on a single specimen.** One model is the sequential multiple assay (SMA) unit, which can be programmed to run a battery of screening tests on one blood sample. Table 24.3 shows a typical SMA-12 **panel** (group of tests) with normal values for each component.

? Think Critically

The patient was admitted with malaise and fever. The ESR was 27 mm/h on admission. Today it is 34 mm/h. What does this indicate?

Serology tests. Serology tests are based on the analysis of blood serum. They are important in diagnosing many diseases stemming from bacterial and viral infections. Diseases such as dysentery, rheumatic fever, typhoid, influenza, rubella, and syphilis produce positive reactions related to antigen antibodies. Radio immunoassays (RIAs), which are based on principles of immunity, use radionuclides (radioactive material; formerly called radioisotopes), such as iodine-125 and iodine-131, to detect minute particles of protein in the blood. Blood typing and identification of blood factors may also be carried out in the serology section of the laboratory. Examples of common serology tests are listed in Box 24.2. Most serology tests can be done without restricting the patient's food or fluid intake. However, some of the RIAs may require the administration of the radionuclide drug at a certain time before drawing blood for the test. For viral infections, two separate specimens are needed to show a rise in titer during the illness.

Urinalysis. Analysis of urine provides valuable information about the kidney function and other biologic processes within the body. Organic compounds found in the urine include urea, uric acid, creatinine, and hippuric acid. Inorganic substances found are sodium, chloride, phosphate, potassium, and ammonia. Urine composition varies according to fluid intake and diet; therefore, the time the specimen is obtained may influence the results.

Clinical Cues

Urine deteriorates rapidly, so specimens should be analyzed soon after collection. Send the specimen to the laboratory quickly or refrigerate it.

Urine specimens can be classified as:

- Single, catheterized, or random specimens that can be collected at any time, with no special preparation required (a specimen of the first voiding in the morning is preferred because it is more concentrated).
- Midstream specimens, in which the external genitalia are cleansed, a small amount of urine is passed, and then a midportion of the voiding is collected in a sterile container and used for a culture.
- Timed, long-period specimens, in which all urine is collected over a 12- or 24-hour period and placed in a container containing some type of preservative.

No special instructions are required for the single, random specimen. Often a urine dipstick test is performed to screen the specimen for abnormalities. Urine dips are performed using test strips or sticks that have various chemicals impregnated in them (Skill 24.3). The Patient Education box in Chapter 29 provides instructions for the midstream specimen. The method for obtaining a specimen from an indwelling urinary catheter is listed in Steps 29.1, in Chapter 29. Consult a laboratory manual for instructions on special types of urine tests. Some tests require restriction of fluid intake; others require that set amounts of fluids be given and urine specimens obtained at specified times. A normal urinalysis is presented in Table 24.4.

Patient Education

Collection of a 24-Hour Urine Specimen

Give the patient a 24-hour urine collection container. Provide the following instructions:

- Empty the bladder into the toilet and begin timing the collection of the specimen.
- For the next 24 hours, add all urine to the collection container.
- Keep the container on ice or refrigerated if instructed to do so (depends on the laboratory and the type of test ordered).
- When the 24 hours is up, empty the bladder and add the urine to the collection container.
- Seal the collection container and return it to the laboratory or the primary care provider's office as directed.

Other laboratory tests. Other laboratory tests performed are bacteriologic, histologic, and cytologic tests. Specimens of blood, urine, feces, and wound drainage, and samples of other body fluids or tissues, may be cultured to identify the disease-causing organism. To obtain a stool specimen, ask the patient to catch some stool in a container suspended in the

Continues on page 416

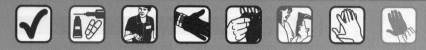

Skill 24.1 Phlebotomy and Obtaining Blood Samples with a Vacutainer System

 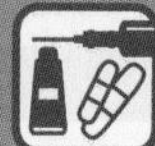 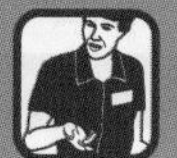 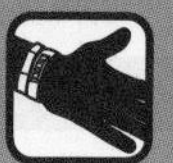 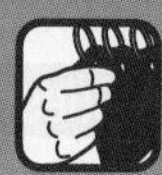 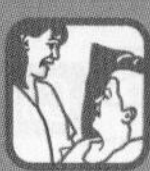 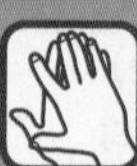 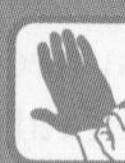

Blood tests are the most commonly ordered diagnostic procedure. Every time a venipuncture is performed for blood sampling, two patient identifiers must be used to verify that the procedure is being performed on the correct patient. The room number cannot be one of the identifiers. Patient name and patient number or birth date are valid identifiers. When there is not a laboratory with a phlebotomist on the premises, the nurse is usually responsible for obtaining the needed blood samples. The Vacutainer system is the most common method used to obtain blood samples. Blood can be drawn using a syringe and needle with the same venipuncture technique. The correct tube, indicated by the color of its top, must be used for the test ordered.

SUPPLIES

- Tube labels
- Pen
- Tape
- Blood-impervious gloves
- Vacutainer tubes
- Vacutainer holder
- Vacutainer needle with needle guard
- Towel, paper towel, or underpad
- Tourniquet
- Alcohol swabs
- 2 × 2 gauze squares
- Bandage
- Cotton balls
- Biohazard sharps container
- Biohazard plastic bag
- Requisition slip

Review and carry out the Standard Steps in Appendix A.

ACTION *(RATIONALE)*

Assessment (Data Collection)

1. Check the medical order for tests to be done. *(Determines the type of tube to be used.)*
2. Ask the patient's name and date of birth or check the wristband. *(Verifies that the right patient will have blood drawn.)*

Planning

3. Check to see that the needed tubes and materials are on hand. *(Prevents having to stop and obtain supplies.)*

Implementation

4. Fill out a label for each tube. *(Ensures that tubes will be correctly labeled.)*
5. Explain the procedure and have patient sit with arm on a table or have patient lie down with the arm stretched out at the side. *(Explaining procedure decreases fear of the unknown. Positioning provides stable access to venipuncture site.)*
6. Perform hand hygiene and don clean gloves. *(Reduces transfer of microorganisms.)*
7. Select an appropriate venipuncture site, avoiding scars, lesions, or a vessel in which intravenous (IV) fluids are infusing. *(Scar tissue is difficult to puncture; a puncture over a lesion may introduce microorganisms into the blood; IV fluids may alter the test results.)*

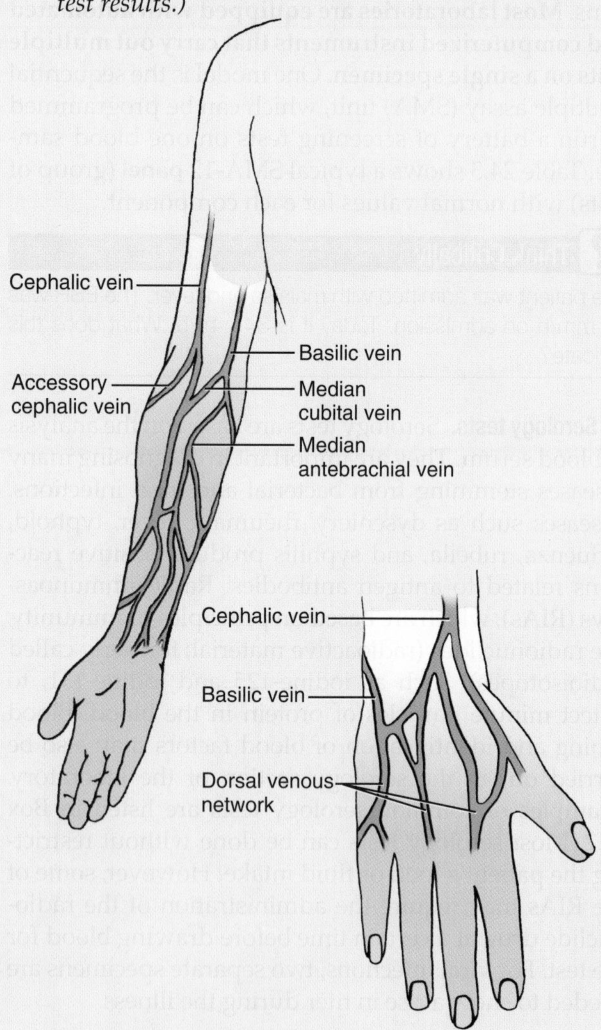

Step 7

8. Place the Vacutainer tube inside the holder, but do not push it onto the needle; position the Vacutainer holder and tubes within easy reach. *(Preparing the system for use allows you to pick up the equipment with one hand after you have stabilized the vessel.)*

9. Lower the extremity so the site is below the heart. *(A dependent position enhances blood flow to the site.)*
10. Apply a tourniquet to the extremity 2 to 4 inches above the venipuncture site. It should be moderately tight. Ask the patient to make a fist (unless a potassium level specimen is being drawn). *(The tourniquet obstructs blood flow out of the vessel and causes the vein to fill with blood. A distended vein is easier to palpate and puncture. Making a fist aids in vein distention, but elevates the reading for potassium by forcing potassium out of cells.)*
11. Cleanse the site with 70% alcohol in a circular motion outward; allow the area to dry. *(Alcohol decreases the number of microorganisms on the skin, preventing their transfer to the blood.)*
12. Pick up the Vacutainer holder and tube in your dominant hand and remove the needle cover. *(Prepares the unit for venipuncture.)*
13. Anchor the vein with the thumb of your nondominant hand, far enough below the site so that the needle will not touch the thumb as it enters the vessel. *(Stabilizes the vein so that it does not roll when venipuncture is performed.)*
14. Hold the Vacutainer unit with the needle bevel facing up and position it at a 30-degree angle over the desired venipuncture site. *(Positions the needle for entry into the vessel.)*

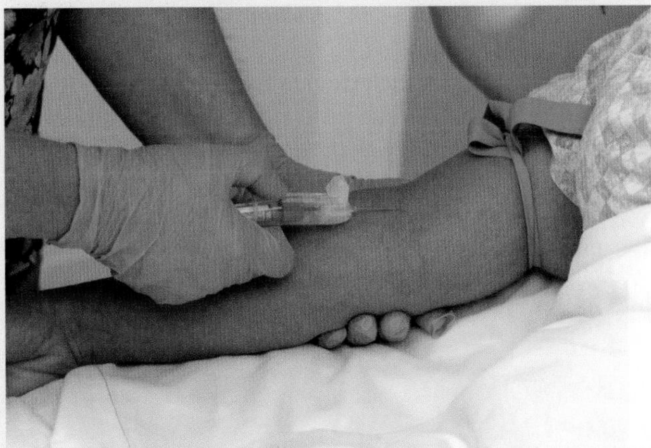

Step **14**

15. Puncture the site, and, while stabilizing the Vacutainer unit, press the tube stopper onto the needle; blood running into the tube indicates successful venipuncture. *(Stabilizing the unit prevents pushing the needle through the vein when pressing the tube stopper onto the Vacutainer needle.)*
16. Allow tube to fill completely. *(Ensures a sufficient quantity of blood to perform the test.)*
17. If further specimens are needed, stabilize the holder and remove filled tube and set safely aside. Place next tube carefully on needle and allow to fill. Repeat until all required tubes are filled. Remove final tube. *(Obtains sufficient blood for all ordered tests. Stabilizing holder prevents pushing needle through vessel wall. Removing last tube before removing needle prevents introducing air into the tube.)*
18. Loosen the tourniquet then withdraw the needle from the vein and secure the needle guard. *(Loosening tourniquet before withdrawing the needle decreases the amount of bleeding that occurs.)*
19. Immediately apply a dry gauze pad with pressure to the vein to stop the bleeding. *(A dry pad aids coagulation of the blood, and pressure constricts the vessel, decreasing bleeding.)*
20. Apply a small adhesive bandage over the puncture site. *(Decreases entrance of microorganisms at the site and helps prevent further bleeding.)*
21. Carefully remove and dispose of the Vacutainer needle in a biohazard sharps container. *(Prevents accidental needle sticks.)*
22. Remove and label the tube(s) of blood, and place in a biohazard bag. *(Labeling tube(s) correctly identifies the patient's blood. A biohazard bag prevents blood contamination should the tube[s] become broken.)*
23. Fill out the laboratory requisition slip, and attach to the blood samples; send to the laboratory. *(Identifies the correct test to be done for the right patient.)*
24. Remove gloves and perform hand hygiene. *(Reduces transfer of microorganisms.)*

Evaluation

25. Check to be certain the correct tubes were used and all samples have been obtained with adequate blood in each tube. *(Ensures that patient will not have to return for another venipuncture.)*

Documentation

26. Note the procedure and samples obtained on the patient's medical record; include how they were sent to the laboratory. *(Verifies that the ordered blood samples were drawn and sent to the laboratory.)*

Documentation Example

1/8 0700 Successful venipuncture; three tubes drawn and sent to lab for CBC, SMA-12, and VDRL. No hematoma at site; bleeding stopped and bandage applied. Patient tolerated procedure without problems. (Nurse's electronic signature)

? Critical Thinking Questions

1. An older adult tells you that technicians and nurses always have difficulty drawing her blood samples because she has tiny veins. What would you do to ensure a successful venipuncture?
2. If you have done three "sticks" on a patient for blood samples and have not been successful, what would you do?

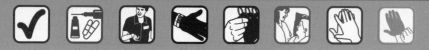

Skill 24.2 Performing a Capillary Blood Test: Blood Glucose

 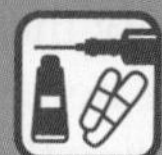 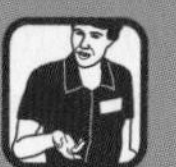 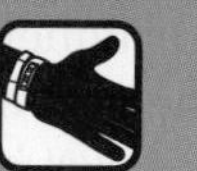 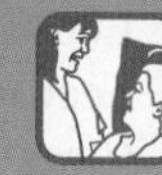 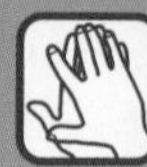 

Random blood glucose tests are performed for known diabetic patients and for patients who are showing signs and symptoms of hyperglycemia or hypoglycemia.

SUPPLIES

- Gloves
- Cotton ball
- Fingerstick device holder
- Bandage
- Lancet
- Alcohol swabs
- Glucometer (Accu-Chek)
- Glucometer strips

Review and carry out the Standard Steps in Appendix A.

ACTION *(RATIONALE)*

Assessment (Data Collection)

1. Gather equipment and assess whether all supplies are on hand. *(Prevents having to stop procedure to retrieve needed items.)*
2. Identify the patient and determine what is known about the procedure. *(Identifies what information needs to be given to patient.)*

Planning

3. Plan which finger to use and ask patient to allow hand to hang downward. If hand is cold, have patient warm it under running warm water, or warm it with your hands. *(Holding hand down and warming it brings blood to the fingertips.)*

Implementation

4. Perform hand hygiene and don gloves. Cleanse the chosen fingertip thoroughly with an alcohol swab. Ask the patient to hold the finger separated from the others and not to touch anything as the alcohol dries. *(Removes bacteria from the finger, preparing it for the puncture. Alcohol will dry while machine is set up, saving time.)*
5. Turn on the machine, place the lancet in the holder, and remove the lancet cover. Cock the lancet device. Check the control number that appears on the screen with the control number on the bottle of test strips. *(Prepares the equipment to puncture the skin. Checking control number ensures that the correct setting is used for the machine because it must match the strip number.)*

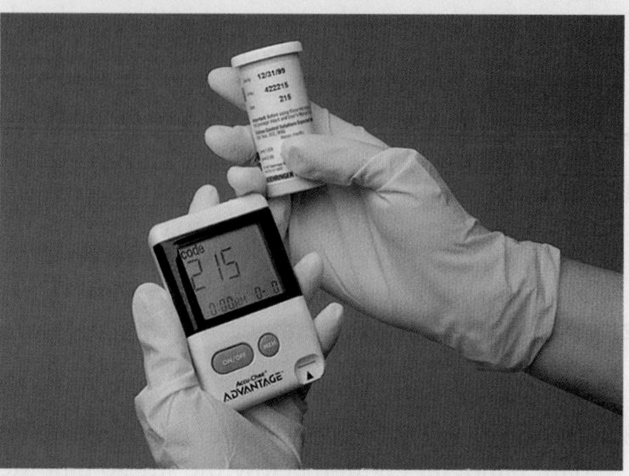

Step 5

6. Remove a test strip from the bottle and insert the end with the metal strips into the machine. (For machines that have intervening steps, check the manufacturer's directions. Some machines require that the specimen be obtained and a certain time period elapse before the strip is placed in the machine.) *(Prepares the machine to read the amount of glucose in the blood.)*
7. Place the fingerstick device firmly on the skin and push the release button, causing the lancet to pierce the skin. *(With the device at a right angle to the fingerprint lines, the needle should pierce the skin deeply enough to provide free blood flow with little pressure.)*

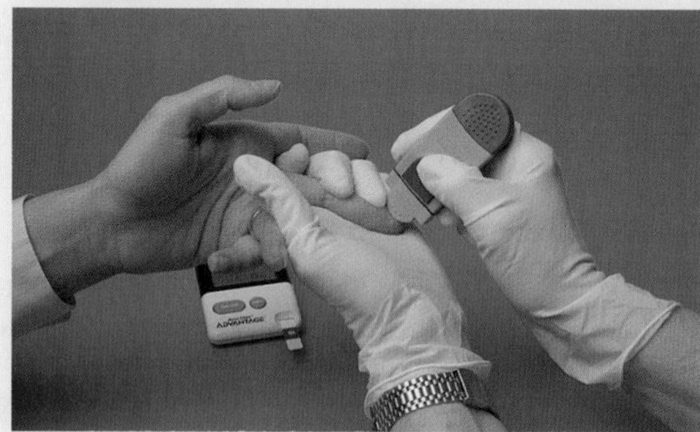

Step 7

8. If machine directions indicate it, wipe away the first drop of blood with a clean cotton ball. *(First drop often contains a large portion of serous fluid that dilutes the specimen, causing a false result.)*
9. Lightly squeeze the finger, gently milking down the finger toward the tip until an appropriate drop of blood has formed on the tip. *(Provides an adequate amount of blood for the specimen.)*

10. Lightly apply the drop of blood to the pad on the test strip and apply a clean cotton ball to the puncture wound with pressure. Ask patient to hold the cotton ball tightly in place. *(Applying blood to test strip begins the test. Pad must be completely covered with blood for accurate results. Pressure and dry cotton ball stop the bleeding.)*

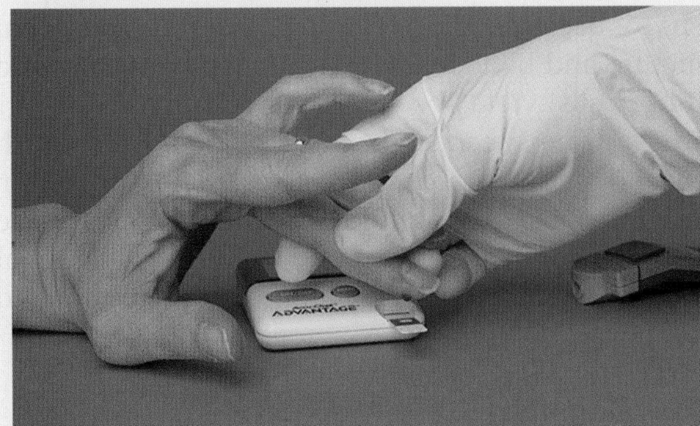

Step **10**

11. For alternate type of glucometer, start the timer and place the test strip on a paper towel beside the timer. At 60 seconds, place the test strip into the machine. See the manufacturer's directions. *(Some machines require different procedures for an accurate result.)*

Evaluation

12. Note the reading on the screen of the machine and record it. Turn the machine off. Share the result with the patient. *(Machine will provide a reading. If "error" appears, turn off the machine and start the procedure over from the beginning. Too much or too little blood on the test strip may cause an error. The patient must know the reading to participate in care.)*

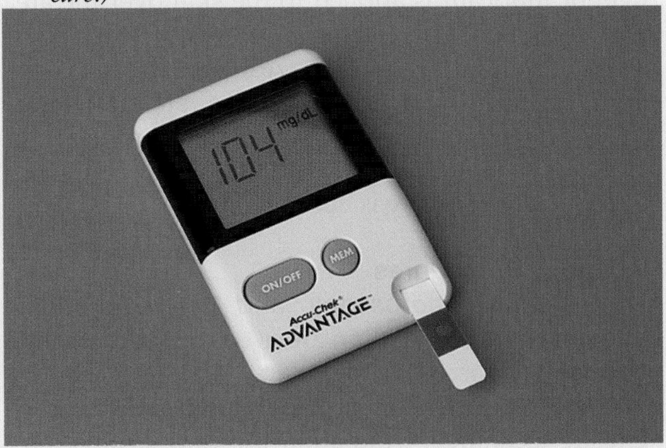

Step **12**

13. Assess whether the patient's finger is still bleeding. Stop the bleeding and apply an adhesive bandage if patient desires one. *(Prevents blood from continuing to flow; prevents transmission of possible blood-borne pathogens.)*
14. Dispose of test strip, lancet, and blood-tinged supplies in the appropriate hazardous materials waste receptacles. Remove gloves and perform hand hygiene. *(Prevents transmission of blood-borne pathogens.)*

Documentation

15. Document the procedure and the reading on the patient's medical record. In the inpatient facility, record the reading on the appropriate medication administration record (MAR) or electronic medication administration record (eMAR). *(Provides a record of the reading; patients on insulin have a place on the MAR or eMAR to record blood glucose readings.)*

Documentation Example

1/6 1030 Fingerstick glucose 126. (Nurse's electronic signature)

Special Considerations

- Warming the patient's hand before attempting the finger stick provides a greater chance of a successful specimen on the first attempt.
- Small children need to be held by the parent or another nurse.
- Children should be told that they will feel "a tiny sting" and that they will see blood. Do not lie to children.
- Having children use a finger puppet on the other hand sometimes will distract them sufficiently from the procedure, and they will hold still.
- Older adults bleed more easily than younger people do and may not need as deep a puncture.
- The puncture depth of the lancet needle can be adjusted by pushing the lancet further in or pulling it out a little from the holder.
- This procedure should never be performed without the use of gloves because of the risk of contamination with blood.

? Critical Thinking Question

1. If you get an error message when performing a finger stick for blood glucose, what would you do?

Table 24.3 Sequential Multiple Assay Panel (SMA-12)

TESTS INCLUDED	NORMAL RANGE[a]
Albumin	3.5-5.0 g/dL
ALP	30-120 units/L
AST	0-35 units/L
Bilirubin, total	0.3-1.1 mg/dL
Calcium, serum	8.4-10.6 mg/dL
Cholesterol	less than 200 mg/dL
Glucose	70-100 mg/dL
LDH	140-280 units/L
Phosphate	2.5-4.5 mg/dL
Total protein	6.0-8.0 g/dL
BUN	11-23 mg/dL
Uric acid	2.2-8.0 mg/dL

[a]Normal range may vary among laboratories depending on the type of test performed and the reagents used. (The SMA-6, SMA-7, and SMA-20 are different panels containing tests for 6, 7, and 20 substances, respectively.)
ALP, Alkaline phosphatase; *AST*, aspartate aminotransferase; *BUN*, blood urea nitrogen; *LDH*, lactate dehydrogenase; *SMA*, sequential multiple assay.

Box 24.2 Examples of Serology Tests

Many different types of serology tests may be ordered. Common examples are:

- Agglutination tests for specific organisms
- Antistreptolysin-O titer
- Blood typing: ABO groups and Rh
- Carcinoembryonic antigen (CEA) assay
- Coombs test
- C-reactive protein antiserum
- Heterophil antibody titer
- Immunoelectrophoresis
- Immunoglobulin (Ig) types: IgG, IgA, IgM, IgE, and IgD
- Radioimmunoassays (RIAs)
- Tests for syphilis
  - *Treponema pallidum*–microhemagglutination (TP-MHA)
  - Venereal Disease Research Laboratory (VDRL)
  - Fluorescent treponemal antibody (FTA)
- Enzyme-linked immunosorbent assay (ELISA) antibody test for human immunodeficiency virus (HIV)
- Western blot

toilet bowl, in a bedpan, or in plastic wrap draped on the rim of the toilet bowl. Transfer a small amount of stool to the appropriate container for a culture or a test for ova and parasites (O & P) or onto cards for the occult blood test (Skill 24.4). Maintain aseptic technique when collecting specimens for culture and sensitivity. In sensitivity tests, the identified organism is subjected to various antibiotic drugs to see which ones are most effective in killing it. With culture media that contain chromogens that interact with bacterial and fungal enzymes, organisms can be identified after only 24 hours of incubation.

Histologic and cytologic tests involve the study of tissues and cells. Confirmation of a diagnosis often depends on viewing tissues under a microscope to see the effects of the disease. Organs and tissues removed at **biopsy** (surgical excision of a small amount of tissue) are studied closely, and a pathology report is prepared. Studies of tissues and cells are performed to detect carcinogenic, metabolic, vascular, and other changes.

A variety of procedures may be used to obtain specimens for bacteriologic or cytologic examinations. Venipuncture and bone marrow **aspiration** (withdrawal of fluid or cells) yield specimens for culture or cytologic studies; urine specimens can be obtained from catheters and by clean-catch procedures. Lumbar puncture is used to obtain spinal fluid for culture. Standard Precautions must be employed and aseptic technique followed to guard against infection or contamination of specimens.

Ultrasonography

Ultrasonography (sonography) is a noninvasive method of visualizing soft tissue structures of the body. **The sonogram is a recording of the reflection of the ultrasonic waves directed into the tissues.** The procedure is used to diagnose many pathologic conditions of female reproductive organs, prostate, heart, kidney, pancreas, gallbladder, lymph nodes, liver, spleen, thyroid, eye, and peripheral blood vessels. It is often used in conjunction with radiography or nuclear medicine scans. The procedure is quick and does not usually produce much discomfort. Sonograms are produced with high-frequency sound waves that pass through the body. Echoes vary with tissue density, and the tracing produced is an echo-reflection map.

Patient preparation depends on the type of sonogram desired. For an abdominal sonogram, the patient is asked to drink a liter of water before the procedure. A gel or lubricant is applied to the skin over the area to be examined. The technician moves the **transducer** (wand emitting the sound waves) over the area with slight pressure. The echo-reflection pattern is displayed on a monitor, and pictures may be recorded or printed. The test takes approximately 35 to 45 minutes. No particular aftercare is needed.

Radiology Procedures

X-ray studies, fluoroscopy, and cineradiography. Different types of radiation are used for diagnosis and treatment of disease: alpha rays, beta rays, gamma rays, and x-rays. The most widely used radiologic diagnostic technique, irradiation by x-ray beams, produces an image of the denser tissues of the body by passing rays through the part to expose a film. The denser tissues block the x-rays and prevent them from exposing the film; therefore, tissues appear as black, gray, or white images depending on the degree of density. X-ray studies of the bony skeleton are examples of this process. Radiopaque solutions and materials can be used in various organs to form shadows on the film

Skill 24.3 Performing a Urine Dipstick Test

 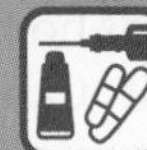 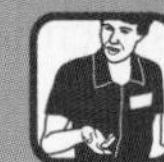 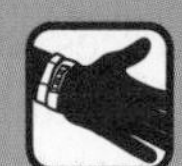 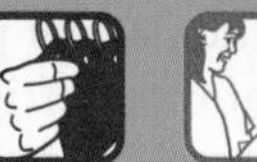 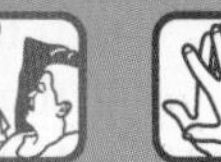 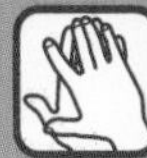 

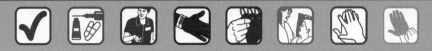

Urine dipsticks are manufactured to test for several substances in the urine. They provide a quick and easy way to screen for abnormalities in the urine in the primary care provider's office, at home, in the clinic, in the long-term care facility, or on the hospital nursing unit. A random or midstream urine specimen is used for the test.

SUPPLIES

- Multistix for urine testing
- Gloves
- Timer or watch
- Urine specimen

Review and carry out the Standard Steps in Appendix A.

ACTION *(RATIONALE)*

Assessment (Data Collection)

1. Assess whether patient can produce urine specimen. *(If patient has recently emptied the bladder, it may be necessary for them to drink some water and wait a while before producing specimen.)*

Planning

2. Determine that gloves and Multistix are available. *(Prevents hunting for supplies when ready to test specimen.)*

Implementation

3. Fill in a laboratory report form with the patient's name, the primary care provider's name, the date, and your initials. *(The sheet is ready for recording of test results.)*
4. Obtain the specimen, don gloves, and wet the dipstick with urine, making certain that each colored square is moistened. Remove the stick from the urine quickly and gently tap it on the side of the container to remove excess urine. *(The stick can be dipped into the urine or a small amount of urine can be poured down the stick while holding it over the toilet or a workroom sink.)*

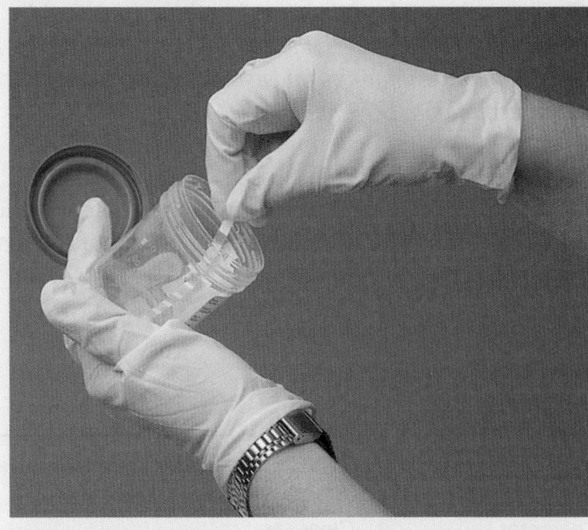

Step 4

5. Start timing the tests immediately after wetting the stick. *(Exact timing is necessary for the accuracy of the test results. Some portions of the test require 30 seconds before reading; others are read at 40 seconds, 45 seconds, or 60 seconds.)*

Evaluation

6. Hold the stick horizontally and compare the color chart on the side of the Multistix bottle with the color on the strip at the correct time interval. *(Allows for close comparison of the colors for each square on the stick with the color chart on the bottle.)*

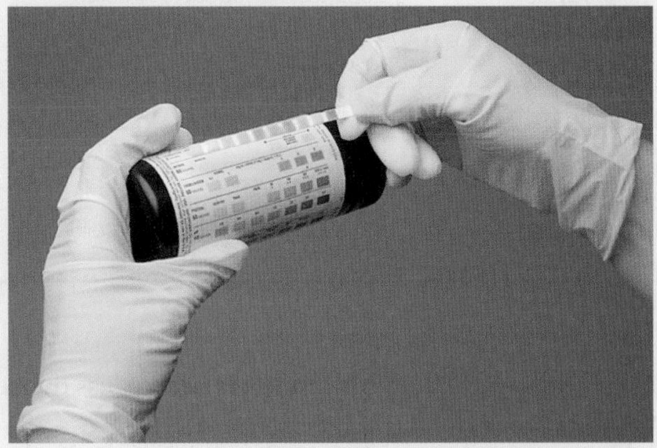

Step 6

7. Document the result for each component of the test on the laboratory report form. *(Records the test results.)*
8. Dispose of urine, container, and used Multistix correctly in the biohazard waste receptacle. Remove gloves and perform hand hygiene. *(Reduces transfer of microorganisms.)*
9. Share results with patient or give the report to the primary care provider. *(Participation of patient in testing and care improves understanding of treatment. Documentation is the completed laboratory slip.)*

Special Considerations

- Certain medications and vitamins may discolor the urine and interfere with accurate reading of the test results.
- Urine specimens must be tested while they are fresh for the result to be accurate.
- If the patient produces the specimen at home, ask that it be refrigerated until it can be brought in for testing.

Critical Thinking Questions

1. If some of the test-strip squares turn an odd color after exposure to urine, what would you do?
2. If a patient's specimen was obtained 2 hours ago and brought to the office, will the test results of a urine dip be accurate?

Table 24.4 Normal Urinalysis

CHARACTERISTIC	NORMAL VALUE
Color	Yellow, straw, dark yellow, amber
Character	Clear
Specific gravity (sp gr)	1.003-1.030
Acetone, ketones	Negative
Glucose (gluc)	Negative
Protein (Alb)	0-0.8 mg/dL
Nitrite	Negative
Occult blood	Negative
pH	4.6-8.0
Odor	Faint (not fruity, musty, fishy, or fetid)
Urobilinogen	Negative or 0.1-1 Ehrlich units/dL
Cells Erythrocytes Leukocytes	 Less than or equal to 2 cells/ high-power field Less than or equal to 4 cells/ high-power field
Casts	None
Crystals	None
Bacteria or fungi	None
Parasites	None
Epithelium	Less than or equal to 10 cells/ high-power field

that show the size, location, and structure of less dense tissues (Fig. 24.1).

Fluoroscopy is used to examine movement. X-rays are passed through the body part and are projected on a fluorescent screen. The dense tissues produce dark shadows on the film, whereas soft tissues appear whiter. To examine movement through organs or soft tissues, the room is made dark, and a radiopaque substance is introduced into the body. For example, to observe movement and structure of the throat, esophagus, and stomach, barium is swallowed. Cineradiography is the method of adding a video camera to the fluoroscope equipment and making a video recording of the procedure so the results can be examined in further detail.

The low intensities of diagnostic x-rays make them safe to use because the exposure is of short duration and the rays do not penetrate deeply into the tissues. Higher intensity doses of radiation are harmful to the cells and are used therapeutically to bombard and kill cancer cells in the body. Commonly performed radiologic procedures include:

- Chest x-ray (CXR) studies
- Barium swallow and upper gastrointestinal (GI) series
- Barium enema and small bowel series
- Kidneys, ureters, and bladder (KUB) x-ray studies
- Gallbladder series and cholangiogram
- Intravenous pyelogram (IVP)
- X-ray studies of the bony skeleton: arthrogram and myelogram
- Radionuclide scans
- Computed tomography scans (CT scans)

Think Critically

The patient asks how a sonogram works. Can you explain the process in easy-to-understand terms?

Radionuclide scans. Radionuclide scans are based on the fact that various organs and soft tissues of the body attract and concentrate certain radionuclides. These studies are carried out in the nuclear medicine department, which is often a division of the radiology department. A radioactive substance is injected into a vein and then, after allowing time for the organ being scanned to absorb the substance, a radioactivity scanner (scintillator) is passed over the area where the organ is located. Serial pictures are then produced at intervals. The radioactive substance is typically passed from the body, in the urine, quickly, depending on the patient's renal function. Only a small amount of radia-

Skill 24.4 Obtaining a Stool Specimen for Occult Blood, Culture, or Ova and Parasites

 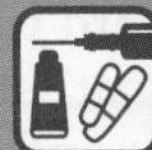 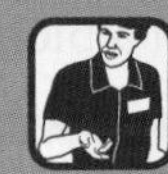 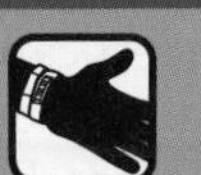 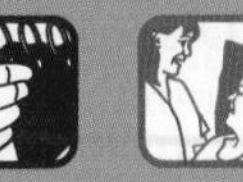 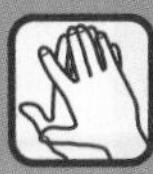 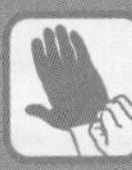

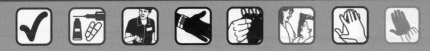

Nurses frequently need to obtain a stool specimen from a patient and test it for occult blood indicating GI tract bleeding. Specimens may also be sent for culture or for tests for ova and parasites or other substances when a GI complaint needs to be diagnosed. Stool for ova and parasites must be sent to the laboratory immediately. In some states, stool testing is permitted only in the laboratory.

SUPPLIES

- "Hat" collection container to place in the toilet
- Bedpan
- Toilet tissue
- Gloves
- Container with culture preservative
- Sterile swab(s)
- Specimen container for ova and parasites
- Test cards for stool for occult blood
- Wooden sticks
- Tongue blades

Review and carry out the Standard Steps in Appendix A.

ACTION *(RATIONALE)*

Assessment (Data Collection)

1. Determine whether the patient understands why the specimen is needed. *(Understanding helps patient accept need for specimen.)*
2. Determine whether patient will need to use a bedpan or can use the toilet to deposit the specimen. *(Identifies equipment needed.)*

Planning

3. Determine when patient usually has a bowel movement. *(Allows nurse to be available to collect the specimen.)*
4. Instruct patient about need for stool specimen. *(Understanding makes patient more cooperative.)*

Implementation

5. Place collection container by toilet or position patient on bedpan. Ask patient to use call button when specimen is ready. *(Container will be at hand when needed. Alerts nurse to collect specimen.)*
6. Instruct patient to void and use tissue before placing the stool collection container in toilet to catch stool specimen; or clean and replace bedpan after voiding. *(Stool specimen should be free of urine or tissue.)*
7. Don gloves; assist patient with cleansing of rectal area if needed. Assist to perform hand hygiene. *(Keeps patient clean and prevents spread of microorganisms.)*
8. Perform hand hygiene and don fresh gloves. *(Protects hands from fecal contamination.)*
9. Take specimen in covered bedpan to bathroom or utility room if bedpan was used. *(Provides a private area in which to transfer the specimen to the laboratory container or onto the stool cards.)*

Stool Culture

10. Open specimen jar containing culture medium, placing lid upside down on the counter. Withdraw sterile swab from culture tube or package and place it into the stool to obtain a stool sample the size of a bean. Place stool into the stool culture container with the culture medium. Taking care not to contaminate the inside of the jar lid, replace it on the container. *(Placing lid upside down prevents contamination of the lid. Prepares stool for laboratory culture.)*

Test for Ova and Parasites

11. Using wooden tongue blade(s), transfer a portion (1 inch [2.5 cm]) from the middle of the stool to the container for the ova and parasite specimen. If the stool is liquid, transfer about 15 mL of liquid stool to the container. Place container in a biohazard bag and seal. *(Readies the specimen for the laboratory.)*
12. Send specimen to the laboratory immediately with a completed requisition slip. Be certain specimen container is properly labeled with the patient's name and room number, the date, and the primary care provider's name. *(Identifies specimen as belonging to the patient; routes laboratory result to the correct care provider.)*

Test for Occult Blood

13. Open the front window(s) of the specimen card. *(Readies the card for receipt of the specimen.)*
14. With wooden stick, obtain a small amount of stool from the middle, interior portion of the specimen. Smear it on the area within the window of the stool card. Repeat if more than one window is to be filled for the test. *(Places specimen within the testing area of the card. Only a small amount of stool is required.)*

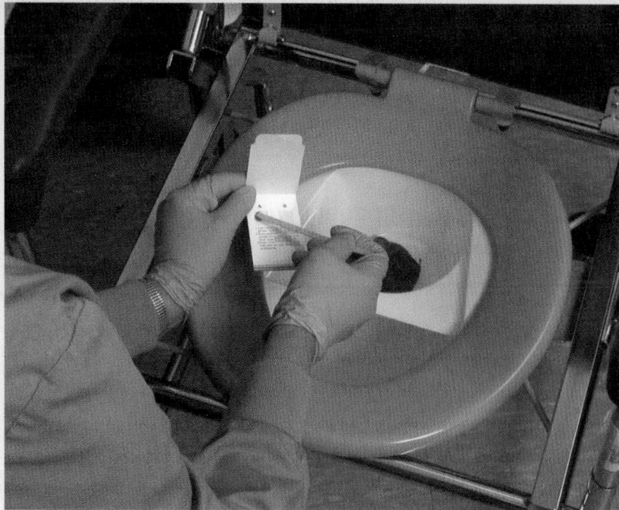

Step **14**

15. Open the occult blood specimen card back window. *(Provides access to the specimen for testing.)*
16. Place two drops of the occult blood specimen reagent on the stool smear and one drop on the control; repeat for each window on the card. (Check test instructions for the number of drops of the reagent; some test instructions differ.) *(Begins the test.)*

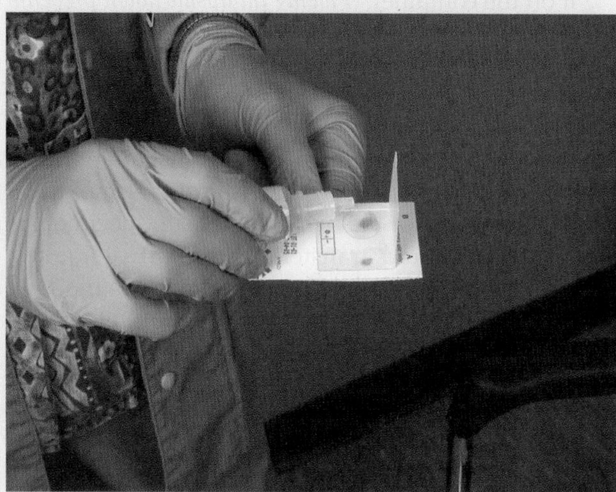

Step **16**

17. Wait 30 seconds. Read the test, looking for blue discoloration in or around the stool smear. Check that the control turned blue. *(Blue color within 30 seconds indicates that blood is present in the stool. Careful timing is essential for test accuracy.)*
18. Dispose of the test card in a biohazard waste container. Cleanse the bedpan or "hat" stool-collection container. Remove gloves and perform hand hygiene. *(Reduces transfer of microorganisms.)*

Evaluation

19. If the test result is positive, be certain that the patient adhered to the diet restrictions before reporting. Determine whether the patient took any medications that could have produced a false-positive test result. *(Ensures accuracy of test result.)*

Documentation

20. Complete the laboratory test form with the patient's name, date, the primary care provider's name, type of test, and the result, or enter the result in the patient's medical record. *(Ensures that the test result is recorded.)*

Documentation Example

1/04 0915 Stool for occult blood negative ×2. (Nurse's electronic signature)

Special Considerations

- False-positive and false-negative results for occult blood tests are prevented by the patient following the recommendations for diet and medication cessation for several days before the test. See the particular test manufacturer's recommendation sheet.
- Stool cultures are often done in a series of three on specimens taken from different bowel movements.
- Newer fecal immunochemical tests can be performed without dietary and medication restrictions (check the manufacturer's product information).

? Critical Thinking Questions

1. Why do you think a stool specimen for ova and parasites needs to be fresh when it reaches the laboratory?
2. Why is it contraindicated to take aspirin for 5 days before obtaining a stool sample for an occult blood test?

tion is given, and the patient is not considered radioactive. Radionuclides are used in scanning the thyroid gland, kidneys, the brain, the liver, lungs, bones, and pericardium and in determining blood volume. The time required for the scan depends on the organ being scanned.

! Safety Alert

NUCLEAR SCANS AND PREGNANCY

Radionuclide tests are contraindicated for pregnant or nursing women. Always verify whether a woman is pregnant, could be pregnant, or is nursing before sending her for a nuclear scan.

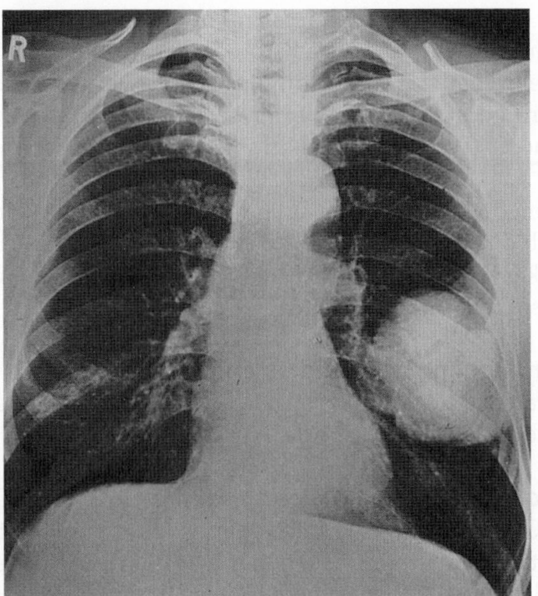

FIGURE 24.1 Chest x-ray film showing a tumor. (From Grainger, R. G., Allison, D. J., Adam, A., & Dixon, A. K. [2002]. *Grainger & Allison's Diagnostic Radiology* [4th ed.]. Philadelphia, PA: Churchill Livingstone.)

Nursing care involves proper disposal of linens, waste materials, and body secretions that have been exposed to radioactive materials. The patient is asked to empty the bladder when imaging is complete to reduce radiation exposure time. Part of patient education is to assure patients that they are not radioactive or a danger to others in the vicinity.

Computed tomography. CT scans of various organs and parts of the body are used to confirm a diagnosis, plan treatment, evaluate the effects of treatment, and guide needle placement for biopsy or aspiration. A computer enhances x-ray images and allows examination of horizontal sections of the body at various angles to define tissue density.

Blood flow is assessed with CT angiography. A contrast medium in used for the procedure. The test is used for suspected pulmonary embolism and arteriovenous malformation, to determine patency of coronary arteries, and to detect blood flow patterns to tumors.

Clinical Cues

If a patient who has diabetes is to have a CT scan with an iodine-based contrast medium and is taking a medication containing metformin, that medication must be discontinued before the test and another means used to control blood glucose, because metformin can significantly alter renal function.

Most CT scans are noninvasive, but consent may be required for scans using any contrast medium. Preparation of the patient depends on the organ or part to be examined. The CT scan requires that the patient be in one position for 10 to 45 minutes. The patient is positioned on a table inside the scanner. The scanning machinery revolves around the body part being scanned. Data are fed into the computer, which produces images in shades of gray that indicate the different densities of the organ.

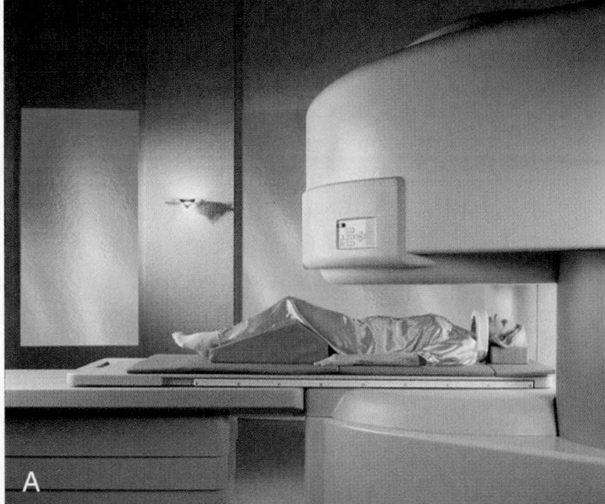

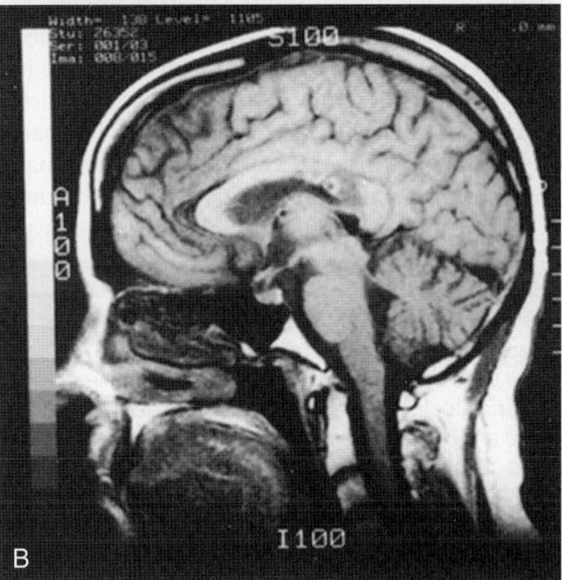

FIGURE 24.2 (A) MRI machine. (B) Midline sagittal view of the brain using MRI. (From Lewis, S. L., Heitkemper, M. M., Dirksen, S. R., O'Brien, P. G., & Bucher, P. [2007]. *Medical-Surgical Nursing: Assessment and Management of Clinical Problems* [7th ed.]. St. Louis, MO: Mosby.)

Think Critically

If your patient expresses fear at receiving a radionuclide for a particular diagnostic test, how could you reassure them?

Magnetic resonance imaging. Magnetic resonance imaging (MRI) is a noninvasive method of differentiating normal from abnormal tissue in the body. MRI is commonly used for the brain, knee joint, spine and spinal cord, and abdominal organs. The patient must lie flat and very still. The patient is placed on a table and then slid inside the large cylinder-shaped machine; the cylinder may be of open or closed design (Fig. 24.2).

As scanning takes place, loud clicks can be heard. The procedure takes up to 1½ hours. The patient can talk through an intercom system to the MRI staff. This may help relieve feelings of claustrophobia. Patients with metal devices implanted in the body, such as cardiac pacemakers, automatic implantable cardiac defibrillators, metal hip prostheses, artificial cardiac valves, vascular clips, or staples from recent surgery, cannot undergo this procedure because the machine emits a strong magnetic field. Patients with tattoos occasionally report burning or swelling of the tattooed area because some inks contain traces of metal. The patient must inform the MRI technician of any tattoos, and if they experience any burning feeling during the procedure.

Magnetic resonance angiography (MRA) is used to visualize arteries, veins, and the heart chambers, using the same technology as MRI. MRA is useful in detecting aneurysm of the aorta and atherosclerotic disease in the arterial system. MRA may be used to assess the arteries that supply a tumor before tumor removal. It is particularly useful in identifying arteriovenous malformations in the brain and alterations of blood flow in the circle of Willis that could contribute to stroke.

Clinical Cues

For patients undergoing MRI, remove any transdermal medication patch, including a nicotine patch because the metal backing may cause a burn from this procedure. Inquire about any internal prosthetic device that contains metal. Many patients become anxious about being placed in an MRI scanner. Obtain an order for sedation, if needed, before the procedure.

Describe the machine and procedure to the patient. The underlying concept is one of changing magnetic fields, and information is translated into images of different densities of tissue in the body.

Nursing care involves obtaining consent and making certain that all surface metal (e.g., rings and watch) is removed from the patient's body. Instruct the patient to lie very still during the procedure and to keep the eyes closed to decrease feelings of claustrophobia. Music of the patient's choice may be provided. Teach the patient deep-breathing and rhythmic breathing relaxation techniques.

Think Critically

The patient scheduled for an abdominal MRI says she does not think she can stand to hold still in a restricted position for more than 10 minutes. What would you do?

Positron emission tomography scans. Positron emission tomography (PET) scans are used to diagnose cancer, heart disease, and some brain disorders. The scan produces digital pictures that show abnormal cells in the body. The scan shows differences in blood flow and oxygen uptake in cells. Problems can be identified earlier with PET than with CT or MRI. The test takes about 2 hours and is noninvasive and painless. Tell patients not to exercise for 24 hours and not to eat or drink anything for several hours before the scan. Metal should be eliminated from clothing, and no jewelry should be worn because it can interfere with the scan. An intravenous (IV) radiotracer is injected before beginning the scan. About 45 minutes later, the scan will be performed. The scanner is a large donut-shaped machine with a table that slides into the opening. The machine makes whirring and clicking sounds. The patient must lie still during the scan.

Cardiopulmonary Studies and Procedures

A battery of tests that range from simple to complex is used to diagnose heart or lung disease (Box 24.3).

Electrocardiogram. The electrocardiogram (ECG or EKG) was one of the first diagnostic tests of heart activity. It remains important because it is quick and easy and it provides an immediate visual record. **The ECG consists of waves and lines that represent the electrical activity during the cardiac cycle** (Fig. 24.3). The ECG tracing shows the P wave, the QRS complex, and the T wave, occurring in a repeating sequence. Sometimes a U wave is present. The person trained in interpreting the tracing can determine whether the waves are normal or abnormal. Nurses in medical offices or clinics often are responsible for obtaining the ECG tracing. Clothing is removed from the upper body to apply the electrodes to the skin (Fig. 24.4). Female patients are given a gown positioned with the ties in the front. Necklaces, bracelets, belt buckles, and watches are removed because they sometimes interfere with the electrical tracing (Steps 24.1).

Cardiac catheterization. Cardiac catheterization is a procedure used to determine the function of the heart, valves, and coronary circulation. During cardiac catheterization, readings can be taken of oxygen concentration at different sites, of pressure in the different heart chambers, and of cardiac output. Abnormal blood flow through the heart and the coronary vessels can be detected. Cardiac catheterization is of great value in diagnosing coronary artery disease and valvular dysfunction.

The patient signs a consent form and must have a complete history and physical examination before the procedure. Nothing is given by mouth for at least 6 hours, and a sedative narcotic may be given to allay apprehension and anxiety.

Cardiac catheterization is a surgical procedure using surgical aseptic techniques. It is carried out in a special cardiac catheterization laboratory, radiology department, or surgical suite. A catheter is inserted into a vein or artery and threaded into the heart for injection of contrast media and to obtain pressure readings. Heart action is observed by fluoroscopy and is continuously monitored by ECG until the tests are completed. A videotape is made to provide records of heart function. Postcatheterization nursing care includes ensuring the patient has bed rest for 2 to 12 hours, frequently checking the

Box 24.3 Common Tests and Procedures for the Heart and Lungs

EXAMINATIONS OF THE HEART

Cardiac catheterization: A complex procedure in which a long catheter is passed through an artery or vein to the heart to obtain information about defects, valves, patency of coronary arteries, pressures, and blood specimens.

Angiocardiography, left: Use of contrast medium to visualize the left side of the heart.

Digital subtraction angiography (DSA): A procedure in which contrast medium is injected into the arteries and the computer performs "digital subtraction" to reveal structures that block clear view of arteries.

Ventriculography, left: Use of contrast medium to define the formation of the left ventricle.

Electrocardiogram (ECG or EKG): Record of the electrical activity of the heart, which normally produces P, Q, R, S, and T waves.

Echocardiogram: A record of the position and motion of the heart produced by ultrasound waves; used to picture the structure of the valves.

Electron beam computed tomography (EBCT): Computed tomography of the heart, a noninvasive procedure that shows calcified plaque in the coronary arteries.

Master two-step test: An ECG made of heart response to the exercise of stepping up and down two steps that are 9 inches high.

Mixed venous oxygen saturation (SvO_2): A pulmonary artery catheter measurement of the oxygen saturation of venous blood as it returns to the right side of the heart.

Phonocardiogram: A graphic record of heart sounds.

Treadmill stress test: A test of the heart's response to graded levels of exercise or stress on a treadmill.

Vectorcardiography: A record of the direction and magnitude of the forces of the heart during one heartbeat.

Nuclear cardiography: A process in which radioisotopes are injected intravenously, and the radioactive uptake is counted over the heart by a scintillation camera; provides information about myocardial contractility, myocardial perfusion, and cellular injury from infarction.

EXAMINATIONS OF PULMONARY FUNCTION

Oximetry: A test that monitors arterial or venous oxygen saturation; venous measurements are noninvasive because the probe is attached to the fingertip, earlobe, nose, or forehead (venous oxygen saturation); arterial readings are done by pulmonary artery catheter (arterial oxygen saturation).

Bronchospirometry: A method of measuring the air entering and leaving each lung separately; a double lumen catheter with two balloons is passed into the bronchus under fluoroscopy.

Capnography: A method of monitoring the partial pressure of carbon dioxide in respiratory gases; assists in detecting beginning hypoxia during anesthesia and in critically ill patients; shows a pattern on a monitor screen with parameters for normal and abnormal.

Plethysmography: A method of measuring blood flow through the pulmonary capillaries, using an airtight "body box."

Radioactive gas perfusion tests: Use of radioactive tracers given intravenously to measure blood flow through the lungs; radionuclides are given for lung scans.

Spirometer: An instrument that measures the amount of air taken into the lungs and expelled.

Ventilation tests: Measurement of air volume moved in and out of the lungs; includes tidal volume, residual volume, minute respiratory volume, inspiratory reserve volume, and expiratory reserve volume.

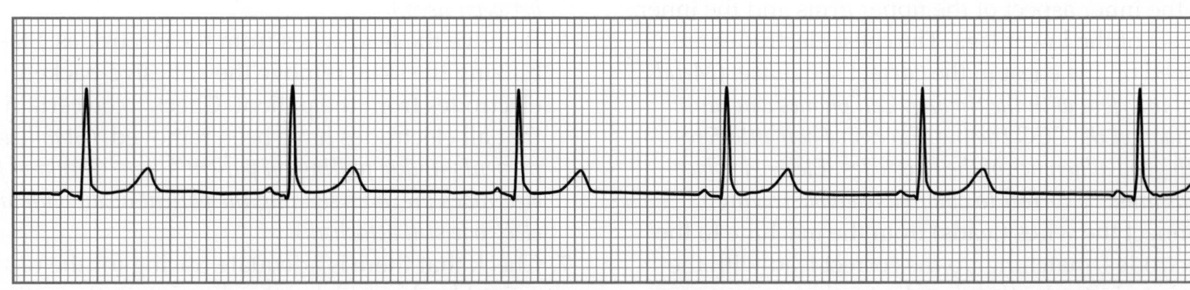

FIGURE 24.3 Normal ECG tracing.

pressure dressing over the insertion point, and measuring vital signs and the distal pulse every 10 to 15 minutes for the first hour and the temperature every 6 hours. When the femoral approach has been used, the patient's leg may be immobilized for several hours to reduce the chance of bleeding. Unless a self-sealing type of catheter is used, immobilization is often done by placing a special pressure device or small sandbags. Observe closely for chest pain, dyspnea, bleeding from the wound, quality of pulses distal to the catheter entry point, abnormal neurologic signs, and any signs of infection.

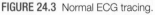

Legal & Ethical Considerations

ASSESSMENTS AFTER CARDIAC CATHETERIZATION

Health care providers have a legal responsibility to check neurologic signs and distal pulses below the site of entry after a cardiac catheterization. Should a hematoma form at the entry site and pressure on the nerves be so great that function is lost in the leg or foot, the nurse would be legally liable if the pulses and sensation had not been regularly assessed. Document the assessment findings to protect against legal ramifications.

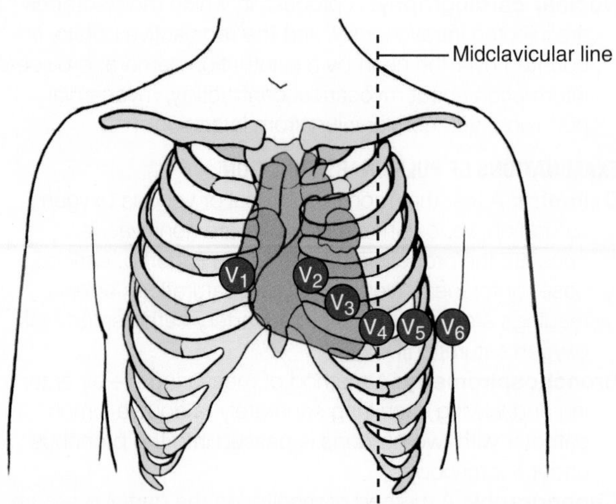

FIGURE 24.4 Positions for placing electrodes.

When a noninvasive procedure to evaluate heart function is advisable, an electron beam tomography test may be performed on the heart. This will show the percentage of calcification present in the coronary arteries. Calcium deposits are part of the atherosclerosis process and can help predict the risk for coronary occlusion or myocardial infarction.

Angiography and arteriography. Angiography and arteriography are used to locate lesions, occluded vessels, tumors, and malformed blood vessels. A contrast medium is injected into an artery, and x-ray studies are taken of the dye spreading through the vessels. The procedure may be used to diagnose problems in arteries anywhere in the body: heart, neck, brain, or extremities.

A consent form is signed and baseline vital signs are obtained. Usually the patient is given nothing by mouth for at least 6 hours, and a mild sedative or tranquilizer is given before the procedure. After the procedure the patient is kept on bed rest for a

Steps 24.1 Obtaining an Electrocardiogram Tracing

Each type of ECG machine has its own set of operating instructions. Consult the manual for the machine on hand for variations in the operating procedure.

ACTION *(RATIONALE)*

1. Ask patient to remove all metal and temporarily turn off cellular devices. After the patient is positioned comfortably, shave or clip hair as needed for electrode placement. The extremity electrodes go on the inner aspect of the upper arms and the inner aspect of the lower legs. The chest electrodes are placed on the chest in the correct sequence. *(Metal may interfere with the tracing. Cell phones can cause artifact on the ECG tracing. Excessive hair interferes with good adherence of the electrodes. Electrode placement must be correct to obtain a readable tracing.)*
2. Connect the wires (leads) from the machine to the electrodes, matching up the correct lead with the correct electrode. *(Labels indicate which wire goes to which electrode. If the wires are not attached to the correct electrode, the tracing will not be correct.)*
3. Turn the machine on; ask the patient to hold still. Press the auto-run button. *(The machine will begin the tracing and automatically stop after recording the beginning leads.)*
4. Press the manual-run button and immediately press the "1-2-3" button. Allow the machine to run through two full sheets of recording paper and press "stop." *(This sets the machine to record the other required leads.)*
5. Press "manual run" again and allow enough paper to run through the machine so that the patient's tracing can be torn off cleanly. Check the tracing for a correct appearance. Roll or fold up the tracing and place it to one side. The tracing should be on an even line and without tiny vibration lines indicating electrical interference. If the tracing is not clear, troubleshoot according to the manual with the machine and retake the tracing. Turn off the machine. *(This method prevents losing some of the patient's tracing. The machine should not be left on between uses.)*
6. Remove the lead wires from the electrodes. Stabilizing the skin, remove the adhesive-backed electrodes from the patient. Check to be certain that all electrodes have been removed. *(Stabilization prevents undue pulling on patient's skin. Checking for electrodes prevents sending the patient away with an electrode still attached.)*
7. Check that there is adequate tracing for the required leads and label the sheets with the patient's name and the required information: age, sex, blood pressure, height and weight, and medications the patient is taking. *(Assists primary care provider in interpreting the tracing correctly.)*
8. Assist patient off the table. Allow the patient to redress. Be certain that all jewelry removed is returned to the patient. *(Shows caring; prevents jewelry from being misplaced.)*
9. Document the procedure in the patient record. Route the tracing for interpretation. *(Provides information that the procedure was carried out. Allows the primary care provider to interpret the tracing.)*

number of hours; an ice pack is applied to the insertion point; and vital signs are measured periodically. The contrast medium insertion point is also checked for bleeding or formation of a **hematoma** (collection of clotted blood). Be alert for any reaction to the dye. The Infraredx LipiScan NIR Coronary Imaging System uses infrared imaging to detect lipid and to assess the quantity of lipid core plaque in the coronary arteries. The catheter has a fiberoptic laser light that provides spectroscopy images based on the fat and other substances in the plaque.

Treadmill stress test. The treadmill stress test measures the cardiac heart rate and blood pressure response to clinically controlled active exercise. It is used to diagnose heart capacity, to guide convalescence from a myocardial infarction (heart attack), and to determine response to medical treatment. While having heart action continuously monitored by ECG, the patient walks on a treadmill, pedals a stationary bicycle, or climbs a set of stairs (Fig. 24.5). The speed and degree of the incline of the treadmill can be changed to increase the amount of work or stress on the heart. The speed and resistance of the exercise bicycle can also be changed to meet the established standards for the test. The test is terminated when the desired heart rate is reached, the patient shows signs of fatigue, or the ECG shows signs of cardiac ischemia. Often thallium-201, a radioisotope, is used to show myocardial perfusion while the patient is exercising during the stress test. A consent form is signed, and the patient may have a light meal 4 to 6 hours before the test and must avoid caffeine and smoking for 4 hours before the test. The patient may be told to discontinue taking certain medications when the test is for diagnostic purposes; medications may be taken when the test is to determine response to treatment. After a period of rest, the patient is able to resume usual activities.

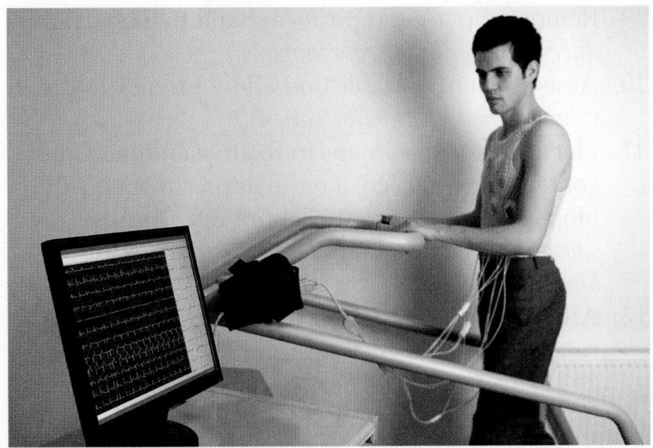

FIGURE 24.5 Cardiac treadmill stress test. (Photo copyright istock.com.)

Pulmonary function tests. Pulmonary function tests provide information about respiratory function, lung capacity, and diffusion of gases. Appointments are made for the tests to be performed in the pulmonary laboratory. Spirometers and other breathing devices may be used. No special preparation is required.

Capnography. Capnography is used to detect respiratory depression, particularly after surgery for patients with epidural analgesia and during diagnostic procedures requiring sedation. It measures end-tidal carbon dioxide ($ETCO_2$). The patient wears a nasal cannula or oxygen mask that contains a sensor. The results are read from a small hand-held device.

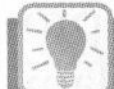 QSEN Considerations: Evidence-Based Practice

Capnography Reduces Opioid-Induced Respiratory Depression

A project study has validated the effectiveness of $ETCO_2$ monitoring (capnography) in helping nurses detect early signs of respiratory depression following opioid analgesia, thereby reducing the number of cases of opioid-induced respiratory depression (Carlisle, 2015).

Endoscopic Examinations

Many procedures are based on the use of an **endoscope** (an instrument used to view inside a body cavity). Endoscopes are small metal or plastic devices or flexible tubes equipped with fiberoptics that provide direct light to the tissues being examined. Preparation of the patient depends on the test to be performed.

Bronchoscopy. A **bronchoscope** is used to inspect the larynx, the trachea, and bronchi. An informed consent is required. The patient is NPO for 4 to 8 hours before the test to decrease the risk of aspiration. Good mouth care should be performed before the procedure to prevent excessive bacteria from entering the airways. Preprocedural sedation is administered. A local anesthetic is sprayed into the throat before insertion of the bronchoscope. Biopsy specimens may be obtained from the structures. After the procedure, the patient should not eat or drink anything for 2 hours or until the gag reflex has fully returned. A fever may occur within 24 hours. A high persistent fever should be reported to the primary care provider.

Gastroscopy. **Gastroscopy** is the visual inspection of the upper digestive tract and the stomach to obtain specimens of gastric contents and perform a biopsy on the stomach tissues. A signed consent form is required. Instruct the patient to take nothing by mouth for 8 hours before the examination. About 30 minutes before the procedure, an injection of an atropine-like drug and a sedative is given.

The test is conducted in the GI laboratory. A local anesthetic is sprayed on the pharynx, and a gastroscope is passed to the stomach. The scope has a fiberoptic system for its lens. The gastroscope may be equipped with a camera to take color photographs. Washings are done to obtain specimens for cytologic studies, or a biopsy specimen is taken.

The patient should take nothing by mouth until the effects of the local anesthetic have worn off and the gag reflex has returned. After resting, the patient can resume usual activities. Observe for signs of bleeding or unexplained pain, which might be due to perforation of an ulcer.

Proctosigmoidoscopy. Proctosigmoidoscopy is the visual inspection of the lower bowel and is used to check the lining for ulceration, **polyps** (growths protruding from a mucous membrane), tumors, inflammation, and other abnormalities. Consent is required for the procedure. The bowel should be clear of fecal material; therefore, a cathartic is given the night before the procedure, and an enema may be ordered. The patient may be restricted to a liquid diet the day before the test. The patient should empty the bladder before the test and then assume a side-lying or Sims position on a table. The sigmoidoscope is inserted. The fiberoptic lens enables the examiner to see the structures, and suction can be used to remove secretions. Air may be introduced to inflate the lower bowel to better view the wall, and biopsy forceps may be used to remove a specimen of tissue. Some abdominal cramping is usually experienced. No special aftercare is required (Steps 24.2).

Colonoscopy. **Colonoscopy** is the inspection of the entire large intestine for polyps, areas of inflammation, and malignant lesions. It confirms suspicious findings of x-ray studies and is used to take biopsy specimens or remove polyps found on other studies or in patients with a known history of polyps. A long, flexible fiberoptic endoscope is inserted anally and slowly advanced through the large intestine.

The patient is placed on a clear liquid diet for 24 to 48 hours before the procedure, avoiding liquids that contain red or purple dye, and given nothing by mouth for at least 8 hours. Sometimes a particular diet is ordered for the 3 days before the test. Bowel cleansing with laxatives, cathartics, and enemas is performed in the 24 hours before the test. Bowel fluid must return clear before colonoscopy can be successfully performed. Sedation is given to promote relaxation and decrease awareness. The procedure takes 30 to 90 minutes.

A signed consent is required. Check the patient's laboratory values for CBC and clotting times to verify

Steps 24.2 Assisting with a Flexible Sigmoidoscopy

Assisting with a sigmoidoscopy is often the duty of the nurse employed in a medical office or clinic.

ACTION *(RATIONALE)*

1. Set up the sigmoidoscopy equipment and check that the light is functioning and the suction functions. Place gloves and lubricant on a prepared field. *(Checking prevents an equipment problem during the procedure.)*
2. Inquire if the patient completed the bowel preparation as instructed. *(Bowel must be clean for visualization of the mucosal walls.)*
3. Have patient empty the bladder before the procedure. *(Prevents added discomfort during procedure.)*
4. Ask patient to remove all clothing from the waist down and put on a gown so that it ties in the back. *(Allows examiner to access the anus.)*
5. Assist patient onto the examining table and into the left lateral or Sims position. *(Positions the rectum for entry of the sigmoidoscope.)*
6. Drape patient so that only the anus is exposed. *(Protects patient's modesty and privacy. Draping prevents unnecessary chilling.)*
7. Ask patient to breathe slowly and deeply through the mouth during the procedure and to try to relax the lower abdominal and rectal muscles. Explain that discomfort is often caused by air instilled to improve visualization. *(Breathing through the mouth slowly helps the patient relax and maintain relaxed muscles. Relaxing the muscles aids in the insertion and progression of the sigmoidoscope.)*
8. After the procedure, don gloves and clean the patient's anal region of excess lubricant using tissue wipes. Allow patient to rest before arising from the table. *(Cleaning prevents lubricant from getting on table or patient's clothes.)*
9. Remove gloves and perform hand hygiene. *(Reduces transfer of microorganisms.)*
10. Assist patient off table and allow privacy to dress. *(Shows consideration for patient.)*
11. Place biopsy specimens in fixative and label the containers; complete a requisition slip. Send biopsy specimens to the laboratory. *(Ensures specimen is labeled correctly and sent to the laboratory.)*
12. After the patient has left the room, clean up the room and cleanse the equipment. *(Prepares room for next patient. Equipment must be disinfected before next use.)*

that they are within normal limits. **Any iron medication, aspirin, and most anti-inflammatory drugs must be withheld for 3 days.** Instruct the patient in the clear liquid diet regimen and bowel-cleansing program. Administer the bowel preparation components as ordered. Give any ordered pretest medications. Teach the patient about the procedure and what to expect. Colonoscopy should not be done sooner than 10 to 14 days after barium GI studies. Obtain baseline vital signs. After the test, monitor the vital signs every half hour for 2 hours and then according to facility protocol. Monitor rectal bleeding. Slight bleeding is expected if polyps were biopsied or removed. Keep the patient on bed rest for the time ordered. Someone must drive the patient home.

Life-Span Considerations

Older Adults

- Older adult patients who are repeatedly kept NPO (nothing by mouth) for various tests and procedures are susceptible to dehydration and electrolyte imbalances. Frequent assessment is needed to determine hydration status.
- A series of enemas can also upset electrolyte balance. Assess for signs of potassium and sodium imbalance after administering enemas.
- Older adults with a cardiac history must be monitored carefully for signs of vasovagal response. Cardiac rhythm is usually monitored during the procedure.

Cystoscopy. **Cystoscopy** is the visual inspection of the interior of the bladder for the collection of biopsy specimens, collection of urine separately from each ureter, and treatment of various conditions. It is valuable in diagnosing urologic ailments. Aseptic technique is used throughout the procedure to avoid introducing microorganisms and causing infections in the urinary tract. With the patient in the lithotomy position, the cystoscope is passed through the urethra, and the bladder is visually inspected. Cystoscopy is often carried out in conjunction with IVP and is used for surgical procedures involved in transurethral resection of the prostate, removal of bladder tumors or polyps, and various other bladder treatments. Local or general anesthetics are used when cystoscopy will cause discomfort or pain.

A signed consent form is needed, and the patient is to be given nothing by mouth after midnight. Usually a cathartic is given the evening before the test to empty the colon of feces. Maintain the patient on bed rest for 3 to 4 hours after the procedure, or until recovered from the effects of anesthesia. Increase fluid intake per orders. It is common for the urine to be pink tinged after the procedure, but red urine and clots should be reported to the primary care provider. Mild analgesics may be given for complaints of backache. Monitor vital signs per protocol, and monitor temperature every 6 hours because some patients experience a fever a day or so after the procedure resulting from the spread of an infection already present in the urinary tract.

Endoscopic retrograde cholangiopancreatography. Endoscopic retrograde cholangiopancreatography (ERCP) is used to identify a cause of biliary obstruction such as stricture, cyst, stones, or tumor. The procedure is usually done because of **jaundice** (yellowness of the skin, mucous membranes, and sclera caused by presence of bile pigments). The patient is placed on the x-ray or endoscopy table, and a local anesthetic is sprayed on the pharynx to help prevent gagging during insertion of the endoscope. The endoscope is inserted through the mouth and down into the duodenum after IV sedation, usually with diazepam or midazolam. Atropine may be given to decrease secretions in the oropharynx. Secretin may also be given when the duodenum is reached to stop peristalsis. A catheter is inserted into the pancreatic duct via the endoscope, and a contrast medium is injected. X-ray films are taken. The procedure takes about an hour. The patient is monitored during the procedure for complications from medications or from perforation by the endoscope.

The patient is given nothing by mouth for at least 6 hours before the test. A signed consent is required. Certain drugs must be discontinued before ERCP as determined by the primary care provider.

QSEN Considerations: Safety

Question About Iodine Allergies

Allergy to iodine or shellfish must be assessed because an iodine-based contrast medium is used during the ERCP test.

After the test, monitor vital signs every half hour for 2 hours, and then hourly for 4 hours or until stable. Ensure that the gag reflex has returned before offering foods and fluid.

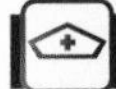

Clinical Cues

Offer a warm saline gargle or throat lozenges to reduce throat soreness.

Observe skin color for increasing jaundice after the test because irritation from the endoscope may make a stricture worse until inflammation subsides.

Aspirations

Aspirations are performed to obtain bone marrow, liver cells, spinal fluid, abdominal fluid, or fluid in the chest cavity. These procedures are usually performed at the bedside or in a procedure room by the physician or other trained care provider (such as nurse practitioner). Most of these procedures are uncomfortable for the patient. Obtain the equipment needed, open sterile supplies as requested, position and drape the patient, and assist the care provider. Pretest analgesia or sedation is administered if ordered. It is essential that the patient remain still during the procedure. Take baseline vital signs before the procedure begins. Table 24.5 provides information on positioning and care of patients undergoing an aspiration.

Electroencephalography

The brain's neurologic and physiologic activity produces electrical charges that can be measured as brain waves. The tracing of the brain waves is an **electroencephalogram (EEG)**. The EEG is done to localize and diagnose brain lesions, scars, epilepsy, infections, blood clots, and abscesses. It is also performed to determine brain death in comatose patients on life support systems.

Patients scheduled for an EEG are to have no stimulants, no sedatives, and no anticonvulsant drugs (such as phenytoin) for 48 hours before the test unless needed to control seizures. It is not necessary to shave any hair, and, generally, no special preparation is required. Some electroencephalography laboratories require that the hair be shampooed and dried before the test.

The patient sits in a chair or remains on a stretcher in a quiet room, and electrodes are attached to the scalp with skin glue or paste, or a mesh cap containing the 19 to 25 electrodes is placed on the head (Fig. 24.6). The equipment detects the electrical energy generated

Table 24.5 Aspiration Procedures

PROCEDURE	EXPLANATION	IMPLEMENTATION
Lumbar puncture (spinal tap)	Insertion of a needle into the subarachnoid space in the spinal canal to obtain specimens of spinal fluid; measure pressure; or instill dye, anesthetic, or medication	Take baseline vital signs. Help patient assume a side-lying, flexed position.
Site of needle puncture		Third lumbar vertebra Distal end of spinal cord Dura mater Subarachnoid space Cauda equina
		Set up sterile tray and supplies for the care provider. Tell patient not to cough and to breathe slowly and deeply. Hold patient's arms and legs in flexed position. Warn patient when discomfort will occur. When procedure is finished, label tubes with correct information. Be certain pressure dressing is intact over the puncture site. Instruct patient to maintain a dorsal recumbent position for 4-12 h; turning side to side is permitted. Medicate for pain as needed. Document the procedure and patient's response.
Bone marrow aspiration	Insertion of a needle into the bone to extract bone marrow cells for laboratory analysis	Take baseline vital signs. Premedicate as ordered. Set up sterile tray and supplies; help patient assume correct position (depends on aspiration site). Warn patient when pressure and discomfort will be felt. Monitor patient's status during the procedure. Note characteristics of aspirate and document the procedure and patient response.
Liver biopsy (aspiration)	Insertion of a needle into the liver for the aspiration of liver cells	Take baseline vital signs. Have patient empty the bladder. Premedicate as ordered. Set up the sterile tray and supplies. Assist the patient to a supine position at the far right side of the bed with the right arm over the head and the head turned to the left. Have patient practice taking a deep breath, blowing it all out, stopping breathing briefly, then breathing normally. Explain that this will need to be done for the procedure. Warn patient when puncture is about to occur. After the procedure, help patient move to the center of the bed and turn onto the right side. Instruct to maintain position for 2 h. Label specimen and send to laboratory with proper requisition. Keep patient on bed rest for 6 h. Assess vital signs q 15 min × 4, then q 30 min × 4; then q 1 h × 4; then q 4 h.
Thoracentesis	Insertion of a needle through the chest wall into the pleural space to remove air, fluid, or blood collected there	Take baseline vital signs. Set up the sterile tray and supplies. Help patient sit up, leaning on an over-the-bed table padded with pillows. Support the patient's body in this position during the procedure. If the patient is unable to sit up, a side-lying position is used.

Table 24.5 Aspiration Procedures—cont'd

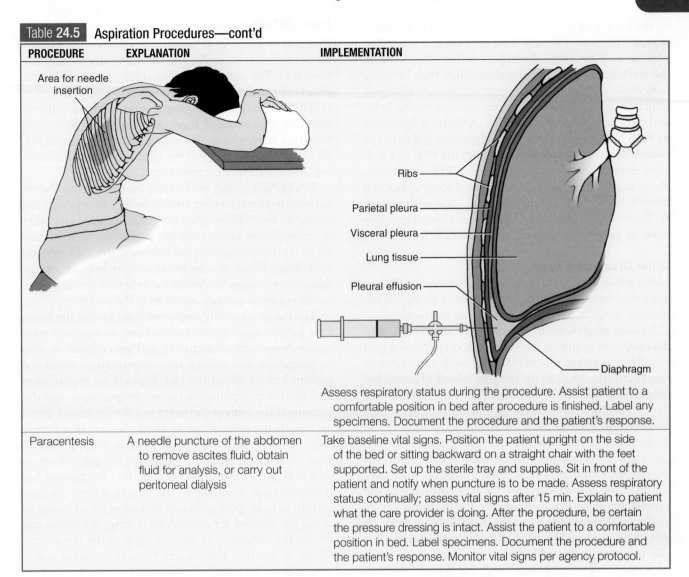

PROCEDURE	EXPLANATION	IMPLEMENTATION
		Assess respiratory status during the procedure. Assist patient to a comfortable position in bed after procedure is finished. Label any specimens. Document the procedure and the patient's response.
Paracentesis	A needle puncture of the abdomen to remove ascites fluid, obtain fluid for analysis, or carry out peritoneal dialysis	Take baseline vital signs. Position the patient upright on the side of the bed or sitting backward on a straight chair with the feet supported. Set up the sterile tray and supplies. Sit in front of the patient and notify when puncture is to be made. Assess respiratory status continually; assess vital signs after 15 min. Explain to patient what the care provider is doing. After the procedure, be certain the pressure dressing is intact. Assist the patient to a comfortable position in bed. Label specimens. Document the procedure and the patient's response. Monitor vital signs per agency protocol.

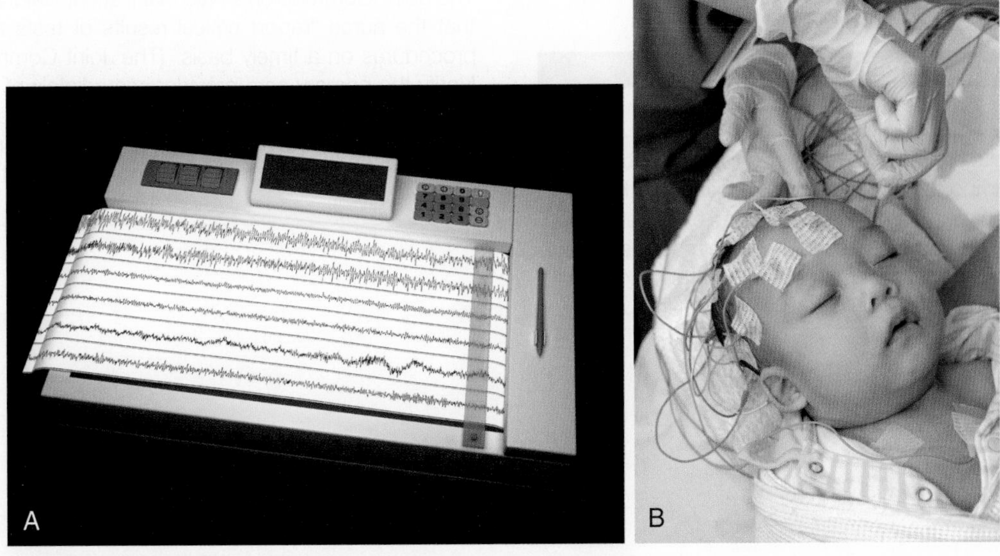

FIGURE 24.6 EEG. (A) EEG machine with waves. (B) Patient undergoing an EEG test with electrodes placed on the scalp. (Photos copyright istock.com)

by the brain and produces a graphic record of the brain waves. The patient should close the eyes and relax. The patient may be asked to hyperventilate for some of the tracings because abnormalities may then be more noticeable. Rapid shallow breathing causes alkalosis, which in turn produces vasoconstriction in the brain and may activate seizure activity. A flashing light may be held over the face to induce abnormal activity. The patient may be sleep deprived before the test, or a sedative may be given when a sleeping EEG is desired. Sleep deprivation is helpful in producing abnormal brain activity, particularly that associated with epilepsy. The test may take up to 1 hour and 15 minutes. Any paste or gel used is washed away after the test.

Other Diagnostic Tests

Many other diagnostic tests are performed each day. They will be encountered in the units of study for the medical-surgical and obstetric nursing courses.

Nurses employed in medical offices, clinics, and hospitals are required to obtain blood specimens and to perform certain diagnostic tests such as wound or throat culture (Skill 24.5), random blood glucose, hemoglobin levels, and urine dips. They also assist with Papanicolaou (Pap) **smears** (application of secretions and cells on a slide) (Skill 24.6) and sigmoidoscopies. It should be noted that there are many models of glucometers. If the machine to be used is different from the one indicated in Skill 24.2, the procedure may vary slightly. The correct steps for the procedure are in the instruction manual accompanying the machine.

An important step is to fill out the laboratory or test requisition slip properly. Information generally required is the patient's name, the primary care provider's name, the date, and the type of test requested. For some tests, names of medications that the patient is taking will be requested. All specimens should be labeled on the container (not lid) with the patient's name, the date, and the primary care provider's name.

Life-Span Considerations

Older Adults

When older adults are taken to another department for a diagnostic test, it is important to send an extra blanket with them in case they have to wait in a holding area for an extended period. Very often these areas are cool, and the cover sheet is not sufficient to keep older adults warm. An attendant should be with the patients or personnel should check on them frequently.

◆ EVALUATION

Evaluation involves determining whether the expected outcomes written for each nursing diagnosis have been met. The patient is assessed for potential adverse effects of the diagnostic procedure. One way to continuously improve patient preparation is to ask patients after the procedure if there was anything they wish they had been told in advance. Obtaining information this way is often helpful for future patient education regarding a particular procedure.

Evaluation is also performed by comparing the results of tests performed from one day to another. For example, the WBC reading on a CBC indicates whether an infection is improving or worsening. If the treatment is effective against the infection, the WBC should be falling. When serum potassium is low, check the laboratory values to determine whether the administration of extra potassium corrects the problem.

The nurse is usually responsible for giving the home care patient appropriate instructions and patient education before scheduled tests and procedures. A visit or telephone call allows for assessment of what the patient knows about the test. Provide an explanation and teaching, explain the pretest preparation, and determine if the patient can carry out the necessary preparation. If the patient needs assistance, enlist a family member to help or schedule a visit at the appropriate time to help the patient prepare for the procedure. In addition, determine ahead of time that the patient has transportation available to the facility where the procedure is to be performed. When samples of blood or urine are needed for laboratory testing, the nurse can obtain the samples and deliver them to the laboratory. Check to see that the consent form is signed if one is required.

! Safety Alert

Critical Laboratory Values

The Joint Commission's National Patient Safety Goals require that the nurse "report critical results of tests and diagnostic procedures on a timely basis" (The Joint Commission, 2016). Notify the primary care provider immediately of any laboratory test result considered "critical" when such a result arrives on the unit. Note in the medical record that the telephone call was made and to whom the laboratory result and the importance of it was given.

Skill 24.5 Obtaining Culture Specimens: Throat and Wound

 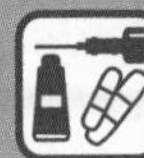 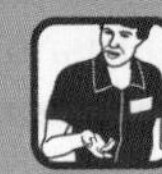 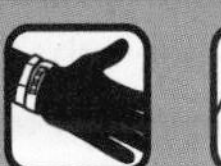 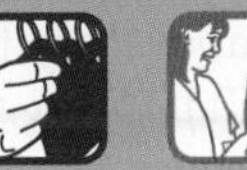 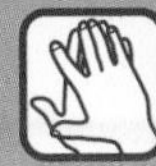 

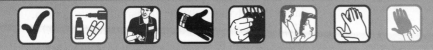

Nurses frequently must obtain specimens for throat cultures when working in medical offices or clinics. Wound cultures are frequently obtained by the hospital, long-term care, and home care nurse. Careful technique is essential to avoid contaminating the sample to be cultured.

SUPPLIES

- Culture tube
- Label
- Requisition slip
- Biohazard plastic bag
- Gloves

For Throat Culture

- Tongue blade

For Wound Culture

- Alcohol swabs
- Dressing supplies

Review and carry out the Standard Steps in Appendix A.

ACTION *(RATIONALE)*

Assessment (Data Collection)

1. Check the primary care provider's order for the specific culture. *(Determines the type of tube to be used.)*
2. Identify the patient by asking her name, or check the ID armband. *(Verifies that the right patient will have the culture specimen obtained.)*

Planning

3. Verify all supplies are on hand and that there is good lighting for the area to be cultured. *(Prevents having to stop and obtain supplies. Good lighting provides a good visual field for obtaining the needed specimen.)*

Implementation

4. Explain the procedure to patient and label the culture tube. *(Prepares patient and identifies the specimen.)*
5. Perform hand hygiene and don gloves. *(Prevents contamination of hands.)*

For Throat

6. Position a light so that the pharynx may be viewed. Withdraw the sterile swab from the tube or package. *(The light from an otoscope works well; otherwise, use an examining light. Pharynx must be visible to obtain the specimen.)*
7. Ask patient to tip her head back slightly and open her mouth wide. Instruct patient to sing a low note ("ah"). *(Allows visualization of pharynx and keeps tongue out of the way.)*
8. Depressing the tongue with a tongue blade and, without touching the teeth, tongue, cheek, or gums, insert sterile swab into the throat and rotate it slightly around the tonsil area and back wall, only touching areas of exudate (fluid with cellular debris from inflammation) or areas of inflammation. Withdraw the swab without touching other structures. *(Obtains secretions that may contain microorganisms from throat area only.)*

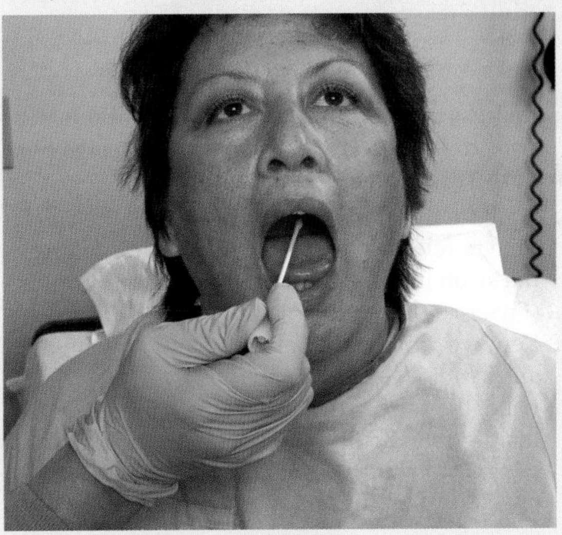

Step 8

9. Place swab into the culture tube without touching any other surface. *(Prevents contamination of specimen.)*

For Wound (Aerobic Culture)

Follow steps 1-5 above

10. Remove dressing, folding the soiled sides together, and dispose of it in biohazard waste container. *(Prevents spread of microorganisms.)*
11. Cleanse area around wound edges with an antiseptic swab. *(Removes old exudate and skin bacteria.)*
12. Remove and dispose of gloves properly. *(Prevents transfer of microorganisms.)*
13. Open sterile gloves and dressing supplies. *(Prepares equipment to take the specimen and redress the wound.)*
14. Don gloves. Take the sterile swab(s) from the culture tube and insert the tip(s) into the wound where drainage is occurring; rotate swab gently. Remove the swab(s) and replace them carefully in the culture tube without touching any other

surface. *(Obtains the specimen from the area most likely to contain microorganisms. Prevents contamination of specimen.)*

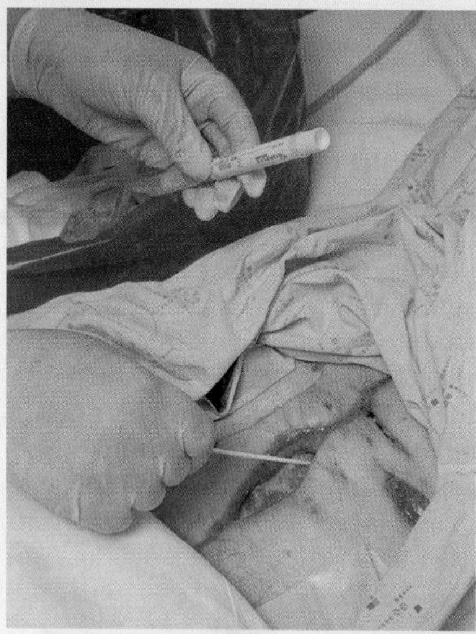

Step **10**

15. Redress the wound using sterile technique. *(Prevents contamination of wound with microorganisms.)*

For Both Throat and Wound Cultures

16. Squeeze the ampule in the bottom of the culture tube to release the preservative solution. Press the swab into the solution to wet it thoroughly. *(Preserves the specimen.)*
17. Remove gloves and perform hand hygiene. *(Reduces transfer of microorganisms.)*
18. Label the tube and complete the laboratory requisition; send culture to the laboratory. *(Prevents culture from being lost or mislabeled.)*

Evaluation

19. Review the report when it is returned from the laboratory to see what organism(s) have grown. *(Type of organism will dictate the correct therapy.)*
20. Check orders to see whether the primary care provider has ordered the appropriate therapy to treat the infection according to the laboratory sensitivity report. If not, call the provider. *(Provides a check to see that treatment has been ordered for the infection.)*

Documentation

Documentation Example: Throat

12/22 1100 Throat culture obtained and sent to lab. (Nurse's electronic signature)

Documentation Example: Wound

12/22 1300 Wound culture obtained from wound on right upper thigh. Wound redressed using sterile technique. Culture sent to lab. (Nurse's electronic signature)

Special Considerations

- Anaerobic cultures require a different culture medium and procedure. Check the facility manual. Anaerobic cultures are performed from deep within wounds for organisms that cannot grow when exposed to air.

? Critical Thinking Questions

1. How would you obtain a throat culture from a crying, squirming 5-year-old child?
2. Considering your daily tasks for the patient, when do you think the best time to obtain a wound culture would be?

Skill 24.6 Assisting with a Pelvic Examination and Papanicolaou Test (Smear)

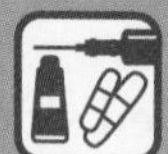
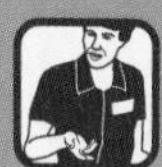
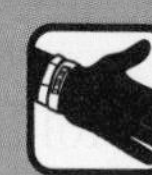
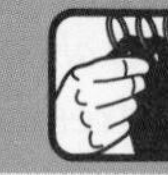
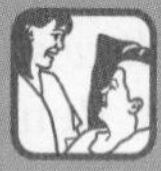
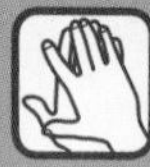

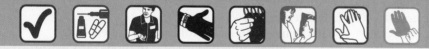

Papanicolaou (Pap) smears are a frequent diagnostic test for cervical, vaginal, or endometrial cancer ordered in a medical office or a clinic. Occasionally a Pap smear may be obtained in the procedure room at the hospital. The Pap smear is done in conjunction with a pelvic examination on the female patient. A chaperone may accompany the patient (and may be required by facility policy). Patients should not use vaginal medication or douche for 24 hours before the test. The specimens are either placed on slides or swished into a special solution in a container (ThinPrep [LBC] type of Pap smear).

SUPPLIES

- Gloves
- Saline solution
- Examination table with stirrups
- Examination light
- Vaginal speculum
- Biohazard waste container
- Cotton-tipped applicator or cytology brush
- Cervical scraper

- Patient gown and drape
- Lubricant
- Examination stool
- Glass slide with a frosted edge or ThinPrep specimen container
- Pencil
- Pathology requisition slip
- Cytology fixative

Review and carry out the Standard Steps in Appendix A.

ACTION *(RATIONALE)*

Assessment (Data Collection)

1. Assess whether patient is familiar with the procedure. *(Determines patient's knowledge base.)*
2. Assess equipment and supplies on hand. *(Aids in determining whether any supplies are missing before starting the procedure.)*

Planning

3. Plan ahead and label the frosted end of the slide with the patient's name and date or label the ThinPrep container. *(Identifies the specimen as belonging to the patient; prevents report error.)*
4. Fill out the requisition slip with the required information. *(Ensures that requisition is ready after smear is taken.)*

Implementation

5. Explain the procedure if patient is unfamiliar with it; answer questions. *(Decreases fear of the unknown, and helps patient relax.)*
6. Set up the table and equipment as the examiner prefers. *(Prepares equipment for patient and examiner.)*
7. Provide patient a gown, and ask that all clothing below the waist be removed and the gown put on so that it ties in the back; provide privacy. *(Allows examiner to access perineal area. If the examiner wishes to do a breast check, ask patient to remove all clothing.)*
8. When patient is ready, assist onto the table, with the lower half of the body covered with a drape. Assist into a lithotomy position with feet in the stirrups and buttocks right at the end of the table. The knees should be apart. The drape can be left free or positioned so that the corners can be wrapped around the lower legs and feet with the third corner hanging over the perineum. *(Lithotomy position allows examiner to visualize the vagina and cervix with the speculum. The drape protects patient's modesty and provides privacy. The third corner of the drape can be folded back when the examiner is ready to begin.)*

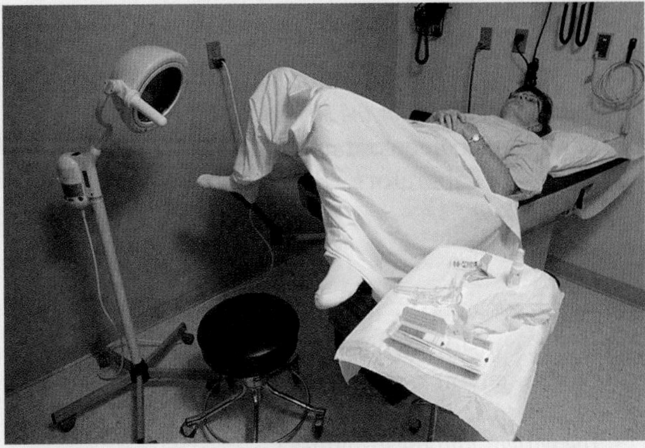

Step 8

9. Reassure the patient and help her relax during the procedure by telling her to take deep, slow breaths through the mouth and to try to relax the abdominal muscles. *(Procedure will go more smoothly if patient is relaxed. Examiner will perform the pelvic examination after the smear has been taken.)*
10. Assist the examiner by passing equipment as requested. *(Helps procedure go quickly and smoothly.)*
11. Apply gloves and fix the slide(s) by flooding them with 95% ethyl alcohol or spraying them with cytology fixative according to the directions on the spray container. If a ThinPrep container and solution was used, just close the container. *(Smears on slides must be fixed within 10 seconds after collection to maintain the normal appearance of cells and to prevent the smears from being exposed to contaminants in the air. Spray lightly from left to right and then from right to left.)*

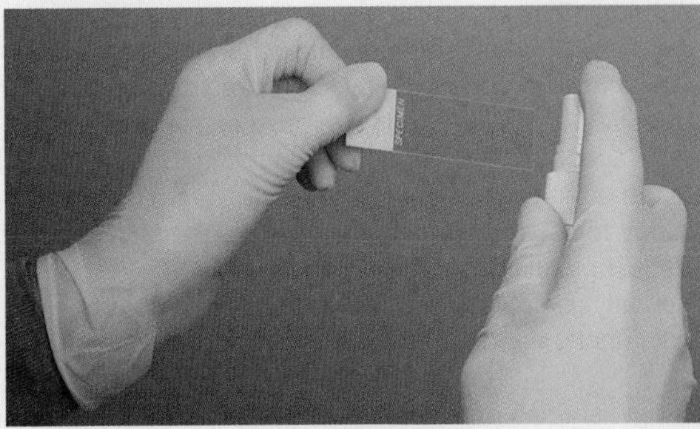

Step 11

12. When the procedure is finished, help the patient slide back, pull out the table extension, and remove the feet simultaneously from the stirrups and lay them straight on the table. Ask patient to slide back slightly onto table. When patient is ready to sit up, assist to a sitting position as you slide the table extension into the table. *(Shows consideration for the patient. Positions the patient to sit up.)*

13. Allow the slide(s), if used, to dry for at least 5 minutes before packaging them in a slide container to send to the laboratory. *(Prevents contamination or disruption of the smear[s].)*
14. Send the labeled container and the requisition slip to the laboratory. *(Ensures that smears reach the laboratory.)*

Evaluation

15. Evaluate whether the procedure went smoothly. If not, consider what should be changed for the next time you assist with the procedure. *(Assists in perfecting technique and improving helpfulness to the patient and the examiner.)*

Documentation

16. If the examiner does not document the procedure on the patient's medical record, note that the procedure was done and the specimen sent to the laboratory. *(Notes the date that the procedure was performed.)*

Documentation Example

6/19 1015 Pap smear and pelvic examination done by Flavio Vanderbilt, NP; tolerated without problems. Smear fixed and sent to pathology lab with requisition. (Nurse's electronic signature)

? Critical Thinking Questions

1. What would you say and do to help a young woman relax during her first pelvic examination and Pap smear?
2. If a patient's legs are visibly shaking during a Pap smear and the examiner is having trouble seeing into the vagina, what would you do?

Get Ready for the NCLEX Examination!

Key Points

- Assess what patients know about the test or procedure they are about to undergo. Perform patient education based on current knowledge.
- Schedule time in the daily work plan for diagnostic test preparation and posttest care.
- Hematology tests are studies of the blood and its components. The CBC is the most commonly ordered hematology test.
- Blood chemistry tests provide information about electrolyte balance; the body's ability to metabolize nutrients; the function of the liver, kidneys, muscles, and the heart; and the accumulation of toxic substances. Chemistry tests are often ordered by SMA panel.
- Serology tests are helpful in diagnosing or confirming bacterial or viral infection.
- The urinalysis provides valuable information about kidney function and other biologic processes within the body.
- Cytologic studies of tissue and cells are performed to detect carcinogenic, metabolic, vascular, and other changes.
- Culture and sensitivity tests of body fluids are done in the bacteriology laboratory to determine the organisms responsible for infection and the drugs that will kill them.
- Sonography uses sound waves and their echoes to picture structures within the body.
- Radiology uses x-rays to obtain pictures of bones and tissues within the body. An opaque contrast medium can be used to outline hollow organs.
- Radionuclide scans help determine abnormalities in the structure or function of different organs.
- CT scans use a computer to enhance x-ray studies and allow visualization of structures within the body. MRI is based on electromagnetic fields, and it can produce clearer images on internal structures than CT scans can.
- The ECG is a tracing of the electrical activity in the heart; the EEG traces the electrical pattern produced by brain waves.
- Cardiac catheterization is an invasive procedure to determine abnormalities in the structure and function of the heart; it is combined with coronary angiography.
- All invasive tests or tests requiring injection of a contrast material or radionuclide require a signed consent form from the patient.
- Evaluation is based on whether the expected outcomes have been met. Laboratory values are compared to see if the patient's condition is improving.

Additional Learning Resources

SG Go to your Study Guide for additional learning activities to help you master this chapter content.

evolve Go to your Evolve website (http://evolve.elsevier.com/Williams/fundamental) for additional online resources. 

Review Questions for the NCLEX Examination

*Choose the **best** answer for each question.*

1. A culture is obtained when a patient has a bladder infection for the purpose of:
   1. Selecting the correct dose of medication.
   2. Determining the prognosis of the disease.
   3. Ruling out an infectious process.
   4. Growing and identifying causative organisms.

2. The sensitivity part of a culture and sensitivity test is for the purpose of:
   1. Identifying the causative organism of the infection.
   2. Determining which medications are ineffective against the causative organism.
   3. Testing anti-infective medications to see which ones are most effective against the causative organism.
   4. Growing colonies of the causative organism on a culture medium.
3. When taking a culture sample from an infected throat, the nurse should: *(Select all that apply.)*
   1. Don sterile gloves to obtain the sample.
   2. Depress the tongue with a tongue blade.
   3. Swab around the back of the throat.
   4. Swab around the tonsil area.
   5. Place the swab in the sterile culture tube and seal it.
4. Correct technique for obtaining a stool specimen for ova and parasites is to use a wooden stick and:
   1. Obtain the specimen from the middle of the stool.
   2. Place the whole stool specimen in the specimen container.
   3. Obtain the specimen from two parts of the stool.
   4. Include any liquid stool.
5. When instructing a patient about an MRI test, you would explain that: *(Select all that apply.)*
   1. It is necessary to hold very still during the test.
   2. Heavy sedation is usually provided before the test.
   3. Loud noise will be heard during the test.
   4. Communication with the technician is possible.
   5. Relaxation is achieved using soft music.
6. When instructing the patient about a colonoscopy, you would include that: *(Select all that apply.)*
   1. The prep for the procedure begins 24 to 48 hours beforehand.
   2. Sedation will be given before the procedure.
   3. It is OK to drive home afterward.
   4. There is often some rectal bleeding afterward.
   5. Cranberry juice is encouraged pre-procedure to minimize the risk of UTI.
7. When caring for the patient who has just undergone a liver biopsy, you must:
   1. Keep the patient positioned on the right side for 2 hours.
   2. Apply pressure to the aspiration site by hand for 30 minutes.
   3. Keep the patient on bed rest for 24 hours.
   4. Turn the patient to the left side afterward.
8. When collecting a blood sample with a Vacutainer system, it is important to:
   1. Replace the tube stopper firmly for each sample.
   2. Release the tourniquet after successful venipuncture.
   3. Withdraw the holder and tube at the same time.
   4. Stabilize the holder when changing tubes.

Critical Thinking Activities

Read each clinical scenario and discuss the questions with your classmates.

Scenario A

The patient underwent a cardiac catheterization this morning.

1. What assessments would you need to make regularly afterward?
2. If you have difficulty finding the dorsalis pedis pulse in the leg where the catheter was inserted, what would you do?
3. What might it mean if the leg in which the catheter was introduced begins to swell?

Scenario B

The patient has blood chemistries ordered every morning. On the third day, she complains that she does not want this done because she is sick and becoming sicker because they are taking all her blood. How would you respond to the patient?

chapter 25

Fluid, Electrolyte, and Acid-Base Balance

http://evolve.elsevier.com/Williams/fundamental

Objectives

Upon completing this chapter, you should be able to do the following:

Theory

1. Discuss the various functions water performs in the body.
2. List the major electrolytes and the function of each.
3. Describe three ways in which body fluids are continuously being distributed among the fluid compartments.
4. Identify the signs and symptoms of the common fluid and electrolyte imbalances.
5. State the main signs and symptoms of acid-base imbalances.

Clinical Practice

1. Assess an assigned patient for signs of fluid and electrolyte imbalance.
2. From patient laboratory results, identify electrolyte values that are abnormal.
3. Implement patient education for someone with hypokalemia.
4. Develop a plan of care for a patient who has a fluid and electrolyte imbalance.
5. Identify patients who might be at risk for an acid-base imbalance.

Skills

Key Terms

acidosis (ă-sĭ-DŌ-sĭs, p. 445)
active transport (p. 440)
alkalosis (ăl-kă-LŌ-sĭs, p. 446)
ascites (ă-SĪ-tēz, p. 442)
dehydration (dē-hī-DRĀ-shŭn, p. 438)
diffusion (dĭ-FŪ-zhŭn, p. 439)
edema (ĕ-DĒ-mă, p. 442)
electrolytes (ĕ-LĔK-trō-līts, p. 438)
extracellular (ĕks-tră-SĔL-ū-lăr, p. 438)
filtration (fĭl-TRĀ-shŭn, p. 440)
hydrostatic pressure (hī-drō-STĂ-tĭk PRĔ-shŭr, p. 440)
hypercalcemia (hī-pĕr-kăl-SĒ-mē-ă, p. 446)
hyperchloremia (hī-pĕr-klōr-Ē-mē-ă, p. 446)
hyperkalemia (hī-pĕr-kă-LĒ-mē-ă, p. 446)
hypermagnesemia (hī-pĕr-măg-nĕ-SĒ-mē-ă, p. 446)
hypernatremia (hī-pĕr-nā-TRĒ-mē-ă, p. 445)
hyperphosphatemia (hī-pĕr-fŏs-fă-TĒ-mē-ă, p. 447)
hypertonic (hī-pĕr-TŎN-ĭk, p. 439)
hyperventilation (p. 449)
hypervolemia (hī-pĕr-vō-LĒ-mē-ă, p. 442)
hypocalcemia (hī-pō-kăl-SĒ-mē-ă, p. 446)
hypochloremia (hī-pō-klōr-Ē-mē-ă, p. 446)
hypokalemia (hī-pō-kă-LĒ-mē-ă, p. 445)
hypomagnesemia (hī-pō-măg-nĕ-SĒ-mē-ă, p. 446)
hyponatremia (hī-pō-nā-TRĒ-mē-ă, p. 442)
hypophosphatemia (hī-pō-fŏs-fă-TĒ-mē-ă, p. 446)
hypotonic (hī-pō-TŎN-ĭk, p. 439)
hypovolemia (hī-pō-vō-LĒ-mē-ă, p. 438)
interstitial (ĭn-tĕr-STĬSH-ăl, p. 438)
intracellular (ĭn-tră-SĔL-ū-lăr, p. 438)
intravascular (ĭn-tră-văs-kū-lăr, p. 438)
isotonic (ī-sō-TŎN-ĭk, p. 439)
osmosis (ŏz-MŌ-sĭs, p. 439)
tetany (TĔT-ă-nē, p. 450)
transcellular (trănz-SĒ-lū-lăr, p. 438)
turgor (p. 441)

Concepts Covered in This Chapter

- Acid-base balance
- Elimination
- Fluid and electrolyte balance
- Metabolism
- Perfusion

COMPOSITION OF BODY FLUIDS

WATER

The two largest constituents of the body fluids are water and electrolytes. Water is present in greater proportion than electrolytes are. Water serves many functions, but the four main functions of water in the body are: (1) to act as a vehicle for the transportation of substances to and from the cells; (2) to aid heat regulation by providing perspiration, which evaporates; (3) to assist in maintenance of hydrogen (H^+) balance in the body; and (4) to serve as a medium for the enzymatic action of digestion.

More than half of the body's weight is water. The amount varies by age, sex, and health status. The adult male body contains about 60% water; the adult female body, because of more fat tissue, contains about 50% water. The greater the amount of fat the body contains, the less the percentage of water it has because fat contains less water than other tissue does. **The infant and the older adult are affected more quickly and seriously by minor changes in their fluid balance and can become rapidly dehydrated.** The infant, because of its large body surface area compared with body weight, loses more fluid through the skin than the adult does. The infant's kidneys are not as efficient as the adult's are, and less fluid is reabsorbed. The older adult has an age-related decline in total body water, diminished thirst sensation, a decrease in urine concentrating ability of the kidney, and a decrease in the effectiveness of antidiuretic hormone (ADH). These factors cause dehydration to occur more quickly than in the younger adult. Dehydration may cause hypovolemia (Concept Map 25.1). If an excess of fluid volume is present in the body, hypervolemia occurs.

Water is critical to maintaining homeostasis because water is the medium in which most metabolic and chemical reactions in the body take place. Without sufficient water, cells cannot function, and death results.

Water is the avenue for transportation within the body. It carries nutrients to the cells and transports waste for excretion. Body water continuously moves in and out of the blood, through the lymph vessels, between the cells, and in and out of the cells. Table 25.1 shows sources of water and avenues of water loss.

? Think Critically

How might NPO (nothing by mouth) status before tests or surgery affect a person's body?

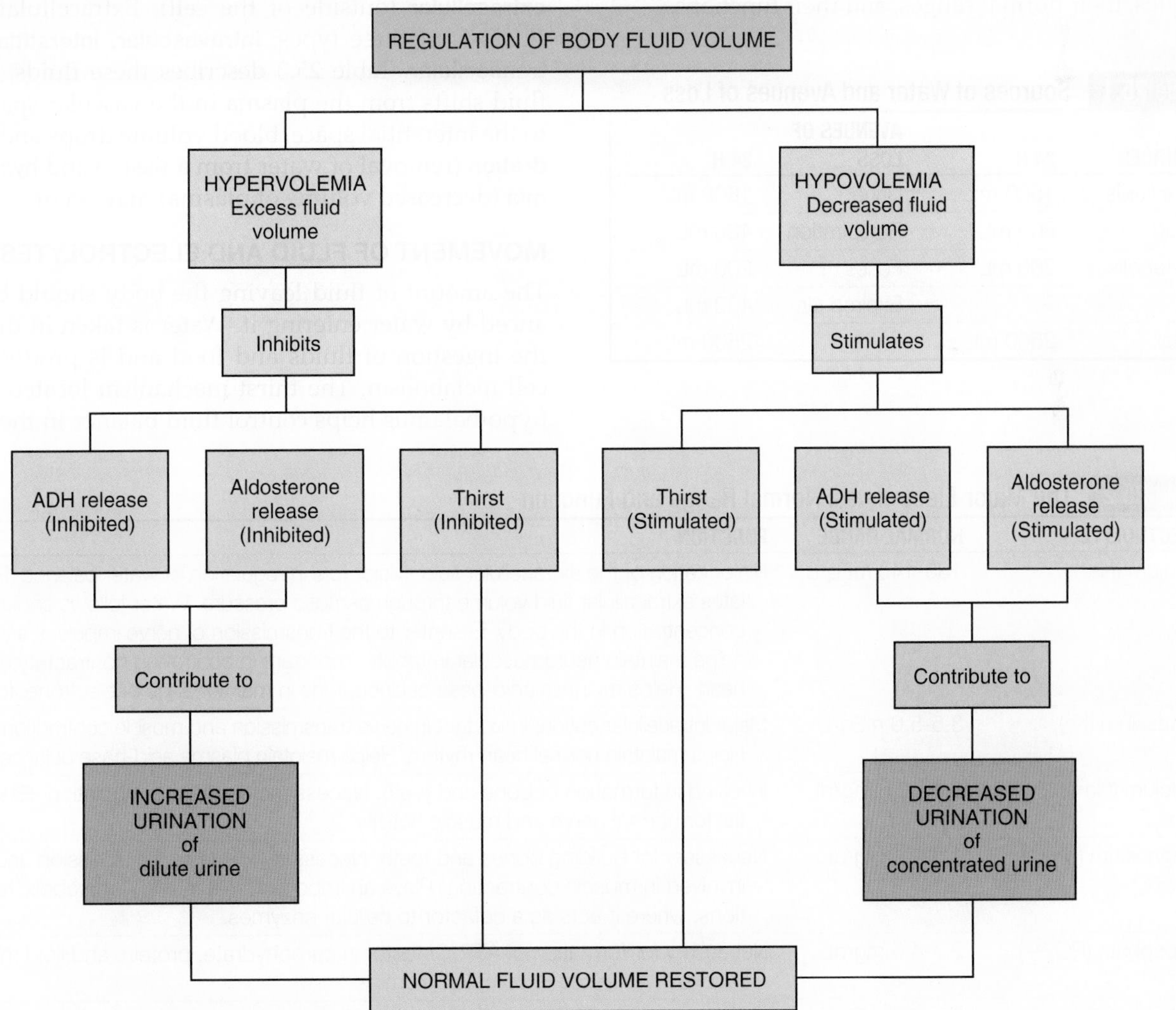

CONCEPT MAP 25.1 Regulation of body fluid volume. *ADH,* Antidiuretic hormone. (Redrawn from Black, J. M., & Hawks, J. H. [2005]. *Medical-Surgical Nursing: Clinical Management for Positive Outcomes* [7th ed.]. Philadelphia, PA: Saunders.) (From White, B. [1994]. Maintaining fluid and electrolyte balance. In V. B. Bolander [Ed.], *Sorensen and Luckmann's Basic Nursing: A Physiologic Approach* [3rd ed.]. Philadelphia, PA: Saunders.)

ELECTROLYTES

Electrolytes are minerals or salts that are dissolved in body fluid. They are measured in milliequivalents per liter (mEq/L), which is a unit of measure of the chemical activity that occurs when the electrolyte reacts with hydrogen. When in solution, they break up into particles known as **ions** that have a tiny electrical charge. The ions develop a positive electrical charge and then they are known as **cations,** or they develop a negative electrical charge and are **anions. For each positively charged cation in a fluid compartment, there must be a negatively charged anion so that balance is maintained.** As fluids move from compartment to compartment, the body works to maintain homeostasis in each compartment by balancing the anions and cations so that there is electrical neutrality. Electrolytes move within the body freely, but each has a primary location. Because disturbances in homeostasis upset the normal balance of electrolytes, the location and function of each electrolyte become important in understanding what is occurring in the body. **The major source of electrolytes is from diet.** Table 25.2 presents the electrolytes, their normal ranges, and their functions.

Table 25.1 Sources of Water and Avenues of Loss

SOURCES	24 H	AVENUES OF LOSS	24 H
Oral fluids	1500 mL	Urine	1500 mL
Food	800 mL	Perspiration	400 mL
Metabolism	200 mL	Feces	200 mL
—	—	Expired air	400 mL
Total	2500 mL	—	2500 mL

NONELECTROLYTES

The intermediate products of metabolism—amino acids (proteins), glucose, and fatty acids—are nonelectrolytes. They remain bound together when dissolved in body fluid. In the healthy individual who is eating normally, the nonelectrolytes circulating in the body fluid remain stable.

BLOOD

The body has 4 to 6 L of circulating blood volume, depending on body size and sex. Erythrocytes (red cells), leukocytes (white cells), and platelets (thrombocytes) are the blood cells that are carried in the plasma. **Any condition that alters body fluid volume also alters the plasma volume of the blood and can affect blood pressure and circulation.** The plasma proteins and colloids contribute to plasma colloid osmotic pressure, which helps keep fluid in the vascular compartment.

DISTRIBUTION OF BODY FLUIDS

Body fluids are either **intracellular** (within the cell) or **extracellular** (outside of the cell). Extracellular fluid (ECF) is of three types: **intravascular, interstitial,** and **transcellular.** Table 25.3 describes these fluids. When fluid shifts from the plasma in the vascular space out to the interstitial space, blood volume drops and **dehydration** (removal of water from a tissue) and **hypovolemia** (decreased volume of plasma) may occur.

MOVEMENT OF FLUID AND ELECTROLYTES

The amount of fluid leaving the body should be balanced by water entering it. Water is taken in through the ingestion of fluids and food and is produced by cell metabolism. The thirst mechanism located in the hypothalamus helps control fluid balance in the body.

Table 25.2 The Major Electrolytes: Normal Range and Function

ELECTROLYTE	NORMAL RANGE	FUNCTION
Sodium (Na^+)	135-145 mEq/L	Major cation of the extracellular fluid. Major role in regulation of water balance. Regulates extracellular fluid volume through osmotic pressure. Water follows sodium concentration in the body. Essential to the transmission of nerve impulses and helps maintain neuromuscular irritability. Important in controlling contractility of the heart. Helps maintain acid-base balance. Aids in maintenance of electroneutrality.
Potassium (K^+)	3.5-5.0 mEq/L	Major intracellular cation. Important in nerve transmission and muscle contraction. Helps maintain normal heart rhythm. Helps maintain plasma acid-base balance.
Calcium (Ca^{2+})	8.4-10.6 mg/dL	Involved in formation of bone and teeth. Necessary for blood coagulation. Essential for normal nerve and muscle activity.
Magnesium (Mg^{2+})	1.3-2.1 mg/dL	Necessary for building bones and teeth. Necessary for nerve transmission and is involved in muscle contraction. Plays an important role in many metabolic reactions, where it acts as a cofactor to cellular enzymes.
Phosphate (PO_4^{3}–)	2.7-4.5 mg/dL	Necessary for formation of ATP. Cofactor in carbohydrate, protein, and lipid metabolism. Activates B-complex vitamins.
Chloride (Cl–)	96-106 mEq/L	Helps maintain acid-base balance. Important in formation of hydrochloric acid for secretion to the stomach. Aids in maintaining plasma electroneutrality.
Bicarbonate (HCO_3–)	22-26 mEq/L	A buffer that neutralizes excess acids in the body. Helps regulate acid-base balance.

ATP, Adenosine triphosphate.

It monitors fluid volume and concentration. Hypothalamic receptors sense when fluid is more concentrated and stimulate nerve impulses that are interpreted in the brain as thirst, which motivates the person to drink. Intake of sufficient water lowers the concentration and the receptors are no longer stimulated.

Fluid is lost in the urine and feces and through **insensible** (invisible) losses via exhaled air and through the skin as perspiration. **The kidney is the main organ through which fluid excretion is achieved.** Urine output is affected by several hormones, particularly ADH, aldosterone, and atrial natriuretic peptide (ANP). ADH is secreted by the posterior pituitary. More ADH is released when the blood becomes more concentrated; circulating blood volume is decreased; or the person is experiencing pain, nausea, or stress. With increased ADH, the renal tubules reabsorb more water, and urine output decreases. Aldosterone is released by the adrenal cortex when ECF volume is low or when sodium concentration is decreased, causing reabsorption of sodium from kidney tubules. This creates an osmotic gradient by which more water is retained. The release of aldosterone is stimulated by the renin-angiotensin-aldosterone system. ANP acts to protect the body from fluid overload, and it is released from sites in the myocardium and the brain. Blood volume and pressure also affect the glomerular filtration rate and urine output.

Water and the substances suspended or dissolved in it must move from compartment to compartment, so that they are normally distributed within the body. They must pass through the semipermeable membranes of the body's cells to do this. The heart circulates blood throughout the body. As the blood flows

Table 25.3 Body Fluid Distribution

BODY FLUID	DISTRIBUTION
Extracellular fluid	Approximately ⅓ of total body water. Transports water, nutrients, oxygen, and waste, to and from the cells. Regulated by renal, metabolic, and neurologic factors. High in sodium (Na^+) content.
Intravascular fluid	Fluid within the blood vessels. Consists of plasma and fluid within blood cells. Contains large amounts of protein and electrolytes.
Interstitial fluid	Fluid in the spaces surrounding the cells. High in sodium (Na^+) content.
Transcellular fluid	Includes aqueous humor; saliva; cerebrospinal, pleural, peritoneal, synovial, and pericardial fluids; gastrointestinal secretions; and fluid in the urinary system and lymphatics.
Intracellular fluid	About ⅔ of total body fluid. Fluid contained within the cell walls. Most cell walls are permeable to water. High in potassium (K^+) content.

through the capillaries, fluid and solutes can move into the interstitial spaces, where substances in every cell of the body can be exchanged. Several processes move fluids, electrolytes, nutrients, and waste products back and forth across the cell membranes.

Passive Transport

Diffusion. **Diffusion** is the process by which substances freely move back and forth across the membrane until they are evenly distributed throughout the available space. Substances move from a high to a low concentration until the concentration on both sides of the membrane is equal. This is called movement down a concentration gradient. Glucose, oxygen, carbon dioxide, water, and other small ions and molecules move by diffusion. It is a process of equalization.

Diffusion may occur by movement along an electrical gradient as well. The attraction between particles of opposite charge and the repellent action between particles of like charge comprise an electrical gradient. Many intracellular proteins have a negative charge that tends to attract the positively charged sodium and potassium ions from the ECF.

Osmosis. **Osmosis** refers to the movement of a pure solvent (liquid) across a membrane. In the body, water diffuses by osmosis. When there are differences in concentration of fluids in the various compartments, water (and other fluids) move from the area of less solute concentration to the area of greater concentration until the solutions in the compartments are of equal concentration. The process takes place via a semipermeable membrane—a membrane that allows some substances to pass through but prevents the passage of other substances. Fluid moves between the interstitial and intracellular and the interstitial and intravascular compartments by osmosis. Cell wall membranes are semipermeable, as are the walls of blood vessels.

When living cells are surrounded by a solution that has the same concentration of particles, the water concentration of the intracellular fluids (ICF) and ECF will be equal. Such a solution is termed **isotonic** (of equal solute concentration). If cells are surrounded by a solution that has a greater concentration of solute than the cells have, the water in the cells moves to the more concentrated solution, and the cells dehydrate and shrink. The solution is **hypertonic** (of greater concentration) in relation to the cells. If the cells are surrounded by a solution that has less solute than the cells have, the solution is **hypotonic** (of less concentration) in relation to the cells. The particles within the cells exert an osmotic pressure, drawing water inward through the semipermeable membrane. The cells swell from the extra fluid (overhydrate). These concepts are important to the administration of intravenous (IV) fluids (see Chapter 36). Solutions are classified as isotonic, hypertonic, or hypotonic according to their concentration of electrolytes and other solutes. **Therefore, by osmosis, water**

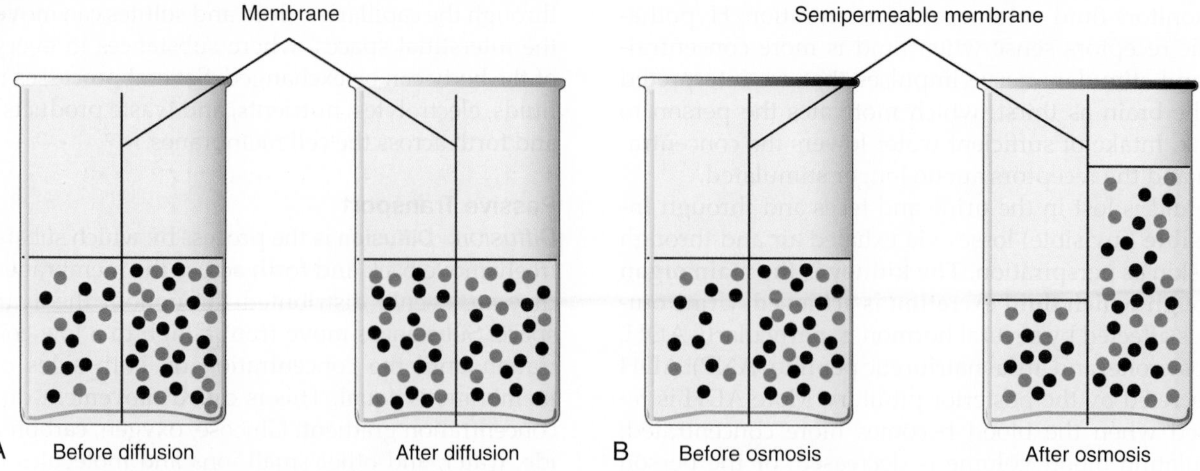

FIGURE 25.1 (A and B) Diffusion and osmosis. (From Lewis, S. L., Heitkemper, M. M., Dirksen, S. R., Bucher, L., & Camera, I. [2011]. *Medical-Surgical Nursing: Assessment and Management of Clinical Problems* [8th ed.]. St. Louis, MO: Mosby.)

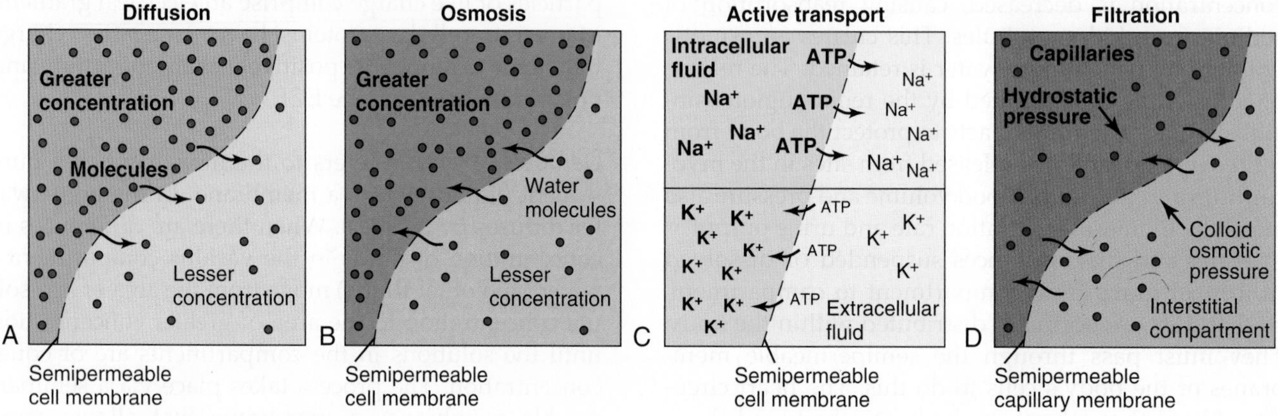

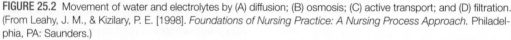

FIGURE 25.2 Movement of water and electrolytes by (A) diffusion; (B) osmosis; (C) active transport; and (D) filtration. (From Leahy, J. M., & Kizilary, P. E. [1998]. *Foundations of Nursing Practice: A Nursing Process Approach.* Philadelphia, PA: Saunders.)

passes rather freely across cell membranes. The process of osmosis is essential to the life of the cells and to the balance of water and electrolytes in the body. Osmotic pressure within vessels helps to keep fluid from leaking out into the interstitial spaces (Fig. 25.1).

Filtration. **Filtration** is the movement of water and suspended substances outward through a semipermeable membrane. The pumping action of the heart creates **hydrostatic pressure** (pressure exerted by fluid) within the capillaries. Hydrostatic pressure causes fluid to press outward on the vessel. That force promotes filtration, forcing movement of water and electrolytes through the capillary wall to the interstitial fluid (see Fig. 25.1B).

Active Transport

Active transport, contrary to diffusion, osmosis, and filtration, requires cellular energy. This force can move molecules into cells regardless of their electrical charge or the concentrations already in the cell. **Active transport may move substances from an area of lower concentration to an area of higher concentration.** The energy source for the process is adenosine triphosphate (ATP). ATP is produced during the complex metabolic processes in the body's cells. Enzyme reactions metabolize carbon chains of sugars, fatty acids, and amino acids, yielding carbon dioxide, water, and high-energy phosphate bonds. Active transport can move amino acids, glucose, iron, hydrogen, sodium, potassium, and calcium through the cell membrane (Fig. 25.2).

FLUID AND ELECTROLYTE IMBALANCES

Healthy people maintain intake and output (I & O) balance by drinking sufficient fluids and eating a balanced diet each day. **The healthy kidney regulates fluid and electrolyte balance by regulating the volume and composition of ECF.** Illness affects fluid balance in many ways. The patient may be unable to ingest food or liquids, may have a problem with absorption from the intestinal tract, or may have a kidney impairment that affects excretion or reabsorption of water and electrolytes. Any disease that affects circulation (e.g., heart failure) ultimately affects the distribution and composition of body fluids. Burns, in which large amounts of body fluid may be lost through open wounds, also present problems of fluid balance. **In fact, any seriously ill patient is at risk for a fluid and electrolyte imbalance.**

Life-Span Considerations

Older Adults

Any patient over age 65 is at risk for confusion from fluid and electrolyte imbalance. Always look for signs of a fluid and electrolyte imbalance when an older adult becomes confused.

A fluid imbalance exists when the body has an excess (too much) or a deficit (too little) of water. When this occurs, there will be an accompanying imbalance in the substances dissolved in the water. When considering sodium imbalances, it is important to remember that **water follows sodium in the body**. The sodium concentration causes an osmotic pull, and water goes to where that concentration is highest.

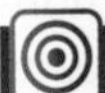

Focused Assessment

Assessing Fluid and Electrolyte Status

For patients admitted with vomiting, diarrhea, high fever, or a history of heart failure, diabetes, renal disease, head injury, thyroid disease, adrenal disease, or inflammatory bowel disease, perform a general head-to-toe assessment and assess for:

- Fatigue
- Weakness
- Tissue turgor
- Edema, dependent or generalized, and degree of pitting
- Dyspnea
- Confusion
- Dizziness
- Blood pressure change
- Rapid pulse
- Cool, dry skin
- Sunken eyeballs
- Mucous membranes for dryness
- Jugular vein distention
- Rapidity of hand vein emptying and refill
- Changes in vital signs
- Changes in daily weight
- Alteration in input and output balance

DEFICIENT FLUID VOLUME

Those at risk for deficient fluid volume are: (1) patients unable to take in sufficient quantities of fluid because of impaired swallowing, extreme weakness, disorientation, coma, or the unavailability of water; and (2) patients who lose excessive amounts of fluid through prolonged vomiting, diarrhea, hemorrhage, diaphoresis (sweating), or excessive wound drainage. Treatments that can cause a fluid deficit are diuretic therapy and gastrointestinal suction without fluid replacement.

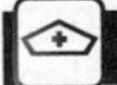

Clinical Cues

Keep an accurate record of the amount of drainage removed by suction so that adequate fluid can be replaced and dehydration can be avoided.

Box 25.1 Signs and Symptoms of Dehydration (Fluid Volume Deficit)

- Complaints of dizziness
- Confusion
- Cool, dry skin
- Dark, concentrated urine
- Decreased blood pressure
- Decreased urine production
- Dry, cracked lips and tongue
- Dry mucous membranes
- Elevated temperature
- Flat neck veins when lying down
- Increased pulse rate
- Poor skin turgor
- Postural hypotension
- Thick saliva
- Thirst
- Weak, thready pulse
- Weakness

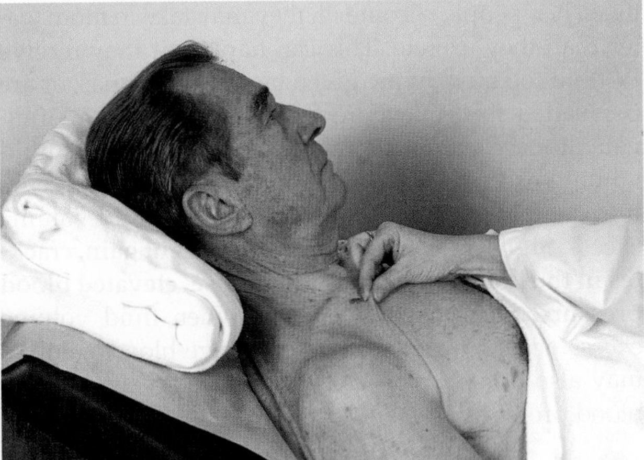

FIGURE 25.3 Testing for tissue turgor and signs of dehydration. (From Seidel, H. M., Ball, J. W., & Dains, J.E., & Benedict W. G. [2003]. *Mosby's Guide to Physical Examination* [5th ed.]. St. Louis, MO: Mosby.)

Burns and drainage from large wounds or fistulas can deplete the fluid volume. Treatment of deficient fluid volume involves remedying the underlying cause and replacing fluids.

Dehydration

When a fluid deficit occurs, it causes loss of water from the cells (dehydration). When there is too little water in the plasma, water is drawn out of the cells by osmosis to equalize the concentration, and the cells shrivel. Dehydration is treated by fluid administration, either orally or intravenously.

Signs and symptoms of dehydration are listed in Box 25.1. Tissue **turgor** (degree of elasticity) is checked by gently pinching up the skin over the abdomen, forearm, sternum, forehead, or thigh (Fig. 25.3). In a person with normal fluid balance, the pinched skin immediately falls back to normal when released. If a fluid deficit is present, the skin may remain elevated or tented for several seconds after the pinch. This test measures skin elasticity, as well, and it is not always a valid indicator of fluid loss in the elderly and infants. Weight loss and dark or limited urine output can also be signs of dehydration. Dehydrated infants may show evidence of sunken eyeballs and a depressed anterior fontanel.

 Life-Span Considerations

Older Adults

The older adult who suffers from nausea, vomiting, or diarrhea is especially prone to dehydration. If the person has a fever, this adds to the fluid loss. Because of the fluid and accompanying electrolyte losses, the person may become confused. Offering the patient small amounts of water frequently or an electrolyte solution such as Gatorade, if it can be kept down, helps prevent additional problems.

EXCESS FLUID VOLUME

Healthy people do not ordinarily drink too much water. When people become ill, they may take in more water than they excrete. This can happen if they receive IV fluid too quickly, are given tap water enemas, or are persuaded to drink more fluids than they can eliminate. If these events happen, the patient suffers a fluid volume excess. Impaired elimination, such as occurs in renal failure, is an important cause of fluid volume excess. **Signs of overhydration are weight gain, crackles in the lungs, slow bounding pulse, elevated blood pressure, and possibly edema.** When fluid volume excess occurs, **hypervolemia** (excessive blood volume) may also occur. Hypervolemia causes an elevation of blood pressure.

Edema

Edema is an excessive accumulation of interstitial (tissue) fluid. It is often a sign of fluid overload, but it may be due to other causes.

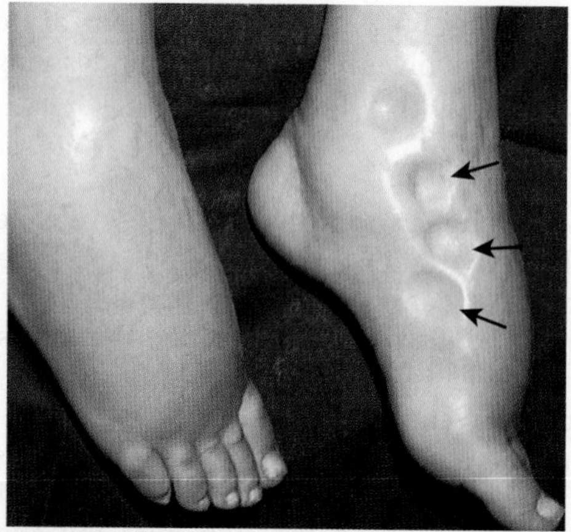

FIGURE 25.4 Example of pitting edema. The finger depressions (arrows) do not refill quickly after pressure has been exerted. (Patton, K. T., & Thibodeau, G. A. [2014]. *The Human Body in Health and Disease* [6th ed.]. St. Louis, MO: Mosby.)

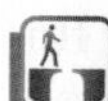 Clinical Pitfall

Recall that plasma proteins are responsible for maintaining colloid osmotic pressure and, thus, for keeping fluid in the vascular compartment. Although we often see peripheral edema and automatically assume *excess* fluid volume, in a patient with severe protein deficiency, it is possible to exhibit peripheral edema in the presence of *deficient* fluid volume, because of decreased colloid osmotic pressure. Remember, what is in the vascular space determines fluid volume deficit versus excess!

In ambulatory patients, the excessive fluid tends to accumulate in the lower extremities (Fig. 25.4). In the bedridden patient, the fluid accumulates in the sacral region. These types of fluid accumulations are termed *dependent edema.* Generalized edema occurs when excess interstitial fluid is spread throughout the body. It is most visible in the hands and face, where swelling is detectable. Causes of generalized edema are: (1) kidney failure, (2) heart failure, (3) liver failure, and (4) hormonal disorders involving the overproduction of aldosterone and ADH (Fig. 25.5). Local edema may be caused by infection or injury and the resulting inflammation.

Treatment involves correcting the underlying cause and assisting the body to rebalance fluid content. The patient may have fluid intake restricted or be given a diuretic drug, which causes the kidneys to increase the excretion of fluid.

 Think Critically

Why should you auscultate the lungs of older adult patients who are receiving IV fluids even if they have no current lung problems?

ELECTROLYTE IMBALANCES

A summary of the normal ranges of the major electrolytes, the causes of imbalances, the signs and symptoms of imbalances, and nursing interventions is provided in Table 25.4.

Sodium Imbalances

Hyponatremia. **A deficit of sodium in the blood is called hyponatremia** (Na^+ less than 135 mEq/L). This can occur from sodium loss or an excess of water. This is the most common electrolyte imbalance patients' experience. Sodium loss may occur from excessive vomiting or diarrhea when the fluid loss is replaced with plain water. Decreased secretion of aldosterone can result in sodium loss. Heart failure, liver disease with **ascites** (abnormal accumulation of fluid within the peritoneal cavity), and sometimes chronic renal failure, result in excessive water retention without concurrent sodium retention. The result of this is hypervolemia combined with hyponatremia. The average intake of sodium is 6 to 12 g/day. If there is a problem with water balance, the patient may be advised to restrict sodium in the diet.

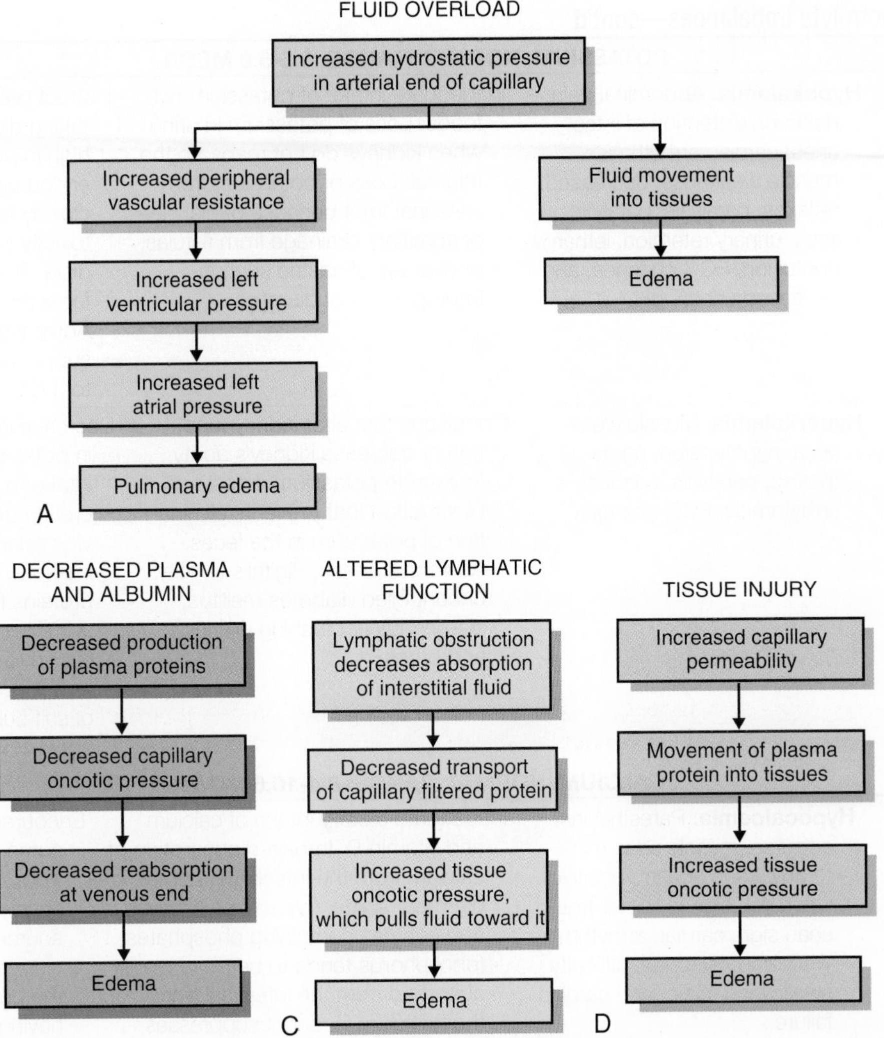

FIGURE 25.5 Mechanisms of edema formation. (A) Fluid overload. (B) Decreased plasma and albumin. (C) Altered lymphatic function. (D) Tissue injury. (From Black, J. M., & Hawks, J. H. [2009]. *Medical-Surgical Nursing: Clinical Management for Positive Outcomes* [8th ed.]. St. Louis, MO: Saunders.)

Table 25.4 Electrolyte Imbalances

SERUM VALUE	SIGNS AND SYMPTOMS	CAUSES AND RISK FACTORS	NURSING INTERVENTIONS
		SODIUM: NORMAL RANGE: 135-145 MEQ/L	
Less than 135 mEq/L	**Hyponatremia.** Central nervous system and neuromuscular changes resulting from failure of swollen cells to transmit electrical impulses. Mental confusion, headache, altered level of consciousness, anxiety, coma, anorexia, nausea, vomiting, muscle cramps, seizures, and decreased sensation.	Inadequate sodium intake, as in patients on low sodium diets. Excessive intake or retention of water (kidney failure and heart failure). Loss of bile, which is rich in sodium, because of fistulas, drainage, gastrointestinal surgery, nausea and vomiting, and suction. Loss of sodium through burn wounds. Administration of IV fluids that do not contain electrolytes.	Restrict water intake as ordered for patients with heart failure, kidney failure, and inadequate antidiuretic hormone production. Liberalize diet of patient on low sodium diet. Closely monitor patient receiving IV solutions to correct hyponatremia. Replace water loss with fluids containing sodium.
Greater than 145 mEq/L	**Hypernatremia.** Dry mucous membranes, loss of skin turgor, intense thirst, flushed skin, oliguria, and possibly elevated temperature; weakness, lethargy, irritability, twitching, seizures, coma, and intracranial bleeding; low-grade fever.	High sodium diet, inadequate water intake as in comatose, mentally confused, or debilitated patient. Excessive sweating, diarrhea, and failure of kidneys to reabsorb water from urine. Administration of high-protein, hyperosmotic tube feedings and osmotic diuretics.	Encourage increased fluid intake; measure I & O; give water between tube feedings; restrict sodium intake; monitor temperature.

Continued

Table 25.4 Electrolyte Imbalances—cont'd

POTASSIUM: NORMAL RANGE: 3.5-5.0 MEQ/L			
Less than 3.5 mEq/L	**Hypokalemia.** Abdominal pain, gaseous distention of intestines; cardiac arrhythmias, muscle weakness, decreased reflexes, paralysis, paralytic ileus, urinary retention, lethargy, confusion, ECG changes, and increased urinary pH.	Inadequate intake of potassium-rich foods. Loss of potassium in urine when kidneys do not reabsorb the mineral. Loss of potassium from intestinal tract because of diarrhea or vomiting, drainage from fistulas, or overuse of gastric suction. Improper use of diuretics.	Instruct patients (especially those taking diuretics) about foods high in potassium content; encourage intake. Observe closely for signs of digitalis toxicity in patients taking this drug. Teach patients to watch for signs of hypokalemia. Administer potassium chloride supplement as ordered. Monitor I & O and cardiac rhythm.
Greater than 5.0 mEq/L	**Hyperkalemia.** Muscle weakness, hypotension, paresthesias, paralysis, cardiac arrhythmias, ECG changes.	Conditions that alter kidney function or decrease kidney's ability to excrete potassium. Intestinal obstruction that prevents elimination of potassium in the feces. Addison disease, digitalis toxicity, uncontrolled diabetes mellitus, insulin deficit, crushing injuries, and burns.	Decrease intake of foods high in potassium. Increase fluid intake to enhance urinary excretion of potassium; provide adequate carbohydrate intake to prevent use of body proteins for energy. Carefully administer proper dose of insulin to diabetic patients. Instruct patient in proper use of salt substitutes containing potassium.
CALCIUM: NORMAL RANGE: 8.4-10.6 MG/DL			
Less than 8.4 mg/dL	**Hypocalcemia.** Paresthesias, seizures, muscle spasms, tetany, hand spasm, positive Chvostek sign, positive Trousseau sign, cardiac arrhythmia, wheezing, dyspnea, difficulty swallowing, colic, and cardiac failure.	Inadequate dietary intake of calcium and vitamin D. Impaired absorption of calcium from the intestinal tract, as in diarrhea, sprue, overuse of laxatives and enemas containing phosphates (phosphorus tends to be more readily absorbed from the intestinal tract than calcium is, and it suppresses calcium retention in the body). The parathyroid regulates calcium and phosphorus levels. Hyposecretion of parathyroid hormone can result in hypocalcemia.	Encourage adults to consume sufficient calcium from cheese, broccoli, shrimp, and other dietary sources. Have 10% calcium gluconate solution at the bedside of the patient having a thyroidectomy in case of surgical damage to the parathyroid glands. Give all oral medicines containing calcium ½ hour before meals to facilitate absorption.
Greater than 10.6 mg/dL	**Hypercalcemia.** Anorexia, abdominal pain, constipation, polyuria, confusion, renal calculi, pathologic fractures, and cardiac arrest.	Excess intake of calcium, as in the patient taking antacids indiscriminately. Excess intake of vitamin D. Conditions that cause movement of calcium out of bones and into extracellular fluid (e.g., bone tumor and multiple fractures). Tumors of the lung, stomach, and kidney and multiple myeloma. Immobility and osteoporosis.	Administer diuretics as prescribed to increase urine output and calcium excretion. Monitor I & O; encourage high fluid intake (3000-4000 mL/day).
MAGNESIUM: NORMAL RANGE: 1.3-2.1 MEQ/L			
Less than 1.3 mEq/L	**Hypomagnesemia.** Insomnia, hyperactive reflexes, leg and foot cramps, twitching, tremors, seizures, cardiac arrhythmias, positive Chvostek sign, positive Trousseau sign, vertigo, hypocalcemia, and hypokalemia.	Chronic malnutrition; chronic diarrhea. Bowel resection with ileostomy or colostomy; chronic alcoholism; prolonged gastric suction; acute pancreatitis; biliary or intestinal fistula; osmotic diuretic therapy; diabetic ketoacidosis.	Diet counseling to help patients at risk increase level of magnesium (e.g., milk and cereals). Monitor closely IV infusions of magnesium. Monitor I & O.

Table 25.4 Electrolyte Imbalances—cont'd

MAGNESIUM: NORMAL RANGE: 1.3-2.1 MEQ/L			
Greater than 2.1 mEq/L	**Hypermagnesemia.** Hypotension; sweating and flushing, nausea and vomiting; muscle weakness, paralysis, respiratory depression; cardiac dysrhythmias.	Overuse of antacids and cathartics containing magnesium; aspiration of seawater, as in near drowning. Chronic kidney disease.	Teach patients to avoid abuse of laxatives and antacids; instruct patients with renal problems to avoid over-the-counter drugs that contain magnesium. Encourage fluid intake to increase urinary excretion of magnesium if not contraindicated. Monitor I & O. Administer diuretics as ordered.
PHOSPHATE: NORMAL RANGE: 2.7-4.5 MG/DL			
Less than 2.7 mg/dL	**Hypophosphatemia.** Confusion, seizures, numbness, weakness, and possible coma. Chronic state may cause rickets and osteomalacia.	Vitamin D deficiency or hyperparathyroidism; use of aluminum-containing antacids.	Assess for vitamin D deficiency, hyperparathyroidism, or overuse of aluminum-containing antacids.
Greater than 4.5 mg/dL	**Hyperphosphatemia.** Anorexia, nausea, and vomiting.	Renal insufficiency.	Assess for restlessness, confusion, chest pain, and cyanosis. Monitor respirations. Check all electrolyte levels.

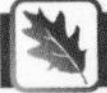

Life-Span Considerations

Older Adults

Older adults are more susceptible to hyponatremia than younger ones are. Those taking thiazide diuretics or selective serotonin reuptake inhibitors (SSRIs) are particularly at risk for hyponatremia. The problem is especially prevalent in long-term care residents.

Hypernatremia. **When the serum sodium concentration rises above 145 mEq/L, a state of hypernatremia exists.** This occurs when there is an excess of sodium or a loss of body water. Excessive administration of sodium bicarbonate for the treatment of **acidosis** (excess of acid or depletion of alkaline substances in the blood and body tissues) is one cause. More commonly, water loss from fever, respiratory tract infection, or watery diarrhea is the cause.

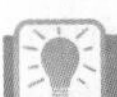

QSEN Considerations: Safety

Long-Term Steroid Risk

Patients on long-term corticosteroids that cause potassium depletion may develop hypernatremia. Observe for signs of edema in these patients.

Decreased water intake may occur in immobile, confused, or dependent patients or in those who have sustained damage to the thirst center in the hypothalamus. The body tries to correct the situation by conserving water through reabsorption in the renal tubules. Hypernatremia causes an osmotic shift of fluid from the cells to the interstitial spaces, causing cellular dehydration and interruption of normal cell processes. Sodium intake is restricted for the patient with hypernatremia.

Patient Education

Foods High in Sodium

The patient who is experiencing a fluid volume excess or who has been advised to decrease sodium intake should avoid the foods listed below. The patient who is low in sodium may add some of these foods to the diet.

- Buttermilk
- Canned meats or fish
- Canned soups (regular)
- Canned vegetables (regular)
- Casserole and pasta mixes
- Cheese (all kinds)
- Dried fruits
- Dried soup mixes
- Foods containing monosodium glutamate (MSG)
- Frozen vegetables with sauces
- Gravy mixes
- Ham
- Hot dogs
- Ketchup
- Lunch meats
- Olives
- Pickles
- Prepared mustard
- Preserved meats
- Processed foods
- Salted nuts
- Salted popcorn
- Salted snack foods
- Softened water high in sodium
- Soy sauce (regular)
- Tomato or vegetable juice

Potassium Imbalances

Hypokalemia. **When the potassium level falls below 3.5 mEq/L, hypokalemia exists.** Extra potassium must be given to help correct the imbalance. Hypokalemia may be a result of malnutrition, illness causing a shift of potassium from ECF to ICF, or increased potassium loss. Hypokalemia can also be related to laxative or enema abuse, and medications such as Amphotericin B, diuretics, and antibiotics, and certain genetic disorders (Thomas, 2015). Vomiting, diarrhea, and prolonged gastrointestinal suction may deplete potassium levels (Lederer, 2014). Potassium-sparing diuretics help restore serum potassium when a diuretic is needed. The patient is encouraged to eat foods high in potassium, and IV replacement may be necessary

 Patient Education

Foods High in Potassium

The patient with hypokalemia should be encouraged to add the foods listed below to the daily diet. Patients in renal failure may need to restrict their intake of these foods.

- Apricots
- Avocados
- Bananas
- Cantaloupe
- Codfish
- Dates
- Meats
- Milk
- Orange juice
- Oranges
- Potatoes
- Raisins
- Salmon
- Tuna

 Safety Alert

Hypokalemia

Severe hypokalemia (K^+ less than 2.5 mEq/L) may cause cardiac arrest. Potassium-wasting diuretics used without potassium replacement can cause hypokalemia. Premature ventricular contractions and changes in the electrocardiogram (ECG) pattern such as ST segment depression, a prolonged Q-T interval, and U wave occurrence may be seen.

Hyperkalemia. **When the serum potassium level rises above 5.0 mEq/L, a state of hyperkalemia exists.** Patients with renal failure, severe burns, or crush injuries and those undergoing major surgery are at risk for hyperkalemia. The mechanical disruption of cell membranes causes a shift of potassium from the ICF to the ECF. Hyperkalemia occurs in overuse of potassium-sparing diuretics, digitalis toxicity, overuse of potassium-containing salt substitutes, uncontrolled diabetes mellitus, and a variety of other illnesses.

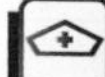 Clinical Cues

Hyperkalemia can cause life-threatening cardiac arrhythmia. Tall or peaked T waves may be seen on the ECG. P waves may be small.

Calcium Imbalances

Hypocalcemia. **When the calcium level drops below 8.4 mg/dL, hypocalcemia occurs.** This can result from nutritional deficiency of calcium or vitamin D. Hypocalcemia occurs in disorders in which there is a shift of calcium into the bone. Metastatic cancer invading bone is one such cause. Removal or injury of the parathyroid glands during thyroidectomy causes parathyroid hormone deficiency and consequent hypocalcemia. Excessive infusion of bicarbonate solution, **alkalosis** (excess of alkaline or decrease of acid substances in the blood and body fluids), blood transfusions, and hypoparathyroidism may cause hypocalcemia.

Hypercalcemia. **Hypercalcemia, a serum calcium level above 10.6 mg/dL,** can occur during periods of lengthy immobilization when calcium is mobilized from the bone or when an excess of calcium or vitamin D is taken into the body. Most cases are related to hyperparathyroidism or malignancy in which there is metastasis with bone resorption. Such malignancies include multiple myeloma and lung or renal cancers.

Magnesium Imbalances

Hypomagnesemia. **Hypomagnesemia, a serum level below 1.3 mEq/L,** can result from numerous situations including decreased magnesium intake from starvation, malabsorption, or alcoholism; pancreatitis; and gastrointestinal losses from diarrhea, vomiting, or gastric suction. Genetic abnormalities in the renal tubules and medications can also be the cause (Fulop, 2014). Uncontrolled diabetes, hypercalcemia, and diuretic therapy can be causes of hypomagnesemia (Lewis, 2013). Recent studies suggest proton pump inhibitors may lead to hypomagnesemia in patients already receiving diuretics (Zipursky et al., 2014). Hypomagnesemia often accompanies hypokalemia.

Hypermagnesemia. **Hypermagnesemia, a serum level above 2.1 mEq/L,** occurs rarely and usually in the presence of renal failure, although magnesium-containing laxatives or antacids or severe dehydration can cause it.

Anion Imbalances

Imbalances of chloride, phosphate, and bicarbonate accompany cation imbalances because of the principle of electroneutrality. **Hypochloremia, a chloride level below 96 mEq/L, is associated with hyponatremia.** It can also occur with severe vomiting and is seen as a compensatory decrease in acid-base disorders. **Hyperchloremia, a chloride level above 106 mEq/L, occurs along with hypernatremia and a form of metabolic acidosis. Hypophosphatemia occurs when the level of phosphate falls below 2.7 mg/dL.** It may result from use of aluminum-containing antacids that bind phosphate, from vitamin D deficiency, or from hyperparathyroidism. **Hyperphosphatemia, a phosphate level above 4.5 mg/dL, commonly occurs in renal failure.**

 Think Critically

Why may some older adults have a low serum calcium even though they take in sufficient calcium in the diet? What type of fluid and electrolyte imbalances can occur in the patient who is undergoing diuretic therapy? Why?

ACID-BASE BALANCE

Acid-base balance is very important to maintaining homeostasis in the body because cell enzymes can function only within a very narrow range of pH.

PH

pH is a measure of the degree to which a solution is acidic or alkaline. Cell metabolism constantly produces carbon dioxide, which combines with water to form carbonic acid (H_2CO_3), which immediately breaks down into hydrogen ions and bicarbonate ions. The concentration of hydrogen ions (H^+) determines the pH reading. **The normal serum pH is 7.35 to 7.45.** Death may occur at a serum pH below 6.8 or above 7.8. Because of the production of acids by the body's metabolic systems, the body tends to become acidic if homeostasis is upset.

BICARBONATE

Bicarbonate is an important substance in maintaining acid-base balance. **The normal range of bicarbonate (HCO_3–) is 22 to 26 mEq/L.** The major function of this alkaline electrolyte is the regulation of the acid-base balance in the body. Bicarbonate acts as a buffer to neutralize the excess acids in the body and maintain the bicarbonate-to-carbonic acid ratio at 20:1, which is needed for homeostasis. The kidneys selectively reabsorb or excrete bicarbonate to regulate serum levels and help maintain acid-base balance.

CONTROL MECHANISMS

For the serum pH to remain within the normal range of 7.35 to 7.45, the ratio of bicarbonate ion to carbonic acid must be 20:1. If one component of the ratio changes, the other must change proportionately to maintain the proper balance for serum pH to be within the normal range. There are three control mechanisms for pH. The first is the blood buffer system, which consists of weak acids and weak bases. These buffer pairs can act quickly to stabilize the serum pH. The buffer pair that is monitored in clinical settings is the sodium bicarbonate–carbonic acid buffer system. When an acid is added to the blood, it combines with the base (bicarbonate) component of the buffer, forming a weaker acid. Because weak acids do not readily release free H^+, changes in serum pH are minimized. When a base is added to the blood, it combines with the acid component of the buffer to form a weaker base. The other blood buffer systems are protein buffers and phosphate buffers. They minimize pH changes but do not remove acid or base from the body.

The second control mechanism for pH is the lungs. In the lungs, the hydrogen ion and the bicarbonate ion dissociation reaction can be reversed, and water and carbon dioxide (CO_2) are reformed. The carbon dioxide and water are expired from the lungs, decreasing the amount of acid in the body. The lungs can either expel more carbon dioxide or conserve it to help balance the pH. The respiratory system can readjust quickly to help control serum pH.

The third control mechanism for pH is the urinary system. In the kidney, enzymes promote the dissociation of carbonic acid to free hydrogen ions, which can be excreted in the urine. The bicarbonate ions are returned to the blood to restore the levels of buffer. The kidneys reduce the acid content of the serum by exchanging hydrogen for sodium with the help of aldosterone, and the kidneys can neutralize acids by combining them with ammonia and other chemicals. When there is excess alkali (base), the kidney can also excrete excess bicarbonate. This compensatory ability of the kidney takes more time to work compared with the compensatory action in the lungs. Figure 25.6 shows the interaction of these control mechanisms.

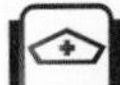 Clinical Cues

Usually about 3 days are needed for the kidneys to stabilize pH within normal range.

 Think Critically

If the blood flow to the kidneys is reduced for a considerable time, what effect might it have on serum pH?

ACID-BASE IMBALANCES

There are four types of acid-base imbalances, as shown in Table 25.5. To determine if an acid-base imbalance exists, the pH, arterial carbon dioxide partial pressure ($PaCO_2$), and bicarbonate ion are measured by arterial blood gas analysis performed on a sample of arterial blood. **An increase in hydrogen ions results in acidosis (decrease in pH). A decrease in hydrogen ions results in alkalosis (increase in pH).** Imbalances may be acute or chronic. An initial change in carbon dioxide is nearly always the result of a respiratory disorder. Disorders that show an initial change in bicarbonate ions are metabolic. The three control mechanisms continually work together to maintain acid-base balance. When an imbalance occurs, the lungs and kidneys try to **compensate** by working to bring the pH back toward normal limits.

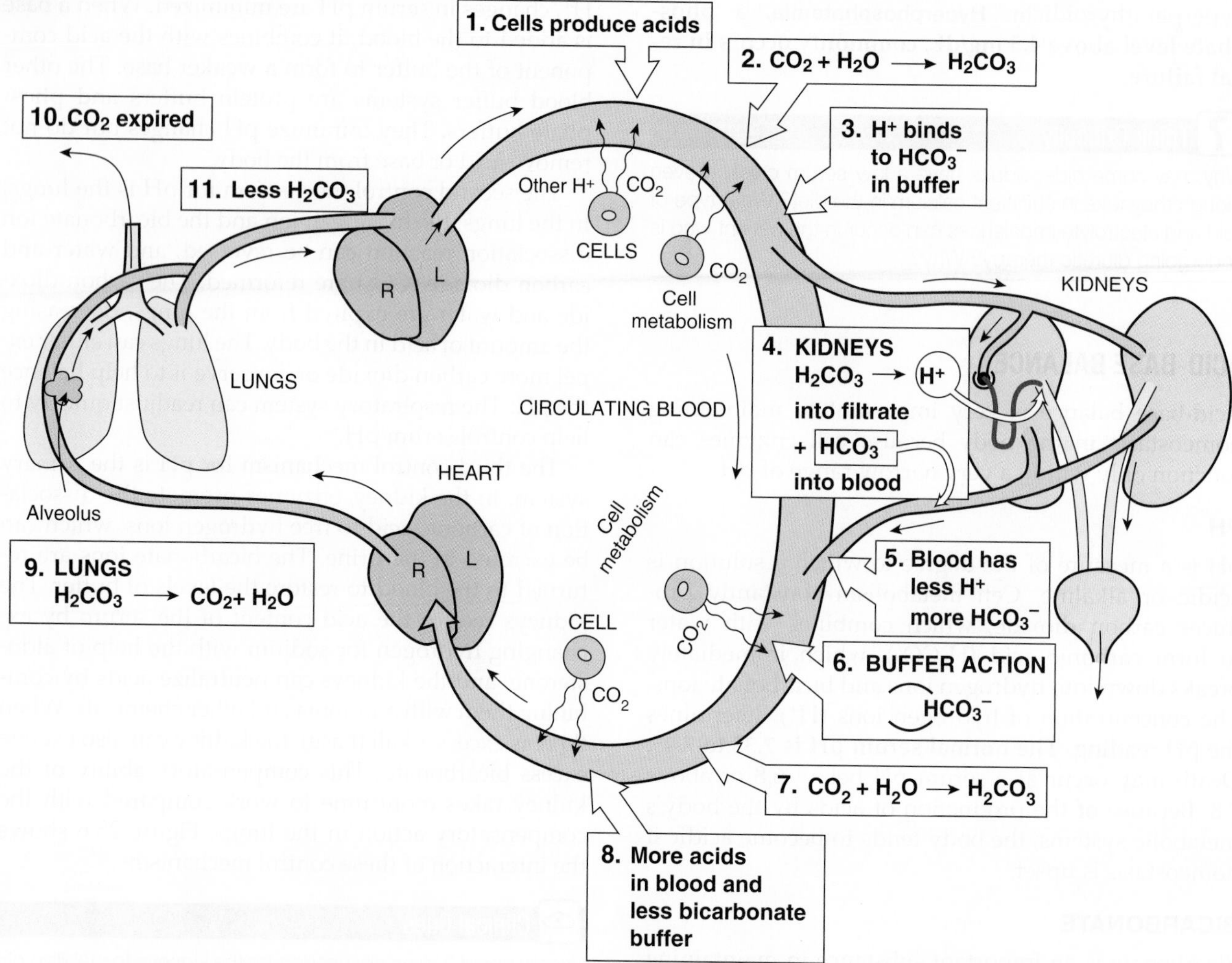

FIGURE 25.6 Regulation of acid-base balance by chemical buffers, respiratory system, and renal system. *CO_2*, Carbon dioxide; *H^+*, hydrogen ion; *HCO_3–*, bicarbonate; *H_2CO_3*, carbonic acid; *H_2O*, water.

Table 25.5 Acid-Base Imbalances

IMBALANCE	CAUSES	SIGNS AND SYMPTOMS	ARTERIAL BLOOD GAS VALUES[a]
Respiratory acidosis	Slow, shallow respirations/hypoventilation; respiratory congestion or obstruction; can be due to COPD, severe pneumonia, or excessive sedation; respiratory muscle weakness	Hypoventilation; dyspnea; anxiety; confusion	pH less than 7.35; $PaCO_2$ greater than 45 mm Hg
Metabolic acidosis	Shock; diabetic ketoacidosis; lactic acidosis; renal failure; diarrhea; starvation	Kussmaul respirations; headache; confusion; malaise	pH less than 7.35 HCO_3; less than 22 mEq/L
Respiratory alkalosis	Hyperventilation caused by anxiety or pain; mechanical ventilation	Hyperventilation; confusion; lightheadedness	pH greater than 7.45; $PaCO_2$ less than 35 mm Hg
Metabolic alkalosis	Vomiting; prolonged gastric suction; hypokalemia; medications: diuretics, antacids or bicarbonate, mineralocorticoids	Hypoventilation; confusion; numbness/tingling; decreased LOC	pH greater than 7.45; HCO_3 greater than 26 mEq/L

[a]Normal blood gas values: pH: 7.35-7.45; PaO_2: 80-100 mm Hg; $PaCO_2$: 35-45 mm Hg; HCO_3–: 22-26 mEq/L.

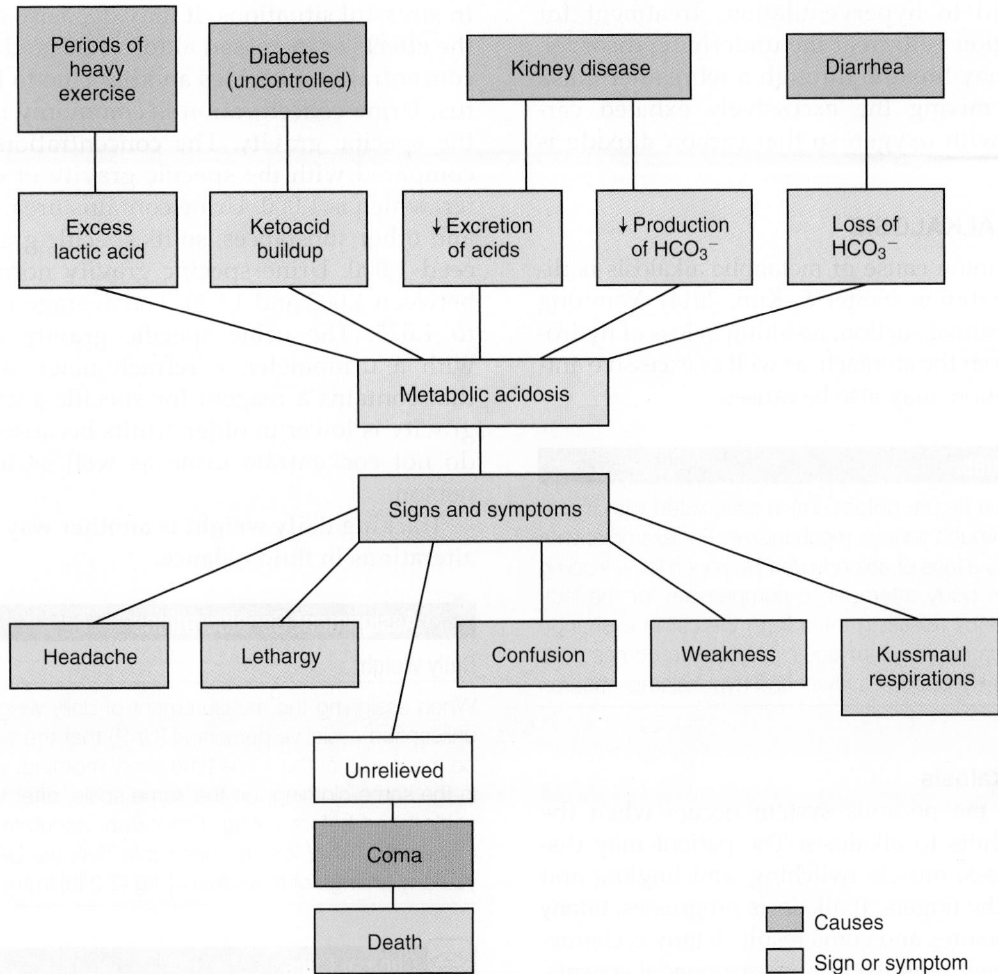

CONCEPT MAP 25.2 Causes, signs, and symptoms of metabolic acidosis. *HCO_3–*, Bicarbonate.

RESPIRATORY ACIDOSIS

Carbon dioxide levels increase in a variety of disorders, including acute problems such as airway obstruction, pneumonia, asthma, or chest injuries. Increased levels are also seen in patients taking opiates, which depress the respiratory rate. Chronic respiratory acidosis is prevalent among people with chronic obstructive pulmonary disease (COPD), also called chronic airflow limitation (CAL).

METABOLIC ACIDOSIS

An excessive loss of bicarbonate ions or an increased production or retention of hydrogen ions leads to metabolic acidosis. The loss of bicarbonate ions with diarrhea is one cause of metabolic acidosis. Metabolic acidosis also occurs when large amounts of acid are produced within the body. This happens when more energy than usual is expended and lactic acid builds up in the body, a condition called lactic acidosis, one type of metabolic acidosis. Lactic acidosis is most commonly caused by poor tissue perfusion in states such as shock (Gunnerson, 2015). The faulty metabolism of a patient with diabetes can cause a buildup of ketoacids, resulting in another type of metabolic acidosis, diabetic ketoacidosis. The other major cause of metabolic acidosis is kidney disease, in which there is decreased excretion of acids and decreased production of bicarbonate (Concept Map 25.2). In this instance, dialysis is required to maintain the pH within life-permitting limits.

Effects of Acidosis

Acidosis depresses the nervous system, causing headache, lethargy, weakness, and confusion. If the acidosis is unrelieved, coma and death will ensue. Evidence that the compensatory mechanisms are at work in metabolic acidosis is deep rapid breathing (Kussmaul respirations) and secretion of urine with a low pH.

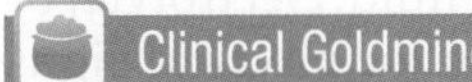

Clinical Goldmine

Kussmaul respiration is the body's attempt to correct acidosis by "blowing off" carbon dioxide, which is an acid.

RESPIRATORY ALKALOSIS

Hyperventilation (a rapid respiratory rate) results in respiratory alkalosis. It is usually caused by anxiety, high fever, or an overdose of aspirin. Head injuries may also lead to hyperventilation. Treatment for hyperventilation is to treat the underlying disorder. The person may breathe through a rebreather mask temporarily, mixing the excessively exhaled carbon dioxide with oxygen so that carbon dioxide is inhaled.

METABOLIC ALKALOSIS

The most common cause of metabolic alkalosis is diuretic administration (Soifer & Kim, 2014). Vomiting and gastrointestinal suction, resulting in loss of hydrochloric acid from the stomach, as well as excessive antacid consumption, may also be causes.

Clinical Cues

Hypokalemia (low serum potassium) is associated with metabolic alkalosis through various mechanisms. For example, with vomiting, there is a loss of chloride and hydrogen ions, leading to alkalosis. The body attempts to compensate for the lack of hydrogen ions by releasing them from the cell in exchange for potassium ions (potassium goes in/hydrogen comes out). Thus, the serum K+ becomes lower and hypokalemia occurs.

Effects of Alkalosis

Irritability of the nervous system occurs when the pH balance shifts to alkalosis. The patient may display restlessness, muscle twitching, and tingling and numbness of the fingers. If alkalosis progresses, **tetany** occurs, and seizures and coma result. Tetany is characterized by severe muscle cramps, carpopedal spasms, laryngeal spasms, and stridor (shrill, harsh sound on inspiration).

? Think Critically

Can you identify the type of imbalance that might result from (1) rapid respiratory rate, (2) out-of-control diabetes, (3) renal failure, and (4) consuming excess antacids for a nervous stomach?

More in-depth information about acid-base imbalances will be covered in your medical-surgical nursing courses and can be found in a medical-surgical nursing textbook.

❖ APPLICATION OF THE NURSING PROCESS

◆ ASSESSMENT (DATA COLLECTION)

First, assess the patient for risk of fluid, electrolyte, or acid-base imbalance. Then assess for physical signs and symptoms of alterations in normal balance. Examine laboratory test results for electrolyte levels that are outside the normal range. Evaluate blood gas levels to determine whether an acid-base imbalance exists, and, if so, what type of imbalance is present. Evaluate I & O records to determine whether there is a fluid imbalance. The urine volume the adult usually excretes in 24 hours is approximately 1500 mL. In stressful situations, it may decrease slightly from the effects of increased aldosterone and ADH. Urine concentration provides another clue to the fluid status. Urine concentration is commonly measured by the specific gravity. The concentration of urine is compared with the specific gravity of distilled water, which is 1.000. Urine contains urea, electrolytes, and other substances, so its specific gravity will exceed 1.000. Urine specific gravity normally ranges between 1.003 and 1.030. The average range is 1.010 to 1.025. The urine specific gravity is measured with a urinometer, a refractometer, or a dipstick that contains a reagent for specific gravity. Specific gravity is lower in older adults because the kidneys do not concentrate urine as well as in a younger person.

Tracking daily weight is another way to assess for alterations in fluid balance.

Assignment Considerations

Daily Weight

When assigning the measurement of daily weight, remind the unlicensed assistive personnel (UAP) that the weight needs to be measured at the same time every morning, with the patient in the same clothing, on the same scale, after the patient has voided and before eating. Otherwise, accurate measurement of weight gain or loss is impossible. Ask the UAP to report to you any change of more than 1 kg (2.2 lb) immediately.

Clinical Cues

A weight gain or loss of 1 kg (2.2 lb) in 24 h indicates a gain or loss of 1 L of fluid.

Skin turgor (elastic condition) is partially dependent on the amount of tissue fluid supporting the skin. Checking skin turgor is useful when assessing fluid balance (see Fig. 25.3), although it is unreliable in older adults. The sternum is one of the most reliable places to check skin turgor.

Edema may be an indicator of fluid volume overload. Look for puffy eyelids and swollen hands. Edema may sometimes be evidenced by a pit developing when a fingertip is pressed into the tissue over a bony prominence, such as the malleolus or tibia, and held for 5 seconds. After the finger is removed, the pit slowly disappears. A better method of assessing the course of peripheral edema is to measure the circumference of the extremity in the same location each day.

Changes in vital signs are pertinent when assessing fluid, electrolyte, and acid-base balance. Fever increases fluid loss and predisposes the patient to fluid-volume deficit. A pulse rate greater than 100 bpm may be an early sign of decreased vascular volume from fluid volume deficit. A weak, thready pulse accompanies fluid volume deficit, and a bounding pulse is associated with fluid volume overload. Potassium and magnesium deficits may cause an irregular pulse rate. Rapid breathing may cause an alkaline blood pH by expelling large amounts of carbon dioxide, or it may be the body's way to compensate for an acidic blood pH. Moist respiratory sounds in the absence of cardiac or respiratory disease are a sign of excess fluid in the lungs from fluid overload. Fluid overload causes a rise in systolic blood pressure.

Clinical Cues

To assess for a fluid deficit, measure the blood pressure and pulse in the lying, sitting, and standing positions. If systolic blood pressure drops 20 mm Hg, or the diastolic blood pressure drops 10 mm Hg, accompanied by a pulse rate increase of 20 bpm at 1 min after the position change, deficient fluid volume is present (see Chapter 21).

Severe fluid volume deficit decreases blood flow to the brain and results in decreased sensorium and confusion. Imbalances in sodium have direct effects on the brain volume and mental function as well.

Neuromuscular irritability is assessed when imbalances in calcium and magnesium are suspected. Deep tendon reflexes may be tested to monitor neuromuscular irritability. Check for Chvostek and Trousseau signs when calcium or magnesium deficit is a possibility. Chvostek sign is assessed by tapping the facial nerve about an inch in front of the earlobe. A unilateral twitching of the face is a positive response. To test for Trousseau sign, place a blood pressure cuff on the arm and inflate it above the patient's systolic pressure for 3 minutes. A spasm of the hand indicates a positive Trousseau sign. Deep tendon reflexes are tested by tapping a partially stretched muscle tendon with a percussion hammer. The extent of the reflex is scored from 0 to 4+, with 0 representing no response, 2+ a normal response, and 4+ a hyperactive response.

Life-Span Considerations

Older Adults

Checking for tenting is not an accurate way to assess dehydration in older adults because their skin loses elasticity with aging and will tent with normal hydration. It is better to check for dry mucous membranes, concentrated urine, and other signs and symptoms in these patients.

◆ NURSING DIAGNOSIS

Using critical thinking, analyze the assessment database, identify problem areas, and choose nursing diagnoses. Nursing diagnoses commonly used for patients with fluid, electrolyte, or acid-base imbalances are as follows:

- Deficient fluid volume
- Excess fluid volume
- Risk for imbalanced fluid volume
- Ineffective peripheral tissue perfusion
- Decreased cardiac output
- Impaired gas exchange
- Ineffective breathing pattern

Other nursing diagnoses may be appropriate because of the fluid, electrolyte, or acid-base imbalance or may be related to the cause of the imbalance, for example, diarrhea.

◆ PLANNING

Collaboration with the patient and family or caregiver allows the best plan to be devised. Priorities of care are set. The goal is to restore the patient's fluid, electrolyte, or acid-base balance. Individual expected outcomes are written as appropriate. Expected outcomes might be as follows:

- Patient will exhibit normal skin turgor.
- Weight will stabilize at patient's baseline.
- Intake and output will be balanced.
- Blood gases will return to normal.
- Breath sounds will be clear on auscultation.
- There will be no evidence of edema.
- Electrolyte values will be within normal limits.

A specific time frame would be incorporated into the expected outcome. Nursing interventions are chosen to help the patient achieve the outcomes. Nursing Care Plan 25.1 presents examples of expected outcomes and nursing interventions.

◆ IMPLEMENTATION

When patients are unable to consume sufficient fluids independently, consult with the primary care provider on strategies for providing adequate fluid and electrolytes. If patients can swallow and retain fluid, assist them frequently with taking small amounts of fluid. Establish a plan for assisting with both hot and cold liquid consumption. With conscientious care, the need for IV feeding can be avoided. Assessment of what the patient prefers is helpful. In addition to water, offer fruit juices, bouillon, Popsicles, soft drinks, or gelatin. For patients who cannot drink and need only short-term assistance, IV therapy is ordered (Table 25.6). See Chapter 36 for more discussion on IV therapies. For those who will be unable to take in fluids or food on their own for an extended period, a feeding tube must be placed or total parenteral nutrition (TPN) started. Care of the patient with a feeding tube and TPN is discussed in Chapter 27. It is important to track the patient's I & O whether there is a risk of fluid volume imbalance, actual deficit, or actual overhydration (fluid volume excess).

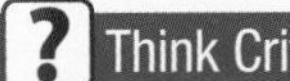

Think Critically

What type of fluid and electrolyte imbalances is the patient who has intestinal flu and suffers from both vomiting and diarrhea likely to have?

Nursing Care Plan 25.1 Care of the Patient With Dehydration

SCENARIO Nina Hiaji, age 76, is placed in the skilled care section of her retirement home. She has been ill for several days with the flu and fever. Her daughter found her confused and lethargic when she came to visit her this morning. Her temperature is 100.8°F (38.2°C), and her blood pressure is 132/72 mm Hg (her normal pressure is 142/88 mm Hg). Her pulse is 96 bpm, and her skin is warm and dry. She is complaining of thirst. Her urine is dark and concentrated. Her oral mucous membranes appear dry, and her saliva is thick and stringy. She is dehydrated and hypernatremic.

PROBLEM/NURSING DIAGNOSIS *Very thirsty with fever and dehydration*/Deficient fluid volume related to fever and lack of intake.

Supporting Assessment Data *Subjective:* Thick saliva. *Objective:* Poor skin turgor at sternum. Dry mucous membranes. Has had flu for several days and has been eating and drinking very little.

Goals/Expected Outcomes	Nursing Interventions	Selected Rationale	Evaluation
Fluid balance will be normal within 24 h.	Encourage intake of 8 oz of fluid every hour.	Fluid intake promotes rehydration.	*Is patient taking fluids?* Yes, took 32 oz by noon. Progressing toward goals.
	Provide mouth care every 4 h and before meals.	Mouth care provides comfort and promotes appetite.	Provided q 4 h and ac.
Patient will not be confused in 32 h.	Reorient to person, place, and time frequently.	Reorientation decreases confusion.	*Is patient confused?* Yes, still confused.
	Monitor fluid intake and output and record it. Assess intake related to output.	Monitoring shows progress toward rehydration.	Intake 2645 mL. Output 2480 mL. Is rehydrating.
	Monitor laboratory values of electrolytes for signs of electrolyte imbalance. Monitor for increasing signs of dehydration; notify primary care provider if they appear.	Monitoring laboratory values indicates success or failure of interventions.	Laboratory values not available yet.
	Monitor IV therapy; prevent fluid-volume excess. Fluid intake promotes rehydration.	Monitoring helps keep fluid therapy on track as ordered. Progressing toward goals.	IV flowing on time. Continue plan.

CRITICAL THINKING QUESTIONS

1. Can you explain the physiologic process of how the flu and fever cause dehydration and hypernatremia?
2. Can you explain the physiologic mechanism of why postural hypotension may occur when a person is dehydrated? What causes the dizziness?

Table 25.6 Why Use This Intravenous Fluid?

CATEGORY OF FLUID	TYPE OF FLUID AND EXAMPLES	ACTION	USE
Crystalloids	Isotonic Fluids		
	0.9% sodium chloride, D_5W solution, Ringer solution, Lactated Ringer solution	Raise intravascular volume without causing cellular fluid shifts or changing the electrolyte concentrations in the plasma.	Used for fluid loss from vomiting and diarrhea, for those waiting for blood products, and for fluid loss during surgery.
	Hypertonic Fluids		
	Concentrated dextrose in water: 20%, 30%, 40%, 50%, 60%, or 70%, 3% or 5% sodium chloride solution	Draw fluid from the intracellular to the extracellular compartment, thereby relieving cellular edema.	Concentrated dextrose solution is often used to lower cerebral edema.
	Hypotonic Fluid		
	0.45% sodium chloride	Expands intravascular volume.	Used to replace hypotonic fluid losses. A maintenance solution.
Colloids	Albumin	Draws fluid from the interstitial and intracellular spaces, replenishing intravascular volume.	Diminish ascites (intraperitoneal fluid), maintain blood pressure, and use in shock when crystalloid solutions are insufficient to maintain vascular volume.

Table 25.7 Measurement Equivalents

HOUSEHOLD MEASUREMENT	METRIC EQUIVALENT (mL)
15 drops	1
1 teaspoon	5
1 tablespoon	15
1 ounce	30
1 cup (8 ounces)	240
1 pint	500
1 quart	1000
5 ice chips to 1 ice cube (1 ice chip = 1 teaspoon)	25 (about ½ volume of chips)

Table 25.8 Common Equivalents of Food Containers[a]

CONTAINER	VOLUME (mL)
Coffee cup	240
Iced tea glass	320
Juice glass	120
Wax drinking cup	180
Styrofoam cup	210
Large glass	230
Cream package	15
Sherbet	90
Soup, clear	120
Soup, thick	180
Gelatin	80
Milk carton	240

[a]Varies from one facility to another.

Recording Intake and Output

Look at the meal tray before it is removed from the room and record the intake on the shift I & O record. Fluids that must be measured include anything that is liquid or will become liquid if left at room temperature (e.g., ice cream, sherbet, milk shakes, gelatin, gruel, and thinned baby cereals). Record amounts in milliliters (Table 25.7). Most facilities provide a list of the amounts contained in the type or size of dish used by the dietary department (Table 25.8). If this information is not available, and for the home care patient, use a graduated container to measure the capacity of various dishes and glasses. Record the amounts the patient drinks between meals as well.

IV fluid infused is recorded as intake. At the beginning of the shift during the handoff report, note how much is left in an IV container that is in progress. Another IV container may be started during the shift when the old one is totally infused. By adding and subtracting, you can calculate the total amount of IV intake. For example, suppose a patient has 350 mL remaining in the IV bag at the beginning of the shift, it infuses, and a new bag is hung at 1:00 pm. At the end of the shift, 200 mL has infused from the new bag. Add 350 mL and 200 mL for a total of 550 mL of IV intake for the shift. Enter this amount on the I & O record as intake under the IV column. Most fluids entering the patient's body are recorded as intake; blood and blood products administered are recorded separately (Fig. 25.7).

Fluid output is also counted and recorded. The average urine output in a 24-hour period is 1000 to 1500 mL; an output of less than 720 mL in a 24-hour period, or less than 30 mL/h, should be reported to the charge nurse or primary care provider. To measure urine output, pour the urine from the bedpan or urinal into a graduated container. (Always wear gloves when handling urine containers.) Place the container on a flat surface and read the level of fluid at eye level. Record the amount on the I & O record under output. For the ambulatory patient, give instructions about saving urine and provide a collection container for the toilet. Ask the patient to call when the container needs emptying or show the patient how to measure and record the urine before disposing of it. Urine drainage bags are emptied before they become full or at least once a shift. The amount is measured and recorded on the I & O record.

Output from all other sources is measured, including drainage from nasogastric tubes, chest tubes, and wound drainage suction devices. If the patient has diarrhea, the liquid stool can be measured in the same manner as urine. Profuse perspiration that requires a change of dampened linen is noted on the I & O record according to agency protocol. Emesis is also measured and recorded as output. At the end of each shift, the total intake and total output are tallied and entered on the 24-hour I & O record in the medical record. You do not need a medical order for instituting the recording of I & O; this is a nursing responsibility (Skill 25.1).

The patient with a fluid volume excess may have an order for fluid restriction. This means that the patient may have only a certain amount of fluid over a 24-hour period. Work out a schedule of fluid intake so that liquids are spaced evenly and the patient does not receive all the allotted liquids in a short time. A typical schedule would be day, 600 mL; evening, 400 mL; night, 200 mL. If not prohibited, hard candies and chewing gum can help relieve thirst. Frequent oral care is essential.

Diuretics are often prescribed, particularly when there is a potential for heart failure or pulmonary edema. Daily weight and electrolyte status must be monitored along with I & O for these patients.

Skin care is particularly important in preventing a breakdown over an edematous area. The stretched skin is extremely fragile, has a decreased blood supply, and is no longer flexible. Keep bed linens dry and smooth, and turn the patient frequently to relieve pressure over

SimChart

Logout

Carlos, Jose

Medical Record Number: 6069804 Room Number: 497 Health Care Provider: P Hartm, MD

Sex: M Weight: 140 lbs Code Status: 01 Isolation: 00 Food Allergies: NKA Diet: 00 Hospital Floor:

Age: 20 Y Height: 5′ 4″ Alerts: 00 Drug Allergies: NKA Env. Allergies: NKA BMI: 24 Medical-Surgical

Charting Day|Time: Monday 12:00

INFO PANEL

Simulations

Set-up Simulation EHR

Intake/Output

Chart inputs

INTAKE:

Oral Intake:

Type: -SELECT- Amount: mL

Intravenous Fluids:

Intravenous #1: -SELECT- Amount: mL

Miscellaneous:

Type: -SELECT- Amount: mL

Meals:

Meals: -SELECT- % Consumed:

OUTPUT:

Entry Type: Volume Frequency

Output Type: -SELECT- Amount: mL

Chart Time	Type	Description	Amount	Entry By
Mon 16:00	Intake	Oral Intake: PO Fluids	280 mL	JK
Mon 16:00	Intake	Intravenous #1: Dextrose 5% in ½ NS	320 mL	JK
Mon 16:00	Output	Urine	550 mL	JK
Mon 12:00	Intake	Oral Intake: PO Fluids	320 mL	JK
Mon 12:00	Intake	Intravenous #1: Dextrose 5% in ½ NS	320 mL	JK

Showing 1 to 5 of 7 entries First Previous 1 2 Next Last

Intake/Output in mL

1500

1000

500

0

Mon

Intake

Output

Day	Input mL	Output mL
Monday	1240	975

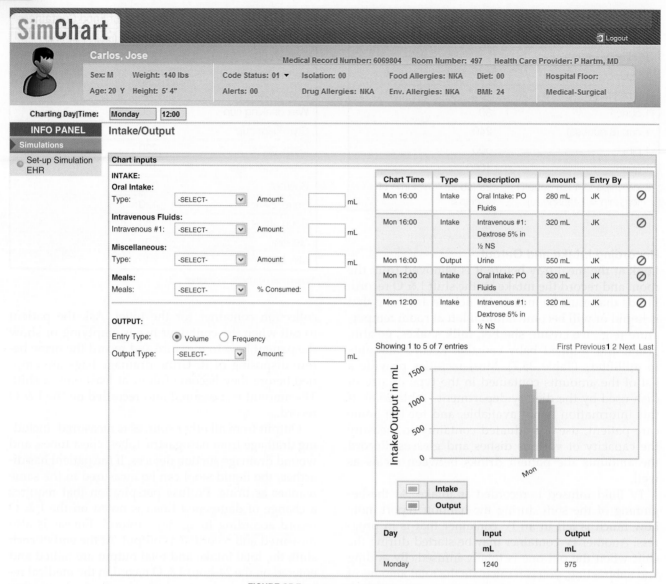

FIGURE 25.7 Intake and output record.

bony prominences. **Be gentle in repositioning and turning the patient to avoid friction on the skin; use a lift sheet. A break in edematous skin can quickly form a pressure injury.**

The patient with a fluid volume excess may be placed on sodium restriction because sodium usually is retained along with water. Table salt is prohibited, and special attention must be paid to the foods and fluids allowed the patient. For items that should be particularly avoided, see Patient Education box on p. 445.

Monitor laboratory values for electrolytes and acid-base balance to determine whether treatment is effective and imbalances are being corrected. When potassium is ordered, check the level before administering the next dose. Assess urine output to ensure adequate flow. Carefully check orders for fluids before a new IV infusion is begun. Assessment for fluid imbalance is ongoing.

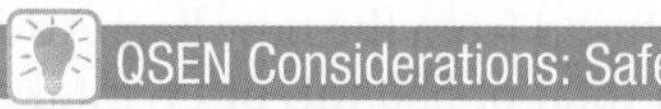

Administering Potassium IV

If urine output is less than 30 mL/h, potassium should not be given. Check IV fluids for added potassium before initiating IV therapy. Check the IV fluid that is in progress. Giving potassium when urine flow is inadequate may cause kidney damage.

For the home care patient, perform thorough patient education so that the patient can meet the requirements for fluid intake or restriction. Monitor adherence to sodium restriction by periodically checking the patient's food intake. Obtaining feedback regarding comprehension of instructions is a vital part of the education. Collaboration with the patient on the plan of care is essential to obtain patient compliance.

When acid-base imbalance occurs, control of the underlying disorder is instituted. Blood gases are monitored, and oxygen and electrolytes are administered as needed. Institute nursing measures to improve pulmonary function as appropriate.

Think Critically

What characteristics would you expect to find in a urine specimen from a patient who is dehydrated? How would it differ from a urine specimen from a patient who has a fluid volume excess?

◆ EVALUATION

Every 24 hours, perform evaluation to see whether the nursing interventions are helping the patient meet expected outcomes. If the patient is not progressing toward achievement of the outcomes, use problem solving and critical thinking to determine why. The plan of care is altered appropriately. When outcomes are met, that portion of the plan is discontinued.

Skill 25.1 Measuring Intake and Output

 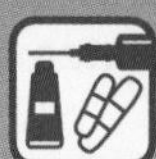 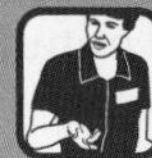 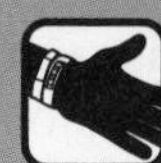 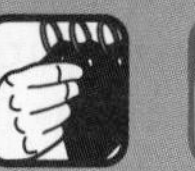 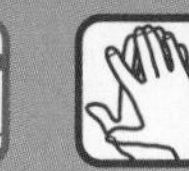 

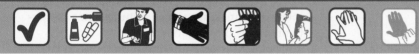

I & O are measured and recorded whenever a patient has a potential or an actual fluid balance problem. The primary care provider may order I & O monitoring, or the nurse may independently decide to monitor the patient's I & O. Usually, I & O are measured and recorded for every patient who is receiving intravenous (IV) therapy or has a nasogastric (NG) tube attached to suction, a urinary catheter, or other drainage tube.

Supplies

- I & O record sheet
- Bedpan or urinal
- Graduated measuring container
- "Hat" toilet collection device
- Gloves
- Pen or pencil

Review and carry out the Standard Steps in Appendix A.

NURSING ACTION *(RATIONALE)*

Assessment (Data Collection)

1. Determine need for recording I & O. *(There may be an order or a need to perform this nursing function.)*
2. Assess what equipment will be needed in the room to measure and record I & O. *(Ensures that measuring container and I & O sheet are in the room when needed.)*

Planning

3. Note on I & O sheet all items that need to be recorded. *(Reminds everyone caring for patient that IV medications, NG tube irrigations, and wound drainage all need to be recorded.)*
4. Place a sign above toilet stating that I & O is to be recorded. Tell personnel to record all intake. *(Sign above the toilet alerts personnel to measure all urine before disposal. Intake will be recorded.)*
5. Ask patient to use the call light when urine has been collected. *(Alerts personnel to measure the urine.)*

Implementation

6. Explain the procedure to patient and ask that each amount of fluid taken between meals be recorded. *(Patient must understand the procedure to adhere to the recording of I & O.)*
7. Calculate fluid intake before removing a food tray from the room. *(A more accurate count is obtained than when relying on memory.)*
8. Assess fluid intake each time you are in the room. *(It is easier for patients to remember what they drank if questioned soon afterward.)*
9. Don gloves and measure and record all output. *(Gloves reduce transfer of microorganisms. Output includes urine, diarrheal stool, emesis, gastric drainage, wound drainage, and excessive perspiration. A graduated container measures all liquid output accurately.)*
10. Dispose of the output in the commode and clean the equipment; remove gloves and perform hand hygiene. *(Removes a medium for growth of pathogens; reduces transfer of microorganisms.)*
11. Note the amount of output in the correct column on the I & O sheet. *(Writing down the amount immediately helps provide an accurate record.)*
12. Note additional types of intake on the I & O sheet as they occur. *(Jotting down the amount of an IV infusion or the amount of gastric irrigant instilled helps maintain an accurate record of intake.)*
13. At the end of the shift, mark and record the amount of gastric suction secretions, wound drainage in collection devices, and chest drainage. Empty the urine collection bag and measure and record the output. If the suction collection container is full, dispose of the canister according to agency protocol and install a new one. Total the amount of output for the shift. *(For accuracy, all output must be recorded on the I & O sheet. Collec-*

tion containers are emptied; the level at the end of the shift is marked with the date and time or containers are replaced if they are full and disposable. All types of output are added together for the shift total.)

14. At the end of the shift, calculate the amount of IV fluid intake and add it to the intake side of the I & O sheet. *(All IV fluid infused is included as intake.)*
15. After the shift totals have been calculated, enter the amounts on the I & O flow sheet. At the end of a 24-hour period, total the amounts for all shifts for both intake and output. *(The total I & O amount over 24 hours presents the most accurate picture of the patient's fluid balance. What constitutes a normal I & O depends on the patient's condition and any restrictions imposed.)*
16. Place a new shift I & O sheet in the patient's room; make certain the name and room number are on the sheet. *(A record form must be available for the recording of the I & O).*

Evaluation

17. Determine whether I & O are within normal limits. Compare the amounts to see if there is any indication of a fluid imbalance. Compare the total with the totals from the previous 2 days to see if either intake or output is increasing. Compare I & O 24 hour totals with daily weights to see that they "match." *(If the output is greater or less than the intake, the patient may have a fluid imbalance. Comparison of the totals shows whether there is an increase in intake or output; 24 hour I & O totals should mirror the trends of daily weight: for example, if a patient is 2 L "fluid positive," you expect to see weight gain of 2 kg.)*

Documentation

18. Documentation is done on the I & O sheet or on the computer flow sheet.

Critical Thinking Questions

1. What would you do if you recorded the patient's intake for breakfast and 30 minutes later, the patient vomits into the toilet?
2. Your patient is on a full liquid diet, has an IV running at 100 mL/h, and receives an IV piggyback medication of 50 mL at 2:00 pm. They have a urinary catheter. What would you include as output on your shift record? What would you include as intake?

I & O, Intake and output.

Get Ready for the NCLEX Examination!

Key Points

- Body fluids are intracellular or extracellular and shift from one compartment to another.
- Fluid moves from compartment to compartment by diffusion, osmosis, filtration, and active transport.
- Fluids are lost from the body through urine, feces, expired air, and perspiration; 24-hour output is approximately 2500 mL.
- Fluid is taken in or produced from liquids, digestion of food, or cell metabolism; this should total 2500 mL/day.
- The kidney is the major organ regulating fluid and electrolyte balance.
- Daily fluid intake in the adult must be at least 1500 mL/day to maintain homeostasis.
- Common causes of fluid volume deficit are vomiting, diarrhea, gastric suction, wound and fistula drainage, and burn injuries.
- A fluid volume deficit results in dehydration.
- The older adults and the very young can become dehydrated quickly; and can present differently.
- Signs of fluid volume excess are weight gain; edema; elevated blood pressure; slow, bounding pulse; and crackles in the lungs.
- Causes of edema include kidney failure, heart failure, liver failure, and hormonal disorders.
- Tracking daily weight is a method of determining fluid-volume excess or deficit.
- Sodium is the predominant electrolyte in the ECF; potassium is the predominant electrolyte in the ICF.
- Whenever a water imbalance exists, there will be an accompanying sodium imbalance.
- Hyponatremia is a frequent cause of hospitalization of older adults.
- It is important to know the causes of electrolyte imbalance, the normal range for the major electrolytes, and the signs and symptoms of imbalance.
- Acid-base balance is necessary to maintain homeostasis in the body.
- Normal serum pH is 7.35 to 7.45.
- Three mechanisms control pH in the body: the blood buffer system, the lungs, and the kidneys.
- An increase in hydrogen ions results in acidosis, as evidenced by a decrease in pH. There are two types of acidosis: respiratory and metabolic.
- Acidosis depresses the nervous system, causing headache, lethargy, weakness, and confusion, and can progress to coma and death.
- A decrease in hydrogen ions results in alkalosis, as evidenced by an increase in pH. There are two types of alkalosis: respiratory and metabolic.
- Alkalosis causes irritability of the nervous system with restlessness, muscle twitching, and tingling and numbness of the fingers; it can progress to tetany, seizures, and coma.

- Dependent edema is assessed by checking for pitting by pressing a fingertip against the tissue at a bony prominence.
- Fluid restriction is often necessary for the patient who has excess fluid volume.
- Accurately recording I & O is essential in caring for a patient with a fluid imbalance.

Additional Learning Resources

SG Go to your Study Guide for additional learning activities to help you master this chapter content.

evolve Go to your Evolve website at http://evolve.elsevier.com/Williams/fundamental for additional online resources.

Online Resources

- *American Association for the History of Nursing*, www.aahn.org
- *Florence Nightingale Museum*, www.florence-nightingale.co.uk
- *National Association for Practical Nurse Education and Service*, www.napnes.org
- *National Council of State Boards of Nursing*, www.ncsbn.org
- *National Federation of Licensed Practical Nurses*, www.nflpn.org
- *American Nurses Association*, www.nursingworld.org

Review Questions for the NCLEX Examination

Choose the ***best*** *answer for each question.*

1. You are starting an intravenous infusion with D5½NS at 150 mL/h. If the IV tubing delivers 15 drops/mL, you would start the infusion at:
   1. 37.5 or 38 gtt/min.
   2. 25 gtt/min.
   3. 31 gtt/min.
   4. 21 gtt/min.
2. The older adult is at greater risk for dehydration than the middle-aged adult is because: *(Select all that apply.)*
   1. Older adults have a diminished sense of thirst.
   2. Older adults have less muscle mass as years advance.
   3. The older adult's body is almost 80% water.
   4. Compensatory mechanisms work less efficiently.
   5. Older adults have increased surface area and more evaporative losses.
3. An 82-year-old male patient is admitted with vomiting and diarrhea. On assessment, you note that he is apprehensive and his skin is cool, dry, and pale. His pulse is rapid, and his blood pressure is lower than normal. These symptoms are indicative of:
   1. Fluid overload.
   2. Electrolyte imbalance.
   3. Dehydration.
   4. Intestinal flu.
4. Your male patient has been ill with pneumonia and was admitted yesterday to start IV antibiotic therapy. He has a history of heart failure and is taking digitalis and furosemide. He has not been eating well the past 3 days because he was feeling so bad. The primary care provider ordered fluids and daily laboratory work yesterday. The patient seems more confused this morning and is very weak. His urine output has fallen. To determine what is causing these symptoms, you would first:
   1. Check the morning electrolyte levels.
   2. Call his primary care provider.
   3. Check yesterday's laboratory results.
   4. Ask for an order for extra potassium.
5. A patient with heart failure has lost 4.6 lb. This represents a fluid loss of approximately:
   1. 1500 mL.
   2. 1 L.
   3. 650 mL.
   4. 2 L.
6. Patients who are undergoing diuretic therapy to decrease excess body fluid tend to lose potassium. If too much potassium is lost, the patient will have which electrolyte and acid-base imbalance?
   1. Hyperkalemia, metabolic acidosis
   2. Hypokalemia, metabolic alkalosis
   3. Hyponatremia, metabolic acidosis
   4. Hypernatremia, metabolic alkalosis
7. One of the best methods to assess whether peripheral edema is increasing or decreasing is to:
   1. Compare intake with output over several days.
   2. Weigh the patient daily and compare weights.
   3. Use a fingertip to assess for pitting edema of the tissue.
   4. Measure the circumference of the affected extremity in the same location each day.

Critical Thinking Activities

Read each clinical scenario and discuss the questions with your classmates.

Scenario A

George Torres is admitted with a head injury. He is comatose and is breathing rapidly. His blood gases show a pH of 7.37, $PaCO_2$ of 32 mm Hg, and HCO_3- of 26 mEq/L. Compare these gases to normal values. What type of acid-base imbalance does this patient have?

Scenario B

Lena Mason, who has diabetes, is admitted in a stuporous condition. Her blood gases show a pH of 7.33, PaCO2 of 40 mm Hg, and HCO3− of 20 mEq/L. What type of acid-base imbalance does this patient have?

Scenario C

Douglas Byrd is on fluid restrictions and is to have no more than 1200 mL of fluid per day. This is his third day on restrictions, and he is complaining bitterly of being thirsty. What creative ways can you think of to decrease his thirst while staying within his fluid allotment?

Scenario D

Ramon Hernandez is admitted in a confused state from his home. His neighbor says he has been ill for several days. What would you do to assess him for dehydration and electrolyte imbalance?

chapter

26 Concepts of Basic Nutrition and Cultural Considerations

http://evolve.elsevier.com/Williams/fundamental

Objectives

Upon completing this chapter, you should be able to do the following:

1. Review the structure and function of the gastrointestinal system.
2. Use the components of the United States Department of Agriculture (USDA) MyPlate website to assist patients in planning their diets.
3. List medical conditions that may occur because of protein, calorie, vitamin, or mineral deficiency or excess.
4. Discuss the function of proteins, carbohydrates, fats, vitamins, minerals, and water in the human body.
5. Identify food sources of proteins, carbohydrates, fats, vitamins, and minerals.
6. Identify a variety of factors that influence nutrition.
7. Explore cultural influences on nutritional practices.
8. Compare nutritional needs throughout life's stages.

Clinical Practice

1. Identify patients at risk for nutritional deficits.
2. Complete a nutritional assessment on an assigned patient.
3. Use therapeutic communication with a patient while discussing needed nutritional modification.
4. Develop a patient education plan for a prescribed therapeutic diet.

Key Terms

amino acids (ă-MĒ-nō, p. 462)
body mass index (BMI) (p. 477)
carbohydrates (kăr-bō-HĪ-drātz, p. 464)
carotenoids (kă-RŌ-tĕ-nŏyds, p. 466)
catabolism (kă-TĂB-ō-lĭzm, p. 459)
cholesterol (kō-LĔS-tĕr-ŏl) (p. 466)
colostrum (kō-LŌ-strŭm, p. 473)
complementary proteins (kŏm-plĕ-MĔN-tă-rē, p. 462)
complete proteins (p. 462)
digestion (dī-GĔS-chŭn, p. 459)
essential amino acids (p. 462)
fat (p. 465)
fiber (FĪ-bĕr, p. 465)
fructose (FRŪK-tōs, p. 464)
glucose (GLŪ-kōs, p. 464)
glycemic index (p. 464)
incomplete proteins (p. 462)
kosher (KŌ-shĕr, p. 472)
kwashiorkor (kwăsh-ē-ŌR-kōr, p. 463)
lacto-ovo-vegetarian (LĂK-tō-Ō-vō-vĕ-jĭ-TĂ-rē-ăn, p. 463)
lactose (LĂK-tōs, p. 464)
lactovegetarian (LĂK-tō-vĕ-jĭ-TĂ-rē-ăn p. 463)
malnutrition (măl-nū-TRĬ-shŭn, p. 463)
marasmus (mă-RĂZ-mŭs, p. 463)
metabolism (mĕ-TĂB-ō-lĭzm, p. 459)
minerals (MĬN-ĕr-ălz, p. 467)
MyPlate (p. 460)
nonessential amino acids (p. 462)
nutrients (NŪ-trē-ĕntz, p. 462)
nutrition (nū-TRĬ-shŭn, p. 458)
obesity (ō-BĒ-sĭ-tē, p. 475)
Omega-3 fatty acid (p. 466)
protein (PRŌ-tēn, p. 462)
saturated fats (săt-ū-RĀ-tĕd, p. 466)
sucrose (SŪ-krōs, p. 464)
unsaturated fats (p. 466)
vegan (VĒ-găn, p. 463)
vegetarians (vĕ-jĕ-TĂ-rē-ănz, p. 463)
vitamins (VĪ-tĭ-mĭnz, p. 466)

Concepts Covered in This Chapter

- Acid-base balance
- Cognition
- Culture
- Fluid and electrolyte balance
- Glucose regulation
- Immunity
- Nutrition
- Patient education
- Tissue Integrity

Nutrition is the sum of processes involved in taking in nutrients and absorbing and using them. Nutrition is concerned with those properties of food that build sound bodies and promote health. A balanced diet containing adequate amounts of the essential nutrients for proper body function must be consumed for good health. The functions of nutrients include providing energy, regulating body processes, and building, maintaining, and repairing tissue.

Nutrients from food are made available to all body cells through the process of **catabolism** (the process by which large molecules are broken down into smaller molecules to make energy available to the organism). The body's **metabolism** enables the absorbed nutrients to enter the blood following **digestion** (the process of converting food into chemical substances that can be absorbed into the blood and used by the body tissue).

OVERVIEW OF THE STRUCTURE AND FUNCTION OF THE GASTROINTESTINAL SYSTEM

WHICH STRUCTURES ARE INVOLVED IN THE GASTROINTESTINAL (DIGESTIVE) SYSTEM?

- The gastrointestinal system is composed of the mouth, tongue, teeth, pharynx, esophagus, stomach, small intestine, large intestine, and anus (Fig. 26.1).
- Accessory organs include the salivary glands, liver, gallbladder, and pancreas.
- The mouth is the first part of the digestive tract. It contains the teeth and the tongue and it receives secretions from the salivary glands.
- The tongue is composed mostly of skeletal muscle. It is the largest, most movable organ of the mouth.
- Adults have 32 permanent teeth. Teeth are categorized as incisors, cuspids, bicuspids, and molars.

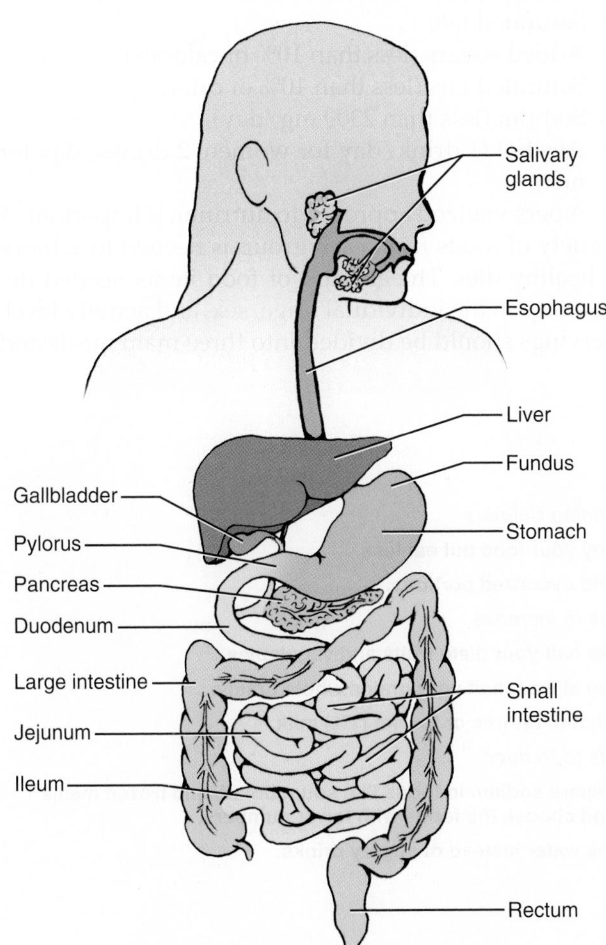

FIGURE 26.1 The gastrointestinal system.

- The parotid glands are the largest of the salivary glands. One is located on each side of the body, anterior and inferior to the ear.
- The pharynx is a fibromuscular passageway that connects the nasal and oral cavities to the larynx and esophagus. Food is forced into the pharynx by the tongue.
- The esophagus is a collapsible muscular tube about 20 cm long. It is the passageway for movement of food to the stomach.
- The stomach is located in the upper left quadrant of the abdomen. The adult stomach has an average capacity of 1.5 L.
- The small intestine includes the duodenum, jejunum, and ileum. It is 2.5 cm in diameter and 6 meters long.
- The large intestine includes the cecum, ascending colon, transverse colon, descending colon, sigmoid colon, rectum, and anus. It is about 2.5 to 7 cm in diameter and 1.5 meters long.
- The liver is a large, reddish-brown organ located in the upper right quadrant of the abdomen.
- The gallbladder is a pear-shaped sac that is attached to the surface of the liver by the cystic duct.
- The pancreas is a flat, elongated organ located along the posterior abdominal wall. The head of the pancreas is on the right side in the curve of the duodenum. The tail is on the left side, next to the spleen.

WHAT ARE THE FUNCTIONS OF THE ORGANS OF THE GASTROINTESTINAL SYSTEM?

- The mouth receives food and breaks it into small particles by chewing and mixing it with saliva.
- The tongue manipulates food in the mouth for chewing and mixing with saliva.
- The tongue helps position food for swallowing. Taste buds are also located on the tongue.
- The teeth are used for grasping, tearing, crushing, and grinding food.
- The salivary glands secrete saliva into the mouth for mixing with food during chewing. Saliva breaks down food for tasting. Saliva plays a role in the chemical digestion of starches.
- The pharynx serves as a passageway for food to enter the esophagus through swallowing.
- The esophagus is the passageway for food to enter the stomach. The lining of the esophagus secretes mucus to ease the passage of food.
- The stomach is a temporary storage place for food. The churning action of muscles of the stomach mixes food with gastric juices. Food is changed to a semiliquid state for passage to the small intestine. Gastric acids begin digestion of proteins. Vitamin B_{12} is absorbed in the stomach through the action of intrinsic factor secreted from the stomach wall.
- The small intestine receives food from the stomach and secretions from the liver and pancreas. The process of digestion is finished in the small intestine.

Nutrients are absorbed and residue is passed to the large intestine.
- The large intestine is the site of absorption of fluid and electrolytes and the elimination of waste products.
- The liver produces and secretes bile into the small intestine for digestion of fats. The liver plays a major role in digestion of fats, carbohydrates, and proteins through its metabolic functions.
- The gallbladder stores and concentrates bile. Fatty foods in the duodenum stimulate the flow of bile from the gallbladder to the duodenum.
- The pancreas secretes digestive juices into the small intestine for digestion of carbohydrates, proteins, and fats. The pancreas also secretes insulin for utilization of glucose.

WHAT CHANGES IN THE DIGESTIVE SYSTEM OCCUR WITH AGING?

- Increased dental caries and tooth loss may lead to decreased ability to chew food normally.
- Decreased sense of taste and smell may lead to loss of appetite.
- Decreased gag reflex may increase the risk of choking and aspiration.
- Decreased muscle tone at sphincters may increase heartburn or risk of esophageal reflux.
- Decreased gastric secretions may interfere with digestion of food.
- Decreased peristalsis may increase the risk of constipation or bowel impaction.

DIETARY GUIDELINES

USDA MYPLATE AND THE 2015 DIETARY GUIDELINES FOR AMERICANS

The **MyPlate** was developed by the USDA's Center for Nutrition Policy and Promotion to promote healthy diets for all Americans. This food guidance system shows the five food groups necessary for good nutrition and explains the use of each component. MyPlate is consumer friendly and easy to remember because it visually demonstrates that about half of your typical plate of food should come from fruits and vegetables (Fig. 26.2). In addition, the US Department of Agriculture (2015) publishes dietary guidelines every 5 years. The 2015-2020 guidelines include the following recommendations:
- Follow a healthy eating pattern across the life span.
- Focus on variety, nutrient density, and amount.
- Limit calories from added sugars and saturated fats and reduce sodium intake.
- Stick to healthier food and beverage choices.
- Support healthy eating patterns for all.

The guidelines further define a healthy eating pattern to include:
- Vegetables: from all subgroups (dark green, red, orange, legumes, and starchy)
- Fruits: especially whole fruits
- Grains: at least half consisting of whole grains
- Dairy: fat-free or low and/or fortified soy beverages
- Protein: including seafood, poultry, eggs, legumes, nuts/seeds, and soy
- Oils

The guidelines further define a healthy eating pattern to *limit*:
- Saturated fats
- Added sugars (less than 10% of calories)
- Saturated fats (less than 10% of calories)
- Sodium (less than 2300 mg/day)
- Alcohol (1 drink/day for women; 2 drinks/day for men)

A personalized approach to nutrition is important. A variety of foods from each group is needed to achieve a healthy diet. The amount of food items needed depend upon the individual's age, sex, and activity level. Servings should be divided into three main meals and

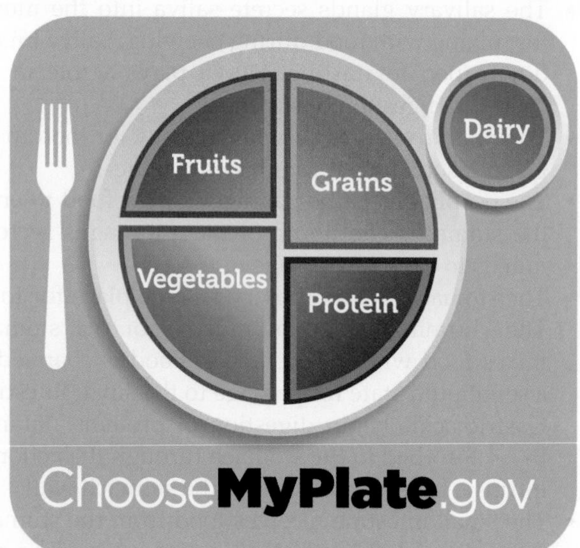

Balancing Calories
- **Enjoy your food but eat less.**
- **Avoid oversized portions.**

Foods to Increase
- **Make half your plate fruits and vegetables.**
- **Make at least half your grains whole grains.**
- **Switch to fat-free or low fat (1%) milk.**

Foods to Reduce
- **Compare sodium in foods like soup, bread, and frozen meals – and choose the foods with lower numbers.**
- **Drink water instead of sugary drinks.**

FIGURE 26.2 The USDA MyPlate. (Copyright US Department of Agriculture [www.choosemyplate.gov].)

two snacks. People of all ages are encouraged to adjust their exercise level and food intake to maintain body weight within the recommended limits. The American Heart Association updated their recommendations for diet and lifestyle in 2015 (Box 26.1).

It is recommended that 8 oz of cooked seafood should be consumed weekly.

An alliance of federal and state agencies, the Healthy People Consortium, revises its nutrition-related objectives every 10 years. The current objectives *Healthy People 2020* address, among other things, the issue of disparities in risk for nutrition-related disease among ethnic minorities and low-income groups. Issues such as obesity and food insecurity (limited access to safe, nutritious food) have been evident in the low-income, Hispanic, African American, Native American, and Asian/Pacific Islander American communities, especially among females. A major focus on meeting the objectives of this area of *Healthy People 2020* includes emphasis on diet and activity for all population groups to ensure that all individuals have access to nutritionally adequate foods (HealthyPeople.gov, 2015).

Box 26.1 American Heart Association 2015 Diet and Lifestyle Recommendations

1. Use up at least as many calories as you take in.
   - Know how many calories you are eating and drinking.
   - Increase physical activity as needed to match number of calories consumed.
   - If you are trying not to gain weight, do not consume more calories than you know you can burn up every day.
   - Plan for 150 minutes of moderate physical activity or 75 minutes of vigorous activity per week (or you can do a combination of both). If you cannot do long periods, try to do a minimum of 10 min sessions of activity spread out over a week to equal the recommended amount.
2. Eat a variety of nutritious foods from all of the food groups. Choose foods such as vegetables, fruits, whole grain products, fat-free or low fat dairy products, and nuts and legumes. Eat skinless fish at least twice a week, especially fish high in omega-3 fatty acids (salmon, trout, and herring), and use non-tropical cooking oils to reduce your risk for coronary artery disease.
3. Eat less of the nutrient-poor foods and limit how much saturated fat, *trans*-fat, cholesterol, and sodium you eat.
   - Choose lean meat and poultry without skin and prepare them without added saturated and *trans*-fat.
   - Select fat-free, 1% fat, and low fat dairy products.
   - Cut back on foods containing hydrogenated vegetable oils to reduce *trans*-fat in your diet.
   - Reduce foods high in dietary cholesterol. Aim to eat less than 300 mg of cholesterol each day.
   - Cut back on foods and beverages high in calories and low in nutrients or with added sugars.
   - Choose and prepare foods with little or no salt; aim to eat less than 1500 mg of sodium per day.
   - If you drink alcohol, drink in moderation. That means one drink per day for females and two drinks per day for males.
   - Follow the American Heart Association recommendations when you eat out, and keep an eye on your portion sizes.

Health Promotion

Healthy People 2020: Objectives for Nutrition and Weight Focus

HEALTHIER FOOD ACCESS

- Increase the number of states with nutrition standards for foods and beverages provided to preschool-aged children in childcare
- Increase the proportion of schools that offer nutritious foods and beverages outside of school meals
- Increase the number of states that have state-level policies that incentivize food retail outlets to provide foods that are encouraged by the Dietary Guidelines for Americans
- Increase the proportion of Americans who have access to a food retail outlet that sells a variety of foods that are encouraged by the Dietary Guidelines for Americans

HEALTH CARE AND WORKSITE SETTINGS

- Increase the proportion of primary care physicians who regularly assess body mass index (BMI) in their adult patients
- Increase the proportion of physician office visits that include counseling or education related to nutrition or weight
- Increase the proportion of worksites that offer nutrition or weight management or counseling

WEIGHT STATUS

- Increase the proportion of adults who are at a healthy weight
- Reduce the proportion of adults who are obese
- Reduce the proportion of children and adolescents who are considered obese
- Prevent inappropriate weight gain in youth and adults

FOOD INSECURITY

- Eliminate very low food security among children
- Reduce household food insecurity and, in doing so, reduce hunger

FOOD AND NUTRIENT CONSUMPTION

- Increase the variety and contribution of fruits to the diet of the population aged 2 years and older
- Increase the variety and contribution of vegetables to the diets of the population aged 2 years and older
- Increase the contribution of whole grains to the diets of the population aged 2 years and older
- Reduce consumption of calories from solid fats and added sugars in the population aged 2 years and older
- Reduce consumption of saturated fat in the population aged 2 years and older
- Reduce consumption of sodium in the population aged 2 years and older
- Increase consumption of calcium in the population aged 2 years and older

IRON DEFICIENCY

- Reduce iron deficiency among young children and females of childbearing age
- Reduce iron deficiency among pregnant females

Source: http://www.healthypeople.gov/2020/topics-objectives/topic/nutrition-and-weight-status/objectives

Six **nutrients** (biochemical substances used by the body that must be supplied in adequate amounts from foods consumed) are essential to normal functioning: proteins, carbohydrates, fats, vitamins, minerals, and water.

PROTEIN

FUNCTIONS OF PROTEIN

A constant supply of **protein** is essential to meet the body's need to build and replace tissue and cells. During times of illness and after surgery, injuries, burns, or blood loss, more protein is required to help rebuild cells and tissues. Protein plays a role in maintaining fluid balance and acid-base balance; transporting nutrients; and producing antibodies, enzymes, and hormones. Protein is also a source of energy for the body. **Protein supplies 4 calories per gram.**

Proteins are composed of **amino acids** (organic compounds that are the chief components of proteins). Amino acids are the building blocks of proteins. Proteins consist of long chains of amino acids linked together. The body can produce some amino acids to build its own proteins. Nine amino acids are considered **essential amino acids** because they must be consumed through food sources. The essential amino acids are indispensable and cannot be synthesized in the body.

The nonessential amino acids are important to health but can be synthesized by the healthy well-nourished body. The liver can manufacture 11 amino acids; these are considered **nonessential amino acids.** For body cells to build proteins, they must have all amino acids. The body only stores protein in the "amino acid" pool. The body protects its protein stores by first using carbohydrates, and then fat, for energy. If these are low or absent, the body uses dietary protein, and then tissue protein, for energy.

FOOD SOURCES OF PROTEIN

Food sources of protein include meats, poultry, fish, eggs, dairy products, cereals, grains, legumes, and most vegetables. Animal sources (red meat, eggs, milk and milk products, poultry, and fish) are **complete (or high quality) proteins** because they contain all nine essential amino acids. The World Health Organization recently classified processed meat, however, as a carcinogen, and red meat as a "probably carcinogen" (Simon, 2015). Plant sources of protein are **incomplete (or low quality) proteins** because they do not contain all essential amino acids. The only plant source of all nine essential amino acids is soybeans. Soybeans and soy products can be a less expensive substitute for meat in the diet while supplying high quality protein. Combining plant sources of foods, or **complementary proteins,** can provide complete protein intake in the diet (e.g., cereal with milk, beans with rice, and peanut butter sandwiches).

Health Promotion

The Essential and Nonessential Amino Acids

ESSENTIAL AMINO ACIDS	NONESSENTIAL AMINO ACIDS
Histidine	Alanine
Isoleucine	Arginine
Leucine	Asparagine
Lysine	Aspartic acid
Methionine	Cysteine
Phenylalanine	Cystine
Threonine	Glutamic acid
Tryptophan	Glutamine
Valine	Glycine
	Proline
	Serine
	Tyrosine

DIETARY REFERENCE INTAKES OF PROTEIN

Dietary Reference Intakes (DRIs) have been developed by the US National Academy of Sciences to provide guidelines for estimating nutrient intake for planning and evaluating diets of healthy people. Healthy adults require 0.8 g of protein per kilogram of body weight. **The average DRI is 46 to 56 g of protein per day for the healthy adult.** This can be achieved through a combination of meat and plant sources. Protein intake should be approximately 10% to 15% of the total daily calories. The typical American diet is high in protein (about 75 g/day). A serving of protein is, for example, a 3-oz portion of meat or a serving of beans equivalent to ½ cup of dry beans. A 3-oz serving is about the size of a deck of cards.

? Think Critically

What size portion of meat is typical in your diet? Do you limit beans to ½ cup dry? Do you eat more than a 3-oz portion of meat?

The DRI for protein may vary depending on activity level, state of health, and availability of protein food sources. Very active adults such as athletes and bodybuilders may raise their DRI to 1.2 to 1.4 g/kg, or up to a maximum of 1.7 to 1.8 g/kg. **The body requires more protein (1) during times of illness or injury, for such processes as cell repair and antibody production, and (2) during times of rapid tissue growth such as pregnancy and lactation.** Individuals who are vegetarians or who live in areas where meat sources of protein are scarce may need to consume up to 1.6 g/kg of complementary proteins to meet complete protein needs by combining foods.

To determine the protein requirement per day for a healthy adult, calculate as follows:

$$\text{Weight in Pounds} \div 2.2 = \_\_\_\_\_\text{kg} \ (1\text{kg} = 2.2\text{lb})$$
$$\_\_\_\_\_\text{kg} \times 0.8 = \_\_\_\_\_\text{g of protein}$$

PROTEIN DEFICIENCY

In many nations throughout the world, the availability of protein-rich food is limited. Millions of children under age 5 are affected by lack of protein intake. This lack of protein can lead to permanent disabilities because of the fast rate of brain growth that occurs during childhood. Extreme protein deficiency results in the conditions of marasmus and kwashiorkor. **Marasmus** is a form of protein energy and nutrient **malnutrition** (a disorder of nutrition related to an unbalanced diet, malabsorption, or a lack of assimilation of nutrients) occurring chiefly in the first year of life, characterized by growth retardation and wasting of subcutaneous fat and muscle. Marasmus is the result of severe starvation. The body uses its carbohydrate and fat sources for energy. When these are depleted, protein muscle mass is used for energy. Catabolism of muscle mass for energy results in heart, lung, and kidney damage. Uncorrected, marasmus can lead to death.

Kwashiorkor is a condition occurring in infants and young children soon after weaning from breast milk. It is due to severe protein deficiency. **Kwashiorkor differs from marasmus in that adequate energy from other nutrients may be consumed; however, the diet is deficient in protein.** Symptoms of kwashiorkor include edema, skin pigment changes, impaired growth and development, distention of the abdomen, and liver changes. Low protein intake leads to changes in water balance, which leads to edema. Protein is the main component of hair; therefore, deficiency results in changes in the color and texture of the hair. The liver becomes fatty and loses its ability to function. Fatty enlargement of the liver results in an enlarged abdomen.

PROTEIN EXCESS

The average American diet supplies 1½ to 2 times the DRI for protein. Athletes and very active individuals may consume higher levels. High protein diets for people who do not require a protein increase may be stressful to the liver and kidneys. The kidneys must rid the body of excess waste products resulting from an increased protein intake. Protein is metabolized by the liver. Liver function may be strained with the excess load of protein to metabolize. High protein diets, especially from meat sources, can lead to excess fat in the diet. High fat diets are associated with increased risk of obesity, heart disease, and certain types of cancer (colon, breast, pancreas, and prostate).

Health Promotion

Although studies are inconclusive, evidence suggests that certain food components can decrease cancer risk, including:

- Phytochemicals (e.g., carotenoids): found in brightly colored or strongly flavored vegetables and fruit
- Antioxidants (e.g., vitamin C, vitamin E, beta-carotene): found in raspberries, strawberries, blueberries, and many other foods
- Omega-3 fatty acids: found in fish, vegetable oil, flax seed, and leafy vegetables

VEGETARIAN DIETS

Many people have become **vegetarians** as a means to maintain desired weight and decrease the amount of animal fat in the diet. Cultural, religious, and personal factors (e.g., objection to the killing of animals for food) also influence a person's choice of a vegetarian diet. The primary types of vegetarian diets are as follows:

- **Lacto-ovo-vegetarian:** Dairy products, eggs, and plant foods are included in the diet.
- **Lactovegetarian:** Eggs are excluded. Dairy products and plant foods are included.
- **Vegan:** All animal food sources, including honey, are excluded.

A vegetarian diet must be planned to include essential nutrients. Individuals choosing this dietary practice should engage in research and consult a nutrition specialist to ensure that nutritional needs are met. The well planned vegetarian diet is believed to offer health benefits such as reduced risk of heart disease, hypertension, diabetes, cancer, and obesity. The challenge is to plan meals that provide adequate levels of complete proteins, vitamins, and minerals. Vegans, in particular, may have a diet deficient in vitamin B_6, vitamin B_{12}, iron, zinc, calcium, riboflavin, and vitamin D. The more limited the vegetarian diet, the greater the risk of nutritional deficiencies.

Nutrient requirements can be met by combining categories of food to meet protein needs by following a modified version of the MyPlate. Some combinations that provide a good protein source are whole grains and legumes; legumes and nuts or seeds; or whole grains, legumes, nuts, or seeds and dairy products. Soybeans are a legume high in protein and contain all nine essential amino acids. Soy products include tofu, legumes, protein powders, and soy milk. Mineral deficits can be avoided by eating dark green leafy vegetables; adding fruits with high levels of vitamin C to meals to aid in absorption of iron; or taking dietary supplements of calcium and vitamin B_{12}, since these may be difficult to obtain in the absence of animal food sources.

Individuals who follow vegetarian diets meet their protein needs without consuming meat products by combining plant sources of food to achieve a complete protein intake. Examples of using complementary proteins include red beans and rice, peanut butter on whole wheat bread, bean soup with cornbread, or stir-fried vegetables with tofu. In the 1970s, it was thought that it was critical for each meal to contain a combination of incomplete proteins to achieve a complete protein intake. Now it is known that a nutritious diet can exist when incomplete proteins are combined over a 24-hour period by eating a variety of protein-rich plant-based foods (Cullum-Dugan, 2014).

 Think Critically

Did You Know?

Plant-based diets have been shown to reduce cholesterol levels and body weight in obese children (Zolot, 2015).

 Think Critically

What nonmeat foods that you like could be combined during a 24-hour period to provide complete and adequate protein?

CARBOHYDRATES

Carbohydrates are the body's main source of energy. Carbohydrates should make up 60% of the daily caloric intake. **Each gram of carbohydrate supplies 4 calories.** The three major forms of carbohydrates are simple carbohydrates, complex carbohydrates, and fiber. Complex carbohydrates should make up about 90% of the total proportion of carbohydrates consumed. This category of carbohydrates contains fiber and other nutrients. Simple carbohydrates tend to be nutrient poor.

FUNCTIONS OF CARBOHYDRATES

Carbohydrates are a quick source of energy and are easily converted to glucose, the fuel for the body's cells. Carbohydrates are important to the function of internal organs, the nervous system, and muscles. Carbohydrates are also needed to regulate protein and fat metabolism. They help to fight infection and promote growth of body tissues. High fiber intake is helpful in treating certain gastrointestinal disorders (e.g., constipation and hemorrhoids) and reducing blood cholesterol synthesis and levels.

SIMPLE CARBOHYDRATES

Glucose is the metabolized form of sugar in the body. It is found in table sugar **(sucrose),** fruit sugar **(fructose),** and milk sugar **(lactose).** Glucose is chemically nearly identical to dextrose; these words are used interchangeably. All of these simple carbohydrates are quickly absorbed into the bloodstream as a ready source of energy for the cells. Sucrose is the major sweetener found in foods such as candy, ice cream, cookies, and cakes. High fructose corn syrup is added to many foods; it adds calories and should be avoided whenever possible. Other forms of sugar added to foods are sucrose, lactose, maltose, and dextrin. The typical American diet is high in simple carbohydrates. Although simple sugars cause a quick rise in blood glucose, the level falls rapidly and can result in a return to a hunger state.

Think Critically

Did You Know?

Many people believe they are being "healthy" drinking (or serving their children) juice every day—but juice actually increases your risk of Type 2 diabetes about 21% because of its high **glycemic index** (the rate at which carbohydrates boost blood glucose) (Roeder, 2013). In fact, Canada is moving away from endorsing juice as equivalent to fruit in its guidelines (Kirkey, 2015). Eating the actual fruit, however, does not pose the same risk, and it provides you with vital fiber and antioxidants. Get rid of those juice boxes and hand the kid a tangerine instead!

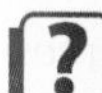 Think Critically

Can you identify hidden sugar content of foods by reading the food label (Fig. 26.3)?

COMPLEX CARBOHYDRATES (STARCHES)

Complex carbohydrates are foods such as breads, pasta, cereal, potatoes, and rice. They are broken down into simple sugars for digestion, absorption, and use by the body. Starches provide a more consistent blood glucose level than simple sugars do. Experts recommend that 85% to 95% of carbohydrates consumed should be complex, and very little should be simple sugars. Carbohydrate content varies dramatically among foods: for example, a half cup of strawberries only has 5 carbs, whereas slice of pecan pie yields a whopping 65 carbs (primarily simple carbohydrate). On the contrary, one-half cup of red beans and rice has 40 carbs but they are primarily complex carbohydrate (balanced with protein), so numbers alone do not tell the entire story.

RECOMMENDATIONS FOR INTAKE

Children and adults need a minimum of 130 g of carbohydrates per day. Weight-loss plans such as the Atkins diet and the South Beach diet stress low carbohydrate consumption. Several studies suggest that there may be benefits to low carbohydrate diets as a means for weight loss. Compared with other meal plans, these diets may be effective for weight loss, maintaining weight loss, and improvement of high-density lipoprotein and triglyceride levels. Recent research is suggesting that simple carbohydrates, particularly fructose and sucrose, may play a greater role in the development of coronary heart disease than do saturated fats (DiNicolantonio et al., 2016). Most Americans need to increase complex carbohydrates and decrease consumption of simple sugar.

 Think Critically

Can you determine your carbohydrate intake? Write down your food intake for the past 24 hours. Calculate total calories. What was the percentage of simple and complex carbohydrates? Divide carbohydrate calories by total calories.

Nutrition Facts

Serving Size 1 cup (228g)
Servings Per Container 2

Amount Per Serving	
Calories 250	Calories from Fat 110
	% Daily Value*
Total Fat 12g	**18%**
Saturated Fat 3g	**15%**
Trans Fat 3g	
Cholesterol 30mg	**10%**
Sodium 470mg	**20%**
Potassium 700mg	**20%**
Total Carbohydrate 31g	**10%**
Dietary Fiber 0g	**0%**
Sugars 5g	
Protein 5g	
Vitamin A	4%
Vitamin C	2%
Calcium	20%
Iron	4%

* Percent Daily Values are based on a 2,000 calorie diet. Your Daily Values may be higher or lower depending on your calorie needs.

	Calories:	2,000	2,500
Total Fat	Less than	65g	80g
Sat Fat	Less than	20g	25g
Cholesterol	Less than	300mg	300mg
Sodium	Less than	2,400mg	2,400mg
Total Carbohydrate		300g	375g
Dietary Fiber		25g	30g

A

EQUIVALENCIES

1 tsp fat/oil	=	5 g fat
1 tsp sugar	=	4 g sugar
¼ cup sugar	=	50 g sugar = 50 g CHO
If fiber >5 g, substract from CHO		
15 g CHO	=	1 slice bread
	=	½ cup fruit
	=	1 cup milk
½ cup beans	=	8 g fiber + 7 g PRO
¼ cup meat (1 oz)	=	7 g PRO + 1-10 g fat
1 cup milk		
1 oz chicken/fish	=	1 g fat
½ cup beans	=	1 g fat
1 oz red meat	=	5 g fat
1 oz cheese	=	10 g fat
1 oz nuts	=	20 g fat

B

FIGURE 26.3 (A) Food nutrition label. (B) Nutritional equivalencies. *CHO*, Carbohydrate; *PRO*, protein. (Peckenpaugh N. J. [2010]. *Nutrition Essentials and Diet Therapy* [pp. 16]. 11th ed. Philadelphia, PA: Saunders.)

FIBER

Dietary **fiber** is the portion of carbohydrates that cannot be broken down by intestinal enzymes and juices. Fiber passes through the small intestine and colon undigested. Food sources of fiber include whole grain cereals and the skins of fruits, vegetables, and legumes. Various types of dietary fiber are polysaccharides.

Fiber increases bulk in the stool, leading to good intestinal function and elimination. The presence of fiber in the colon also is beneficial in delaying absorption of carbohydrates and cholesterol from the intestine. This delay may be beneficial to diabetic patients by decreasing blood glucose levels. Some properties of fiber may also decrease absorption of fat. **Health experts recommend 21 to 38 g of fiber per day for adults.** Fiber content in the diet can be increased by such practices as replacing white bread with whole wheat bread and white rice with brown rice, or eating whole grain cereals and pasta. Increasing intake of fresh fruit and vegetables, beans, and peas also increases fiber intake. Fiber content of selected foods is listed in Table 26.1. It is not desirable to use concentrated fiber supplements in place of dietary fiber because dietary fiber contains many needed vitamins and minerals.

FATS (LIPIDS)

Health promotion strategies emphasize the negative effect of fat on health. High fat intake has been linked to obesity, breast and colon cancer, hypertension and other cardiovascular diseases, and stroke. Triglycerides are the major lipid found in both foods and the body.

FUNCTIONS OF FAT

Fat is an essential nutrient. Fat supplies a concentrated form of energy. It also spares protein from being burned for energy. **Fat supplies 9 calories per gram consumed.** Other functions of fat include:

- Provides a source of fatty acids
- Adds flavor to foods and contributes to texture
- Dissolves and transports fat-soluble vitamins and fat-soluble phytonutrients (carotenoids)
- Insulates and controls body temperature
- Makes food smell appetizing

Table 26.1 Fiber Content of Selected Foods

FOOD	QUANTITY	FIBER (G)
Fruits		
Apple, unpeeled	1 small	3.0
Apple, peeled	1 small	2.0
Banana	1 medium	2.0
Orange	1 medium	1.7
Cantaloupe	½	3.0
Grapefruit	1 cup	3.0
Strawberries	1 cup	4.0
Grains and Cereals		
Biscuit	1	1.0
Bread, white	1 slice	1.0
Bread, wheat	1 slice	2.0
All Bran	½ cup	9.0
Oatmeal, cooked	½ cup	4.0
Shredded wheat	¾ cup	4.0
Vegetables		
Green beans	1 cup	1.9
Broccoli, raw	1 cup	3.5
Cauliflower, raw	1 cup	2.3
Celery, raw	1 cup	1.8
Corn, whole kernel	½ cup	3.0
Potato, with skin	1 medium	2.5
Sweet potato, baked	1 medium	3.0
Legumes, Cooked		
Kidney beans	1 cup	19.0
Pinto beans	1 cup	20.0
Black-eyed peas	1 cup	16.0
Lima beans	1 cup	16.0
Black beans	1 cup	21.0

- Cushions and protects body organs
- Facilitates transmission of nerve impulses
- Gives a feeling of fullness after eating

Fats are made up of fatty acids and glycerol called triglycerides. Fatty acids are classified as either **saturated fats** or **unsaturated fats,** depending on the amount of hydrogen they contain. Fats can be of liquid or solid consistency. Fats that are liquid at room temperature are called *oils.* Most oils are unsaturated fat: examples include olive oil, corn oil, safflower oil, sunflower oil, soybean oil, and canola oil. **Omega-3 fatty acid** (found in salmon, trout, halibut, sardines, tuna, canola oil, soybean oil, omega-3–rich chicken eggs, and walnuts) is the most unsaturated form of fatty acid. These foods should be added to the diet as sources of unsaturated fat. Solid fats, which are saturated fats, include shortening, margarines, and lard.

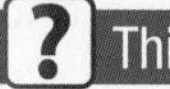 **Think Critically**

How much saturated and unsaturated fat is used in your home per day?

FOOD SOURCES OF FAT

Animal food sources provide the most saturated fatty acids, and vegetables, nuts, or seeds supply unsaturated fatty acids. Two saturated vegetable fats are coconut oil and palm oil. **There are three essential fatty acids: linoleic acid (found in corn oil, safflower oil, and sunflower oil), oleic acid (found in olive oil and beef), and linolenic acid (found in green leafy vegetables, walnuts, pecans, soybean oil, and soybean products).** These three fatty acids are necessary for the production of healthy blood cells, healthy arteries, nerve function, and skin maintenance. Deficiencies of these three fatty acids may lead to illness or skin problems.

Most Americans consume more fat in the diet than is needed to maintain health. The recommended daily allowance of fat is 20 to 30 g/day. Saturated and polyunsaturated fats should be limited to 10% of total fat intake. Some cardiologists recommend diets of 20% fat for individuals at risk for heart disease and as low as 10% fat for individuals with a history of heart disease. Research has shown a marked reduction of risk for further complications of heart disease and, in some instances, reversal of cardiac pathologic conditions. A very low fat intake will not be beneficial to heart health, however, if the fat is replaced with simple carbohydrates.

A component of fat, **cholesterol,** is linked to heart disease and hardening of the arteries. Cholesterol is only found in animal products and oils such as palm and coconut. Increased cholesterol level places the individual at risk for heart disease and stroke. Cholesterol, however, has an important role in the structure of essential hormones and in the conversion of vitamin D by the action of sunlight on the skin. Cholesterol is also essential to the production of bile in the liver. Table 26.2 lists the fat content of selected foods. Coconut oil, although a saturated fat, is unique and healthy because it is composed mostly of medium-chain triglycerides.

VITAMINS

Vitamins are organic compounds essential to proper function of the body. They are best consumed through food sources; however, vitamin supplements can provide the nutrients needed. Vitamins are classified as *fat soluble* or *water soluble.* Water-soluble vitamins are easily absorbed into the bloodstream for use by the body. Fat-soluble vitamins are absorbed in the small intestine the same as other fats by action of bile in the duodenum, and they are stored in the liver.

The fat-soluble vitamins are vitamins A, D, E, and K. These vitamins, because they are stored in the body, can cause toxic effects if ingested in excessive quantities. Guidelines for the intake of vitamin D can be found in Table 26.3. Vitamin A can be produced in the body by **carotenoids** (e.g., beta-carotene). Carotenoids act as antioxidants, protecting the cells and tissues from damage from free radicals, and have been shown to increase immunity, improve vision, and have a role in cancer prevention.

Table 26.2 Fats

SATURATED FATS	QUANTITY	FAT (G)
Limit the Following:		
Saturated Fats (Solid at Room Temperature)		
Butter	1 Tbsp	12
Shortening	1 Tbsp	12
Fat in Meat		
Beef	3 oz	26
Bacon	3 oz	9
Ham	3 oz	14
Pork Chop	3 oz	19
Chicken, with skin	1/2	18
Lard	1 Tbsp	13
Coconut oil	1 Tbsp	12
Palm oil	1 Tbsp	11
Less-Saturated Fats (Soft at Room Temperature)		
Tub margarine	1 Tbsp	11
Squeeze margarine	1 Tbsp	6
Ice cream	1 cup	14-38
Trans Fats (Used in Processed Foods)		
Hydrogenated liquid oils	1 Tbsp	12
Stick margarine	1 Tbsp	11
Packaged snack foods		
Crackers	1 serving	1-4
Chips	1 serving	1-4
Microwave popcorn	1 serving	1-3
Fried foods	1 serving	1-12
Candy	1 oz	2-10
Baked Goods, commercial	1 serving	1-27

HEALTHY FATS:	QUANTITY	TOTAL FAT (G)	SATURATED FAT (G)
Unsaturated Fats (Liquid at Room Temperature)			
Monounsaturated			
Olive oil	1 Tbsp	14	2
Canola oil	1 Tbsp	14	1
Peanut oil	1 Tbsp	14	2
Sunflower oil	1 Tbsp	14	2
Avocado	1 med	21	3
Nuts			
Almonds	1 oz	14	1
Peanuts	1 oz	14	2
Macadamia	1 oz	21	3
Pecans	1 oz	20	2
Hazelnuts	1 oz	17	1
Cashews	1 oz	12	2
Polyunsaturated			
Corn oil	1 Tbsp	14	2
Safflower oil	1 Tbsp	14	1
Soybean oil	1 Tbsp	14	2
Flaxseed oil	1 Tbsp	14	2
Fish			
Salmon	3 oz	10	2
Tuna (in water)	3 oz	5	1
Mackerel	3 oz	34	10
Herring	3 oz	8	2
Trout (Rainbow)	3 oz	5	1
Sardines (in oil)	3 oz	10	1

Commercially made baked goods (cookies, cupcakes, doughnuts, muffins, cakes, and pizza dough).

Table 26.3 Recommendations for Vitamin D Intake

AGE	RECOMMENDED DAILY INTAKE
Birth-12 months	400 IU
Children 1-13 years	600 IU
Teens 14-18 years	600 IU
Adults 19-70 years	600 IU
Adults age 71 and older	800 IU
Pregnant and breastfeeding teens and women	600 IU

Office of Dietary Supplements, National Institutes of Health. Available at https://ods.od.nih.gov/factsheets/VitaminD-Consumer/.

The water-soluble vitamins include the B-complex vitamins (thiamine, riboflavin, niacin, vitamin B_6, folic acid, vitamin B_{12}, pantothenic acid, and biotin) and vitamin C. Vitamin C is thought to be beneficial in healing wounds. Some of these vitamins (especially niacin, vitamin B_6, and folate) accumulate in toxic amounts if a person is taking large quantities of them as supplements or is suffering from kidney failure.

Although vitamins do not have caloric value, they are essential to the body for building tissue, promoting proper cellular function, and facilitating the reactions that release energy from carbohydrates, proteins, and fats. Table 26.4 summarizes the function, common food sources, signs of deficiency, and signs of toxicity of fat-soluble and water-soluble vitamins.

MINERALS

Minerals are inorganic substances contained in animals and plants. They are essential for metabolism and cellular function. Minerals are categorized as major minerals (macro minerals) or trace minerals (micro minerals). The major minerals are calcium, magnesium, sodium, potassium, phosphorus, sulfur, and chlorine. Selected foods with high sodium content are listed in Table 26.5. Trace minerals are iron, copper, iodine, manganese, cobalt, zinc, molybdenum, selenium, fluoride, and chromium. **Minerals are necessary for proper muscle and nerve function, and they act as catalysts for many cellular functions.** They combine to form salts and are largely responsible for the acid-base balance of the body. Because mineral actions are

Table 26.4 Vitamins

VITAMIN	MAJOR FUNCTION	FOOD SOURCE	DEFICIENCY	EXCESS
Fat-Soluble Vitamins				
Vitamin A (retinol)	Maintenance of epithelial cells and mucous membranes; important for night vision Necessary for adequate immune response	Liver, dark green leafy vegetables, deep-orange vegetables and fruit	Night blindness; rough, dry skin; dry mucous membranes; xerophthalmia (an eye disease)	Appetite loss, hair loss, dry skin, bone and joint pain, enlarged liver and spleen, and fetal malformations
Vitamin E	Protects red blood cells from rupture; prevents destruction of vitamin A in the intestine Helps maintain normal cell membranes	Vegetable oils, wheat germ, legumes, nuts, fish, and green leafy vegetables	Breakdown of red blood cells	Decreased thyroid hormone level and increased triglycerides
Vitamin K	Necessary for blood clotting	Dark green leafy vegetables, cauliflower, soybean oil, green tea, and synthesis of intestinal bacteria	Hemorrhage	None known
Vitamin D	Aids in absorption of calcium and phosphorus; regulates blood levels of calcium; promotes bone and teeth mineralization	Fortified milk, fish with bones, and cod liver oil	Rickets (children); osteomalacia (adults)	Calcification of soft tissues, hypercalcemia, renal stones, and growth failure in children
Water-Soluble Vitamins				
Vitamin B_1 (thiamine)	Carbohydrate metabolism; assists function of the heart, muscles, and nervous system; promotes appetite and good function of the digestive tract	Whole grains, wheat germ, organ meats, pork, legumes, and brewer's yeast	Polyneuritis, beriberi, fatigue, depression, poor appetite, edema, nervous instability, Wernicke encephalopathy, Korsakoff psychosis, spastic muscle contractions, mental confusion, and metabolic acidosis	Rare with IV thiamine
Vitamin B_2 (riboflavin)	Essential for certain enzyme systems that aid in the metabolism of carbohydrate, proteins, and fats	Milk and milk products, eggs, green leafy vegetables, organ meats, peanuts, whole grains, and soybeans	Tongue inflammation, scaling and burning skin, sensitive eyes, cataracts, and anemia	Inhibition of zinc absorption
Vitamin B_3 (niacin, nicotinic acid)	Part of the enzymes that aid in the metabolism of carbohydrates, proteins, and fats; needed for healthy skin, lips, tongue, and digestive system	Meats and organ meats, whole grain flour, mushrooms, turkey, chicken, tuna, and halibut	Pellagra if severe, gastrointestinal disturbances, photosensitive dermatitis, and depressive psychosis	Flushing caused by vasodilation; nausea and vomiting; abnormal glucose metabolism; abnormal plasma uric acid levels; abnormal liver function; gastric ulceration, anaphylaxis, and circulatory collapse
Vitamin B_6 (pyridoxine)	Metabolism of proteins, amino acids, carbohydrates, and fats; essential for proper growth and cell membrane function	Liver and red meats, whole grains, potato, green vegetables, chickpeas, tuna, pork, lentils, and sweet potato	Believed to lead to convulsions, peripheral neuropathy, secondary pellagra, possible depression, and oral lesions	Sensory nerve damage, numbness of extremities, ataxia, bone pain, and muscle weakness

Table 26.4 Vitamins—cont'd

VITAMIN	MAJOR FUNCTION	FOOD SOURCE	DEFICIENCY	EXCESS
Vitamin B_{12} (cobalamin)	Aids in hemoglobin synthesis, normal functioning of all cells, and folic acid metabolism; important in energy metabolism	Meats, organ meats, dry milk and milk products, eggs, sardines, and clams	Pernicious anemia, anorexia, degeneration of the spinal cord, various psychiatric disorders, and contributes to osteoporosis	None known
Folic acid	Formation of red blood cells and normal functioning of gastrointestinal tract Aids in metabolism of proteins and DNA	Glandular meats, yeast, dark green leafy vegetables, legumes, whole grains, enriched rice, and wheat germ	Impaired cell division, megaloblastic anemia, possible neural tube defect, and various psychiatric disorders	None known
Vitamin C (ascorbic acid)	Helps protect the body against infections Aids in wound healing; important for tooth dentin, bones, cartilage connective tissue, and blood vessels	Citrus fruits, tomatoes, strawberries, cantaloupe, peaches, papaya, kiwi, broccoli, cabbage, potatoes, green peppers, and green leafy vegetables	Scurvy, anemia, swollen and bleeding gums, loose teeth, poor wound healing, and easy bruising from ruptured small blood vessels	Urinary stones, diarrhea, hypoglycemia, and inhibition of zinc absorption

Adapted from Peckenpaugh, N. J. (2010). *Nutrition Essentials and Diet Therapy* (11th ed.). Philadelphia, PA: Elsevier Saunders.

Table 26.5 Selected Foods with High Sodium Content

FOOD	QUANTITY	SODIUM (MG)
Prepared Foods		
Cream of potato soup	1 cup	1422
Tomato soup	1 cup	1022
Chili, no beans	1 cup	1024
Cheese ravioli	1 cup	1280
Cream of chicken soup	1 cup	1047
Chicken noodle soup	1 cup	1000
Fast Food		
Burger King Whopper	1	1105
Arby's Beef and Cheddar	1	1801
Subway Cold Cut Sub	6 inch	1651
Supreme pizza	1 slice	1313
Miscellaneous Foods		
Pickle	1 slice	56
Olive	1	75
Table salt	1 tsp	2300
Sausage link	1	643
Cheese	1 oz	264
Soy sauce	1 Tbsp	1000
Taco seasoning	2 tsp	480

interrelated, a deficiency of one mineral will affect the action of another mineral in the body. Other functions of minerals include:

- Maintaining rigidity and strength in teeth and bones
- Facilitating contraction and relaxation of muscles
- Assisting in blood clotting and tissue repair and growth

DRIs have been created for every mineral. Generally, sufficient minerals can be supplied by a balanced diet. Extra iron is needed when blood loss from surgery or trauma has occurred. The body does not manufacture its own minerals; therefore, all must be provided through food sources or supplements. Table 26.6 lists minerals, their function, food sources, signs of deficiency, and signs of toxicity.

WATER

Water is the most essential of all nutrients. The adult body is 50% to 60% water by weight. The proportion of water depends on body composition, age, bone density, body weight, and hormone status. **The water requirement for adults is approximately 1 mL/calorie of intake** (or 35 mL/kg in adults, 30 mL/kg in older adults). Water requirements are increased for patients who are immobile, have a fever, or have diarrhea.

Water is used in every body process, from digestion to absorption to elimination or secretion. Most foods contain water, and the body obtains a substantial amount of the water needed directly from food. Water is not stored in the body, and what is lost during 24 hours must be replaced. **A general rule is that the patient should take in an amount equal to the recorded fluid output plus 500 mL.**

FACTORS THAT INFLUENCE NUTRITION

To help patients reach their optimum nutritional state, you must consider a variety of factors that may influence an individual's ability to meet nutritional needs. A dietitian should be consulted if malnutrition or risk of malnutrition is suspected.

Table 26.6 **Minerals**

MINERAL	FUNCTION	FOOD SOURCE	DEFICIENCY	EXCESS
Calcium	Muscle contraction and relaxation, coagulation; building of strong bones and teeth; plays a role in nervous system function; aids in blood coagulation	Milk and milk products, dark green leafy vegetables, soybeans, sardines, salmon with bones, tofu and other soy products, hard water	Poor bone growth and tooth development, poor blood clotting, osteoporosis, rickets in children, osteomalacia in adults, and possible hypertension	Kidney stones in predisposed individuals
Chloride	Maintenance of fluid and acid-base balance; aids in activation of gastric enzymes	Table salt, fish, and vegetables	Disturbances in acid-base balance; possible growth retardation, psychomotor defects, and memory loss	None known
Magnesium	Builds strong teeth and bones, protein synthesis, lipid metabolism, regulation of heartbeat, and involved in hormonal reactions	Raw dark green leafy vegetables, nuts and soybeans, whole grains, bananas, apricots, seafood, coffee, tea, cocoa, hard water, and milk	May lead to hypertension, ischemic heart disease, arrhythmia, preeclampsia, and asthma	Increased calcium excretion
Phosphorus	Helps build strong bones and teeth, present in the nuclei of all cells, acid-base balance, and a factor in energy metabolism	Milk and milk products, eggs, meats, legumes, fish, turkey, sunflower seeds, whole grains, and soft drinks	With malabsorption can cause anorexia, weakness, stiff joints, and fragile bones	Hypocalcemia, tetany
Potassium	Acid-base and fluid balance; transmits nerve impulses and helps control muscle contractions and regulation of heartbeat; necessary for enzyme reactions	Apricots, bananas, oranges, grapefruit, green beans, broccoli, carrots, potatoes, meat, milk, peanut butter, legumes, molasses, coffee, tea, cocoa, and tomato and orange juice	May cause impaired growth, hypertension, bone fragility, central nervous system changes, renal hypertrophy, diminished heart rate, arrhythmias, and death	Hyperkalemia, with cardiac disturbances
Sodium	Acid-base balance, fluid balance, transmits nerve impulses and helps control muscle contractions	Salt (major source), processed foods, milk, milk products, and several vegetables	Hyponatremia, edema of the lower extremities	May cause hypertension, can lead to renal disease and cardiovascular disease
Chromium	Activates enzymes and enhances removal of glucose from the blood	Liver and other meats, whole grains, cheese, legumes, and brewer's yeast	Weight loss, abnormalities of the central nervous system; possible aggravation of diabetes mellitus	Liver damage
Fluoride	Aids in formation of bones and teeth and decreases cavities	Fluoridated water, fish, tea, and gelatin	Increased risk of dental caries	Mottling of teeth
Iodine	Helps regulate metabolism as a part of thyroid hormones; helps keep skin, hair, and nails healthy	Iodized salt, saltwater fish, seaweed products, and vegetables grown in iodine-rich soils	Goiter; cretinism in children born to iodine-deficient mothers	Possible thyroid dysfunction

Table 26.6 Minerals—cont'd

MINERAL	FUNCTION	FOOD SOURCE	DEFICIENCY	EXCESS
Iron	Formation of hemoglobin; part of several enzymes	Liver, red meats, dark green leafy vegetables, fortified cereals, legumes, whole grains, almonds, and eggs	Iron deficiency anemia	Idiopathic excess hemoglobin, which can lead to cirrhosis, diabetes mellitus, and cardiac enlargement
Zinc	Component of 50 enzymes, protein synthesis and DNA repair, normal growth and sexual development, wound healing, immune function, and smell acuity	Whole grains, wheat germ, crabmeat, oysters, liver, brewer's yeast, legumes, pork, yogurt, and milk	Depressed immune function, poor growth, delayed sexual maturation, decreased myelination of nerve fibers, and low level of alkaline phosphatase enzyme	Severe anemia, nausea, vomiting, cramps, diarrhea, malaise, fatigue, fever, renal damage, low blood serum copper, and impaired immunity
Selenium	Part of the enzyme system, acts as antioxidant with vitamin E, helps fertility, promotes immunity and thyroid function, plays a role in glucose metabolism, and helps prevent inflammatory, cardiovascular, and neurologic diseases	Nuts, turkey, herring, oysters, sardines, and beef	Cardiomyopathy, osteoarthropathy, reduced production of sperm, and flagellar defects	Defects of nails, hair loss, nausea, abdominal pain, diarrhea, peripheral neuropathy, fatigue, and irritability
Manganese	Normal bone structure, reproduction, normal central nervous system function, and is a component of some enzymes	Nuts, pineapple, whole wheat products, chickpeas, spinach, and blackberries	None	Parkinson disease–like symptoms when on long-term TPN
Molybdenum	Component of three enzymes, needed for normal cell functioning	Milk, organ meats, legumes, whole grains, and dark green vegetables	Vomiting, tachypnea, tachycardia, coma, and possible neurologic dysfunction	None known
Copper	Aids in production and survival of red blood cells and plays a role in enzymes involved in respiration and a role in lipid metabolism	Molasses, beef liver, cashews, oysters, legumes, pears, and soy milk	Anemia, neurologic problems, abnormal ECG, bone fragility, impaired immune responses, and a possible factor in failure to thrive in premature infants	Neuron and liver cell damage in Wilson disease
Cobalt	Essential component of vitamin B_{12} and activates enzymes	Figs, cabbage, spinach, lettuce, watercress, and beet greens	Pernicious anemia	Polycythemia, hyperplasia of bone marrow, and increased blood volume

ECG, Electrocardiogram.
Adapted from Peckenpaugh, N. J. (2010). *Nutrition Essentials and Diet Therapy* (11th ed.). Philadelphia, PA: Elsevier Saunders.

AGE

Infants are dependent on others to meet their nutritional needs. Nutrition may be provided by breast milk or formula. As the child grows, nutritional needs change based on the stage of development. Parents and caregivers face the challenge of experimenting with a variety of foods and meal strategies to meet the needs of growing children.

Adolescents are strongly influenced by their peers. Food choices are often of the fast-food and pizza variety. Growth spurts during this time may result in voracious appetites, leading to concerns about weight management. Eating disorders are a concern during this growth period, especially among adolescent girls, but the prevalence of such disorders in adolescent boys is increasing.

Physiologic changes and physical limitations may influence the eating habits of older adults. Poor dentition or difficulty swallowing often affects an older person's food intake. Older adults may be at risk for inadequate nutrition because of income limits, loneliness, and difficulty obtaining and preparing food. Malnutrition can often mimic dementia, and older patients showing signs of dementia should be evaluated for nutritional deficiencies.

Clinical Cues

Older adults may be overweight because of decreased activity and high fat intake. A method of accurately assessing if a person is overweight is to determine the waist-to-hip ratio. Measure the waist at the narrowest point and the hips at the widest point. Divide the waist measurement by the hip measurement to determine the ratio. A ratio of 0.7 for women and 0.9 for men is considered healthy. The higher the ratio, the greater the risk for heart disease and other conditions related to overweight and obesity.

ILLNESS

Nutritional needs usually increase during illness. Patients with diseases such as cancer and human immunodeficiency virus/acquired immunodeficiency syndrome (HIV/AIDS) experience loss of muscle mass, resulting in the need for more calories and protein. A loss of appetite may occur because of pain, nausea, vomiting, and stomatitis. Achieving optimal nutrition in these patients is a special challenge to health care workers.

Nutrition Considerations

Three types of malnutrition, based on etiology, are:

- Starvation-related malnutrition without inflammation: for example, anorexia nervosa (discussed in Chapter 27)
- Chronic disease-related malnutrition: for example, cancer
- Acute disease-related malnutrition: for example, burns or sepsis (Mauldin & O'Leary-Kelley, 2015)

EMOTIONAL STATUS

An individual's emotional state has a strong influence on eating habits. Some people tend to overeat during times of emotional distress, whereas others lose their appetite. Be aware of the patient's response to stress and take opportunities to intervene if nutrition is compromised.

ECONOMIC STATUS

Sufficient income does not guarantee optimum nutrition; however, it does provide the opportunity to make healthy choices. Individuals with limited income can benefit from patient education related to good nutritional choices because a balanced diet is affordable even with low income. In addition, patients should be referred to community and government programs (e.g., Women, Infants, and Children [WIC] Special Supplemental Nutrition Program) for assistance in meeting nutritional needs. Social workers and dietitians can be helpful in recommending community resources providing nutritional interventions and programs.

RELIGION

Religious practices and affiliations influence nutrition by dictating food preparation, foods allowed, and those to avoid. You must develop an awareness of and respect for patients' religious beliefs related to food to promote good nutrition effectively. Some common religious food practices include:

- **Islam:** No pork or pork products. No alcohol.
- **Judaism:** Foods grown, harvested, or processed in a **kosher** manner (prepared for use according to Jewish law). Separate dishes, pans, and silverware must be used to prepare and serve meat and dairy food. Meat and milk may not be eaten at the same meal. Pork, shellfish, crustaceans, and birds of prey are not allowed. Orthodox Jews follow stricter guidelines than others do.
- **Seventh-Day Adventist:** No stimulants (coffee or tea). Shellfish, pork, and alcohol must be avoided. Many are lacto-ovo-vegetarians, with an emphasis on whole grain foods.

CULTURE

Cultural influences, both ethnic and environmental, have an important effect on nutrition. Individuals are more likely to consume foods with which they are familiar. Most traditional ethnic diets can be modified to meet required nutritional needs.

FOOD SAFETY

Food safety in the United States has become a serious issue because several incidents of illness and death have been linked to contamination with foodborne pathogens. The most common culprits are *Salmonella, Shigella,* and *Campylobacter* organisms and *Yersinia enterocolitica* (Riddle et al., 2013). In addition, *Clostridium botulinum* sometimes contaminates canned and bottled foods. Food safety inspections have decreased considerably since 2003, and imports of foods from countries where food safety is less of a concern have increased dramatically. Fruits and vegetables should be washed thoroughly before preparation. Ground beef must be cooked until well done (no longer pink at all). Chicken must be thoroughly cooked because it frequently is contaminated with *Campylobacter* organisms. Condiments, especially salsa, are frequently contaminated when left out on tables unrefrigerated. All surfaces and utensils should be washed with hot soapy water after meat or poultry preparation to prevent cross-contamination with other foods or utensils. Additionally, the use of household bleach, 1 tablespoon to 1 gallon of water, is acceptable for decontaminating utensils and surfaces.

CULTURAL INFLUENCES ON NUTRITION

American society is composed of multiple cultures. Ethnicity, culture, and region of residence have a strong influence on nutrition. Awareness of nutritional preferences of different ethnic groups can enhance your ability to provide effective nutritional counseling.

Clinical Cues

Consult with or refer patients to the dietitian or nutritionist to provide foods the patient will find acceptable to eat. Allowing family to prepare and provide food for the patient may be a means to ensure proper nutrition. Family members can be advised of any restrictions required because of specific medical needs.

AFRICAN AMERICAN

The African American diet closely resembles food preferences of the southern region of the United States. African and West Indian influences are also prevalent, as evidenced by inclusion of foods such as okra, black-eyed peas, and peanuts and peanut products in the diet.

Typical foods in the traditional African American diet include a variety of greens (collard, mustard, turnip, and kale), dry beans, cornbread, sweet potatoes, pork, catfish, and chicken. Most meats and fish are prepared by frying. Seasonings for vegetables include smoked bacon, ham, and salted pork. Desserts may include sweet potato pie, peach cobbler, and fried pies. These preferences often contribute to high fat, sugar, and salt content in the traditional African American diet.

HISPANIC AMERICAN

The Hispanic population is one of the fastest growing in the United States. Several groups are represented including Mexican, Puerto Rican, and Cuban. Nutrition preferences have a Spanish and American Indian influence. The Hispanic diet is high in carbohydrates such as beans, rice, corn, and tortillas. Meats and meat dishes are heavily seasoned and spicy. The diet can be high in fat because of the use of lard in the preparation of fried foods. Desserts are very sweet and may be prepared with syrup-like sauces. Preferences for fried foods lead to high fat in the diet.

ASIAN AMERICAN

The popularity of Asian American cuisine is evident throughout the United States. The traditional Asian diet is high in carbohydrates and vegetables and low in meat and fish. Mung beans and soybeans and products such as sprouts are also used. Vegetables are rarely eaten raw. They are stir-fried with small amounts of added meat and served with rice or noodles. The practice of adding monosodium glutamate (MSG) to enhance flavor has decreased. However, dishes may still have a high sodium and high fat content.

MIDDLE EASTERN AMERICAN

Food preferences among Middle Eastern cultures include fermented dairy products such as yogurt, meats, grains in the form of wheat or rice at each meal, fresh fruits, and vegetables. Some foods are specially prepared if the individual practices the Muslim religion. Food preparation includes grilling, frying, grinding, and stewing.

NUTRITION COUNSELING

The nurse and dietitian can help patients modify diets to meet nutritional requirements. Dietary counseling should include modification of the culture's traditional diet to accomplish a more healthy composition and preparation while maintaining the diet's basic components. Meals can be made healthier by teaching patients to prepare food with less fat and sodium. Use of herbal, low sodium seasoning can maintain the desired flavor. A summary of food patterns of American cultural groups can be found in Table 26.7.

NUTRITIONAL NEEDS THROUGHOUT THE LIFE SPAN

INFANTS

The first year of life marks the fastest growth period in human development. By 6 months of age, the birth weight of the normal newborn should double. By the end of the first year, the birth weight should triple. The American Academy of Pediatrics recommends that infants be breastfed or receive breast milk for the first full year of life. Emphasis on the importance of breastfeeding is a major component of prenatal education programs. In addition to providing complete nutrition, breast milk also provides immunity to most childhood diseases through the first few months of life. The first breast fluid, **colostrum**, is available at delivery. Colostrum also contributes to passage of meconium stool and growth of normal bacterial flora in the bowel. Within 7 to 10 days of delivery, the composition of breast milk changes. Protein and fat-soluble vitamin content decreases, and water-soluble vitamins, fat, and calories increase. By the 14th day, mature milk is produced. Breast milk rarely causes allergic responses in the infant.

Infant formulas are similar in composition to breast milk; however, nutrients in human milk are more easily digested and absorbed. Formulas are a modified form of cow's milk, made more digestible and with

Table 26.7 Culturally Diverse Food Patterns of Americans

CULTURE	HISTORICAL DIETARY PATTERN[a]
African American	All meats, fish, and chicken; pork often consumed (spareribs, bacon, and sausage); vegetables cooked in salt pork for a long time; grits and cornbread muffins; some lactose intolerance. Popular vegetables include collard greens, beet greens, and sweet potatoes.
Chinese American	Rich in vegetables (bean sprouts, broccoli, bamboo shoots, and mushrooms). Vegetables cooked until crisp; meat consumed in small portions with other food. Soy sauce, tofu, peanut butter; limited milk and cheese; fish baked with native spices; soups with egg, meat, and vegetables. Tea is China's national beverage. Rice is a staple of the diet.
Jewish American	Diet varies according to whether family is Orthodox, Reform, or Conservative. For the Orthodox family, food must be kosher (clean); meat is soaked in salt water to remove blood; the only meat eaten is that of divided hoofed animals that chew a cud; fish without scales (shellfish) and pork are prohibited; milk and meat cannot be combined. Favorites are gefilte fish, lox (smoked salmon), herring, eggs, bagels, cream cheese, and matzo.
Laotian American	Numerous varieties of freshwater fish and shellfish (eaten fresh, dried, or salted); pork, beef, chicken, rabbit, often mixed with vegetables and spices; eggs, peanuts, black-eyed peas; vegetables eaten raw, as juice, or cooked with meat or fish and preserved by drying or pickling; sticky rice, rice or bean thread noodles, and legumes are often used in desserts; soybean drink, sugar cane drink, tea, and coconut juice. Popular seasonings include padek, chilies, curry, tamarind, and red and black pepper.
Italian American	All meats, fish, and chicken, including cold cuts (e.g., salami and mortadella) and Italian pork sausage; pasta (a staple of the diet), breads, olive oil, wine, cheese, and all varieties of fruits and vegetables.
Japanese American	Fish and seafood (fresh, smoked, and raw) and beef. Food is cut into small portions. Principal fruit is nasi, which tastes like a pear. Many vegetables are eaten such as seaweed, bamboo shoots, onions, beans, and dried mushrooms (shitake); pickled vegetables. Rice is the national staple. Beverages include tea and sake. Little cheese, milk, butter, or cream is consumed. Chief cooking fat is soybean oil or rice oil.
Mexican American	Chicken, pork chops, wieners, cold cuts, hamburger, eggs (used frequently), beans (eaten mashed or refried with lard), potatoes (basic item, usually fried), chilies, fresh tomatoes, corn (maize—often used as basic grain), tortillas, packaged cereals; little milk because of lactose intolerance.
American Indian	Acorn flour, a staple food made into mush or bread; salmon, fresh or dried; other varieties of fish, deer, duck, geese, and other small game; nuts such as buckeye and hazel; wild berries, seeds, and roots.
Puerto Rican American	Meat cooked in stews; poultry, pork, fish, dried beans or peas mixed with rice; milk in combination with coffee (café con leche), a variety of fruits, starchy vegetables (e.g., plantains, cassava, and sweet potatoes), salad, and soft drinks.
Vietnamese American	Pork is the most common meat; meats cut into small pieces and fried, boiled, or steamed; all types of freshwater and saltwater fish and shellfish, often fried and dipped in fish sauce; eggs, soybeans, legumes, and a wide variety of fruits and vegetables; rice is often eaten with every meal. Seasonings including oyster sauce, soy sauce, monosodium glutamate, ginger, garlic, nuoc mam sauce; tea, coffee, soft drinks, and soybean milk.
Middle Eastern American	Lamb is the most common meat; pork is prohibited for Muslims and Jews; legumes such as black beans, chickpeas, and lentils; feta cheese is a favorite dairy product; unleavened bread and pita bread; eggplant is commonly eaten; fruits and vegetables, preferred raw; preferred spices and herbs include dill, garlic, mint, cinnamon, oregano, parsley, pepper, and olive oil.

[a]Eating patterns become more diverse as future generations of a culture become assimilated.
Adapted from Leifer, G. (2015). *Introduction to Maternity and Pediatric Nursing* (7th ed.). Philadelphia, PA: Elsevier Saunders; data from Mahan, L. K., & Escott-Stump, S. (2008). *Krause's Food, Nutrition and Diet Therapy* (12th ed.). Philadelphia, PA: Elsevier Saunders; and other sources.

added carbohydrate and fat content. Infants with allergy to modified cow's milk may use soy-based formulas (unless soy allergy is a concern) or special hypoallergenic formulas. An advantage of bottle-feeding is the opportunity to share the feeding responsibility with other caregivers. Feeding can be a time to build an emotional bond with the infant. Fathers, grandparents, and older siblings can also establish this bond. Breastfeeding mothers can pump their breasts so that the infant can be bottle-fed by other caregivers.

A milestone for infants is the introduction of solid foods. Pediatricians prefer adding solid foods to the diet at 4 to 6 months of age; however, some health care professionals encourage later introduction of solid foods (starting at 9 to 12 months) to decrease further the risk of food allergy or sensitivity. Eggs and fish are not recommended during the first year because of potential allergic reactions. Many parents add solid foods earlier in the belief that solid foods will satisfy the infant and result in the infant sleeping through the night. This practice should be discouraged because the infant's gastrointestinal system is still immature and is unable to digest cereals before 3 months of age. **Introducing solid foods before 4 to 6 months of age also increases the risk of the infant developing food allergies as the immune system matures.**

Solid foods should be introduced gradually, one item at a time. This provides the opportunity to identify allergic responses. A single grain cereal such as rice or oatmeal is a good initial choice. These cereals are easily tolerated, and they provide additional iron and calories. Another new food can be introduced in about 1 week. Each new food should be a single item. Introduction of combination foods decreases the ability to identify foods that may be responsible for an allergic response should one occur. After the first year, as the child shows evidence of tolerating solid foods, weaning from the bottle or breast should be considered. Parents and caregivers should allow children to develop their own healthy food preferences and to decide when and how much to eat.

TODDLERS AND PRESCHOOL CHILDREN

During the toddler and preschool years (ages 2 to 5 years), the growth rate tends to level off. The child consumes less milk and increases intake of solid foods. Toddlers' food choices may change frequently. They seem to have a hearty appetite at times and then show lack of appetite at other times. Specific food preferences may be evidenced (e.g., mashed potatoes and gravy); then the child suddenly refuses these items. Parents and caregivers become frustrated with these reactions and are often concerned that the child is not obtaining adequate nutrition. Parents can use some of the following guidelines to assist toddlers to eat:

- Provide a pleasant environment at mealtimes.
- Avoid combination foods. Toddlers prefer single-item foods that do not touch each other on the plate.
- Provide plates and utensils in a size that can be easily handled by the small child.
- Provide small servings.
- Include finger foods for active toddlers.
- Use dishes that are colorful or contain pictures of favorite characters.
- Avoid forcing a child to eat.
- Offer foods that are easy to chew.
- Try colorful foods (e.g., peas and carrots).

SCHOOL-AGE CHILDREN

School-age children may be influenced by their peer group when making food choices. They are susceptible to advertisements for fast food that show toys as prizes and children in play areas when eating. Children at this age may desire sweet, non-nutritive foods such as soda, candy, cake, and ice cream. Parents and caregivers should serve as role models by eating nutritious meals and snacks and providing healthy meals and snacks for school time. Children should be served a well-balanced breakfast before leaving for school. Studies have shown that a healthy breakfast increases a child's ability to concentrate and achieve in school. Lunches could be taken from home or selected from the school cafeteria menu. Children should be taught to make wise choices from the school menu. Children from lower-income families may be able to take advantage of government-sponsored school breakfast and lunch programs.

An increasing number of children come home after school to an environment without adult supervision. Parents can provide nutritious after-school snacks such as fruit and raw vegetables. Snacks high in sodium and sugar should be minimized or avoided. Because of the high calorie and high sodium preferences of many young children, **obesity** (excessive accumulation of body fat) is becoming a health issue during the school-age years.

ADOLESCENTS

Many physiologic changes occur during the adolescent years. Of these changes, the growth spurt and social and emotional changes related to puberty have a great effect on nutrition and eating habits. Adolescents tend to consume many fast foods, from either fast-food restaurants or vending machines. Fast-food restaurants also serve as a social gathering place for many adolescents.

During the growth spurt (girls ages 10.5 to 14 and boys ages 12.5 to 14), the body requires more calories and nutrients such as B vitamins, calcium, and iron. Adolescent girls require increased levels of iron after the menstrual cycle begins. Calcium and vitamin D (for calcium absorption) are also very important for adolescents to prevent future osteoporosis because future bone health depends greatly on bone deposition from early adolescence (Donaldson, 2013). Many pediatricians recommend considering a calcium supplement. Adolescent girls are very aware of their appearance. Concern about weight may lead to eating disorders resulting in inadequate calories and nutrients for growth. Parental supervision and intervention may be critical in helping the adolescent meet appropriate nutritional needs. Parents can assist by:

- Providing snacks high in calcium, iron, and protein
- Decreasing preparation of high fat foods
- Teaching how to select more healthful choices from fast-food restaurants and preparing healthier versions at home with friends
- Keeping sparkling water and low fat milk available instead of high calorie sodas
- Keeping vegetable sticks and fresh fruit available as snack choices

ADULTS

Child-rearing, work, and family responsibilities influence the eating habits of most adults. Many adults rely on fast food or convenience foods to meet their nutritional needs. Studies have shown that adults eat many of their meals, especially breakfast and lunch, from fast-food restaurants. Often the only meal consumed at home is the evening meal, and even that may not be prepared at home. Medical problems such as obesity and hypertension are prevalent during early and middle adulthood. This can be attributed to stress, poor eating habits, and lack of exercise. Lifestyle and dietary recommendations for adults include:

- Decreasing fat and sodium intake
- Decreasing intake of simple sugars
- Increasing fruits, fresh vegetables, and whole grains in the diet
- Preparing more meals at home, where fat and sodium content can be controlled
- Increasing activity

Communication

THE PATIENT WITH HYPERTENSION

Mrs. Hernandez is readmitted to the hospital with a blood pressure of 190/120 mm Hg. She is sitting in a chair looking out the window. You notice she has been crying.

Nurse: "Good morning, Mrs. Hernandez. I'm Lisa, your nurse today."

Mrs. Hernandez: *(Continues to look out the window. Sobs quietly.)*

Nurse: "You seem upset, Mrs. Hernandez. How can I help you?"

Mrs. Hernandez: "This disease is going to kill me!" *(Continues to cry. Grasps arms of chair tightly.)*

Nurse: "Your disease is going to kill you?"

Mrs. Hernandez: "Yes! My blood pressure has gotten so high, and it's all my fault!"

Nurse: "Tell me more." *(Places hand on patient's shoulder, pulls up a chair, and sits next to her.)*

Mrs. Hernandez: "I take my medicine, but I just can't stop eating and lose weight. Look at my hands and feet. They are so swollen." *(Points at hands and feet.)*

Nurse: "Yes, I see they are swollen. Tell me about your diet at home."

Mrs. Hernandez: "I like a lot of salt in my food. My favorite foods are cheese, enchiladas, burritos, and chips. They don't taste good without lots of salt."

Nurse: "Seasoning is very important to making food taste good. Let's discuss ways to season the foods you like without using too much salt. The excess salt in your diet may be the cause of the swelling in your hands and feet."

Mrs. Hernandez: *(Looks up at nurse.)* "You can do that? I really want to learn to do this. I'm not ready to die!"

Nurse: "I hear you are afraid you will die from this disease. Uncontrolled blood pressure can put you at risk for serious complications including death; however, managing your diet and taking your medications are ways to reduce those risks."

Mrs. Hernandez: *(Smiles at nurse.)* "Thanks for talking to me. Let's start talking about the things I need to know."

Patient education about good nutrition and making healthy choices is important. Many want to change habits, but may not have the needed information.

Nutrition Considerations

Obesity is a complex problem and not simply a calorie supply versus demand issue. Behavioral interventions such as tracking foods eaten, eating more slowly, and limiting portion size have been shown to help individuals trying to lose weight (Budd, 2015). There are strong psychological factors involved in obesity, and many obese and overweight people desperately wish to lose weight but face numerous physical and psychological obstacles. It is important for the nurse to maintain a nonjudgmental attitude.

OLDER ADULTS

Older adults are the group most at risk for inadequate nutrition. Many factors influence eating habits of older adults. Economic status, physical disabilities, chronic disease, access to food sources, and physiologic changes must be considered when planning nutrition for this group. **Nutrient requirements do not change with aging except in the presence of disease or illness, although calorie needs decrease each decade after age 50.** Physical activity, including strength training and flexibility activities, should be encouraged to promote muscle mass, maintain functional abilities, and promote appetite and a sense of well-being. Physiologic changes such as a decrease in taste and smell may decrease the appetite of many older adults. The taste of sweets remains strongest and may contribute to older adults consuming more sweets than is advisable. Physical limitations such as chronic lung disease and arthritis make food preparation more difficult and may result in reliance on convenience foods that may not be nutritious. Many older adults have lost spouses and friends through death. Eating alone is unpleasant for many individuals. If possible, arrange for companionship during meals, such as sitters or attendance at senior centers for a mid-day meal. At least one meal a day is served at most centers. Some older adults have limited incomes and must limit food choices. Programs such as Meals on Wheels (Fig. 26.4), the Supplemental Nutrition Assistance Program (SNAP), and community food banks, as well as family intervention, can help older adults to meet nutritional needs. Social workers and dietitians can assist in making these referrals. Families can prepare meals that can be frozen and easily heated by older adults.

Patient Education

Improving Nutrition of Older Adults

Mrs. Lewis, a 76-year-old, has lived alone since her daughter and grandchildren moved away 3 months ago. She chose not to move and live with her daughter's family. For the past month, Mrs. Lewis has experienced a progressive decrease in appetite. She states that she does not enjoy eating alone and that it is too much trouble to cook for one person. Mrs. Lewis should be taught to:

- Prepare several portions of favorite foods at one time and place the foods in freezer containers for easy reheating.
- Keep nutritious snacks available, including fruit, vegetable slices, and soft nutritious desserts such as yogurt.
- Participate in church or community senior citizen social activities to increase socialization.
- Serve food in an attractive setting, even when eating alone.
- Listen to favorite music during mealtimes to serve as a stimulant when eating alone.
- Add flavorful low sodium seasoning and spices to food. Many spices have proven health benefits.
- Maintain adequate fluid intake.
- Engage in exercise such as gardening or walking to stimulate appetite and provide a feeling of general well-being.

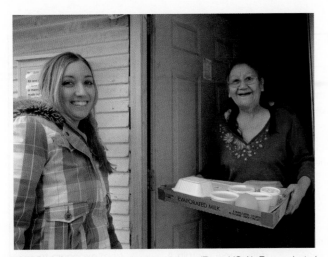

FIGURE 26.4 A meals on wheels recipient. (From US Air Force photo/ Airman 1st Class Katrina Heikkinen.)

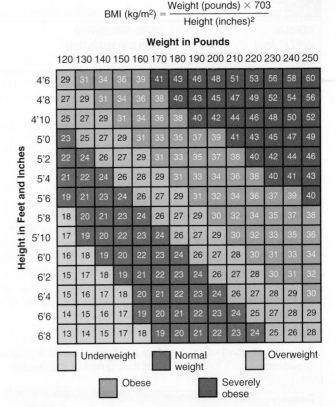

Another concern for older adults living alone is senility. Many older adults with memory loss may not remember eating or may not eat for long periods. Family intervention to provide supervision of meal preparation and eating can help ensure that the person is eating nutritionally and preparing foods safely.

$$\text{BMI (kg/m}^2) = \frac{\text{Weight (pounds)} \times 703}{\text{Height (inches)}^2}$$

Weight in Pounds

Height in Feet and Inches	120	130	140	150	160	170	180	190	200	210	220	230	240	250
4'6	29	31	34	36	39	41	43	46	48	51	53	56	58	60
4'8	27	29	31	34	36	38	40	43	45	47	49	52	54	56
4'10	25	27	29	31	34	36	38	40	42	44	46	48	50	52
5'0	23	25	27	29	31	33	35	37	39	41	43	45	47	49
5'2	22	24	26	27	29	31	33	35	37	38	40	42	44	46
5'4	21	22	24	26	28	29	31	33	34	36	38	40	41	43
5'6	19	21	23	24	26	27	29	31	32	34	36	37	39	40
5'8	18	20	21	23	24	26	27	29	30	32	34	35	37	38
5'10	17	19	20	22	23	24	26	27	29	30	32	33	35	36
6'0	16	18	19	20	22	23	24	26	27	28	30	31	33	34
6'2	15	17	18	19	21	22	23	24	26	27	28	30	31	32
6'4	15	16	17	18	20	21	22	23	24	26	27	28	29	30
6'6	14	15	16	17	19	20	21	22	23	24	25	27	28	29
6'8	13	14	15	17	18	19	20	21	22	23	24	25	26	28

Underweight · Normal weight · Overweight · Obese · Severely obese

FIGURE 26.5 Body Mass Index Chart. Healthy weight: BMI 18 to 24.9 kg/m^2; overweight: BMI 25 to 29.9 kg/m^2; obesity: BMI 30 kg/m^2. BMI = weight (kg)/height (m^2). (From: Lewis, Sharon, Shannon Dirksen, Margaret Heitkemper, Linda Bucher. (2013). *Medical-Surgical Nursing: Assessment and Management of Clinical Problems.* 9th ed. Mosby, VitalBook file.

❖ APPLICATION OF THE NURSING PROCESS

◆ ASSESSMENT (DATA COLLECTION)

Determine factors that may have a negative effect on the patient's nutritional status. Observe for potential nutritional problems during the admission assessment. Admitting diagnoses such as cancer, kidney disease, liver disease, gastrointestinal disease, HIV/AIDS, obesity, diabetes mellitus, or hypertension indicate a need to address nutritional issues. Surgical procedures such as gastrectomy or colon resection also indicate the need to address nutrition. Dietary consults should be ordered for any of these diagnoses. When a patient is admitted to an acute care facility, the Joint Commission dictates that a nutritional screening must be performed within 24 hours.

The nutritional assessment begins with a complete medical, family, and social history. Information can be obtained from the family if the patient is unable to respond. Consider the patient's income level, education, activity, and family status.

Begin physical examination with observation of the patient's general appearance. Is the patient obese? Is there muscle wasting? Examine the patient's skin, hair, nails, eyes, mouth, and extremities. Assess neurologic function as well. Measure height and weight, noting weight gain or loss. Determine excessive thinness or fatness using the patient's **BMI**. The BMI uses height and weight to estimate fat values at which the risk for disease increases. The BMI may provide more useful information than body weight alone does because ideal body weight formulas do not take into consideration individuals with large muscle mass.

A BMI chart is used (Fig 26.5). The chart is not all-inclusive. Use of a more extensive chart or calculations is required for patients whose weight is outside the limits of the chart.

The recommended range for BMI is 18.5 to 24.9. A BMI below 18.5 is considered underweight, between 25 and 29.9 overweight, above 30 obese, and above 40 morbidly obese and at severe risk for disease. Waist circumference may also be a determining factor for risk of disease. A waist size greater than 35 inches for women and 40 inches for men is associated with increased risk for disease. The BMI serves as a screen only. Results should be evaluated with other assessment information to determine the patient's risk for disease.

Review results of laboratory studies as part of the nutritional assessment. Serum albumin (protein), hemoglobin, and hematocrit indicate whether the patient is at risk for malnutrition, is anemic, or is dehydrated. Table 26.8 summarizes physical signs of malnutrition.

Table 26.8 Physical Signs Indicating Possible Malnutrition

NORMAL APPEARANCE	SIGNS ASSOCIATED WITH MALNUTRITION	DISORDERS, NUTRITIONAL DEFICITS	NON-NUTRITIONAL PROBLEMS
Hair			
Shiny, firm, and well rooted	Lack of natural shine: dull and dry, thin and sparse, dyspigmented, and easily plucked (no pain)	Kwashiorkor and, less commonly, marasmus protein deficiency	Excessive bleaching of hair, alopecia
Face			
Skin color uniform, smooth, healthy appearance, and not swollen	Scaling of the skin around the nostrils; swollen face (moon face)	Riboflavin	Acne vulgaris
Eyes			
Bright, clear, and shiny; no sores at the corners of the eyelids; membranes are a healthy pink and moist; no prominent blood vessels or mound of tissue or sclera	Pale conjunctiva; conjunctival xerosis (dullness); corneal xerosis; keratomalacia (softening of cornea); redness and fissuring of eyelid corners; corneal arcus (white ring around eye); xanthelasma (small yellowish bumps around the eyes)	Anemia (e.g., iron deficiency) vitamin A, riboflavin, and pyridoxine; hyperlipidemia	Bloodshot eyes from exposure to weather, lack of sleep, smoke, or excessive alcohol consumption
Lips			
Smooth, not chapped or swollen	Angular cheilosis (white or pink lesions at the corners of the mouth)	Riboflavin	Excessive salivation from improper-fitting dentures
Tongue			
Deep red in appearance, not swollen or smooth	Magenta tongue (purplish); filiform papillae atrophy or hypertrophy (red tongue)	Riboflavin, folic acid, and niacin	Leukoplakia
Teeth			
No cavities, no pain, and bright	Mottled enamel, caries (cavities), and missing teeth	Fluoride excess; excessive sugar	Malocclusion, periodontal disease, and poor dental hygiene
Gums			
Healthy, red, do not bleed, and not swollen	Spongy, bleeding, and receding gums	Scurvy (vitamin C deficiency)	Periodontal disease
Glands			
Not swollen	Thyroid enlargement (front of the neck swollen); parotid enlargement (swollen cheeks)	Iodine starvation; bulimia nervosa	Allergic or inflammatory enlargement of thyroid
Nervous System			
Psychological stability and normal reflexes	Psychomotor changes; mental confusion; sensory loss; motor weakness; loss of position sense; loss of sense of vibration; loss of ankle and knee jerks; burning and tingling of hands and feet (paresthesia); dementia	Kwashiorkor, (protein deficiency), thiamine niacin, and vitamin B_{12}	

Adapted from Mahan, C. K., & Arlin, M. (2008). *Krause's Food, Nutrition and Diet Therapy* (10th ed., p. 375). Philadelphia, PA: Elsevier Saunders; and Peckenpaugh, N. J. (2010). *Nutrition: Essentials and Diet Therapy* (11th ed., pp. 34-35). Philadelphia, PA: Elsevier Saunders.

Focused Assessment

Assessment of Nutrition

The health care facility may have a nutritional assessment tool. If not, ask questions to assess the patient's nutritional patterns.

- What foods do you like or dislike?
- Are there foods that cause you discomfort (e.g., indigestion, diarrhea, constipation, or stuffy nose)?
- What types of snacks do you eat? How often do you snack?
- What types and amount of fluids do you drink?
- What milk products do you use? How often?
- Do you eat bread at each meal? What type?
- How much fruit do you eat each day?
- Do you add salt to your food? How much?
- How often do you eat desserts?
- Do you use sugar or salt substitutes? What types?
- Do you drink alcohol? How much? How often? What type(s)?
- What types of meat do you eat (chicken or red meat)? How much do you eat each day?
- Do you eat fish? How often? How is it prepared?
- How much sugar do you add to foods and fluids?
- Have any members of your family been told they have diabetes?
- Are any immediate family members overweight?
- Is food prepared by anyone other than you? If so, do you make suggestions concerning meal planning?
- Do you read the labels of prepared foods to determine fat and sodium content?

After completing the nutritional assessment, determine whether a nutritional problem is present. Document the findings and conclusions. Documentation should include a summary of the findings and indicate any problem identified and the course of action taken. Make a nutritional referral to the dietitian, with the primary care provider's permission, if malnutrition or other nutritional problems are identified so that early intervention can be started.

◆ NURSING DIAGNOSIS

After data collection, nursing diagnoses and goals/expected outcomes should be formulated. Some nursing diagnoses related to nutrition include:

- Imbalanced nutrition: less than body requirements
- Ineffective coping
- Readiness for enhanced nutrition
- Deficient fluid volume
- Excess fluid volume
- Deficient knowledge
- Impaired swallowing
- Risk for aspiration

◆ PLANNING

Some examples of goals and expected outcomes for the above nursing diagnoses are as follows:

- Patient will consume 2200 calories/day.
- Patient will restrict caloric intake to 1800 calories/day.
- Patient will verbalize methods to manage stress such as relaxation exercises.
- Patient will consume 1500 mL of fluid per day.
- Patient with edema in upper and lower extremities will experience its decrease by day of discharge.
- Infant will gain 5 oz by day of discharge.
- Patient will choose appropriate foods from the hospital menu for a low fat, low cholesterol diet.
- Patient will consume at least 50% of a pureed diet.
- Patient will have breath sounds that remain clear with no evidence of aspiration on repeat swallow studies.

◆ IMPLEMENTATION

Interventions for nutritional care include assisting patients with the meal tray, feeding when necessary, providing enteral nutrition or total parenteral nutrition when needed, performing patient education about proper diet, encouraging adherence to a therapeutic diet, and monitoring the patient's nutritional status.

Before serving a meal, provide for elimination by offering the bedpan or urinal or assisting the patient to the bathroom. Help the patient wash the hands and face as needed. Provide oral hygiene if desired. Create an attractive and pleasant environment for eating. Remove distracting articles such as an emesis basin or a urinal, and use a spray or deodorizer to remove unpleasant odors in the room if not contraindicated. Position the patient comfortably for the meal with the head of the bed elevated (if allowed), or help the patient sit up in a chair and prepare the over-the-bed table for the diet tray.

When serving trays from the dietary kitchen, serve those patients first who are able to feed themselves. Check each tray against the unit dietary order list to verify that the correct diet tray has been prepared. Deliver the trays as quickly as possible to prevent food from cooling.

When dietary personnel deliver meal trays, the nurse is responsible for positioning the patient and setting up the tray to promote food and fluid intake. Many people have difficulty opening the sealed packages of eating utensils and condiments. For the patient with an intravenous cannula in the hand, milk cartons and other sealed food items should be opened and prepared for eating. Attending to these details quickly after the trays are served helps the patient enjoy a warm meal.

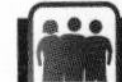

Assignment Considerations

Assigning of Feeding Responsibilities

Feeding patients may be delegated to unlicensed assistive personnel (UAPs) such as certified nursing assistants or patient care technicians. Knowledge of the skill level of the UAP is essential to provide a pleasant and safe environment for the feeding experience.

Patient and Family Education

Depending on the patient's nutritional problem and type of diet prescribed, the following points may be included in the patient's education plan:

- Ideal weight for body height and build
- Caloric intake needed to maintain ideal weight
- Need for added calories, proteins, and vitamins to promote healing
- Foods high in iron and vitamin C that are used to build iron stores
- Use of frozen or "low salt" or "no salt" canned vegetables
- How to read food labels to determine the content and caloric value of various foods
- Use of a variety of herbs and spices to enhance the taste of food
- Use of frequent small meals, which may be more appealing when appetite is diminished
- Methods of increasing the amount of vegetables and fruit in the diet
- Methods of shopping wisely for prepared frozen foods when limited time is available for food preparation
- Resources such as community food banks, SNAP, and WIC for patients with limited financial resources

◆ EVALUATION

Evaluation is based on the achievement of the expected outcomes. Review the goals and expected outcomes. Did the patient achieve them? Did she partially achieve them? If problems were not resolved, why not? While evaluating a patient's achievement of outcomes, you may need to work with the patient to change, modify, or eliminate some expectations (Nursing Care Plan 26.1).

Sample evaluation statements include:

- Patient gained 1 lb in 1 week.
- Patient lost 1 lb in 1 week.
- Patient consumed 90% of food and fluids at each meal.
- Patient made appropriate food choices from an 1800-calorie menu.

Nursing Care Plan 26.1 Care of the Patient with Malnutrition

SCENARIO Emily Montgomery is a 55-year-old woman admitted with a diagnosis of pneumonia and malnutrition. Mrs. Montgomery was brought to the emergency department by a friend. She lives alone and does not work outside the home. Her husband of 30 years died about 1 year ago. She has a son and a daughter; both are married and live about 100 miles away. Physical examination reveals a thin, frail-appearing woman in mild respiratory distress. She is receiving oxygen at 2 L/min, intravenous fluids of 5% dextrose, and water with 40 mEq of potassium added. She is on a full liquid diet with orders to push oral fluids. She is 5′6″ tall and weighs 103 lb. She states she has had a poor appetite for the past year and usually eats one small meal daily. Mrs. Montgomery reports a 40-lb weight loss. Laboratory values: hemoglobin 9.7 g/dL, hematocrit 30.1%, albumin 2.8 g/dL.

PROBLEM/NURSING DIAGNOSIS *Considerable weight loss with malnutrition*/Imbalanced nutrition: less than body requirements related to loss of appetite.

Supporting Assessment Data *Subjective:* States "I haven't had much of an appetite since my husband died. I usually eat one meal a day." ***Objective:*** Height 5′6″, weight 103 lb. Hemoglobin 9.7 g/dL, hematocrit 30.1%, albumin 2.8 g/dL. Muscle wasting in the abdomen and all extremities, 40-lb weight loss.

Goals/Expected Outcomes	Nursing Interventions	Selected Rationale	Evaluation
Weight gain of at least 2 lb by date of discharge	Obtain daily weights; teach proper weight for height	Provides information on patient progress and potential need for more interventions	*Did the patient gain at least 2 lb by discharge?* Gained 3 lb by date of discharge. Outcome met.

PROBLEM/NURSING DIAGNOSIS Husband of 30 years died 1 year ago/Depression, isolation/Ineffective coping related to death of husband.

Supporting Assessment Data *Subjective:* States loss of appetite since death of husband; eats one meal daily. *Objective:* Thin, frail appearing, depressed, withdrawn appearance.

Goals/Expected Outcomes	Nursing Interventions	Selected Rationale	Evaluation
Verbalizes feeling of well-being by time of discharge	Assess economic and social factors that may hinder achievement of optimal nutrition	Provide subjective data concerning resources available to the patient	*Did patient express improvement in well-being?* States, "I feel better but I still get tired sometimes." Progressing toward expected outcome.
Energy level increased to perform activities of daily living with assistance by date of discharge	Assess level of activity	Promotes the patient's self-care abilities	*Did the patient complete activities of daily living with limited assistance by time of discharge?* Completes daily hygiene with minimal assistance. Requires occasional rest periods. Progressing toward expected outcome.

Nursing Care Plan 26.1 Care of the Patient with Malnutrition—cont'd

PROBLEM/NURSING DIAGNOSIS *Eats only one small meal each day/Lack of understanding of appropriate food choices/*Deficient knowledge related to choosing diet with adequate calories and nutrients.

Supporting Assessment Data *Subjective:* States poor appetite; eats one meal per day. *Objective:* 40-lb weight loss, muscle wasting.

Goals/Expected Outcomes	Nursing Interventions	Selected Rationale	Evaluation
Demonstrates the ability to choose a balanced diet from a hospital menu by date of discharge	Teach components of nutritious diet Provide daily menus to choose appropriate foods Involve family in discussion concerning nutritional needs	Provides information concerning the patient's ability to care for self, as well as the level of adherence	*Can the patient verbalize a plan to increase nutritional intake?* Is working on formulating a plan to meet nutritional needs. Working with a dietitian and a social worker. Progressing toward outcome.
The patient formulates a 2500-calorie healthy diet plan by discharge	Assess the level of activity tolerance	Provides the tools needed to formulate an acceptable diet	*Did the patient formulate an appropriate 2500-calorie diet plan?* Has formulated 3 days' worth of menus for the 2500-calorie diet plan.
Demonstrates the ability to choose a balanced diet from a hospital menu by date of discharge	Teach components of nutritious diet and calories needed daily Provide daily menus to choose appropriate foods Involve the family in discussion concerning nutritional needs	Provides information concerning the patient's ability to care for self, as well as the level of compliance	*Can the patient choose appropriate foods from hospital menus?* Choosing appropriate foods from the hospital menu with assistance. Progressing toward expected outcomes.

CRITICAL THINKING QUESTIONS

1. The patient is ready for discharge. What strategies could the family use to ensure that the plan of care is followed?
2. What are some signs and symptoms the patient should be taught to report to the health care provider?

Get Ready for the NCLEX Examination!

Key Points

- To achieve good nutrition, individuals should consume a balanced diet containing all essential nutrients: proteins, carbohydrates, fats, vitamins, minerals, and water.
- USDA MyPlate divides foods into five groups, and it contains recommendations for daily portions of each group.
- General dietary recommendations include:
  - Increase total complex carbohydrates.
  - Decrease saturated fats and *trans*-fatty acids.
  - Decrease sugar intake.
  - Eat more fiber, especially soluble fiber.
  - Decrease sodium intake.
  - Consume alcohol in moderation or not at all.
- Protein is needed for tissue building, regeneration of cells, tissue healing, and energy. It supplies 4 calories/g.
- Carbohydrates are the main source of energy for the body, and they supply 4 calories/g.
- Functions of carbohydrates include a quick source of energy and regulation of protein and fat metabolism.
- Dietary fiber is the portion of carbohydrates that cannot be broken down by intestinal enzymes and juices. Food sources include whole grain cereals and skins of fruit, vegetables, and legumes.
- Fiber increases bulk in the stool, leading to good intestinal function and elimination.
- High fat intake has been linked to obesity, breast and colon cancer, hypertension and other cardiovascular diseases, and stroke.
- Fats are classified as saturated (solid at room temperature) and unsaturated (liquid at room temperature). Fat provides a concentrated source of energy, supplying 9 calories/g.
- Functions of fat include absorbing fatty acid, adding flavor to foods, absorbing fat-soluble vitamins, and providing insulation and controlling body temperature.
- Vitamins are classified as fat soluble or water soluble. Fat-soluble vitamins are A, D, E, and K. Water-soluble vitamins are the B-complex vitamins and vitamin C.
- Minerals are essential for metabolism and cellular function. Major minerals (dietary needs are more than 100 mg/day) include calcium, magnesium, sodium, potassium, phosphorus, sulfur, and chlorine. Iron, zinc, fluoride, chromium, selenium, iodine, and copper are called trace minerals because the body requires less than 100 mg/day of each.
- Minerals also play a role in maintaining strong teeth and bones and in blood clotting.

- Water is involved in all of the body's chemical processes, and it is the most essential of all nutrients.
- Awareness of a patient's economic status and religious and cultural preferences can help the nurse individualize patient care.
- The first year of life marks the fastest growth period of human development. Birth weight should double by the end of 6 months and triple by the end of 1 year.
- Infant nutrition usually consists of breast milk or formula for the first year, with solid foods introduced gradually, one food at a time, at 4 to 6 months of age so that symptoms of allergy or sensitivity can be noted.
- Children at risk for poor nutrition should be referred to school breakfast and lunch programs.
- Puberty and the adolescent growth spurt increase nutritional requirements of protein, calcium, vitamin D, and iron.
- Teaching adolescents how to make wise choices at fast-food establishments can be important.
- Eating disorders, especially among adolescent girls, are prevalent during this developmental stage.
- Adults should be taught to make wise choices in food selection to help avoid conditions such as obesity, hypertension, diabetes mellitus, and cardiovascular disease.
- Older adults may be at risk for malnutrition. Chronic disease and physical disability or limited income may interfere with older adults meeting nutritional needs.
- Patients with gastrointestinal disorders, cancer, HIV/AIDS, abdominal surgery, and immobility are at risk for malnutrition and should be evaluated by the dietitian.
- The recommended BMI range is 18.5 to 24.9 for an adult.

Additional Learning Resources

SG Go to your Study Guide for additional learning activities to help you master this chapter content.

evolve Go to your Evolve website at http://evolve.elsevier.com/Williams/fundamental for additional online resources.

Online Resources

- *Choose MyPlate*, www.choosemyplate.gov
- *Dietary Reference Intakes*, http://iom.nationalacademies.org/~/media/Files/Activity%20Files/Nutrition/DRIs/5_Summary%20Table%20Tables%201-4.pdf.

Review Questions for the NCLEX Examination

*Choose the **best** answer for each question.*

1. A patient has had a hysterectomy. She needs to increase her protein and vitamin C intake to promote healing. Which foods would be best to include in her diet? *(Select all that apply.)*
   1. Steak
   2. Carrots
   3. Tomatoes
   4. Eggs
   5. Muffins
2. The major nutrient involved in fluid balance is:
   1. Fat.
   2. Protein.
   3. Niacin.
   4. Carbohydrates.
3. The major component necessary for metabolism of carbohydrate is (are):
   1. Pancreatic enzymes.
   2. Insulin secreted by the pancreas.
   3. Bile secreted by the liver.
   4. Mucus secreted from the duodenum.
4. The hospital dinner menu includes broiled pork chop with brown gravy, mashed potatoes, peas, and a green salad with apple pie for dessert. This choice would not be appropriate to serve a(n) ____________ patient.
   1. American Indian
   2. African American
   3. Middle Eastern Muslim
   4. Hispanic
5. A patient who weighs 185 lb is placed on a 2200-calorie diet. How many grams of protein should the diet contain to meet the maximum recommended daily requirement of this nutrient?
   1. 56 g
   2. 67 g
   3. 75 g
   4. 82 g
6. The dietitian recommends an increase of fiber in the diet. Which meal would provide the most fiber?
   1. Meat loaf, mashed potatoes, and steamed spinach
   2. Chicken breast with gravy, rice, and asparagus
   3. Milk, instant oatmeal, and orange juice
   4. Beans, rice, corn tortillas, and a mixed green salad
7. During a physical examination of a patient, which might indicate malnutrition?
   1. Red cheeks
   2. Absence of gray hair
   3. Ridged nails
   4. Pale conjunctiva

Critical Thinking Activities

Read each clinical scenario and discuss the questions with your classmates.

Scenario A

Ray Brown, age 28, is 6′1″ and weighs 250 lb. He states he has had difficulty remaining on the 2500-calorie diet prescribed by the dietitian. History reveals Mr. Brown's diet is mainly a traditional African American diet, including many high fat and high sodium foods.

1. Determine Mr. Brown's BMI.
2. What medical conditions is Mr. Brown at risk for because of his present weight and eating habits?
3. How can Mr. Brown's diet be modified to help him meet his weight loss goal and dietary needs?

Scenario B

Tina Aquirre, age 19, is a student at a local community college. She frequently skips breakfast and lunch or grabs a sweet roll and soda mid-morning and a candy bar and soda mid-afternoon. She is experiencing fatigue and inability to concentrate during late afternoon classes.

1. How do you explain Tina's fatigue in the late afternoon?
2. What nutritional strategies would you suggest to help Tina meet her nutritional needs and provide needed energy for her classes?

Scenario C

Sam Minor, a 56-year-old accountant, is diagnosed with hypertension. His blood pressure is 164/100 mm Hg when he comes to the primary care provider's office for a checkup.

1. What additional assessment data do you need to develop a patient education plan for Mr. Minor to meet his nutritional needs?
2. Develop a patient education plan for Mr. Minor.

Scenario D

Marian Chou, age 50, is undergoing chemotherapy for liver cancer. She is experiencing loss of appetite, nausea, and abdominal pain.

1. What nursing diagnoses are appropriate for Mrs. Chou?
2. What nursing interventions would you implement to help stimulate Mrs. Chou's desire to eat and take fluids?

chapter 27

Nutritional Therapy and Assisted Feeding

http://evolve.elsevier.com/Williams/fundamental

Objectives

Upon completing this chapter, you should be able to do the following:

Theory

1. Identify the nurse's role related to nutritional therapy and special dietary needs.
2. Compare and contrast a full liquid diet with a clear liquid diet.
3. Explain the different dietary modification levels: pureed, mechanically altered, advanced, and regular.
4. Describe health issues related to nutrition.
5. List disease processes that may benefit from nutritional therapy.
6. Verbalize the rationale for assisted feedings and tube feedings.
7. List the steps for the procedure to insert, irrigate, and remove a nasogastric tube.
8. Discuss the procedure for tube feeding.
9. Identify the medical rationale and nursing care for a patient receiving peripheral parenteral nutrition (PPN) and total parenteral nutrition (TPN).
10. Understand the possible complications associated with modified diets, tube feedings, PPN, and TPN.

Clinical Practice

1. Using therapeutic communication, assist a patient who requires a special diet.
2. Develop a patient education plan for nutritional therapy.
3. Demonstrate insertion, irrigation, and removal of a nasogastric tube.
4. Demonstrate feeding a patient through a nasogastric tube or percutaneous endoscopic gastrostomy (PEG) tube.
5. Know your facility's policies, procedures, and protocols for nutrition-related problems and complications with tube feedings.

Skills & Steps

Skills

Steps

Key Terms

anorexia nervosa (ăn-ō-RĔK-sē-ă nĕr-VŌ-să, p. 488)
atherosclerosis (ăth-ĕr-ō-sklĕ-RŌ-sĭs, p. 491)
binge eating (p. 488)
body mass index (BMI) (p. 489)
bulimia nervosa (bū-LĒ-mē-ă, p. 488)
diabetes mellitus (dī-ă-BĒ-tēz MĔL-ĭ-tĭs, p. 491)
dysphagia (dĭs-FĀ-jē-ă, p. 495)
enteral (ĔN-tĕr-ăl, p. 495)
feeding pump (p. 501)
gastrostomy tubes (găs-TRŌS-to-mē, p. 495)
glycosuria (glī-kōs-ŬR-ē-ă, p. 504)
heart failure (HF) (p. 491)
homeostasis (hō-mē-ō-STĀ-sĭs, p. 487)
hyperosmolality (HĪ-pĕr-ŎS-mō-LĂ-lĭ-tē, p. 504)
hypertension (p. 489)
jejunostomy or duodenal tubes (jĕ-jūn-ĂW-stō-mē, dū-ă-DĒ-năl, p. 495)
myocardial infarction (MI) (p. 491)
nasogastric (NG) tubes (nā-zō-GĂS-trĭk, p. 495)
NPO (p. 487)
parenteral (pă-RĔN-tĕr-ăl, p. 504)
percutaneous endoscopic gastrostomy (PEG) tubes (pĕr-kū-TĀ-nē-ŭs găs-TRŎS-tō-mē, p. 495)
peripheral parenteral nutrition (PPN) (pă-RĔN-tĕr-ăl, p. 504)
postoperative (p. 487)
preoperatively (prē-ŎP-ĕr-ă-tĭv-lē, p. 487)
residue (p. 487)
total parenteral nutrition (TPN) (pă-RĔN-tĕr-ăl, p. 504)

Concepts Covered in This Chapter

- Acid base balance
- Care coordination
- Cellular regulation
- Clinical judgment
- Collaboration
- Communication
- Culture
- Health promotion
- Nutrition
- Elimination
- Fluid and electrolyte balance
- Glucose regulation
- Patient education
- Safety
- Tissue integrity

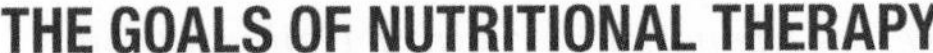

THE GOALS OF NUTRITIONAL THERAPY

The goals of nutritional therapy are to treat and manage disease, prevent complications, and restore or maintain health through appropriate diet. Patients in health care facilities have multiple dietary needs related to disease processes; surgical procedures; physical health; and cultural, religious, and individual preferences. The specific diet for each patient is prescribed on the primary care provider's order. Some patients may have diets without restrictions that are similar to meals eaten at home. For other patients, nutritional therapy is a significant factor in their medical treatment. **You can assist patients in meeting their nutritional goals by completing thorough nutritional data collection.** Monitor the patient's food and fluid intake and document the response to therapy.

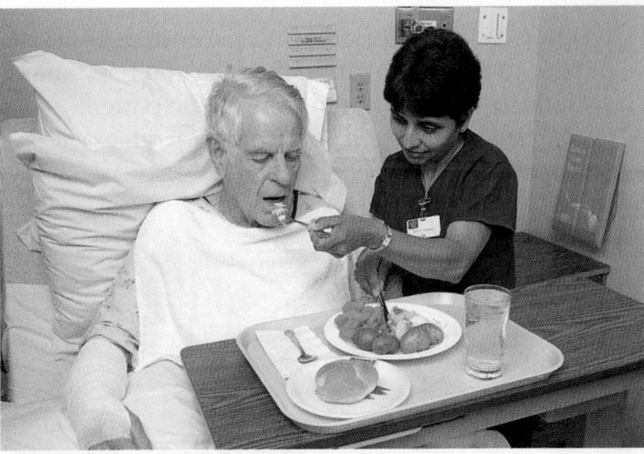

FIGURE 27.1 Assisting with feeding.

Weight gain or loss, percentage of meals eaten, and ability to tolerate the diet should be included in the documentation.

 QSEN Considerations: Teamwork and Collaboration

Nutritional Modification

Modification of the diet to increase the effectiveness of therapy can be accomplished through discussion with the patient, the primary care provider, and the registered dietitian. Collaboration with the patient is key.

Patients who may need assistance with food and fluid intake include those who have paralysis of the arms, visual impairment, intravenous lines or other devices in their hand or arm, problems breathing or swallowing **(dysphagia)**, or severe impairments or weakness (Fig. 27.1). You may delegate this task to the nursing assistant or a family member, if appropriate (Skill 27.1).

Skill 27.1 Assisting a Patient with Feeding

 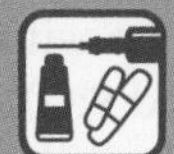 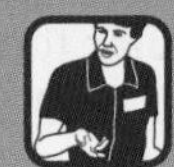 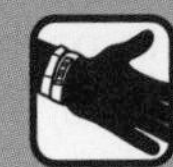 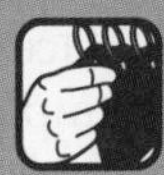 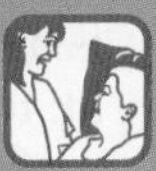 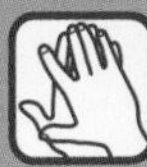 

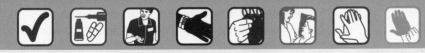

Assisting a patient with feeding is a nursing responsibility. Patients with physical or mental impairment may require the expertise of a nurse to ensure that a safe feeding procedure is followed.

SUPPLIES

- Tray with dishes of food
- Over-the-bed or tray table
- Utensils
- Napkin
- Straw
- Small towel or extra napkin (clothing protector)

Review and carry out the Standard Steps in Appendix A.

ACTION *(RATIONALE)*

Assessment (Data Collection)

1. Assess patient's need for assistance with feeding. *(Guides type of assistance to be given.)*

Planning

2. Check the diet on the tray with the diet sheet. *(Ensures that patient receives the correct diet.)*
3. Clear the over-the-bed table and place the diet tray on it. Position patient in as high a Fowler

position as is comfortable and permitted, or assist patient to a chair. Position the over-the-bed table with the diet tray on it in front of the patient. *(Swallowing is enhanced by an upright position.)*

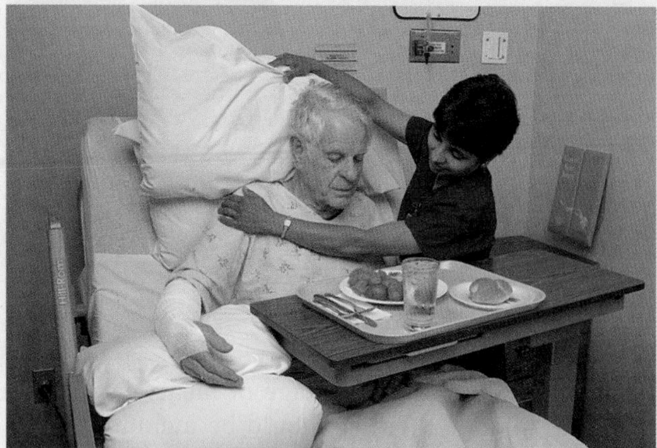

Step **3**

4. Protect patient's clothing and bed linens with a towel, clothing protector, or napkin. *(Protects clothing or bed linens from soiling if food is spilled.)*

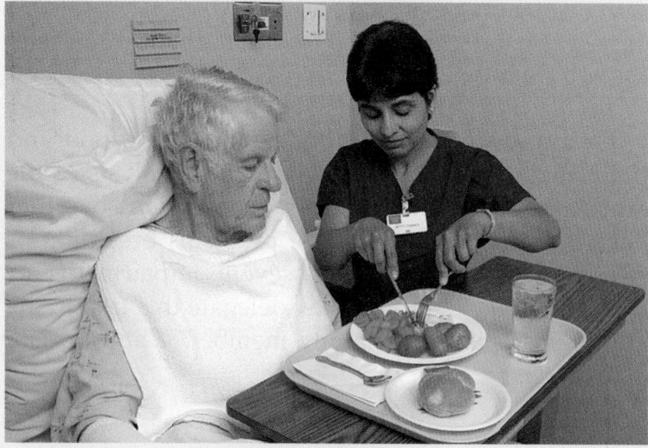

Step **4**

5. Open the containers of food, fluids, condiments, and eating utensils. *(Prepares food for feeding the patient.)*

Implementation

6. Ask which foods the patient prefers to begin with; alternate foods. Add condiments as desired by the patient. Offer small bites, and wait until the patient has chewed and swallowed before offering the next bite. *(A relaxed, unhurried manner will encourage the patient to eat more of the meal.)*
7. Offer fluids when the patient desires. Place a flexible straw in the fluid container and hold the container steady to allow the patient to grasp the straw with his lips. Be certain the liquid is not too hot. *(Liquids help wash down food. Do not offer too much to drink because this will interfere with digestion. A straw masks the degree of heat in the fluid, and patients may burn their mouths if the liquid is too hot.)*

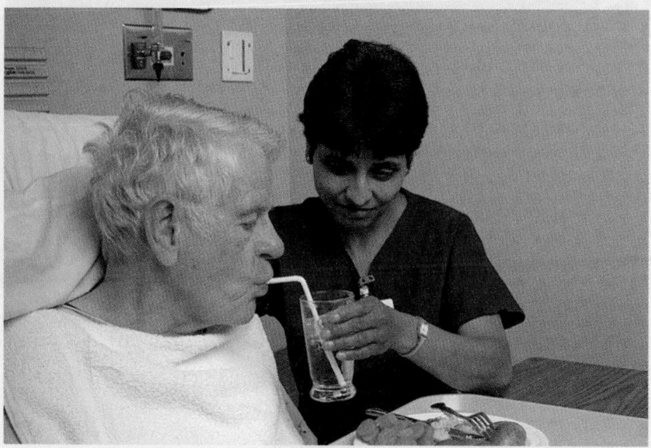

Step **7**

8. Wipe the mouth at intervals as needed. Talk with the patient during the meal. Do not appear rushed. *(Removal of food particles from the sides of the mouth preserves the patient's dignity. Conversation adds to the social atmosphere and can improve food intake.)*
9. Encourage patients who are physically capable to feed themselves as much as possible. *(Self-feeding increases self-esteem.)*
10. Refrain from insisting that patient finish entire meal. *(Gentle persuasion to take just another bite is appropriate for the patient who is taking a smaller amount of nutrients than required, but patient's wishes must be respected.)*
11. When the meal is finished, remove the tray; offer hand hygiene and oral hygiene. *(The patient's hands may have become soiled if the patient participated in feeding. Oral hygiene refreshes the mouth and removes retained food particles.)*

The Visually Impaired Patient

12. For the patient who is visually impaired but able to self-feed, describe what foods are on the plate and tray. Orient the patient to the position of the foods on the plate by describing the plate as if it is a clock face with particular foods positioned at: for example, 12:00, 3:00, 6:00, and 9:00. *(Many patients who have their eyes bandaged or who are blind are still able to feed themselves if given adequate orientation to the plate and tray.)*
13. Complete procedure as listed for the patient who needs assistance. *(Patients with additional impairment may need nursing assistance for feeding.)*

Evaluation

14. Assess the patient's tolerance of the meal, the amount consumed, and any difficulty experienced. *(Provides information for modification of diet if necessary.)*

Documentation

15. Document the amount and type of food consumed during the feeding and patient's response. *(Documents nutritional intake and how it is tolerated. Communicates progress to the health care team.)*

Documentation Example

2/16 1200 Fed lunch; ate 50% of meal. Had difficulty chewing and swallowing meats. Occasional coughing when swallowing. Discussed with primary care provider. Diet changed to pureed meats. (Nurse's electronic signature)

Critical Thinking Questions

1. The patient requires assistance with feeding, but is reluctant to allow the nurse to help. Identify strategies the nurse might use to make the procedure more acceptable.
2. The patient is recovering from a stroke. Right-sided weakness is noted on assessment. What safety measures might the nurse use to reduce the risk of complications during assisted feeding?

THE POSTOPERATIVE PATIENT

Patients scheduled for surgical procedures may have special nutritional needs. Ideally, the surgical patient should be well nourished **preoperatively** (before surgery) to facilitate **postoperative** (after surgery) healing and recovery.

Preoperative patients usually placed on **NPO** (take no food or fluids by mouth) status for up to 12 hours before the procedure. This practice decreases the risk of vomiting while under anesthesia, which could lead to aspiration of stomach contents. Aspiration can result in serious respiratory complications. Always check with the surgeon for exceptions to NPO orders. These exceptions may include diabetic, cardiac, and/or any other medications (with a "sip" of water) that ensure patient stability during surgery.

Think Critically

How does the anatomy of the gastrointestinal tract relate to the risk of aspiration when a patient is under anesthesia?

Postoperative patients progress from a clear liquid diet to a full liquid diet. Solid foods are added when the patient can tolerate them without nausea, vomiting, or other abdominal discomfort.

Clear liquids are started when the patient has a return of bowel sounds detected by auscultation. Clear liquids primarily maintain fluid **homeostasis** and relieve thirst. The goal is to introduce fluids that have low **residue** (remains after digestion), are easily digested, and have low risk of causing abdominal discomfort. Abdominal distress, such as vomiting and distention, can cause injury to surgical interventions.

Foods that are clear fluids at room temperature (e.g., gelatin and Popsicles) and liquids that are clear are included on the clear liquid diet. Some care providers restrict use of cola drinks on a clear liquid diet, but allow carbonated drinks that are clear, such as ginger ale. Clear liquid diets are used short term because the diet is deficient in most nutrients. Bouillon (broth) added to the diet provides small amounts of protein and some electrolytes.

A full liquid diet may be used as a step between clear liquid and mechanical soft or regular diet. Full liquid is used following surgery, long-term fasting, or for those with chewing or swallowing problems. Full liquid diets include all fluids, custards, ice cream, sherbet, puddings, and cooked refined cereals. Full liquids can be used for longer-term nutritional management because protein and other essential nutrients, vitamins, and minerals are available from the foods allowed. The full liquid diet is, however, low in iron, vitamin A, vitamin B12, and thiamine; therefore, vitamin and mineral supplements must be provided for longer-term use. Foods allowed in clear liquid diets and full liquid diets are compared in Box 27.1.

Patients recovering from surgical procedures that involved manipulation of or surgical incision into the stomach or bowel may progress to a soft diet before attempting a general or regular diet. Soft diets are low in fiber, and foods are softened by cooking, mashing, or chopping. Foods allowed on a soft diet include eggs; breads without seeds; boiled or mashed potatoes; soups; fruit; juices; tender cooked vegetables; meat that is stewed, boiled, or ground; cooked cereals; mashed bananas; applesauce; and milk products. As the patient's condition progresses, the diet is advanced to general. This diet has no specific restrictions unless required because of a patient's specific disease process.

Think Critically

Your patient is scheduled for a bowel resection. How would you discuss dietary goals with your preoperative patient? What would you include in the expected dietary progression and explanation to your patient?

HEALTH ISSUES RELATED TO NUTRITION

FEEDING AND EATING DISORDERS

Feeding and eating disorders are comprised of categories of disorders that occur across the life span. In adolescence and young adulthood, individuals can develop conditions related to dietary intake. These are diagnosed as mental health disorders and include anorexia nervosa, bulimia nervosa, and binge eating.

Box 27.1 Full Liquid and Clear Liquid Diets

FOOD ALLOWED ON A CLEAR LIQUID DIET	FOOD ALLOWED ON A FULL LIQUID DIET
• Grape, apple, and cranberry juices • Strained fruit juices • Vegetable broth • Carbonated water (preferably clear) • Clear fruit-flavored drinks • Sweetened gelatin and ices • Clear candies • Popsicles • Tea or coffee • Clear broth	• Milk and milk beverages • Yogurt, eggnog, and pudding • Custard and ice cream • Pureed meats and vegetables in cream soups • Strained fruit juices • Vegetable juices • Sweetened plain gelatin • Cooked refined cereals • Strained or blended gruel • All other beverages • Cream, margarine, and butter • Sherbet • Popsicles

Anorexia Nervosa

Anorexia nervosa is a psychological disorder characterized by restriction of caloric intake, a very low body weight for the developmental stage, a pathological fear of becoming fat, and a severe disturbance in body image. It is prevalent among adolescent and young women; however, adolescent and young men may also be affected. They view themselves as obese despite being extremely underweight. Patients with anorexia nervosa severely restrict caloric intake and focus on moderate to vigorous physical activity. **If not corrected, anorexia nervosa can be fatal.** Treatment is a combination of nutritional intervention, behavioral modification, and psychological counseling.

QSEN Considerations: Patient-Centered Care

Considering Patient and Family Values

Collaboration among the patient, family, primary care provider, mental health professional, nurse, and dietitian is crucial. A nutritional plan to be implemented should always be acceptable to the patient.

The treatment goals are to plan and achieve a nutritious, healthy eating pattern and to attain a body weight that is at least 85% of expected weight for height. The patient must be willing to remain in psychological therapy and follow nutritional recommendations to achieve treatment success.

Communication

The Patient With Anorexia Nervosa

Terri Mashburn is a 16-year-old high school junior admitted with a diagnosis of anorexia nervosa. Terri has lost 30 lb over the past 3 months because of extreme caloric restriction and excessive exercise. She is observed during all meals. You are assigned to sit with Terri during her lunch.

Nurse: "Hello, Terri. Your lunch is here. I'm going to sit with you while you eat."

Terri: *(Moves from chair to bed.)* "You can take that away. I can't eat that stuff! I'm not hungry anyway." *(Curls up in bed; hides face in pillow.)*

Nurse: *(Places tray on table. Sits on bed next to Terri.)* "You seem upset, Terri. Tell me what's bothering you." *(Places hand on Terri's shoulder.)*

Terri: "Nothing is bothering me. I just don't want to eat."

Nurse: "Tell me about that."

Terri: "The nurse weighed me this morning. I've gained 2 lb since I've been here. This food is making me fat!"

Nurse: "I know you are concerned about your weight. Let's talk about the medical plan concerning your weight."

Terri: *(Sits up in bed.)* "OK, but you are not going to make me eat all that food."

Nurse: *(Brings tray to beside.)* "Tell me which foods you will eat. If you do not like any of them, I can get whatever you want from the dietary department."

Terri: *(Raises cover on food.)* "None of that will do. It will make me fat. I'll eat a salad and an apple. Sprite to drink will be all right."

Nurse: "I will call dietary now." *(Calls dietary department to order food.)* "Now, let's review your medical plan while we wait."

Bulimia nervosa. **Bulimia nervosa** is an eating disorder characterized by episodic binge eating, followed by behaviors designed to prevent weight gain, including purging, fasting, using laxatives, and exercising excessively. Women with bulimia nervosa are aware of their problem and often feel ashamed of the behavior. Treatment of bulimia nervosa is usually easier because of this awareness. Psychological and nutritional counseling is necessary. The treatment plan may include nutritional supplements and monitoring of patients after eating to ensure purging does not occur. Medical conditions such as esophageal and peptic ulcers, depressed gag reflex, and dental issues may accompany bulimia because of the gastric acid exposure during frequently induced vomiting. This condition must be treated with behavioral modification to stop these practices.

Binge eating disorders. **Binge eating** is defined as recurrent episodes of consuming significantly more food in a defined period of time than most people would eat under similar circumstances. Binge eating disorder is one of the most common eating disorders; however, it often goes undiagnosed. Binge episodes are marked by feelings of lack of control. An individual with binge eating disorder may consume foods rather quickly and often do this when they are not hungry. Women are most often affected by this disorder. Many individuals experiencing binge eating generally hide their habit as it is characterized by feelings of guilt, embarrassment, or disgust (American Psychiatric Association, 2013).

Clinical Cues

The patient with a feeding and eating disorder requires careful observation and skilled therapeutic communication. You should observe the patient for evidence of "hoarding" food and structure communication to achieve compliance with the treatment regimen.

Nursing interventions for patients with feeding and eating disorders include nutritional management, behavioral modification, patient education, and monitoring progress. Patient education should include principles of healthy weight maintenance; components of a healthy diet; the dangers of fasting, purging, and binging; and the availability of community support groups. Nurses should document the patient's weight, compliance with nutritional recommendations, and behaviors, as well as the effectiveness of the diet and need for modification of any aspect of the treatment plan.

OBESITY

Obesity rates continue to rise, and obesity (excessive accumulation of body fat) has become a national health threat. The Centers for Disease Control and Prevention (2015) estimates that about 34.9%, or 78.6 million, of adult Americans are obese. Poor diet and limited physical activity are major factors contributing to the epidemic levels of overweight and obese Americans. Obesity is the second leading cause of preventable death in the United States. Many factors contribute to obesity, including genetics, environment, poor eating habits, lack of knowledge about good nutrition, medications, body physiology, age, and gender. Nutritional modifications and physical activity to manage obesity must be individualized and incorporate all factors relevant to the patient.

It is well documented that obesity is responsible for putting people at risk for 30 chronic health conditions, including cardiovascular disease, stroke, diabetes, **hypertension** (abnormally elevated blood pressure), gallbladder disease, joint disease, and some forms of cancer. The goal of obesity treatment is to improve health and quality of life. Long-term success of weight management programs is low. **Approximately 5% of obese people who reach their desired weight management goal can maintain their weight status over a 2- to 5-year period.** Reaching a specific weight status should not be the only measure of success; a lifestyle change is key.

Nutrition Considerations

LET'S MOVE!

The Let's Move program was launched by Michelle Obama, the First Lady of the United States. The goal of this program is to eliminate childhood obesity within a generation. The program encourages the promotion of healthy families and healthier choices at home, to set everyone up for success. Recommendations include:

- Eat five fruits and vegetables each day
- Have healthy choices available at home
- Eat meals together as a family
- Reduce snacks; offer fruits and vegetables when snacking
- Be mindful of portion size
- Reduce fat, sugar, and sugary drinks

To accomplish weight loss, the individual must expend more energy than is consumed through intake of calories. Physical activity designed to match the patient's ability is usually a component of weight management programs. Nutritional therapy depends on the patient's degree of obesity. Obesity is characterized as mild to extreme. Obesity is determined using the **body mass index (BMI)** chart (see Chapter 26). The BMI is a mathematical calculation of height and weight; it may not be as reliable for individuals with very lean bodies or those who are pregnant or lactating. Excessive body fat is present in all instances of obesity. Obesity treatments include consultation and follow up with a health care provider, medically supervised special meal plans, medications (including appetite suppressants and nutrient absorption blockers), and surgical interventions. Effective nursing activities for weight reduction assistance include encouragement of low-calorie diets, plant-based or vegetarian diets, appropriate portion size, activity recommendations, and behavior modification. The American Heart Association has diet and lifestyle recommendations for Americans (see Chapter 26).

Bariatric surgery, which reduces stomach size and/or reduces calorie and nutrient absorption, is currently touted as the most effective treatment to provide long lasting weight loss for people with extreme obesity (American Society for Metabolic and Bariatric Surgery, 2013); however, there are serious potential complications, even death. Very-low-calorie diets (500 calories/day or less) are used only under close medical supervision because they can produce harmful complications.

Nutrition Considerations

BMI classifications

Below 18.5—Underweight
18.5-24.9—Normal weight
24.5-29.9—Overweight
30 and greater—Obese
40 and greater—Morbid or extreme obesity

Table 27.1 Recommendations for Total and Rate of Weight Gain During Pregnancy, by Prepregnancy Body Mass Index

PREPREGNANCY BMI[a]	BMI+ (KG/M²) (WHO)	TOTAL WEIGHT GAIN RANGE (LB)	RATES OF WEIGHT GAIN[b] 2ND AND 3RD TRIMESTER (MEAN RANGE IN LB/WK)
Underweight	Less than 18.5	28-40	1 (1-1.3)
Normal weight	18.5-24.9	25-35	1 (0.8-1)
Overweight	25.0-29.9	15-25	0.6 (0.5-0.7)
Obese (includes all classes)	30.0 and greater	11-20	0.5 (0.4-0.6)

BMI, Body mass index.
[a]Body mass index is calculated as weight in kilograms divided by height in meters squared or as weight in pounds multiplied by 703, divided by height in inches.
[b]Calculations assume a 0.5 to 2 kg (1.1 to 4.4 lbs) weight gain in the first trimester.
Modified From Institute of Medicine (2009). Reprinted with permission from the National Academies Press. Copyright 2009, National Academy of Sciences.

Table 27.2 Changes in Nutrient Requirements During Pregnancy and Lactation

MYPLATE GROUPS[a]	NONPREGNANT WOMEN	PREGNANT WOMEN (SECOND HALF OF PREGNANCY)	LACTATING WOMEN
		MILK[b]	
Adult/Adolescent	3 or more cups/4 or more cups	3 or more cups/5 or more cups	4 or more cups/5 or more cups
Vegetable and fruit			
Citrus and other vitamin C foods	1 serving	2 servings	2-3 servings
Dark green leafy or deep-orange vegetable	1 serving at least every other day	1 serving daily	1-2 servings daily
Other fruits or vegetables, including potatoes[c]	3-4 servings	2 servings	2 servings
Meat or alternate protein	2 or more servings	3 or more servings (6 or more oz cooked)	3 or more servings (6 or more oz cooked)
Cereal and bread, whole grains	6 or more servings	6 or more servings	6 or more servings

[a]Additional servings of these or any other food may be added as needed to provide the necessary calories and palatability. Use iodized salt. Use water or other beverages—at least 6 to 8 cups daily.
[b]If fortified milk is not used, obtain the primary care provider's instructions for vitamin D supplementation.
[c]Total vegetable and fruit intake advised to be at least 4½ cups daily.
Adapted from Peckenpaugh, N. J. (2011). *Nutrition essentials and diet therapy* (11th ed.). Philadelphia: Elsevier Saunders.

PREGNANCY

Nutritional status before and during pregnancy can influence the health of the mother and the fetus. Nutritional data collection and counseling are important throughout the pregnancy to reduce the risk of complications such as low-birth-weight infants, gestational diabetes, and pregnancy-induced hypertension. Factors to consider when counseling a pregnant woman include her nutritional status before pregnancy, her age, the number of prior pregnancies, and her BMI at the onset of pregnancy. An increase in nutrients is needed for healthy growth of fetal and maternal tissues. Counseling should emphasize management of maternal weight gain and the taking of prenatal supplements, as prescribed. The guidelines for weight gain in pregnancy (Table 27.1) are more individualized because pregnant women now tend to be older and overweight or obese at the onset of pregnancy, and multiple pregnancies have become more common (American College of Obstetricians and Gynecologists, 2013, reaffirmed 2015). Table 27.2 summarizes dietary needs during pregnancy and lactation.

SUBSTANCE-RELATED AND ADDICTIVE DISORDERS

Individuals who use alcohol, smoking, and other substances often present with nutritional deficits when entering health care facilities. Substance use interferes with food intake by decreasing appetite, decreasing financial resources for food, and substituting calories in alcohol for calories in food. Substance use may also lead to impaired absorption and reduced storage and use of nutrients, along with increased metabolic needs. Patients with a history of substance use should be assessed for nutritional deficits.

Thiamine deficiency is often present with alcohol use. Medical treatment usually includes fluid and electrolyte supplements; vitamin and mineral supplements, especially thiamine; and a high calorie, high carbohydrate diet. Liver damage is common in patients with substance use because of the increased stress of metabolizing excessive alcohol and other substances. Dietary fat should be restricted if liver function is impaired. The nurse plays a vital role in evaluating nutritional status and the progress of treatment.

DISEASE PROCESSES THAT BENEFIT FROM NUTRITIONAL THERAPY

CARDIOVASCULAR DISEASE

Cardiovascular disease includes diseases of blood vessels, hypertension, **myocardial infarction (MI)** (loss of blood supply to the heart muscle), and **heart failure (HF)** (pump failure of the right or left ventricle). Nutritional therapy is focused on reduction of saturated and *trans*-fat, cholesterol, sodium intake, and red meats. Excessive saturated and *trans*-fat intake leads to development of **atherosclerosis** (accumulation of fatty deposits on the walls of blood vessels). This process narrows the vessel diameter, resulting in decreased blood supply throughout the body and specifically to the major organs. Narrow blood vessels increase the workload of the heart, resulting in hypertension as the heart attempts to circulate blood. Dietary management includes reduced intake of saturated fats (less than 7% of total calories), *trans*-fats (less than 1% of total calories), and cholesterol (less than 300 mg/day).

The blood contains three types of cholesterol. **High-density lipoprotein (HDL),** known as "good cholesterol," tends to cleanse vessels of fatty deposits. **Low-density lipoprotein (LDL)** increases fatty deposits on vessel walls. **Very-low-density lipoprotein (VLDL)** serves as a carrier for **triglycerides** in the blood (a type of fat linked to atherosclerosis and coronary artery disease); therefore, levels should be kept low. Consumption of *trans*-fats also increases levels of triglycerides. Increased levels of triglycerides can also signal a risk for diabetes or poor control of diabetes. Red meats, eggs, and high fat dairy products contain large amounts of saturated fat. Convenience foods, such as prepackaged or frozen foods, chips, and fast foods, usually have high levels of *trans*-fats. Consumption of low fat dairy products, vegetable oils, poultry, and fish is desirable to lower cholesterol levels.

Recent research is suggesting that concentrated sugars may play a greater role in the development of heart disease than the consumption of saturated fats. Studies have linked a diet high in sugars to a 3-fold increase in death from cardiac disease, with fructose and sucrose posing the greatest risk (DiNicolantonio et al., 2016).

Vitamin D may prevent cardiovascular disease, but three out of four Americans do not have adequate levels (30 to 40 ng/mL). How much vitamin D the body produces in response to sunlight exposure depends on many factors such as time of day (11 am to 3 pm is the best), time of year (summer is better), pigmentation in the skin (lighter skinned people produce it faster); yet it appears that 10 to 15 minutes of sunshine exposure is sufficient to produce sufficient vitamin D for people with lighter skin (National Health Service [NHS], 2013). Several studies identified that calcium supplements with vitamin D decrease the inflammatory response, thereby decreasing the risk of cardiovascular disease (Carvalho & Sposito, 2015). Still, food is the best source of calcium (National Institutes of Health, 2013).

Control of dietary sodium is also therapeutic in prevention and management of cardiovascular disease. Large amounts of sodium cause fluid retention. Increased fluid volume in patients with HF increases the workload of the heart and results in increased respiratory distress and edema in the legs and feet. Increased fluid volume and edema can also lead to hypertension. Research shows that Dietary Approaches to Stop Hypertension (DASH)—diets low in sodium and high in fruits, vegetables, nuts, seeds, legumes, and low-fat dairy products—can lower blood pressure even in healthy people (Mayo Clinic Staff, 2013). This might prevent hypertension later in life. The health care provider may prescribe a regular diet with no added salt, or sodium restriction from 250 mg to 4 g. Sodium content is concentrated in many foods, and limits can easily be exceeded. Teach and encourage patients to read food and beverage labels for sodium content and avoid adding salt to foods during cooking. Salt substitutes and no-salt seasonings may be used in cooking. Patients should consult with the primary care provider or dietitian before using salt substitutes because many contain ingredients that should be avoided by some people.

? Think Critically

Do you know how much sodium you consume? Read the labels for sodium content of your favorite snack foods. Develop an awareness of the amount of salt you add to foods at the table or during meal preparation.

DIABETES MELLITUS

Diabetes mellitus is a disturbance of the metabolism of carbohydrates and other nutrients and the use of glucose by the body. There are two main types of diabetes. **Type 1 diabetes,** or T1DM, occurs when the beta cells of the pancreas stop secreting insulin. Insulin is needed to transport glucose across the cell wall. Type 1 diabetes usually develops at an early age. **Type 2 diabetes,** or T2DM, accounts for 90% to 95% of all cases of diabetes; it occurs when glucose receptors on the cell membrane lose their sensitivity to insulin. Insulin is secreted in normal or excessive amounts; however, the receptor sites do not allow most glucose to enter the cell. Although it used to appear primarily after age 40, type 2 diabetes is now appearing frequently in younger people; even children.

The incidence of diabetes is increasing at an alarming rate in the United States. Of particular concern is the prevalence of type 2 diabetes among children, adolescents, and young adults. According to the American Diabetes Association (2014) African Americans, Mexican Americans, American Indians, Native Hawaiians, Pacific Islanders, and Asian Americans are at higher risk for T2DM, heart disease, and stroke. The goal of nutritional therapy for patients with diabetes is to control the amount of carbohydrates in the diet to maintain the blood glucose level at 70 to 120 mg/dL. The American Diabetes Association (ADA) does not endorse any one percentage of nutrients or any one meal plan for diabetes. The ADA does recommend a diet of moderate complex carbohydrates, including pasta, beans, whole grains, rice, and fruit. Patients should distribute carbohydrate intake

Box 27.2 Dietary Strategies for Patients with Diabetes

- **Individualization:** Arrange individualized medical nutritional therapy with a registered dietitian to tailor dietary strategies and goals for the person with diabetes.
- **Energy requirements:** Match calories with physical activity; calories may be restricted if the person is overweight.
- **Variety:** Eat a variety of foods, including fresh fruits and vegetables, complex carbohydrates, whole wheat pasta, legumes, whole grains, and brown rice.
- **Salt:** Limit the amount of salt added to the diet.
- **Unusual physical activity:** With T1DM, increase calories to meet increased metabolic demands.
- **Sick day plan:** Maintain calorie intake and insulin dosages (for T1DM); the person may need to have small frequent feedings.
- **Travel:** Continue the treatment plan regarding foods, medication, and blood glucose monitoring while away from home, and plan for the unexpected.
- **Eating out:** Plan, determine appropriate choices beforehand, and modify the meals before and after the outing to ensure a balanced daily intake of carbohydrates.

throughout the day and avoid ingestion of large amounts of carbohydrates at one meal. Complex carbohydrates usually contain more nutrients and higher fiber content. Research suggests that fiber delays the absorption of glucose, resulting in lower blood glucose levels. Dietary counseling related to reducing fat and sodium in the diet should be a part of the meal plan. People with diabetes are advised to reduce saturated fats to less than 10% of calories, minimize *trans*-fats, and restrict cholesterol to 300 mg/day (American Diabetes Association, 2015). A summary of general dietary strategies for patients with diabetes is provided in Box 27.2.

Patients with diabetes are at higher risk for cardiovascular disease, hypertension, kidney disease, blindness, and stroke. Careful management of blood glucose levels can prevent or delay the onset of these complications. The nurse should encourage patients with diabetes to monitor their blood glucose closely, especially the effect of carbohydrate intake on blood levels. Individuals with diabetes should consult with and follow the dietary recommendations of a dietitian or nutritionist.

Instruct patients in ways to include favorite foods into the diet and remain within their individual dietary plan. Develop the plan taking into consideration the type of diabetes, the patient's activity level, and whether the patient is overweight. Every person with diabetes responds differently to carbohydrate intake. A serving of carbohydrates is 15 g regardless of the type of food. A patient can monitor his response to particular carbohydrates by measuring the blood glucose 1½ to 2 hours after eating. A blood glucose level of 180 mg/dL or below usually indicates an acceptable level following meals. Teach patients to read food labels to determine the amount of carbohydrates in a specific food and include that food in the diet as part of the overall meal plan. A patient may consume simple carbohydrates such as ice cream or candy if they are included as part of the daily allowance of carbohydrates. Including these food items should depend on good diabetes control as determined by the health care provider. (Nursing Care Plan 27.1).

Nursing Care Plan 27.1 Nutritional Therapy for a Patient with Type 2 Diabetes

SCENARIO Teresa James is a 46-year-old African American diagnosed with type 2 diabetes 3 months before admission. She is an attorney in a busy law firm. She states she rarely has time to plan and prepare meals. "I just grab something on the run or eat out." Mrs. James's blood glucose level is 413 mg/dL on admission. She is 5′3″ and weighs 187 lb.

PROBLEM/NURSING DIAGNOSIS *Risk for unstable blood glucose level* related to unwillingness or inability to make lifestyle adjustments.

Supporting Assessment Data *Subjective:* Patient states, "I don't have time for meal planning and preparation. I just grab something on the run or eat out." ***Objective:*** Blood glucose 413 mg/dL. Weight 187 lb.

Goals/Expected Outcomes	Nursing Interventions	Selected Rationale	Evaluation
Patient will lose 2 lb by discharge date.	Assess knowledge of disease process.	Establishes knowledge base about disease process.	*Has weight loss occurred?* Loses 2 lb by discharge date. Goal met.
	Assess willingness to make lifestyle changes.	Provides baseline data for patient compliance.	
	Refer to dietitian for diet planning.	Provides resource for component of needed lifestyle changes.	
Patient's blood glucose level will be below 130 mg/dL by second day of admission.	Assess patient skill in measuring blood glucose.	Establishes patient's ability to complete skill.	*Has blood glucose dropped?* Blood glucose 128 mg/dL by second day of admission. Outcome achieved.
	Provide instruction as needed.	Patient must monitor blood glucose to assess diabetes control and response to carbohydrates in diet.	

Nursing Care Plan 27.1 Nutritional Therapy for a Patient with Type 2 Diabetes—cont'd

Goals/Expected Outcomes	Nursing Interventions	Selected Rationale	Evaluation
Patient will verbalize understanding of relationship of medications to diet.	Teach about medications, their use, administration, and side effects. Teach signs and symptoms of hypoglycemia and hyperglycemia. Teach interventions for episodes of hypoglycemia and hyperglycemia.	Encourages patient compliance with dietary and pharmacotherapeutic management of disease process.	*Does patient understand about medication and diet?* Verbalizes relationship of medications to diet. Outcome achieved.

PROBLEM/NURSING DIAGNOSIS *Acknowledges inability to make appropriate food choices*/Risk-prone health behavior related to meal planning for diabetes; relationship of diet to management of disease.

Supporting Assessment Data *Subjective:* Patient states, "I don't have time for meal planning and preparation. I just grab something on the run or eat out." ***Objective:*** Blood glucose 413 mg/dL. Weight 187 lb.

Goals/Expected Outcomes	Nursing Interventions	Selected Rationale	Evaluation
Patient will demonstrate ability to choose appropriately from a variety of fast-food and restaurant menus.	Provide variety of fast-food and restaurant menus.	Provides patient with flexibility in meal planning. Promotes understanding of carbohydrate counting.	*Does patient choose appropriate foods?* Demonstrates ability to choose appropriate foods from fast-food and restaurant menus. Outcome achieved.
Patient will demonstrate ability to develop a 24-h meal plan.	Provide a list of a variety of foods to compile menu.	Demonstrates patient's understanding of meal plan.	*Can patient develop a 24-h meal plan?* Demonstrates development of a 24-h meal plan. Outcome achieved.
Patient will verbalize a weight management plan.	Advise of proper weight.	Weight management is a critical component in control of disease process.	*Has patient developed a weight loss plan?* Verbalizes she will begin an exercise program to assist with weight management. Progressing toward outcome.

CRITICAL THINKING QUESTIONS

1. You are asked to provide a list of dietary recommendations to a patient with diabetes. What will you include in the list?
2. Your patient states that she does not understand how to use the American Diabetes Association carbohydrate counting. Briefly describe the use of the carbohydrate counting and its implications for the diabetic patient.

? Think Critically

Do you have a close family member who has diabetes? Genetics play an important role in the development of T2DM. What steps can you take to prevent the onset of T2DM?

HIV/AIDS

Human immunodeficiency virus (HIV) and acquired immunodeficiency syndrome (AIDS) are associated with severe diarrhea, profound weight loss, and muscle wasting. Some patients lose as much as 50% of their body weight because of treatment, multiple infections, loss of appetite, malignancies, and gastrointestinal disorders. Nutritional therapy is directed toward replacing fluids and electrolytes, fostering weight gain, replacing muscle mass through protein intake, and maintaining the strength of the immune system. Patients should be referred to the dietitian as soon as they are diagnosed as HIV positive. An older research study suggested the multivitamin supplements might delay the onset of full-blown AIDS (Fawzi et al., 2004). A more recent study demonstrated benefits of vitamins B, C, and E in delaying disease progression in pediatric AIDS patients (Zgambo et al., 2012). Although more research is needed, good nutrition is important for the patient living with HIV/AIDS.

Calorie intake should be increased for patients with HIV/AIDS, with emphasis on protein intake. Infections, an impaired immune system, and medical treatment may result in painful lesions in the mouth and ulcerations in the esophagus and stomach. Solid food may be difficult to eat. Offer milkshakes with added calories and supplements such as Ensure Plus or Boost Plus to provide calories and protein. Fluids and electrolytes are best replaced orally, but per medical orders, may be replaced intravenously. Dietary considerations include:

- Maintaining high calorie intake
- Increasing protein intake to maintain or increase muscle mass
- Offering bland, soft, or pureed foods when the mouth is painful
- Adding thickening agents to liquids if indicated by the swallowing evaluation
- Adding seasonings to help food taste more appealing
- Encouraging small, frequent meals

Note: If thickening agents are used, assess for adequate hydration, because research has shown they may lead to inadequate fluid intake. Complete assessment of health and nutritional status is important for patients diagnosed with HIV/AIDS. Typical nursing diagnoses for HIV/AIDS patients are:

- Impaired oral mucous membrane related to altered immune system
- Imbalanced nutrition: less than body requirements related to anorexia and oral lesions
- Deficient fluid volume related to prolonged diarrhea and decreased fluid intake

Table 27.3 provides a summary of nutritional recommendations for diseases and disorders of various body systems.

ASSISTED FEEDING

Patients who have high care needs, malnutrition, cardiovascular or nervous system disorders, or dementia may be unable to tolerate oral fluid and food intake.

Table 27.3 Nutritional Therapy for Specific Diseases and Disorders

CONDITION	NUTRITIONAL THERAPY
Gastroesophageal reflux disease (GERD): Reflux of gastric contents into the esophagus, causing irritation	Assess foods that are best or least tolerated. Decrease alcohol, chocolate, and fat intake. Avoid cigarette smoking. Increase protein intake for healing. Lose weight if appropriate.
Peptic ulcer: loss of tissues lining the esophagus, stomach, and duodenum	Increase iron in the diet because of blood loss from ulcers. Increase protein and vitamin C. Avoid snacks that stimulate gastric acid. Eat small, frequent meals. Avoid medications that irritate the mucosa (e.g., aspirin or ibuprofen).
Dumping syndrome: nausea, weakness, sweating, palpitations, and diarrhea, occurring after a patient has had a gastrectomy	Eat small, frequent meals. Decrease intake of simple carbohydrates. Drink fluids 45-60 min before or after meals. Lie down for 15-20 min after meals to decrease dumping.
Inflammatory bowel disease: inflammation of the bowel causing malabsorption of nutrients (e.g., Crohn disease or ulcerative colitis)	Avoid foods that cause symptoms. May be NPO for bowel rest; TPN in severe cases. High calorie, high protein, low fat, low fiber, lactose-restricted diet.
Diverticulosis or diverticulitis: formation of small sacs protruding through the bowel wall	Clear liquid diet during acute phase. Progress to a high fiber diet. Management: Avoid nuts, seeds, and foods with skin or undigested particles.
Liver disease: cirrhosis and hepatitis	Document intake and output. High protein diet to increase lean mass; restrict protein in advanced stages. High calorie diet for energy. Fat-restricted diet. Nutritional supplements. Avoid foods that irritate the esophagus because of esophageal varices. NPO during the acute phase.
Nausea and vomiting	Avoid food during the acute phases of nausea and vomiting. Limit foods to bland, low fat choices when they can be tolerated (e.g., dry toast and crackers). Clear liquids in small amounts. Eat small, frequent meals.

Table 27.3 Nutritional Therapy for Specific Diseases and Disorders—cont'd

CONDITION	NUTRITIONAL THERAPY
Kidney failure	High calorie, high carbohydrate, low protein diet. Control sodium, potassium, and phosphorus in the diet.
Renal calculi	Calcium- or oxalate-restricted diets may be ordered (restrict legumes, nuts, dark green leafy vegetables, and citrus fruits). Modified calcium restriction may be ordered. High fluid intake is usually indicated.
Celiac disease	Avoid wheat, barley, rye, and triticale (wheat–rye cross) products. Carefully scrutinize processed foods ingredient list for gluten. Avoid sharing utensils when preparing food.

GERD, Gastroesophageal reflux disease; *NPO,* no food or fluids by mouth; *TPN,* total parenteral nutrition.

One in five older adults residing in long-term care facilities may experience **dysphagia** (difficulty swallowing) (van der Maarel-Wierink et al., 2015). Some patients may show common signs of swallowing problems such as coughing when drinking, drooling, or having food remaining in the mouth. A physician and a speech-language pathologist may conduct a formal swallowing evaluation and develop a management plan. **More than half of patients who aspirate show no obvious signs or symptoms such as coughing** (Macht et al., 2013). The aspiration may cause a voice change or feeling of food being stuck in the throat. For these patients, it is important to match dietary modifications to the patient's swallowing, motor, and cognitive ability. Liquids can be thickened to help prevent aspiration. Solids can be ordered at four different texture levels: *level I,* pureed (pudding texture); *level II,* mechanically altered (moist and minced to ¼ inch maximum); *level III,* advanced (moist and bite sized; no hard or crunchy foods); and *level IV,* regular (all foods). Some patients recover and advance to level IV, whereas others may progress in their aging or disease process and may no longer tolerate oral intake of any kind. Once this happens, a feeding tube can be considered.

NASOGASTRIC AND ENTERAL TUBES

There are several types of **enteral** tubes. Tubes may be placed through the nose into the stomach **(nasogastric tubes [NG] tubes),** placed directly into the stomach **(gastrostomy tubes** or **percutaneous endoscopic gastrostomy [PEG] tubes),** or placed into the intestine **(jejunostomy or duodenal tubes)** (Fig. 27.2).

Nasogastric tube placement is usually a temporary measure to provide nutritional support. The tube is placed through the nose and esophagus into the stomach. The NG tube may be used for other purposes, such as (Fig. 27.3):

- Stomach decompression, such as removing stomach contents before or after surgery
- Obtaining laboratory specimens
- Gastric lavage for patients with gastrointestinal bleeding or for removal of ingested toxins
- Medication administration (see Chapter 34, Skill 34.4)

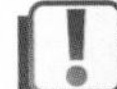

Safety Alert

Tubing Misconnections

The Joint Commission has issued several Sentinel Event Alerts involving tubing misconnection, including NG infusions inadvertently connected to IV tubing, and vice versa. **Patient death has resulted from tubing misconnections**. Luer-Lok connectors can cause many of these issues because they allow functionally dissimilar tubes to be connected. Always follow your facility's policies.

When enteral (intestinally absorbed) nutrition is needed over an extended time, small-bore feeding tubes (8 to 10 Fr.) may be inserted. Small-bore tubes are soft, flexible tubes that must be inserted by a skilled person using a guidewire or stylet. Active patients may find the tube restrictive and inconvenient.

Nursing care of patients with NG tubes involves insertion, irrigation, administration of tube feeding, checks for placement, checks for residual volume, and removal of the tube. Success in inserting the tube is more likely if the patient's confidence is gained first. Tube insertion is more difficult if the patient is unable to cooperate, such as patients who are unconscious or have impaired cognitive function (Skill 27.2). Explain the procedure and its benefit to the patient before beginning insertion. Proper placement of small-bore tubes must be verified by x-ray examination. A tube that is not correctly positioned or poor body position can cause aspiration. Elevate the head of the bed for 30 to 60 minutes after a feeding to ensure residual volume is not aspirated.

QSEN Considerations: Safety

Check Tube Placement and Residual Volume

Check tube placement and residual volume before feeding or administering medications, returning residuals per your facilities policies.

Patients with decreased level of consciousness or a decreased cough or gag reflex may not exhibit expected symptoms if the tube is displaced into the respiratory tract. Placement of the tube in the respiratory tract can lead to severe respiratory complications if misplacement is not detected before feeding or medication administration.

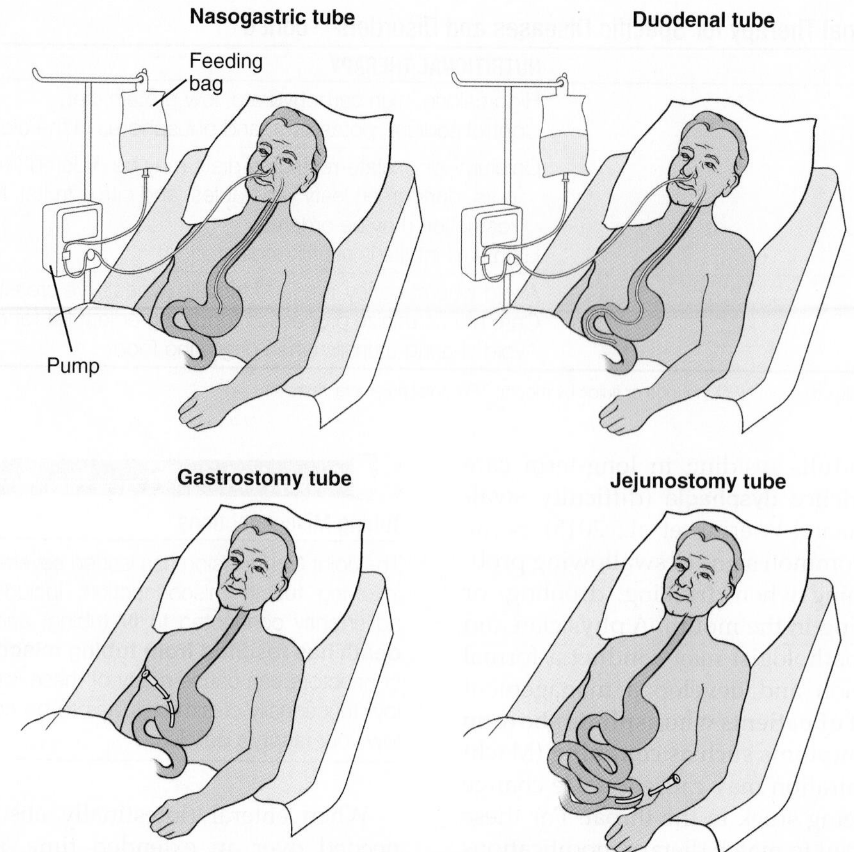

FIGURE 27.2 Anatomic locations for nasogastric, duodenal, gastrostomy, and jejunostomy tubes.

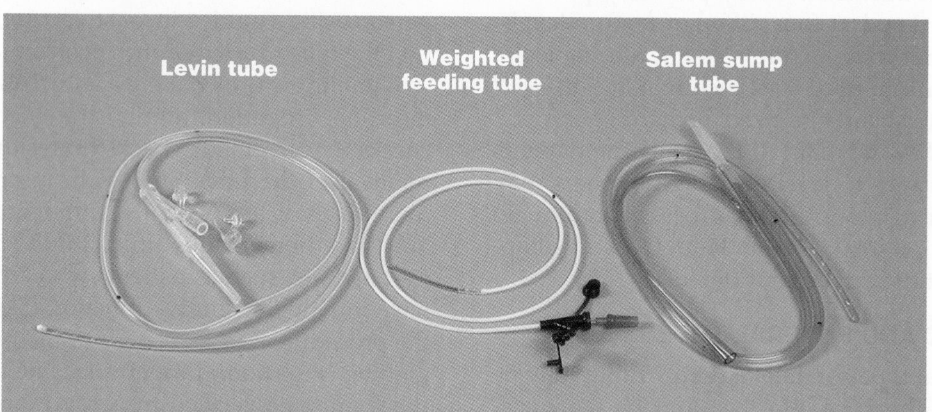

FIGURE 27.3 Nasogastric and enteral feeding tubes.

Monitor NG tubes frequently. Irrigate the NG tube with 30 to 60 mL of sterile water solution to ensure it is patent. Count the amount used for irrigation as part of the recorded intake (Steps 27.1, p. 499). Monitor for complications such as constipation, nausea, diarrhea, hyperglycemia, and electrolyte imbalances. When therapy is completed or the patient is able to tolerate oral feedings, remove the NG tube (Steps 27.2, p. 500.

PERCUTANEOUS ENDOSCOPIC GASTROSTOMY OR JEJUNOSTOMY TUBES

A PEG or PEJ tube is used when a patient requires long-term nutritional support and cannot take oral nutrition. The PEG/J tube has replaced surgical gastrostomy tube placement in most situations. The tube is placed via endoscopy. The PEG/J tube allows patients more freedom of ambulation and allows the patient to administer his own feeding easily. A PEG/J tube can be removed easily when it is no longer indicated.

Care of the PEG/J tube is similar to that of the NG tube. **Check tube placement at least every shift and before feeding or administering medication.** Check the medical record for the placement measurements. Measure the tube length from skin level to the end of the placement adapter; compare the measurements. Higher measurements indicate the tube has migrated outward. If the tube becomes dislodged, notify the charge

Skill 27.2 Inserting a Nasogastric Tube

 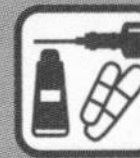 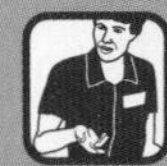  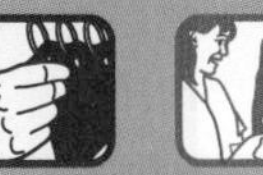 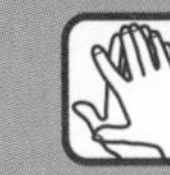 

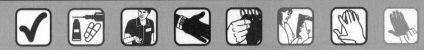

A nasogastric (NG) tube is inserted per a care provider's order, and is used with suction when a patient is experiencing excessive vomiting, needs stomach decompression after intestinal surgery, or is at risk for aspirating stomach contents because of decreased level of consciousness. If the patient needs enteral feedings, the tube is either attached to a feeding pump or left unattached and plugged off for intermittent feedings.

SUPPLIES

- Emesis basin
- Stethoscope
- Gloves
- Drape or towel
- Tongue blade
- Measuring tape
- NG tube
- Flashlight
- Glass of water, straw
- Tape
- Water-soluble lubricant
- Plug for tube
- Irrigation syringe and solution container
- Safety pin
- Tissues, paper towel
- Sterile water solution
- pH indicator strip (scale 1 to 11)
- Wall suction or suction machine and connecting tubing, or feeding pump and tubing

Review and carry out the Standard Steps in Appendix A.

ACTION *(RATIONALE)*

Assessment (Data Collection)

1. Assess patient's understanding of procedure. *(Patients can be more cooperative when they understand what is happening to them.)*

Planning

2. Check airflow through the nostrils: close one side of the nose, and check airflow through the other. *(Determines which nostril is most patent and should be used for tube's passageway.)*
3. Gather all equipment needed. Position patient with the head of the bed elevated 30 to 90 degrees. Raise head of bed to working height. *(Demonstrates good time management. Elevating head of the bed enables the tube to move by gravity down the digestive tract.)*
4. Hand the emesis basin and the tissues to the patient. Otherwise, place emesis basin close beside the patient's face with the tissues near the pillow. Agree on a hand signal that will instruct you to stop if the patient experiences too much discomfort. *(Basin will catch emesis if patient vomits. The signal allows the patient some control of the procedure.)*
5. Don gloves. *(Barrier protection is needed in case patient vomits or there is spillage of gastric contents.)*
6. Measure the distance the tube is to be inserted by measuring from the tip of the nose to the tip of the ear and then to the xiphoid process. Mark the distance on the tube with a piece of tape. *(Some tubes have approximate target markings on them: one black band indicating the length of the tubing needed to reach the stomach, two bands for the pylorus, and three bands for the duodenum. Marking the tube after measurement individualizes the tube length.)*

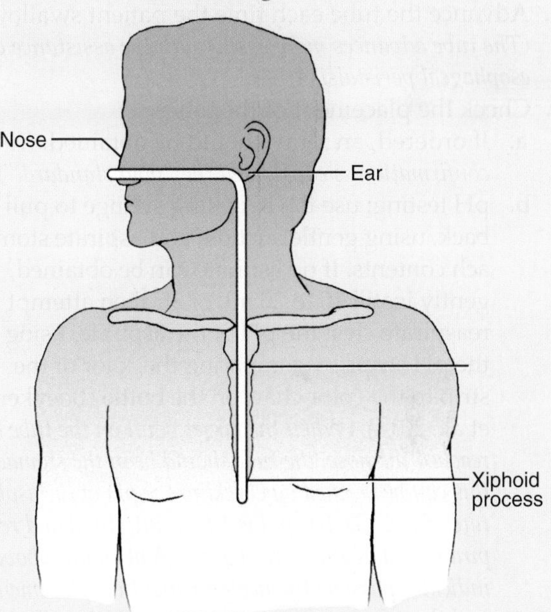

Step 6

7. Chill or warm the tube to desired stiffness for insertion. *(A too limp or too stiff tube is difficult to insert. Placing a soft rubber tube in a basin of ice will stiffen it; placing a stiff plastic tube in a basin of warm water will soften it.)*

Implementation

8. Lubricate the tip of the tube and insert it through the nostril with the best airflow. If changing the NG tube, insert it in the nostril other than the one previously used to avoid further irritation of the tissue. With patient's head hyperextended, aim the tube down and toward the ear. Twist tube slightly as you advance it. If you encounter severe resistance, withdraw the tube and insert in the other nostril. Do

not forcibly push it because you could injure tissue and cause bleeding. *(Using the largest passageway for insertion of the tube decreases tissue trauma. For easier insertion, use water or a water-soluble lubricant to moisten the tip of the tube. Do not use an oil-based lubricant because of the possibility of lipid aspiration.)*

9. As the tube reaches the back of the throat, have patient take sips of water through the straw, drop the head forward, and begin to swallow. *(Offer encouragement by saying, "swallow, swallow," when advancing the tube.)*
10. Check the position of the tube as it passes down the back of patient's throat by having the patient open his mouth and hold down the tongue with a tongue depressor. If the tube is coiled up in the mouth, withdraw it into the nose and begin again by having the patient bend head forward and swallow. The patient can signal you to stop for a moment to rest, if necessary, but avoid waiting too long. *(Difficulty with the tube entering the esophageal opening sometimes occurs.)*
11. Advance the tube each time the patient swallows. *(The tube advances more easily with the assistance of esophageal peristalsis.)*
12. Check the placement of the tube:
    a. If ordered, an x-ray should be obtained. *(X-ray confirmation is considered the "gold standard.")*
    b. pH testing: use the irrigating syringe to pull back, using gentle suction, and aspirate stomach contents. If no aspirate can be obtained, gently instill 10 to 20 mL of air then attempt to reaspirate. Test the pH of the aspirate, using the pH strips by comparing the color of the strip to the color chart on the bottle (Boeykens et al., 2014). *(When the target point on the tube has reached the nose, the tube should be in the stomach; this can be verified by checking the pH of the aspirated fluid. Gastric pH is 1 to 4; intestinal and respiratory pH values are above 6. A pH value above 6 indicates possible tracheobronchial tube placement, and the primary care provider should be notified.)*
    c. Observe for changes in the volume and appearance of feeding tube aspirate *(Gastric aspirates are typically grassy green or colorless; intestinal aspirates may be bile or yellow colored; respiratory aspirates are usually tan or off-white and mucoid.)*
13. Tape the tube securely to the face. Clean the bridge of the nose with a prep pad or apply tincture of benzoin to it. Cut a 4-inch long piece of 1-inch tape; split it up the middle for 3 inches. Place the solid piece of tape on the bridge of the nose, and spiral the split ends down the tube. Secure the tape with one more piece across the bridge of the nose. Be certain the tube is not rubbing the side of the naris because it can cause necrosis. *(The tube must be secured so that it is not easily dislodged. Commercially made NG tube holders are available and may be used in your facility.)*

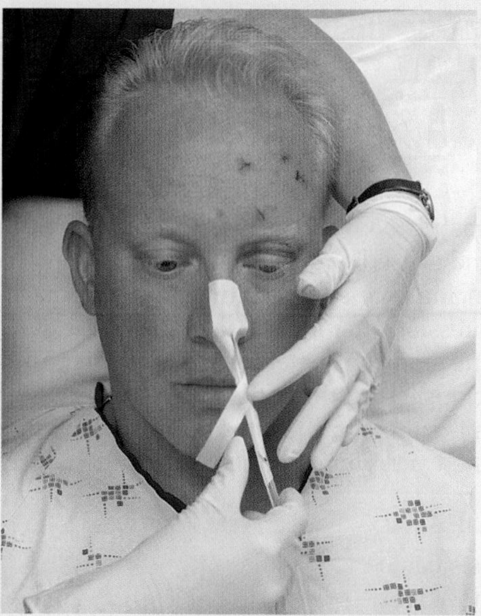

Step **13**

14. Measure the tube from the insertion point at the nare, to the end of the tube. Document the length. *(This assists with verifying placement and can determine if the tube has migrated.)*
15. Attach the free end of the tube to the connecting tubing attached to the suction machine or feeding tube. Turn the suction machine or wall unit to low intermittent suction for a patient who needs stomach decompression. If using a feeding pump, adjust the drip rate to the rate prescribed by the primary care provider, connect the tubing, and turn on the pump. When the patient is up and not attached to the suction machine or feeding pump, loosely loop the tube in a circle, secure the loop with adhesive tape, and pin the tube to the gown. *(Low, intermittent suction is usually ordered to prevent damage to the stomach mucosa. Securing the tube to the gown helps prevent pulling the tube, which is uncomfortable for the patient and can dislodge the tube.)*
16. Remove gloves. Position the tube by looping it above the stomach level, placing a piece of tape around it to make a tab, and fastening the tab to the gown with a safety pin. *(Prevents the tube from becoming dislodged.)*
17. Perform hand hygiene. *(Prevents transmission of organisms to others.)*

Evaluation

18. For a patient who needs stomach decompression, ask the patient if nausea is relieved. Assess abdomen for distention. Note the flow of stomach contents into the suction canister. *(Determines effectiveness of procedure.)*
19. If feeding tube is inserted and feeding has started, assess residual stomach contents in 4 hours. If patient is able to communicate, ask if there is any abdominal discomfort. Assess abdomen for distention and patient for nausea and vomiting. *(Evaluates patient's tolerance of tube feeding.)*

Documentation

20. Document procedure on the nurse's notes. Document intake on the intake and output record. Documentation should include:
    - Reason for tube insertion
    - Time of procedure
    - Type of procedure
    - Type and size of tube
    - Patient's tolerance of procedure
    - Length from insertion point at nares to tip of nasogastric tube
    - pH of gastric aspirate
    - Amount and characteristics of stomach contents

    (Provides members of the health care team with description of the procedure and the patient's response.)

Documentation Example

2/13 1300 Number 16 Levin tube inserted in right nostril. 500 mL dark green fluid returned, pH of 2. Vomited 200 mL dark green fluid during tube insertion. Tube taped to nose. Measured at 18.5 cm from nares to tip of tube. States nausea and abdominal pain relieved after tube insertion. Tube connected to low, intermittent suction. (Nurse's electronic signature)

Special Considerations

- Insertion of NG tube in patients who are unconscious or have endotracheal tubes in place may require assistance. Seek the help of another nurse to ensure patient safety.
- Consult with the primary care provider before inserting an NG tube into the nostril of a patient who has had nasal or throat surgery or trauma to the nose. Special care is usually required.
- Patients with cognitive impairment may attempt to pull out the feeding tube. Restraints may be applied (with a medical order and correct documentation, after attempting other alternatives) to prevent pulling out the tube.
- Keeping the suction connecting tubing above the entrance to a portable suction unit helps the suction to work more efficiently.

Critical Thinking Questions

1. The nurse inserts an NG tube and checks for placement. The nurse aspirates 10 mL of fluid from the tube. The pH strip test is 7.0. What action should the nurse take?
2. The patient has an NG tube inserted postoperatively. The nurse notes that there has been no drainage from the tube in the past hour. List appropriate nursing actions.

Steps 27.1 Nasogastric Tube Irrigation

Nasogastric tubes are irrigated to verify patency and keep them from clogging. They may be irrigated every few hours or once a day depending on the situation and the medical orders.

Review and carry out the Standard Steps in Appendix A.

ACTION (*RATIONALE*)

1. Check primary care provider's order for frequency of irrigation and amount and type of solution. *(Ensures following procedure as ordered.)*
2. Assess color, amount, and characteristics of gastric secretions. *(Provides baseline information.)*
3. Assess bowel sounds. *(Bowel sounds are evidence of return or improvement of bowel function.)*
4. Assess patient for complaints of discomfort. *(Information may indicate potential complications.)*
5. Position patient in semi-Fowler position at 30 to 60 degrees. *(A slightly upright position helps prevent reflux.)*
6. Perform hand hygiene and don gloves. *(Possible contact with body fluids requires the use of gloves.)*
7. Verify proper placement of the tube. *(Prevents instilling irrigation fluid into lungs.)*
8. Fill the syringe with irrigating solution, usually normal saline or sterile water, by holding the syringe between your index finger and thumb. Place the tip of the syringe in the solution, and pull the plunger up to obtain at least 30 mL of solution. *(Normal saline is isotonic and will not upset electrolyte balance.)*
9. Disconnect the gastric tube from the suction tubing on the machine; hold the connecting tubing between the last two fingers of your nondominant hand; hold the gastric tube in a fist-like grasp with the other fingers of that hand. *(The tube may be irrigated only if disconnected from suction.)*
10. Attach the filled syringe to the free end of the gastric tube and instill the solution. *(Assists in clearing the tube.)*
11. When irrigation is completed, attach gastric tube to the suction tubing; restart the suction. *(Checking that the suction machine or unit is turned on will ensure correct function.)*
12. Remove gloves and perform hand hygiene; ensure patient comfort. *(Performing hand hygiene prevents spread of microorganisms.)*
13. Add amount of irrigating solution to intake record. *(Documents intake.)*

Steps 27.2 Nasogastric Tube Removal

When the condition for which the NG tube was inserted has resolved, the tube is discontinued.

Review and carry out the Standard Steps in Appendix A.

ACTION (*RATIONALE*)

1. Check care provider's order sheet for order to remove NG tube. *(Prevents removal of the tube while still needed.)*
2. Assess amount, color, and character of drainage in suction canister. *(Amount, color, and character of drainage must be documented in the medical record.)*
3. Explain procedure to patient. *(Helps gain patient's confidence and cooperation.)*
4. Elevate head of bed to 30 degrees. *(Position is more comfortable for patient.)*
5. Perform hand hygiene and don personal protective equipment (PPE). *(Protects against exposure to body fluids.)*
6. Turn off suction or the tube feeding pump if present. Place the towel or basin where the withdrawn tube can be placed into it quickly. Flush the tube with 20 mL of sterile water followed by 20 mL of air. Pinch off the tube and pull out gently but quickly. *(Flushing the tube clears gastric content from the tube that may leak into the esophagus and cause irritation. Instillation of air pushes tube away from stomach lining and reduces risk of trauma during removal. Pinching off the tube prevents spillage of any residual fluid.)*
7. Offer mouth care. *(Removes unpleasant taste from the mouth.)*
8. Measure and record the gastric drainage. Rinse or dispose of the drainage container and tube following facility policy. *(Gastric drainage is recorded as part of output for the shift.)*
9. Remove PPE and perform hand hygiene. *(Prevents spread of microorganisms.)*
10. Assess every 2 hours for signs of nausea, vomiting, or abdominal distention. Assess bowel sounds. *(Provides for early recognition of intolerance to removal of NG tube.)*
11. Document the time the tube was removed and the patient's response to the procedure. If the tube was used for suction, record amount and characteristics of drainage. *(Documentation provides communication to other health care personnel concerning the care provided to the patient.)*

nurse and the primary care provider. Follow the facility policy and licensure regulations regarding reinsertion of the tube. The tube may be reinserted by a licensed practical nurse/licensed vocational nurse (LPN/LVN) if permitted by the scope of practice and facility policy. Document your findings and report them to the primary care provider if discrepancies are present.

Daily care of the tube involves washing the tube insertion site with soap and water. Use a cotton swab moistened with saline to remove encrustation. Inspect the skin for evidence of irritation, maceration, or infection. Dry the site and rotate the external disk to prevent sticking to the skin. Document the appearance and treatment of the site. Observe the patient for abdominal distention or aspiration. Abdominal pain, vomiting, or respiratory distress may be signs of complication. Before feeding or administering medications, measure the amount of residual fluid in the stomach. If a continuous feeding is in progress, stop the infusion before checking for residual volume. Use an irrigation syringe to withdraw stomach contents. If the residual volume is greater than 250 mL (or per agency policy), replace the withdrawn fluids, document the residual, and notify the registered nurse (RN) or primary care provider (promotility medications may be ordered), and delay further feeding for 1 to 2 hours if facility policy states to do so. **Keep the patient's bed elevated at least 30 degrees at all times if the patient is on continuous feeding, to facilitate stomach emptying and prevent aspiration.** Further information can be found in your medical-surgical textbook.

FEEDING TUBES AND PUMPS

Tube feedings can be continuous or intermittent. Continuous feeding is effective for patients who cannot tolerate large amounts of fluid at one time. Intermittent feeding is beneficial for patients who are able to feed themselves or when beginning to reintroduce oral feeding. Intermittent feeding more closely resembles regular meals. Feelings of hunger stimulate appetite and aid in the transition from tube to oral feeding.

The type and amount of tube feedings are prescribed by the primary care provider and usually ranges from 240 mL to 360 mL per feeding. It may be necessary to start with smaller amounts and increase the feeding amount as the patient is able to tolerate the formula. A daily amount of 2000 mL is generally sufficient to meet the patient's nutritional requirements. High concentrations of carbohydrates are needed to increase the caloric content of the formula above this amount, but this often leads to diarrhea. If a syringe is used, it should be 30 mL or larger, and the formula should flow in by gravity; it should not be pushed in as a bolus or in large amounts. Allow about 10 minutes for an intermittent feeding to flow into the tube. Flush the tube with 30 mL of water after each feeding to prevent clogging.

Skill 27.3 Using a Feeding Pump

 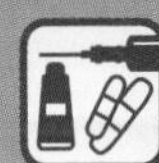 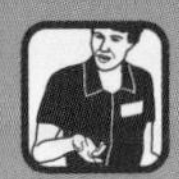  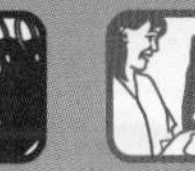 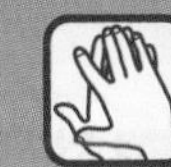 

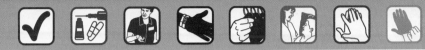

Continuous feeding via a feeding pump is usually prescribed when a patient requires long-term nutritional support or cannot tolerate large volumes of feeding formula at one time.

SUPPLIES

- Feeding formula
- Irrigating syringe
- Feeding pump
- Stethoscope
- Tubing for pump
- Gloves
- Feeding tube bag
- Sterile water or tap water

Review and carry out the Standard Steps in Appendix A.

ACTION (*RATIONALE*)

Assessment (Data Collection)

1. Check the primary care provider's order for type, amount, and flow rate of feeding. *(Ensures correct feeding formula is administered.)*
2. Don gloves. Assess tube placement or residual if PEG tube is in place. *(Possibility of coming in contact with body fluids requires wearing gloves. Assessing placement determines nasogastric [NG] tube is in the stomach and prevents infusion of feeding into respiratory tract. Check residual to determine whether stomach is emptying effectively.)*

Planning

3. Elevate head of bed at least 30 degrees. Keep bed elevated at all times. *(Assists in preventing gastric reflux and/or aspiration of feeding.)*
4. Open tubing and feeding bag and connect to feeding pump with tubing clamp closed. Open formula and pour enough to infuse over a 4- to 6-hour period. If using commercially prepared feeding container, close the roller clamp on the tubing, spike the infusion port, and fill the drip chamber. *(Small amount of feeding formula in the bag prevents spoilage of formula. Some formulas are prepared in an administration container. These formulas are prepared to hang for up to 24 hours.)*
5. Open the clamp and prime the tubing by allowing the formula to fill the length of the tubing. *(Prevents air from entering the stomach and causing abdominal distention and discomfort.)*

Implementation

6. Attach the tubing to the NG tube or PEG tube. Set the flow rate and turn on the pump. *(Begins administration of feeding formula.)*
7. Observe the infusion for 2 to 3 minutes before leaving patient. *(Determines whether formula is infusing properly.)*
8. Remove gloves and perform hand hygiene. *(Prevents spread of microorganisms.)*

Evaluation

9. Assess patient for signs of complications, including abdominal distention, abdominal pain, nausea, or vomiting. *(Determines patient's tolerance of tube feeding.)*
10. Assess stomach residual every 4 hours by aspirating contents. *(Determines whether stomach is emptying properly.)*

Documentation

11. Document the time the infusion was started, type of formula, amount, and flow rate. Include checking for tube placement or checking for residual. Document patient's response to the infusion. *(Verifies nutritional intake and patient response.)*

Documentation Example

2/14 1000 Feeding via pump initiated with 200 mL formula at 50 mL/h. Tube patent and in place with return of gastric secretions. Positioned at 30 degrees. Bowel sounds present all 4 quads. (Nurse's electronic signature)

? Critical Thinking Questions

1. The nurse discovers the feeding solution bag empty and the pump continuing to infuse. Identify nursing interventions.
2. The home care nurse discovers the patient resting on the left side with the head on a pillow and the head of the bed flat. A continuous tube feeding is infusing at 30 mL/h. What action, if any, should the nurse take?

Continuous feedings are instilled into the tube drop by drop in much the same manner as an intravenous feeding. For this purpose, a **feeding pump** and a tube feeding set is used (Skill 27.3). Set the rate on the pump, or regulate the drops through the drip chamber to control the amount given; this device can be used with NG tubes, PEG tubes, or jejunostomy tubes (Skill 27.4).

Tube feedings contain a high level of glucose to provide the necessary calories. They should be given

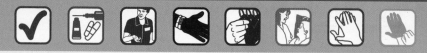

Skill 27.4 Administering a Nasogastric, Duodenal, or Percutaneous Endoscopic Gastrostomy Tube Feeding

 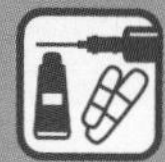 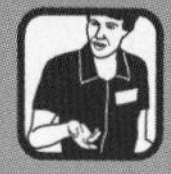 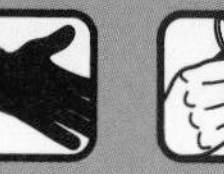 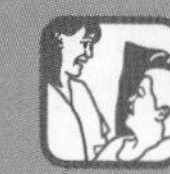 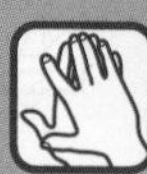 

Tube feedings are administered to patients who cannot ingest food orally but do not have a problem with absorption of nutrients from the intestinal tract. They may be used for short-term or long-term nutritional support. Intermittent feedings should be used only with stomach tubes.

SUPPLIES

- Large syringe or feeding bag and feeding formula
- Tubing
- Feeding pump (if needed)
- Stethoscope
- Gloves
- Adaptor for syringe for small-bore tubes
- Sterile water or tap water

Review and carry out the Standard Steps in Appendix A.

ACTION (*RATIONALE*)

Assessment (Data Collection)

1. Check the primary care provider's order for type of feeding, amount, and strength of solution. (*Ensures feeding is given according to primary care provider's order.*)
2. Assess abdomen for distention or tenderness. (*Identifies discomfort before feeding to avoid complications.*)

Planning

3. Elevate head of bed 30 degrees. (*Elevation allows gravity to help flow of the formula into the stomach and thus helps prevent reflux. The position should be maintained at least 30 to 60 minutes after the feeding.*)
4. Perform hand hygiene. Don gloves. (*Possible contact with body fluids requires the use of gloves.*)

Implementation

5. Pinch off the tube and remove the plug, cap, or clamp. (*Pinching the tube prevents fluid leaking from the tube.*)
6. Check placement of the tube. For a NG tube, attach a syringe and aspirate a small amount of stomach contents (5 to 10 mL); if no fluid is obtained, instill 10 to 20 mL of air and attempt to reaspirate; for a small-bore feeding tube, verify that placement has been checked by x-ray examination. Reinstill aspirated fluid. (*Obtaining gastric or intestinal contents is the best evidence of proper tube placement. Small-bore feeding tubes frequently collapse when aspiration is attempted, and nothing can be obtained. Checking residual with a small bore or PEG/PEJ will increase the tube's tendency to become clogged. Stomach or intestinal contents are high in electrolytes, and removal depletes electrolytes. When more than 250 mL of residual formula are obtained, notify the primary care provider because it indicates that the feeding is not well tolerated.*)

For Intermittent Feedings

7. Pinch off the tube and pour the formula into a gavage bag or the barrel of the syringe, keeping it no more than 18 inches above the level of entry into the stomach or intestine. If a gavage bag is used, fill it with the prescribed amount of formula and regulate it to run in slowly over 30 minutes. (*The formula should be given over 10 minutes or longer; gravity pull will draw it in. Flow can be regulated by raising and lowering the container.*)

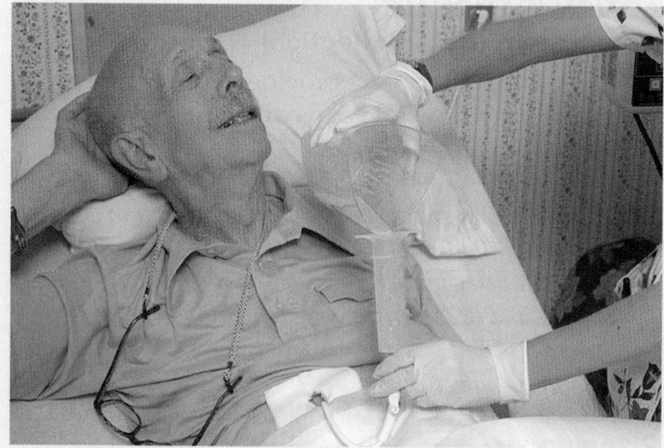

Step 7

8. Add formula to keep the neck of the syringe filled. Continue adding formula to the syringe until prescribed amount is given. Flush the tube with 30 to 60 mL of sterile water. (*If the formula level falls below the neck of the syringe, air will enter the tubing and the intestinal tract, causing distention and discomfort. Flushing tube with sterile water helps prevent clogging. Tap water flushes are related to infections.*)

For Continuous Tube Feeding

9. Fill the feeding bag with the prescribed amount of formula, clear the tubing of air, and attach it to an intravenous pole or infusion pump. Thread the tubing into the programmable feeding pump if used (Step 9A). Set the rate according to the primary care provider order (Step 9B). (*Feeding bag can be hung at room temperature for 4 hours within the hospital environment. A feeding pump delivers a controlled flow of formula. Some gavage bags have a pocket in which to place ice, which allows the formula to hang up to 6 hours.*)

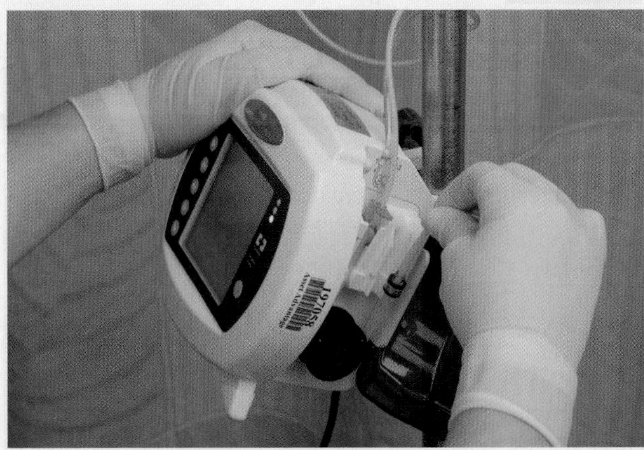
Step **9A**

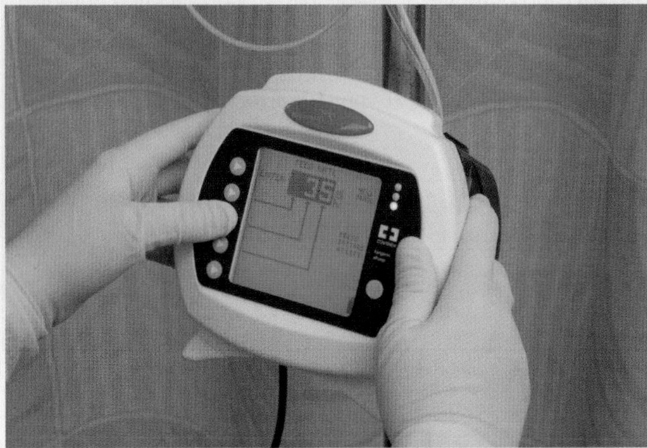
Step **9B**

10. Verify enteral, gastrostomy, or jejunostomy tube placement. *(Aspirating usually will not produce fluid from the jejunum; air cannot be easily detected when instilled into the jejunum. If the tube is not in place, the feeding could spill into the abdominal cavity, causing a chemical peritonitis.)*
11. Check the amount of residual from the previous feeding for the gastrostomy tube by aspirating with a syringe; reinstill the fluid. *(Residual should be checked every 4 hours for continuous gastrostomy tube feedings.)*
12. Attach the tubing from the feeding bag to the enteral, gastrostomy, or jejunostomy tube using an adaptor as needed. Turn on the pump and check the drip rate; begin feeding. *(Check the drip rate frequently. Assess patient tolerance of the feeding hourly while the patient is awake. Increasing abdominal distention or pain indicates a problem.)*
13. Follow the formula with 30 to 60 mL of sterile water to clear the tube. Keep the liquid level above the neck of the syringe or bag to prevent air bubbles from collecting in the system or in the patient's intestinal tract. *(Sterile water helps clear the tubing and prevents clogging.)*

For Both Intermittent and Continuous Tube Feeding

14. Remove the syringe or connecting tubing, and clamp the tube by inserting the plug and covering with a cap protector or with a 2 × 2 gauze secured with a rubber band; a clamp may also be used (for intermittent feedings). *(This prevents backflow of the formula or stomach fluid.)*
15. In the home, wash the bag and tubing or other equipment with soap and water every 8 hours; change the bag and tubing or syringe every 24 hours. *(In home setting, equipment is washed with soap and water every 8 hours but may be reused for 3 to 7 days. Equipment is rinsed thoroughly after each feeding in the hospital and in the home.)*
16. Remove gloves and perform hand hygiene. *(Prevents spread of microorganisms.)*

Evaluation

17. Assess patient for evidence of discomfort or complications such as nausea, vomiting, and respiratory distress. *(Provides evidence of patient's tolerance of tube feedings.)*
18. Monitor laboratory values and weight daily. *(Assesses evidence of resolution of malnutrition.)*

Documentation

19. Documentation should contain type of formula given, amount (including flush), verification of tube placement or securing sutures, amount of residual if obtained, and any signs of intolerance of the feeding. *(Documents nutritional intake and any problems.)*

Documentation Example

5/16 1300 240 mL Jevity given via PEG tube. Abdomen soft, bowel sounds present in all quadrants. Tolerated feeding without evidence of discomfort. Head of bed remains at 30 degrees. (Nurse's electronic signature)

Home Care Considerations

Nursing support for the patient and family is essential. Patient education should involve the patient and family if possible. The education plan should include the following:

- Type of feeding
- Amount of feeding
- Operation of the feeding pump if used
- Checking for tube placement
- Signs and symptoms of complications
- Positioning the patient
- Procedure for manual feeding
- Safety factors during feeding
- Signs of problems to report

Critical Thinking Questions

1. The patient is receiving continuous tube feeding at 70 mL/h. The nurse evaluates the patient who is positive for abdominal distention and auscultates hypoactive bowel sounds. The nurse then checks residual and returns 500 mL. What action(s) should the nurse take?
2. The caregiver reports to the home care nurse that the patient has been coughing, and 'milk-like' drainage has been noted around the patient's nose. List appropriate nursing interventions.

Box 27.3 Principles of Tube Feeding

Follow these principles when giving patients tube feedings:

- Elevate the head of the bed 30 to 90 degrees before feeding and leave it up for 30 to 60 minutes after the feeding.
- Keep the head of the bed elevated at least 30 degrees at all times if the patient is receiving continuous feeding.
- Assess bowel sounds at least once every 8 hours.
- Assess abdomen for distention.
- Check the tube position within the gastrointestinal tract before each feeding is started or at least once each shift.
- Check for gastric residual by aspirating via the gastric tube before each intermittent feeding or at least every 4 hours if the patient is receiving continuous feeding. If the gastric residual is greater than 250 mL (or per agency policy), replace the residual, document and notify the RN or primary care provider, and delay the next feeding for 1 to 2 hours.
- Perform fingerstick for blood glucose every 4 to 6 hours as ordered for hyperglycemia until the patient demonstrates a normal blood glucose level.
- If nausea occurs, stop the feeding and notify the primary care provider.
- Maintain an accurate intake and output record. Dehydration can occur because of diarrhea or the high glucose content of the formula.
- If persistent diarrhea occurs, notify the primary care provider.

slowly to prevent diarrhea and **glycosuria** (glucose in the urine). The preferred method is to give the feedings slowly over a 24-hour period. When feedings are ordered for four or more times a day, the patient is usually given 150 to 240 mL per feeding and advanced at a rate of 50 mL/day until the desired volume is tolerated. Principles to observe when administering tube feedings are summarized in Box 27.3.

TOTAL PARENTERAL NUTRITION

Total parenteral nutrition (TPN) is a method of delivering complete nutrition through a catheter placed in a large central vein (e.g., subclavian vein). A large, central vein with high blood flow is needed to dilute the solution rapidly. The solution may also be infused through a port implanted in the patient's chest wall or through a **peripherally inserted central catheter (PICC).** These options are used for patients receiving long-term therapy, such as those with massive burns, intestinal obstruction, inflammatory bowel disease, AIDS, and cancer, or chemotherapy. For shorter-term uses, a peripheral vein (usually in the arm) may be used; it is called **peripheral parenteral nutrition (PPN).** Parenteral nutrition does not involve the digestive system, and it is absorbed directly through the bloodstream.

Maintain aseptic technique when performing TPN administration to reduce the risk of catheter-related infection. Both PPN and TPN are composed of high concentrations of carbohydrates as the main source of energy. Protein is provided through solutions of all amino acids. Solutions of other essential nutrients are also added to the infusion. Fatty acids are administered through lipid solutions that are infused daily or several times per week. PPN and TPN solutions are started slowly to allow the body to adjust to the solution's high glucose concentration and **hyperosmolality** (increased concentration of solutes within the fluid). Usually 1000 to 2000 mL is administered in the first 24 hours. After the first 24 hours, the infusion is increased until the desired volume is met. Monitoring of PPN and TPN should be ongoing. Carefully begin the infusion rate and monitor it throughout the shift. If the rate is lower or higher than the prescribed rate, adjust the infusion to the correct flow rate. **Never attempt to catch up if the rate has slowed. The rapid infusion of glucose can be harmful to the patient.** Table 27.4 summarizes the steps for monitoring PPN and TPN.

Table 27.4 Monitoring Peripheral Parenteral Nutrition and Total Parenteral Nutrition[a]

ITEM TO ASSESS	WHEN TO ASSESS
IV site (PICC, central line, MediPort, peripheral IV)	Every 4 h. Observe for redness, swelling, or drainage from the site.
Patient response	Every shift. Observe for signs of restlessness or discomfort.
Blood glucose	Every 6-8 h. Report abnormal levels to the primary care provider.
Vital signs	Every 4-8 h. Abnormal vital signs may signal development of complications.
Weight	Daily or weekly as ordered. Evaluates the patient's response.
Intake and output	Every shift. Abnormal urine output may signal hyperglycemia or altered kidney function.
Flow rate	Every 4 h. Prescribed flow rates should be followed to prevent hyperglycemic intolerance to TPN.
Electrolytes, CBC, and BUN	Daily or as ordered. Evaluates the patient's response.
Nutritional status	Ongoing. Includes weight, albumin levels, and status of muscle mass.

PICC, Peripherally inserted central catheter.
[a]Baseline levels of blood chemistry, vital signs, weight, and nutritional status should be completed before beginning peripheral parenteral nutrition (PPN) or total parenteral nutrition (TPN) infusion. Compare ongoing monitoring to baseline results.

Life-Span Considerations

Older Adults

Older adult patients are at risk for fluid overload when receiving large volumes of intravenous fluids. Patients should be assessed for symptoms of fluid overload, including increased pulse rate, cough, respiratory distress, crackles on auscultation of the lungs, and imbalance in intake and output.

❖ APPLICATION OF THE NURSING PROCESS

The steps of the nursing process are applied when caring for patients with NG or intestinal tubes.

◆ ASSESSMENT (DATA COLLECTION)

The first step in assessment is to determine the reason for the tube. This information is necessary for evaluating the tube's effectiveness. Determine patient understanding of the procedure before beginning. Once the tube is in place, assess the function of the tube at least every 4 hours for the first 48 hours of feeding, followed by once a shift thereafter (Abbott Laboratories, 2015). Monitor for signs of complications such as nausea, vomiting, abdominal distention, abdominal pain, and respiratory distress.

◆ NURSING DIAGNOSIS

After data collection, nursing diagnoses and goals/expected outcomes should be formulated. Nursing diagnoses appropriate for patients requiring nutritional assistance are:

- Self-care deficit: feeding related to inability to take food from plate to mouth
- Risk for deficient fluid volume related to diarrhea or excessive vomiting
- Imbalanced nutrition: less than body requirements related to anorexia or NPO status
- Risk for injury related to aspiration of stomach contents into the respiratory tract from difficulty swallowing
- Impaired swallowing related to neuromuscular difficulties

◆ PLANNING

Establish goals/expected outcomes based on the nursing diagnoses chosen. Examples of goals/expected outcomes are:

- The patient will tolerate food and fluids without vomiting.
- The patient will consume at least 90% of all meals.
- The patient's breath sounds will remain clear, without evidence of aspiration of food or fluids.
- The patient will gain 2 lb by time of discharge.
- The patient's stools will be formed.

◆ IMPLEMENTATION

Nursing measures include frequent mouth care to prevent drying and cracking of the mucous membranes. To keep the mouth and lips moist, swab the oral cavity with a gauze pad or cotton swab that has been moistened with normal saline or water.

The nostrils often become dry and tender. If not contraindicated, a room humidifier can be helpful for the patient who is experiencing nose and throat discomfort. Cleanse the nares with a swab and warm water daily or as needed. Use water-soluble lubricant on the nares. Other nursing actions include:

- Securing the tubing to the patient's clothing to permit maximum activity without pulling on the nares.
- Preventing kinking of the tubing.
- Keeping the environment clean, quiet, and well ventilated.

Patient Education

Patient with a Nasogastric or Intestinal Feeding Tube

Discuss the need for and advantages of having an NG or intestinal tube in place. Teach the patient or primary caregiver to:

- Perform oral care every 2 hours while the patient is awake to decrease mouth dryness; keep lips moistened.
- Observe for side effects from tube feeding, such as abdominal distention, nausea, diarrhea, constipation, vomiting, or hyperglycemia.
- Tape the tube to the nose or face and attach to gown or clothing so that it does not hang lower than the stomach or point of entry into the patient's body.
- Keep the patient sitting upright at an angle of at least 30 degrees for 1 hour after feedings to prevent reflux and possible aspiration.
- Administer tube feedings at room temperature. Keep open formula refrigerated between feedings.
- Discard prepared or open refrigerated formula after 24 hours.
- Use a two-method confirmation, such as pH testing of gastric fluid and measuring for placement verification, before administering each feeding. Check the gastrostomy or jejunostomy tube entrance site before feeding.
- Irrigate the tube with a small amount of sterile water before and after each feeding.
- Clear the tube with sterile water between each medication and after the last medication is given. Use 30 mL of water first, then give one medication, instill 5 mL of water, give next medication, instill 5 mL of water, and so on. When all medications are given, instill 30 mL of water to clear the tube.
- **Never** mix medications together, because this causes clumping, which clogs tubes, and causes medication interactions and absorption issues.
- Clamp tubing when not in use.
- Clean the area around the gastrostomy or jejunostomy tube with warm water. Do not use hydrogen peroxide because it is corrosive to the skin.
- Turn the bumper of the gastrostomy or jejunostomy tube daily and if a dressing is ordered, place the dressing over the bumper to prevent tension on the tube.

◆ EVALUATION

Determine whether goals were met, partially met, or unmet. Collaborate with the registered nurse to retain, revise, or terminate nursing diagnoses, goals, or nursing interventions as appropriate. Evaluate the patient's ability to take food by mouth without nausea or vomiting. Evaluate nutritional parameters to ascertain success of tube feeding. Reassess abdominal peristalsis, signs of intestinal bleeding, or their absence.

Examples of evaluation statements are:

- The patient takes food by mouth without nausea or vomiting.

- The patient gained ½ lb/wk while receiving tube feedings.
- The patient takes food by mouth without aspiration of stomach contents into the airway.
- The patient has formed stools.

Documentation

Document the following:

- Size of tube inserted and how the patient tolerated the procedure.
- Amount of formula and fluids given, and the result of tube feeding or medication administration.
- Measurement of the tube.
- How placement of the tube was checked (2 methods recommended), as well as the amount of and character of gastric residual at each feeding.
- Presence or absence of bowel sounds each shift.
- How the patient tolerated the procedure, including problems with nausea, constipation, or diarrhea.
- Date and time of tube removal.

Get Ready for the NCLEX Examination!

Key Points

- Nursing knowledge and understanding of nutritional therapy are important to assist patients in meeting their nutritional needs.
- Nutritional therapy may involve progressive introduction of foods.
- Dietary management of eating disorders must include behavioral management and psychological and nutritional counseling.
- Obesity is an increasing health care problem. Success of nutritional therapy for obese patients is low. Interventions include education, behavior modification, calorie control, appetite suppressants, surgery, and psychological counseling.
- Maintaining optimum nutrition during pregnancy is critical to maternal health and healthy development of fetal tissues.
- Nutritional deficits are common in patients with substance abuse and require a nutritional assessment and plan.
- Nutritional therapy can be beneficial in managing many disease processes, including gastrointestinal disorders, cardiovascular diseases, diabetes, nausea and vomiting, urinary disorders, cancer, and HIV/AIDS.
- Enteral tubes are sometimes prescribed when patients are unable to eat or when food in the digestive tract aggravates a disease process. Enteral tubes may be used short or long term.
- Nursing responsibilities when tubes are in place include patient education, tube insertion and removal, verification of placement, irrigation of tube, administration and management of tube feedings, and assessment for the development of complications.
- Patients experiencing severe malnutrition related to disease or treatment may require long-term and extensive nutritional support. PPN or TPN may be prescribed to meet those needs.
- Nursing knowledge concerning management of PPN and TPN is essential for success of treatment. Nurses are responsible for evaluating the patient for potential complications and ensuring that the fluids are administered as ordered.

Additional Learning Resources

SG Go to your Study Guide for additional learning activities to help you master this chapter content.

evolve Go to your Evolve website at http://evolve.elsevier.com/Williams/fundamental for additional online resources.

Review Questions for the NCLEX Examination

*Choose the **best** answer for each question.*

1. When performing patient education about a clear liquid diet, what would the nurse instruct the patient to include in the meal plan? *(Select all that apply.)*
   1. Milk
   2. Ginger ale
   3. Chicken broth
   4. Gelatin
   5. Popsicles
2. A 70-year-old stroke patient needs assistance with feedings and begins coughing when drinking water. What should the nurse do first?
   1. Advise the dietitian to change the patient's diet to thickened liquids.
   2. Assess whether the patient's airway is clear and any water was aspirated.
   3. Check patient's gag reflex and consult with speech and language therapist for diet change.
   4. Position patient in an upright position and administer the Heimlich maneuver.
3. A patient is admitted to the hospital with a diagnosis of heart failure (HF). Patient education related to nutritional therapy for HF should include:
   1. Reduction of fat and protein.
   2. Increasing calories and fluids.
   3. Reduction of sodium intake.
   4. Increasing simple carbohydrates.

4. A patient with diabetes asks if a slice of cake can be added to the meal for dessert. The best response by the nurse would be:
   1. "Diabetic patients should not eat cake."
   2. "Yes, but you must omit other carbohydrates of equal value from the meal."
   3. "You will have to check with your primary care provider."
   4. "Yes, but don't do this too often."
5. A patient is receiving TPN. The night nurse reported that the infusion rate had been increased to 75 mL/hour. When you make your rounds at 8 am, you discover the rate is still infusing at 50 mL/hour. The appropriate nursing action is to: *(Select all that apply.)*
   1. Increase the rate to 75 mL/hour now.
   2. Notify the primary care provider of the error.
   3. Change the rate to 125 mL/hour for 4 hours to catch up.
   4. Leave the rate at 50 mL/hour because the patient is tolerating oral fluids.
   5. Verify the medical orders.
6. The nurse teaches a patient with diabetes to limit saturated fat and sodium intake because:
   1. All diabetic patients are at risk for obesity.
   2. These foods contribute to higher glucose levels.
   3. These nutrients are nonessential.
   4. Diabetic patients are at risk for cardiovascular disease.
7. An older adult patient has just started TPN at 70 mL/hour and at assessment is found to have a high pulse rate, crackles in the lungs, and shortness of breath. Which nursing action is most important?
   1. Lower the TPN rate to 40 mL/hour and contact the primary care provider.
   2. Stop the TPN infusion and contact the primary care provider.
   3. Provide the patient with oxygen.
   4. Check the TPN administration site for signs of blockage or infection.

Critical Thinking Activities

Read each clinical scenario and discuss the questions with your classmates.

Scenario A

Martin Stevens is admitted with exacerbation of symptoms of inflammatory bowel disease. He is placed on NPO status. Laboratory studies reveal severe electrolyte imbalance and malnutrition. TPN is ordered.

1. What are indications for TPN?
2. What is the composition of TPN?
3. Describe nursing interventions for patients receiving TPN.

Scenario B

Flora Smith, age 87, is cared for in her home following a stroke. She is unable to swallow and has a PEG tube in place. Her daughter administers continuous tube feeding using a feeding pump.

1. What parameters will you evaluate when you visit Mrs. Smith?
2. What factors will indicate tolerance of the feeding?
3. What complications may occur?
4. What patient education points will you review with Mrs. Smith's daughter?

Scenario C

James Kelly, age 42, is newly diagnosed with type 2 diabetes.

1. Differentiate between the types of diabetes.
2. What is the goal of dietary management of diabetes?
3. What are the recommendations for distribution of calories for a patient with diabetes?

Scenario D

Maria Torres, age 32, visits a health clinic for advice concerning weight loss. She is 5'9" tall and weighs 288 lb. She states she has been walking for 30 minutes three times a week for the past 2 weeks.

1. Ms. Torres is at high risk for which medical conditions?
2. How would you determine her dietary needs?
3. What diagnostic tests would be appropriate?
4. Develop a patient education plan for Ms. Torres.

chapter

28 Assisting with Respiration and Oxygen Delivery

http://evolve.elsevier.com/Williams/fundamental

Objectives

Upon completing this chapter, you should be able to do the following:

Theory

1. Explain how the respiratory system functions.
2. Identify three causes of hypoxia.
3. Outline procedures to follow in the event of respiratory or cardiac arrest.
4. Describe the various methods used for oxygen delivery.
5. List safety precautions to be observed when patients are receiving oxygen therapy.

Clinical Practice

1. Prepare to assist patients in clearing the airway via coughing, postural drainage, suctioning, abdominal thrusts (Heimlich maneuver), and inhalation therapy.
2. Regulate oxygen flow and correctly apply an oxygen delivery device.
3. Prepare to provide care for the tracheostomy patient.
4. Prepare to care for the patient who has a chest tube and drainage system.

Skills & Steps

Skills

Steps

Key Terms

anoxia (ă-NŎX-ē-ă, p. 510)
apnea (ĂP-nē-ă, p. 529)
atelectasis (ă-tē-LĔK-tă-sĭs, p. 532)
cannula (KĂN-ū-lă, p. 518)
cyanosis (sī-ă-NŌ-sĭs, p. 511)
dyspnea (DĬSP-nē-ă, p. 510)
endotracheal (ĔN-dō-TRĀ-kē-ăl, p. 526)
expectorate (ĕk-SPĔK-tō-rāt, p. 518)
expiration (p. 509)
humidifier (hū-MĬ-dĭ-fī-ĕr, p. 519)
hypercapnia (hī-pĕr-KĂP-nē-ă, p. 510)
hypoxemia (hī-pŏx-SĒ-mē-ă, p. 510)
hypoxia (hĭp-ŎX-ē-ă, p. 510)
inspiration (p. 509)
nebulizer (NĔ-bū-lī-zĕr, p. 518)
obturator (ŎB-tŭ-rā-tŏr, p. 537)
retractions (p. 511)
stridor (STRĪ-dŏr, p. 510)
tachypnea (tă-KĬP- nē-ă, p. 510)
tenacious (tē-NĀ-shŭs, p. 525)
tracheostomy (trā-kē-ŎS-tō-mē, p. 526)

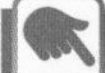

Concepts Covered in This Chapter

- Acid Base Balance
- Anxiety
- Collaboration
- Gas Exchange
- Infection
- Inflammation
- Mobility
- Pain
- Patient Education
- Safety

OVERVIEW OF THE STRUCTURE AND FUNCTION OF THE RESPIRATORY SYSTEM

WHICH STRUCTURES ARE INVOLVED IN RESPIRATION?

- The nose, mouth, pharynx, larynx, and trachea comprise the upper respiratory system (Fig. 28.1).
- The trachea divides into the right and left main bronchi, which lead to the right and left lungs.
- The right lung has three lobes, and the left lung has two lobes.

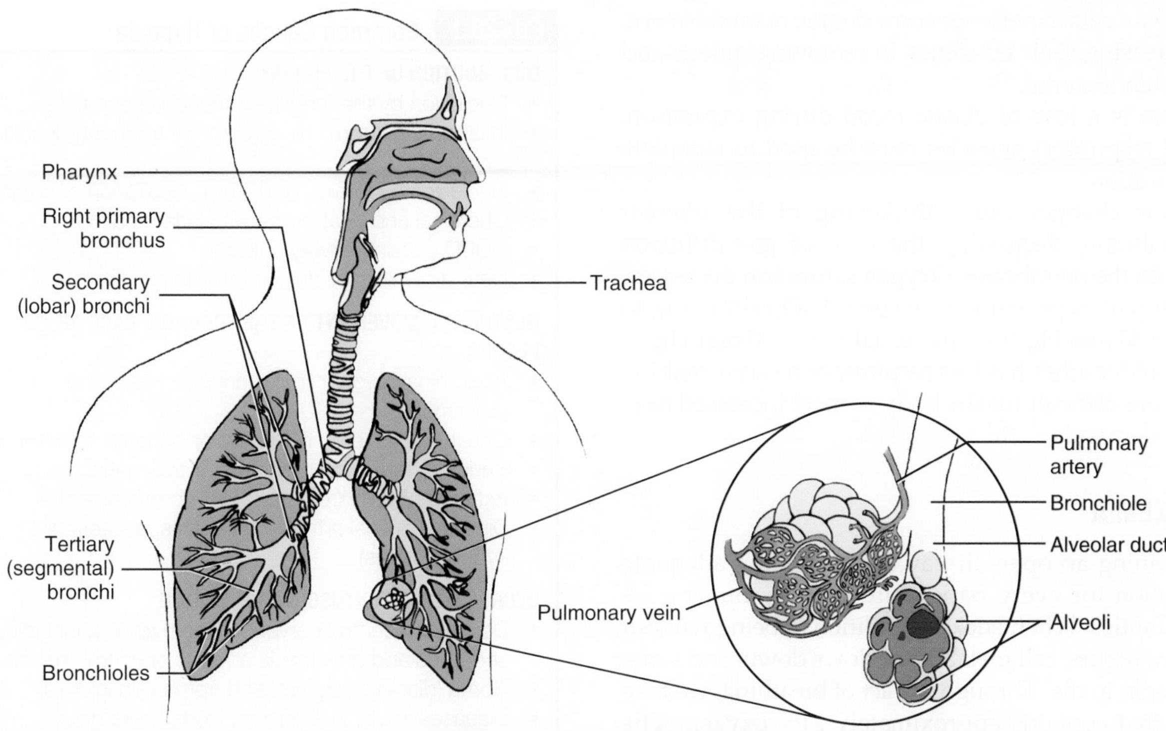

FIGURE 28.1 The respiratory system.

- Within each lung, the bronchi divide into smaller and smaller branches and then divide into bronchioles attaching to the alveoli.
- The **alveoli** (air sacs) are the terminal respiratory units of the lung and are lined with mucous membrane. There are between 300 million and 1 billion alveoli in the lungs.
- The diaphragm beneath the lungs moves, causing enlargement of the thoracic cavity. Because of negative pressure within the cavity, **inspiration** (movement of air into the lungs) occurs. When the diaphragm muscle relaxes, the thoracic cavity space is decreased and air is forced out of the lungs in **expiration** (movement of air out of the lungs).
- The chest muscles combine with diaphragm action to move air in and out of the lungs.
- The respiratory muscles depend on nerve impulses from the spinal cord.
- The thoracic cage allows the respiratory muscles to function correctly.

WHAT ARE THE FUNCTIONS OF THE RESPIRATORY STRUCTURES?

- The upper respiratory pathways carry air to and from the lungs.
- Air is warmed and humidified as it passes through the upper airway passages.
- The bronchi channel air to and from the lungs. The mucous membrane lining the bronchial tree contains tiny hairlike projections, or **cilia,** to trap and help remove small foreign particles that are inhaled.
- The mucous membrane secretes mucus that assists cilia in cleansing foreign substances from the respiratory tract.
- The alveoli contain macrophages that quickly phagocytize inhaled bacteria and other foreign particles.
- The mucus and cilia propel the foreign substances toward the entrance of the respiratory tract; the cough reflex works to expel the secretions.
- The central nervous system controls respiration.
- Chemoreceptors located in the aorta and carotid arteries sense changes in oxygen or carbon dioxide and send signals to the brainstem.
- Changing levels of hydrogen ions (indicated by pH), carbon dioxide, and oxygen in the blood trigger the respiratory center in the medulla to send signals through the spinal cord to the nerves that control the respiratory muscles, causing an increased or decreased rate of respiration.
- During normal breathing, about 500 mL of air moves in and out of the lungs with each breath.
- Oxygen diffuses across the alveolar membrane into the blood; carbon dioxide diffuses across the alveolar membrane from the blood to the alveoli.
- The blood transports oxygen to the cells and carries carbon dioxide from the cells to the lungs. Most of the oxygen is transported attached to the hemoglobin molecule in the red blood cells. Most of the carbon dioxide is transported to the lungs in the plasma portion of the blood.

WHAT CHANGES OCCUR WITH AGING THAT AFFECT RESPIRATION?

- After age 70 there is decreased elasticity of the thorax and respiratory tissues.
- Total body water decreases 50% after age 70, leading to dry respiratory membranes and thicker mucus.

- Airway cilia experience some degree of impairment, decreasing their efficiency in removing mucus and foreign material.
- There is a loss of elastic recoil during expiration, and respiratory muscles must be used to complete expiration.
- Tissue changes cause thickening of the alveolar membrane, decreasing the ease of gas diffusion across the membrane. Oxygen saturation decreases, with partial pressure of oxygen (PaO_2) dropping to 75 to 80 mm Hg from the usual 80 to 100 mm Hg.
- The older adult has less respiratory reserve, making it more difficult for the body to meet increased oxygen demands.

HYPOXEMIA

Maintaining an open airway and providing adequate ventilation for every patient are primary nursing responsibilities. When **anoxia** (condition of being without oxygen) occurs, cell metabolism slows down, and some cells begin to die. Through the act of breathing, we take in air that contains approximately 21% oxygen. **The most common cause of respiratory insufficiency is airway obstruction.** Fortunately, obstruction is often easily reversed with positioning and suctioning techniques.

Nurses must identify patients with breathing problems, take appropriate nursing actions to help relieve airway obstructions, and competently initiate or maintain oxygen therapy when it is used in the patient's treatment.

The foremost problem of the respiratory system is a disturbance in the levels of the gases oxygen and carbon dioxide in the bloodstream. This disturbance causes **respiratory insufficiency,** the body's inability to meet its oxygen needs and remove excess amounts of carbon dioxide. The decreased amount of oxygen in the bloodstream is called **hypoxemia** and leads to less oxygen available to meet cellular needs, or **hypoxia**. The increased level of carbon dioxide in the blood is called **hypercapnia**.

 QSEN Considerations: Safety

Hypoxemia

Hypoxemia poses a dangerous threat to patients.

The onset of hypoxemia may be rapid and obvious, or it may be insidious and gradual, with no clear-cut symptoms of **dyspnea** (difficulty breathing) or shortness of breath (SOB). The nurse must promptly recognize the problem and act swiftly when airways become obstructed. Box 28.1 lists common causes of hypoxia.

 QSEN Considerations: Teamwork and Collaboration

Teamwork for Hypoxic Patients

Persistent hypoxic states require the collaboration of a team consisting of a physician, a respiratory therapist, a laboratory technologist, and a nurse.

Box 28.1 Common Causes of Hypoxia

OBSTRUCTION OF THE AIRWAY
- Occlusion by the tongue or mucous secretions
- Inflammation from croup, asthma, tracheobronchitis, or laryngitis
- Occlusion by foreign body (e.g., aspiration or vomitus)
- Chemical and heat burns with inflammation
- COPD causing airway collapse
- Near drowning: occlusion by water

RESTRICTED MOVEMENT OF THE THORACIC CAGE OR THE PLEURA
- Abdominal surgery (incisional pain restricting movement)
- Chest injuries (e.g., flail chest or penetrating wounds)
- Pneumothorax (spontaneous or traumatic)
- Extreme obesity (restricts thoracic movement)
- Diseases (spinal arthritis, peritonitis, ascites, or kyphoscoliosis)

DECREASED NEUROMUSCULAR FUNCTION
- Depressed central nervous system (drugs, including sedatives and anesthesia agents; brain trauma; stroke)
- Coma (diabetic, uremic, and from brain injuries)
- Diseases (multiple sclerosis, myasthenia gravis, poliomyelitis, or Guillain-Barre syndrome)

DISTURBANCES IN DIFFUSION OF GASES
- Diseases (pulmonary fibrosis or emphysema)
- Trauma (contusion)
- Emboli, fat embolus
- Tumors, benign or malignant
- Respiratory distress syndrome

ENVIRONMENTAL CAUSES
- High altitude (decreased oxygen in the atmosphere)

SYMPTOMS OF HYPOXIA

The symptoms of hypoxia result from decreased oxygenation of various organs. The tissues of the body differ in their ability to survive by means of anaerobic (without oxygen) metabolism. Brain cells, however, cannot withstand deprivation of oxygen and very quickly show the effects of hypoxia. The areas of memory, judgment, and intellectual ability are most quickly affected. The heart and the retina of the eye are also highly vulnerable to hypoxia. Other organs are also affected, such as the kidneys, which retain more sodium when hypoxic.

Because the brain, the retina, and the heart are most susceptible to slight changes in oxygenation, the earliest signs of hypoxia involve these organs. Patients just do not "seem right" even though the vital signs are within normal limits. There may be signs of confusion. Patients who have difficulty breathing often become anxious, and their anxiety increases the respiratory rate, although the higher rate may not increase the oxygenation. **Tachypnea** (fast breathing rate) or **stridor** (high pitched, harsh, or musical sounds on inspiration) may be present. Arrhythmias (irregular heartbeats) develop as the amount of oxygen supplied to the heart muscle is reduced. Patients with labored breathing, as

Table 28.1 Signs of Hypoxia and Respiratory Insufficiency

EARLY SIGNS	INITIALLY	LATER	LATEST
Sits up to breathe	Increased blood pressure	Decreased blood pressure	Cyanosis
Complains, "I can't catch my breath"	Increased pulse	Decreased pulse	Muscle retractions
Memory lapse	Increased respirations	Arrhythmia	—
Mental dullness	—	Use of accessory muscles	—
Restlessness	—	Stridor	—

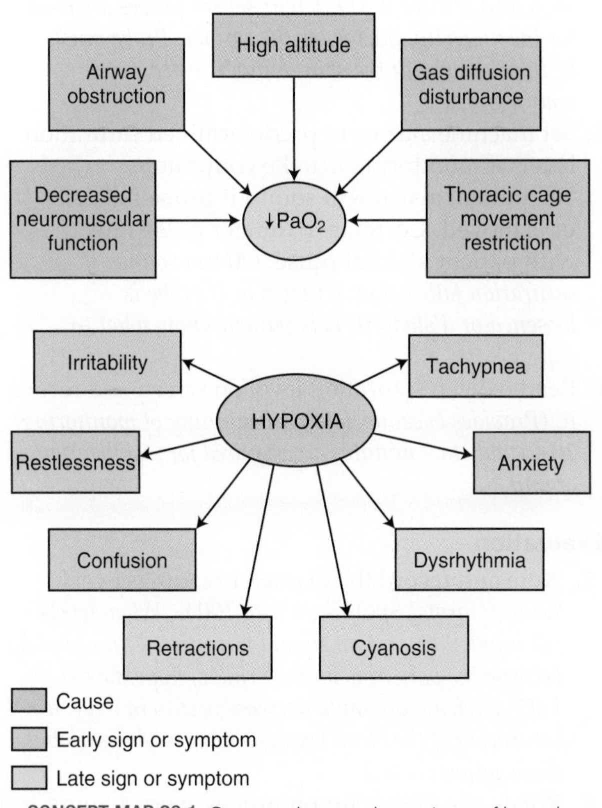

CONCEPT MAP 28.1 Causes, signs, and symptoms of hypoxia.

seen in obstructive pulmonary disease or lung fibrosis, use 30% to 50% of their energy just to breathe. **Cyanosis** (blue tinge to skin or mucous membrane) and **retractions** (muscles moving inward on inspiration) of accessory muscles of the neck, chest, and abdomen are late signs of respiratory insufficiency (Table 28.1 and Concept Map 28.1). Hypoxia depresses body functions and disturbs the body's acid base balance. Less oxygen in the bloodstream leads to respiratory acidosis (Chapter 25). Hypoxia is treated by administering oxygen and correcting the cause. Blood gases are a valuable tool for determining the degree and possible cause of hypoxia.

Patients suffering from hypoxia are highly susceptible to respiratory tract infections. Inadequate inflation of the lungs results in pooling of secretions and provides a medium for growth of microorganisms. It is essential to protect the respiratory patient from hospital-acquired infections. Keep personnel and visitors with respiratory tract infections out of the patient's environment.

Think Critically

How would you know that a patient is in respiratory distress? What signs and symptoms might be present?

PULSE OXIMETRY

Pulse oximetry is used for any patient thought to be at risk of hypoxia. With the pulse oximeter, changes in arterial oxygen saturation can be continuously monitored. The device measures oxygen saturation by determining the percentage of hemoglobin that is bound with oxygen. A sensor or probe is attached to the patient on an appendage through which infrared and red light can reach the capillary vascular bed (Skill 28.1, Fig. 28.2). Oxyhemoglobin absorbs more infrared than red light. A microprocessor in the monitor receives the information from the sensor or probe, computes the saturation value, and displays it on the monitor screen.

Adhesive sensors can be applied to the nose or the forehead. Clip-on probes are used on the earlobe, the fingertip, the toe, or an infant's foot. Adhesive sensors are generally disposable, whereas clip-on probes may be reusable. Pulse oximetry is not recommended in certain situations.

Clinical Cues

If the patient has on nail polish, the sensor may function best if the polish is removed or the sensor is positioned on the sides of the finger. Sensor misplacement, cyanosis, cold fingertips, reduced peripheral pulses, ambient light, and anemia are other factors that may cause inaccurate readings.

Another way to measure oxygenation is by determining oxygen saturation. This is an invasive procedure usually done in the critical care unit (see Chapter 24).

AIRWAY OBSTRUCTION AND RESPIRATORY ARREST

Sometimes the airway becomes obstructed with a foreign object or food that is swallowed incorrectly. If a person seems to be choking and cannot breathe, there are specific procedures that must be performed. In some cases the person will exhibit the universal signal for choking, signaling for help (Fig. 28.3). In this event, you should perform abdominal thrusts (Heimlich

Skill 28.1 Using a Pulse Oximeter

 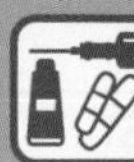 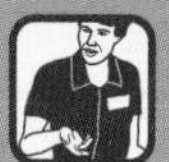  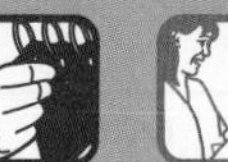 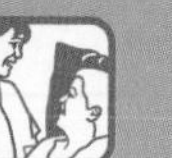 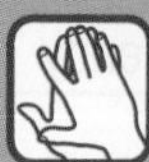 

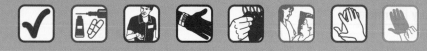

Pulse oximetry provides the pulse oxygen saturation level (SpO_2), which is a reliable measure of oxygen saturation of the blood. It is a noninvasive measurement of the amount of oxygen carried by hemoglobin. In this manner, intermittent or continuous monitoring of oxygen saturation can be obtained. This is a painless procedure that allows immediate evaluation of the patient's response to treatment for hypoxia. The procedure may not be accurate if the patient has had recent tests using intravenous dye, or is jaundiced. The oximeter sensor contains both red and infrared light-emitting diodes (LEDs) and a photodetector. The photodetector registers light passing through the vascular bed, and the microprocessor determines oxygen saturation from the data received. It is most accurate when there is no direct sunlight or fluorescent light on the patient. The normal SpO_2 is greater than 90%. The sensor should be placed on a site that is free of moisture and has good local circulation.

SUPPLIES

- Pulse oximeter
- Probe (clip-on or adhesive)

Review and carry out the Standard Steps in Appendix A.

ACTION *(RATIONALE)*

Assessment (Data Collection)

1. Assess for an appropriate site for placement of the sensor. *(The fingertip is the most common site because light easily passes through the tissue.)*

Planning

2. Set up the oximeter; plug in machine, turn on the power, and check for proper function. *(Prepares machine to measure oxygen saturation. Check the manufacturer's instruction book.)*

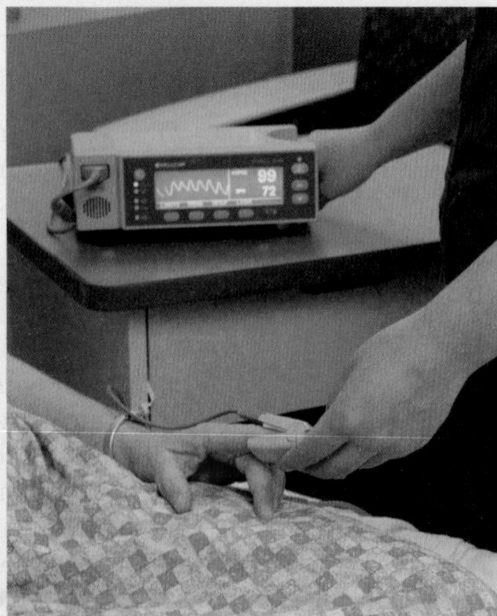

Step 2

Implementation

3. Remove dark nail polish or artificial nail if using a fingertip sensor. *(Dark nail polish or artificial nails may distort readings.)*
4. Attach the correct sensor for the site flush to the skin and secure it. *(Different sensor probes are used for the fingertip, the toe, or the earlobe. Probe must be in contact with the skin to produce accurate readings.)*
5. Set machine alarms to predetermined saturation levels if monitoring is to be continuous. Tell patient alarm will sound if probe falls off or is moved. Correlate oximeter pulse rate with patient's radial pulse. *(Alarm sounds if saturation falls below set level or if probe is loosened or dislodged. Lets patient know what to expect.)*
6. Read oxygen saturation level on screen and record it. *(Provides baseline data for beginning of monitoring; 10 seconds to 2 minutes are required for stabilization of unit.)*

Evaluation

7. Note and record the oximeter readings every hour. *(Normal SpO_2 is 90% to 100%. When levels fall below 90%, action should be initiated immediately because the patient is on the brink of hypoxia; as PaO_2 falls, a more rapid decrease occurs in oxygen saturation of the blood because of the oxyhemoglobin dissociation curve.)*
8. Rotate site of the clip-on probes every 4 hours and disposable probes at least every 24 hours. *(Skin breakdown can occur with prolonged use of a probe. Apply skin cream to previously used areas if skin dryness occurs.)*
9. Adjust oxygen flow according to readings and primary care provider's orders. *(Oxygen flow rate may be increased or decreased per orders depending on the SpO_2 level.)*
10. Check the oximeter's calibration per manufacturer's directions at least once a day. *(Ensures that saturation readings are accurate.)*
11. When the order for pulse oximetry is discontinued, take a final reading, remove the probe, disconnect the machine, and clean the sensor site and the equipment. *(Prepares equipment for next use.)*
12. Record the time that procedure is discontinued and final oximetry reading. *(Verifies that testing has been discontinued.)*

Documentation

Documentation Example

10/12 1400 SpO_2 92%; O_2 by nasal cannula at 4 L/min. (Nurse's electronic signature)

Special Considerations

- A small portable oximeter can be used to spot-check a patient's oxygen saturation. The probe is applied in the same manner as in this skill.

Critical Thinking Questions

1. What are two nursing actions you could take if your patient, who has had trauma to the ribs and a leg fracture, develops a PaO_2 of 86%?
2. What simple measures can a patient take that might increase the PaO_2 when it begins to decrease?

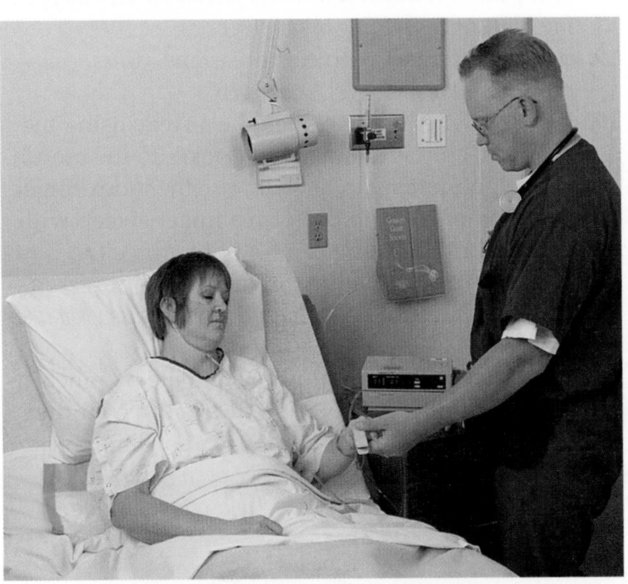

FIGURE 28.2 Monitoring oxygen saturation with the pulse oximeter.

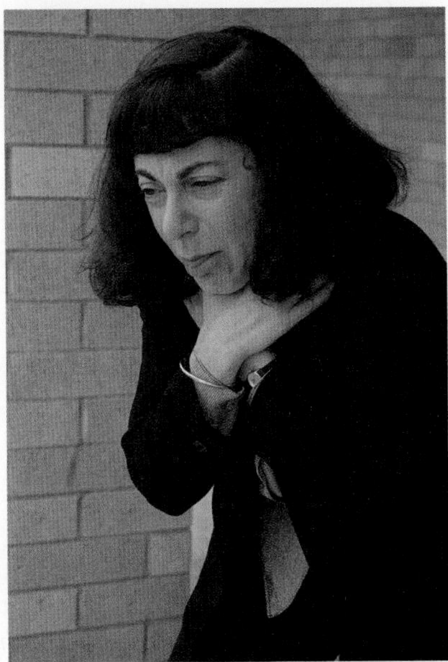

FIGURE 28.3 The hand grasping the throat is the universal signal for choking.

maneuver) on adults and children older than 1 year of age. For the infant less than 1 year, back slaps and chest thrusts should be delivered (Skill 28.2). For an infant, the ability to cry is the best sign that the airway is unobstructed. **In the unconscious person, the most common cause of airway obstruction is the tongue.**

For a choking victim who becomes unconscious, start cardiopulmonary resuscitation (CPR) (Skill 28.3). Current guidelines for performing adult CPR for the health care worker and lay rescuer are listed in Table 28.2. CPR trained community bystanders are to give 30 chest compressions for every two rescue breaths. For those not CPR trained, Hands-Only (compression-only) CPR should be performed on the adult who collapses, which emphasizes the need to "push hard and fast" on the center of the chest (American Heart Association, 2015).

Think Critically

What are two advantages of pulse oximetry over arterial blood gases for monitoring oxygenation?

CLEARING RESPIRATORY SECRETIONS

THE EFFECTIVE COUGH

Mucus and secretions of the respiratory tract are typical causes of obstruction of the free passage of air. **The simplest method of clearing the air passages is to cough effectively.** Deep breathing and coughing are two standard measures used to clear secretions and prevent hypoxia. Deep breathing increases oxygenation, opens alveoli, and may precipitate coughing. Many patients with lung disease or the inability to expel forcibly a volume of air need to be taught how to cough effectively. They must learn to make the most of their air volume to remove the obstructing materials. Ineffective coughing spasms may produce additional hypoxia, lead to the rupture of alveoli, or even precipitate the collapse of air passages. Although forceful exhalation can be used with patients who are lying down, it is more effective in the sitting position. For forceful exhalation, the patient takes two deep breaths, inhales deeply again, then rapidly, and forcefully exhales with the mouth open. This moves secretions up the bronchial tree. Repeated forceful exhalation can bring the secretions up to a point where they can be more easily coughed up.

Patient Education

Deep Breathing and Coughing

Have the patient sit up on the side of the bed or in a chair leaning slightly forward. If the patient cannot sit up, raise her to a high Fowler position. Demonstrate the following steps and then

Text continues on page 517

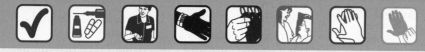

Skill 28.2 Administering Abdominal Thrusts (Heimlich Maneuver)

 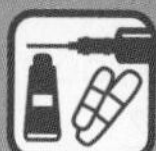 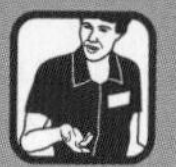  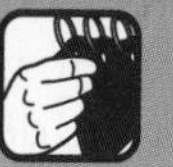 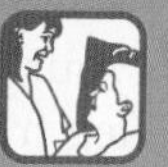  

Abdominal thrusts below the diaphragm, also called the Heimlich maneuver, are administered to a conscious victim with an airway obstruction. The purpose of the maneuver is to dislodge whatever is obstructing the airway and reestablish normal respiration.

ACTION *(RATIONALE)*

For a Conscious Person

1. Ask person if she can speak. *(Establishes whether person can get air into and out of the lungs.)*
2. If person is unable to talk or coughing is proving ineffective, position her to deliver abdominal thrusts. *(Person needs assistance to dislodge obstruction.)*
3. Stand behind the person and place arms around her waist. *(Places hands at correct height to deliver the thrusts.)*
4. Make a fist with one hand and place the other hand over the fist. *(Prepares the hands to deliver a solid thrust.)*
5. Place the hands slightly above the umbilicus and well below the sternum with the thumb of the fist inward. *(Locates correct position for thrust delivery.)*
6. Using an upward rotating motion of the fist, forcefully thrust the hands into the abdomen at an upward angle. *(Creates an artificial cough, making the diaphragm move and forcing air out of the lungs.)*

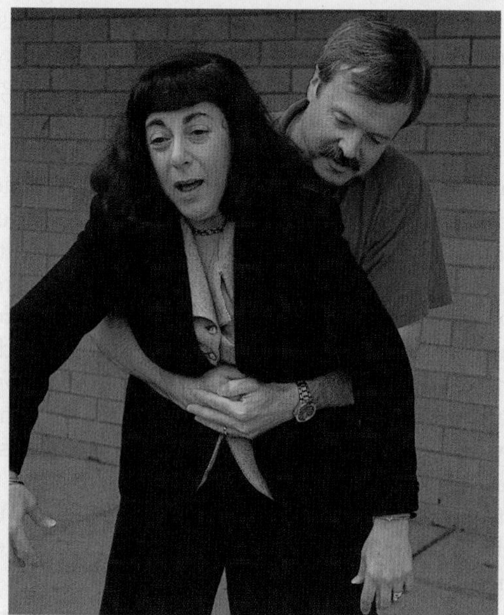

Step 6

7. Repeat the thrusts until the foreign body is expelled or the person becomes unconscious. *(The person cannot get air into the lungs until the obstruction is removed.)*

For an Unconscious Person

8. Call for help and/or activate emergency medical services (EMS) and slide the victim to the floor and place on back. *(Positions victim for airway opening maneuver and finger sweeps.)*
9. Begin CPR. Start with compressions. *(Chest compressions may dislodge the object.)*
10. Before giving breaths, open the airway using the head tilt–chin lift maneuver. Look into the mouth. If foreign matter can be seen, use the index finger of the other hand to perform a finger sweep with a hook motion, being careful not to force the object farther down the throat. *(Allows rescuer to visualize the object in the mouth; finger sweep removes the object.)*
11. Open airway and attempt to ventilate by pinching off the nose and placing the mouth over the patient's mouth; if unsuccessful, reposition head and try again. *(Airway must be open for air to enter the lungs. Repositioning will often open the airway.)*

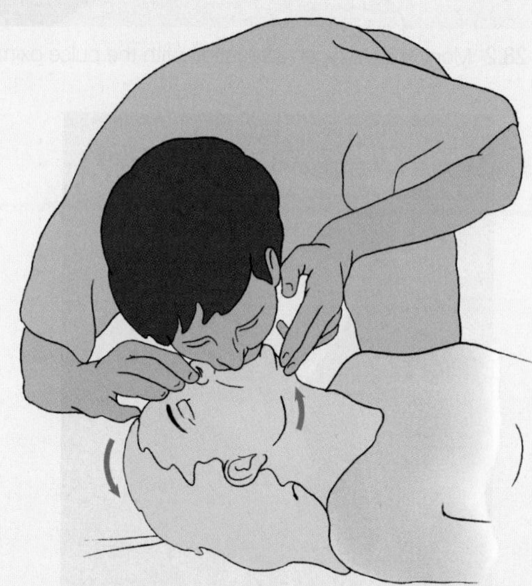

Step 11

12. If ventilation is still unsuccessful, continue CPR with compressions. *(Chest compressions increase airway pressure and may dislodge the object.).*
13. Open the airway. If a foreign object is seen, sweep with a curved finger down inside of the cheek toward the base of the tongue, sweeping debris out the other side of the mouth. *(Removes any dislodged object.)*
14. Attempt to ventilate. *(If airway is open, breaths will go into victim's lungs. If airway is still obstructed, the attempt to ventilate will be unsuccessful.)*

15. If ventilation is not successful, repeat steps 12 to 1. Repeat sequence until foreign object is dislodged. If person resumes breathing, turn to side with arms in front of the body. *(Person cannot breathe if obstruction is present. Side-lying recovery position aids continued respiration and prevents aspiration if person vomits.)*

For the Conscious Infant

16. Place the infant face down straddling your arm, keeping the head lower than the trunk. Place your hand under the chest and around the jaw for support. *(Positions the infant for effective back blows. This position helps object move up into or out of mouth and protects the infant's head and neck.)*
17. Deliver five blows between the shoulder blades. *(Force of the blows should dislodge foreign body.)*
18. Sandwich the infant between your arms and turn her over. Hold the back of the head for support. With the head down, deliver five chest thrusts using two fingers over the lower half of the sternum. *(Helps dislodge object. Protects the head and neck.)*
19. Repeat steps 17 to 18 until object is dislodged or the infant becomes unconscious. *(Infant cannot breathe when object is in airway.)*

For the Unconscious Infant

20. Call for help and/or activate EMS. Turn the infant onto her back and place on a firm, hard surface preferably above the ground. *(Positions victim for airway opening and chest compressions.)*
21. Begin CPR starting with 30 compressions. *(Chest compressions increase airway pressure and may dislodge the object.)*
22. Perform the head tilt–chin lift to open the airway. If you can see an object, carefully perform a finger sweep to remove it. *(This position allows visualization of the object in the mouth; finger sweep removes object.)*
23. Attempt to ventilate with your mouth over the infant's mouth and nose. *(If airway is unobstructed, the chest will rise.)*
24. If the chest does not rise, reposition the head and attempt to ventilate again. *(Airway is obstructed; repositioning may open it.)*
25. If still unable to ventilate, continue CPR with 30 chest compressions. *(No air can reach the lungs if the airway is obstructed.)*
26. Perform head tilt–chin lift and, if you can see an object, finger sweep it out. *(Removes the obstructing object.)*
27. Attempt to ventilate. *(If airway is open, breaths will go into victim's lungs. If airway is still obstructed, the attempt to ventilate will be unsuccessful.)*
28. If ventilation is not successful, repeat steps 25 to 27 until object is dislodged. If alone, activate EMS after 2 minutes of CPR. *(Repeating sequences will dislodge the object. EMS activation will bring help.)*

Special Considerations

- If the victim is pregnant, use chest thrusts rather than abdominal thrusts to dislodge the obstruction; make a fist with one hand and place it on the lower half of the sternum with the other hand on top of the fisted hand. Press straight back to administer the chest thrusts.
- If the victim is obese, chest thrusts may be more effective.

? Critical Thinking Questions

1. What do you think are the most common causes of choking in adults?
2. What should you teach parents of young children regarding types of foods to avoid serving and supervision when children are eating?

Skill 28.3 Cardiopulmonary Resuscitation

 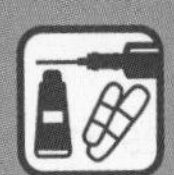 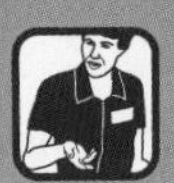 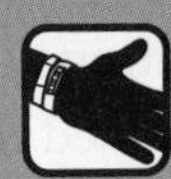 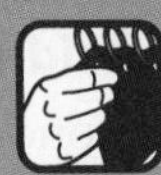 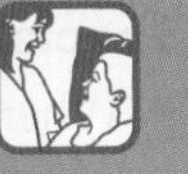 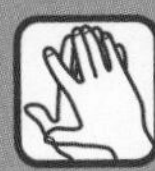 

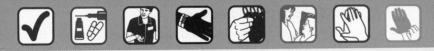

CPR must be started whenever someone is found in respiratory or cardiac arrest, meaning without breathing or without a heartbeat. It is vitally important to call for help while beginning to assess the victim. The following method is appropriate for adults, and it reflects the 2015 American Heart Association guidelines to focus on circulation (compressions) first, followed by airway and breathing (C-A-B).

ACTION (RATIONALE)

1. Check the scene for safety. (*A rescuer cannot help if he or she is injured.*)
2. Shake victim and shout name or "Are you OK?" (*Arouses the victim if conscious.*)
3. Call for nearby help. (*It is reasonable to check for breathing and a pulse before fully activating emergency medical services [EMS].*)
4. Check for breathing and signs of cardiac arrest for no more than 10 seconds. Kneel beside the person, locate the victim's larynx with two fingers, and then slide your fingers slightly laterally with gentle pressure to locate the carotid pulse. (*Positions the fingers over the carotid artery to assess pulse activity.*)
5. Activate EMS and get an automated external defibrillator (AED) as soon as possible. (*Emergency assistance and supplies for advanced life support should arrive within minutes.*)
6. Place the victim supine on a firm surface.
7. If there is a pulse but victim is not breathing, perform rescue breathing at a rate of 1 breath every 5 to 6 seconds. (*Circulation of blood does not improve patient outcome if it does not carry oxygen.*)
8. If there is no pulse and no breathing, place the heel of one hand on the lower half of the sternum. Place the heel of the other hand on top of the first hand, keeping the fingers off the chest. (*Positions hands for effective chest compressions and prevents damage to the liver.*)
9. With your body aligned directly over the hands, depress at least 2 inches (5 cm) but no more than 2.4 inches, with equal time for compression and release. Give 30 compressions at a rate of 100 to 120/min and minimize interruptions to <10 seconds. Push hard and fast. (*Pumps blood out of the heart at a rate sufficient to provide adequate oxygenation to maintain tissue life.*)

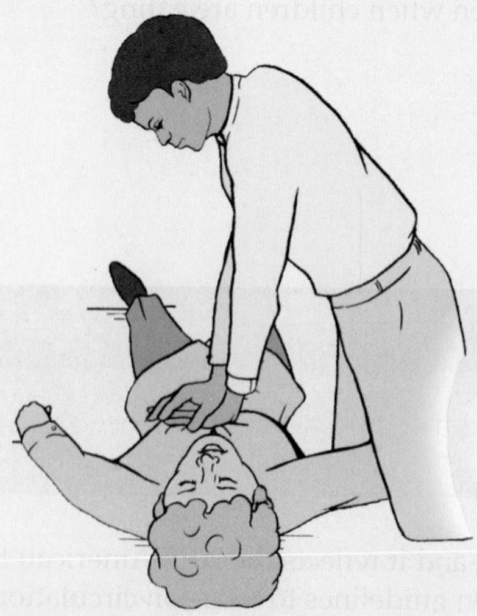

Step 9

10. Stop compressions. **Open the airway** by placing the heel of one hand on the forehead and two fingers of your other hand on the bony prominence of the chin; lift the chin to open the airway. If a mask is available, place it over the victim's nose and mouth with the bridge of the nose as a guide. If no mask is available, maintain the head tilt and pinch the nose with your fingers. Take a deep breath and, forming a seal around the victim's mouth with your own, **give two breaths.** If the first breath does not go in, the airway may have become obstructed; reposition with the head tilt–chin lift and try to deliver the breaths again, watching for the chest to rise and fall. If the breath still does not go in and the chest does not rise, the airway is obstructed, begin compressions. (*Rescue breathing opens airway and provides oxygen.*)

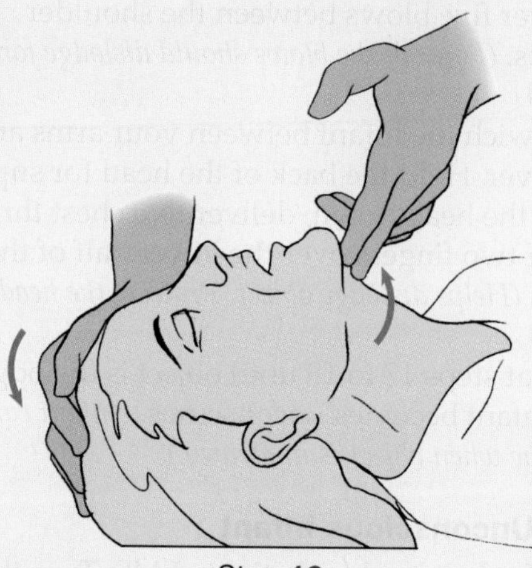

Step 10

11. When the AED arrives, place it by the victim's side. Turn the AED on and place the pads on victim's bare chest to assess victim's status and defibrillate as needed. Continue as instructed by the AED. (*Allows for monitoring of heart and administration of shock if needed.*)
12. If there is no pulse or signs of circulation (e.g., movement) or the victim is only gasping, continue CPR sequence of 30 compressions to 2 breaths until patient responds; you are relieved or you are too exhausted to continue; or if the scene becomes unsafe. If possible, compressors should rotate every 2 minutes to prevent fatigue and ensure quality compressions. (*Compressions circulate oxygenated blood, and rescue breathing opens airway and provides oxygen.*)

Special Considerations

- When a second trained rescuer is present, and the patient is intubated or has an advanced airway (i.e., a tracheostomy): perform two-rescuer CPR with continuous chest compressions at a rate of 100 to 120/min. Breaths are simultaneously delivered at a rate of 1 breath every 6 seconds, or 10 breaths/min. The second person is positioned directly above the victim's head to deliver the breaths with

a bag-mask device. Interruptions in CPR should be brief and as few as possible to maximize cardiac output. Rescuers should switch roles after every 5 cycles. Communication during CPR is important. The first rescuer should count aloud while performing compressions so that the second rescuer knows when to give breaths and when to switch roles.
- For chest compressions when the victim is an infant up to 1 year of age, use 2 fingers on the lower half of the sternum and depress at least one-third the chest depth, approximately 1.5 inches (4 cm).

Critical Thinking Questions

1. What do you do if the victim vomits while you are performing CPR?
2. What do you do if you come upon a motor vehicle accident victim who is still in the car, has no signs of respiration or circulation, and might have a spinal injury?

Table 28.2 Cardiopulmonary Resuscitation for Adults

COMPONENT	ACTION FOR LAY RESCUER	ACTION FOR HEALTH CARE PROVIDER
Recognize symptoms and need for assistance	You find an unresponsive victim and call for help. If help arrives, have that person call 911 and get an AED if available. If no one responds, call 911 and get an AED, if available. Check the victim for breathing. If the victim is not breathing or only gasping, start CPR. As soon as an AED is available, turn the AED on. Apply pads and defibrillate, if necessary.	You find an unresponsive victim and call for help. Check for breathing and a pulse simultaneously. If help arrives, have that person call 911 and get an AED if available. If no one responds, call 911 and get an AED, if available. If no pulse, start CPR. As soon as an AED is available, turn the AED on. Apply pads and defibrillate, if necessary. If the victim has a pulse but is not breathing, begin rescue breathing.
Pulse check	Lay rescuers are not taught this step.	Less than 10 seconds, carotid.
CPR sequence	C-A-B.	C-A-B.
Compression rate	100 to 120/min. Pushing hard, pushing fast, and allowing the chest to recoil between compressions has been found to be the most effective.	100 to 120/min. Pushing hard, pushing fast, and allowing the chest to recoil between compressions has been found to be the most effective.
Compression depth	At least 2 inches but no more than 2.4 inches for an average-sized adult (differs for children and infants).[a]	At least 2 inches but no more than 2.4 inches for an average-sized adult (differs for children and infants).[a]
Compression interruption	Minimize interruptions in chest compressions.	Limit interruptions to less than 10 seconds (i.e., rotating compressors, delivering shock, and pulse check). Rescuers should change compressors q 2 min to prevent fatigue and decreased efficiency of compressions.
Airway	Untrained lay rescuers should not delay compressions to perform airway maneuvers. Trained lay rescuers perform head tilt–chin lift.	Head tilt–chin lift; use jaw thrust if cervical injury is suspected.
Compression-to-breaths ratio (no advanced airway placed)	30:2 Compressions only for untrained lay rescuers.	For adults, 30:2 for one or two health care rescuers For infants and children, 15:2 for two health care rescuers.
AED use	Use as soon as possible.	Use as soon as possible.

AED, Automated external defibrillator; *C-A-B*, compression-airway-breathing; *CPR*, cardiopulmonary resuscitation; *EMS*, emergency medical services.
[a]Consult a pediatrics text and the American Heart Association guidelines for additional data that are specific to children and infants.
Adapted from deWit, S. C., & Kumagai, C. K. (2013). *Medical Surgical Nursing: Concepts and Practice*. St. Louis: Elsevier Mosby.

coach the patient through the steps. These exercises should be performed for at least 72 hours after surgery and during treatment and recovery from a respiratory illness.

Deep Breathing
- Splint an abdominal or chest incision with a small pillow.
- Inhale through the nose; hold the breath for 3 to 5 seconds and then exhale through pursed lips. Keep the shoulders level and use the diaphragm and abdominal muscles to bring air into the lungs.
- Repeat the sequence four more times, breathing slowly.
- Take 5 to 10 deep breaths every 2 hours while awake.

Effective Coughing
- Take a deep breath through the nose, hold it for 3 to 5 seconds, and then exhale through pursed lips.
- Take another deep breath and, in short segments, forcibly exhale in a "huff-cough" with the mouth open. In a huff-cough, the patient performs a series of coughs while saying the word "huff" which prevents the glottis from closing and helps clear secretions. Expel one-third of the expiratory volume with each huff-cough. Use a tissue to cover the mouth.

- Perform the sequence three times or until all secretions have been cleared.
- Expectorate the secretions into a tissue; dispose of the tissue in a sealable plastic bag.
- Use the huff-coughing technique at least once every 2 hours while awake, preferably once an hour.

Patient Education

Obtaining a Coughed Sputum Specimen

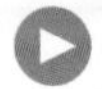

A sputum specimen is best obtained just after the patient awakens or after a nebulizer treatment, because this is when mucus is more available or easier to cough up. Provide a sterile sputum cup. Instruct patient to:

- Rinse the mouth with water.
- Open the sputum cup and place the lid upside down on the counter or table.
- Take several deep breaths, forcefully huff-cough to move secretions up, and expectorate produced sputum into the cup.
- Take several more deep breaths, force another huff-cough, and expectorate produced sputum into the cup.
- Repeat until about a half teaspoon of sputum is in the cup.
- Place the lid on the cup without contaminating the inside of the lid or the lip of the cup.
- Cleanse the mouth.
- Ring for the nurse, who will collect the specimen and send it to the laboratory.

POSTURAL DRAINAGE

Although the respiratory therapist usually is responsible for this procedure in the inpatient setting, in community and home settings the nurse must teach patients the procedure. Different positions are used to drain different segments of the lungs so that secretions can be cleared (Fig. 28.4). As specific segments of the lung are drained into the bronchi, the patient is able to cough more effectively and **expectorate** (cough up and spit out) secretions. The lungs are auscultated before and after the procedure. Generally, the patient should assume each position for 5 to 15 minutes, two to four times a day as tolerated. To prepare a patient for postural drainage, a **nebulizer** (a device that dispenses liquid in a fine spray) with bronchodilator or liquefying medications may be used as inhalation therapy to thin out secretions and relax spasms within the bronchial tree. Best results occur when the procedure is carried out in the morning and 45 to 60 minutes before a meal.

Clinical Cues

Be certain to offer mouth care after postural drainage so that the appetite is not affected by a bad taste in the mouth from coughing up secretions.

Secretions and mucus plugs may be loosened by percussion of the chest. Percussion is the rhythmic clapping with cupped hands over the thoracic area, but not over the spine or sternum. After percussion and postural drainage, the patient is assisted to cough effectively and expectorate the secretions.

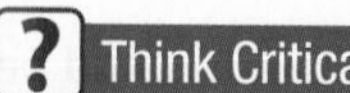

Think Critically

Why do you think postural drainage and percussion should not be done right before a meal or within an hour afterward?

OXYGEN ADMINISTRATION

When the patient cannot maintain a sufficient amount of oxygen in the body, supplemental oxygen is often ordered. Oxygen can be administered by **cannula** (a tube for insertion into a cavity), mask, tent, Croupette, or catheter. Although respiratory therapists are usually responsible for setting up and supervising oxygen equipment, nurses often need to initiate therapy or supervise its use on a PRN (as needed) basis (Skill 28.4).

Oxygen is a colorless, tasteless, and odorless gas that is present in the air. Oxygen is considered a drug, and it should be administered following a prescribed order, noting flow rate, frequency, and route. Oxygen supports combustion. High concentrations of oxygen can cause fires to burn rapidly, and when oxygen is used in patient care, great caution must be taken to prevent fires. Another disadvantage associated with the use of the gas is that it dries the tissues of the respiratory tract. Unless moisture is added, the dried tissues may become cracked and provide less resistance to infection. Overuse of oxygen can create damaging free radicals or physiologic changes in breathing. Thus, oxygen should never be administered if not needed. Patients should be monitored and weaned from oxygen as quickly as possible.

QSEN Considerations: Safety

Safety Alert

OXYGEN THERAPY SAFETY

- Place a "No Smoking: Oxygen in Use" sign on the patient's door and at the foot of the bed or over the head of the bed.
- Remind visitors about the hazard of smoking when oxygen is in use. Teach the family to smoke only far away (outside the building) from the room where oxygen is in use.
- Check all electrical devices for frayed wires, and to see that they are in good working order, to prevent short-circuit sparks that could cause a fire.
- Avoid the use of bedclothes and pajamas that are made of material that can generate static electricity. Cotton fabrics are best.
- Do not use oils, grease-based ointments, alcohol, ether, acetone, or other flammable materials on or near the patient when oxygen is in use.
- If oxygen cylinders are being used, handle with care. Be certain they are strapped securely into stands and transport devices to prevent them from falling. Situate the cylinders away from heat and heavy traffic pathways.
- Monitor the patient for skin irritation from the oxygen delivery device.
- Assess for dry mucous membranes, indicating a need for humidification to prevent tissue breakdown and increased risk for infection.

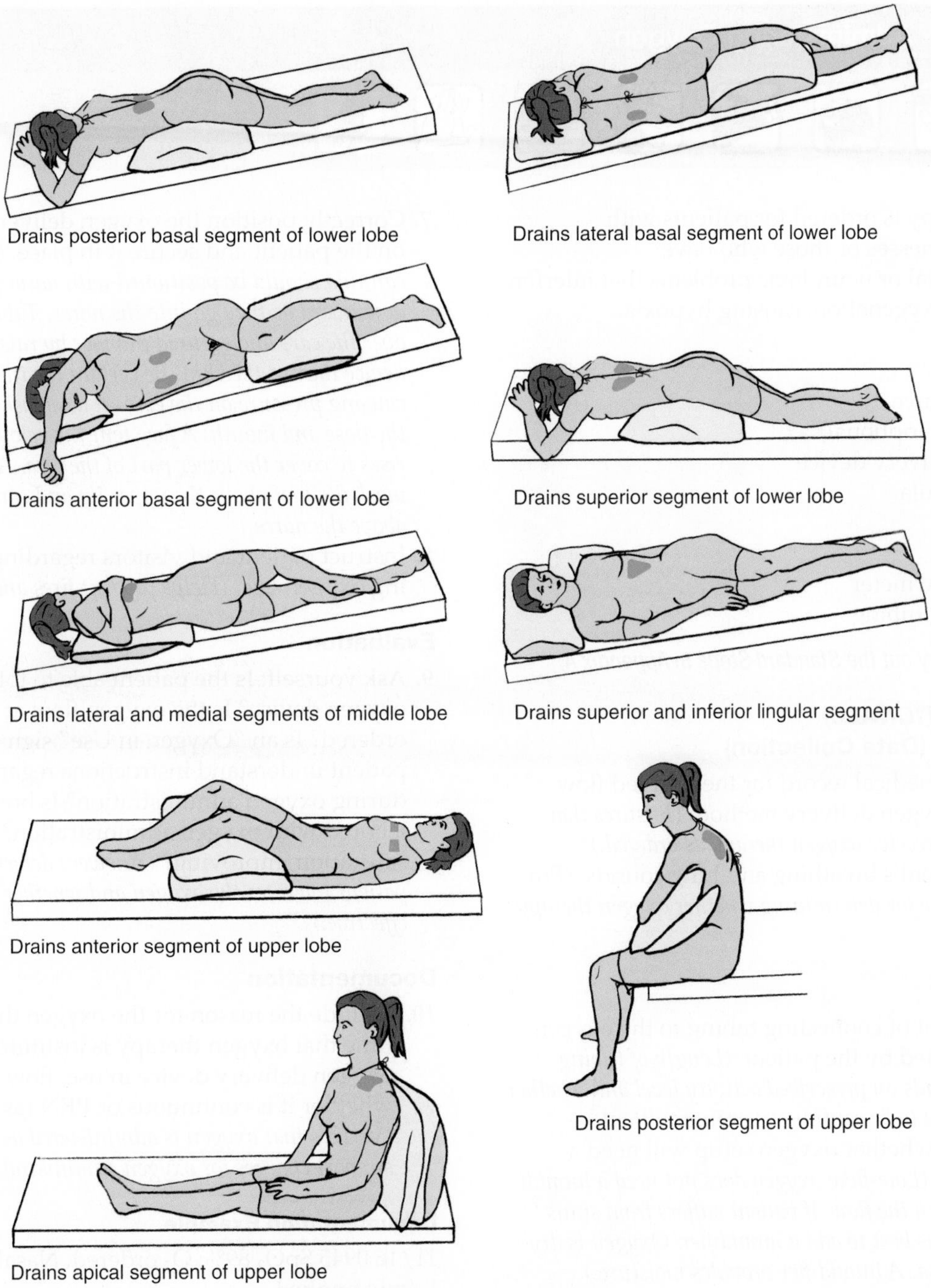

Drains posterior basal segment of lower lobe

Drains lateral basal segment of lower lobe

Drains anterior basal segment of lower lobe

Drains superior segment of lower lobe

Drains lateral and medial segments of middle lobe

Drains superior and inferior lingular segment

Drains anterior segment of upper lobe

Drains posterior segment of upper lobe

Drains apical segment of upper lobe

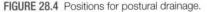

FIGURE 28.4 Positions for postural drainage.

The pieces of equipment needed for oxygen therapy are the oxygen source, the flowmeter, the **humidifier** (device supplying moisture), the tubing, and the appropriate appliance for the method ordered. Most hospitals have a central oxygen supply with outlets mounted in the wall near the patient's bed. The flowmeter is attached to the piped-in oxygen, and it regulates the amount given (Fig. 28.5). The rate of flow is prescribed by the primary care provider and may range from 2 to 12 L/min. The flow rate is based on the patient's condition and on the blood gas report or pulse oximetry. Rates of 4 to 6 L/min are common. The flow rate is adjusted by turning the valve to the "on" position and continuing to turn it until the desired flow level is indicated in the gauge just above the flow adjustment valve (Fig. 28.6).

QSEN Considerations: Safety

Safety Alert

SAFE OXYGEN FLOW RATES

Patients with obstructive lung diseases should be given only 2 to 3 L/min because higher concentrations of oxygen reduce the respiratory rate. This is because their incentive to breathe comes from lower oxygen levels rather than higher carbon dioxide levels in the blood. (These patients commonly have a continuous high level of carbon dioxide.) Check orders for oxygen carefully and always verify high flow rates with the prescribing care provider.

Skill 28.4 Administering Oxygen

 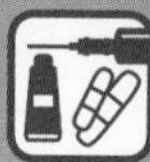 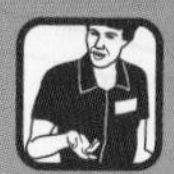 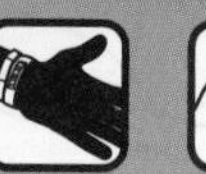 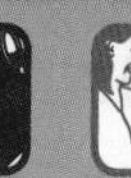 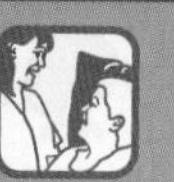 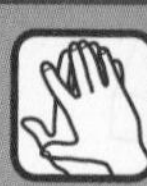 

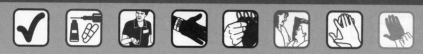

Oxygen therapy is ordered for patients with respiratory illnesses or those who have musculoskeletal or neurologic problems that interfere with proper oxygenation, causing hypoxia.

SUPPLIES

- Oxygen source
- Humidifier (optional)
- Oxygen delivery device
- Nasal cannula
- Face mask
- Face tent
- Oxygen flowmeter
- Connecting tubing

Review and carry out the Standard Steps in Appendix A.

ACTION *(RATIONALE)*

Assessment (Data Collection)

1. Check the medical record for the ordered flow rate and oxygen delivery method. *(Ensures that patient will receive oxygen therapy as ordered.)*
2. Assess patient's breathing and lung sounds. *(Provides baseline for determining whether oxygen therapy is effective.)*

Planning

3. Plan amount of connecting tubing to the oxygen source needed by the patient. *(Length of tubing needed depends on prescribed activity level and whether oxygen needs to be continuous or intermittent.)*
4. Determine whether oxygen setup will need a humidifier. *(Low-flow oxygen does not need a humidifier to moisten the flow. If patient suffers from sinus problems, it is best to add a humidifier. Oxygen is drying to mucosa. A humidifier provides moisture.)*

Implementation

5. Connect the flowmeter to the piped-in oxygen outlet on the wall by pressing it firmly into the outlet. Alternately, attach the flowmeter to the oxygen cylinder. *(Prepares oxygen to be dispensed in a regulated flow.)*
6. Attach the humidifier and the connecting tubing to the oxygen delivery device and turn on the oxygen, adjusting the flow to the ordered rate. Check for flow through the oxygen delivery device. *(Prepares delivery system for the patient. When knob is turned on the flowmeter, the metal ball inside the glass graduated gauge rises, indicating the rate of flow being delivered. The delivery rate is ordered by the primary care provider, and is commonly between 2 and 5 L/min. Feel for the flow with your fingertips.)*
7. Correctly position the oxygen delivery device on the patient and secure it in place. *(An oxygen cannula should be positioned with nasal prongs curved downward as they go into the nares. Tubing is looped over the ears and secured in place by raising the cinch device toward the chin. Be certain the tubing is not causing pressure on the ears. A facemask should fit over the nose and mouth. A face tent fits below the chin and rises to cover the lower part of the face. A small tent-mask fits just above the upper lip and comes to a point above the nares.)*
8. Instruct patient and visitors regarding safety during oxygen use. *(Helps prevent fires and injury.)*

Evaluation

9. Ask yourself: Is the patient able to tolerate the oxygen device? Is the oxygen flow at the level ordered? Is an "Oxygen in Use" sign posted? Does patient understand instructions regarding safety during oxygen administration? Is breathing less labored with oxygen administration? Is oxygen saturation improving? *(Answers determine whether patient tolerates the oxygen and whether procedure is effective.)*

Documentation

10. Include the reason for the oxygen therapy, the time that oxygen therapy is instituted, type of oxygen delivery device in use, flow rate, and whether it is continuous or PRN (as needed). *(Verifies that oxygen is administered as ordered; data support charges for oxygen administration.)*

Documentation Example

11/16 0945 SpO_2 89%; O_2 ordered. Nasal cannula at 3 L/min applied.

1100 SpO_2 94%. Tolerating flow by cannula without complaint; no evidence of redness on ears. (Nurse's electronic signature)

Special Considerations

- If patient does not tolerate oxygen delivery by one method, an order to change to another device may be needed.
- If oxygen is delivered PRN by cannula, instruct the patient that it is desirable to use the oxygen after meals and during activity, when oxygen demands are higher.
- Cleanse the nares regularly when oxygen is in use to prevent excessive crusting.
- It is important that the patient understands the reason for and potential benefits of using the oxygen

before you apply the delivery device; otherwise, compliance with use may be low.

- Check the flow rate each time you enter the patient's room; the patient or a visitor may change it from what is prescribed.
- Oxygen delivery devices should be turned off when not in use; instruct the patient with PRN oxygen how to do this.

QSEN Considerations: Safety

Safety Education

- Teaching safety precautions for the home care patient is especially important because there is no medical supervision after the nurse's visit.

Critical Thinking Questions

1. If you have a patient with a history of frequent sinusitis who is receiving oxygen by nasal cannula at 3 L/min and that patient complains about nasal stuffiness and sinus discomfort, what actions could you perform to alleviate the problem?
2. You have a postoperative patient who is receiving oxygen by nasal cannula. The patient keeps taking off the oxygen cannula. What might you say to convince the patient to leave the oxygen cannula in place?

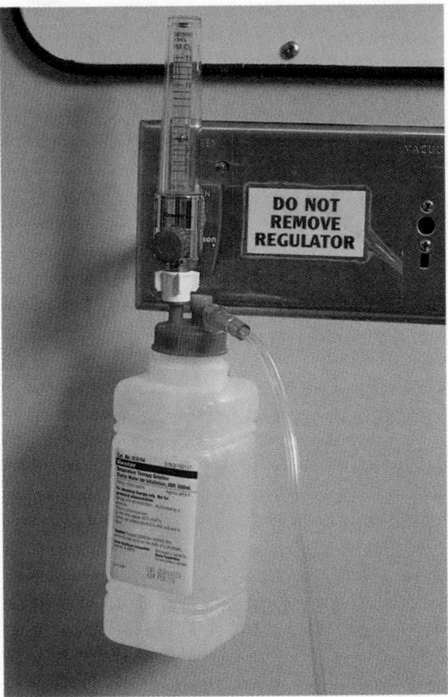

FIGURE 28.5 Wall oxygen flowmeter and humidifier setup.

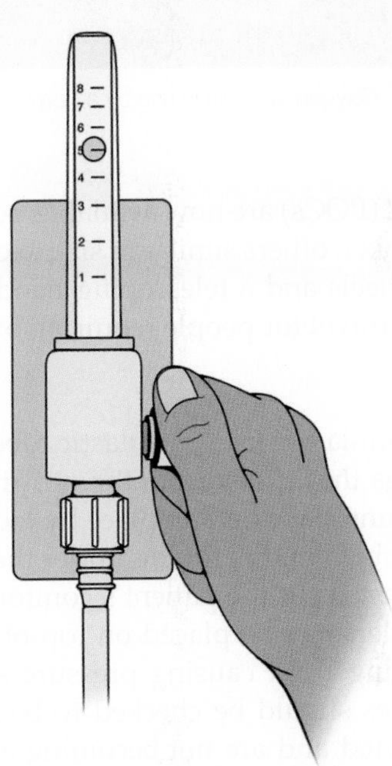

FIGURE 28.6 Adjusting the oxygen flowmeter valve control.

The humidifier is attached to the flowmeter and is usually situated between the flowmeter and the tubing. The oxygen bubbles through the container of water and is moisturized before entering the air passages. Check the level of fluid in the container periodically during the day to ensure that it is working. When the fluid level is low, notify the respiratory care department so that the unit can be replaced or refilled.

In the home setting, a portable oxygen tank may be used. Portable oxygen is also used when transporting oxygen-dependent patients within the hospital. An oxygen concentrator is frequently used in the home or long-term care setting (Fig. 28.7). The machine collects and concentrates oxygen from room air, storing it for use. The machine must be plugged into an electrical outlet. Portable (battery operated) oxygen

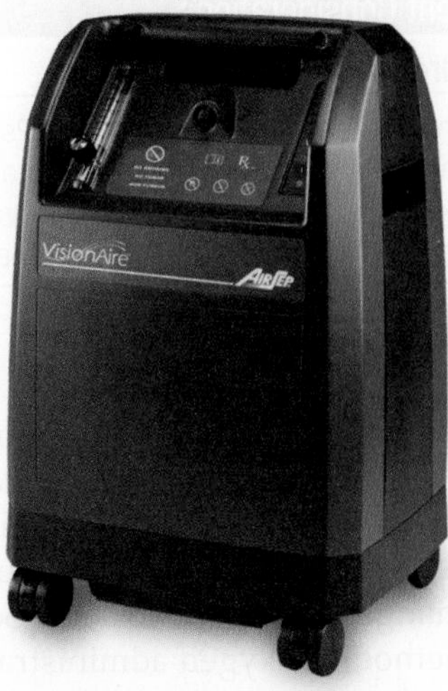

FIGURE 28.7 Oxygen concentrator. (Courtesy AirSep Corp., Buffalo, NY.)

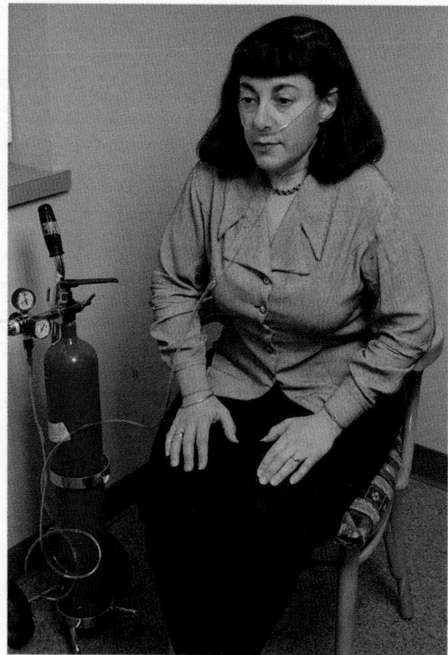

FIGURE 28.8 Oxygen cannula in use by a home care patient.

concentrators (POCs) are now available, some as small as a coffee maker, others similar in size to carry-on luggage with wheels and a telescoping handle, allowing mobility and travel for people requiring oxygen.

CANNULA

The nasal cannula consists of a plastic tube with short, curved prongs that extend into the nostril about ¼ to ½ inch. The cannula is held in place by looping it over the ears and cinching the tubing under the chin; it can be easily adjusted for the patient's comfort (Fig. 28.8). A Velcro holder may be placed on top of the head to keep the tubing from causing pressure sores on the ears. The nares should be checked to be certain they are unobstructed and are not becoming excoriated. A cannula is useful for patients requiring oxygen during meals.

 **Assignment Considerations**

Detecting Skin Irritation

Ask the unlicensed assistive personnel (UAPs) to check the backs of the ears and the nares for tissue irritation when they assist the patient with morning care. This is especially important for older adults, who have thin, easily damaged skin.

MASKS

Various types of masks are available for the administration of oxygen in concentrations ranging from 24% to 55% at flow rates of 3 to 7 L/min (Fig. 28.9). Oxygen concentrations above 60% are rarely used because of the danger of oxygen toxicity. Some patients dislike this method of oxygen administration because the mask must be placed over the face, and they feel claustrophobic.

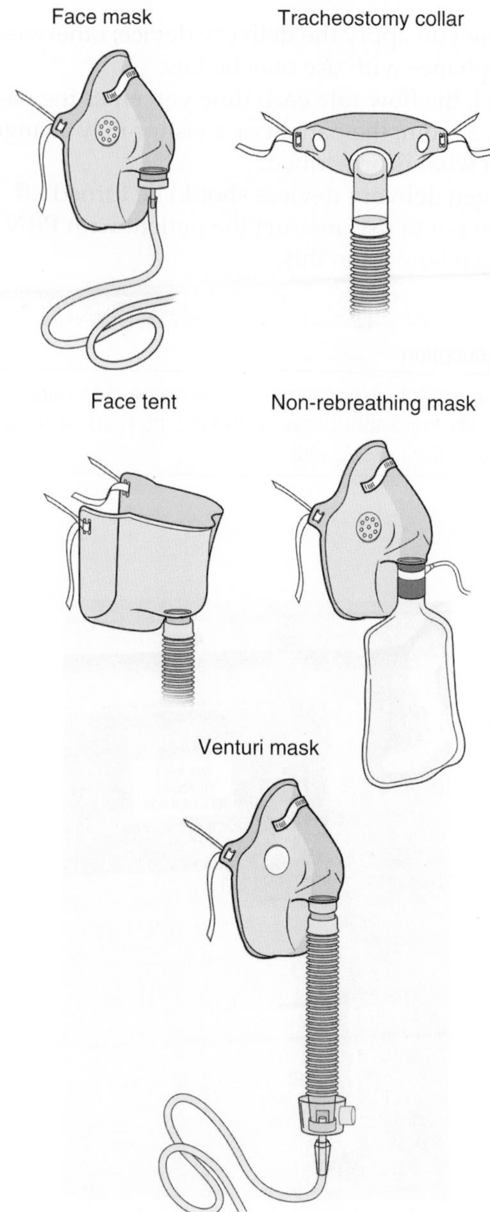

FIGURE 28.9 Various oxygen delivery devices.

Advantages and disadvantages of various oxygen devices are listed in Table 28.3. Oxygen tents are still sometimes used, particularly for small children. Oxygen halos, Oxyhoods, or Croupettes are used for infants.

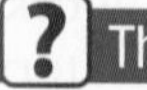 **Think Critically**

How would you explain to a patient who has oxygen ordered by cannula PRN when to use the oxygen?

ARTIFICIAL AIRWAYS

Artificial airways are used for several purposes: to relieve an obstruction, to protect the airway, to facilitate suctioning, and to provide artificial ventilation.

There are two types of pharyngeal airways: the nasopharyngeal airway and the oropharyngeal airway.

Table 28.3 Advantages and Disadvantages of Common Oxygen Administration Devices

METHOD	O_2 DELIVERY	ADVANTAGES	DISADVANTAGES	NURSING IMPLICATIONS
Nasal cannula (nasal prongs)	Low concentrations; dependent on rate and depth of breathing *Flows:* 1 L = 24% O_2 2 L = 28% O_2 3 L = 32% O_2 4 L = 36% O_2 5 L = 40% O_2 6 L = 44% O_2	Patient can move about, eat, and talk while receiving oxygen. Most COPD patients can tolerate 2 L/min flow.	Restless patients can easily dislodge the prongs. Risk of skin irritation at the nares, ears, and cheeks. Flow rate 3 L and above requires humidification because it will dry and irritate nasal mucosa.	Prongs should be curved downward when inserted in the nose; check frequently because patients tend to replace the prongs incorrectly. Clean prongs every few hours.
Simple face mask	Low to medium concentrations; 35%-50% can be achieved with a flow rate of 6-12 L/min.	The mask provides adequate humidification; delivers oxygen quickly for short-term therapy.	Discomfort and risk of pressure necrosis caused by a tight seal between the face and mask. The device must be removed for the patient to eat, drink, or take medications. Muffles the voice when talking. Requires at least 5-L flow to prevent accumulation of expired air in mask.	Wash and dry under the mask and wipe out the mask q 1-2 h. The mask must fit snugly. The straps at the ears may need to be padded to prevent necrosis.
Partial rebreathing mask	Higher concentrations; 40%-60% at flow rates of 6-10 L/min.	The mask is lightweight; the reservoir bag traps a portion of exhaled breath that is high in oxygen for rebreathing.	Risk of pressure necrosis with long-term use. Cannot be used with high humidity.	The bag should not be allowed to deflate during inspiration. Check the skin under the straps frequently.
Non-rebreather mask	Highest concentrations; 60%-90% can be achieved.	Delivers a high concentration of oxygen accurately.	Cannot be used with high humidity. The flow rate must be sufficient to prevent the bag from deflating during inspiration.	The mask should fit snugly; check skin contact areas for pressure necrosis.
Venturi mask ("Venti mask")	Delivers consistent FIO_2 regardless of the breathing pattern. Concentration and liter flow are marked on the mask apparatus; available for 24%, 28%, 31%, 35%, 40%, and 50% O_2.	The mask can provide good humidification; good for delivering low, constant (yet precise) oxygen concentrations to the patient with COPD.	Discomfort and risk of skin irritation. Must be removed for eating, drinking, and taking oral medications. Talking is muffled.	Air ports must not be occluded. Check skin contact areas frequently.
Transtracheal catheter	Delivers oxygen efficiently.	The flow requirement is reduced 60%-80%, increasing the time that oxygen is available from the portable source. The catheter is less visible. Less nasal irritation occurs.	Catheter replacement is an invasive procedure. Not appropriate for someone with excessive mucus production.	Patient and family education about catheter replacement.

Continued

Table 28.3 Advantages and Disadvantages of Common Oxygen Administration Devices—cont'd

METHOD	O_2 DELIVERY	ADVANTAGES	DISADVANTAGES	NURSING IMPLICATIONS
Tracheostomy collar	Delivers O_2 and humidification via the tracheostomy; must be connected to a nebulizer with FIO_2 set at 24%-100%.	Adds humidity to help liquefy secretions. Loses some O_2 flow because the collar is not tight fitting.	Must drain the condensation in the tubing often. Risk of respiratory infection.	Drain condensation from tubing into the receptacle, being careful not to allow fluid to go into the tracheostomy. Remove and clean the collar device and check the skin under the straps at least q 4 h.
T-bar (Briggs adapter)	Delivers O_2 and humidification to the tracheostomy; must be connected to a nebulizer with FIO_2 set at 24%-100%.	Fits more tightly compared with tracheostomy collar. Adds humidity to liquefy secretions.	Must drain the condensation in the tubing often. Risk of respiratory infection.	Drain condensation from the tubing into the receptacle; be careful not to get fluid into the tracheostomy. Remove and clean the T-bar device q 4 h.

From deWit, S. C. & Kumagai, C. K. (2013). *Medical Surgical Nursing: Concepts and Practice* (2nd ed., pp. 323). St. Louis: Elsevier Mosby.

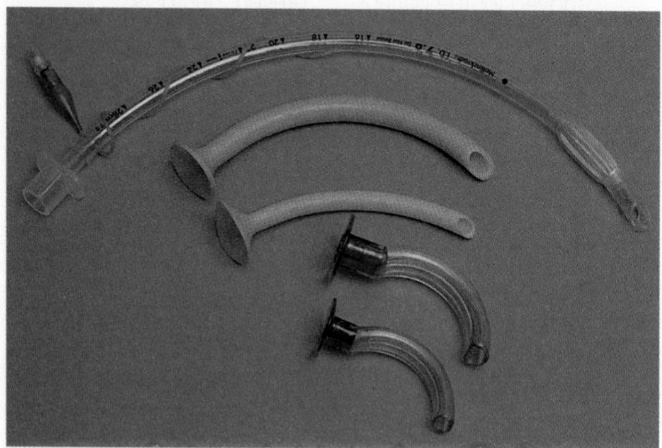

FIGURE 28.10 Types of airways *(top to bottom):* endotracheal, nasal, and oropharyngeal.

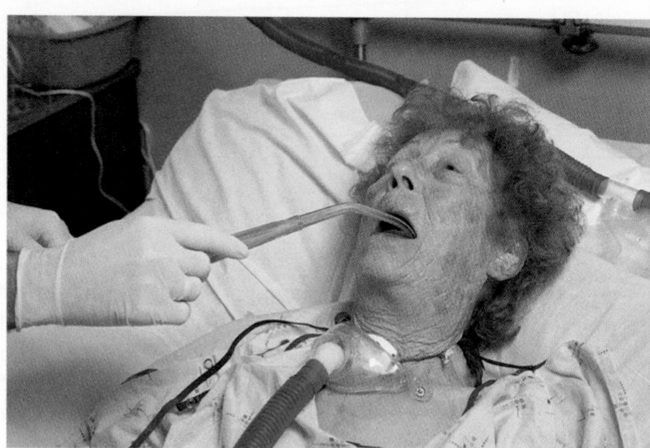

FIGURE 28.11 Yankauer suction tip is used for oral suction.

These are used to keep the tongue from falling back into the throat and are frequently required for postoperative patients until they have recovered from anesthesia (Fig. 28.10). These airways are used for patients who can breathe on their own; however, you must never leave the bedside of a patient with this type of airway in place.

Endotracheal tubes (ETTs) maintain an airway in those patients who are unconscious or unable to breathe on their own. The tube is inserted by a physician or an advanced practice nurse certified in the procedure; intubation is often done under emergency circumstances. The tube is generally removed after 48 to 72 hours, but it may be left in place for a week or more. The patient with an endotracheal tube is unable to speak because the tube sits between the vocal cords; therefore, you must find alternate means of communication such as a communication board or writing utensils. If intubation is needed for an extended period, the patient should have a tracheostomy performed. An endotracheal tube may cause a mucosal ulcer after 5 to 7 days of use, depending on cuff pressures or type of cuff used.

NASOPHARYNGEAL SUCTIONING

The purpose of suctioning is to maintain a patent airway by removing accumulated secretions. When air passages are obstructed by emesis or secretions, suctioning may be a lifesaving procedure. Pharyngeal suctioning involves the upper air passages of the nose, mouth, and pharynx.

Among those who may require suctioning to remove obstructing fluids are infants, gravely debilitated or unconscious patients, and those with an ineffective cough. When possible, the patient should be stimulated to cough because this moves secretions up into the trachea.

Oral suctioning is usually tried before nasopharyngeal suctioning because it is a more comfortable procedure for the patient. A Yankauer suction tip is attached to the suction connecting tubing, and the mouth and top of the pharynx are suctioned (Fig. 28.11). If this does not remove secretions adequately, nasopharyngeal suctioning is performed. **The suction pressure should be set between 80 and 120 mm Hg.**

Select the suction catheter based on the size of the patient's tube and the thickness of the secretions to be removed. Use a smaller 8- to 12-Fr. catheter for thin secretions; use a size 14- or 16-Fr. catheter for an adult with **tenacious** (sticky) or thick secretions. To control the amount of pressure for suctioning, place the thumb over the suction port of the catheter or the open end of a Y connector between the tubing and the catheter.

When suctioning, make every effort to prevent the introduction of pathogens into the airways. Countless microorganisms are found in the upper respiratory tract, and it is virtually impossible to maintain sterility when suctioning the nose or pharynx. Clean technique and thorough hand hygiene are essential for pharyngeal suctioning of the oral and nasal cavities, but aseptic technique is mandatory for suctioning the trachea. **It is best to use aseptic technique for all suctioning of the airway structures.**

Disposable sterile suctioning sets are widely used. A set contains a plastic catheter, a carton to hold a small amount of solution to moisten and rinse the catheter and tubing, and a sterile glove. You may use tap water to clear secretions from the tubing in pharyngeal suctioning (Skill 28.5). **Never reuse a catheter that has been used in the mouth for nasopharyngeal or tracheobronchial suctioning.** Once the catheter has been in the mouth, it is contaminated.

Skill 28.5 Nasopharyngeal Suctioning

 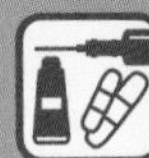 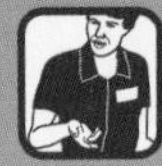 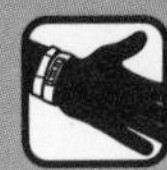  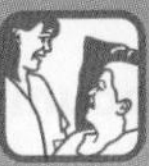 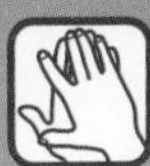 

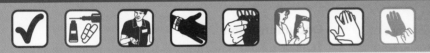

Nasopharyngeal suctioning is performed when the patient is unable to adequately clear secretions from the pharynx or when a patient cannot expectorate sputum for a diagnostic test. Suction equipment is kept at the bedside.

SUPPLIES

- Disposable sterile suction catheter
- Towel or sterile drape
- Solution container
- Suction connecting tubing
- Sterile gloves
- Sterile water or normal saline
- Suction source
- Water-soluble lubricant
- Protective eyewear

Review and carry out the Standard Steps in Appendix A.

ACTION *(RATIONALE)*

Assessment (Data Collection)

1. Auscultate the lungs to locate retained secretions. Help patient cough and expectorate if possible. If secretions cannot be cleared, continue with procedure. *(Determines necessity for suctioning. If secretions are cleared, suctioning is not necessary.)*

Planning

2. Position the patient in the semi-Fowler position if possible. *(Permits an unobstructed view of mouth and nose for correct suctioning.)*
3. Have patient deep breathe for several breaths before suctioning or preoxygenate. *(Helps prevent hypoxia during suctioning.)*
4. Set up and check equipment to see that suction is functioning correctly. Think about placement of supplies to maintain sterility during the procedure. *(Suction must be functioning for procedure to be effective. Planning can help prevent contamination of sterile supplies.)*

Implementation

5. Open the catheter suction kit and pour the solution into the solution container; open the water-soluble lubricant. Open the catheter package; squeeze the lubricant onto the inside of the package. *(Prepares the equipment for sterile suctioning.)*
6. Put on sterile gloves, or one sterile glove on the dominant hand and a nonsterile glove on the other hand. *(Reduces transfer of microorganisms.)*
7. Pick up the sterile catheter with your gloved dominant hand and attach the suction port to the connecting tubing held by your other hand (glove on nondominant hand is no longer sterile). *(Prepares catheter for suctioning procedure. Connecting tubing is not sterile; therefore, the glove that touches it is no longer sterile.)*
8. Moisten 6 to 8 cm of the catheter with water-soluble lubricant and insert the catheter through the right naris into the nasopharynx, about 6 to 8 cm, without suction. If you meet an obstruction, remove the catheter and try the left naris. Do not force the catheter; seek assistance if you meet resistance on the left side also. *(Moistening catheter makes passage through the nasal passages easier.)*
9. While withdrawing the catheter, intermittently open and close the suction port with the thumb of your nonsterile hand. Suction no more than 10 seconds at a time. Rotate catheter while withdrawing it. *(Suctioning extracts oxygen from the patient's airway. Rotating the catheter pulls up secretions from various parts of the airway.)*

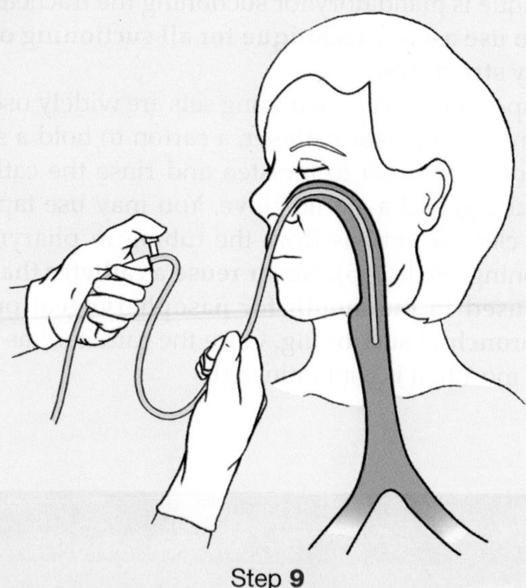

Step 9

10. Rinse the catheter by placing it in a container of solution and applying suction to draw the solution through the catheter. *(Removes secretions from catheter and connecting tubing.)*
11. Suction the other naris. Repeat the entire process if needed. Allow patient to rest for 1 minute between suction sessions. Observe for signs of hypoxia. Talk calmly to reassure the patient and inform of each step before doing it. *(Secretions may be copious, and several short suction sessions may be needed to clear them completely.)*
12. Ask the patient to cough. *(Brings secretions into the back of the nose and throat, where they can be easily suctioned.)*
13. Rinse and moisten the catheter with the solution, insert it into the oral cavity toward the pharynx, and suction the pooled secretions. Suction along the outer gums and cheeks and at the base of the tongue as needed, using 5 to 10 seconds of suction at a time for the throat area. *(Once the catheter has been introduced into the mouth, it is **never** used to enter the nasopharynx area because it is now contaminated. Suctioning in all of these areas clears pooled secretions.)*
14. Rinse the catheter and tubing by placing the tip in the water container and applying suction briefly; turn off the suction. Roll catheter into the palm of one hand and remove the glove, pulling it over the catheter; dispose of the glove and catheter. Remove other glove. *(Rinsing clears suction tubing of secretions. Pulling glove over used catheter disposes of contaminated catheter and gloves using Standard Precautions. If catheter is used only in nasopharynx and therefore can be reused, rinse with sterile water and place it in a closed container according to agency protocol. The catheter should be replaced every 8 hours.)*

Evaluation

15. Auscultate the lungs and listen to see if there is any noise indicating retained secretions. *(Determines whether secretions have been adequately removed.)*

Documentation

16. Document date, time, reason for suctioning, size of catheter used, type of technique, and how patient tolerated procedure. *(Notes reason for invasive procedure and patient's tolerance.)*

Documentation Example

10/20 1015 Noisy respirations 24/min and congested nasal passages. States cannot get secretions out. 16 Fr. catheter used to suction nasopharynx and oral cavity. Caused considerable coughing. Moderate amount of yellow secretions obtained. Respirations quiet; lungs without crackles or wheezes. Resting quietly. (Nurse's electronic signature)

? Critical Thinking Questions

1. Why do you think that moistening the suction catheter well with the lubricant makes the nasopharyngeal suctioning procedure more comfortable for the patient?
2. Why can't you substitute petroleum jelly for the water-soluble lubricant if none is on hand? What would you do if you had no water-soluble lubricant and the patient was becoming severely hypoxic?

TRACHEOBRONCHIAL SUCTIONING

Deep suctioning of the lower respiratory passages stimulates the cough reflex and removes secretions from the trachea and bronchi. This is most frequently performed when a patient has been intubated or has a **tracheostomy** (opening into the trachea) (Skill 28.6). **Sterile technique is mandatory for deep suctioning in the tracheobronchial tree and for the intubated patient.** Use sterile saline or sterile water to wet the catheter when **endotracheal** (within the trachea) or bronchial suctioning is necessary. Because the patient is not receiving oxygen when you are suctioning, do not suction for longer than 10 seconds at a time.

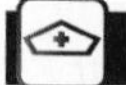
Clinical Cues

Holding your own breath while suctioning is one way to judge how long you can safely suction the patient. Another way is to count "1-1000, 2-1000," etc. to "10-1000" for determining a 10 second period.

Skill 28.6 Endotracheal and Tracheostomy Suctioning

 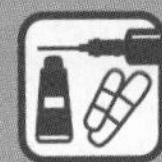 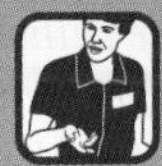 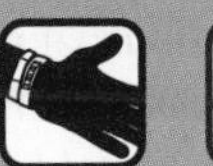 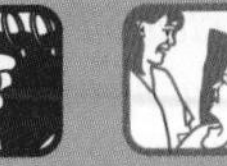 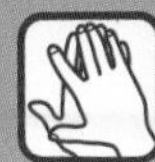 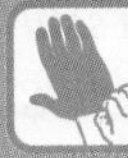

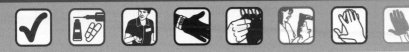

Because it is often difficult for a patient to cough secretions out via an endotracheal or tracheostomy tube, the tube must be periodically suctioned. The tracheostomy tube must be kept free of secretions for the patient to breathe or receive oxygen. To determine when suctioning is needed, auscultate the lungs. A face shield or goggles and mask should be used when suctioning because the patient may spray sputum when coughing.

SUPPLIES

- Suction source
- Face shield
- Sterile normal saline
- Sterile catheter suction kit
- Solution container
- Sterile gloves
- Sterile suction catheter
- Resuscitation bag
- Connecting tubing

Review and carry out the Standard Steps in Appendix A.

ACTION *(RATIONALE)*

Assessment (Data Collection)

1. Auscultate the patient's lungs to determine whether retained secretions are present. *(Moist breath sounds, including gurgles and bubbling, indicate a need for suctioning.)*
2. Measure patient's vital signs. If patient is on a cardiac monitor, note cardiac rate and rhythm. *(This establishes a baseline to assess tolerance of procedure later.)*

Planning

3. Be certain all equipment is at hand and think through the procedure before opening sterile supplies. *(Ensures that the procedure will go smoothly.)*
4. Obtain a partner to preoxygenate the patient with the resuscitator bag if possible. *(The patient should be preoxygenated before suctioning so that oxygen is not seriously depleted by suctioning. The procedure is easier to perform with an assistant.)*
5. Attach the connecting tubing to suction source and turn on suction; check the pressure. Place the connecting tubing nearby. *(Verify that the suction is functioning by occluding end of suction tubing with your thumb and watching pressure on gauge rise. Set pressure according to agency protocol. Wall suction unit pressure is generally set between 80 and 120 mm Hg maximum. Placing tubing nearby prepares tubing to be easily connected to the suction catheter.)*

Implementation

6. Perform hand hygiene; open supplies and put on sterile gloves. Set up the water container. Place sterile drape, if available, across patient's chest. Pour about 100 mL sterile water into the container with the nondominant hand. With gloved dominant hand holding the catheter, attach the catheter to the connecting tubing. Be careful not to contaminate the glove holding the catheter. The hand holding the connecting tubing is no longer sterile. *(Provides sterile field on the chest. Prepares the water for use and maintains sterility of dominant hand. Supplies the catheter with suction.)*
7. Have an assistant oxygenate patient by resuscitator bag with two or three large-volume inspirations while you prepare to suction, or do this yourself. If working alone and the patient is receiving oxygen, increase the concentration to 100% for a short time, keeping a hand on oxygen adjustment, or give two or three sigh breaths with the ventilator. Check agency protocol for desired way to preoxygenate the patient. *(Preoxygenation prevents hypoxia during suctioning.)*

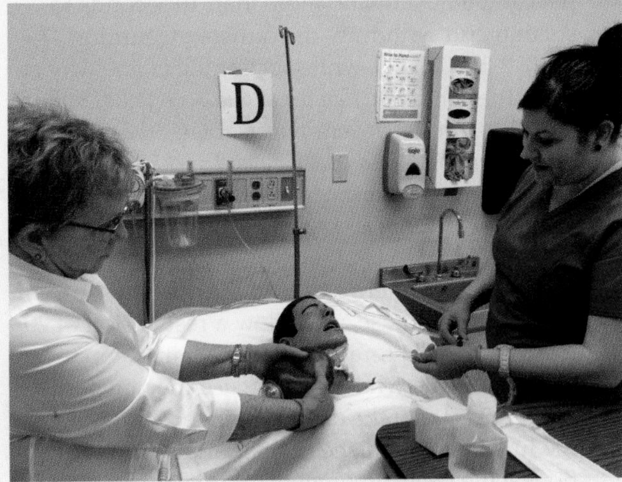

Step 7

8. Moisten the catheter tip in the sterile saline solution and suction up a small bit of the solution to test the system. Disconnect the ventilator tubing if ventilator is in use, and immediately introduce the catheter into the endotracheal tube or tracheostomy tube using only sterile gloved hand; do not use suction while placing the catheter.

Advance catheter until resistance is met, then pull back 1 cm. *(Moisture lubricates the catheter and makes it easier to introduce; testing with solution ensures suction is working properly. Holding the catheter at a 90-degree angle to the tube to enter it helps prevent contaminating the catheter by touching the patient's face or neck. Suction applied on entry draws out oxygen. Resistance occurs when the catheter reaches the carina [junction of main bronchi].)*

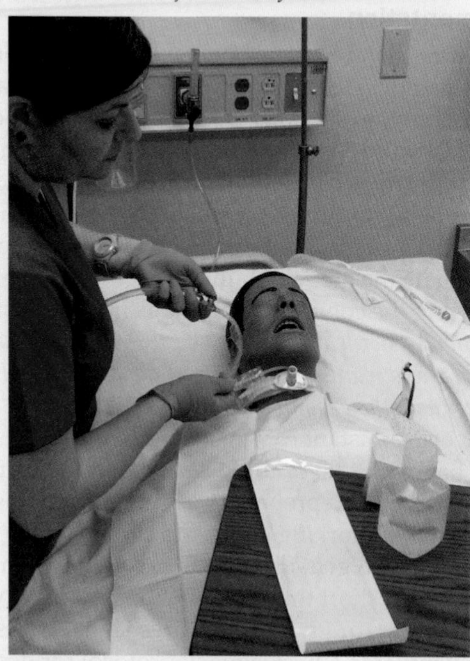

Step 8

9. Apply suction while rotating and withdrawing the catheter. Allow no more than 10 seconds to suction and withdraw the catheter. Counting "1-1000, 2-1000," etc., while suctioning is one way to track the time. *(Suction draws out secretions. Rolling the catheter between your fingers rotates the catheter openings at the tip so that they will suck up secretions around the circumference of the trachea. Suctioning for more than 10 seconds seriously depletes the patient's oxygen.)*
10. Reattach the patient's tube to the oxygen source if one has been in use, and allow a rest period of 20 to 30 seconds before suctioning again. Keep the catheter sterile while waiting; use the nonsterile hand to reattach the oxygen source. Auscultate the lungs when finished to be certain that secretions have been adequately cleared. *(Suction draws out oxygen and secretions and may cause hypoxia. Hyperoxygenation should be done again before each suctioning.)*
11. Suction the nasopharynx if needed. *(Secretions may collect above the cuffed tracheostomy tube and need to be removed.)*
12. Rinse catheter and connecting tubing by suctioning up more solution. Discard the catheter by coiling it in your gloved hand and pulling the glove off over it. *(Connecting tubing should be cleared of secretions. A sterile catheter must be used each time tracheobronchial suctioning is performed. Sterile catheters must be kept at the bedside for immediate use. Pulling glove over the used catheter prevents spread of microorganisms.)*

Suctioning with a Sleeved Catheter

13. Open catheter package without disturbing protective sleeve covering the catheter. Attach catheter to endotracheal tube or tracheostomy adaptor and to suction tubing. *(Sleeve maintains sterility of catheter so that it can be reused several times.)*
14. As catheter is inserted via endotracheal tube or tracheostomy, the sleeve slides back; advance the catheter as far as possible. *(Positions catheter within trachea to the carina.)*
15. Apply suction while rotating and withdrawing the catheter. Allow the sleeve to re-cover the catheter as it is withdrawn; pull it back out of the tube opening. *(The sleeve prevents the catheter from becoming contaminated from environment outside the trachea. Pulling it out of the tube prevents catheter from occluding the airway.)*
16. Remove gloves and perform hand hygiene. Turn off suction. *(Performing hand hygiene reduces transfer of microorganisms. Suction may remain off between suctioning sessions.)*
17. Measure vital signs. *(This assesses the patient's tolerance of procedure.)*

Evaluation

18. Ask yourself: Did patient tolerate the procedure without drastic changes in vital signs? Were there changes to cardiac rhythm? Are the lungs clear to auscultation? Did suctioning remove secretions? Was sterility maintained? *(Answers provide data to determine whether procedure was effective.)*

Documentation

19. Include the number of times the patient received suctioning, type of technique used, characteristics of secretions, and any problems encountered. *(Documents procedure and any problems encountered.)*

Documentation Example

10/24 1430 Coughing; gurgling sounds auscultated. Suctioned × 2 with sterile technique and preoxygenation. Moderate white secretions obtained; lungs clear, tubing reattached to ventilator; no signs of arrhythmia. (Nurse's electronic signature)

Special Considerations

- Some patients can cough secretions out; allow the patient to try before suctioning.
- Holding your breath while you apply suction helps judge the time the patient is without oxygen.
- Empty the suction container at the end of each shift or at least every 24 hours; check agency protocol.
- Do not suction unnecessarily because the procedure is irritating to tracheal tissues.
- Do not instill saline into the tracheobronchial tree; repeated studies have shown an adverse effect on oxygen saturation (Ackley & Ladwig, 2014).
- In the home care situation, suction catheters can be cleaned, sterilized, and reused.
- Perform patient education to the home care patient regarding the suctioning procedure. The patient education plan should be consistently used by all home care nurses working with the patient.

Critical Thinking Questions

1. What is one way to hold the suction catheter to introduce it into an endotracheal tube so that it does not kink and hit the patient's skin or your hand and become contaminated?
2. What would you need to do before suctioning a patient if you know that this patient frequently forcibly coughs out secretions when being suctioned?

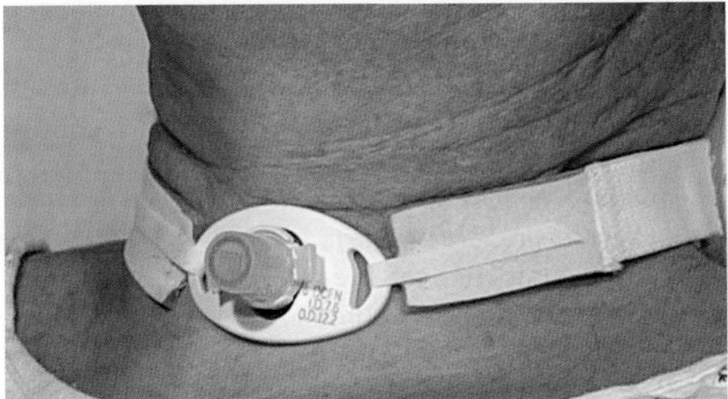

FIGURE 28.12 Patient with a tracheostomy tube and commercial tube holder. (Courtesy Dale Medical Products, Inc., Plainville, MA.)

TRACHEOSTOMY

A tracheostomy consists of a surgical incision into the throat and insertion of a tube to aerate the lungs (Fig. 28.12). It is performed on patients who have **apnea** (absence of breathing) or respiratory obstruction. The procedure is done to prevent aspiration of secretions and blood and to provide easier access to the lower airways. Intubation of the trachea with the endotracheal or tracheostomy tube is performed frequently, often to provide mechanical ventilation. Various types of tracheostomy tubes are used depending on the purpose and the patient's condition.

When a tracheostomy tube has a cuff, it is inflated to seal the space between the tube and the tracheal wall, to prevent fluid from being aspirated into the lungs, and to allow only minimal leakage of air. The tube may have either a foam cuff or a soft balloon cuff. Patients on a positive-pressure ventilator to treat respiratory failure must have a cuffed tracheostomy or endotracheal tube for effective use of the ventilator. When an inflated cuff is present, check cuff pressure at least every 8 hours. **Perform pharyngeal suctioning before deflating the cuff.** Never leave the patient alone when the cuff is deflated because of the danger of aspirating fluid. When the cuff is reinflated, check for air leakage by holding a hand in front of the patient's nose and mouth and asking her to blow. If air movement is felt, the cuff seal is underinflated.

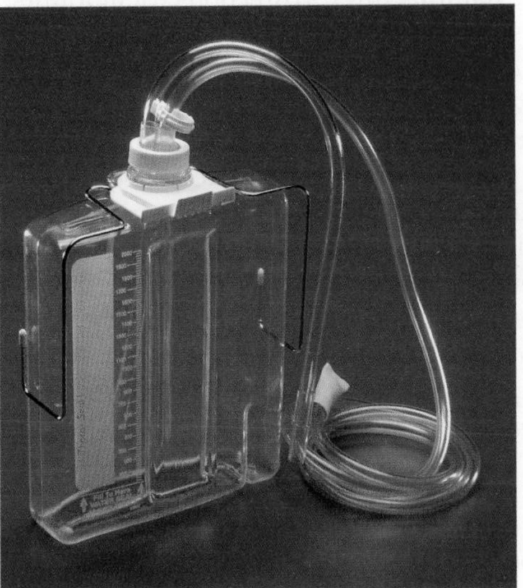

FIGURE 28.13 Disposable chest drainage unit. (ARGYLE is a trademark of Covidien AG. Copyright Covidien. All rights reserved.)

CHEST DRAINAGE TUBES

A chest tube is inserted by the physician or advanced practice nurse as an emergency treatment or at the completion of intrathoracic surgery. It is connected to a disposable pleural drainage system (Fig. 28.13). Drainage systems are used to drain air or fluid out of the pleural space and to keep the air or fluid from being sucked back into the chest. When gravity drainage is inadequate to remove air and fluids from a patient with a large pleural leak, suction can be applied using either wall suction or a portable suction machine. The disposable chest drainage unit has a suction control chamber to prevent excessive negative pressure in the pleural space, as well as a water-seal chamber and a drainage chamber (Steps 28.1). If suction is used in the water-seal system, there should be constant bubbling in the suction chamber. There is also a waterless system that uses a one-way valve in the suction chamber (Fig. 28.14). Some patients are given a mobile chest drainage unit so that they can be discharged home (Fig. 28.15). The mobile devices are designed so that the drainage

Steps 28.1 Maintaining a Disposable Water-Seal Chest Drainage System

Disposable chest drainage systems are frequently used with chest tubes. The nurse must check to ensure the unit is functioning properly.

Review and carry out the Standard Steps in Appendix A.

ACTION *(RATIONALE)*

1. Position the unit below the level of the chest tube; the tubing should hang straight, without looping, from the chest tube to the container. *(Ensures proper drainage, especially when suction is not applied.)*
2. Fill the water-seal chamber to the correct level; refill with sterile water as needed. The suction chamber may also require sterile solution. Check the manufacturer's directions for amounts; some systems are waterless. *(Provides adequate water seal to act as a one-way valve and keep room air from entering the intrapleural space.)*
3. Attach the unit to the wall suction, and set suction to measure 20 cm on the suction control chamber gauge, or to the amount ordered; there should be mild continuous bubbling in the suction chamber. *(Suction is not always ordered. Too much suction pressure may damage the lung. Bubbling indicates that suction is working.)*
4. Tape all connections. *(Prevents accidental disconnection.)*
5. Ensure there are no kinks in the chest tube or connecting tubing. *(Kinks prevent proper function of the unit and allow pooling of fluid in the intrapleural space.)*
6. Lift the tubing and use gravity to drain any blood in the tubing frequently. *(Removing stagnant fluid maintains patency of tubing. The tube can be blocked by blood clots left in the tubing.)*
7. Do not milk or strip the tubing unless there is a medical order. If ordered and necessary, gently squeeze the tube between the thumb and forefinger. Use a gentle pulling motion with the other hand and then release it while gradually working your way down the tubing. *(Provides gentle, intermittent suction to the chest tube. Stripping can increase negative pressures within the chest cavity. It is not needed when suction is continuous to the tube and is not frequently ordered.)*
8. Mark and record the drainage output each shift. *(Measure drainage at eye level and place a mark on the drainage chamber. If drainage exceeds 100 mL/h, report to the primary care provider.)*
9. Help the patient deep breathe and cough and change positions at frequent intervals. *(Assists in re-expanding the lung.)*
10. Assess pain level and medicate as ordered when needed. *(The patient will deep breathe more effectively if kept comfortable. Chest tubes are uncomfortable.)*

chamber can be emptied. A Heimlich valve may be used in place of the chest drainage unit for a small, uncomplicated pneumothorax with little or no drainage and no need for suction. The Heimlich valve, a flutter valve, allows the escape of air but prevents reentry of air into the pleural space (Fig. 28.16). After surgery a drainage set for autotransfusion may be used so that the blood drained can be processed and returned to the patient.

Chest tubes are removed by the physician (and in some states, RNs with special training) when the lung has reinflated, as demonstrated by x-ray examination, and the pleural space has decreased. A suture set is used to take out the suture holding the chest tube in place. After the tube is pulled out, an occlusive dressing is applied. Studies confirm greater patient comfort with premedication with an analgesic before chest tube removal.

APPLICATION OF THE NURSING PROCESS

ASSESSMENT (DATA COLLECTION)

Basic respiratory assessment is covered in Chapter 22. Auscultate the lungs each shift along with assessment of other respiratory status parameters. Carefully document findings to allow other nurses to compare later data and detect subtle trends or deterioration. Respiratory assessment is intertwined with cardiac assessment because, if the heart is not functioning properly, oxygenated blood will not be delivered to the tissues in adequate amounts. Check equipment and settings of respiratory equipment at least once a shift.

Focused Assessment

Guidelines for Interviewing the Patient With a Respiratory Problem

Ask the following questions of any patient who has nursing diagnoses or medical diagnoses indicating a respiratory problem:

- When did the respiratory problem begin? Were you exposed to infection? What are the symptoms? Do you have shortness of breath?
- Do you have allergies? Sinusitis? Asthma? Emphysema? Chronic bronchitis? Exposure to dust or other irritants?
- Do you smoke? How many packs per day and for how many years? Have you had exposure to industrial air pollutants? Have you been exposed to tuberculosis?
- What type of cough do you have? When does it occur? Is it productive of sputum? What color is the sputum?
- When does shortness of breath occur? Is there wheezing?
- What measures ease your breathing or your cough? What medications are you taking?
- How much fluid are you drinking?
- Do you have any heart problems?

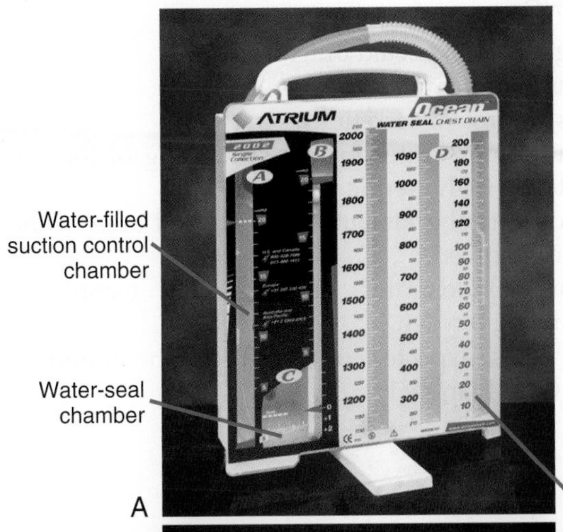

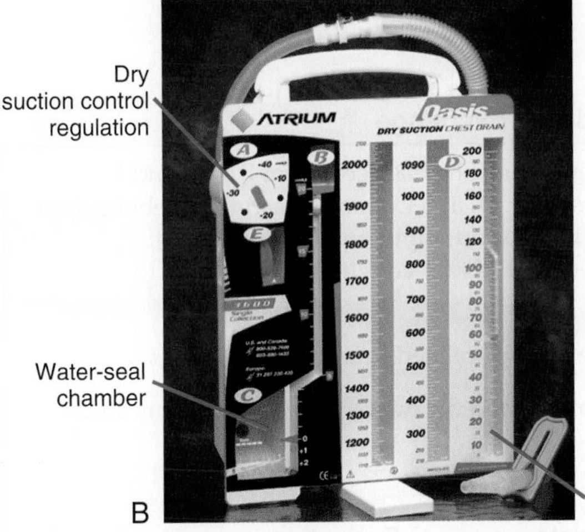

FIGURE 28.14 Disposable chest-drainage devices. (A) Suction chamber with a water-seal chamber and drainage chamber. (B) Dry suction with a self-compensating regulator and drainage chamber. (From Atrium Medical Corporation, Hudson, NH.)

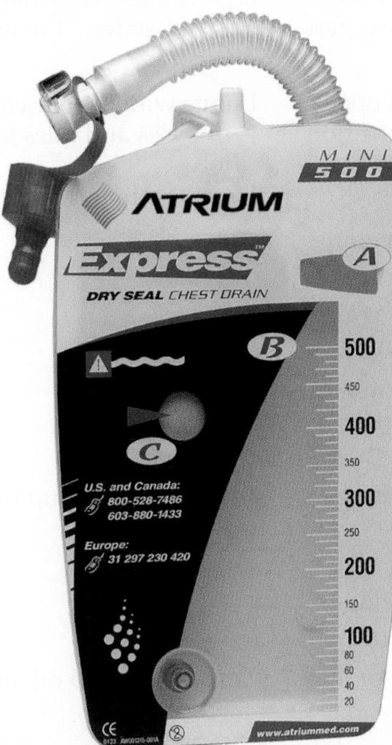

FIGURE 28.15 Small portable closed-chest drainage system allowing the patient mobility. (Courtesy Atrium Medical Corporation, Hudson, NH.)

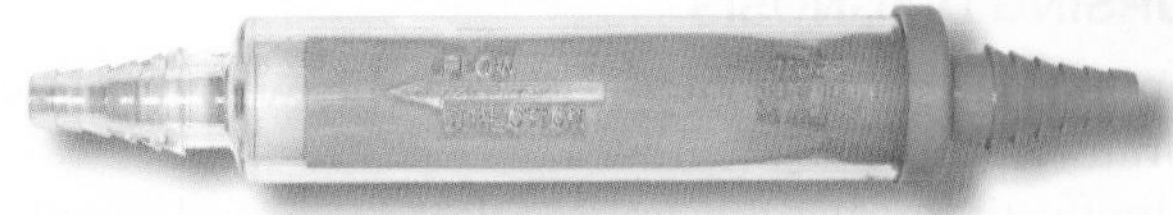

FIGURE 28.16 Heimlich chest-drain valve. (Courtesy and copyright Becton, Dickinson & Co., Franklin Lakes, NJ.)

Focused Assessment

Respiratory System

ASSESSMENT	RATIONALE
Assess respirations: rate, depth, and character.	Although the rate may be within normal limits, the patient may be breathing shallowly and not oxygenating well.
Auscultate the lungs to assess the patency of the airways.	Secretions may be present that interfere with gas exchange, or areas of the lung may not be inflating.
Assess for subtle signs of hypoxemia.	Restlessness, confusion, combativeness, decreased ability to concentrate, lethargy, and headache can all indicate that the patient is not obtaining enough oxygen. Slight hypoxia may be reversed with turning, coughing, and deep breathing.
Assess the mucous membranes and nail beds for signs of cyanosis.	Inside the mouth is the best place to assess for signs of cyanosis in dark-skinned people. Hypoxia may be discovered before the patient experiences respiratory failure.
Assess the character of the cough, if present.	A deep rattling cough indicates retained secretions, whereas a shallow, raspy cough may indicate throat irritation.
Assess the amount and character of sputum and times at which it is produced.	Sputum produced only in the morning may indicate sinus drainage rather than a problem in the lungs.
Assess the patient's ability to cough effectively.	Ineffective coughing will not clear secretions or open lower airways.
Assess for factors that restrict respiratory effort.	Fractured ribs, severe arthritis, and many diseases can cause restrictive respiratory disorders and thus compound the problems of a respiratory illness.

Think Critically

What is the best way to develop skill in detection of all types of breath sound abnormalities?

◆ NURSING DIAGNOSIS

Common nursing diagnoses for patients who have respiratory problems include:

- Ineffective airway clearance related to muscle weakness and impaired cough, decreased level of consciousness, or thick secretions.
- Impaired gas exchange related to retained respiratory secretions.
- Risk for infection related to alteration in airway (tracheostomy).
- Deficient knowledge related to use of oxygen equipment, tracheostomy, ventilator, or incentive spirometer.
- Risk for injury related to improper safety precautions when using oxygen.

◆ PLANNING

Sample goals or expected outcomes are:

- Patient demonstrates effective cough.
- Lungs are free of secretions.
- Patient demonstrates proper suctioning of the tracheostomy with aseptic technique.
- Area of left lobe **atelectasis** (collapsed area of the lung) is resolved.
- Patient demonstrates proper safety techniques when using oxygen.

More goals/expected outcomes can be found in Nursing Care Plan 28.1.

Nursing Care Plan 28.1 Care of the Patient with Impaired Gas Exchange

SCENARIO Susan Tamara, age 72, has been admitted with a bacterial pneumonia. She has been ill for 7 days and is weak because she lives alone and has not felt like preparing meals. Orders read: O_2 at 5 L/min per cannula; nebulization with albuterol q 4 h while awake; TC&DB, incentive spirometer q 2 h, up in chair tid; input and output (I & O); ofloxacin 400 mg intravenous piggyback (IVPB) q12 h; guaifenesin 30 mL q 4 h PRN for cough; increase fluids to 2400 mL/24 h.

PROBLEM/NURSING DIAGNOSIS *Severe chest congestion*/Impaired gas exchange related to secretions in lungs.

Supporting Assessment Data *Subjective:* Patient states, "I am short of breath and dizzy." *Objective:* Chest x-ray study reveals bilateral lower lobe pneumonia. Oxygen saturation 86%.

Goals/Expected Outcomes	Nursing Interventions	Selected Rationale	Evaluation
Oxygen saturation will reach 95% within 12 h.	Provide oxygen by nasal cannula at 5 L/min continuous.	Increases oxygen saturation of blood.	*Is oxygen saturation at 95%?* Oxygen saturation varies from 90% to 92%. Continue to monitor.
Patient will exhibit no SOB by discharge.	Place in semi-Fowler position except when sleeping.	Helps lungs expand more fully so that more oxygen can be absorbed.	*Is patient short of breath?* Yes, but states, "I'm less short of breath."
	Assist to TC&DB q 2 h; use incentive spirometer q 2 h.	Clears secretions and opens alveoli; changing position prevents pooling and stagnant secretions.	Lungs with decreased sounds in bases and rales in middle lobes. Expectorating secretions.
	Provide albuterol nebulizer treatment q 4 h while awake.	Albuterol assists in keeping airways open.	
	Administer ofloxacin 400 mg IVPB q 12 h.	Ofloxasin is effective against the bacterial pneumonia.	
	Monitor oxygen saturation via oximeter q 4 h.	Monitoring will alert nurse if oxygen saturation is dropping.	
	Sit patient up in chair tid for meals.	Sitting upright helps lungs expand completely.	Tolerating being up for meals.
	Auscultate lungs q shift.	Tells nurse whether condition is improving or deteriorating.	
	Encourage fluids at regular intervals to provide intake of 2400 mL/24 h.	Helps thin secretions so they can be coughed up.	Consumed 1875 mL on day shift.

Nursing Care Plan 28.1 Care of the Patient with Impaired Gas Exchange—cont'd

Goals/Expected Outcomes	Nursing Interventions	Selected Rationale	Evaluation
	Offer guaifenesin for cough as needed.	Guaifenesin helps thin secretions.	Gave guaifenesin × 2.
	Encourage to expectorate secretions in tissue and to discard tissue in plastic bag.	Secretions can spread bacteria from the lungs. Plastic bag contains the bacteria.	Expectorating secretions and containing tissues in bag.
	Offer mouth care q 4 h while awake.	Infected secretions have an unpleasant taste. Mouth care improves appetite.	Mouth care provided before meals and at bedtime.
	Inspect ears for pressure areas from cannula q 4 h.	Oxygen cannula may cause pressure areas on ears.	No signs of skin breakdown. Continue with current plan of care. Goal partially met.

CRITICAL THINKING QUESTIONS

1. What is the physiologic reason that increasing fluids will help this pneumonia patient?
2. The patient is weak. Although this care plan only deals with the respiratory problems discussed in this chapter, what other nursing actions do you think would help the patient conserve energy and oxygen?

Other planning involves fitting in time for appropriate care of the respiratory patient in the daily work plan. **Each patient with a respiratory problem or the potential for one should turn, cough, and deep breathe (TC&DB) every 2 hours.** Note the times for this to be done on the shift work organization sheet. Procedures such as postural drainage or tracheostomy care take time, and should be scheduled. If a patient has copious secretions that need frequent suctioning, plan time for this activity. Ensure that necessary supplies for respiratory care are at the bedside.

◆ IMPLEMENTATION

The nurse has an active role in helping the patient perform respiratory exercises, teaching respiratory care, maintaining patient safety, and offering encouragement. Your attention to respiratory care for every patient can prevent complications and nosocomial infection and assist in recovery.

First and foremost, maintain an open airway. Remove secretions by encouraging effective coughing, turning, and deep breathing. Splinting an incision with a small pillow and sitting on the side of the bed allows for a more effective cough (Fig. 28.17). Encourage fluid intake of 1500 to 2000 mL/day to help thin secretions. Use suction to remove secretions and mucus when the patient is unable to cough them out. Be alert to wet, gurgling respirations in the unconscious patient and suction aseptically. For the unconscious or comatose patient, use an oral airway or nasal trumpet airway to keep the tongue from falling back into the throat and obstructing the airway. If the patient cannot breathe deeply enough to maintain adequate oxygenation, a manual resuscitator bag can be used to increase oxygenation (Fig. 28.18). Use proper positioning; turn the patient frequently. Yawns and sighs are two forms of deep breaths that help expand the alveoli in the lung. A yawn is a deep, long inspiration usually because of mental or physical fatigue; a sigh is a prolonged

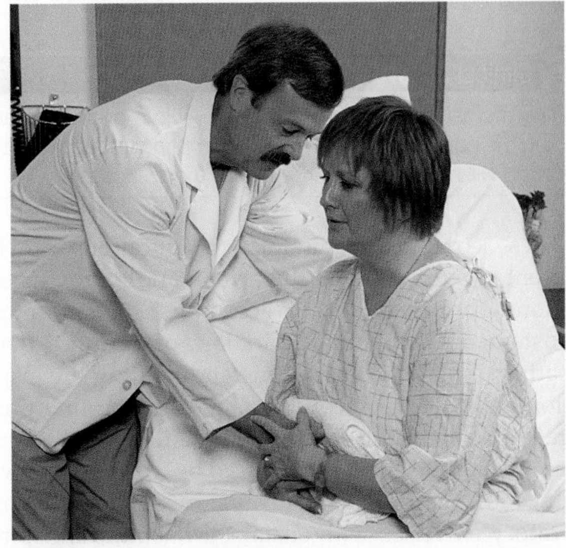

FIGURE 28.17 Teaching the patient to splint an incision while coughing.

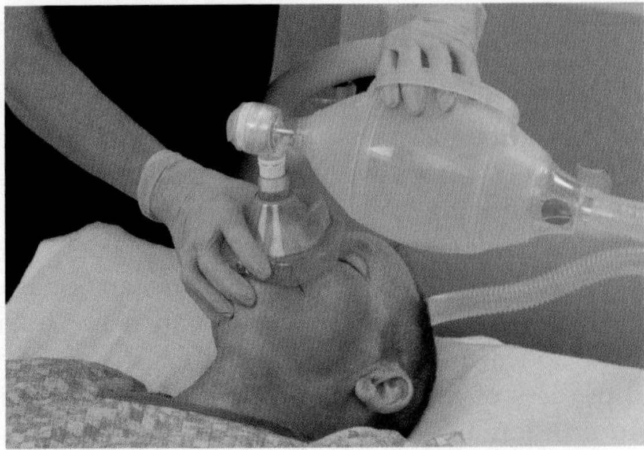

FIGURE 28.18 Use of a manual resuscitator bag.

inspiration followed by a long expiration. Encourage the use of an incentive spirometer to open alveoli and prevent or relieve atelectasis.

Clinical Cues

Restlessness and irritability may be the first signs of hypoxia. In the older adult, confusion often is seen as oxygen levels fall. Observe patients with respiratory problems closely for these early symptoms.

Patients who have undergone abdominal or chest surgery may avoid using muscles in the affected areas because deep breathing and coughing can cause pain. However, these muscles are necessary to take deep breaths or to cough effectively to remove accumulated secretions. Be certain to medicate your postoperative patients adequately for pain, so deep breathing and coughing are more comfortable. Hypoxia, pneumonitis, and atelectasis are risks of inadequate ventilation that can prolong hospitalization. In atelectasis, the alveoli collapse and fail to fill with air. The condition may be acute or chronic and involve a part or the entire lung.

Clinical Cues

Making a small "pillow" with a large towel in a pillowcase and helping the patient splint well when attempting to deep breathe or cough will make the patient's efforts more successful.

These common respiratory complications can be prevented by reinflating the alveoli and removing secretions. The best method to accomplish this is through a sustained maximum inspiration, or taking a deep breath to inflate the entire lung and holding the inspiration for at least 3 seconds so that the resulting pressure will keep the alveoli from immediately collapsing again. The same effect is produced by a sigh or a yawn.

Incentive spirometers encourage patients to do respiratory exercises with sustained maximum inspiration (Fig. 28.19). When the patient takes a deep breath, a ball moves upward, or the amount of air is measured so the results are visible to the user. The incentive is to reach a certain volume of air and hold it for 3 seconds. Patients at risk of developing respiratory complications should be instructed to use the device and take 10 slow, deep breaths every hour when awake.

Use positioning and relaxation techniques to optimize respiratory exchange. Additional energy and oxygen are needed when patients are anxious and have tense, rigid muscles. Nurses can help patients with dyspnea to relax, expand the chest more fully, and use less of their limited oxygen supply by using good positioning. Place bed patients with dyspnea in proper alignment and in high Fowler position unless otherwise contraindicated. Place the patient's forearms on pillows at the sides to relax the shoulder muscles. Patients with obstructive diseases such as emphysema breathe easier when they sit at the side of the bed or in a chair, hunch the upper body over, and rest their arms on two or three pillows placed on a table or nightstand in front of them (orthopneic position, Fig. 28.20). Turning to one side helps prevent the pooling of secretions in the back of the throat of unconscious, weak, or helpless patients. Assist with postural drainage to promote the removal of secretions from the lungs.

When administering oxygen therapy, give the amount as ordered by the primary care provider. When oxygen is in use, perform oral hygiene every 3 to 4 hours because oxygen therapy is drying to the tissues,

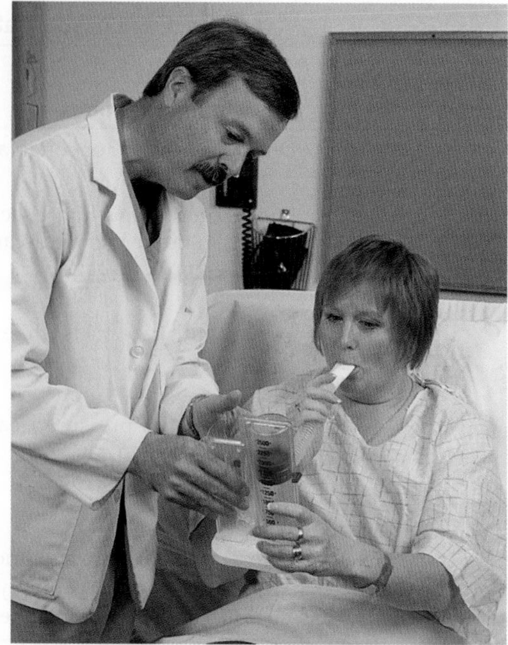

FIGURE 28.19 Teaching use of the incentive spirometer.

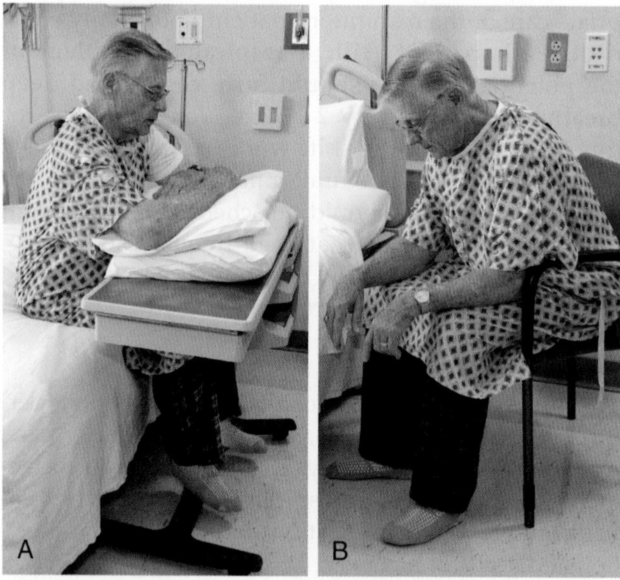

FIGURE 28.20 Position the person who is very short of breath in the orthopneic position, using pillows on the over-the-bed table and in a chair. (From Ignatavicius, D. & Workman, M. [2013]. *Medical-Surgical Nursing: Patient-Centered Collaborative Care* [7th ed.]. St. Louis: W.B. Saunders Company)

which often makes the mouth smell or taste unpleasant. Inspect the skin around the nose and mouth for irritation from the equipment. Prevent infection by changing oxygen delivery equipment per agency policy. Take temperature measurements tympanically, over the temporal artery, or rectally, so that the patient's breathing is not impaired by an oral thermometer.

Monitor the activity of the patient with a respiratory problem. Activity may produce SOB, dizziness, or complaints of chest pain because activity uses up oxygen more quickly than the body at rest does. Space activities and provide sufficient rest periods between activities of daily living and exercise. For the patient who is on PRN oxygen, do not discontinue the oxygen and then immediately ask the patient to get up and move to the chair or go to the bathroom. Allow time for the patient to adjust to room air before activity is increased.

QSEN Considerations: Safety

Oxygen Safety

Observe safety measures to prevent explosion or fire.

Tracheostomy Care

When a patient has either a temporary or a permanent tracheostomy, daily care is needed. Care consists of suctioning and cleaning the skin around the stoma, changing the dressing, cleaning the inner cannula if there is one, and replacing the ties that hold the tube in place when soiled. Tracheostomy care (Skill 28.7) is done every 8 hours or as frequently as needed to keep

Skill 28.7 Providing Tracheostomy Care

 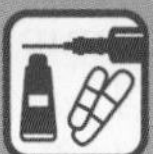 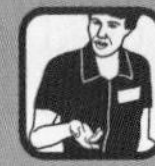 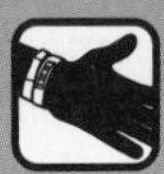 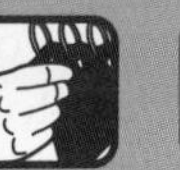 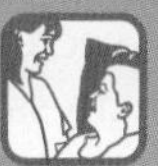  

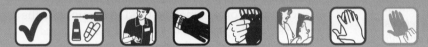

Tracheostomy care is performed every 8 hours. The tracheostomy patient is taught to do this procedure before being sent home with a new tracheostomy. The soiled dressing is removed; the area around the stoma is cleaned; and, if needed, the tape or ties holding the tracheostomy tube in place are changed. If there is an inner cannula, it is removed, cleaned, and replaced.

SUPPLIES

- Normal saline
- Forceps
- Sterile gloves
- Hydrogen peroxide
- Precut tracheostomy dressing
- Brush or pipe cleaners
- Tracheostomy tape or tube fastener
- Scissors
- Sterile 4 × 4 gauze pad
- Cotton swabs
- Solution containers (2)
- Discard bag

Review and carry out the Standard Steps in Appendix A.

ACTION *(RATIONALE)*

Assessment (Data Collection)

1. Suction as needed before beginning the procedure. *(Clears airway. Movement of the tracheostomy tube during cleaning and care may make patient cough, loosening secretions that could block the airway.)*

Planning

2. Set up the equipment on a table close to the patient and plan the order in which to perform the tasks. *(Planning makes work more efficient.)*

Implementation

3. Place patient in the supine position. Perform hand hygiene, open the supplies, and put on one glove. Separate basins with the gloved hand; pour solutions with the ungloved hand. Use one part hydrogen peroxide to one part normal saline for the wash solution; use normal saline to rinse. *(Positioning makes visualization of tracheostomy site clear; opening supplies prepares them for use. Gloves prevent transfer of microorganisms. Some plastic cannulas are harmed by hydrogen peroxide; check manufacturer's instructions.)*
4. Put on the second glove. Undo the lock on the outer cannula, stabilizing the tube flange with the index finger and thumb, and remove inner cannula by gently pulling it out toward you. *(Latch must be unlocked to remove inner cannula. If the tube moves, patient will cough. If difficulty is encountered, obtain assistance.)*
5. Place the reusable inner cannula in the basin of wash solution and clean the lumen thoroughly with pipe cleaners or a small brush. Cleanse the outer surface with the brush. Rinse in the basin of normal saline or sterile water. Place on 4 × 4 gauze

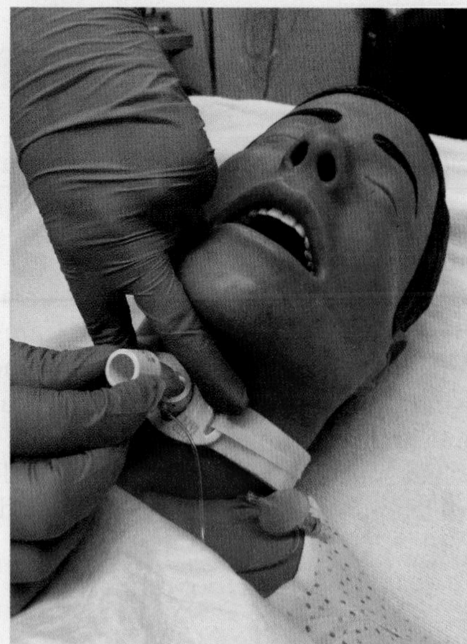

Step 4

pad to drain. Handle silver cannulas carefully because they dent easily. *(Pushing the pipe cleaner all the way through the cannula removes secretions. Some patients have a second inner cannula available to place into the tracheostomy tube while the one removed is cleaned. In that case, store the removed cannula after cleaning.)*

6. Reinsert the cannula after excessive moisture has been removed. Hold the faceplate of the outer tube securely and, using aseptic technique, insert the inner cannula into the lumen of the outer cannula. Lock in place by turning the latch on the outer cannula one-quarter turn counterclockwise. Check to see that it is properly latched. Many hospitals use disposable inner cannulas that eliminate the need for cleaning. *(Excessive moisture may make the patient cough as the cannula is replaced. Cannula must be firmly locked into place so that it is not coughed out.)*
7. Remove the soiled dressing and dispose of it in the discard bag. Clean around the tube with saline (Nance-Floyd, 2011). Move the tube as little as possible during the cleaning process. *(Soiled tracheostomy dressings are changed as needed. The area around the tube is cleaned every 8 hours or per agency protocol. Moving the tube causes irritation to the trachea and is uncomfortable for the patient.)*
8. Replace soiled tracheostomy ties or tube holder. Ask an assistant to help if possible. Punch a hole in the end of the tie with the closed points of the forceps, pass the end through the flange on the side of the tracheostomy tube, and thread the tie through the hole, pulling it taut. Remove the old tie. Repeat for the other side, and tie the tapes at the side of the neck with a double square knot so that the patient need not lie on the knot. The knot should be rotated from one side of the neck to the other with each change. Commercial tracheostomy tube holders may be used in place of tracheostomy tape ties. *(Ties are replaced when soiled or at least once every 24 hours. Ties are easier to replace if done before the new dressing is applied.)*

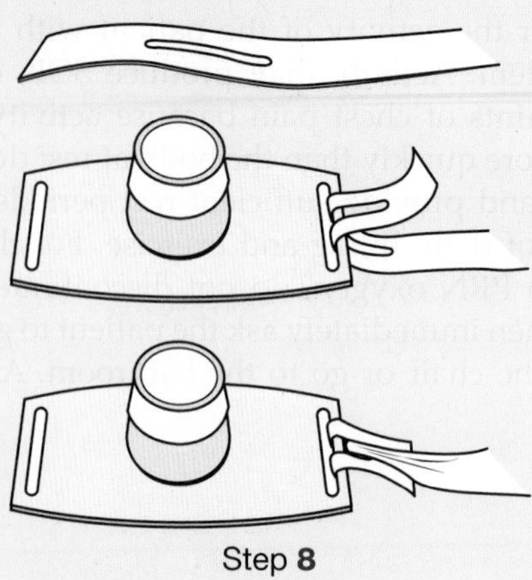

Step 8

9. Apply precut dressing or a V-folded gauze. Place it under and around the outer cannula to catch secretions. Forceps may be used to manipulate the dressing into place. *(Do not cut a 4 × 4 gauze pad to use as a tracheostomy dressing because the loose gauze may fall into the tracheostomy tube and be aspirated by the patient.)*

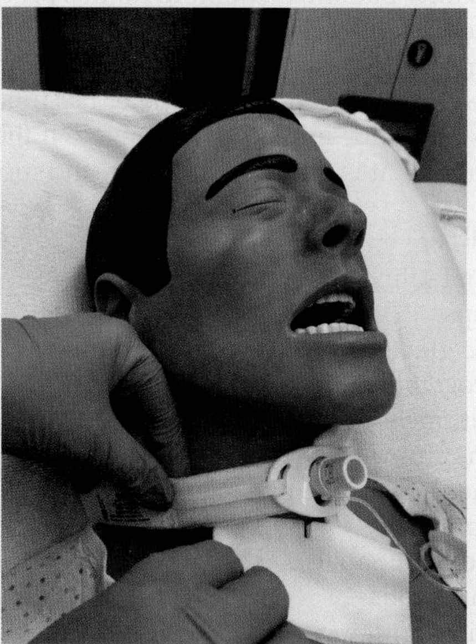

Step 9A

Evaluation

10. Ask yourself: Did the procedure go smoothly? Was the tube moved too much, making the patient cough excessively? Are the ties smooth? Is the dressing sitting properly in place? *(Answers to these questions determine whether the procedure was done properly and efficiently.)*

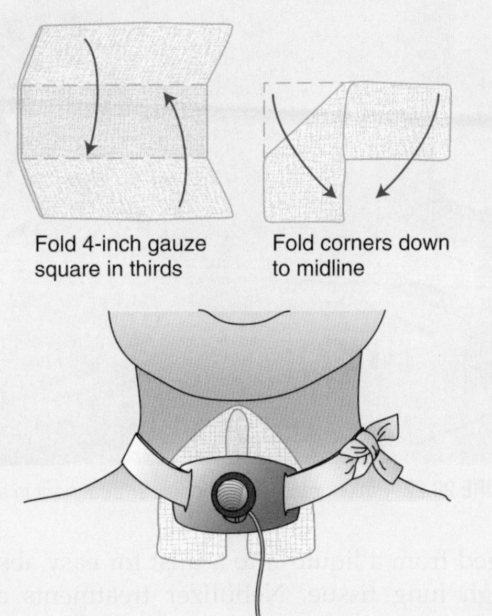
Fold 4-inch gauze square in thirds
Fold corners down to midline

Step 9B (Redrawn from Black, J. M., & Matassarin-Jacobs, E. [1993]. *Luckmann and Sorensen's Medical-Surgical Nursing: A Psychopathologic Approach* [4th ed.]. Philadelphia: Saunders.)

Documentation

11. Documentation may be in narrative form or on a flow sheet. Note the care given and the condition of the tracheostomy site. *(Notes that this nursing care was administered.)*

Documentation Example

10/25 1045 Tracheostomy care given with aseptic technique; reddening 1.5-cm diameter around tube, no complaints of discomfort. Inner cannula cleaned and replaced. (Nurse's electronic signature)

Special Considerations

- With a permanent tracheostomy, patient education should include all steps of tracheostomy care and suctioning. Proceed by explaining the rationale for a step and then demonstrate the step. Teach only a few steps at a time. Have patient demonstrate the procedure with coaching. Obtain a return demonstration of the entire procedure before patient is discharged.
- Assess for skin breakdown each time you provide tracheostomy tube care.

Critical Thinking Questions

1. What could happen if you do not perform oral suction before deflating an inflatable tracheostomy cuff?
2. Why is it best to prepare the tracheostomy tube ties by cutting a slit in each tie before beginning tracheostomy care?

the secretions from becoming dried, blocking the airway (Fig. 28.21).

A tracheostomy tube is a curved, hollow cannula made of plastic or metal. Some have an inner and an outer cannula so that the inner one can be removed for cleaning while the outer one stays in place. All tracheostomy tubes come with a piece called an **obturator,** a curved guide that facilitates tube placement when it is inserted; after insertion of the tube, the obturator is removed. An extra tube and obturator are often taped to the head of the bed so that they are handy should the tracheostomy tube somehow be dislodged and need to be replaced in an emergency.

Because the tracheostomy tube sits below the larynx, the patient cannot speak naturally. Provide for communication with paper and pencil, magic slate, communication board, or other device.

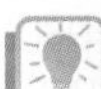 QSEN Considerations: Safety

Call Bell

It is vitally important for this patient to have the call bell at hand at all times.

It is frightening not to be able to call for help should it be needed. Check on the patient frequently.

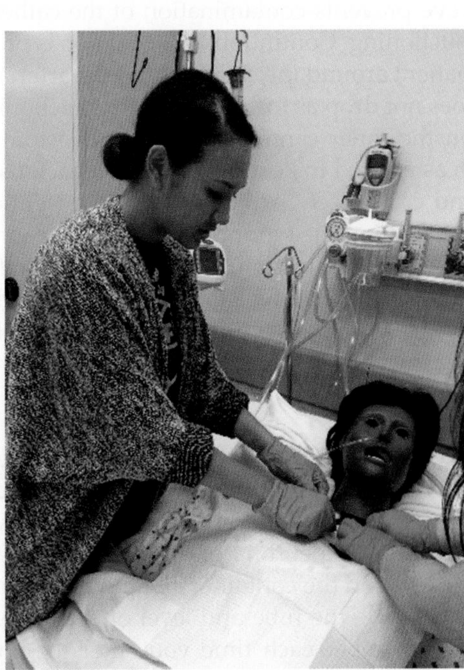

FIGURE 28.21 Nursing student practicing tracheostomy care in the college skills lab.

Assignment Considerations

The Intubated Patient

Remind the UAPs to ensure the call bell is within reach whenever they reposition an intubated patient. The patient with an endotracheal or tracheostomy tube cannot call out for help.

Suctioning secretions after a tracheostomy is performed is of prime importance in maintaining airway patency. Patients with tracheostomies cannot cough effectively. Before suctioning, observe the patient's rate and quality of respiration and auscultate lung sounds. Frequency of needed suctioning varies; in the new tracheostomy patient, it may be needed as frequently as every 15 to 30 minutes. Older tracheostomies have less inflammation and therefore less secretion production and need to be suctioned only periodically. **Suctioning is carried out only as needed, and need is indicated by audible respirations or dyspnea** (see Skill 28.6).

Use strict aseptic technique and use separate catheters and solution when both the nasopharyngeal area and the trachea are suctioned. Suctioning should be no longer than 10 seconds in length. Preoxygenate the patient well before performing tracheal suctioning because hypoxemia produced by prolonged suctioning can lead to sudden death. You may reuse sleeved or in-line catheters several times for tracheobronchial or endotracheal suctioning. These catheters have an outside plastic sleeve covering that slides up to allow the catheter to be introduced into the trachea for suctioning, which then slides over the catheter as it is withdrawn. The sleeve prevents contamination of the catheter between suctioning. Continuous oxygenation is provided to the patient around the catheter, and the arterial PaO_2 level does not drop as low as with other suctioning.

Clean the inner cannula of the tracheostomy tube as often as needed to keep it free from tenacious secretions and crusts (see Skill 28.7). Employ aseptic technique in cleaning the wound and the inner cannula to reduce the risk of infection. Work calmly and efficiently. Remember that having a tracheostomy is a traumatic experience. **Always suction the nasopharynx before deflating the cuff.**

Chest Tube Care

When the patient has a chest tube, auscultate the lungs frequently to assess re-expansion of the involved lung. Accurately measure the amount of drainage every 1, 2, 4, or 8 hours, depending on the situation; mark the drainage level on the container along with the time recorded. Observe the tube and level of drainage in the collection chamber each time you enter the patient's room (see Steps 28.1). Immediately report drainage of more than 100 mL/h.

Nebulizer Treatments

If the patient is having difficulty bringing up mucous secretions trapped in the lung, a nebulizer treatment may be ordered. With nebulization, medication is changed from a liquid into a mist for easy absorption through lung tissue. Nebulizer treatments are also used to deliver bronchodilators to the lung to relieve bronchospasm. Nurses often give these treatments in clinics and medical offices (Fig. 28.22).

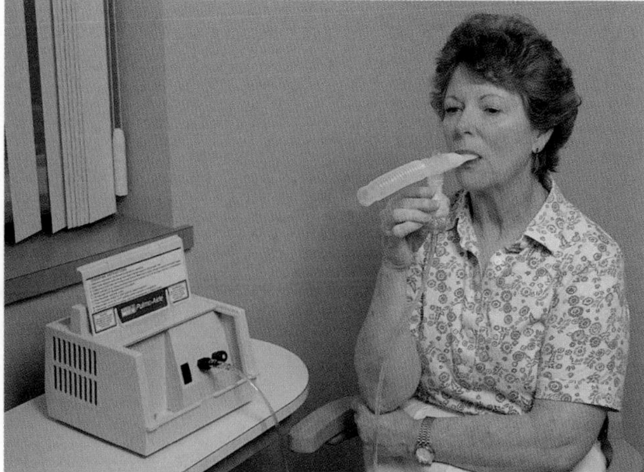

FIGURE 28.22 Patient receiving a nebulizer treatment in a clinic.

Patient Education

Because many respiratory patients have chronic problems, patient education for self-care is important for them to achieve independence. Teach the patient with a permanent tracheostomy to suction properly in an aseptic manner and to care for the tube, the stoma, and the skin. Teach all patients to deep breathe and cough effectively.

 **Home Care Considerations**

Preventing Respiratory Tract Infection

Remind respiratory patients to:

- Avoid places where they will be exposed to flu or respiratory tract infections. Crowded theaters, shopping malls, and other places where people sit close together place the person with compromised respiration at risk.
- Sit a good distance away from anyone who is coughing or sneezing.

Teach home care patients to reduce air pollutants in the home and to avoid them elsewhere as much as possible.

 **QSEN Considerations: Safety**

Memory Jogger

Teach safety measures to the patient and family regarding oxygen use. Explain ways to conserve energy to promote independence. Educate patients and family on suctioning techniques.

 **Home Care Considerations**

Suctioning at Home

- In the home care situation, teach the caregiver and family members how to suction the patient using aseptic technique. Instruct them in signs that indicate suctioning is needed.

- Some patients can learn to suction themselves, but the procedure is uncomfortable and many cannot clear secretions adequately.
- After a suctioning session, if secretions still are not totally cleared, wait approximately 10 minutes to allow the patient to become fully oxygenated before resuming suctioning.
- Note the date and time on the covered catheter container so that the catheter will be changed on schedule after 8 hours.

In the home, teach the patient and the caregiver to clean suction equipment with hydrogen peroxide, gentle soap and water, or a household bleach solution, depending on the type of equipment; rinse it with sterile water; and store it in a clean container until the next use.

◆ EVALUATION

It is vitally important to evaluate the patient's respiratory status continually when the patient is suffering from a respiratory disorder. Evaluate the lungs at least once a shift. Evaluate the success of respiratory treatments and medications each day. Sample evaluation statements are:

- Effectively coughing up secretions.
- PaO_2 increased to 88 mm Hg.
- $PaCO_2$ decreased to 38 mm Hg.
- Patient able to ambulate length of hall without SOB.
- Lungs clear, no sign of respiratory infection.
- Patient turns off oxygen when not using it.
- Atelectasis cleared as evidenced by x-ray.

Documentation

Documentation should include:

- Data from the respiratory assessment
- Oxygen flow rate and method of delivery
- Amount of time PRN oxygen is used
- Time and location of the blood gas sampling
- Location of the oximetry probe and range of oxygen saturation
- Description of the sputum expectorated
- Times the patient deep breathes and coughs
- Time and result of any respiratory treatments

Constantly evaluate suction technique, considering ways to improve in delivering respiratory care. It takes considerable practice to suction efficiently.

Get Ready for the NCLEX Examination!

Key Points

- Respiratory insufficiency is the body's inability to meet its oxygen needs and remove excess amounts of carbon dioxide.
- Airway obstruction is a frequent cause of hypoxia.
- One of the first signs of hypoxia is irritability or restlessness.
- Hypoxia depresses body functions, disturbs the body's acid-base balance, and makes patients susceptible to respiratory tract infections.
- Pulse oximetry is used for continuous, noninvasive monitoring of arterial oxygen saturation.
- Abdominal thrusts are used to dislodge an airway obstruction when the patient suddenly cannot breathe. If the obstruction is not relieved, anoxia occurs, and the heart may stop, necessitating CPR.
- Teach patients to cough effectively; forced exhalation coughing helps bring up secretions.
- Perform postural drainage to drain different segments of the lung.
- Perform nasopharyngeal suctioning aseptically; tracheobronchial (and tracheostomy) suctioning is a sterile procedure.
- Oxygen may be administered by mask, cannula, tent, catheter, Croupette, or ventilator.
- High concentrations of oxygen can cause fires to burn rapidly.
- When a patient cannot maintain respiration in a normal manner, a tracheostomy may be performed to provide an artificial airway.
- A chest drainage tube may be placed in the intrapleural space when the patient has a pneumothorax, hemothorax, or hemopneumothorax. A chest tube may drain air or fluid.
- Every respiratory patient should TC&DB every 2 hours.
- Incentive spirometry assists in regaining or maintaining open airways.
- The patient with chronic obstructive pulmonary disease (COPD), also termed *chronic airflow limitation,* should not be given oxygen at more than 3 L/min because it may depress the respiratory drive.
- All respiratory patients should avoid people with respiratory tract infection and avoid areas where air pollutants occur.
- Evaluation is based on assessment findings, pulse oximetry, and arterial blood gas measurements.

Additional Learning Resources

SG Go to your Study Guide for additional learning activities to help you master this chapter content.

evolve Go to your Evolve website at http://evolve.elsevier.com/Williams/fundamental for additional online resources.

Review Questions for the NCLEX Examination

*Choose the **best** answer for each question.*

1. You observe an older adult patient with pneumonia for early signs of hypoxia. You know that the first signs of hypoxia include: *(Select all that apply.)*
   1. Increasing restlessness or irritability.
   2. Increased respiratory rate.
   3. Cyanosis of the nail beds of the fingers.
   4. Retraction of muscles used in breathing.
   5. Cyanosis around the lips.

2. In providing nursing care for a patient who has undergone a thoracotomy, has a chest tube, and has pain and dyspnea, it is important to reduce her anxiety because it:
   1. Increases the pulse and blood pressure.
   2. Causes tense muscles, which need more oxygen.
   3. Causes needless fear and worry.
   4. Delays recovery and healing of injured tissues.
3. Your patient has undergone a thoracotomy with resection of the right lung. She is receiving oxygen by cannula at 5 L/min and has a chest tube in place attached to a disposable chest drainage system with suction. There is continuous bubbling in the suction chamber of the disposable water-seal chest drainage unit, with 120 mL of drainage in the last hour. What should you do?
   1. Document the drainage and continue to monitor the patient.
   2. Check the suction tubing for air leaks.
   3. Check your patient's vital signs.
   4. Call the primary care provider.
4. When performing nasopharyngeal suctioning, you should: *(Select all that apply.)*
   1. Raise the head of the bed 30 to 45 degrees.
   2. Set suction at 100 mm Hg.
   3. Deflate the cuff before deciding to do nasopharyngeal suctioning.
   4. Moisten the catheter before attempting suctioning.
5. When administering oxygen by nasal cannula, it is important to: *(Select all that apply.)*
   1. Monitor the patient's PaO_2 and $PaCO_2$ levels in the blood.
   2. Increase the flow rate when the patient becomes short of breath.
   3. Decrease the flow rate, per order, when oxygen levels are in normal range.
   4. Verify the care provider's orders and recognize oxygen as a drug treatment.
   5. Educate the patient about the need for oxygen and when to use it.
6. A nurse finds a patient who is unresponsive and calls for help. The patient is not breathing and does not have a pulse. The nurse begins CPR with 30 chest compressions and attempts to ventilate. The chest does not rise. The head is re-tilted and another attempt to ventilate is unsuccessful. What does the nurse do next?
   1. Performs abdominal thrusts
   2. Continues CPR with chest compression
   3. Re-tilts the head and attempts to ventilate again
   4. Performs a blind finger sweep
7. Older adults are more prone to respiratory problems because aging causes which change? *(Select all that apply.)*
   1. Thinning of the alveolar membrane
   2. Decreased elasticity of respiratory tissues
   3. Increased secretion production
   4. Decreased efficiency of the immune system

Critical Thinking Activities

Read each clinical scenario and discuss the questions with your classmates.

Scenario A

Clara Johnson has had upper abdominal surgery. She is reluctant to deep breathe or cough.

1. How would you explain to her the importance of deep breathing and coughing after this surgery?
2. What could you do to make deep breathing and coughing less painful?
3. Being very specific, how would you teach her to use an incentive spirometer?

Scenario B

Paul Suarez has a new tracheostomy. He is receiving oxygen by tracheostomy collar (a device placed over the tracheostomy tube to deliver oxygen).

1. Describe the steps you would use to suction Mr. Suarez's tracheostomy.
2. Because Mr. Suarez cannot speak, how would you communicate with him? He is very weak and has difficulty writing.
3. Create a plan for patient education of Mr. Suarez on how to care for his tracheostomy at home.

chapter 29

Promoting Urinary Elimination

http://evolve.elsevier.com/Williams/fundamental

Objectives

Upon completing this chapter, you should be able to do the following:

Theory

1. Review the structure and functions of the urinary system.
2. Determine abnormal appearance of a urine specimen.
3. Describe three nursing measures to help patients urinate normally.
4. Compare and contrast the purposes and principles of indwelling and intermittent catheterization.
5. Summarize the rationale for using a continuous bladder irrigation system.
6. Analyze different methods of managing urinary incontinence.

Clinical Practice

1. Assess a patient's urinary status.
2. Perform a urine dipstick test accurately.
3. Teach a patient how to obtain a "clean-catch" (midstream) specimen.
4. Assist patients with toileting.
5. Insert an indwelling catheter using sterile technique.
6. Perform catheter care.
7. Teach a patient how to perform Kegel exercises.

Skills & Steps

Key Terms

anuria (ă-NŪ-rē-ă, p. 543)
catheterization (kă-thĕ-tĕr-ĭ-ZĀ-shŭn, p. 553)
commode chair (kō-MŌD, p. 548)
condom catheter (KŎN-dŏm KĂ-thĕ-tĕr, p. 554)
Credé maneuver (krā-DĀ mă-NŪ-vĕr, p. 553)
cystitis (sĭs-TĪ-tĭs, p. 544)
dysuria (dĭs-Ū-rē-ă, p. 544)
glycosuria (glī-kōs-Ū-rē-ă, p. 545)
hematuria (hĕm-ă-TŪ-rē-ă, p. 545)
instillation (p. 544)
ketonuria (kē-tō-NŪ-rē-ă, p. 545)
micturition (mĭk-tū-RĬSH-ŭn, p. 543)
nocturia (nŏk-TŪ-rē-ă, p. 543)
oliguria (ŏl-ĭ-GŪ-rē-ă, p. 544)
polyuria (pŏl-ē-Ū-rē-ă, p. 544)
proteinuria (prō-tēn-YŪR-ē-ă, p. 545)
pyuria (pī-Ū-rē-ă, p. 545)
residual urine (rĕ-ZĬ-dū-ăl Ū-rĭn, p. 543)
stricture (STRĬK-chŭr, p. 553)
suprapubic (SŪ-pră-PYŪ-bĭk, p. 553)
urinary incontinence (ĭn-KŎN-tĭ-nĕns, p. 543)
urinary retention (rē-TĔN-shŭn, p. 543)
urination (ūr-ĭ-NĀ-shŭn, p. 542)
urinometer (yūr-ĭ-NŎ-mĕ-tĕr, p. 544)
urostomy (yūr-Ŏ-stō-mē, p. 569)
void (VŎYD, p. 543)

Concepts Covered in This Chapter

- Acid-base balance
- Anxiety
- Communication
- Culture
- Elimination
- Evidence
- Infection
- Inflammation
- Mobility
- Pain
- Patient education
- Perfusion
- Safety
- Stress

OVERVIEW OF STRUCTURE AND FUNCTION OF THE URINARY SYSTEM

WHICH STRUCTURES ARE INVOLVED IN URINARY ELIMINATION?

- The kidneys are bean shaped, approximately 2½ inches wide, 5 inches long, and 1 inch thick (6 × 12 × 3 cm^3), and are located at the level of L1 on each side of the spine (Fig. 29.1).
- Each kidney contains approximately 1 million nephrons, which are the working units.
- Within each nephron is a glomerulus consisting of a cluster of capillaries, surrounded by Bowman capsule, and a system of tubules.
- The ureters are hollow tubes about 10 to 12 inches (25 to 30 cm) long in the adult, and they connect each kidney to the bladder.
- The bladder is a hollow, muscular organ located in the lower pelvis.
- The urethra is a tube attached to the base of the bladder extending to the outside of the body. In the male, it is about 8 inches (20 cm) long and goes through the penis, ending at its tip. This exit point is the urinary meatus (Fig. 29.2). In the female, the urethra is from 1½ to 2½ inches (4 to 6.5 cm) in length, and it goes to the urinary meatus located beneath the clitoris, between the folds of the labia.
- The internal and external urinary sphincters control the flow of urine out of the body.

WHAT ARE THE FUNCTIONS OF THE URINARY STRUCTURES FOR ELIMINATION?

- The kidneys filter blood through the nephrons, and metabolic waste and excess water are extracted. The kidneys regulate electrolytes in the body by excreting excess amounts, and assist in acid-base balance by retaining or excreting hydrogen ions (H^+) and bicarbonate ions (HCO_3-). The waste products are diluted with water and excreted as urine. The tubules secrete, excrete, or reabsorb electrolytes, water, and other substances.

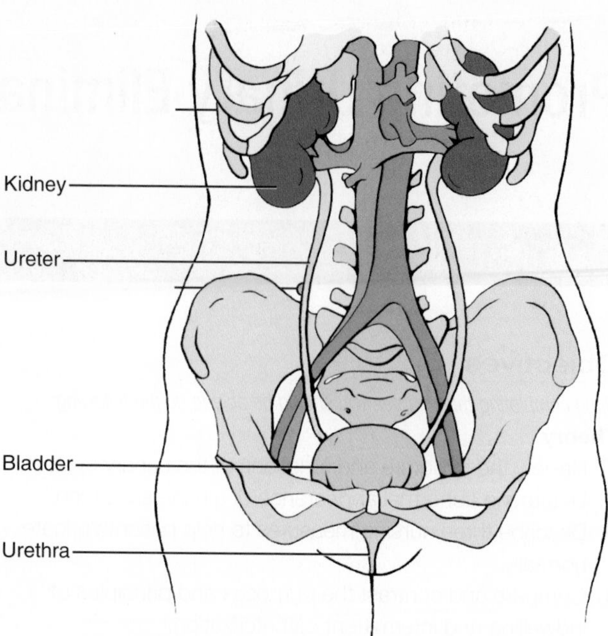

FIGURE 29.1 Structures of the urinary system.

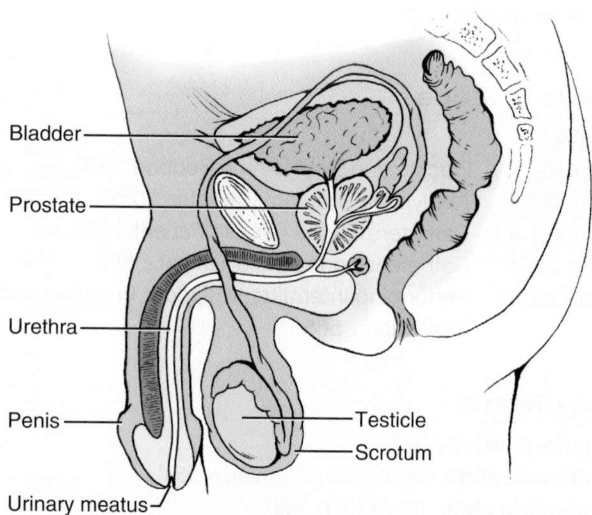

FIGURE 29.2 Tract of the male urethra.

- The kidneys manufacture 1 to 1.5 L of urine on average in 24 hours. Urine output is related to the amount of fluid intake and it can vary considerably.
- The ureters carry urine from the kidneys to the bladder.
- The bladder stores urine and sends a signal to the spinal cord when it becomes full to signal the need for emptying. The signal usually occurs when the bladder contains between 250 and 400 mL of urine.
- The bladder can hold 1000 to 1800 mL of urine. **Average urine output is 1000 to 1500 mL/day.**
- The urethra carries urine from the bladder to the outside of the body.
- The urinary meatus is the exit point for **urination** (expelling urine) and the entrance point for a catheter.

- The internal sphincter relaxes in response to the **micturition** (urination) reflex.
- Voluntary contraction of the external sphincter stops the expulsion of urine. Relaxing the external sphincter starts the flow of urine for excretion.

WHAT FACTORS CAN INTERFERE WITH URINARY ELIMINATION?

- Total loss of the kidney's ability to manufacture urine (kidney failure) may result in **anuria** (absence of urine).
- Decreased kidney perfusion (e.g., from shock or severe dehydration) can lead to kidney damage.
- Blockage of the ureters prevents the urine from traveling to the bladder. Blockage may occur because of the presence of a stone in the ureter, pressure from a tumor in the abdominal cavity, or trauma to the lower abdomen.
- Disruption of the bladder by tumor or trauma may impede the flow of urine out of the bladder or decrease its holding capacity.
- Pressure on the urethra from an enlarged prostate can make emptying the bladder difficult. Trauma to the urethra from any cause can impede the elimination of urine. Childbirth sometimes alters the position of the bladder and urethra and predisposes the woman to incidences of **urinary incontinence** (inability to prevent passing urine).
- Infection in any part of the urinary system causes inflammation and may alter the flow of urine.
- Neurologic damage to the nerves that control the internal and external sphincters or the muscular wall of the bladder may cause alteration in urinary patterns.
- Prostate surgery may damage the external urinary sphincter and cause temporary or permanent urinary incontinence in the male.

WHAT CHANGES IN THE SYSTEM OCCUR WITH AGING?

- There is a decrease in the number of functioning nephrons and a reduction in the rate of renal filtration with aging. Because of these changes, even minor body stress can cause a decrease in renal function.
- The bladder muscle tone decreases, and its capacity lessens, causing **nocturia** (urinating during the night). Decreased muscle tone may interfere with the external urinary sphincter and predispose the person to incontinence. **Incontinence is not a normal part of aging.**
- Decreased bladder and muscle tone may cause incomplete bladder emptying and **residual urine** (urine left in the bladder after urination). Residual urine becomes stagnant and predisposes the person to infection.
- Lower estrogen levels in women can result in tissue atrophy in the urethra, the vagina, and the bladder, which predisposes the person to infection and incontinence.

NORMAL URINARY ELIMINATION

The frequency of urination varies. Infants **void** (excrete urine) from 5 to 40 times a day. The preschool child may void every 2 hours. The adult voids from 5 to 10 times a day. On average, the adult male voids 300 to 500 mL each time, and the adult female voids 250 mL. **There should be at least an hourly urine output of 30 mL. This reflects adequate kidney perfusion.**

People usually have the urge to void on awakening in the morning, after each meal, at bedtime, and after drinking extra fluid. Urine production is decreased during sleep, and many people can sleep through the night without voiding, but voiding once during the middle of the night is considered normal.

FACTORS AFFECTING NORMAL URINATION

Urinary elimination is affected by neurologic and muscle development; alterations in spinal cord integrity; the volume of fluid intake; the amount of fluid lost by perspiration, vomiting, or diarrhea; and the amount of antidiuretic hormone (ADH) secreted by the pituitary gland. Anxiety may increase muscle tension and cause a more frequent urge to void. Most people need privacy for urination to occur freely.

Life-Span Considerations

Older Adult

The older adult male is likely to experience **urinary retention** (urine retained in the bladder after voiding), as the prostate gland undergoes hyperplasia with aging. Retention may predispose the man to episodes of urinary tract infection (UTI). If your patient is receiving medication but continues to have persistent retention, report your findings to the primary care provider, because prostate surgery may be considered to prevent kidney damage.

CHARACTERISTICS OF NORMAL URINE

Color

Urine is normally some shade of yellow, with the average being straw colored or amber. The color may darken when the urine is more concentrated. Smoky red or dark brown urine may indicate the presence of blood or myoglobin, which is a by-product of muscle tissue injury. Very dark amber urine may be due to the presence of bilirubin. Other color variations may occur from medications the patient is taking or from water-soluble dyes consumed in food.

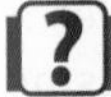
Think Critically

Your older adult patient is upset and concerned because his urine is a different color. What questions could you ask him to obtain more information about the color change?

Clarity

Urine should be transparent or only slightly cloudy. Cloudy urine may contain bacteria or large amounts of protein.

Odor

Normal urine smells faintly like ammonia. If the odor is foul, infection may be present. If the odor resembles acetone, ketones are probably present. Other odors may occur depending on what foods or vitamins the person has ingested.

Specific Gravity

Specific gravity is the thinness or thickness of the urine. It may be measured by a **urinometer,** an instrument that reads the amount of light the urine absorbs, or by a chemical dipstick. **The normal range is 1.010 to 1.030, but conditions such as dehydration and fluid excess may extend the range slightly in either direction.**

pH. The acidity or alkalinity of urine is measured in units called *pH.* **The pH of normal urine is slightly acidic, ranging from 5.5 to 7.0.**

Health Promotion

How to Prevent Recurrent Cystitis

Cystitis and other UTIs may be avoided by:

- Increasing fluid intake to 2500 to 3000 mL/day.
- Avoiding citrus fruits and juice (if prone to frequent reoccurrence) because they cause alkaline urine; bacteria grow more readily in alkaline urine.
- Always wiping the rectal area from front to back after a bowel movement. This is especially important in female patients.
- For the female patient, avoiding wearing tight clothing and nylon pantyhose that cause continual perineal moisture; wearing cotton underwear.
- Not sitting around in a wet bathing suit for extended periods.
- For the female patient, not using bubble bath or feminine hygiene sprays.
- For the female patient, emptying the bladder promptly after intercourse and drinking two glasses of water to flush out microorganisms that may have entered the bladder.
- Bathing or showering daily (both females and males).
- Emptying the bladder every 2 to 3 hours to prevent stasis and potential for bacteria to multiply if present.

ALTERATIONS IN URINARY ELIMINATION

Alterations in urinary elimination patterns are listed in Box 29.1. Urine is normally sterile, but provides a good medium for the growth of infectious organisms if they are introduced into the bladder.

A common UTI is **cystitis** (inflammation of the bladder). Cystitis may be caused by irritation of highly concentrated urine, pathogenic bacteria, injury, or **instillation** (putting in a solution) of an irritating substance. A break in aseptic technique when inserting or caring for an indwelling catheter is a frequent cause of cystitis. Often the *Escherichia coli* bacterium is responsible for cystitis, especially in females.

Symptoms of cystitis are frequency, urgency, dysuria (painful urination), burning, malaise, foul-smelling urine, and a slight temperature elevation (Foxman, 2014). Episodes of recurrent cystitis predispose the patient to kidney infection and consequent kidney damage. In accordance with *Healthy People 2020,* measures should be taken to prevent long-term kidney disease.

Box 29.1 Alterations in Urinary Elimination Patterns

- **Anuria** is present when less than 100 mL of urine is excreted in 24 hours. It may be caused by **urinary suppression** (the kidneys are not forming urine) or to the retention of urine (all urine is not expelled from the bladder during voiding).
- **Dysuria** (painful or difficult urination) occurs when there is inflammation present in the bladder or urethra, usually because of infection or trauma.
- **Incontinence** (involuntary release of urine) occurs with a variety of pathologic conditions. When it is due to decreased muscle tone, special exercises (see Patient Education, p. 569) may prevent it.
- **Nocturia** occurs when the person must get up to urinate during the night more than once or twice.
- **Oliguria** (decreased amount of urine output) occurs when urine output falls below 400 mL/24 h. It may be a sign of kidney failure, blockage of urine outflow somewhere in the system, or retention.
- **Polyuria** (excessive urination) occurs when large amounts of urine are voided, with an output of greater than 1500 mL/24 h. It is usually associated with either diabetes mellitus, in which there is an absence of insulin, or diabetes insipidus, in which there is decreased production of ADH.

Life-Span Considerations

Older Adult

Your older adult patient may develop an infection and not manifest a fever. In fact, the temperature may be lower than normal. Subtle changes in mental status may be the first symptom of an infection, so monitor the older adult closely for changes in alertness and orientation.

QSEN Considerations: Evidence-Based Practice

Complementary and Alternative Therapies

CRANBERRY PRODUCTS TO PREVENT BLADDER INFECTIONS

Cranberries have long been recommended in the prevention of UTIs. Evidence-based practice indicates that cranberry products, specifically juice and tablets, are particularly effective (Geerlings et al., 2014).

Complementary and Alternative Therapies

Probiotics for Urinary Tract Infections

In a study focused on preventing UTIs, the use of a vaginal suppository containing *Lactobacillus crispatus* reduced recurrence of urinary tract infections (Geerlings et al., 2014).

QSEN Considerations: Evidence-Based Practice

Vaginal Estrogen

Evidence-based practice indicates that if a postmenopausal woman experiences recurrent UTIs, she should be offered vaginal estrogen (Mody & Juthani-Mehta, 2014).

APPLICATION OF THE NURSING PROCESS

ASSESSMENT (DATA COLLECTION)

Obtain a history of the patient's usual urinary elimination pattern. Inquire about any incidences of incontinence. Ask if there is a need to urinate frequently, burning when urinating, or a sense of urgency in finding a toilet. Does the patient frequently need to get up to urinate at night? Has the appearance of the urine changed? At what times of the day does the patient usually void? Does the bladder usually feel completely empty after urinating, or does the patient need to void again in less than 2 hours? How much fluid is taken in a 24-hour period? Is there a urinary catheter in place? Is there a history of urinary problems? What is the total 24-hour intake and output? Is it normal? Assess the patient's mobility to determine whether it is safe to allow ambulation to the bathroom unassisted. Note when the patient last voided. **Each patient should void at least every 8 hours unless an indwelling catheter is in place.** If voided amounts are small and intake is normal, gently palpate the bladder to see if it is distended. To do this, feel with the palm of the hand for a bulge indicating a full bladder above the symphysis pubis.

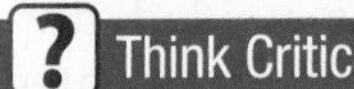

Think Critically

Your patient is voiding only 100 mL of urine at a time. What further assessments should you make? What questions should you ask this patient?

Urine Specimen Collection

Voided Specimen for Urinalysis. Inspection of the urine is the next step in the assessment. For a simple voided specimen for urinalysis, ask the patient to void into a clean bedpan, urinal, collection bottle, or plastic "hat" collection device placed inside the front of the toilet (Fig. 29.3). Provide privacy for the patient. Explain to the female how to hold the urine bottle or cup so that it surrounds the urethra. She should stand in a slightly squatting position, or sit over the toilet and hold the collection container steady to catch the urine as she voids. Explain to both men and women that only about 1½ inches of urine is needed. If the specimen is to go to the laboratory, transfer it to the specimen container, label it properly, and send it to the laboratory within 5 to 10 minutes. **Urine that stands for 15 minutes or more changes characteristics, and the urinalysis will not be accurate.** Box 29.2 shows some common abnormalities found by urinalysis.

Dipstick tests, containing chemical reagents, are routinely performed in most medical offices and outpatient clinics. They may test for a variety of components,

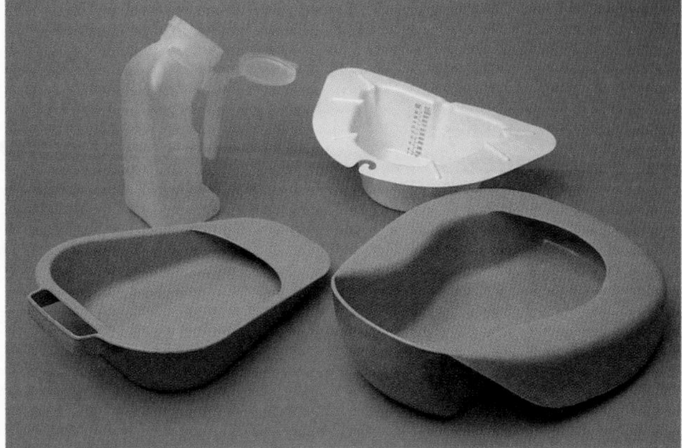

FIGURE 29.3 Urine collection devices. Fracture pan *(left front),* standard bedpan *(right front),* urinal *(left rear),* and in-toilet "hat" *(right rear).*

Box 29.2 Abnormalities Commonly Found in Urinalysis

- **Glycosuria** (glucose in the urine) is present when there is too much glucose in the blood (hyperglycemia) or when the renal threshold for glucose is lowered for some reason.
- **Proteinuria** (protein in the urine) occurs at times of stress, when infection is present, after strenuous exercise, or when there is a disorder of the glomeruli.
- **Hematuria** (blood in the urine) occurs from bleeding somewhere in the urinary system.
- **Pyuria** (purulent exudate in the urine) occurs when there is a bacterial infection in the kidney or the bladder. Bacteria will be present in the urine in large numbers.
- **Ketonuria** (ketones in the urine) occurs when the patient is in ketoacidosis. This occurs in uncontrolled diabetes mellitus.
- **Casts** occur in increased numbers in the presence of bacteria or protein and indicate urinary **calculi** (stones) or kidney disease.
- **Red blood cells** in the urine greater than 0 to 2 cells/high-power field may indicate a stone, tumor, glomerular disorder, **cystitis** (bladder inflammation), or bleeding disorder.
- **White blood cells** in the urine mean there is an infectious or inflammatory process somewhere in the urinary tract.
- **Bilirubin** in the urine suggests liver disease or obstruction of the bile duct.

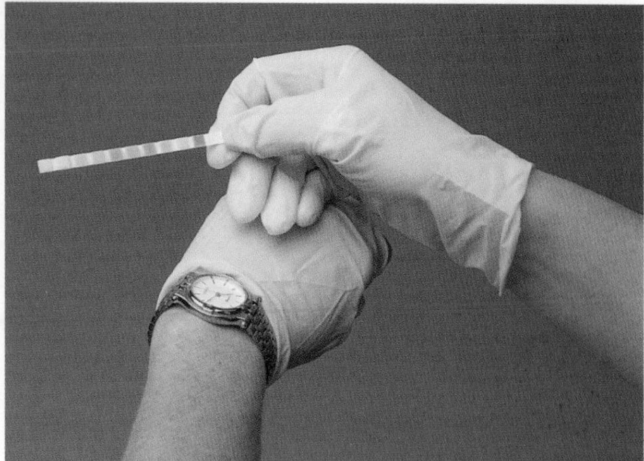

FIGURE 29.4 Timing the reading of a urine dipstick.

including glucose, ketones, protein, blood, specific gravity, pH, nitrate, bilirubin, and leukocytes. To perform a dipstick test, follow the directions on the side of the bottle of test strips. **Exact timing for checking each component is essential for accuracy of the result** (Fig. 29.4).

Midstream (Clean-Catch) Urine Specimen. This procedure is used to obtain a specimen for a culture and sensitivity test when a UTI is suspected. The purpose is to obtain a specimen that is relatively free from external contamination.

 Patient Education

How to Obtain a Midstream Urine Specimen

FOR THE FEMALE PATIENT

- Perform hand hygiene.
- Open the midstream kit and remove the lid of the specimen container, being careful not to touch the inside of the container. Place the lid upside down on the sink or counter.
- Sit on the toilet.
- Open the packets of cleaning swabs.
- With the index finger and thumb of the nondominant hand, spread the labia apart. The labia need to be held apart during cleaning and until the specimen is obtained.
- Clean the right side of the area from front to back in one stroke; discard the swab.
- With a new swab, clean the left side of the area from front to back in one stroke; discard the swab.
- With another swab, clean down the center of the area from front to back in one stroke; discard the swab.
- Pick up the specimen container by the outside; void a small amount of urine into the toilet; catch the middle portion of urine by moving the container into the stream. Collect about 1 oz of urine. Do not let the specimen container touch the skin or pubic hair. Set the container on the sink or on a paper towel, being careful not to touch the inside or the rim. Finish voiding into the toilet.
- Place the lid on the container tightly; do not touch the inside of the lid.
- Rinse and dry the outside of the container.
- Perform hand hygiene.

FOR THE MALE PATIENT

- Perform hand hygiene.
- Open the midstream kit; remove the lid of the specimen container and place it on the sink or counter upside down; be careful not to touch the inside of the container or the lid.
- Open the packets of cleansing swabs.
- If you are uncircumcised, retract the foreskin. Cleanse the end of the penis: start at the urinary meatus (opening) and work outward in circles; discard the swab.
- Repeat the cleansing process with one more swab.
- Pick up the specimen container; with the foreskin still retracted, begin urinating and pass a small amount of urine.
- Move the specimen container into the stream and collect about 1 oz of urine without touching the container to the skin. Put the container down on the sink or on a paper towel.
- Finish urinating into the toilet. Replace the foreskin.
- Replace the lid on the container, being careful not to touch the inside of the container or lid.
- Rinse and dry the outside of the container.
- Perform hand hygiene.

FOR THE PATIENT AT HOME

- After collecting the specimen, label the container with name, date, time, and primary care provider's name.
- Take the specimen to the medical office or laboratory, or place it in a plastic bag and refrigerate until the specimen can be transported.

Specimen from an Indwelling Catheter. A specimen may be obtained from the self-sealing port of an indwelling catheter system (Fig. 29.5, Steps 29.1).

Sterile Catheterized Specimen. When a sterile specimen is ordered and the patient does not have an indwelling catheter in place, the patient is catheterized with a straight catheter (no balloon) that may be attached to a small collection bag, or the urine may be collected by placing the distal end of the catheter into a sterile specimen container.

24-Hour Urine Specimen. All urine voided during the 24-hour period is collected in the designated container and stored on ice if necessary. The laboratory analysis is done to determine the amount of a specified chemical that is excreted through the urine in a 24-hour period. If some urine is accidentally thrown out, the test is invalid and must be started over. A sign should be posted over the bed and over the toilet, indicating that all urine is to be saved. The patient's bladder should be empty at the beginning and at the conclusion of the test. **The patient empties the bladder just before beginning the collection, and that urine is discarded. At the ending time the patient voids, and that urine is added to the collection container.** Check with the laboratory before beginning the test to be certain the right container with preservative is on hand and to see whether the specimen must be kept cold during the 24-hour period (see Chapter 24).

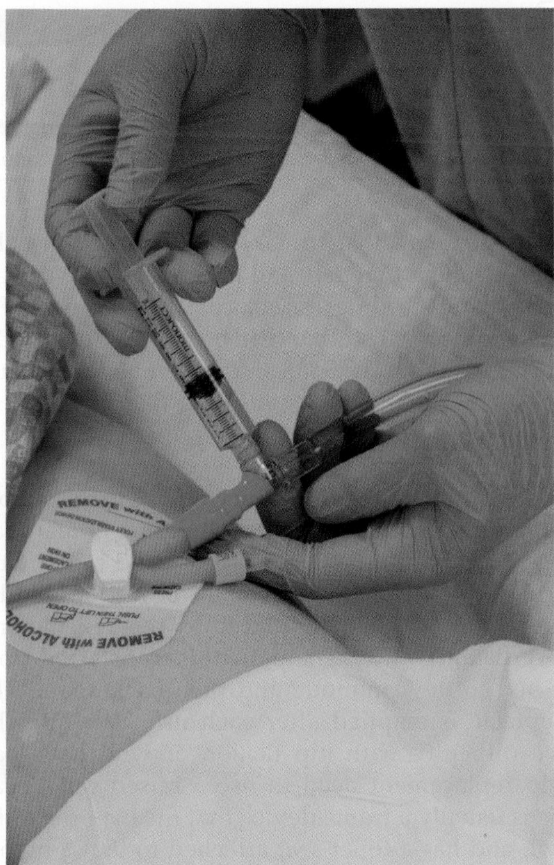

FIGURE 29.5 Aspirating urine from drainage port.

Urinary Collection Bag. This device is used to obtain a urine specimen from an infant or toddler. The skin is cleaned, and then the device is attached to the skin by an adhesive backing and is placed so that it surrounds the genitalia. When sufficient urine has collected in the bag for a specimen, the bag is carefully removed and the urine is poured into a specimen container.

Strained Specimen. If patient is suspected of having a urinary stone, all urine is strained when voided. Usually a fine sieve is used. If a stone is found, it should be saved and sent to the laboratory for analysis.

◆NURSING DIAGNOSIS

Nursing diagnoses for patients with problems of urinary elimination are as follows:

- Urinary elimination, impaired
- Urinary retention
- Urinary incontinence (urge, stress, reflex, overflow, or functional)
- Body image, disturbed
- Infection, risk for
- Pain (acute or chronic)
- Injury, risk for (to kidney from urine blockage)
- Self-care deficit, toileting
- Risk for impaired skin integrity
- Knowledge, deficient

The specific defining characteristics are added to the diagnosis stem for the individual patient.

Steps 29.1 Obtaining a Urine Specimen from an Indwelling Catheter

If it is suspected that the patient is developing a urinary tract infection, the primary care provider may order a urine culture and sensitivity test. The specimen is taken from the port on the catheter or connecting tubing using sterile technique. **The specimen should not be taken from the drainage bag or the tube used to empty the bag.**

Review and carry out the Standard Steps in Appendix A.

ACTION *(RATIONALE)*

1. Clamp the tubing below the aspiration port with a clamp, or double it over and secure with a rubber band. Note the time. Leave it clamped for 15 to 30 minutes per agency policy. *(Ensures there will be fresh urine near the port for the removal of the specimen.)*
2. Perform hand hygiene and don gloves. Scrub the aspiration port of the drainage tubing with alcohol or antimicrobial swab. *(Maintains asepsis and prevents contamination of catheter.)*
3. Insert a 25-gauge needle (or a needleless connector) attached to a 5- to 10-mL syringe into the aspiration port at a 30- to 45-degree angle. *(Use of small-bore needle and angle decreases coring. Needleless connectors are safer, but some aspiration ports may require a needle. Ask for assistance before starting the procedure.)*
4. Aspirate 3 mL of urine by gently pulling back on the plunger of the syringe. Remove the needle or connector from the port. Swab the aspiration port with the alcohol or antimicrobial pad. *(Pulling hard on the plunger may collapse the catheter and prevent urine from flowing into the syringe.)*
5. Empty the syringe into the sterile specimen container without touching inner surface of the container. Dispose of syringe in sharps container. Close and label the specimen container. **Unclamp the catheter.** *(Keeps specimen sterile. Unclamping catheter allows free flow of urine again.)*
6. Ensure the specimen goes to the laboratory within 15 minutes, or refrigerate the specimen. *(Changes can occur in urine that sits at room temperature for more than 15 minutes.)*
7. Remove gloves and perform hand hygiene. *(Reduces transfer of microorganisms.)*

◆ PLANNING

If a patient has been prone to UTIs, plan to increase fluids, unless contraindicated, and reinforce patient education regarding ways to prevent further UTIs. When you need a specimen, inform the patient in advance so he is able to produce the urine. In planning care for your patient, remember to be culturally sensitive in helping your patient meet his toileting needs.

 QSEN Considerations: Patient-Centered Care

Toileting Preferences

CULTURAL AWARENESS FOR TOILETING PREFERENCES

Rather than using toilet paper, patients from other cultures may feel more comfortable if a source of flowing water (e.g., pericare bottle or bidet) is available to clean the perineal area after toileting.

For the patient prone to urinary retention, note the amount of each voiding and palpate the bladder for distention if output falls below normal.

If the patient needs assistive devices for toileting, place a bedpan and/or urinal in the bedside stand or obtain an order for the device needed. Discharge planning includes ensuring that arrangements are made before the patient goes home for devices such as grab bars by the toilet, a **commode chair** (chair with a container inserted to catch urine or feces), or a raised toilet seat (Fig. 29.6).

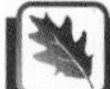 Life-Span Considerations

Older Adult

Plan additional time in your schedule; older adult patients ambulate at a slower pace and may need assistance with clothing fasteners before toileting.

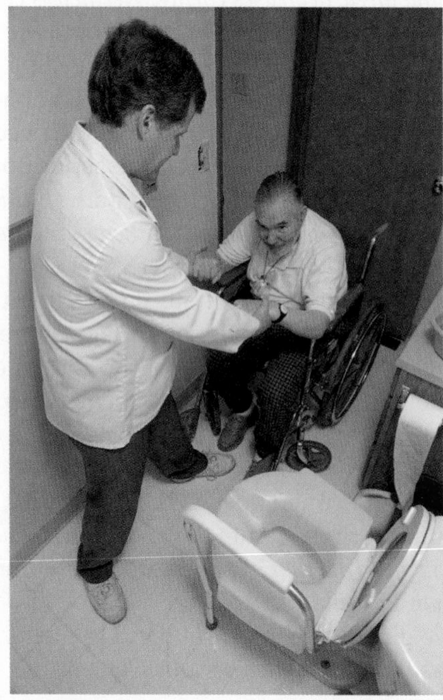

FIGURE 29.6 Grab bars and raised toilet seat in home.

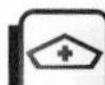 Clinical Cues

Every patient who has an abnormality of urinary elimination should be placed on intake and output (I & O) recording. Place an I & O recording sheet by the patient's bed, and record the I & O in the medical record. All urine voided is recorded as output.

Keep in mind that urinary elimination is usually an independent function, and most people are embarrassed about needing assistance. The insertion of a catheter causes a disturbance in body image even if the catheter is temporary. Some examples of expected outcomes can be found in Nursing Care Plan 29.1.

◆ IMPLEMENTATION

Assisting patients with urinary elimination is a basic nursing function. Patients who can ambulate can be assisted to the bathroom to use the toilet. Others may use a commode chair for bowel or bladder elimination. It is usually placed by the bedside or a short distance away. The patient is transferred from the bed to the commode and then back again. The receptacle is emptied after each use. Patients who have difficulty with hip flexion or who have had a hip replacement need to use a raised toilet seat. This is usually a frame device that fits over the toilet bowl, and has a toilet seat attached to it at a higher point than is usual.

 QSEN Considerations: Safety

Falls

RISK FOR FALLS

An important Joint Commission National Patient Safety Goal is to identify preemptively patients at risk for falls. Patients who need assistance with toileting are likely to have physical or cognitive deficits that increase their fall risk. For example, a commode chair can tip over if an unsteady patient suddenly grabs one handle of the chair.

 Life-Span Considerations

Older Adult

The older adult may experience incontinence because of mobility problems or neurologic deficits. Timed toileting can be helpful in keeping these patients dry.

Patients on bed rest are provided with a bedpan for elimination (see Fig. 29.3). Each patient has an individual bedpan stored in the bedside stand during the hospital stay. The female uses it for both urine and bowel elimination, whereas the male uses it for bowel elimination only. The bedpan should be covered if it must be carried outside the patient's room. Paper towels or a small hand towel may be used.

The **fracture pan** (see Fig. 29.3) is used when patients are unable to sit on a regular-sized bedpan. It is smaller in surface area and height compared with the regular bedpan. It is used for patients with musculoskeletal

Nursing Care Plan 29.1 Care of the Patient With Cystitis

SCENARIO Ms. Juarez, age 33, comes to the outpatient clinic. She states that she has been experiencing burning, urgency, and lower pelvic discomfort for 3 days. She needs to urinate several times an hour. She has had a bladder infection before and is afraid that she has one again. "How do I get these infections? What should I do?" Her blood pressure and pulse are normal, but her temperature is 100.8°F (38.2°C). You ask her to obtain a midstream urine specimen and provide the instructions for obtaining the specimen. You check her urine with a dipstick, and it shows that she has leukocytes in the urine. The primary care provider examines the patient and concludes that she does have cystitis. Trimethoprim-sulfamethoxazole and phenazopyridine HCl are prescribed.

PROBLEM/NURSING DIAGNOSIS *Burning and lower pelvic discomfort*/Pain related to cystitis with urination and lower pelvic discomfort.

Supporting Assessment Data *Subjective*: Discomfort in lower pelvic area for 3 days. States, "It burns." *Objective*: Facial expression shows discomfort.

Goals/Expected Outcomes	Nursing Interventions	Selected Rationale	Evaluation
Pain will be lessened within 6 h.	Review instructions for taking phenazopyridine HCl and trimethoprim-sulfamethoxazole.		*How did patient respond to the treatments?*
Pain will be relieved within 72 h.	Explain that phenazopyridine HCl will turn the urine red or orange.	Patient might be frightened if red or orange urine is not expected.	After taking the medications and fluids for 24 h, patient stated in follow-up phone call that discomfort is almost gone.
	Encourage patient to take trimethoprim-sulfamethoxazole exactly as directed to kill the causative organism.	Patient will feel better after several days of antibiotic; however, failure to complete the full course creates resistant strains of bacteria.	
	Encourage patient to increase fluid intake to 3000 mL/day to keep urine dilute and lessen bladder irritation.	Increasing fluid intake flushes the bladder and decreases bacteria population; thus, irritation is decreased.	
	Explain that sitting in a hot sitz bath with water up to the umbilicus for 20 min two or three times a day will help to increase blood flow to the bladder and lessen bladder irritation and pain.	Hot water increases circulation in the pelvic area.	Meeting expected outcomes.

PROBLEM/NURSING DIAGNOSIS *Does not know how to prevent infection*/Deficient knowledge related to factors that predispose to UTI.

Supporting Assessment Data *Subjective*: Asks, "How do I get these infections? What should I do?" *Objective*: Unable to state how much fluid she should drink in a day. Unable to identify any factors that predispose her to UTI when asked.

Continued

Nursing Care Plan 29.1 Care of the Patient With Cystitis—cont'd

Goals/Expected Outcomes	Nursing Interventions	Selected Rationale	Evaluation
Patient will verbalize five ways to help prevent recurrence of UTI at the follow-up visit in 10 days.	Instruct patient to continue to drink at least 2500 mL of fluid per day.	Understanding risk factors and measures to prevent infection is essential to prevent another bladder infection.	*Was patient able to verbalize ways to prevent recurrent UTIs?* Verbalized five measures to prevent UTIs during follow-up visit. Urine is clear of bacteria. Met expected outcomes.
	Void immediately after intercourse and drink at least a full glass of water.	Voiding after intercourse flushes bacteria from the urethra.	
	Refrain from wearing clothing that is tight in the groin area.	Tight clothing creates a warm, moist environment for bacteria growth.	
	Bathe daily and thoroughly cleanse the perineal area.	Keeping perineal area clean decreases bacteria that can travel up the urethra.	
	Always wipe perineum from front to back only.	Prevents feces from coming into contact with the urethra.	
	Drink cranberry juice.	Acidifies the urine, which discourages growth of bacteria.	
	Empty the bladder at least every 3 h while awake.	Stagnant urine creates a medium for bacterial growth.	

CRITICAL THINKING QUESTIONS

1. Why do you think that many women develop cystitis after having intercourse?
2. What is the rationale for asking a patient to have another urine specimen checked a day after finishing a course of treatment for cystitis?

problems. The flat end with the wide rim is placed under the patient by separating the patient's legs and slipping the pan under the buttocks. The greater depth at the front of the pan helps keep the urine from spilling on the bed. Remove the pan carefully to avoid spilling urine. Skill 29.1 presents instructions on how to place and remove a bedpan.

For the ambulatory patient who needs urine output recorded, place a plastic "hat" device toward the front of the toilet bowel between the bowl and the seat. The inside is graduated to allow recording of the amount of output. After each voiding empty, rinse, and replace the container so that it is ready for the next voiding.

Whatever method is used for urinary elimination, provide an opportunity for hand hygiene after toileting. Leave the patient comfortable, with side rails up and the call bell within reach.

Cultural Considerations

Hand Hygiene

For nurses, hand hygiene is second nature, but for many people, this is not an automatic behavior. For example, a study was conducted with families giving hands-on care to patients in Bangladesh. Although they perceived that washing hands with soap reduced transmission of disease, they rarely were observed washing their hands after contact with bodily fluids. (Islam et al., 2014). In accordance with *Healthy People 2020*, improvements in personal and domestic hygiene are needed to reduce the global incidence of disease.

Assisting With Use of a Urinal

When a male requires assistance to use a urinal, the nurse assists the patient to stand beside the bed, if possible. The male urinal is a bottle with a round neck, a handle, rectangular sides, and a flat base (see Fig. 29.3). It may or may not have a lid. The patient who is confined to bed can use the urinal in any one of four positions: lying supine, lying on either the right or the left side, or lying in Fowler position. Provide privacy by closing the door or curtain, don gloves, lower the side rail, and ask the patient to spread his legs. Hold the urinal by the handle and direct it at an angle between the legs so that the flat side rests on the bed. Lift the penis and place it well within the urinal. After urination, carefully remove the urinal and empty it immediately, measuring and recording the urine voided. Be certain the penis is dry. Clean the urinal and return it to the proper place.

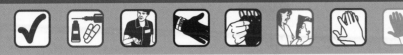

Skill 29.1 Placing and Removing a Bedpan

 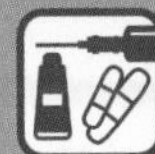 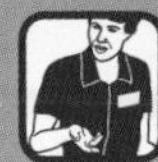 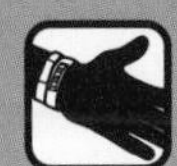 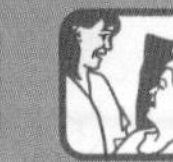 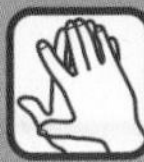 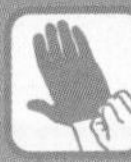

The female patient who is very weak or who has bed rest ordered uses a bedpan to void or to have a bowel movement. The male uses a urinal to void, but uses the bedpan to evacuate the bowel.

Supplies

- Bedpan
- Toilet tissue
- Gloves
- Underpad

Review and carry out the Standard Steps in Appendix A.

NURSING ACTION *(RATIONALE)*

Assessment (Data Collection)

1. Inquire if the patient needs to void. *(Checks for bladder distention and establishes need to void.)*
2. Determine mobility to see if the patient can use a full-size bedpan or if fracture pan is needed. *(Fracture pan use prevents further injury from turning or raising the hips.)*

Planning

3. Gather equipment. Raise the bed to proper working height. *(Facilitates work organization. Prevents back strain.)*
4. Close the door and/or the privacy curtains. *(Protects privacy.)*

Implementation

5. Perform hand hygiene and don gloves. *(Reduces transfer of microorganisms.)*
6. Lower the side rail if up, and raise the top linen enough to determine location of the hips and buttocks. *(Provides access to place bedpan.)*
7. Ask patient to bend the knees and press down with the feet while you slip one hand under the lower back for assistance; place an absorbent pad under the hips and buttocks. Ask the patient to repeat this maneuver and place bedpan under the patient with the back rim at the end of the sacrum. *(Placing your hand palm up under the small of the back and your elbow on the mattress helps lift the patient onto the bedpan. The buttocks will form a seal along the rim of the pan.)*

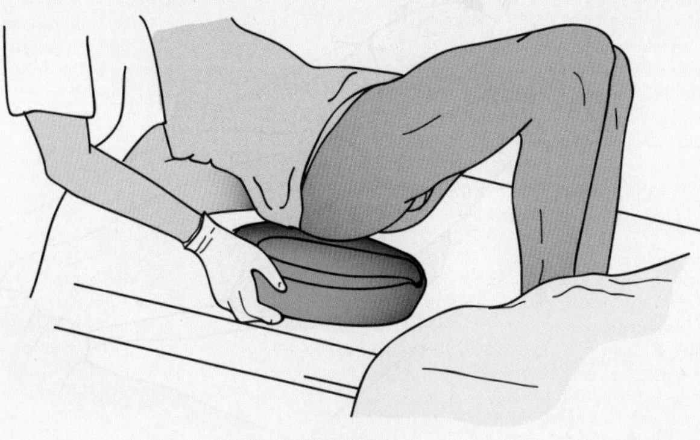

Step 7

8. Raise the head of the bed to 30 degrees if not contraindicated. Place the toilet tissue and call light within reach. If urine is to be measured, instruct patient to put used toilet tissue in wastebasket. *(A sitting position makes voiding easier. Patient can signal for assistance. If toilet tissue is left in the bedpan, it is more difficult to get an accurate output measurement.)*
9. Ask the patient to flex the knees, place the feet on the mattress, and raise the hips. Remove bedpan. Place it on the chair or the floor. *(Allows for removal of the bedpan.)*

For the Helpless Patient

10. Turn the patient on one side; place the bedpan firmly against the buttocks with the top of the bedpan at the top of the fold of the buttocks. Place one hand on the hip and hold the bedpan in place with the other hand. Roll the patient onto the bedpan and check position for comfort. *(The weak patient cannot assist.)*
11. Raise the head of the bed to 30 degrees if not contraindicated. *(Sitting is an easier position for voiding.)*
12. When the patient is finished, lower the head of the bed and assist the patient to turn to the far side of the bed. Hold the bedpan to prevent spilling. Remove the bedpan and set it on the floor. *(Lowering the head and then turning the patient is easier than trying to lift the patient off the pan.)*

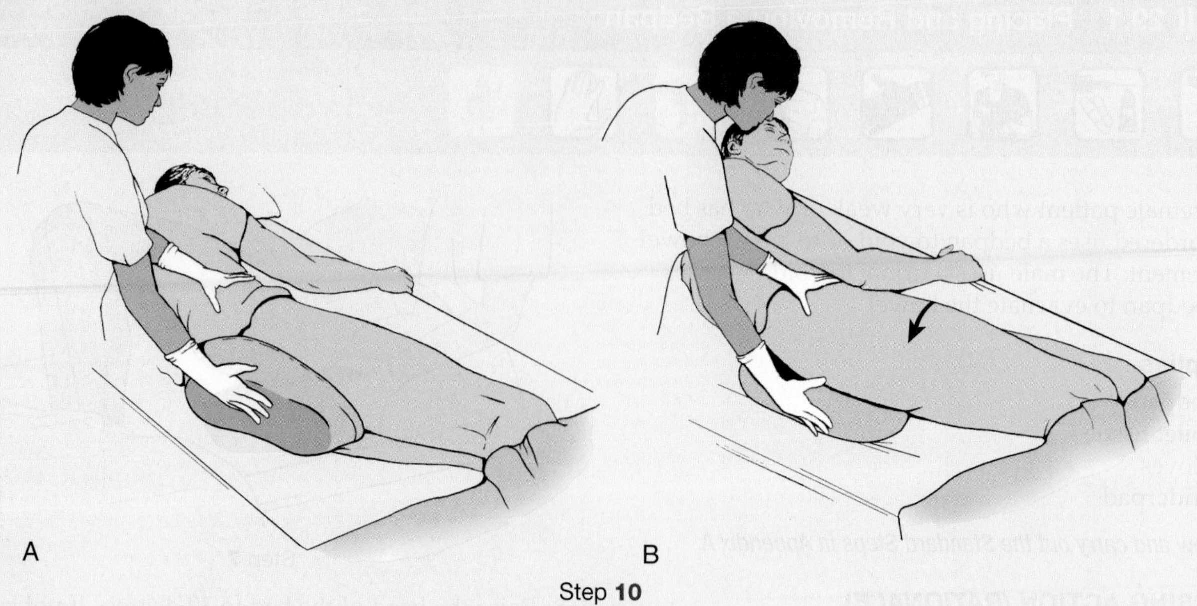

Step 10

13. Wipe the perineal area dry with toilet tissue, stroking from the front of the vulva to the anus. *(Cleansing from front to back prevents contamination of urinary meatus and vaginal area.)*
14. Measure the urine, note unusual characteristics, and record the amount on the intake and output record as needed. Discard the urine and clean and dry the bedpan and store it in its proper place. *(Output and characteristics are documented for trends. Dirty bedpans have an odor and are a source of infection.)*
15. Have patient perform hand hygiene. Remove gloves and perform hand hygiene. *(Reduces transfer of microorganisms.)*
16. Lower the bed and restore the unit. Place call light within reach; raise side rails. *(Makes patient comfortable and institutes safety measures.)*

Evaluation

17. Ask patient if bladder feels empty. Did any urine spill? If so, what would you do differently next time? Has the patient performed hand hygiene? Is the patient comfortable? *(Determines whether procedure went smoothly and accomplished the goal.)*

Documentation

18. Document on the flow sheet or in the nurse's notes depending on agency policy. Note time, amount of voiding, and characteristics of the urine. *(Verifies patient's voiding pattern.)*

Documentation Example

Voided 240 mL clear, pale yellow urine in bedpan. (Nurse's electronic signature)

Special Considerations

- When the patient cannot raise the hips or turn to the side, a fracture pan is used. It can be slid into place from between the patient's legs. The flattened portion of the pan is slipped under the buttocks. A trapeze bar requires upper arm strength, but the patient can self-position on the pan.

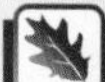

Life-Span Considerations

Older Adult

- The older adult patient may be especially reluctant to have the nurse cleanse the perineum. Be matter of fact and protect dignity, but ensure that the patient is clean.

? Critical Thinking Questions

1. What would you do to make it as easy as possible to place and remove a bedpan for a patient who has an external fixation device on his lower leg?
2. How would you make certain the patient who cannot turn to the side is properly cleansed after a bowel movement?

Helping a Patient Urinate

Patients often have difficulty urinating after surgery and anesthesia, childbirth, or other trauma to the perineum. All efforts are made to help the patient void naturally before resorting to **catheterization** (insertion of a tube into the bladder). Some methods of helping patients initiate the voiding reflex are:

- Run water in a nearby sink so the patient hears the sound.
- Have the patient deep breathe, relax, and visualize a peaceful place with a bubbling brook. Encourage the patient to drink a cup of warm caffeinated coffee or tea.
- Help the male stand by the side of the bed (with a documented order).
- Have the female blow through a straw in a glass of water, causing bubbling, while sitting on the toilet or bedpan.
- Measure several cups of warm water, then pour the water over the perineum while the patient attempts to void. Subtract the measured amount from the total volume to determine how much the patient voided.
- With an order, gently but firmly use **Credé maneuver** over the bladder (massage from top of bladder to bottom by starting above the pubic bone and rocking the palm of the hand steadily downward). This is primarily used for patients with neurogenic urinary dysfunction.
- Obtain an order for a sitz bath and have the patient sit in the warm water. Encourage the patient to void while in the bath. Cleanse the perineum afterward.

When a patient cannot empty the bladder naturally for a period longer than 8 hours, a bladder scan may be performed using an ultrasound machine designed for that purpose (Fig. 29.7). If the bladder contains a large amount of urine, an order is obtained for catheterization. The bladder scan can also disclose the amount of residual urine in the bladder after voiding. This tells the primary care provider whether the bladder is emptying sufficiently. If needed, the care provider orders either a straight "in-and-out" catheterization or the insertion of an indwelling urinary catheter. Other reasons for catheterization include:

- Preparing a patient for a surgical procedure or obstetric delivery.
- Keeping the genitalia and perineum clean after obstetric or surgical procedures.
- Dilating a urethral **stricture** (narrowed lumen).
- Splinting the urethra following surgery on the urethra (the catheter is inserted by the surgeon).
- Measuring the amount of residual urine in the bladder (also accomplished by using a portable ultrasound bladder scanner).
- Monitoring hourly urine output or obtaining exact measurements of total output.

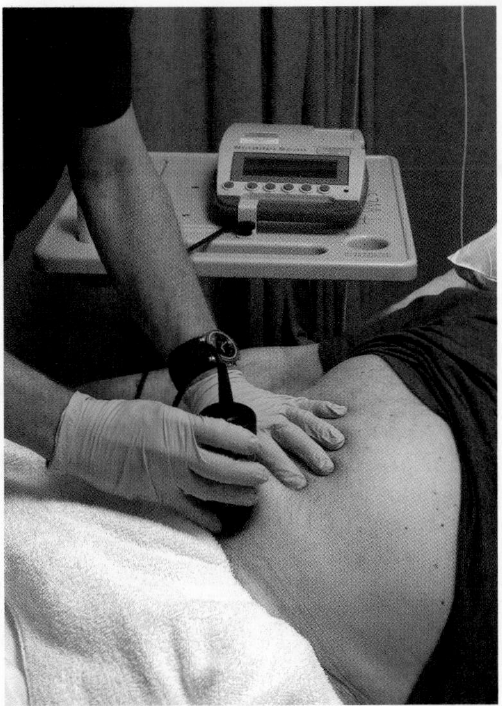

FIGURE 29.7 Using a bladder scanner to determine the amount of urine in the bladder.

- Performing irrigation or instillation and drainage of chemotherapeutic solutions into the bladder.
- Assisting with the re-toning of the bladder muscle after surgery on the bladder.

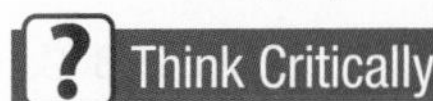

Think Critically

Your patient returned from surgery at 10:30 am and is awake and alert. She had spinal anesthesia, but has recovered the feeling in her lower extremities. It is now 7:00 pm, and she still has not voided since her return to the unit. What would you do to help her void? If she has not voided by 8:00 pm, what would you do?

Types of Urinary Catheters

Catheters come in several sizes and shapes and are either rubber or plastic. Some are Teflon coated. They are sized using the French system, with the average size used for an adult woman being 14 to 16 Fr. and for the man 18 to 20 Fr. (Fig. 29.8). A straight catheter (e.g., the Robinson) is used (1) to relieve retention when a patient is temporarily unable to void or (2) to obtain a sterile specimen. The Foley (retention catheter) is the most common indwelling catheter; it can remain in the bladder for an extended period. A Foley catheter has two lumens, one to drain urine and one for inflation of the balloon holding the catheter in the bladder to prevent it from slipping out the urethra. The balloon usually holds 5 to 10 mL of sterile water. This catheter is used for continuous drainage, particularly after surgery, and it can also be used for **suprapubic** (above the pubic bone) drainage.

The Coudé catheter, a variation of the Robinson catheter, is curved and has a rounded or bulbous tip that is

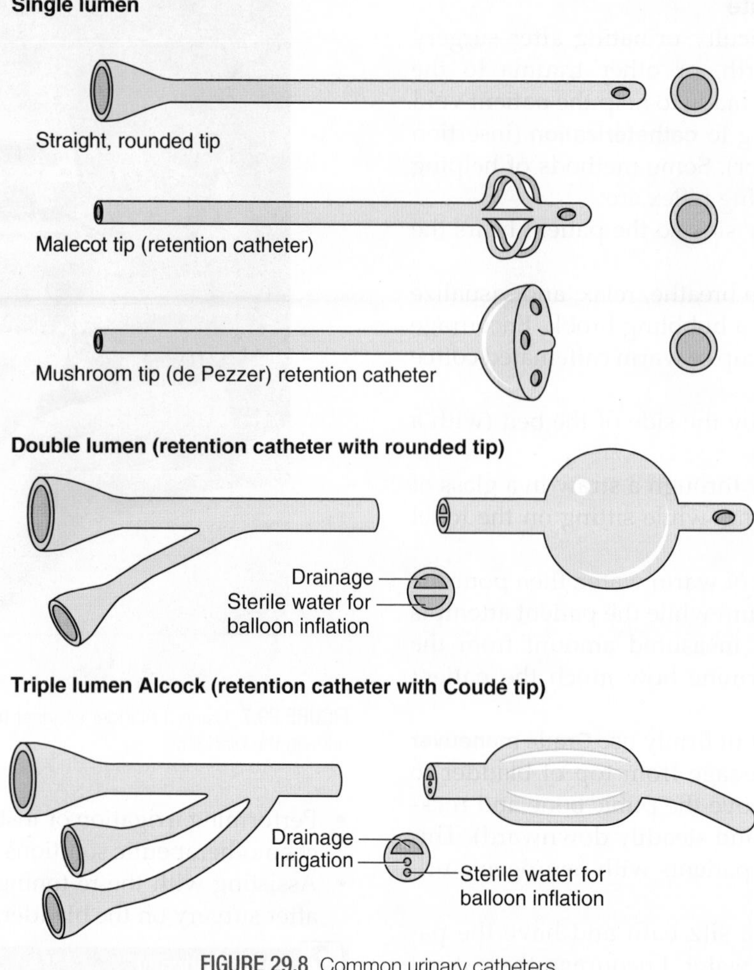

FIGURE 29.8 Common urinary catheters.

easier to insert into the male urethra when the prostate is enlarged. It is usually inserted by a urologist.

The Alcock catheter, used for continuous bladder irrigation following prostate or bladder surgery, is a Foley-type catheter with two drainage eyes. It has three lumens, one for urine drainage, one for inflation of the balloon, and one for instillation of irrigation fluid.

The de Pezzer catheter, which has a tip shaped like a mushroom, is used for suprapubic drainage. The Malecot catheter, which has a large single tube with a tip shaped like wings, is often used as a nephrostomy tube; it is placed into the pelvis of the kidney.

A **condom catheter** consists of a condom with a tube attached to the distal end that is attached to a drainage bag. It is used to provide continuous urine drainage for the male in a noninvasive manner. Read the directions that come with the specific catheter. See Skill 29.2 for additional information.

Performing Catheterization

Sterile equipment and strict aseptic technique must be used to catheterize a patient. **Any break in aseptic technique causing contamination must be corrected before continuing with the procedure.** One of the National Patient Safety Goals is to follow protocols that protect patients from infection. Catheter kits can be used for males or females. The procedure for male and female catheterization is similar except for variations in the positioning, draping, and cleansing of the urinary meatus. In the male, the catheter is inserted farther (about 7 to 8 inches). **When inserting a catheter, gently insert until you see the urine flow and then insert 1 to 2 more inches.** This will ensure the balloon will not damage the urethra during inflation. Skills 29.3 and 29.4 give the steps for catheterization of the female patient and the male patient, respectively.

Communication

Talking to the Patient About Catheter Insertion

James Stanton is suffering from urinary retention. He is in the emergency department because he cannot urinate and is in pain. His primary care provider ordered an indwelling urinary catheter to be inserted. Mr. Stanton has expressed reluctance about having a catheter. The nurse explains the procedure to him.

Nurse: "Hi, Mr. Stanton; I'm Karen. How are you feeling?"
Mr. Stanton: "I'm very uncomfortable."
Nurse: "Can you tell me about your discomfort?"
Mr. Stanton: "I can't pee and I have an ache down low."
(Nurse gently palpates the lower abdomen above the symphysis pubis.)

Continued on page 562

Skill 29.2 Applying a Condom Catheter

 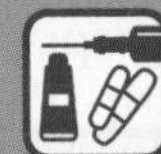 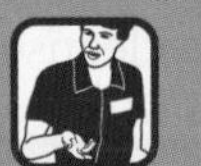 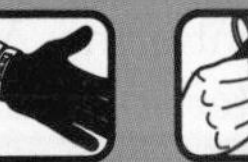 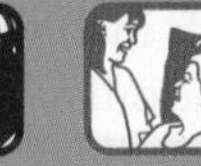 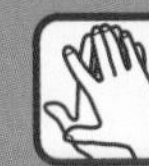 

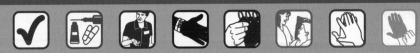

A condom catheter is used for the male who is able to pass urine, but is incontinent. It is preferable to use a condom catheter rather than an indwelling catheter because bladder infection is less likely to occur. **There are different brands of condom catheters and different methods of attachment; follow the specific directions on the package.**

Review and carry out the Standard Steps in Appendix A.

Supplies

- Condom catheter
- Gloves
- Adherent elastic tape strip
- Basin, warm water, soap, washcloth, and towel
- Skin prep pads or solution
- Clippers for hair removal if needed
- Urine collection bag with drainage tubing or leg bag and straps

ACTION *(RATIONALE)*

Assessment (Data Collection)

1. Assess need for and patient's willingness to use a condom catheter. *(Condom catheters are easily detached.)*
2. Assess condition of skin on penis. *(Urine incontinence places the skin at risk for breakdown.)*

Planning

3. Gather equipment and prepare the working space by raising bed to the proper height. *(Promotes work efficiency and prevents back strain.)*
4. Close the door and/or draw the privacy curtains. *(Protects the patient's privacy.)*
5. Explain the procedure. *(Promotes cooperation and reduces anxiety.)*
6. Lower the side rail if up. Place patient in a supine position, drape the upper torso with a bath blanket, and then fold the sheet down so it covers the legs and can be lowered to expose the genitalia. *(Provides comfort, conserves body heat, and prevents unnecessary exposure.)*
7. Prepare the urinary drainage collection system by clamping the drainage bag discard spout and positioning the bag for easy attachment to the condom catheter. Roll the wider tip of the condom sheath toward the narrower tip. *(If the discard spout is not clamped, urine can spill out. Rolling the condom downward will prepare the condom for rolling it upward over the penis.)*

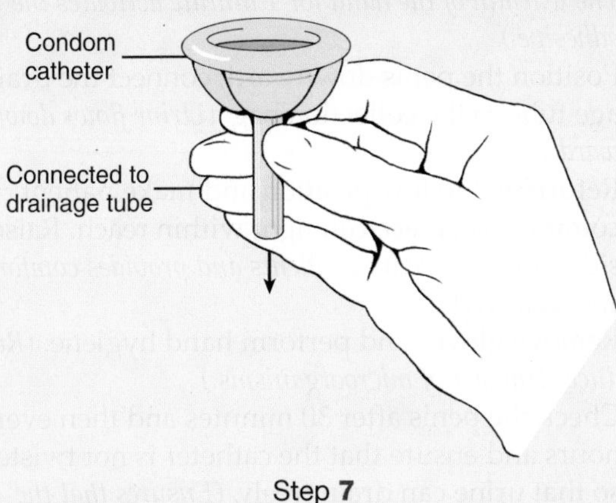

Step 7

Implementation

8. Perform hand hygiene and don gloves. *(Prevents transfer of microorganisms.)*
9. Wash and dry the penis and surrounding skin, clip the hair at the base of the penis, apply the skin prep, and allow to dry. *(Cleansing and skin prep protects the skin and provides an adherent surface.)*
10. Apply the double-sided elastic tape in a spiral fashion from the base of the penis downward. *(Provides a surface on which the condom catheter can be attached without impeding circulation in the penis. Some condom catheters attach with a Velcro strip over the sheath.)*
11. Grasp the penis along the shaft with the nondominant hand. Hold the condom sheath at the tip of the penis and smoothly roll the sheath onto the penis, leaving 1 to 2 inches of space between the tip of the penis and the drainage tube of the condom sheath. *(Positions the condom catheter on the penis. Allows free passage of urine into the collecting tube and drainage bag. Keeps penis away from collecting urine.)*

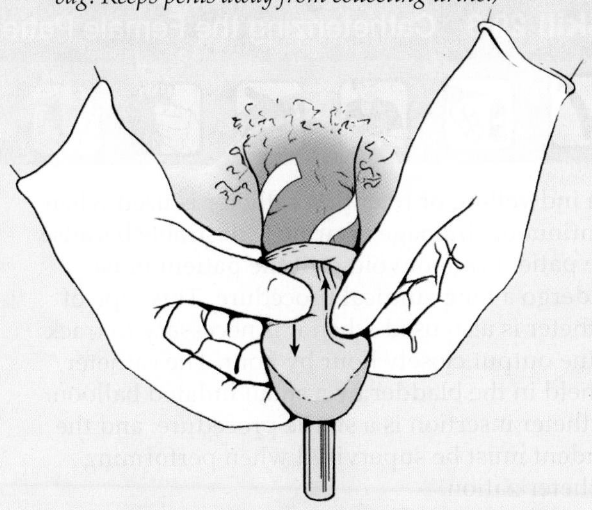
Step 11

12. Gently press the sheath to the underlying adhesive strip with the palm of the hand in a grasp, being careful not to wrinkle the rubber sheath. Hold for 1 minute. Explain the rationale for holding. *(Wrinkles in the sheath may cause urine leakage. The warmth of the hand for 1 minute activates the adhesive.)*
13. Position the penis downward; connect the drainage tube to the collection bag. *(Urine flows downward.)*
14. Return bed to low position and make patient comfortable; place call light within reach. Raise side rails. *(Prevents accidents and provides comfort and security.)*
15. Remove gloves and perform hand hygiene. *(Reduces transfer of microorganisms.)*
16. Check the penis after 30 minutes and then every 2 hours and ensure that the catheter is not twisted so that urine can drain freely. *(Ensures that the catheter is not too tight and impairing circulation.)*
17. If a leg bag is used, empty it when it is partially filled with urine. *(Weight can pull the catheter off.)*

Evaluation

18. Does the catheter fit smoothly and adhere firmly to the penis? Is there evidence of irritation to the skin or impaired circulation? Is urine draining into the bag? Is there any leakage of urine? *(Determines whether system is functioning effectively without problems.)*

Documentation

19. Note date, condition of genital area, size and type of catheter applied, type of skin prep used, type of drainage collection attached to catheter, amount of urine obtained in bag and its color and character, and patient's tolerance of the procedure. *(Documents use of condom catheter.)*

Documentation Example

Skin on genitalia slightly reddened from contact with incontinent urine. Area cleansed, prepped, and condom catheter applied with Velcro strip. Patient states does not feel too tight. Attached to leg bag. Draining clear, yellow urine. (Nurse's electronic signature)

Special Considerations

- If the condom catheter is the newer self-adhesive type, apply catheter as in Step 11 and apply gentle pressure around the penile shaft for 10 to 15 seconds to secure the catheter.
- The catheter must be checked frequently because the end of the sheath is prone to twist, preventing the urine from flowing into the drainage tube. Do not allow any pull on the drainage tubing when repositioning or ambulating the patient because this may dislodge the catheter.
- Remove and change the catheter daily or more often if it fits improperly.
- Wash the used catheter and collection bag with mild soap and water, rinse with a 1:7 strength vinegar solution, and allow it to dry completely.
- If the rolled-over portion at the base of the penis seems too tight, clip the roll a tiny bit to loosen it. It should not constrict the penis and interfere with blood flow.
- Check for swelling, discoloration of the penis, and complaints of discomfort.

? Critical Thinking Questions

1. If an older adult man resists the idea of a condom catheter and the only other option is to insert an indwelling catheter, what might you say to him that might make him accept the condom catheter?
2. How would you tell if the condom catheter is too tight?

Skill 29.3 Catheterizing the Female Patient

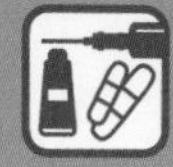
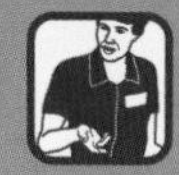

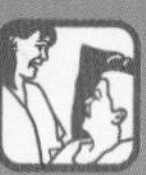
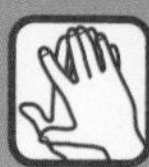

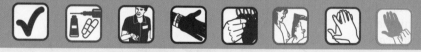

An indwelling or retention catheter is used when continuous drainage of urine is desirable because the patient cannot void or if the patient must undergo a long surgical procedure. This type of catheter is also used when it is necessary to track urine output closely hour by hour. The catheter is held in the bladder by a small inflated balloon. Catheter insertion is a sterile procedure, and the student must be supervised when performing catheterization.

Supplies

- Indwelling urinary catheter kit with appropriate size catheter (adult female: 14 to 16 Fr.)
- Sterile 4 × 4 gauze
- Bath blanket
- Basin with warm water
- Towel and washcloth
- Mild soap
- Catheter securing device
- Extra light (standing lamp or flashlight)

Review and carry out the Standard Steps in Appendix A.

ACTION *(RATIONALE)*

Assessment (Data Collection)

1. Check the primary care provider's order for type of catheter. *(Catheterization requires a medical order.)*
2. Assess patient's knowledge of catheterization and use of a catheter. *(Patient education is based on knowledge deficit.)*
3. Assess whether patient is allergic to iodine or tape. *(Povidone-iodine is often used to cleanse the perineum before catheterization.)*
4. Assess woman's ability to assume the dorsal recumbent (lithotomy) position. *(If the female patient cannot assume the dorsal recumbent position, a side-lying position may be used.)*

Planning

5. Check the patient's identification band, gather equipment, and prepare the working space by raising the bed to proper height and positioning the over-the-bed table for use. *(Ensures the procedure is performed on the correct patient; promotes work efficiency and prevents back strain.)*
6. Close the door and/or privacy curtains. *(Protects the patient's right to privacy.)*
7. Explain the procedure. *(Patient's cooperation is necessary to maintain sterility during procedure.)*

Implementation

8. Perform hand hygiene and don disposable gloves. *(Reduces transfer of microorganisms.)*
9. Help patient assume the dorsal recumbent position, with thighs relaxed so that hips can externally rotate, and drape with a bath blanket or sheet. *(Positions patient for ease of viewing the meatus and inserting the catheter into the bladder.)*
10. With the use of good lighting, inspect the perineum. Wash the area if needed. Spread the labia with your nondominant hand and locate the urinary meatus. *(An assistant may be needed to hold a flashlight with the beam directed at the perineum.)*

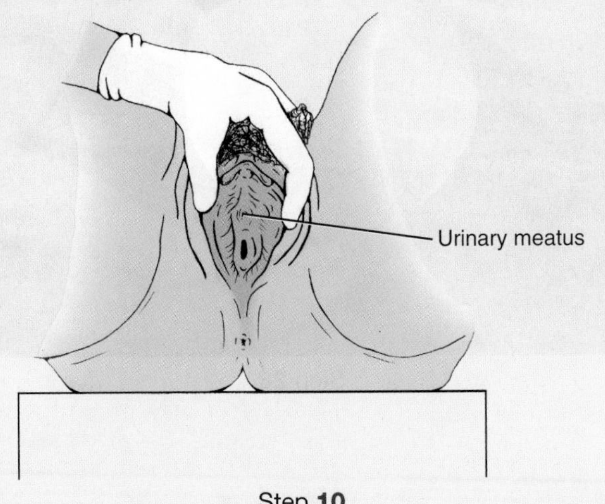

Step **10**

11. Remove gloves and perform hand hygiene. *(Reduces transfer of microorganisms.)*
12. Open the plastic covering of the catheter kit by tearing along the lined perforated edge. Use the plastic cover as a discard bag and place it to the side of the field or toward the foot of the bed for waste disposal. *(Provides a receptacle for used supplies.)*
13. Remove the paper-wrapped catheter tray and place it on the bed between the patient's legs, near the perineum (8 to 12 inches away). *(Provides a workspace.)*
14. Fold back the corner of the bath blanket drape to expose the perineum. With clean hands, using sterile technique, open the wrapper and use it as a sterile field. *(Provides a sterile field.)*
15. Pick up the sterile absorbent underpad by one corner. Hold two corners turned over your fingers, slip it under the patient's buttocks, plastic side down, while patient lifts buttocks. Touch only the corners and underside of the sterile underpad. *(Top and center of the pad are sterile. The underside and edges are considered nonsterile.)*
16. Put on the sterile gloves and separate the two containers in the kit, placing the tray with the cotton balls in front of the box containing the catheter and drainage bag. *(Interior of the tray and all equipment within tray must be kept sterile.)*
17. Place the drape with the opening over the genital area, exposing the labia. *(Sterile drape helps prevent catheter from touching the skin on the thighs as the meatus is approached.)*
18. Loosen the cotton balls from one another, open the antiseptic solution pack, and drizzle antiseptic solution evenly over the cotton balls. *(Cotton balls will stick together if they are not separated.)*
19. Open the package of lubricant, or remove the stopper from the syringe containing it, and squirt it into an open area of the tray. *(Catheter tip can be rotated in the lubricant.)*
20. Place the sterile specimen bottle on the side of the tray or discard it. *(Bottle may be discarded if no specimen is required. Specimen can also be collected after the procedure is completed.)*
21. Remove the plastic sleeve on the catheter by tearing it down the perforated side while carefully controlling the catheter. Place the catheter within the sterile tray where it can be easily reached. *(The catheter is rubbery and can "flip or jump" and strike a nonsterile surface if you do not control it. Wrapping the catheter around a gloved hand while tearing the sleeve helps prevent a break in sterile technique.)*
22. Attach the sterile water-filled syringe to the balloon port on the catheter, and leave the syringe attached to the catheter balloon port. Do not pretest the balloon. *(If the syringe is detached now, later you will have to reattach it with one hand. Pretesting of the balloon before insertion can distort the catheter and lead to trauma upon insertion.)*

23. With the forefinger and thumb of the nondominant hand, separate the labia minora, exposing the meatus. Pull slightly upward (see figure with Step 10). Leave this hand in place, holding the labia open until the catheter is inserted. *Remember:* The hand holding open the labia is now contaminated and must not be used to handle sterile objects. *(Exposes urinary meatus so that catheter can be introduced. Using a sterile 4 × 4 gauze between the fingers and the inner labia helps prevent the fingers from slipping.)*

24. Using forceps, pick up one saturated cotton ball at a time and cleanse down one side of the labia majora and then the other, discarding each used cotton ball after one stroke. Cleanse one side of the labia minora and then the other. Cleanse last over the meatus with a slow downward stroke. **Do not allow the labia to close over the meatus after cleansing.** *(Removes microorganisms from perineal area and urinary meatus. Do not pass over the sterile field with used cotton balls when discarding them because this contaminates the sterile field.)*

a. If solution is obscuring the meatus, a dry sterile cotton ball can be used to sponge up the excess solution. *(This allows better visualization of the meatus.)*

b. Dispose of the forceps in the discard bag. *(Contaminated materials must be discarded.)*

25. Pick up the catheter about 3 inches from the tip, lubricate it well, and gently insert it into the meatus while pointing the catheter slightly toward the umbilicus. Insert it about 2 to 3 inches or until you visualize urine flow. After you see the urine flow, insert the catheter an additional 1 to 2 inches. There may be slight resistance as the catheter passes the internal urethral sphincter. If urine does not flow, rotate the catheter gently and carefully insert it another inch farther. Do not use force. If resistance is encountered, ask the patient to take a deep breath, and twist and advance the catheter as the patient does so; this relaxes the sphincter. If the catheter has been inserted into the vagina by mistake, leave it there as a marker for the vaginal opening; perform hand hygiene and begin the procedure again with a sterile kit. *(Patient will feel a pinch as the catheter passes through the sphincter and may report the urge to urinate. Leaving marker catheter in place ensures vaginal opening is not repeatedly mistaken for urinary meatus.)*

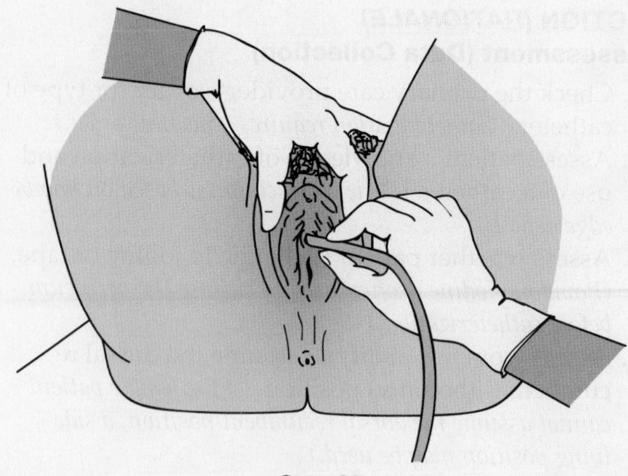

Step **25**

26. Hold the catheter in place with the dominant hand while instilling the water into the balloon with the nondominant hand. Remove the syringe from the port after inflation and discard. Gently pull on the catheter to see if it is anchored securely, and then gently push it back slightly. **Watch the patient's face for an expression of discomfort while inflating the balloon; if there is pain, stop immediately because the balloon may be in the urethra, not the bladder.** *(If the balloon is inflated while in the urethra, the pressure could cause damage that would require surgical repair.)*

27. Cleanse the antiseptic solution from the perineum and remove the underpad. *(Prevents antiseptic solution from irritating the skin and makes the patient more comfortable.)*

28. Attach the drainage bag to the stationary part of the bed frame along the side of the bed close to the middle. Remove the drapes, dry the genital area, dispose of used supplies, remove gloves, and perform hand hygiene. *(Do not attach the bag to the side rail or any moveable part of the bed frame.)*

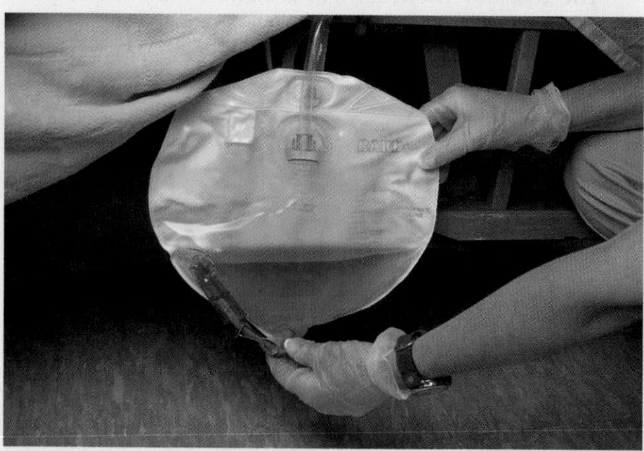

Step **28**

29. Attach the catheter to the thigh with a catheter-securing device. *(Tension on the catheter causes pressure on the internal urethral sphincter and may damage it. Use tape if a commercial device is not available.)*

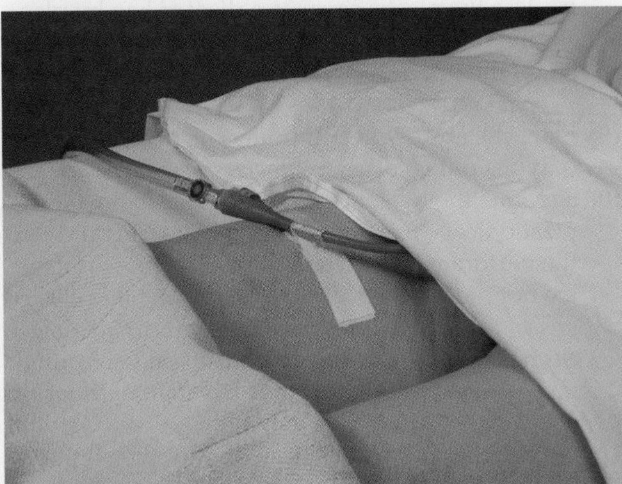

Step **29**

30. Coil the excess drainage tubing on the bed so that the last portion hangs straight to the drainage bag and secure it. *(The catheter will drain better if no tubing is hanging below the level of entry of the bag.)*
31. Restore the unit, lower the bed, and place the call light within reach. *(Protects the patient.)*

Evaluation

32. Ask yourself: Was sterile technique maintained? Is urine draining, indicating proper placement in the bladder? Is the patient having any pain associated with the procedure? Is there anything you would do differently next time? *(Determines whether procedure was done correctly and whether catheter system is patent. Helps improve technique.)*

Documentation

33. Note date, time, size and type of catheter, amount of water instilled into balloon, type of technique used, and color and characteristics of the urine. *(Documents catheter insertion.)*

Documentation Example

No. 16 Fr. urinary catheter inserted with sterile technique; balloon filled with 10 mL of water. Closed drainage system attached. Pt expressing slight discomfort with catheter in place. Approximately 230 mL of dark yellow, clear urine obtained in bag. Catheter secured to inner right thigh. Bed into lowest position; call light within reach. (Nurse's electronic signature)

Special Considerations

- Once the catheter has touched the patient's skin, it should not be introduced into the urinary meatus because it is contaminated. Anytime the catheter becomes contaminated, the procedure is stopped and begun again with a sterile catheter and kit.
- **For straight catheterization:** There is no balloon to inflate and no drainage bag. The distal end of the catheter is left in the tray so that urine will drain into it. If a specimen is required, prepare the specimen bottle by labeling and opening it; place the lid upside down on a clean surface. After urine has started to flow, pinch off the catheter with the nondominant hand and place the end of the catheter above the specimen container. Allow 1 to 2 oz of urine to flow into the container. Pinch off the flow, replace the catheter in the tray, and drain the remaining urine from the bladder. Pinch off, remove, and discard the catheter. Measure and record the amount of urine on the intake and output record. Place the lid on container, label, and send to laboratory.

Home Care Considerations

- The working height of the bed may be awkward.
- If necessary, have the caregiver assist by steadying the legs and holding the knees apart.
- Catheters and drainage bags may be reused. Cleanse with mild soap and rinse well. Deodorize the drainage bag with a rinse of 1 part vinegar to 7 parts water and allow to dry. The catheter should be boiled for 20 minutes. When dry, it may be stored in a closed container.

Critical Thinking Questions

1. If you cannot tell where the urinary meatus is located by looking for it, what would you do?
2. If you have a patient who has difficulty keeping her knees apart for the catheterization procedure, what would you do?

Skill 29.4 Catheterizing the Male Patient

 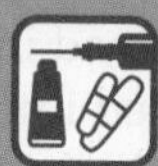 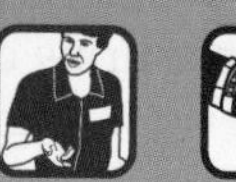  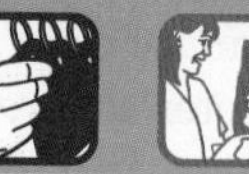 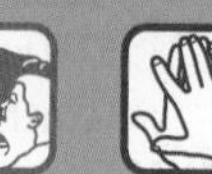 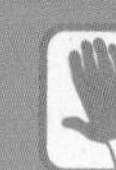

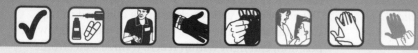

An indwelling or retention catheter is used when the patient cannot void or when it is necessary to track urine output closely. A small inflated balloon holds the catheter in the bladder. Supervision of the student is required for this sterile, invasive procedure.

Supplies

- Indwelling urinary catheter kit with the appropriate size catheter (adult male: 18 to 20 Fr.)
- Basin with warm water
- Bath blanket
- Mild soap
- Towel and washcloth
- Catheter securing device
- Extra light if needed

Review and carry out the Standard Steps in Appendix A.

ACTION *(RATIONALE)*

Assessment (Data Collection)

1. Check the primary care provider's order for type of catheter. *(Ensures the correct type of catheter is used.)*
2. Assess patient's knowledge of catheterization and use of a catheter. Assess whether patient is allergic to iodine or tape. *(Povidone-iodine must not be used for cleaning if the patient is allergic to iodine.)*

Planning

3. Check the patient's identity wristband, gather equipment, and prepare the working space by raising the bed to proper height and positioning the over-the-bed table for use. *(Ensures the procedure is performed on the correct patient. Promotes work efficiency and prevents back strain.)*
4. Close the door and/or privacy curtains. *(Protects the patient's right to privacy.)*
5. Explain the procedure. *(Male patients are often apprehensive about catheter insertion; an explanation helps decrease anxiety.)*

Implementation

6. Perform hand hygiene. *(Reduces transfer of microorganisms.)*
7. With the patient supine and knees slightly apart, drape by fanfolding the bedcovers down to cover the lower legs, exposing the perineal area. Use a bath blanket to cover the trunk. *(Bunching the blanket obstructs patient's view and may decrease embarrassment. An erection can occur when the penis is handled.)*
8.
   a. Open the catheter tray by tearing open the plastic cover at the perforated line. Place the kit on the bed between the legs. *(Supplies must be within reach.)*
   b. Use the plastic cover as a discard bag by placing it to the side of the field or toward the foot of the bed. *(Provides a receptacle for used supplies.)*
9. Place the absorbent pad under the penis; touch only the outer corners. *(Provides a sterile field.)*
10. Separate the two parts of the kit and remove the plastic sleeve from the catheter by tearing it down the perforated side while controlling the catheter. Do not pretest the balloon. *(Controlling the catheter prevents it from touching contaminated surfaces and ensures sterility. Pretesting of the balloon before insertion can distort the catheter and lead to trauma upon insertion.)*
11. Loosen the cotton balls from one another, open the antiseptic solution pack, and drizzle antiseptic solution evenly over the cotton balls. *(Cotton balls will stick together if they are not separated.)*
12. Lubricate around the first 3 to 4 inches (5 to 7 cm) of the catheter if the lubricant comes in a foil package. If it is in a syringe, squirt it directly into the urethra. *(It is recommended practice to place the lubricant into the urethra of the male. If insertion is difficult, obtain an order for lidocaine gel. Squirting this into the urethra relaxes muscle spasm and allows easier entry for the catheter.)*
13. Retract the foreskin if necessary to expose the head of the penis. *(Foreskin interferes with adequate cleansing.)*
14. Using forceps and a saturated cotton ball, grasp the glans below the tip with the nondominant hand, hold the penis erect, and cleanse the glans in a circular motion moving outward from the meatus. *(It is not necessary to clean the full length of the shaft, but cleaning the meatus and the glans decreases bacteria.)*

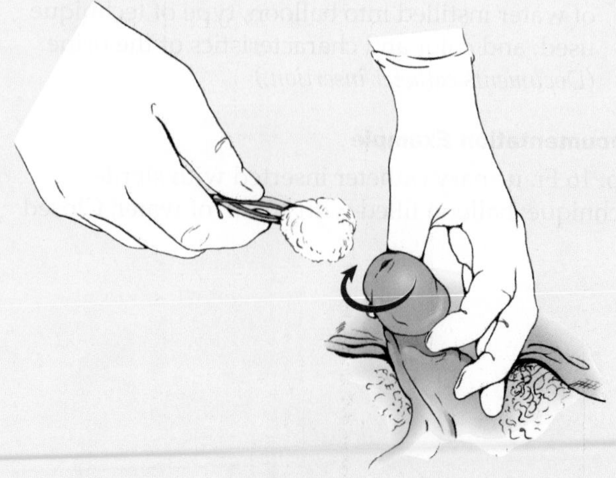

Step 14

15. Discard the used cotton ball and cleanse again with two more cotton balls. Continue to hold the shaft of the penis. *(Crossing the sterile field with used cotton ball contaminates the field.)*
16. Pick up the catheter with the dominant hand 3 to 4 inches (8 to 10 cm) below the tip. With the penis perpendicular to the body, pull it slightly upward; ask the patient to bear down as if trying to urinate; and, using a rotating motion, insert the catheter into the meatus until you reach the catheter bifurcation. Urine should flow. *(Elevating and putting slight traction on the penis straightens the urethra and makes it easier to insert catheter into the bladder.)*

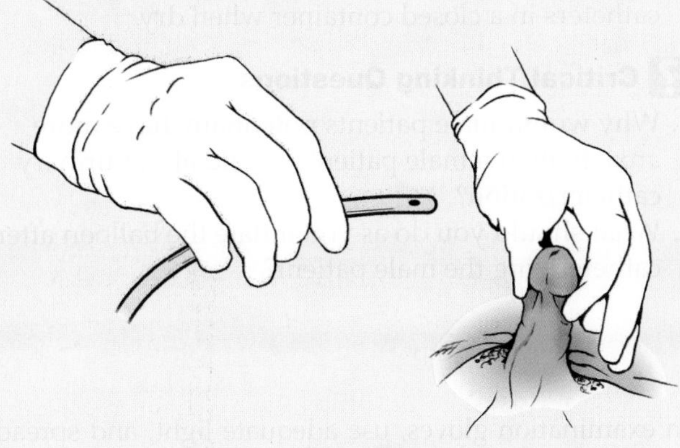

Step **16**

17. If resistance is met, pause and ask the patient to take a deep breath, and then try to twist the catheter or instruct the patient to turn feet soles inward and wiggle the toes to relax the muscles. If resistance persists and the catheter will not advance without difficulty, remove it and notify the primary care provider. *(The internal sphincter relaxes with a deep breath. Forcing the catheter against resistance may cause trauma.)*
18. **After urine starts to flow, insert the catheter an additional 1 to 2 inches** and then hold the catheter in place, inject the contents of the prefilled syringe into the balloon, and detach the syringe while holding the plunger all the way down. *(If you do not hold the catheter in place, it can slip out of position. Filling the balloon keeps the catheter in the bladder. Releasing the plunger allows the water to flow back into the syringe.)*
19. Pull gently on the catheter to check that the balloon is inflated. Then push it back in slightly. *(Relieves pressure on the internal sphincter.)*
20. Clean the antiseptic solution from the penis and remove the drape by tearing it toward the penis on one side. *(Prevents irritation of the skin and makes the patient comfortable.)*
21. Reposition the foreskin if it was retracted. *(If not repositioned, the foreskin can constrict the penis, causing circulation difficulties and swelling.)*
22. Secure the catheter to the abdomen if it is to remain in place for an extended period. Alternatively, it may be positioned on top of the thigh for short-term use. *(Secures the catheter so there is no tension on the internal urinary sphincter. Positioning catheter on the abdomen decrease pressure on the penoscrotal angle.)*

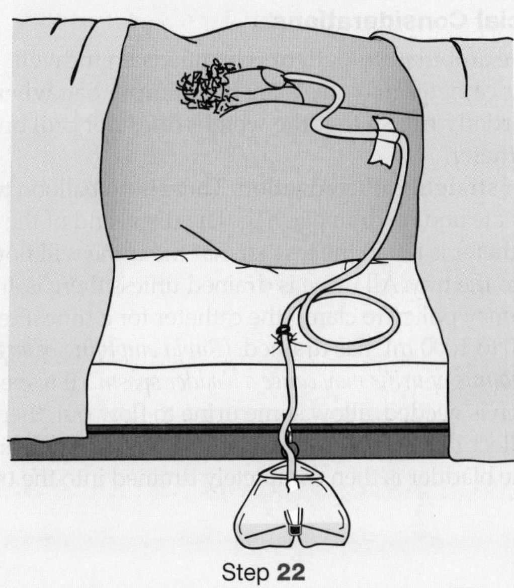

Step **22**

23. Attach the drainage bag to a nonmovable part of the bed frame (not the side rail). Coil the excess drainage tubing on the mattress and secure it. *(Bladder drains more readily when bag is lower and tubing is not below the bag.)*
24. Remove the drape, make the patient comfortable, lower the bed, and restore the unit, placing the call light within reach. *(Provides for patient comfort and safety.)*
25. Dispose of used supplies in the appropriate waste container. *(Used supplies are a source of infection.)*
26. Note the initial amount and character of urine in the bag. *(Provides a baseline for further assessments of urine character and output.)*
27. Remove gloves and perform hand hygiene. *(Reduces transfer of microorganisms.)*

Evaluation

28. Was sterile technique maintained? Was urine obtained? Were any problems encountered? Would you do anything differently next time? *(Self-evaluation helps to improve technique.)*

Documentation

29. Note date, time, size and type of catheter inserted, amount of water in balloon, any problems encountered, and amount and character of urine obtained initially. *(Documents procedure, catheter size, and amount of water in balloon for future reference.)*

Continued

Documentation Example

18-Fr. indwelling urinary catheter inserted with sterile technique; balloon filled with 10 mL of water. Slight resistance encountered, but catheterization successful. Approximately 300 mL dark yellow, cloudy urine obtained. Bed in lowest position; call light in reach. (Nurse's electronic signature)

Special Considerations

- The ambulatory patient who needs an indwelling catheter may use a leg bag. Empty bag when partially full so that the weight does not pull on catheter.
- **For straight catheterization:** There is no balloon to inflate and no drainage bag. The distal end of the catheter is left in the tray so that the urine will flow into the tray. All urine is drained unless there is an agency policy to clamp the catheter for a time after 800 to 1000 mL has drained. *(Rapid emptying of large amounts of urine may cause a bladder spasm.)* If a specimen is needed, allow some urine to flow out, then collect 1 or 2 oz of urine in the specimen container. The bladder is then completely drained into the tray. The catheter is pinched off, removed, and discarded. The urine is measured and recorded as output. The specimen is labeled and sent to the laboratory.
- Evidence-based practice supports catheterization in the home using a clean technique rather than a sterile one with no increased risk for catheter-associated urinary tract infection (Newman & Willson, 2011). The patient's bladder should be resistant to the organisms normally found in the home. The drainage bag can be washed in mild soap and water, rinsed, and rinsed again with a solution of 1 part vinegar to 7 parts water to deodorize it. It should be allowed to dry before reuse. Catheters should be washed with mild soap, rinsed well, and allowed to dry before boiling for 20 minutes. Store catheters in a closed container when dry.

? Critical Thinking Questions

1. Why would male patients potentially have more anxiety than female patients would about urinary catheterization?
2. What should you do as you inflate the balloon after catheterizing the male patient?

Nurse: "Mr. Stanton, your bladder is very full. Your primary care provider has ordered a catheter so that the urine can drain. Have you ever had a catheter inserted before?"
Mr. Stanton: "No; isn't that like a tube of some sort?"
Nurse: "Yes, it is a tube. Since you've been having so much trouble urinating, the primary care provider wants me to insert the catheter and leave it there so urine will drain. In addition, we will be trying to determine why you are having trouble passing your urine."
Mr. Stanton: "Will I have to have the catheter forever? I don't want that."
Nurse: "Usually medication or surgery can correct the problem, and then the catheter won't be needed."
Mr. Stanton: "Will it hurt?"
Nurse: "It may be a little uncomfortable when it is put into the bladder. You can help by relaxing and by doing some deep breathing when I instruct you to do so. The catheter will relieve the pain you are feeling from not being able to urinate and the discomfort will go away. When the urine drains, there is no backup that could damage your kidneys."
Mr. Stanton: "OK. Then let's just get it over with. I sure don't want to damage my kidneys."
Nurse: "I'm sorry you are having this problem, Mr. Stanton. The catheter should bring you some relief. I will drape your groin area; cleanse the penis with iodine solution, which feels cool; and then insert the catheter. It will be hooked up to a bag to collect the urine. Are you allergic to iodine?"
Mr. Stanton: "No, I'm not."
Nurse: "OK, then I'll go ahead and get started."

It is a good idea to identify the urethral meatus in the female before beginning the procedure. When the patient is in the dorsal recumbent position and draped, put on examination gloves, use adequate light, and spread the labia minora to reveal the inner anatomy. The urethral meatus is usually slightly above the vaginal opening and often looks like a dimple or fold in the mucous membrane. If you have difficulty identifying the urinary meatus, ask the patient to cough or bear down. The meatus will usually pucker. If there is still doubt, you can explore the folds of tissue very gently with a sterile cotton swab.

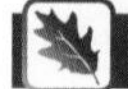

Life-Span Considerations

Older Adult

In the older adult female, the urinary meatus is sometimes found just inside the opening of the vagina. If the patient has difficulty with the dorsal recumbent position, place her on her side with the knees flexed and the upper leg supported by pillows, then approach the meatus from the rear (Fig. 29.9).

QSEN Considerations: Evidence-Based Practice

Lidocaine

Retrograde injection of lidocaine gel into the urethra before catheter insertion is recommended to decrease discomfort in male patients (Bardsley, 2015). In most facilities, you will need an order from the primary care provider for lidocaine injection.

The catheter is secured to the thigh of the female, preferably the inner thigh, and to the top of the thigh or the abdomen of the male. Allow a little slack in the

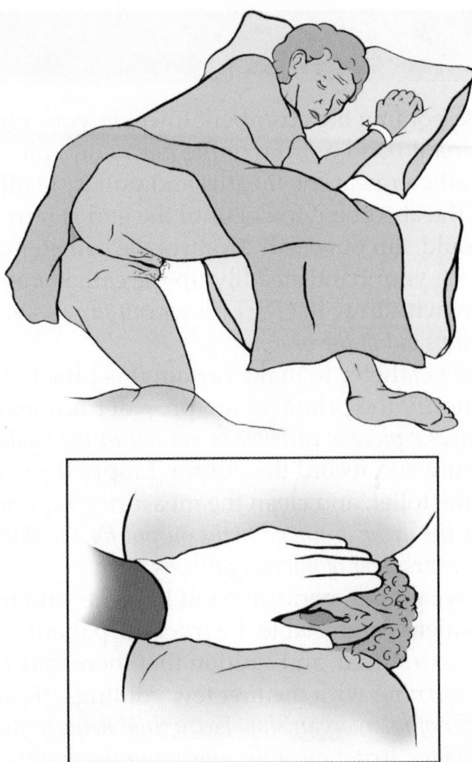

FIGURE 29.9 Side-lying position for catheterization.

catheter before securing it to the skin so that there is not constant tension on the internal sphincter by the balloon. All patients with an indwelling catheter are placed on I & O recording.

The perineum is cleaned during the daily bath, and the external portion of the catheter is washed at that time if it is soiled. No special cleansing of the urinary meatus is recommended (Halm & O'Connor, 2014). Box 29.3 provides suggestions for caring for the patient with an indwelling catheter.

The Nurse's Role in Preventing Catheter-Related Urinary Tract Infections

In performing catheterization and providing daily care, nurses should be aware that catheter-related UTI (CAUTI) results in 30% to 40% of hospital-acquired infections every year (Halm & O'Connor, 2014). In addition, Medicare and Medicaid no longer reimburse for this complication because CAUTI is viewed as an indicator of poor care (Kennedy et al., 2013). Nursing interventions such as maintaining basic infection control procedures including handwashing, utilizing bladder ultrasounds, and placing condom catheters or other alternatives have been proven to reduce the number of UTIs. Another UTI-preventing intervention is the use of a checklist, which includes the reason for the catheter and the number of days that the catheter has been in place. Based on the checklist data, the nurses remind the care providers to consider removal of the catheter. Toileting schedules and intermittent catheterization are incorporated whenever possible (Chenoweth et al., 2014).

Box 29.3 Care of an Indwelling Urinary Catheter

- Ensure that the patient takes in adequate fluid to flush bacteria and sediment from the urinary system.
- Maintain a closed drainage system (Chenoweth et al., 2015).
- Accurately measure and record the urine output at least every 8 hours.
- Wash hands before and after working with a patient's catheter. Wear clean, nonsterile gloves (Bardsley, 2015).
- Empty the urine bag via the spout at the bottom, being careful not to contaminate the spout. Wipe the spout with a clean antiseptic swab before returning it to the storage sleeve. Use a separate collection container to empty the bag for each patient (Gokula & Gaspar, 2014).
- Observe the drainage tubing and amount of urine in the bag each time the patient is seen. Keep the drainage tubing above the level of entrance to the collection bag. Check to see that the patient is not lying on the catheter or tubing.
- Keep the drainage bag below the level of the bladder. Clamp the tubing before raising the bag above the level of the bladder when moving the patient to avoid urine backflow into the bladder. (Remember to unclamp the tube after patient is repositioned.)
- Provide perineal care at least twice daily. Cleanse the genitalia and perineum, and also cleanse 7 to 10 inches down the catheter with soap and rinse well, or follow the agency's policy for cleansing.
- Keep the catheter firmly attached to the leg or to the abdomen of the male to prevent pulling on the catheter at the meatus, which causes irritation.
- Cleanse the insertion site of the suprapubic catheter twice a day according to agency policy.
- Expect at least 30 mL/h urine output. Less than this is abnormal unless there is a known physiologic reason, such as chronic kidney disease. Check for kinked tubing, bladder distention, or a wet bed. If no reason is found, report the decreased flow to the primary care provider.

 **QSEN Considerations: Evidence-Based Practice**

Automatic Stop Orders

REMOVAL OF AN INDWELLING CATHETER

Evidence-based practice indicates that automatic stop orders would reduce the incidence of CAUTIs (Huber et al., 2015). 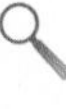

If the facility does not use the automatic stop-order system, then it is the nurse's responsibility to obtain an order for removal as needed. The patient is kept on I & O recording for 12 to 24 hours after catheter removal to ensure that the bladder is draining adequately. Steps 29.2 give the steps and rationale for this removal.

The Suprapubic Catheter

A suprapubic catheter may be used for urine drainage following gynecologic and bladder surgery. It is

Steps 29.2 Removing an Indwelling Catheter

When the primary care provider writes the order to discontinue an indwelling catheter, the catheter is removed. The catheter and bag should be disposed of in a biohazard bag or container and not left in the trash can in the patient's room.

Review and carry out the Standard Steps in Appendix A.

ACTION *(RATIONALE)*

1. Check the order in the patient's medical record. *(An order is required for this procedure.)*
2. Obtain a 10-mL syringe and an absorbent towel. *(Water in the balloon must be withdrawn before removing the catheter. Some balloons may hold as much as 25 mL of water.)*
3. Perform hand hygiene, don gloves, and check the patient's identity wristband while explaining the procedure. Warn the patient that there may be slight discomfort as the catheter is removed. *(Correctly identifies the right patient; reduces fear of the unknown.)*
4. Place the absorbent towel on the mattress under the catheter, and attach the syringe to the balloon port. Withdraw the water from the balloon until resistance is met. **Never cut the catheter.** *(Protects the mattress; deflates the balloon. Cutting the catheter will sever the access to the balloon. If the catheter does not come out, it will have to be surgically removed.)*
5. While holding the absorbent towel in your nondominant hand in front of the perineum, pinch off the catheter near the meatus and pull it steadily out onto the absorbent towel until the end is retrieved. It should slip out easily. Control the catheter by moving your hand steadily up the catheter as you gently withdraw it. *(The catheter can flip or spill urine as it slips out of the urethra.)*
6. Inspect catheter to make certain it is intact. If it is not, notify the primary care provider immediately. *(Ensures a piece of catheter is not left in the bladder.)*
7. Measure and record the output. Empty the urine into the toilet, and clean the measuring equipment. *(Adds the urine drainage to the output for the shift. Reduces transfer of microorganisms.)*
8. Remove gloves, perform hand hygiene, and make the patient comfortable. Instruct the patient to drink extra fluid, and caution that there may be mild burning with the first few voidings. *(Reduces transfer of microorganisms. Extra fluid helps to flush the bladder. Irritation of the mucosa in the urethra may cause burning with voiding.)*
9. Document the time of removal and time limit for the next voiding. *(Sets guideline so all nurses know when to check to see if the patient has voided.)*

inserted through the abdominal wall by the surgeon. The suprapubic catheter is sutured to the skin at the time of insertion (Fig. 29.10).

Intermittent Self-Catheterization

Intermittent self-catheterization is used for patients who regularly experience incontinence or urinary retention. In accordance with National Patient Safety Goals, patients should be taught and encouraged to participate in their own care. Often these patients have a spinal cord problem that prevents proper function of the nerves that control the bladder and urinary sphincters.

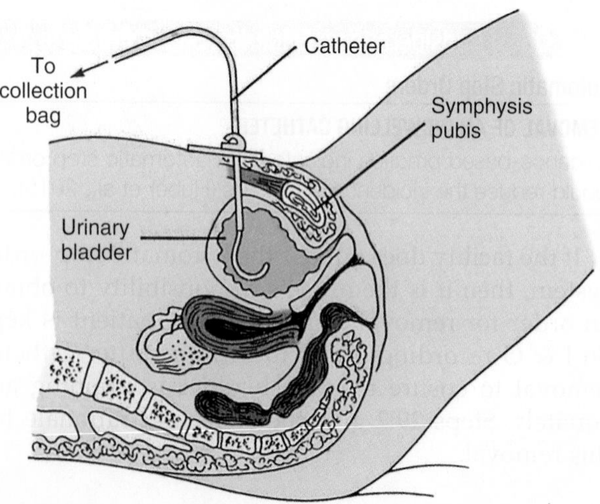

FIGURE 29.10 Suprapubic catheter. (From Elkin, M. K., Perry, A. G., & Potter, P. A. [2007]. *Nursing Interventions and Clinical Skills* [4th ed.]. St. Louis, MO: Mosby.)

 Patient Education

Self-Catheterization

- Catheterize as frequently as necessary to reduce residual urine volume as indicated by your physician or nurse.
- Gather equipment, use a good light source, and (for females) remove a tampon if one is in use.
- Perform hand hygiene.
- Squeeze some lubricant on a paper towel and then roll the catheter in the lubricant to lubricate at least 2 inches of the catheter (female); inject lubricant into the meatus (male). Place supplies within reach.
- Assume a comfortable position such as semireclining in bed or sitting on a chair or the toilet. Men may wish to stand.
- Cleanse the urinary meatus with a towelette or a soapy washcloth; rinse with a wet washcloth; pat dry. If female, hold the inner labia open and stroke down and back to prevent fecal contamination of the meatus.
- For the female, locate the meatus by touch. Place the index finger of your nondominant hand on the clitoris.

Place the third and fourth fingers at the vaginal opening and locate the meatus between the index and third fingers. Separate the labia.

- For the male, lift the penis to a 60- to 90-degree angle to straighten the urethra before inserting the catheter.
- With the drainage end over a basin or the toilet, insert the catheter into the meatus. For the female, direct the angle toward the umbilicus. Twist the catheter as you advance it. If resistance is met, take a deep breath while trying to advance the catheter.
- Hold the catheter in place until all urine stops draining.
- Pinch and withdraw the catheter slowly.
- Wash the catheter in warm soapy water, rinse, and dry with a clean towel. Place it in a plastic container. Reusable catheters may be boiled in water for 20 minutes to kill bacteria.

QSEN Considerations: Evidence-Based Practice

Clean Procedure

Self-catheterization, primarily performed outside the hospital, is considered to be a "clean" rather than a "sterile" procedure, and it does not require the use of a sterile catheter (Shaw & Logan, 2013).

Bladder Irrigation or Instillation

Irrigation or instillation (Skill 29.5) is performed on patients with indwelling catheters to:

- Wash out residual urine or sediment from the bladder.
- Remove clots and stop oozing of blood after prostate or bladder surgery.
- Soothe irritated bladder tissues and promote healing.
- Ensure that the lumen of the indwelling catheter is open and draining.
- Instill medication into the bladder.

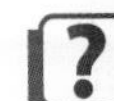

Think Critically

The nurse applies a clamp to a urinary catheter after instilling a medication, but forgets to remove the clamp at the designated time. In fact, she leaves the hospital at the end of her shift without remembering to undo the clamp. What are the patient complications that could result from this error?

Continuous irrigation is performed after prostate or bladder surgery via the three-way indwelling (Foley) catheter system where the irrigation solution is hooked up to the irrigation port of the catheter. The solution container is positioned on an intravenous (IV) pole. Using sterile technique, solution is run through the tubing to remove air, and then the tubing is connected to the irrigation port of the catheter. When using a three-way catheter, consult the package instructions to determine which port should be attached to the irrigating solution, and which port is designated for the drainage bag connection. (Note: The inner lumen with the largest diameter should be used for the drainage because of the potential for clots or debris washed from the bladder.) The third port is for inflating the balloon and appears similar to a standard indwelling catheter port. Check the order for the flow rate. Generally, the irrigation solution is set to flow just fast enough to prevent clots from

Continued on page 568

Skill 29.5 Performing Intermittent Bladder Irrigation and Instillation

 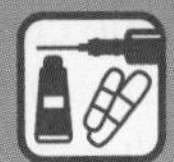 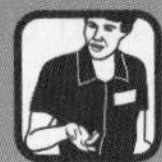  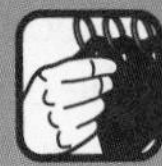 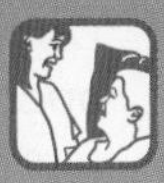 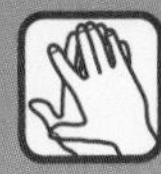 

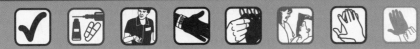

Bladder or catheter irrigation is performed when urine will not drain because debris is blocking the catheter. A bladder instillation is performed to place a medicated solution in the bladder. The catheter and drainage system should not be opened for irrigation unless all other methods have been considered.

Supplies

- Sterile irrigation set
- Basin
- Clean and sterile gloves
- Absorbent pad
- Antiseptic swabs
- Sterile normal saline or ordered irrigation solution
- Sterile 30- to 50-mL syringe with a sterile insertion connector
- Tubing clamp
- Bath blanket

Review and carry out the Standard Steps in Appendix A.

ACTION *(RATIONALE)*

Assessment (Data Collection)

1. Check the order and the patient's care plan. *(Dictates the type and amount of solution to be used.)*
2. Determine what the patient knows about bladder irrigation or instillation. *(Guides patient education.)*

Planning

3. Check the patient's identity wristband. *(Verifies that correct patient is to receive the irrigation.)*
4. Gather the equipment and set up the workspace, raising the bed to working height. *(Promotes work efficiency and prevents back strain.)*
5. Plan sufficient time to perform the irrigation without neglecting other patients. *(Demonstrates good work organization.)*
6. Explain the procedure to the patient. *(Decreases fear of the unknown and elicits patient's cooperation.)*
7. Close the door and/or privacy curtains. *(Protects patient's privacy.)*

Continued

Implementation

8. Perform hand hygiene and lower the side rail if up. *(Reduces transfer of microorganisms.)*
9. Have patient assume a dorsal recumbent position and fanfold the linen to expose the catheter without exposing the patient. Use a bath blanket to cover the trunk of the body. *(Protects dignity.)*
10. Check the bladder for distention by palpation. *(Ensures fluid will not overdistend the bladder.)*
11. Open the sterile irrigation set and place it beside the patient's thigh or between the legs. Maintain sterility. *(Keeps supplies within reach.)*
12. Place the absorbent pad under the catheter drainage tubing connection, handling only the corners of the pad. *(Provides a field within which to work. Protects the bedding.)*
13. Don gloves. *(Reduces transfer of microorganisms.)*
14. For a bladder irrigation or instillation, clamp the drainage tubing distal to the catheter connection. *(Clamping directs solution toward the bladder and prevents solution from draining into collection bag.)*
15. Determine the amount of urine in the drainage bag before beginning the irrigation. *(The amount of urine must be subtracted from the total drainage at the end of the procedure to determine if all the irrigation solution is returned.)*
16. Pour 100 to 200 mL of irrigating solution into the sterile container using aseptic technique. *(Amount depends on medical order or agency policy.)*
17. Draw up 30 to 40 mL of solution into syringe while maintaining sterility. Expel air and attach syringe to sterile insertion connector. *(For irrigation of the adult bladder, 30 to 40 mL is acceptable. Injecting air into the bladder causes discomfort.)*
18. With an antiseptic swab, scrub the port on the drainage tubing for instilling solution. *(Reduces contamination of the system by microorganisms.)*
19. Attach the sterile insertion connector into the port and gently instill the solution. *(Gentle instillation prevents injury to the lining of the bladder and helps prevent bladder spasms.)*
20. Remove the insertion connector from the port and cleanse the port with an antiseptic swab. Place the cap on the connector to maintain sterility of the insertion tip. *(Sterility must be maintained until the entire amount of irrigant has been instilled.)*
21. a. For irrigation, immediately unclamp the tubing and lower the catheter so that the fluid runs into the drainage tubing. *(Irrigating fluid and debris that clog the catheter must flow out.)*
    b. For a bladder instillation, leave tubing clamped for ordered amount of time, then unclamp it and allow the fluid to run into the drainage container. *(Medicine must contact bladder wall before draining.)*

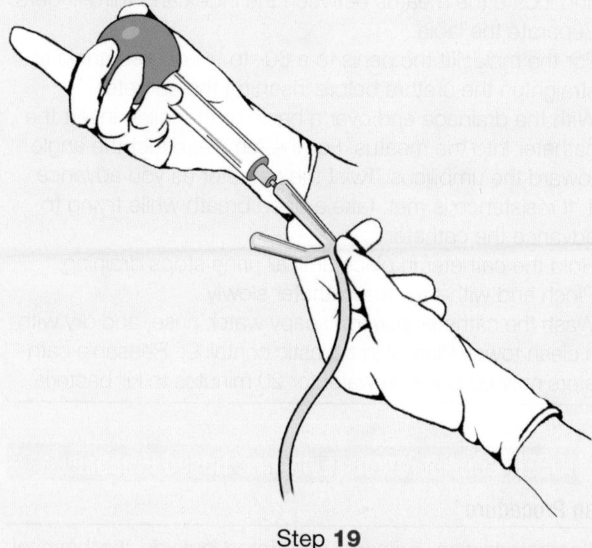

Step 19

22. Repeat the process until all of the ordered solution has been used or until the catheter is clear and the bladder is draining clear urine. *(Accomplishes purpose of the irrigation or instillation.)*
23. Empty the urine drainage bag and measure the output. Note the color and characteristics of the drainage. Enter the amount on the intake and output record. *(Irrigation solution must be deducted from total output to determine actual urine output. Urine color and clarity are compared to baseline.)*
24. Dispose of used equipment, remove gloves, and perform hand hygiene. *(Equipment cannot be reused.)*
25. Make the patient comfortable, lower the bed, raise side rails, and place the call light within reach. Double-check to make certain that the clamp is open at the end of the treatment. *(Urine must flow into drainage bag to prevent blockage that could damage kidneys.)*

Evaluation

26. Assess for changes in discomfort. Ask yourself: Is the catheter draining properly now and is the urine clear and without clots? *(Determines whether the procedure was effective.)*

Documentation

27. Note date, time, irrigation method, amount of solution used each time, appearance of return fluid, how patient tolerated the procedure and whether catheter is patent. *(Verifies procedure was carried out.)*

Documentation Example

Urinary catheter tubing clamped and catheter irrigated ×4 per orders with 40 mL sterile saline using sterile technique. Unclamped between irrigations. Return cloudy with debris ×2, then cleared. Draining adequate urine; no bladder distention. Voiced only mild discomfort with first irrigation. Resting comfortably; bed into lowest position; call light in reach. (Nurse's electronic signature)

Variation: Open System Irrigation

28. Obtain a sterile connector cap. After patient and workspace are prepared (Steps 1 through 16, pp. 565 to 566), perform hand hygiene and don sterile gloves. Be certain there is an order or valid reason for performing an open irrigation. *(Catheter drainage system should not be opened unless there is no other option.)*
29. With an antiseptic swab, disinfect the junction of the catheter and drainage tubing. *(Reduces contamination of the catheter or drainage tubing.)*
30. Placing your fingers at least 1 inch from the junction, separate the catheter and tubing and place a sterile tube cap over the end of the drainage tubing. *(Keeps the end of the drainage tubing sterile.)*
31. Draw up 30- to 40-mL of solution into the sterile irrigation syringe, and carefully fit the tip into the end of the catheter. *(If the syringe is not snug, the pressure of injection may cause disconnection.)*

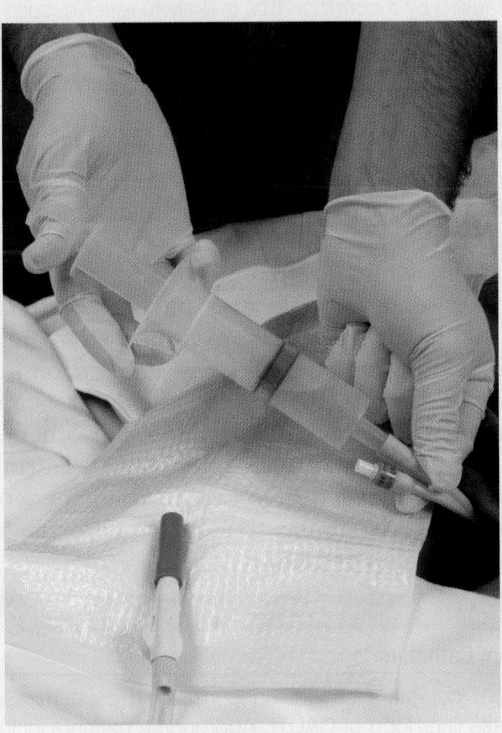

Step 31

32. Gently instill the solution into the catheter by pressing on the plunger. *(Too much force may damage the bladder lining or cause bladder spasms.)*
33. Remove the syringe and allow the fluid to run from the catheter into the sterile drainage receptacle. Repeat until the fluid is running freely or the purpose of the irrigation is accomplished. *(Provides avenue for fluid drainage. A clogged catheter may take several irrigations before it is unclogged.)*
34. Carefully remove the cap on the drainage tubing and reattach it to the catheter, keeping both ends sterile. Swab the connection with an antiseptic swab. *(Sterility of the system must be maintained.)*
35. Remove gloves, perform hand hygiene, and follow the remaining steps as for closed irrigation. *(Reduces transfer of microorganisms.)*

Special Considerations

- When there is no specific solution or amount of solution ordered for the irrigation, check the agency's policy and procedure manual for the accepted protocol.
- Although it is always preferable to use a closed irrigation technique, using the open irrigation method in the home is less likely to lead to an infection than if done in the hospital because there are fewer resident microorganisms in the average home.

Critical Thinking Questions

1. What could happen if the irrigation solution is introduced into the bladder too rapidly?
2. Where should you clamp the indwelling catheter system when doing a closed bladder irrigation?

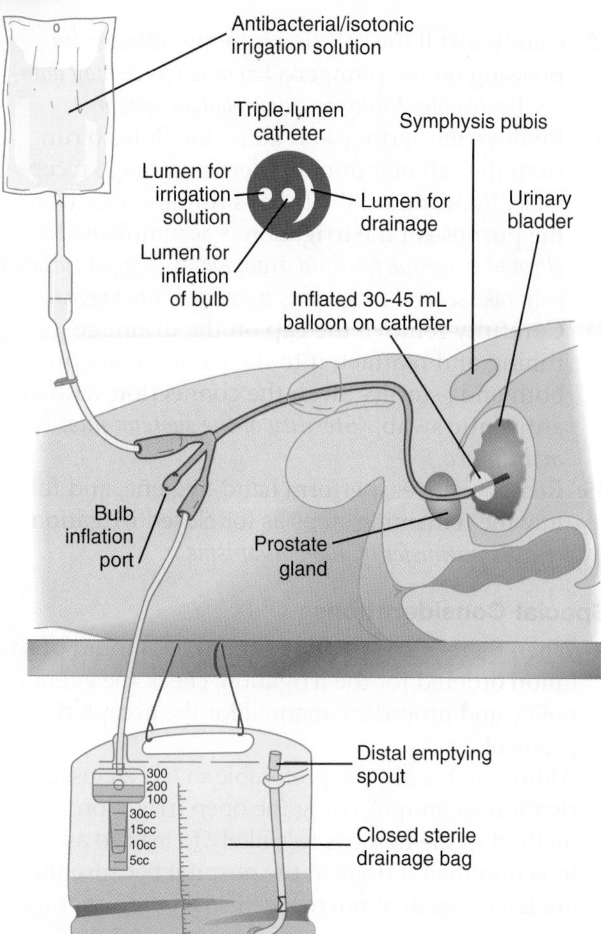

FIGURE 29.11 Continuous bladder irrigation. (From Black, J. M., & Hawks, J. H. [2009]. *Medical-Surgical Nursing: Clinical Management for Positive Outcomes* [8th ed.]. Philadelphia, PA: Saunders.)

forming in the bladder (Fig. 29.11). The return should be pink to light red. The irrigation solution container is changed at least every 24 hours. All irrigation fluid is subtracted from the amount of output.

QSEN Considerations: Evidence-Based Practice

Closed Versus Open Irrigation

Evidence-based practice indicates that closed irrigation is preferable over opening the system (Chenoweth et al., 2015).

When the drainage system must be opened for irrigation, **strict asepsis must be maintained.** Take special care not to contaminate the end of the drainage tubing or the end of the catheter.

Assisting the Patient Who Is Incontinent

There are different types of incontinence: urge, stress, overactive bladder, overflow, functional, mixed, or transient (National Kidney and Urologic Diseases Information Clearinghouse, 2012) (Box 29.4). The incontinent patient suffers a body image disturbance over the loss of a normal function. There is risk of skin breakdown from moisture and waste products in the urine, as well as worry over being wet and smelling of urine. There is also the risk of infection because urine is a medium for bacterial growth. Urinary incontinence may be temporary or permanent.

Management and treatment of incontinence is complex; some patients may have more than one form of incontinence. For example, stress incontinence is often accompanied by urge incontinence. For some patients, better and quicker assistance to the toilet will resolve the problem. For others, continence training may help (Steps 29.3). During the night, incontinence briefs can be used for women. Absorbent pads similar to sanitary napkins can be used for women or men.

Box 29.4 Types of Incontinence

- **Urge incontinence:** Involuntary loss of urine in response to a strong sensation of need to empty the bladder (urinary urgency). This type can be a result of diabetes, a stroke, an infection, or another medical condition.
- **Stress incontinence:** Urethral sphincter failure that is often associated with increased intra-abdominal pressure, as occurs with sneezing, laughing, coughing, and aerobic exercise.
- **Mixed incontinence:** A combination of different types such as stress and urge incontinence.
- **Overactive bladder:** Powerful, immediate urges to urinate frequently and possibly urge incontinence.
- **Overflow incontinence:** Poor contractility of the detrusor muscle of the bladder and obstruction of the urethra may be related to prostate enlargement in the male or genital prolapse or abnormality in the female.
- **Functional incontinence:** Caused by cognitive inability to recognize the urge to urinate, extreme depression, or dementia. Inability to reach the bathroom because of restraints, side rails, or physical impairment can also result in this type of incontinence.
- **Transient incontinence:** Temporary urinary loss caused by a condition that is likely to resolve, such as taking a new medication or coughing because of a cold.

QSEN Considerations: Evidence-Based Practice

Condom Catheters

Condom catheters should be considered as a measure to decrease likelihood of CAUTI. Appropriate patients include incontinent men who are able to understand the purpose of the condom device and who do not have problems with postvoid residual (Chenoweth et al., 2014).

QSEN Considerations: Teamwork and Collaboration

Nursing Assistants Helping With Continence Training

If continence training is in progress, time must be planned to work with the patient and the nursing assistant on this task. Instruct the nursing assistant about timed interval toileting, and work together as a team to clean up accidents.

Steps 29.3 Continence Training

When a patient is experiencing incontinence that is possibly correctable, continence training is implemented to try to correct the problem.

ACTION *(RATIONALE)*

1. Determine the cause of urinary incontinence and whether a continence program is appropriate. *(Bladder training is not appropriate for all types of incontinence.)*
2. Keep a record of actual voiding times for 3 days. *(Provides data about patient's usual voiding times.)*
3. Establish a 2-hour voiding schedule timed before the patient's usual voiding times. *(Having patient void before the bladder overfills prevents incontinence.)*
4. Encourage the intake of 2000 to 3000 mL of fluid between awakening and 6 pm *(Provides sufficient urine for hydration and scheduled voidings. Stopping liquids at 6:00 pm decreases nighttime incontinence.)*
5. Toilet just before bedtime; do not awaken for toileting except before the time when the patient has been consistently incontinent during the night. *(Empties bladder and prevents nighttime incontinence.)*

 QSEN Considerations: Evidence-Based Practice

Kegel Exercises

Regularly performing Kegel exercises may greatly reduce or stop incontinence for some patients (Hall & Woodward, 2015). Several surgical procedures can be used for patients who choose to correct a specific physiologic problem.

 Patient Education

Pelvic Muscle (Kegel) Exercises to Correct Female Incontinence

- Concentrate on stopping the flow of urine when voiding by tightening the pelvic muscles. If you cannot identify the correct muscles this way, place a finger inside your vagina or rectum and try to squeeze around the finger. These are the same muscles you use to keep from expelling gas or a bowel movement. If you are contracting your abdominal muscles, you are doing the exercise incorrectly. Do not hold your breath while contracting and holding.
- To do the exercise, squeeze the muscle you identified and hold for a count of 10 seconds. Relax for a count of 10 seconds. At first you may not be able to hold the contraction for the full 10 seconds. With practice you will build up to the full 10 seconds, usually over a 2-week period.
- Do the exercise three times a day. Try to do 15 repetitions in the morning, 15 in the afternoon, and 20 at night. Or exercise for 10 minutes three times a day. Set a timer. Try to work up to 25 repetitions at one time. It will take at least 2 weeks of consistent exercise to notice a difference. Within a month of regular exercise, you should notice a decrease in instances of incontinence.

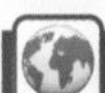 Cultural Considerations

Differences in Musculature and Structure of the Pelvic Floor

Derpapas et al. (2012) detected racial differences in black versus white female anatomy via ultrasound. The researchers concluded that racial differences in musculature and structure of the pelvic floor may affect urinary incontinence. Other studies have demonstrated cultural differences in female anatomy between Caucasian and East Asian pregnant women as well (Cheung et al., 2015).

For those incontinent patients for whom there is no cure, such as people with neurologic damage that prevents sphincter control, you must help the patient stay dry and clean and preserve his dignity.

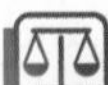 Legal and Ethical Considerations

Preserving Patients' Dignity and Rights in Toileting

The Patients Association and Nursing Standard launched a campaign in 2011 (Buswell, 2013) that addressed the primary concerns that patients and their families have about care. They focused on helping with toileting while maintaining dignity, especially for patients with impaired sight and dementia. One of their recommendations was to improve signage so that patients could more easily find the toilets. In addition, patients deserve to use clean facilities or equipment in a timely, safe fashion, and attention should be given to their views and preferences.

Urinary Diversion Care

Urinary diversion is necessary when the bladder must be removed or bypassed for some reason. When urinary diversion is performed, one or both ureters are implanted into the abdominal wall, the bowel, or a portion of bowel that forms a pouch. When the ureter exits on the abdominal wall, discharging urine through the opening, it is called a **urostomy** (opening through which urine drains). Collection of the draining urine and care of the skin around the urostomy are nursing responsibilities. Unless the urostomy is constructed with an internal pouch and valve, urine drains constantly. When changing the urostomy bag, place a tampon in the opening while you clean the skin and prepare the clean urostomy bag. The urostomy with an internal pouch is emptied by the insertion of a catheter. Urine contains ammonia, which is irritating to the skin, and a skin barrier is applied before attaching the collection appliance. Because bowel ostomies are more common than urostomies, particulars of skin care and changing the ostomy bag (appliance) are presented in Chapter 30.

◆ EVALUATION

Review the expected outcomes written during the planning phase to properly evaluate the effectiveness of interventions for the patient's problems. Determine whether the patient can urinate normally without urgency, dysuria, or frequency. A urinalysis may be performed after treatment is complete or when an indwelling urinary catheter is removed, to check for presence or resolution of infection. Recording I & O and comparing data from day to day indicate whether fluid intake is sufficient and output is adequate. Noting the perineal skin condition of the incontinent patient provides information as to whether measures to protect the skin are sufficient. Evidence that the patient has had fewer episodes of incontinence over time indicates that the continence training program is helpful. Checking the urine appearance for normal characteristics is another evaluation tool.

Obtain feedback for all patient education performed. Can the patient tell you measures to take to prevent UTIs? Can the patient who needs intermittent self-catheterization successfully perform the procedure? Does the patient, or the family member of the patient at home, know how to care for the catheter and empty the collection bag properly? Is the patient in the long-term care facility who has functional incontinence now receiving the needed assistance? Nursing Care Plan 29.1 provides some specific examples of evaluative statements for expected outcomes.

Documentation

When a patient voids normally and without problems in adequate amounts, include a short note of "voiding quantity sufficient and without verbalized complaints." If a patient has problems with urinary elimination, document the number of voidings per day, the amount of urinary output, and the appearance of the urine. When a patient is catheterized, note the appearance of the urine returned from the catheter and any problems encountered during the procedure. The size and type of catheter are documented, along with the amount of water instilled in the catheter balloon. A description of the urine should be documented at least once a day when a patient has an indwelling catheter; include signs of infection or resolution of infection.

For the incontinent patient, note the number of normal voidings and the time and circumstances of incontinent voidings. The assessment of the perineal skin is documented at least once a shift.

All patient education is documented in the medical record, as are all diagnostic tests and specimens obtained, urostomy care, and the condition of the stoma and the surrounding skin.

If a bladder irrigation or instillation is performed, document the amount of solution instilled, whether aseptic technique was maintained, the time the fluid remained in the bladder, the amount and description of the outflow, and any problems encountered. When an indwelling catheter is removed, document the time, the date, and the amount of urine in the drainage bag; include the time by which the patient should void (within 8 hours). Document any problems the patient has voiding after catheter removal and any follow-up measures that were performed.

Get Ready for the NCLEX Examination!

Key Points

- The kidneys, the ureters, the bladder, and the urethra make up the urinary system, which functions to rid the body of waste and excess fluid. Fluid balance is a primary function of the kidneys.
- Infection, severe dehydration, shock, destruction of tissue, blockage, pressure, and lack of neurologic innervation can interfere with proper function of the urinary system.
- Kidney function and bladder muscle tone decrease with age. In males, the prostate gland can enlarge and may lead to urethral obstruction.
- Urination is under voluntary control. The adult voids 5 to 10 times a day, ridding the body of an average of 1 to 1.5 L of urine a day.
- Symptoms of urinary dysfunction are dysuria, urgency, anuria, polyuria, oliguria, retention, and difficulty starting the urinary stream.
- Urine specimens are obtained in different ways (e.g., clean catch and catheterization) for a variety of diagnostic tests (e.g., culture and sensitivity).
- An indwelling urinary catheter is inserted for a variety of reasons (e.g., urinary stricture and bladder irrigation). The closed urinary catheter and drainage system should be kept sterile.
- It is best to perform closed intermittent irrigation, rather than opening the drainage system, to prevent microorganisms from entering the bladder.
- There are different types of incontinence: urge, stress, overactive bladder, overflow, functional, mixed, or transient; interventions must be tailored to the cause.
- When the patient has a urinary diversion, the focus is on collection of the urine and care of the skin around the urostomy.
- Comparison of daily I & O is part of the evaluation process.

Additional Learning Resources

SG Go to your Study Guide for additional learning activities to help you master this chapter content.

evolve Go to your Evolve website at http://evolve.elsevier.com/Williams/fundamental for additional online resources.

Online Resources

- *Urodry (example of new design of condom catheter),* www.urodry.com
- *National Association for Continence,* www.nafc.org

Review Questions for the NCLEX Examination

*Choose the **best** answer for each question.*

1. A nurse is caring for a patient who is incontinent. What is the **priority** action?
   1. Help the patient void every 2 hours.
   2. Decrease the fluid intake, especially in the evening.
   3. Gather data to find the cause of incontinence.
   4. Encourage expression of feelings of embarrassment.
2. The nurse has just collected a midstream urine specimen from a patient. Which urine characteristic would be of the **greatest** concern?
   1. Urine smells slightly of ammonia.
   2. Urine is dilute.
   3. Urine is slightly cloudy.
   4. Urine is dark brown.
3. A patient is admitted with urinary retention. There is an order to insert an indwelling urinary catheter into his bladder. He attempts to void and passes 100 mL of urine. Before catheterization, the nurse should:
   1. Use a condom catheter with a leg bag.
   2. Wait 2 hours and have him try to void again.
   3. Have him drink two to three glasses of water.
   4. Perform a bladder scan to determine the amount of urine retained.
4. The nurse is catheterizing a male patient. Resistance is met. The nurse should:
   1. Apply more pressure with a twisting motion to insert the catheter.
   2. Obtain a new sterile kit and try again with a sterile Coudé catheter.
   3. Ask him to take a deep breath and slowly exhale as the catheter is inserted.
   4. Discontinue the procedure and try again after the patient relaxes.
5. The nurse must perform a bladder irrigation to instill medication. During the procedure, the tube will have to be clamped. What is the **best** rationale for clamping the tubing?
   1. Follows the standard procedure
   2. Ensures that sterility of the system is maintained
   3. Prevents the solution from going directly into the bag
   4. Prevents urine from being drawn back into the catheter
6. Which statement by the patient indicates an understanding of how to perform the clean-catch method for a urine specimen?
   1. "I should clean my genital area first, pee into the cup, and then clean myself."
   2. "I should fill the cup completely and save it in the refrigerator."
   3. "I should keep the contents of the kit sterile at all times."
   4. "I should clean myself first, pee a little into the toilet, and then pee into the cup."
7. The patient had a resection of the prostate gland yesterday and has a three-way catheter for continuous irrigation. The draining urine is increasingly red. This means that the nurse needs to:
   1. Notify the surgeon immediately.
   2. Increase the rate of flow of the irrigation solution.
   3. Increase his fluid intake to 4000 mL/24 hour.
   4. Empty the drainage bag to prevent clotting.
8. A 24-hour urine specimen is ordered for a patient. The nursing assistant discards some of the urine that should have been saved. Which is the most appropriate nursing action?
   1. Verbally reprimand the nursing assistant.
   2. Make a note to extend the urine collection period.
   3. Continue the urine collection and label the specimen.
   4. Notify the charge nurse and restart the test.

Critical Thinking Activities

Read each clinical scenario and discuss the questions with your classmates.

Scenario A

A patient comes into clinic and says to you, "I think I have a urinary tract infection. Can I get a prescription for antibiotics?" What assessment data would you need to determine whether the patient has a UTI?

Scenario B

You are caring for a patient who needs to have an indwelling urinary catheter inserted before going to radiology for diagnostic testing. How would you explain to a patient what a catheterization procedure is like?

Scenario C

Mrs. Jones returned from surgery 6 hours ago. She states, "My bladder feels full, but I can't urinate." What measures would you use to help a patient urinate?

Scenario D

You are caring for two older adult patients, Mr. Borders and Mrs. Pendragon. Both patients need to have a retention catheter inserted. Mr. Borders needs a catheter because he is having trouble passing urine because of an enlarged prostate. He is slightly confused, but is cooperative with repetitive coaching. Mrs. Pendragon needs a retention catheter because she is scheduled for surgery. She is very obese, but cooperative and coherent. Compare and contrast the issues that you will need to address related to catheter insertion for these two patients.

chapter

30 Promoting Bowel Elimination

http://evolve.elsevier.com/Williams/fundamental

Objectives

Upon completing this chapter, you should be able to do the following:

Theory

1. Describe the process of normal bowel elimination.
2. Identify abnormal stool characteristics.
3. Summarize the physiologic effects of hypoactive bowel, as well as nursing interventions to assist patients with constipation.
4. Analyze safety considerations related to giving a patient an enema.
5. Analyze the psychosocial implications for a patient who has an ostomy.
6. Discuss the stoma and periostomal assessment and skin care.
7. Describe three types of intestinal diversions.

Clinical Practice

1. Summarize nursing measures to promote regular bowel elimination in patients.
2. Collect a stool specimen.
3. Perform a focused assessment of bowel function.
4. Write a nursing care plan for a patient with bowel problems.
5. Prepare to administer an enema.
6. Assist and teach a patient with a bowel retraining program for incontinence.
7. Evaluate the performance of a patient who is self-catheterizing a continent diversion.
8. Provide ostomy care, including irrigation and changing the ostomy appliance.

Skills & Steps

Skills

Steps

Key Terms

anus (Ā-nŭs, p. 573)
appliances (p. 585)
atrophy (Ă-trō-fē, p. 574)
bile (BĪL, p. 574)
bowel training program (p. 584)
chyme (KĪM, p. 573)
colostomy (kŏ-LŎS-tō-mē, p. 587)
constipation (p. 575)
defecate (DĔF-ĕ-kāt, p. 573)
diarrhea (dī-ă-RĒ-ă, p. 576)
effluent (ĕ-FLŪ-ĕnt, p. 587)
excoriation (ĕks-kŏr-ē-Ā-shŭn, p. 579)
fecal impaction (FĒ-kăl ĭm-PĂK-shŭn, p. 576)
fecal incontinence (ĭn-KŎN-tĭ-nĕns, p. 576)
feces (FĒ-sēz, p. 573)
flatus (FLĀ-tŭs, p. 575)
gastrocolic reflex (găs-trō-KŎL-ĭk RĒ-flĕks, p. 573)
hemorrhoid (HĔM-ō-rŏyd, p. 574)
ileostomy (ĭl-ē-ŎS-tō-mē, p. 587)
melena (MĔL-ĕh-nă, p. 574)
occult (ŏ-KŬLT, p. 574)
ostomy (ŎS-tō-mē, p. 585)
paralytic ileus (păr-ă-LĪ-tĭk ĭl-e-ŭs, p. 574)
periostomal (pĕr-ĭ-Ŏ-stō-mŭl, p. 587)
peristalsis (pĕr-ĭ-stăl-sĭs, p. 573)
rectum (RĔK-tŭm, p. 573)
sphincter (SFĬNK-tĕr, p. 573)
steatorrhea (STĒ-ă-tŏ-RĒ-ă, p. 574)
stoma (STŌ-mă, p. 585)
stool (p. 573)
vagal response (VĀ-găl rĕ-SPŎNS, p. 584)
Valsalva maneuver (văl-SĂL-vă mă-NŪ-vĕr, p. 573)

Concepts Covered in This Chapter

- Anxiety
- Culture
- Elimination
- Evidence
- Fluid and electrolyte balance
- Infection
- Inflammation
- Mobility
- Pain
- Patient education
- Safety

The term *bowel* refers to the intestine. Bowel elimination, the excretion of solid waste, is the final step in the process of digestion. The processing of nutrients through digestion is discussed in Chapter 26. There are ways to assist the patient in achieving and maintaining regular elimination of **stool** (waste matter from the bowel) and procedures to alleviate problems related to alterations in elimination. When an alternative for waste elimination is needed because of disease of the intestine, an ostomy (opening into the intestine for outflow) may be performed.

OVERVIEW OF THE STRUCTURE AND FUNCTION OF THE INTESTINAL SYSTEM

WHICH STRUCTURES OF THE INTESTINAL SYSTEM ARE INVOLVED IN WASTE ELIMINATION?

- The small intestine—consisting of the duodenum, the jejunum, and the ileum—carries **chyme** (liquefied food and digestive juices) from the stomach to the large intestine.
- The small intestine attaches to the large intestine at the cecum. The ileocecal valve controls the progress of substances into the large intestine.
- The large intestine has four main sections: the ascending colon, transverse colon, descending colon, and sigmoid colon. It is larger in diameter than the small intestine but only about 59 inches (1.5 meters) long (Fig. 30.1).
- The **rectum** (distal portion of the large intestine where feces are stored) connects to the **anus** (opening of the rectum at the skin).
- The walls of the intestines have four layers: mucosa, submucosa, muscular layer, and a serous layer called the serosa.

WHAT ARE THE FUNCTIONS OF THE INTESTINES?

- The small intestine further processes chyme into a more liquid state. Food substances are absorbed into the bloodstream from the villi on the walls of the small intestine.
- In the large intestine, water, sodium, and chlorides are reabsorbed, and waste material is propelled to the anus.
- The large intestine contains bacteria that break down waste products. Water is extracted from the waste during transit.
- **Peristalsis** (wavelike movement through the intestines) moves chyme and gas formed by bacterial action through the intestines. The circular, longitudinal, and oblique muscle layers of the intestine expand and contract to accommodate and move the chyme.
- The movement of liquid and gas causes the rumbling noise of bowel sounds. It takes about 18 to 72 hours for food to move from the mouth to the anus.
- **Feces** (intestinal waste material) are stored in the sigmoid colon until they move into the rectum for expulsion through the anus.
- As the rectum fills, the pressure on the **sphincter** (circular muscle that closes an orifice) of the anus increases until the urge to **defecate** (expel feces) occurs.
- The abdominal muscles contract to help force the evacuation of the rectum.
- The internal anal sphincter, located at the top of the anal canal, is under involuntary control; the external anal sphincter at the end of the anal canal is controlled voluntarily.
- The **gastrocolic** (stomach to colon) **reflex** initiates peristalsis, which in turn initiates the urge to defecate; it is stimulated by eating. Reflex emptying of the rectum can be stopped by tightening the voluntary anal sphincter.
- Intra-abdominal pressure increases when a person holds the breath, closes the glottis, and tightens the abdominal muscles. This initiates voluntary defecation and is called the **Valsalva maneuver**.
- The vermiform appendix attaches to the cecum of the ascending colon, and it has no known digestive function.

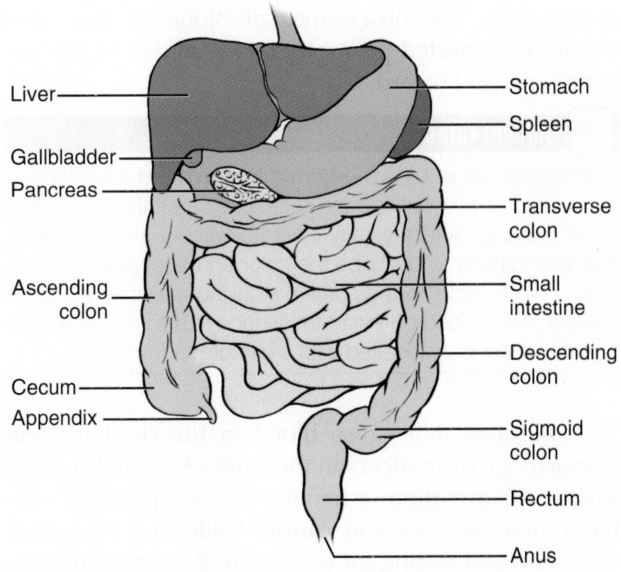

FIGURE 30.1 The intestinal system.

WHAT EFFECT DOES AGING HAVE ON THE INTESTINAL TRACT?

- **Atrophy** (decrease in size) of the villi in the small intestine may decrease the total absorptive surface. However, it has not been proven that decreased absorption of nutrients, other than fats and vitamin B_{12}, actually occurs.
- Sometimes twisting of blood vessels supplying the large intestine compromises the blood flow to the large intestine. Motility in the large intestine may decrease in some individuals, but bowel habits do not change with aging in the healthy individual.

CHARACTERISTICS OF STOOL

Stool is another term for *feces.* Normal feces are one-quarter solid material and three-quarters water. The solid material consists of about 30% dead bacteria and 70% undigested roughage from carbohydrate, fat, protein, and inorganic matter. The appearance of stool is influenced by diet and metabolism.

NORMAL CHARACTERISTICS OF STOOL

Normal stool is light to dark brown, soft, and formed in children and adults. Infant stool may be dark yellow and unformed, depending on the type of feedings. The light to dark brown color is caused by **bile** (orange or yellow digestive fluid produced by the liver). The color of feces may be changed by certain vitamins, drugs, or diet. Stool is usually tubular in shape and has a diameter of about 1 inch (2.5 cm).

ABNORMAL CHARACTERISTICS OF STOOL

The most serious abnormality is blood in the stool. Fresh blood in the stool is easily visible as bright red on the surface of the stool. **Occult** (hidden) or old blood is suspected when the stool changes from a normal brown appearance to a dark black color with a sticky appearance. The observance of blood in the stool should be reported promptly and recorded in the patient's medical record.

Clinical Cues

A small amount of bleeding from a **hemorrhoid** (an enlarged vein inside or just outside the rectum) or an irritation caused by straining to defecate may clear up without any treatment. Ask your patient to describe the color and appearance of the stool. For example, formed brown stool (normal) that has small streaks of red blood on the outer surface of the stool suggests that the blood is associated with a hemorrhoid.

Conditions that cause blood in the stool include hemorrhage from ulcers in the stomach or duodenum; severe inflammation or irritation, as in ulcerative colitis or diverticulitis; and cancer. Collection of a stool specimen and testing for occult blood are presented in Chapter 24.

Bright red blood mixed in the stool is a sign of a recent gastrointestinal (GI) bleeding that has occurred in the large intestine. The color indicates that the blood has not undergone digestion in the upper part of the bowel, nor has it been in the intestinal tract for a prolonged time. Eating red foods, such as beets, may make the stool appear red, so a dietary assessment is essential. As blood moves through the stomach or small intestine, it undergoes partial digestion, which changes it to a dark, tarry substance **(melena)**.

Pale white or light gray stool indicates an absence of bile in the intestine. This is usually due to an obstruction in the bile or common duct leading to the intestine from the liver and gallbladder.

Other abnormal characteristics of feces are the presence of large amounts of mucus, fat, purulent matter, or parasites, such as worms. Unusual amounts of mucus in the stool indicate an irritation or inflammation of the inner surface of the intestines. The mucus coats the stool and gives it a slimy appearance. Stools with an abnormally high fat content **(steatorrhea)** are usually foul smelling and float on water. The presence of purulent material indicates drainage of an ulcer that is inflamed or infected. The most common parasitic worms found in the intestines are the tapeworm, pinworm, and roundworm.

Clinical Cues

Pinworms

Younger children may get pinworms, but may be unable to describe the itching sensation in the anal area. One way for parents to check for pinworms is to use a flashlight and observe the anus at night. The worms will appear as small threadlike filaments around the anus and will withdraw when exposed to a flash of light.

The first signs of colorectal cancer are changes in bowel patterns and stool characteristics. In accordance with the *Healthy People 2020* objectives to reduce colorectal cancers, patients should be encouraged to report these changes and to participate in colon cancer screening programs, which include an annual stool test for occult blood. Evidence-based practice indicates that, beginning at the age of 50, colonoscopy is recommended every 10 years (Hande, 2014). Those with risk factors may need more frequent testing starting at an earlier age (American Cancer Society, 2013). 

HYPOACTIVE BOWEL AND CONSTIPATION

An absence or reduction of peristaltic movement of the bowel results in a hypoactive bowel. Some injuries and diseases cause a hypoactive bowel, but often this condition is a complication of immobility. In addition, after abdominal surgery, patients can develop a **paralytic ileus;** peristalsis stops because the bowel has been manipulated during surgery. In the normal person, lack of sufficient dietary fiber and decreased exercise may produce a sluggish or hypoactive bowel. Encouraging an increase in fiber sources, such as fruit, vegetables, and whole grains, is in accordance with *Healthy People 2020* objectives. Sometimes irritable bowel syndrome (IBS) causes hypoactivity of the bowel, although hyperactivity is more common.

Health Promotion

Promoting Regular Bowel Elimination

Instruct the patient to:

- Pay attention to the urge to defecate; frequently postponing defecation can lead to constipation.
- Eat a diet high in fiber. Foods that provide fiber are bran, whole grain cereals, nuts, prunes, and other raw fruits and vegetables; cooked vegetables provide some fiber (Hall, 2014) (see Table 26.1). Avoid excessive amounts of constipating foods such as cheese, pasta, eggs, and lean meat.
- Drink at least eight 8-oz glasses of liquid each day.
- Exercise every day; walking is excellent for stimulating bowel function.
- Attempt to defecate when the gastrocolic reflex is strongest (e.g., after breakfast).
- Use aids such as drinking a hot cup of coffee, hot water and lemon juice, or prune juice to aid defecation.
- Establish a pattern by attempting defecation at the same time each day.

Constipation (decreased frequency of bowel movement or passage of hard, dry feces) is the most common problem of a hypoactive bowel. With constipation, feces become more compacted and hardened, making them more difficult to expel. Feces tend to back up into the colon. Constipation may occur when muscle tone is lacking; when bowel movements are irregular; or when excessive worry, anxiety, or fear is present.

Box 30.1 Medications that May Cause or Contribute to Constipation

- **Narcotic analgesics,** especially codeine, morphine, and meperidine, depress central nervous system (CNS) activity and slow peristalsis.
- **General anesthetics** slow peristalsis by depressing CNS activity.
- **Diuretics** rid the body of fluid.
- **Sedatives** slow CNS activity and peristalsis.
- **Antidepressants** alter CNS activity and have a drying effect.
- **Anticholinergics** interfere with muscle activation, causing decreased tone in and motility of the gastrointestinal tract, and have drying effects.
- **Calcium channel blockers** cause a blockade of calcium channels, which affects the smooth muscle of the intestine.

Nurses must be aware of the potential of illness-induced constipation. **Any patient restricted to bed rest is at risk for constipation.** Many medications (Box 30.1), barium x-ray studies, or recovery from surgery can contribute to constipation. Patients at risk for constipation should be identified early (Concept Map 30.1).

Abdominal distention is caused by **flatus** (gas) accumulation in the intestinal tract when peristalsis is reduced or absent. Just as fecal matter will collect in the hypoactive bowel, so will flatus. Distention and gas pains occur frequently after abdominal surgery. The discomfort and pain are caused by the stretching of the intestinal wall and spasm of the muscle layers.

Think Critically

Your older female patient had abdominal surgery yesterday. You need to know when she starts passing gas and the frequency and consistency of bowel movements, but she says she would be too embarrassed to talk about this, even with a nurse. What could you say to her?

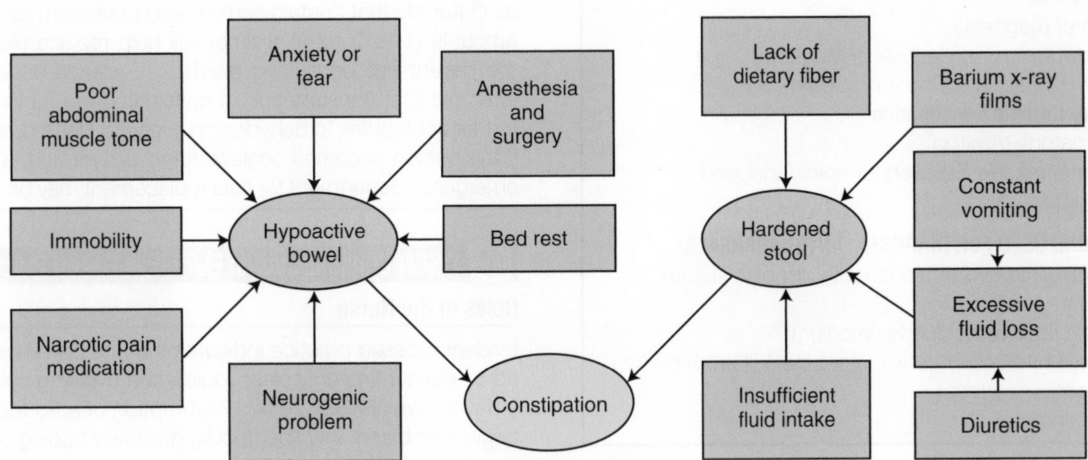

CONCEPT MAP 30.1 Factors contributing to constipation.

Life-Span Considerations

Older Adult

- Older adults who live alone tend to eat more processed convenience foods and do not take in sufficient fiber; therefore they may be more prone to constipation.
- Many older adults decrease fluid intake because they have urinary urgency or stress incontinence. The underlying problem may have to be addressed to establish better fluid intake and softer stool.
- Evidence-based practice indicates that older adult patients should be assessed for polypharmacy, which contributes to constipation. Older adults are also more likely to use over-the-counter laxatives to treat themselves (Rao, 2015).
- Older adults who have been regularly taking mineral oil to aid evacuation must be told that mineral oil interferes with vitamin absorption. Bulk-forming laxatives containing psyllium are a better choice.
- Products such as Metamucil and Benefiber are readily available without prescription. **A large amount of fluid should be taken with these products to prevent constipation and fecal impaction** (the rectum and sigmoid colon becoming filled with hardened fecal material). Box 30.2 lists common medications used for constipation.

Box 30.2 Common Medications Used for Constipation or Diarrhea

MEDICATIONS USED FOR CONSTIPATION

Stool Softeners

- Docusate sodium (Colace)
- Docusate calcium (Surfak)
- Docusate potassium (Dialose)
- Polyethylene glycol–electrolyte solution (MiraLAX)

Bulk-Forming Laxatives

- Polycarbophil (FiberCon)
- Psyllium (Metamucil)
- Methylcellulose (Citrucel)

Irritant or Stimulant Laxatives

- Bisacodyl (Dulcolax and Correctol)
- Cascara sagrada
- Senna (Senokot)
- Sennosides (Ex-Lax)

Saline Laxatives

- Citrate of magnesia
- Magnesium hydroxide (Milk of Magnesia)
- Sodium phosphate (Phospho-Soda)

Laxative for Chronic Constipation

- Lubiprostone (Amitiza)*
- Methylnaltrexone (Relistor) for opioid-induced constipation

MEDICATIONS USED FOR DIARRHEA (ANTIDIARRHEALS)

- Diphenoxylate hydrochloride with atropine sulfate (Lomotil)
- Loperamide hydrochloride (Imodium)
- Difenoxin hydrochloride with atropine sulfate (Motofen)
- Paregoric
- Opium tincture

*Research suggests that Lubiprostone (Amitiza) may be appropriate for opioid-induced constipation without reduction in dosage pain medication (Prichard and Bharucha, 2015)

HYPERACTIVE BOWEL AND DIARRHEA

Increased motility of the GI tract or increased peristalsis results in a hyperactive bowel. Causes of a hyperactive bowel include inflammation in the GI tract, certain drugs, infectious agents, and diseases such as diverticulitis, ulcerative colitis, Crohn disease, and IBS. Patients who have gastric bypass surgery may also experience **diarrhea** (frequent loose stool).

Diarrhea occurs when increased peristalsis pushes food through the intestinal tract too quickly. The increased speed does not allow enough time for the absorption of nutrients, electrolytes, and water, and the feces are liquid or semiformed. Evacuations are more frequent, with an increased number of stools per day. Often, diarrhea is simply the body trying to rid itself of pathogens or toxins from spoiled food. Moderate diarrhea lasting a couple of days usually clears up by itself. At times, diarrhea can lead to temporary **fecal incontinence** (the lack of voluntary control over the anal sphincter) and inability to retain feces. See Box 30.2 for a list of common antidiarrheal medications.

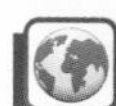

Cultural Considerations

Hand Hygiene to Prevent Diarrhea

According to the Centers for Disease Control and Prevention (CDC, 2013), 2195 children die of diarrheal disease every day. Preventing transmission of diarrheal organisms through good handwashing is essential. Kamm et al. (2014) conducted a study to determine the relationship between providing handwashing stations and soap and preventing diarrhea in Kenya. They found that having soap available reduced diarrhea, whereas handwashing stations alone did not decrease diarrhea. Most homes had soap, but almost none had a handwashing station. Use of culturally relevant information is important when conducting patient education, even for basic measures such as good handwashing with soap.

Life-Span Considerations

Older Adult

Older adults become dehydrated more quickly than younger adults do. Observe closely for signs of dehydration and fluid imbalance when diarrhea occurs. Commercial beverages such as Gatorade that contain sodium and potassium taken in small amounts (1 to 2 oz at a time) will help replace electrolytes if the patient has continuing diarrhea. Evidence-based practice indicates that consumption of caffeinated tea, coffee, or soda further contributes to dehydration (Harvard Health Letter, 2014). If the person becomes confused and dehydrated, a trip to the emergency department for fluid replacement may be necessary.

QSEN Considerations: Evidence-Based Practice

Roles of the Nurse

Evidence-based practice indicates that the bowel can be rested by consuming only clear liquids and avoiding solid food for a day or two (IFFGD, 2014). Resumption of solid foods should begin with bland, low fiber foods, gradually adding other foods as tolerated. Cottage cheese, gelatin, applesauce, and bananas are usually tolerated well.

FECAL INCONTINENCE

People of all ages may become incontinent of feces because of illness such as a stroke, traumatic injury, or neurogenic dysfunction. Incontinence is a distressing condition that causes a loss of dignity, embarrassment, or anxiety. People can also experience loss of self-respect or fear of loss of control. It is important to reassure them that there are measures available to assist them with the problem.

Life-Span Considerations

Older Adult

Older adults have a higher incidence of fecal incontinence related to medications, constipation, or impaired neurologic or cognitive function. Institutionalized older adults are more likely to have problems compared with those who live at home (Gillibrand, 2012). Be aware that prolonged constipation can cause fecal impaction. Small amounts of watery incontinence that seep from around the stool plug can be a sign of impaction.

❖ APPLICATION OF THE NURSING PROCESS

◆ ASSESSMENT (DATA COLLECTION)

Every patient is assessed regarding bowel status every day in an inpatient facility. Home care nurses assess bowel status at each visit. The patient is questioned about the regularity of bowel evacuation, problems, and any abnormal characteristics of the stool. If possible, the stool is visually examined. The Focused Assessment box provides guidelines for bowel assessment. Many people think that it is abnormal not to have a bowel movement every day, but having a bowel movement only every 2 or 3 days is normal for some people. Look at all the factors that affect bowel function and the patient's normal pattern before determining whether there is a problem.

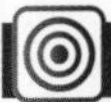

Focused Assessment

Assessment of the Bowel

Use the following points or questions in assessing bowel function and habits.

HISTORY

- Determine the usual bowel pattern, time of defecation, and measures used to promote defecation, if any (e.g., a cup of coffee, breakfast, dose of Metamucil).
- Inquire about use of enemas, laxatives, suppositories, and stool softeners.
- Assess for changes in stool characteristics: alternating diarrhea and constipation, changes in stool shape, changes in stool color, stool floating in commode, or foul odor.
- Determine usual eating habits and dietary intake. Is there sufficient fiber in the diet? Does the patient drink sufficient fluids?
- How much exercise does the patient get?
- Is the patient taking medications that may cause constipation or diarrhea?
- Does the patient have a chronic disorder that contributes to constipation or diarrhea?
- Has there been any exposure to parasites or helminths (especially during travel outside the United States)?
- Does diarrhea occur after eating milk products (may indicate lactose intolerance)?
- Does diarrhea occur after eating wheat and other gluten products (may indicate sprue or gluten intolerance)?
- Does the patient have any food sensitivities? Do spicy foods cause gas discomfort or diarrhea?
- Has incontinence been brought on by a neurologic condition or stroke?
- Is the incontinent patient receptive to a bowel training program?

PHYSICAL ASSESSMENT

- Observe the shape of the abdomen with the patient supine.
- Auscultate for bowel sounds in all four quadrants.
- Percuss for presence of excessive air (gas) in the bowel.
- Gently palpate for masses or tenderness in all four quadrants.

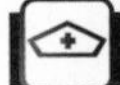

Clinical Cues

Place the patient in a supine position. Auscultate for bowel sounds in all four quadrants. Absent or few bowel sounds indicate decreased motility and potential for constipation, or may signal an abnormal bowel blockage. Active bowel sounds are associated with the increased motility that occurs after eating. Loud hyperactive sounds, called borborygmi, can occur with diarrhea (IFFGD, 2015).

Distention is revealed by an abdomen that is rounder and tighter in appearance than normal. The patient's abdomen is assessed for distention by percussion, and the nurse gently palpates the four quadrants of the abdomen to check for tenderness and masses (Lewis et al., 2014). The patient may complain of abdominal discomfort and often describes it as gas pain. Percussion is used to detect abnormal amounts of gas. Areas of gas produce a drum-like, hollow tone. Review assessment of the abdomen in Chapter 22.

◆ NURSING DIAGNOSIS

When assessment data indicate an intestinal problem, nursing diagnoses are based on the North American Nursing Diagnosis Association-International (NANDA-I) list. Possible choices include:

- Constipation related to hypoactive bowel
- Diarrhea related to food intolerance
- Bowel incontinence related to loss of anal sphincter control
- Acute pain related to abdominal distention
- Self-care deficit, toileting related to body cast
- Disturbed body image related to bowel incontinence
- Deficient knowledge related to factors that contribute to constipation

◆ PLANNING

A care plan is developed by writing short- or long-term expected outcomes for each nursing diagnosis chosen.

Sample expected outcomes for the previous nursing diagnoses are:

- Constipation will be relieved by walking 1 mile each day.
- Episodes of diarrhea will decrease within 3 days.
- Patient will improve bowel control within 2 months of starting a retraining program.
- Pain from distention will be decreased within 24 hours.
- Patient will use an over-the-bed trapeze and a urinal during this shift.
- Body image will improve as incontinence lessens.
- Patient will identify foods to add to the diet to increase fiber during this shift.

See Nursing Care Plan 30.1 for further examples of expected outcomes.

Ordered treatments, such as enemas, may take extra time. When an incontinent patient is assigned, more time must be allotted for attempts at toileting, for cleaning the patient after accidents, and for bowel training, if appropriate.

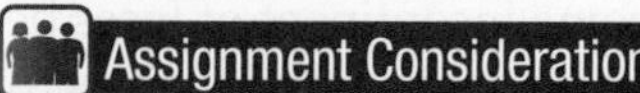

Patient Ambulation

The task of assisting with ambulation is frequently assigned to the nursing assistant. If the patient resists the idea of getting out of bed or ambulating, support the nursing assistant by giving the patient some concrete examples of the benefits (e.g., getting up and walking decreases the risk of pneumonia, deep vein thrombosis, pressure injuries, and constipation). Remember to thank the assistant for his hard work and contributions to the patient's well-being.

◆ IMPLEMENTATION

You must assist the patient on bed rest with use of the bedpan or bedside commode. **Privacy is important.** Patients are often embarrassed by the sounds and smells accompanying defecation of feces. Patients should be

Nursing Care Plan 30.1 Care of the Patient with Constipation

SCENARIO Martina Svoboda, age 64, fractured her left hip in a fall a month ago. Her hip is healing, but she still has difficulty walking. While in the hospital, her usual bowel pattern became disrupted. She has had difficulty with constipation ever since *("having difficulty with bowels")*. She is currently staying at her daughter's home. The stool is hard and dry; she normally has a bowel movement every third day.

PROBLEM/NURSING DIAGNOSIS *Bowel movement pattern changed since hospitalization*/Constipation related to immobility.

Supporting Assessment Data *Subjective:* States … "is having difficulty with bowels." *Objective:* Stool is hard and dry.

Goals/Expected Outcomes	Nursing Interventions	Selected Rationale	Evaluation
Constipation will be relieved by medication within 2 days. Usual bowel pattern will be reestablished within 2 to 3 weeks.	Obtain history of bowel pattern before accident and hip fracture.	History provides baseline for choosing interventions.	*Is the patient making progress toward reestablishing the usual bowel pattern?*
	Assess dietary and fluid intake.	Assists in determining whether enough fluid and fiber is being consumed.	
	Teach ways to increase fiber in the diet (e.g., raw fruits and vegetables; whole grain breads).	Knowledge promotes correct food choices.	States will have oatmeal for breakfast with fresh fruit.
	Increase fluid intake to 1500 mL/day.	Fluid keeps stool soft.	Dislikes drinking too much water: "I don't like plain water."
	Use stool softeners at bedtime for 1 week.	Stool softeners promote softer stool.	Taking stool softener each evening.
	Encourage walking and abdominal muscle-setting exercises.	Muscle strengthening assists with evacuation efforts.	Attending physical therapy three times a week. Starting exercise program.
	Work with family in providing regular, unhurried bathroom time.	Helps to establish a daily evacuation pattern.	Progressing toward expected outcomes. Continue plan.

CRITICAL THINKING QUESTIONS

1. Because the patient still has trouble walking, how could you promote exercise that will strengthen abdominal muscles and assist with bowel evacuation?
2. Ms. Svoboda tells you she does not like to drink water. She loves tea. What would you suggest in the way of increased fluid intake?

helped into as much of a sitting position as their condition allows. The abdominal muscles and gravity can then assist with defecation. Always wear gloves when helping the patient off the bedpan. Check to see that the patient is thoroughly cleaned, especially if the patient cannot lift up off the pan to clean the anus and surrounding area. The bedpan should be thoroughly cleansed, dried, and put away. The bedside commode should be emptied and cleaned promptly after use.

When the average patient has not experienced bowel evacuation within 3 days, measures should be taken to assist elimination. Assessment data guide the measures to be implemented. The least invasive measures are used first. Encouraging and monitoring activity, adequate fluid intake, and a diet with sufficient fiber may lead to regular bowel elimination.

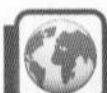 Cultural Considerations

Toileting Practices

Using a bedpan, a bedside commode, or even a typical American-style toilet may be unfamiliar or uncomfortable for your patient because in many other countries, squatting is a more typical position for elimination. A careful cultural assessment will help identify potential issues. With the help of a translator, explain the use and purpose of required and available equipment.

 QSEN Considerations: Safety, Evidenced-Based Practice

Dangers of Safety Rails

Side rails are intended to be a safety measure; however, evidence-based practice indicates that side rails can actually increase the risk for injury for confused patients, as they attempt to crawl around or over the side rails to get out of bed (Shanahan, 2012). Be aware that many incontinent patients are reluctant to call for help even if they understand and acknowledge the use of the call button because, "I didn't want to bother you again." Check on patients every 2 hours, or offer toileting on a set schedule, to decrease attempts to get out of bed unassisted.

Noninvasive measures that can be used to promote bowel elimination include the consumption of 1 to 3 tablespoons of bran mixed with applesauce, small amounts of prune juice, warmed prune juice and cola, hot water with lemon juice, or stewed or dried prunes. Be careful because some people are particularly sensitive to the effects of prunes, and diarrhea may develop.

If these actions are not successful, implement more invasive measures to promote bowel elimination. These measures include the administration of medications to soften the stool, suppositories to stimulate the urge to defecate, laxatives to stimulate bowel activity, and enemas to empty the rectum. All of these measures require a medical order for hospitalized patients. **Measures to rid the bowel of barium are essential after a patient has had a barium x-ray examination.** Encourage an increase in fluid intake of 3500 mL/day for the next 24 hours unless contraindicated. A laxative is often recommended.

Encourage home care patients to telephone the nurse if they have not had a bowel movement in 3 days. Impaction may be prevented if constipation is treated early. The patient's caregiver is taught how to insert a suppository or how to give a small-volume enema in case less invasive measures do not work.

When the patient experiences incontinence, cleansing should occur as soon as possible. Skin care must be thorough and gentle because feces irritate the skin and can cause **excoriation** (abrasion of the skin). The patient who is having diarrheal stools may need a skin protectant around the anus to prevent skin breakdown. Products such as petroleum jelly, A & D ointment, cod liver oil ointments with zinc oxide, and commercial skin barriers are helpful to protect the skin. Gentle washing with soap and water, rinsing, and patting dry are essential. Moist cleansing wipes are useful during diarrheal episodes.

 QSEN Considerations: Teamwork & Collaboration

Teamwork for Better Hygienic Care

Hygienic care is usually assigned to the nursing assistant; however, when a bedridden patient has continuous diarrhea, help the assistant to clean the patient. The task of repeated cleaning is exhausting for the caregiver and the patient; it is much easier for two people to accomplish the job. In addition, the patient's skin needs frequent assessment, and this is a nursing responsibility that cannot be delegated.

When diarrhea is thought to be caused by bacteria or a virus, the primary care provider may want to let it run its course for at least 24 hours so that the body has a chance to rid itself of the offending organism. Diarrhea from other causes simply leads to fluid and electrolyte loss and should not be allowed to continue for long periods. Treatment involves placing the patient on a clear liquid diet to rest the bowel, replacing fluids and electrolytes, and seeking medication to stop the loose stools. **Observe for signs of dehydration when the patient has severe diarrhea: decreased skin turgor, dry mucous membranes with thick saliva, and increased thirst. Self-medication for diarrhea should not continue for more than 48 hours without consulting a primary care provider.**

 Patient Education

Foods to Assist a Patient with Diarrhea

Many antibiotics kill the normal bacteria that reside in the bowel, leading to diarrhea. Teach patients who experience diarrhea from antibiotics to eat yogurt, drink buttermilk, or take probiotics when they begin taking antibiotics. Replacing the normal bacteria with those contained in these food products reestablishes the right balance and stops the diarrhea (Hempel et al., 2012).

◆ EVALUATION

Evaluation for patients with problems of bowel function is based on whether expected outcomes and goals have been met. If outcomes and goals are not being met, reconsider and revise the plan. Examples of evaluation statements are:

- Patient is walking 1 mile a day.
- Patient has increased fluid intake to 3500 mL and is producing stool every other day.
- Patient is participating in a bowel program and is assisted with toileting q 2 hr.
- Patient reports less pain and abdominal distention compared with yesterday.
- Patient is able to use the trapeze to lift self onto bedpan.
- Patient feels better about self since bowel regimen has produced continent stool for 3 days in a row.
- Patient recognized that white bread and noodles are contributing to constipation.

Nursing Care Plan 30.1 provides other examples of evaluation.

Documentation

Document any changes in bowel habits, stool characteristics, episodes of constipation or diarrhea, and measures taken to remedy the problem. Document the patient education plan, times of each teaching session, and material covered. Evaluation of patient education is also noted. All measures to promote bowel elimination must be documented. Document the number and approximate amount of diarrheal stools on the appropriate flow sheets (I & O and daily activity sheets).

RECTAL SUPPOSITORIES

Rectal suppositories used to promote bowel movements are glycerin and bisacodyl suppositories. Suppositories that promote bowel evacuation do so by (1) stimulating the inner surface of the rectum and increasing the urge to defecate, (2) forming gas that expands the rectum, or (3) melting into a lubricating material to coat the stool for easier passage through the anal sphincter. See Chapter 34 for the procedure to insert a rectal suppository.

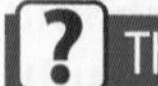 **Think Critically**

What time of day would be best for administering a rectal suppository to stimulate defecation?

ENEMAS

An enema is the introduction of fluid into the rectum and colon by means of a tube. Enemas are given to stimulate peristalsis and the urge to defecate or to wash out waste products or feces. Cleansing enemas are given when the bowel is to be examined by x-ray, colonoscopy, or sigmoidoscopy, or when the bowel is distended by flatus. The volume of a cleansing enema depends on the patient's age: infant or toddler, 50 to 150 mL (normal saline only); ages 3 to 5 years, 200 to 300 mL; school age, 300 to 500 mL; adult, 500 to 1000 mL. Figure 30.2 shows the equipment used for a cleansing enema. An enema kit contains either a bag or a bucket for the solution. The commercially disposable enema, such as the Fleet enema, is convenient and easy to use when only a small amount of fluid is needed to stimulate a bowel movement. Enemas can be given at any time, but it is best to try to give them before the morning bath and bed linen change.

TYPES OF ENEMAS

The type of enema to be given is prescribed by the primary care provider, and it varies depending on the patient's age and condition, the purpose of the enema, and the primary care provider's preference (Table 30.1). The commercially packaged enema may require more lubricant on the nozzle; other supplies needed are the same as for any type of enema. When other types of enemas are ordered, consult the facility's procedure manual for the ingredients and the proportions to use.

Retention Enema

Often an oil-retention enema is ordered for a patient with constipation. The oil must be retained in the rectum to soften and coat the hardened feces. Instill between 120 and 180 mL of warm oil rectally in the same manner as the cleansing enema, except that **the oil should be retained for at least 20 minutes.** Prepackaged enemas are usually used for this purpose, but mineral oil or olive oil can be used.

AMOUNT AND TEMPERATURE OF SOLUTION

Disposable enema units contain about 240 mL of solution (Fig. 30.3). They may be given at room temperature, but work best when slightly warmed. No special

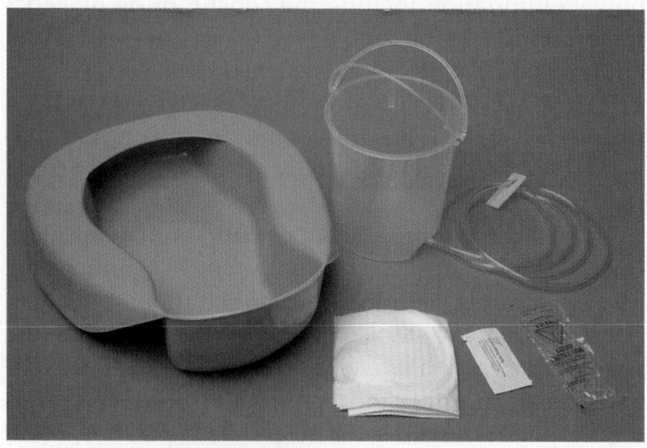

FIGURE 30.2 Enema equipment.

TABLE 30.1 Types of Enemas and Their Actions

TYPES OF ENEMAS	EXAMPLES	ACTIONS
Retention enema	Mineral oil	Softens stool as oil is absorbed
Cleansing enema	Soapsuds (5 mL castile soap in 1000 mL of water), tap water, and saline (500-1000 mL normal saline)	Stimulates peristalsis through distention and irritation of colon and rectum
Distention reduction enema	Carminative (30 g magnesium sulfate, 60 g glycerin, and 90 mL warm water)	Relieves discomfort from flatus causing distention
Medicated enema	Sodium polystyrene (Kayexalate) (removes potassium) and neomycin (reduces bacteria)	Solution with drugs to reduce bacteria or remove potassium
Disposable enema (small volume)	Sodium phosphate (Fleet)	Stimulates peristalsis by acting as an irritant

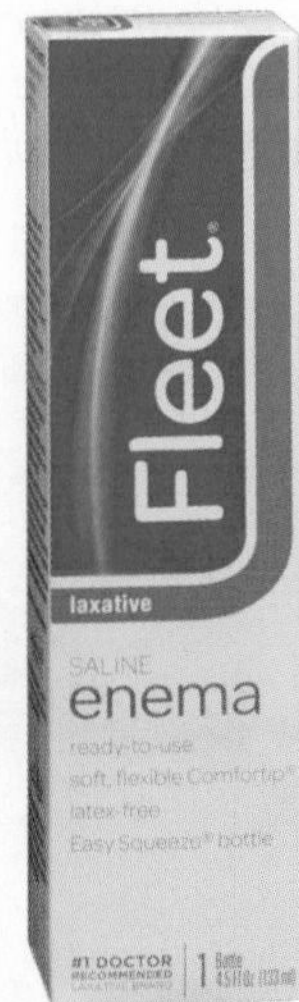

FIGURE 30.3 Disposable enema. (Courtesy C.B. Fleet Co., Lynchburg, VA.)

preparation is needed; they are ready for use when taken from the package. With the patient in the left Sims position, insert the prelubricated nozzle into the rectum, and instill the solution by squeezing the flexible plastic bottle. Rolling the bottle up from the bottom aids in instilling the entire contents.

 **QSEN Considerations: Safety**

Not Too Hot, Not Too Cold

The temperature of the enema solution should be about 105°F (40.5°C). If a bath thermometer is not available, test the temperature of the fluid by pouring a small amount over the inner wrist. It should be warm to the touch but not hot. Solution that is too cool usually cannot be retained; hot solutions may damage the tissues of the rectum.

The amount of solution used for a cleansing enema for adults is between 500 and 1000 mL. Hold the container approximately 12 to 18 inches above the patient's anus and allow the warm solution to run in slowly; a greater height creates too much pressure because the fluid runs in too rapidly and causes painful distention of the rectum and colon. This stimulates the urge to defecate immediately, so that the patient cannot retain the fluid.

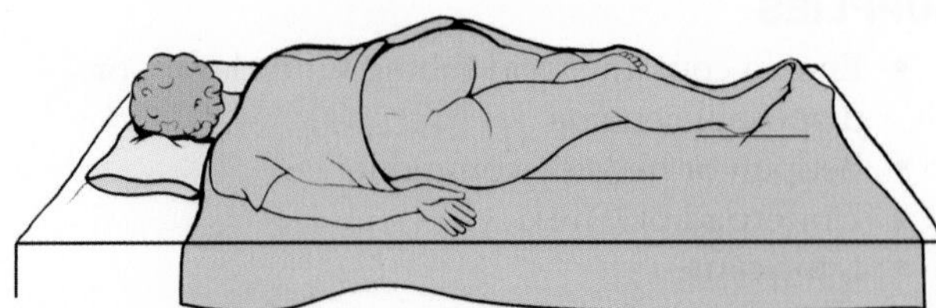

FIGURE 30.4 Position for giving an enema.

 **QSEN Considerations: Safety**

Be Careful with "Enemas until Clear"

When an order to "give enemas until clear" is written, it means that the return fluid must not have any fecal matter in it; however, **no more than three large-volume enemas are given without checking with the primary care provider.** Repeated enemas may deplete electrolytes and can be dangerous.

Clinical Cues

If your older adult patient has trouble holding an enema, take a baby bottle nipple, cut off the tip and insert the enema tube through the nipple. Gently support the outer rim of the nipple with your gloved hand; this provides a temporary "plug" that helps the patient retain the enema.

RECOMMENDED POSITION

The position of choice when giving an enema is the left Sims position, with the hips slightly elevated (Fig. 30.4). This allows the fluid, aided by the force of gravity, to flow downward along the natural curve of the rectum and descending colon. If the patient is unable to turn to the side, the supine position can be used (Skill 30.1).

RECTAL TUBE

When a patient is uncomfortable because of flatus in the lower bowel, a rectal tube can be inserted in the anus. The tube is similar to the enema tubing. This allows the gas to be expelled without the patient straining to open the anal sphincter. Oral medications to reduce gas have mostly eliminated the use of this tube.

Skill 30.1 Administering an Enema

 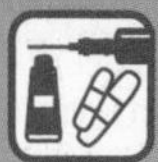 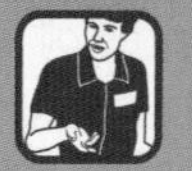  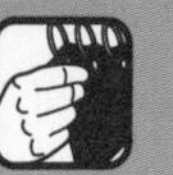 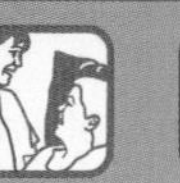 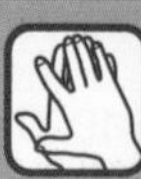 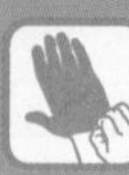

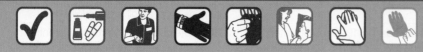

An enema is given to evacuate the bowel. Tap water, soapsuds, or saline solution of 500 to 1000 mL is given to the adult with an enema bucket or bag. A disposable enema, consisting of 120 mL of hypertonic solution, may be ordered. An oil-retention enema may be required to soften stool for ease of evacuation.

SUPPLIES

- Enema container and tubing with clamp, or disposable enema
- Bedpan or bedside commode
- Underpad or Chux
- Lubricant
- Gloves
- Enema solution and additives as ordered
- Bath blanket
- Paper towel and toilet tissue

Review and carry out the Standard Steps in Appendix A.

ACTION (*RATIONALE*)

Assessment (Data Collection)

1. Check the primary care provider's order. Determine what patient knows about the enema procedure. Check to see that a bedpan or bedside commode is on hand. (*Ensures an enema order has been written. Determines how much explanation is needed. Bedpan or bedside commode may be needed immediately.*)

Planning

2. Plan time to give a large-volume enema without interruption. (*A large-volume enema procedure may take as long as 30 minutes if the order is "enemas until clear."*)

Implementation

3. If possible, place the patient in the left Sims position and drape with a bath blanket. Place the underpad under the buttocks. (*Solution travels up the colon when the patient is lying on the left side.*)

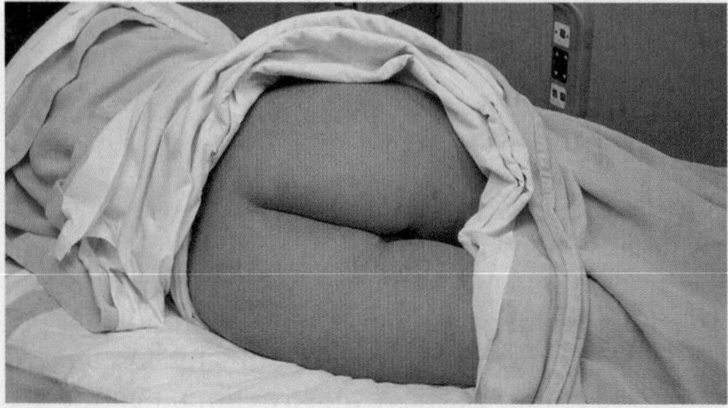

Step 3

For Large-Volume Enema

4. Put on gloves. Fill the enema bag with the correct solution; temperature of the water should be between 100 and 105°F (37.8 and 40.5°C). Expel air from the tubing by opening the clamp and allowing the solution to run through. Use the bedpan or sink to collect the solution; reclamp the tube. (*Water too hot may burn the patient; water too cool may cause cramping. Expelling air from tube prevents air from being introduced into the colon, which could cause the patient discomfort.*)

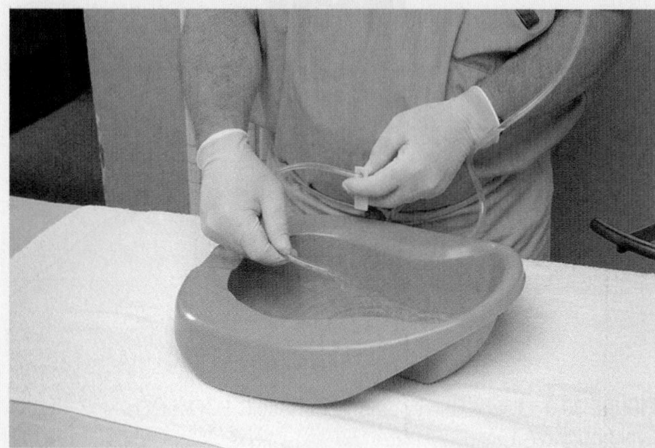

Step 4

5. Position the bedside commode or put the bedpan nearby. Generously lubricate the end of the enema tube and, while the patient takes a deep breath, gently insert it about 4 inches in the adult anus. Direct the tube toward the umbilicus. Ask the patient to take a deep breath through the mouth to relax the anal sphincter. Twisting the tube gently helps it pass through the sphincter. (*There is a small amount of discomfort as the tube passes through the sphincter; deep breathing helps the patient relax. Excessive force may cause perforation of the rectum.*)
6. With the container about 12 to 18 inches above the anus, open the clamp on the tube, steady the tube in place, and allow the solution to flow slowly into the bowel over 5 to 10 minutes. Lowering slightly and again raising the container to this height will regulate the speed of the flow. Slight pressure on the tubing with the clamp can also slow the flow. When the patient expresses discomfort, stop the flow by kinking the tubing or clamping it, and instruct the patient to take deep breaths by mouth until the cramping and urge to expel the fluid pass. Continue until the patient can retain no more or the container is empty. Clamp the tubing and withdraw it, asking the patient to squeeze the sphincter

shut; place the soiled tube on a paper towel. *(Instilling fluid slowly prevents cramping and usually obtains the best result with the least discomfort. Some patients can hold only a few hundred milliliters of solution at a time; others can tolerate the entire volume.)*

For Disposable or Oil-Retention Enema

7. Add extra lubricant to the tip if the amount of prelubrication seems insufficient. Insert the tip into the anal opening as directed previously. Gently and slowly squeeze the bottle, and roll it up from the bottom as the contents enter the bowel. Squeeze as much of the fluid into the patient as possible. Remove the tip slowly and hold the buttocks together. *(The lubricant on the tip sometimes dries out. Disposable enemas contain approximately 120 to 240 mL of solution. An oil-retention enema is given in the same manner, but the patient should retain it for 20 minutes to 2 hours so that it will soften the stool.)*

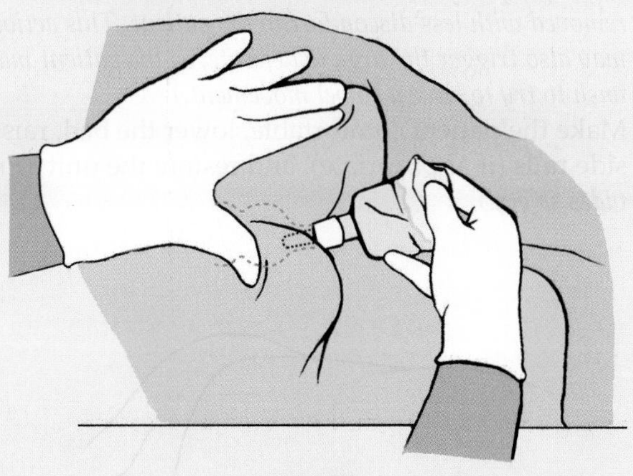

Step 7

For Both Types of Enema

8. Assist the patient onto the bedpan or bedside commode. If the patient uses the toilet, request to see the result before flushing. If a bedpan is used, raise the head of the bed to a sitting position. Place call bell and toilet paper within reach. *(Patient is likely to flush the toilet unless otherwise instructed.)*
9. When the bowel contents have been expelled, assist the patient in cleaning the anal area; observe the results of the enema, noting the color, amount, and consistency of the stool. Remove and clean the bedpan or bedside commode. *(Results of the enema are judged by the stool expelled.)*
10. Restore the patient unit, lower the bed, and place the call bell within reach. *(Provides safety.)*

Evaluation

11. Ask yourself: Was the patient able to hold sufficient enema fluid to flush the bowel? Did all the fluid seem to return? Was there a normal amount of stool expelled? Does the patient feel relief from fullness and flatus? *(Answers determine whether enema was successful.)*

Documentation

12. Note date, time, type of enema, and amount of fluid instilled; describe the result, as well as how the patient tolerated the procedure. *(Documents the procedure and the results.)*

Documentation Example

10/12 0930 1000-mL tap water enema, given 500 mL at a time. No c/o severe cramping. Produced large amount of brown formed stool and returned fluid. States feels much better. Bed into lowest position, call bell in reach. Resting. (Nurse's time-stamped electronic signature.)

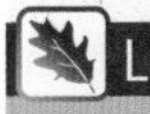 **Critical Thinking Questions**

1. Why do you think that a patient who is taking a diuretic and is now in the hospital may become constipated and need an enema?
2. When an enema is ordered, how would you organize your work for the day if you were working the day shift?

FECAL IMPACTION

Fecal impaction means that the rectum and sigmoid colon become filled with hardened fecal material. The most obvious sign of fecal impaction is the absence of (or only a small amount of) bowel movement for more than 3 days in a patient who usually has a bowel movement more frequently. Impaction occurs in patients who are very ill, are on bed rest, or are not fully aware of their surroundings because of a state of confusion. The very young and very old are more prone to fecal impaction.

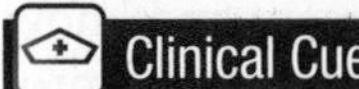 **Clinical Cues**

Passage of small amounts of liquid or semisoft stool onto the bed linens is a sign of fecal impaction. Bacterial action on the hardened surface of the fecal material causes liquefaction.

Life-Span Considerations

Older Adult

- The older adult who becomes dehydrated is very prone to fecal impaction.
- Some medications also contribute to impaction, including narcotic pain medication and diuretics.

Nursing responsibility includes prevention of fecal impaction by daily assessment of bowel patterns of all patients. Fecal impaction is easier to remove when an oil-retention enema is ordered and given, followed by a cleansing enema 2 to 3 hours later. Sometimes the primary care provider orders the impaction to be digitally broken up after the oil has had time to soften the stool (Steps 30.1).

Steps 30.1 Removing a Fecal Impaction

When a patient has impacted stool that cannot be flushed out with an oil-retention enema followed by cleansing enemas, manual removal of the impaction is required. The patient should be given analgesia before this procedure because it is painful.

Review and carry out the Standard Steps in Appendix A.

ACTION (RATIONALE)

1. Assess when the last bowel movement occurred, check risk factors that contribute to constipation, assess the abdomen, and determine whether small amounts of liquid stool have been passed. *(Assessment data help in determining whether fecal impaction has occurred.)*
2. Have patient assume a left lateral or Sims position. Perform hand hygiene, put on gloves, and arrange the bedpan and toilet tissue on a chair by the bed within reach. Lubricate the index finger. *(Generous lubricant makes it easier for the finger to slide up and around the hardened stool and decreases patient discomfort. An oil-retention enema 20 minutes to 3 hours before impaction removal is helpful.)*
3. Insert the index finger into the anus and along the wall of the rectum in a slightly curving motion. As the finger meets feces in the rectum, move the finger into the lower portion of the fecal mass, noting the consistency. *(This action is uncomfortable for the patient, but you must assess the consistency of the fecal matter.)*
4. With the examining index finger, dislodge or break off a small amount of fecal material and gently remove it, placing it in the bedpan. Re-lubricate the finger as needed. Continue removing as much fecal material as you can reach with your finger or until the patient's discomfort or adverse effects such as palpitations or dizziness warrant discontinuing the procedure. After the patient has rested, re-glove and remove the remaining fecal material. Cleanse the rectal area. Remove gloves and dispose of them properly. *(The stool is broken up so that it can be removed with less discomfort to the patient. This action may also trigger the urge to defecate, so the patient may wish to try to have a bowel movement.)*
5. Make the patient comfortable, lower the bed, raise side rails (if appropriate), and restore the unit. *(Provides safety.)*

Digital removal of a fecal impaction must be done gently, and the patient must be watched for signs of **vagal response** (activation of the vagal nerve) from stimulation of the sphincter and rectal wall (Fig. 30.5). **The vagal response may cause a slow pulse and cardiac arrhythmia, and an alteration in blood pressure may develop. Should this occur, immediately stop the procedure, place the patient in a supine position, monitor vital signs, and notify the primary care provider.** A dose of atropine may be ordered to counteract the vagal response.

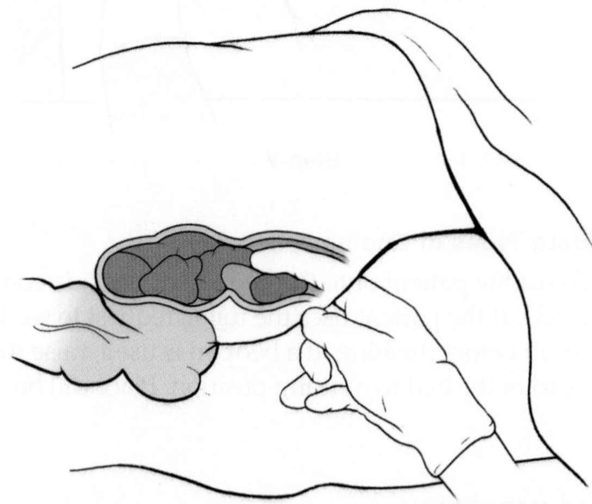

FIGURE 30.5 Removing a fecal impaction.

BOWEL TRAINING FOR INCONTINENCE

The treatment for incontinence is training for bowel control. This is a long process, but it helps the patient regain self-esteem. A special effort should be made to help the very old patient overcome incontinence. Patients who require bowel training may be physically disabled or confused. In accordance with National Patient Safety Goals, ensure the safety of these patients and assist as needed to move to and from the toilet.

A **bowel training program** is based on the principles for establishing regular bowel elimination: adequate diet, sufficient fluids, adequate exercise, and sufficient rest (Box 30.3). A regular time for evacuation should be established. A reasonable goal is to achieve defecation within 1 hour of the established time. Factors that help establish the time include the patient's prior bowel habits or the nurse's observation of when incontinent movements tend to occur. Many bowel retraining programs are timed around a triggering meal when gastrocolic reflexes are the strongest, most commonly breakfast.

After establishing a regular time for evacuation, provide the patient with an environment conducive to evacuation. Privacy and adequate time are only two parts of the environment that are considered. The patient must also feel safe in the environment and know that, if a problem occurs, the nurse is available to provide assistance. Provide the patient with toilet tissue, and remember to encourage hand hygiene after the evacuation.

Box 30.3 Interventions for Bowel Training

- Assess for fecal impaction and remove if present (impaction may cause incontinent diarrhea).
- Ensure the patient's diet is high in bulk and fiber. If teeth or improperly fitting dentures prevent the consumption of high fiber foods, refer to a dentist.
- Increase fluids to 1500 mL/day unless contraindicated by heart failure, chronic kidney disease, potential for increased intracranial pressure, or another disorder.
- Perform a thorough assessment for 1 week to determine intake and output patterns, usual time of incontinent stool, and previous bowel pattern before incontinence began, including frequency of bowel movement, time of day, and surrounding events (e.g., while drinking coffee; use of commode, toilet, or bedpan).
- Encourage regular toileting after meals. Toileting should be performed just before the time at which incontinent defecation has been occurring.
- Use positive reinforcement for continent defecation. Refrain from use of negative reinforcement (e.g., shaming or scolding) at any time.
- Provide privacy for toileting; position the patient comfortably on the commode, toilet, or bedpan with feet supported.
- If diarrhea is present, assess and remedy the cause with diet or medications as ordered.
- Begin an exercise program for the patient to strengthen abdominal muscles.
- If other measures do not work, obtain an order for a suppository or an enema every 2 or 3 days to stimulate peristalsis and produce controlled defecation.

QSEN Considerations: Safety

Hand Hygiene

To comply with The Joint Commission National Patient Safety Goals, nurses should practice and encourage hand hygiene, which is evidence-based practice, according to Centers for Disease Control and Prevention guidelines. Use alcohol-based cleaning agents and/or soap and water. Wash before and after gloving and avoid artificial nails. Additional information can be obtained from the CDC at: www.cdc.gov/handhygiene/Guidelines.html.

Some patients with a neurogenic dysfunction may require digital stimulation to relax the anal sphincter. Using a gloved and lubricated finger, insert the finger 1 to 2 cm into the rectum and gently rotate the finger for 30 to 60 seconds.

Suppositories, stool softeners, and bulk laxatives may be used to assist in establishing a normal, regular bowel pattern. The primary care provider's order dictates the type of suppository. Suppositories are usually inserted about 1 hour before the triggering meal or the established evacuation time. In some bowel retraining programs, a suppository is used every day for the first week, every other day for the second and third weeks, and, thereafter, only as needed to maintain a regular movement every 2 or 3 days. To avoid intestinal obstruction, bulk-forming laxatives must be taken with sufficient fluid, and they generally should not be taken at bedtime (Gardiner & Hilton, 2016). In most cases, stronger laxatives and enemas are not considered part of a bowel training program.

BOWEL OSTOMY

Disease or trauma can damage the intestinal system and require surgical intervention, which alters the process of elimination. A diversion of intestinal contents from the normal path is called an **ostomy**. An ostomy results in the formation of an external **stoma** (opening) or an internal tissue pouch with a valve nipple opening. The internal pouch forming the continent ostomy is usually constructed from a segment of bowel (Fig. 30.6). This type of ostomy is emptied with a catheter (Steps 30.2). Patients with stoma ostomies use various **appliances** (devices to gather and contain output) and special procedures to aid in effective, controlled elimination through the stoma.

Human elimination is a subject that many adults view with embarrassment or distaste. Physical conditions that create the need for an ostomy carry a heavy psychosocial burden for the patient and many new demands in handling elimination. Soiling, wetness, and odor from feces are all socially unacceptable in adult society, and such possibilities are often of grave concern to the new ostomy patient. There is also concern about ability to care for oneself and to return to work and recreational activities performed before surgery. Focus on keeping your body language neutral and not displaying any sign of distaste (even unconsciously) when caring for the ostomy patient. An attitude of acceptance is important.

Conditions that can require ostomy include cancer, abdominal trauma, congenital bowel malformation, and severe chronic Crohn disease or ulcerative colitis. Patients facing an ostomy frequently experience fear, concern, and denial, followed by information seeking. Fear may focus on the loss of a normal body function and change in body image, the possibility of rejection by others, the loss of physical or sexual attractiveness, or the prospect of death from the underlying disease.

The patient may be helped by a visit from a member of the United Ostomy Associations of America, which is a support network of people with ostomies. The patient needs a support system in place before discharge from the hospital. The local office of the American Cancer Society and the United Ostomy Associations are good sources of information about ostomy support groups or visitors in the area.

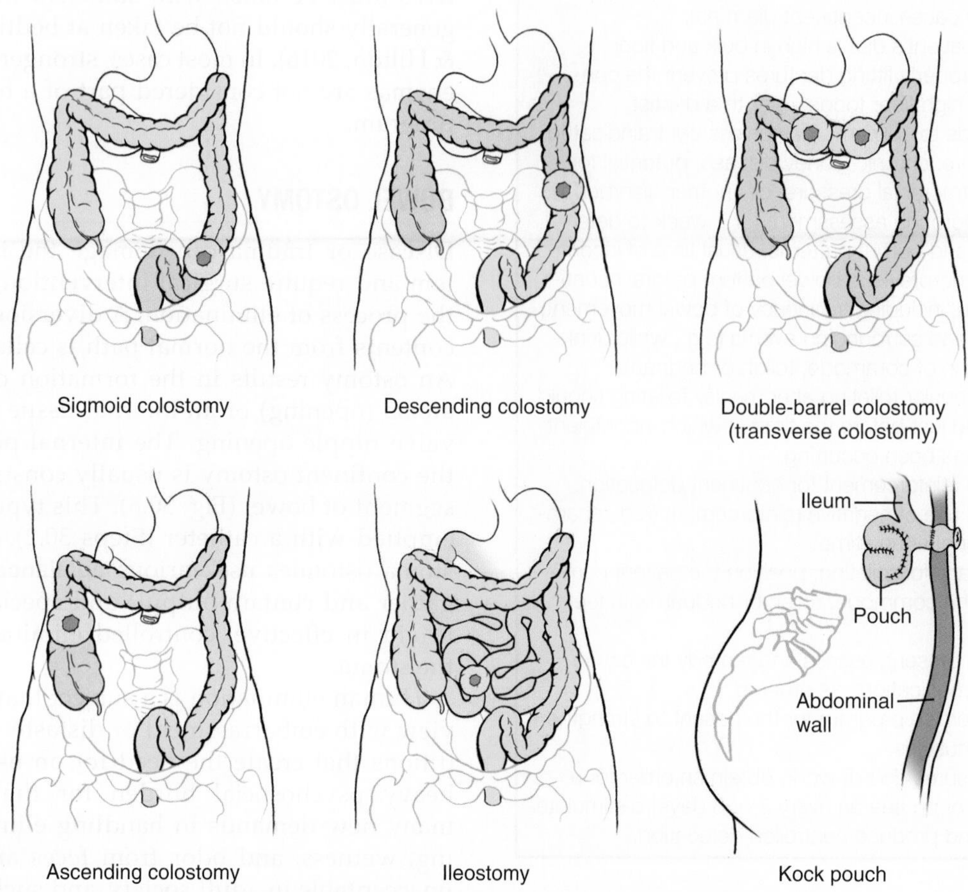

FIGURE 30.6 Types of bowel ostomies and intestinal diversions.

Steps 30.2 Catheterizing a Continent Ileostomy

A continent bowel diversion, such as a Kock pouch, has a nipple valve attached to the abdomen through which the waste contents of the internal reservoir can be drained of stool. Initial catheterization of a fresh continent ileostomy should be done only by a trained enterostomal therapist (ET) nurse or the primary care provider. Thereafter, another nurse may assist the patient as needed.

Review and carry out the Standard Steps in Appendix A.

ACTION (RATIONALE)

1. Assist patient to comfortable position on toilet, commode, or chair. *(Patient will be able to relax abdominal muscles if comfortably positioned.)*
2. Perform hand hygiene, put on gloves, and remove and discard any covering over nipple valve. *(Reduces transfer of microorganisms; prepares nipple valve for catheterization.)*
3. Lubricate the catheter with water-soluble lubricant. *(Allows easier entry of catheter into pouch.)*
4. Place distal end of catheter into waste drainage container or toilet. Slowly insert the catheter through the nipple valve and into the internal reservoir until stool begins to drain. *(When catheter meets resistance of the internal valve, ask patient to take a deep breath and apply gentle pressure to open valve.)*
5. Allow about 5 minutes for the catheter to drain the stool in the reservoir fully. *(Empties the reservoir.)*
6. Ask the patient to cough three or four times to expel any remaining waste. Remove the catheter and rinse in warm water, then wash in mild soap and rinse again. Lay catheter on a towel to dry. *(Prepares the catheter for the next use.)*
7. Clean the nipple valve and surrounding area with water or towelette as necessary and cover with 4 × 4 gauze if needed. *(Cleanses the area and prevents dripping.)*

 Cultural Considerations

Care of Stoma

If your patient is Muslim, it is important to talk with them about the placement of their stoma. When given a choice of left- or right-sided placement, the left is often chosen because acts considered "dirty" are to be performed with the left hand (Iqbal et al., 2013).

OSTOMY CARE

An **ileostomy** is an opening surgically created at the ileum to divert intestinal contents. This is performed because lower portions of the bowel have been surgically removed. **Effluent** (discharged fecal matter) from an ileostomy is liquid. A **colostomy** is an opening into the colon. The stoma is the entrance to the opening. An appliance is the apparatus that attaches to the skin plus a pouch (bag) worn over the stoma to collect effluent (Fig. 30.7). Colostomy effluent is more formed. Patient care involves providing skin care around the stoma and applying the appliance or, if there is a continent ileostomy, draining it with a catheter. Diet can adversely affect the ostomy patient, and thus it is an important topic in patient education (Cronin, 2013). Evaluation of care includes a review of whether the patient is experiencing problems with the ostomy, the skin around the stoma, or the appliance. Care of the ostomy patient is covered more thoroughly in medical-surgical nursing texts.

Skin Care

Periostomal (around the stoma) care includes assessment of the health of the stoma and skin surrounding it. The stoma should appear pink or red, which indicates adequate blood supply. It should look like healthy mucous membrane, such as the membrane inside the mouth (Scemons, 2014).

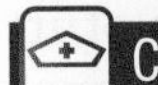 Clinical Cues

A pale or dusky stoma indicates compromised blood supply, and it should be reported to the primary care provider.

 Patient Education

Dietary Guidelines for the Ostomy Patient

ILEOSTOMY

- Eat a diet high in protein, calories, and vitamins.
- Avoid foods that irritate the intestine or require excessive intestinal activity, such as milk products, spicy or fried high residue foods, raw vegetables and fruits, and whole grain cereals.
- Avoid carbonated, caffeinated, and alcoholic beverages because they increase intestinal activity.
- Avoid extremely hot or cold foods and fluids because they cause gas.
- Eat small, frequent meals.
- Drink 8 to 10 cups of fluid per day.

COLOSTOMY

- Control the consistency of the stool with diet.

To Control Diarrhea, Increase Intake of

- Ripe bananas
- Rice
- Creamy peanut butter
- Cheese
- Potatoes (no skin)
- Applesauce
- Tapioca

To Soften the Consistency of the Stool, Increase Intake of

- Beans
- Caffeinated beverages
- Leafy vegetables
- Apple juice
- Prune juice or prunes
- Fresh fruits (except bananas)
- Raw vegetables
- Spicy or highly seasoned foods
- Green beans
- Broccoli
- Fluids

These Foods May Increase Stool or Urine Odor

- Beans
- Fish
- Eggs
- Asparagus
- Coffee
- Onions
- Cabbage
- Turnips
- Cucumbers
- Broccoli
- Beer

These Foods May Decrease Stool Odor

- Parsley
- Beet greens
- Buttermilk
- Yogurt

These Foods Increase Flatus

- Beer
- Carbonated beverages
- Dried beans and peas
- Strong flavored cheeses
- Onions
- Broccoli, cabbage, and brussels sprouts
- Radishes
- Cucumbers
- Eggs
- Turnips
- Corn
- Spicy foods

Avoid These Foods Because They May Cause Obstruction

- Popcorn
- Chinese vegetables (e.g., bok choy or Chinese broccoli)
- Raw fruits
- Pineapple
- Whole kernel corn
- Celery
- Tomatoes
- Nuts
- Coconut
- Fruits with seeds
- Tough meats, shrimp, and lobster

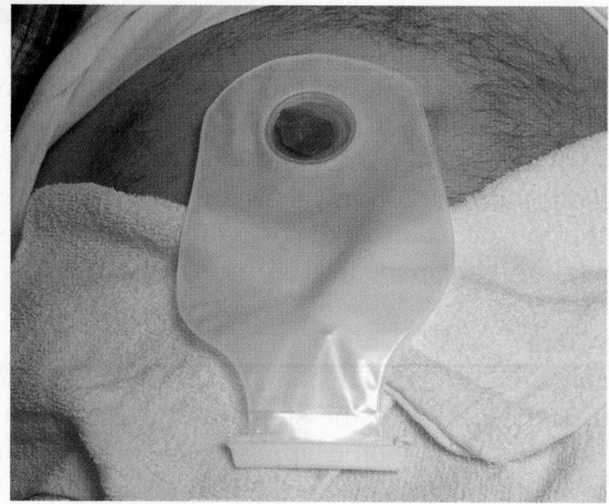

FIGURE 30.7 Ostomy collection device in place.

Assess the skin around the stoma for signs of irritation or breakdown. With an ileostomy, enzymes in the effluent can quickly cause excoriation. When changing the faceplate (every 3 to 5 days), wash the stoma and skin with mild soap and water and pat dry. Apply a skin barrier paste, with care, to prevent any of it from getting on the stoma. Skin barriers are commercially available along with other ostomy supplies (Fig. 30.8). A karaya ring may be attached to the skin to hold the faceplate in place; it is often part of the faceplate. Karaya is a plant material that becomes gelatinous (soft and sticky) when wet; it helps prevent excoriation.

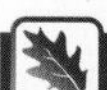 Life-Span Considerations

Older Adults

Older adults are more likely to have periostomal skin complications, such as infection or poor healing. As the body ages, the skin becomes more frail and prone to damage, which significantly slows the healing process. Diabetes and other disease processes can also affect the skin and healing of the skin (Burch, 2014b). Consult the clinical nurse specialist or enterostomal therapy specialist if you need assistance in developing a good wound care plan.

Applying an Ostomy Appliance

Ostomy appliances come in many different sizes and types. All appliances have a faceplate, or disk, that attaches to the abdomen, and a pouch for collecting effluent. Flushable appliances may appeal to some patients (Burch, 2014c). The appliance is positioned with the stoma protruding through the opening in the center of the faceplate. **It is essential that the appliance be the correct size for the patient's stoma.** The stoma must be measured so that the right-size appliance can be chosen. The pouch attaches over the stoma and is fastened onto the faceplate. Some patients wear a belt

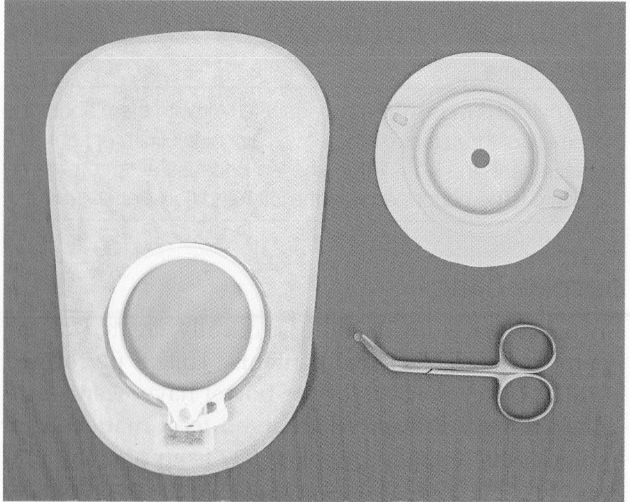

FIGURE 30.8 Ostomy application and supplies. (Photo copyright istock.com.)

that also supports the pouch so that it is not pulled loose from the faceplate as effluent fills the pouch. A clamp at the bottom of the pouch allows effluent to be drained. Pouches are emptied and rinsed as needed and are detached and replaced only every few days. It is best to empty stool from the pouch when it becomes one-third to one-half full so that the weight of the effluent does not pull the appliance loose (Skill 30.2).

 Life-Span Considerations

Older Adult

The body contours change with age. If your older adult patient has had the ostomy for a long time, the sizing and fit of the appliance may have changed if the patient has lost or gained weight or developed wrinkles (Burch, 2014a). Assess for appropriate fit and teach the patient accordingly.

 Life-Span Considerations

Older Adult

Assess your older patient's manual dexterity and vision. Velcro fasteners and one-piece collection pouches may be easier for your patient to manipulate independently (Bowles and Redding, 2013).

Irrigating a Colostomy

To irrigate a colostomy, instill a solution into the colon via the stoma; it is similar to giving an enema (Steps 30.3).

 Think Critically

What concerns do you have about caring for an ostomy patient for the first time?

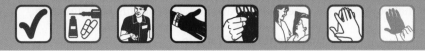

Skill 30.2 Changing an Ostomy Appliance

 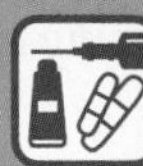 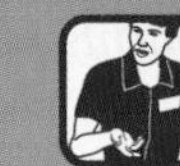   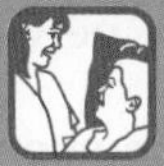 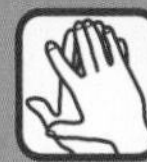 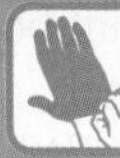

An ostomy pouch is changed when adherence to the skin is no longer adequate or, more commonly, when skin condition is at risk for compromise. The type of pouch applied depends on the type of ostomy.

SUPPLIES

- Washcloth or premoistened towelettes
- Plastic disposal bag
- Clear plastic stoma measuring template
- Clean pouch and faceplate with pouch closure device
- Gloves
- Skin barrier paste
- Scissors
- Tissues or portion of tampon
- Tape or belt

Review and carry out the Standard Steps in Appendix A.

ACTION (*RATIONALE*)

Assessment (Data Collection)

1. Assess for type of ostomy and location. Assess stoma for color and appearance, and assess skin condition around stoma. Assess size of stoma using stoma measuring device. *(If the stoma is more than 6 months old, a precut appliance of the correct size may be used. Red or dark pink color indicates adequate blood supply. Stoma should not be receding or protruding. Skin breakdown may be caused by stool, improperly fitting pouch, perspiration, irritation from appliance, allergic reaction, or bacterial or fungal infection.)*

Planning

2. Gather appropriate supplies needed to apply the new pouch/appliance. *(Facilitates workflow.)*

Implementation

3. Measure the stoma with the stoma measuring device. Prepare the skin barrier or pouch with faceplate by cutting an opening in the center approximately ⅛ inch (for urostomy) to ¼ inch (for colostomy) larger than the stoma. Smooth the cut edges with your finger to prevent irritation or leakage around the stoma. *(If the opening is too small, there may be irritation or restricted blood flow.)*
4. Put on gloves. Empty old pouch. *(Heavy weight of the pouch can cause loosening or spillage.)*
5. Remove old pouch by stabilizing the skin with one hand and pulling the backing with the other hand; discard the old pouch. Save the closure clip. *(The skin should be assessed for irritation or breakdown.)*
6. Clean the stoma and skin gently with warm water and a soft cloth. Dry the skin well by patting. Place tissue or piece of tampon at stoma opening to prevent leakage. *(Cleaning the stoma may cause some slight bleeding, which is considered normal. Persistent bleeding or bloody discharge from the stoma should be immediately reported [Scemons, 2014].)*
7. Change gloves. Remove paper from skin barrier on back of appliance. Apply skin barrier paste to periostomal area. Wet fingers, and spread paste around the stoma, but not on it. *(Prepares an adhesive surface on the skin for attachment of pouch appliance.)*
8. Center and carefully apply the pouch appliance while having patient push out the abdomen. *(Avoids skin wrinkles while pressing pouch into place.)*
9. Gently press down the skin barrier ring around the stoma while the patient pushes out the abdomen. Check that seal is wrinkle free. *(Good adherence prevents leakage.)*

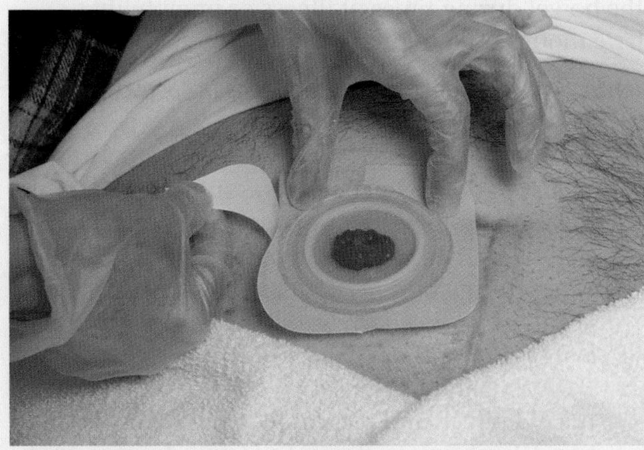

Step 9

10. Reinforce ring with tape as needed. *(Prevents edges from loosening during showers.)*
11. Instruct patient to lie quietly or sit still for 5 minutes to allow body heat to seal pouch well. *(Body heat activates the skin barrier and causes it to adhere to the skin.)*

12. Place deodorant inside pouch if patient desires. *(Ostomy deodorants are available commercially.)*
13. Attach and secure pouch tail closure so that bow of clip fits curve of abdomen. Allow a 1-inch fold-over of pouch before closing the clip. *(When bow fits curve of abdomen, clip is less noticeable under clothes.)*
14. Attach belt to faceplate of pouch if belt is to be worn. *(If stoma is flush to the skin, a belt may be needed to prevent leakage from the pouch.)*
15. Remove gloves and perform hand hygiene. *(Reduces transfer of microorganisms.)*
16. Assist patient in replacing gown or clothing and position for comfort. Restore the area. *(Provides safety.)*

Evaluation

17. Ask yourself: Is the appliance applied without wrinkles? Is it attached securely? Is the bottom of the pouch closed securely? Was the old pouch disposed of properly? Is there any leakage from the pouch? *(Determines whether appliance/pouch was applied correctly.)*

Documentation

18. Note the date, time, and condition of the stoma and periostomal area. Indicate the type of skin barrier used, the size of the opening cut for the new appliance, the treatment of the skin, and the new pouch applied. *(Documents nursing action.)*

Documentation Example

10/14 0920 Colostomy stoma red and moist; periostomal skin intact; cleaned with warm water and dried. Stomahesive applied around stoma; 2⅛" opening cut in faceplate; new pouch applied without wrinkles. (Nurse's time-stamped electronic signature.)

Special Considerations

- The old pouch must be securely closed and disposed of as hazardous waste.
- Some pouches can be washed and reused. Rinse with tepid water, wash with warm soap and water, rinse with vinegar solution (1 part water to 7 parts vinegar), and allow to dry.

? Critical Thinking Questions

1. How would you handle a patient with a new colostomy who does not even want to look at the stoma, much less change the appliance?
2. What are possible consequences of using an ostomy appliance that is too small?

Steps 30.3 Irrigating a Colostomy

When the colostomy patient has difficulty evacuating the bowel during times of illness or immobility, irrigation is used to promote evacuation.

Review and carry out the Standard Steps in Appendix A.

ACTION (RATIONALE)

1. Assist patient as needed to assume comfortable position on the toilet or commode chair. Place patient on bed, resting in side-lying position. *(If patient is confined to bed, assisting into a side-lying position will permit irrigation with evacuation into a bedpan or bedside commode.)*
2. Perform hand hygiene, don gloves, and remove the old pouch and place it in a plastic disposable bag. *(Pouch may be cleansed and reused or discarded. Supporting the skin around the appliance during removal will prevent pulling.)*
3. Cleanse skin and stoma with tepid water and pat dry. Observe the condition of skin and stoma. *(Determines whether any problems with stoma or skin exist.)*
4. Apply irrigating sleeve and secure with belt. Direct the sleeve between the thighs or over side of the bed and into the toilet, bedside commode, or bedpan. *(The sleeve is the correct length if it reaches water level in the toilet; cut off any excess.)*
5. Hang irrigation container filled with approximately 1 quart of warm water so that the base of the container is level with the patient's shoulder or 18 inches above bed. *(Cold water causes cramping, and hot water can burn the intestinal mucosa. More than 1000 mL of water overdistends the bowel. Hanging the container too high results in too much force and cramping. If the container is too low, there will not be sufficient flow to irrigate adequately.)*
6. Allow enough water to flow through irrigation tubing to remove air. Close the clamp. *(Air entering the colon can cause gas pains.)*
7. Lubricate the cone tip and gently insert it through hole in top of irrigation sleeve into stoma; use gentle pressure to hold the cone in place. *(Lubrication makes insertion easier. Cone should fit snugly to hold water in the bowel and prevent backflow.)*

8. Open control clamp, and allow solution to flow into the patient (takes about 5 to 10 minutes). If there is no flow, rotate the cone. Initially 500 mL may be used. If water will not flow, the cone may be against the bowel, requiring repositioning. If repositioning does not result in better flow, there may be kinks in tubing or hard stool blocking the stoma. *(A slow flow gently distends the bowel without causing cramping.)*
9. If cramping occurs, slow or stop the flow of fluid. *(When cramps occur, fluid must be stopped until they subside. Have patient take deep breaths through the mouth to relax the abdominal muscles.)*
10. When all irrigation fluid has been instilled, close the flow control clamp and remove the irrigation cone from the stoma. Close the top of the irrigation sleeve. The end of irrigation sleeve should be in toilet or appropriate container. *(Return of stool takes 10 to 20 minutes. Proper positioning of sleeve prevents spillage of feces.)*
11. After initial evacuation is complete, close end of irrigation sleeve with the clip. Patient may get up and walk around, shower, shave, etc. *(Further evacuation occurs in about 30 minutes. Exercise stimulates evacuation.)*
12. Have patient resume position on toilet and open sleeve into the bowl or container until drainage is complete. *(Directs feces and fluid into toilet.)*
13. Remove the irrigation sleeve, rinse it well, and hang up to dry if it is reusable. Cleanse the skin as needed, apply skin barrier, and clean the pouch as appropriate (see Skill 30.2). *(Many irrigation sleeves are reusable. Pouch prevents accidental leakage of feces.)*
14. Remove gloves and perform hand hygiene. *(Reduces transfer of microorganisms.)*
15. Assist patient in replacing gown or clothing and position for comfort. Restore the area. *(Provides safety.)*

Get Ready for the NCLEX Examination!

Key Points

- The small and large intestines are involved in waste production and elimination.
- The appearance of stool is affected by diet and metabolism; normal stool is light to dark brown, soft, and tubular in shape, with a diameter of about 1 inch.
- Black, sticky stool indicates bleeding in the upper intestinal tract; red blood indicates bleeding in the large intestine or rectal area. Pale white or light gray stool indicates an absence of bile in the intestine.
- Constipation is the most common problem of a hypoactive bowel; feces become compacted and hardened. Any patient restricted to bed rest is at risk for constipation.
- The older adult may develop constipation from a lack of fiber or from decreasing fluid intake. If a laxative is needed, a bulk-forming type is best.
- Diarrhea occurs when increased peristalsis pushes food through the intestinal tract too fast; infants or older adult patients with diarrhea can become dehydrated very quickly.
- Fecal incontinence may affect people of all ages because of illness, injury, or neurogenic dysfunction.
- Bowel status should be assessed for every patient every day.
- The average patient may need assistance with elimination if there is no bowel movement for 3 days.
- To promote regular bowel movements, encourage exercise, dietary fiber, and at least 1500 mL of fluid per day.
- Patients undergoing barium x-ray examinations need to flush the bowel after the test to prevent impaction.
- Diarrhea caused by a virus or bacteria is usually not treated with medication for 24 to 48 hours. The patient is given clear fluids and allowed to rest.
- If diarrhea does not clear within 48 hours after starting medication, consult the primary care provider.
- Rectal suppositories are used to stimulate a bowel movement. Enemas are given to cleanse the bowel, deliver medication, relieve distention, or soften stool.
- Fecal impaction is first treated by oil-retention enema followed several hours later by a cleansing enema; if this does not relieve the impaction, obtain an order for digital removal.
- Notify the primary care provider if the patient is not clear after three large-volume enemas.
- A bowel training program takes 2 to 3 months or longer.
- A bowel ostomy is performed when fecal diversion is necessary. An ileostomy produces liquid effluent, whereas a colostomy produces more formed stool.
- A pale or dusky stoma indicates compromised blood supply, and it should be reported to the primary care provider.

Additional Learning Resources

SG Go to your Study Guide for additional learning activities to help you master this chapter content.

evolve Go to your Evolve website at http://evolve.elsevier.com/Williams/fundamental for additional online resources.

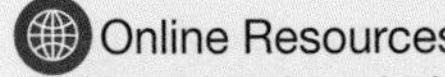

Online Resources
- *Hand Hygiene in Healthcare Settings,* www.cdc.gov/handhygiene/Guidelines.html
- *United Ostomy Associations of America,* www.ostomy.org

Review Questions for the NCLEX Examination

*Choose the **best** answer for each question.*

1. The nurse is doing preprocedural education with a patient who is scheduled to have a barium enema. Which statement by the patient indicates a need for additional patient education?
   1. "I will have to increase my fluid intake after the procedure."
   2. "The barium increases my risk for diarrhea."
   3. "I may receive a laxative after the procedure."
   4. "My stool may be chalk-colored for several days."
2. The nurse is administering an enema to the patient. Immediately after the nurse starts the flow of enema solution, the patient complains of cramping and discomfort. Which action should the nurse take **first**?
   1. Increase the flow rate so that the procedure can be finished sooner.
   2. Call the primary care provider and report that the patient cannot tolerate the procedure.
   3. Discontinue the flow of enema solution and offer the patient a bedpan.
   4. Slow the flow rate and check the temperature of the solution.
3. Which abnormal stool characteristic is the cause for the **greatest** immediate concern?
   1. Dark black, sticky stool
   2. Pale white or light gray stool
   3. Mucus coated and slimy appearance
   4. Foul smelling and floating
4. Which statement by the patient indicates an understanding of the information that was taught for self-care related to diarrhea?
   1. "I should consume clear liquids for 2 days and then try applesauce."
   2. "I should increase my consumption of fruits and vegetables."
   3. "I should eat small, frequent meals that include high-quality proteins."
   4. "I should try over-the-counter antidiarrheals for at least 3 days."
5. The nurse is attempting to remove a fecal impaction manually. The nurse notes that the patient is having a vagal response. What is the **most** appropriate action?
   1. Discontinue the procedure because the patient is having severe pain in the rectal area.
   2. Place the bedpan because the patient is about to expel semiliquid stool and flatus.
   3. Obtain an order for an oil-retention enema because the stool is too hardened.
   4. Check the patient's pulse and blood pressure and attach to a cardiac monitor.
6. The discharge patient education plan for a colostomy patient should include: *(Select all that apply.)*
   1. Emptying the pouch when it is ⅓ to ½ full.
   2. Applying sterile gloves for appliance changes.
   3. Cutting the barrier to size.
   4. Inspecting skin for irritation.
   5. Washing and drying skin when changing appliance.
7. An older adult living in an extended care facility has a nursing diagnosis of bowel incontinence related to confusion. Which intervention would be the **best** for this patient?
   1. Use positive reinforcement for incontinence episodes.
   2. Obtain a primary care provider's order for a low fiber diet.
   3. Have the patient drink 1000 mL of fluid unless contraindicated.
   4. Assist the patient to the toilet, especially after meals.

Critical Thinking Activities

Read each clinical scenario and discuss the questions with your classmates.

Scenario A

Lana Jakubowsky had a stroke and has been incontinent of feces. Her condition is improving and she is regaining muscle tone in her left arm and leg.

1. How would you go about devising a bowel training program for her?
2. How long do you think it might take her to be continent of stool again?

Scenario B

Von Troung, age 78, has had the flu and diarrhea for 3 days. He is confused, and the skin around his anus is inflamed.

1. How would you determine whether Mr. Troung is experiencing an electrolyte imbalance?
2. What would you do about skin care for Mr. Troung?
3. What measures should be taken to treat Mr. Troung's diarrhea?

Scenario C

Carol Tweed is to have a hip replacement. She also has a colostomy.

1. Create a care plan for her risk of developing constipation because of her intestinal diversion, narcotic analgesics, and NPO status.
2. What extra precautions would need to be taken in the early postoperative period for this patient?

Scenario D

Virgil Sunsweet is an older person who has chronic constipation. He is obese and seldom goes out of the house. He is able to ambulate independently, but expresses reluctance to go anywhere.

1. What assessment questions would you use to gather data about this patient?
2. What dietary recommendations would you make to alleviate constipation?
3. Discuss the use of laxatives for a person such as Mr. Sunsweet.

chapter 31

Pain, Comfort, and Sleep

http://evolve.elsevier.com/Williams/fundamental

Objectives

Upon completing this chapter, you should be able to do the following:

Theory

1. Discuss the application of The Joint Commission pain standards in planning patient care, including the clarification of the standards.
2. Give the rationale for why pain is considered the "fifth vital sign."
3. Illustrate the physiology of pain using the gate control theory.
4. Describe the use of a variety of nursing interventions for pain control, including biofeedback, distraction, guided imagery, massage, and relaxation.
5. Analyze the need for normal sleep.
6. Recognize how the need for sleep changes over the life span.
7. Delineate factors that can interfere with sleep.
8. Recognize the sleep disorders insomnia, sleep apnea, and narcolepsy.

Clinical Practice

1. Assist the patient in accurately describing sensations of pain and discomfort.
2. Accurately and appropriately, record the patient's report of pain using clear, descriptive terms.
3. Teach the patient to use a transcutaneous electrical nerve stimulation (TENS) unit.
4. Evaluate the effects of various techniques used for pain control.
5. Care for patients receiving patient-controlled analgesia (PCA) or epidural analgesia.
6. Evaluate the effects of pain medication, and accurately report and record observations.
7. Gather data regarding a patient's sleep difficulties.
8. Develop a plan designed to assist the patient in getting adequate sleep.

Skills & Steps

Skills

Steps

Key Terms

analgesic (ăn-ăl-JĒ-zĭk, p. 604)
biofeedback (BĪ-ō-FĒD-băk, p. 602)
bolus (BŌ-lŭs, p. 605)
continuous positive airway pressure (CPAP) (p. 610)
distraction (dĭs-TRĂK-shŭn, p. 603)
endorphins (ĕn-DŎR-fĭnz) (p. 595)
epidural analgesia (ĕ-pĭ-DŬ-rŭl ă-năl-JĒ-sē-ă, p. 607)
gate control theory (GĀT KŎN-trōl, p. 595)
guided imagery (Ĭ-măj-rē, p. 603)
hypnosis (hĭp-NŌ-sĭs, p. 603)
insomnia (ĭn-SŎM-nyă, p. 610)
massage (mă-SĂJ, p. 604)
meditation (mĕd-ĭ-TĀ-shŭn, p. 603)
narcolepsy (NĂR-cō-lĕp-sē, p. 611)
non–rapid eye movement (NREM) sleep (p. 609)
nonsteroidal anti-inflammatory drugs (NSAIDs) (nŏn-stē-RŎY-dăl ĂN-tī-ĭn-FLĂ-mă-tŏ-rē, p. 604)
pain (PĀN, p. 594)
patient-controlled analgesia (PCA) (p. 605)
rapid eye movement (REM) sleep (p. 609)
relaxation (rē-lăk-ZĀ-shŭn, p. 602)
sleep apnea (SLĒP ĂP-nē-ă, p. 610)
transcutaneous electrical nerve stimulation (TENS) (trănz-kū-TĀ-nē-ŭs, p. 599)

Concepts Covered in This Chapter

- Addiction
- Anxiety
- Communication
- Culture
- Infection
- Inflammation
- Mobility
- Pain
- Safety
- Stress

PAIN AND DISCOMFORT

Pain (a feeling of discomfort strong enough to be intrusive and to affect or interfere with normal activity) is experienced by the majority of patients sometime during their health care experience. Surgical patients experience postoperative pain, and the condition requiring surgery may cause pain. Many medical conditions, ranging from a headache to a myocardial infarction (heart attack), can cause pain. Fever causes generalized discomfort. Cancer, infection, fractures, cuts, and abrasions—indeed the majority of illnesses and conditions—are accompanied by varying degrees and types of pain.

There is no accurate objective measurement of pain. It can only be assumed that patients will experience pain based on their diagnosed condition. Pain has historically been regarded as a symptom of a condition to be diagnosed and treated, thus eliminating the pain. For example, based on experience, it was understood that patients with appendicitis experience severe pain. After surgery, they were expected to experience significant incisional pain for the first day or two, with the degree of pain steadily decreasing with each passing day until it ceased altogether. Using this model, continued severe pain was judged either as an indication of complications or, in the absence of such complications, as drug-seeking behavior in a patient who has become addicted to the pain medication. Now, however, experts in the field regard pain as a condition rather than a symptom, and ideas about pain and its management are changing.

In the past, pain control measures were based on the health care providers' understanding of how much pain the patient *should* have, based on the diagnosis. The primary care provider ordered what was believed to be an appropriate amount of pain medication, and it was dispensed in response to the patient's request and the nurse's assessment of the actual degree of need. For example, the primary care provider might order hydromorphone 2 to 4 mg every 4 to 6 hours subcutaneously for pain as needed, and the nurse would then determine how frequent and how large a dose within these limits would keep the patient comfortable.

The approach to pain control has changed. The establishment of pain assessment and treatment standards and the expansion of pain management options are two factors that have contributed to these changes. In 2014, The Joint Commission clarified the standards related to pain in effect that focus on the patient. The revisions focused on including both pharmacologic and nonpharmacologic methods, in addition to the benefits and risks to patients, when deciding the most effective pain management strategy (The Joint Commission, 2014). The standards relative to direct patient care state:

- Patients have the right to appropriate assessment and management of pain.
- Pain is assessed in all patients.
- Patients are educated about pain and managing pain as part of treatment, as appropriate.
- The discharge process provides for continuing pain care based on the patient's assessed needs at the time of discharge.

Pain assessment is performed along with each assessment of vital signs, and pain is considered the "fifth vital sign." Documentation of the findings must occur. Hospitalized patients frequently use patient-controlled analgesia (PCA) pumps. These allow patients to self-administer medication within safe boundaries based on their perception of pain. There is also an increased use of nonpharmacologic methods of pain relief, such as biofeedback, distraction, guided imagery, massage, and relaxation techniques, each of which is discussed in this chapter. Other complementary treatments, such as chiropractic, acupuncture, and acupressure, are also being used (see Chapter 32).

The fentanyl patch is a newer method for controlling chronic pain. It is replaced every 72 hours and can be managed at home by the patient. Fentanyl nasal spray can be used for breakthrough pain in adult cancer patients, but it comes with a warning that it should only be prescribed by physicians experienced in treating pain in patients with cancer because it can be extremely dangerous otherwise (National Institutes of Health, Medline Plus, 2012). For postsurgical patients the ON-Q pain relief system is a pump with a tiny catheter at the incision site, allowing the patient to administer local anesthetic directly into the site.

THEORIES OF PAIN

Pain is defined as a feeling of discomfort, distress, or suffering caused by the stimulation of nerve endings. Acute pain is often a warning of potential or actual tissue damage, and it allows the sufferer to withdraw from the source or to seek help in relieving symptoms.

Pain is transmitted to the brain through the nervous system. This is done through afferent (sensory) neurons leading to the spinal nerves, and then to the brain. Once the signal is interpreted, the brain sends out a message to the body to respond (Fig. 31.1).

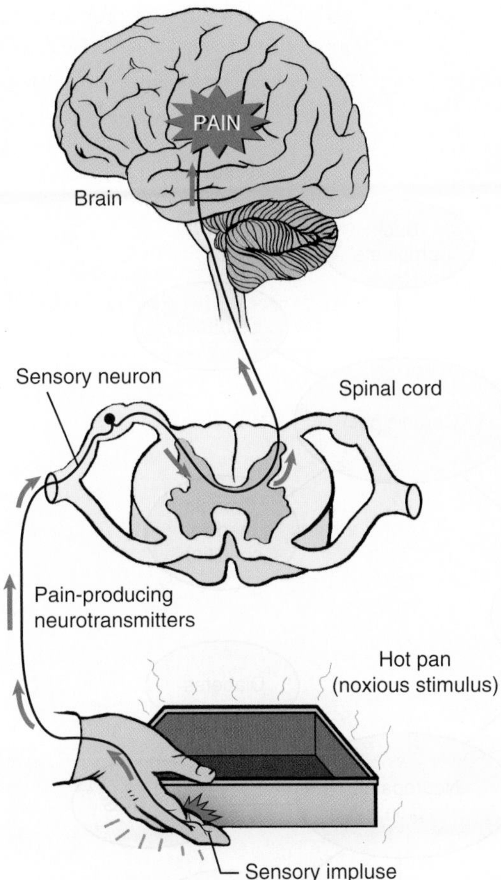

FIGURE 31.1 Pain transmission.

Gate Control Theory

The **gate control theory** was first described by Melzack and Wall in 1965 (Moayedi & Davis, 2013). Pain transmission is viewed as being controlled by a gate mechanism in the central nervous system (Fig. 31.2). Stated in the simplest terms, opening the gate allows the transmission of pain sensation, and closing the gate blocks this transmission. Several ideas that affect nursing practice are part of the gate control theory, including:

- The gate may be opened by activity in the small-diameter nerve fibers from such things as tissue damage. Activity in the large-diameter nerve fibers, such as that provided by massage or vibration, seems to close the gate.
- Brainstem impulses caused by a high sensory input seem to close the gate, whereas a lack of this input allows the gate to open. This may be why people who are bored or lonely can experience more intense pain than when they are occupied or distracted by visitors or an interesting program or activity.
- The cerebral cortex and thalamus play a role by opening the gate with impulses originating from an increase in anxiety, or by closing it with impulses originating from a decrease in anxiety. For example, fear that the pain will get worse and that it will not be controlled can increase the intensity; knowing that pain can be and is being controlled can reduce the intensity.

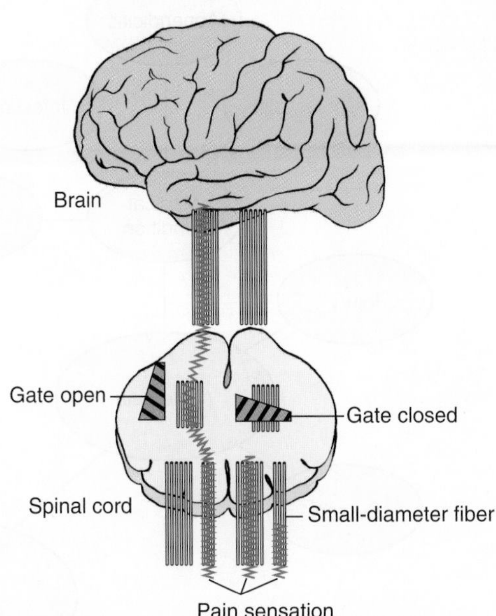

FIGURE 31.2 The gate control theory of pain.

Endorphins

Endorphins are endogenous, naturally occurring, opiate-like peptides that reduce or block the perception of pain. The word *endorphin* comes from *morphine* and *endogenous* (from within). Like morphine, endorphins attach to nerve endings in opioid receptors and block pain transmission. Both physiologic and psychologic stressors can release endorphins, resulting in a reduction in pain and an increase in the sense of well-being.

TYPES OF PAIN

Determining the type and intensity of pain the patient is experiencing assists in selecting methods that will best relieve that discomfort. The patient's verbal description of pain, nonverbal signs of pain, and physiologic indicators of pain may vary according to the type of pain the patient is experiencing. **Treatment decisions should be based on assessment that considers all these factors.** Concept Map 31.1 depicts the various types of pain. Often pain is referred from one deep organ in the body to another place on the body's surface (Fig. 31.3).

Acute Pain

Acute pain is usually associated with an injury, medical condition, or surgical procedure. It is of short duration, lasting from a few hours to a few days. Injuries causing acute pain may include burns, bone fractures, and muscle strains. Medical conditions causing acute pain may include pneumonia, sickle cell crisis, angina, herpes zoster, inflammations, infections, and blockages. Acute pain may be described as aching, throbbing, or searing. The patient may be agitated or restless and may protect the painful area

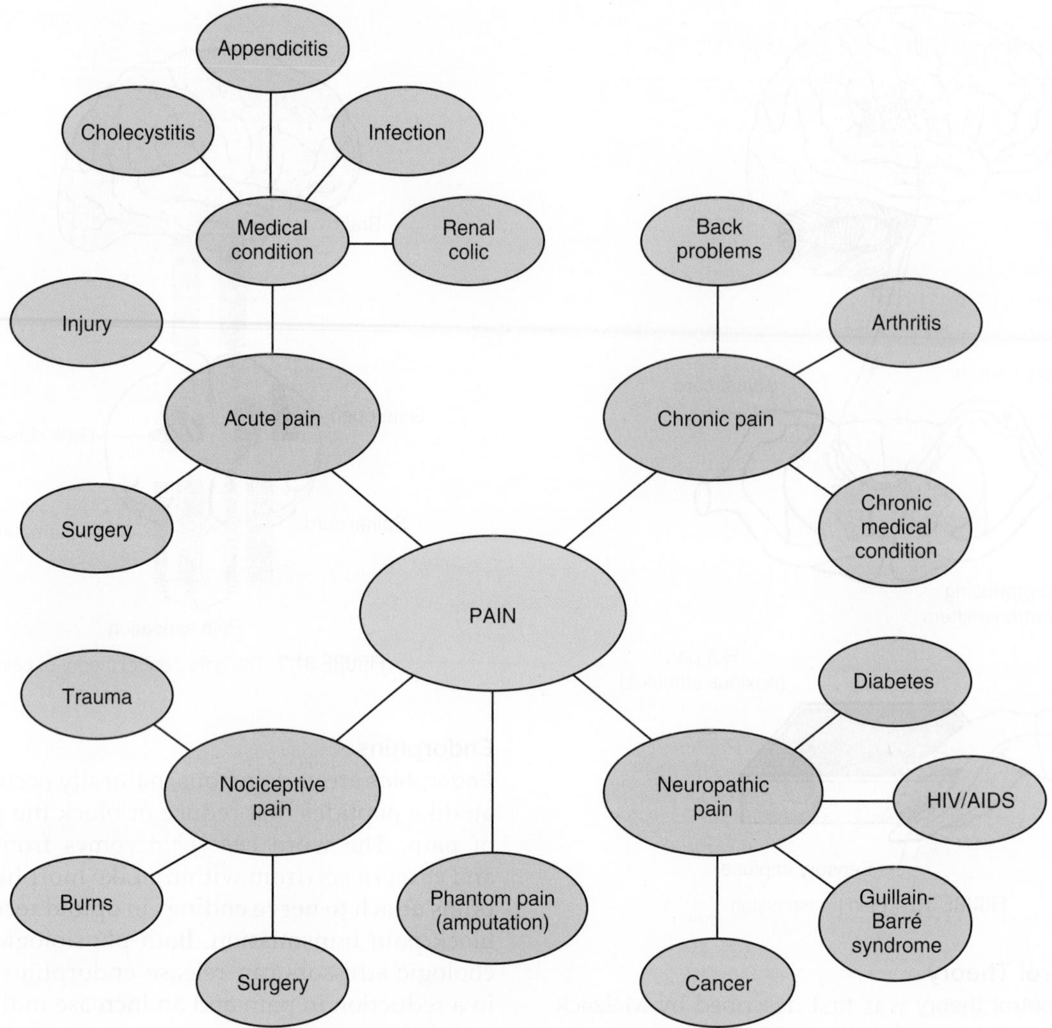

CONCEPT MAP 31.1 The various types and causes of pain.

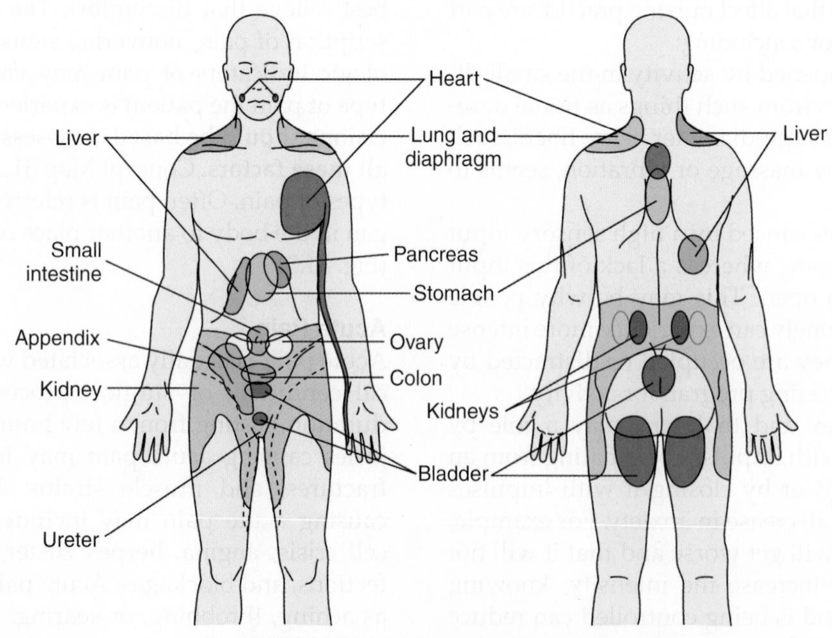

FIGURE 31.3 Usual sites of referred pain.

by **splinting,** or supporting the area. Pain may also be accompanied by an increase in heart rate, blood pressure, and respiratory rate. **Acute pain may worsen in the presence of anxiety or fear.** The cause is usually easily determined, and the pain is well controlled with analgesics (pain medications), surgery, or other techniques. Once the cause is removed, acute pain will be relieved.

Chronic Pain

Chronic pain may continue for months or possibly years. Chronic pain is associated with ongoing conditions, such as arthritis and back problems. Many medical problems can cause chronic pain. The limitations imposed by chronic pain can cause long-lasting psychosocial effects for the patient because of necessary changes in lifestyle. Chronic pain may be described as dull, constant, shooting, tingling, or burning. The increased heart rate, blood pressure, and respiratory rate seen with acute pain are often absent with chronic pain. A combination of pharmacologic and nonpharmacologic treatments is recommended to alleviate chronic pain. This would include combining medication with treatments such as guided imagery, application of heat and cold, and massage.

Nociceptive Pain

Nociceptive pain involves injury to tissue in which receptors called **nociceptors** are located. Nociceptors may be found in skin, joints, or organ viscera. Injuries triggering nociceptive pain may be caused by trauma, burns, or surgery. Nociceptive pain involves four phases: (1) **transduction** begins when tissue damage causes the release of substances that stimulate the nociceptors and start the sensation of pain, (2) **transmission** involves movement of the pain sensation to the spinal cord, (3) **perception** occurs when pain impulses reach the brain and the pain is recognized, and (4) **modulation** occurs when neurons in the brain send signals back down the spinal cord by release of neurotransmitters.

Treatment of nociceptive pain may be directed toward one or all of the four phases. Nonsteroidal anti-inflammatory drugs (NSAIDs) work by blocking the production of the substances that trigger the nociceptors in the transduction phase. Drugs that interfere with the transmission phase include opioids. Nonpharmacologic treatments such as distraction and guided imagery may be effective during the perception phase. Drugs that block neurotransmitter uptake work in the modulation stage.

Neuropathic Pain

Neuropathic pain is usually associated with a dysfunction of the nervous system, specifically, an abnormality in processing sensations. Pain receptors in the body become sensitive to stimuli and send pain signals more easily. Nerve endings grow additional branches that send stronger pain signals to the brain. As the branches grow, they influence touch and warmth receptors, and these receptors begin to send pain signals. In some cases, the pain signal that normally moves from the periphery toward the brain reverses and is sent in the opposite direction. These changes in the nervous system are often associated with medical conditions rather than tissue damage. Diabetes, Guillain-Barré syndrome, multiple sclerosis, cancer, HIV, and nutritional deficiencies are examples of medical conditions associated with neuropathic pain. Analgesics and opioids alone usually do not relieve neuropathic pain. Neuropathic pain is sometimes managed with common analgesics such as those in the NSAID family, but also increasingly with adjuvant medications such as tricyclic antidepressants, anticonvulsants, and corticosteroids.

Phantom Pain

Phantom pain occurs after the loss of a body part from amputation. The patient may "feel" pain in the amputated part for years after the amputation has occurred. If this cannot be controlled with conventional methods, pain may be controlled by the use of continuous electrical stimulation from electrodes surgically implanted in the thalamus.

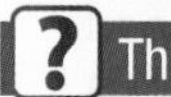
Think Critically

What conditions might involve chronic pain, and what might cause acute pain?

❖ APPLICATION OF THE NURSING PROCESS

◆ ASSESSMENT (DATA COLLECTION)

According to pain specialists, McCaffery and Pasero, **"pain is whatever the experiencing person says it is," existing whenever he says it does** (Kumar & Elavarasi, 2016). In other words, only the patient knows what hurts and how much, and interventions must be based on the patient's own assessment of the degree of pain and the need for pain relief.

Perception of Pain

One of the most difficult aspects of pain management is the assessment of pain and the evaluation of the effectiveness of interventions. Cultural background influences how people show pain. Some cultures teach that outward expressions of pain are to be avoided. Men in some cultures may believe that denying the presence of pain shows bravery and strength. Care must be taken to ensure that adequate pain management is provided. The older adult may not express pain because they mistakenly believe it is a logical consequence of aging, because they do not want to be a bother, or because they have been culturally trained not to complain about pain.

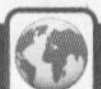 Cultural Considerations

Perception of Pain

People from other cultures may have differing ideas about pain, both how to react to pain and what to do about it. It is important to understand these differences, and equally important not to assume someone believes a certain way because they belong to a particular cultural group.

Observable indicators of pain include moaning, crying, irritability, inability to sleep, grimacing or frowning, restlessness, and a rigid posture in bed. Remember that these things can also indicate sorrow, worry, fear, and fatigue. In addition, some stoic patients may show none of these outward expressions of pain. Other detectable signs of pain can be an elevation in blood pressure, heart rate, and respirations or the presence of nausea or diaphoresis. Fully assess the patient's pain, and encourage the patient to express the perception of the pain being experienced. **Some patients may perceive pain to be less than or greater than what you may have seen before for the same condition.**

 Focused Assessment

Pain Assessment

- **History of pain:** Events or factors that precipitated the pain, location and radiation, intensity, quality (what the pain feels like), aggravating factors, relieving measures, past episodes, past successful treatments, surgery, fracture, burns, and injury
- **Medications:** Present treatment and past treatment, including prescriptions, over-the-counter medications, herbal preparations or supplements, and alcohol or other drug use
- **Verbal indicators:** Severity of pain (pain scale assessment), words used to describe pain; moaning, grunting, crying, as well as the timing of when the pain began, and whether it has changed
- **Nonverbal indicators:** Grimacing, guarding, splinting, evident muscle tension, pacing, rocking, fetal positioning, wincing, inability to sleep, restless movements, and withdrawal from others
- **Social or psychologic factors:** Fear or anxiety, extreme stress, worry, or depression
- **Treatments used:** Medications, heat, cold, massage, vibration, acupuncture, chiropractic adjustment, brace or splint, or aromatherapy
- **Contributing factors:** Constipation, sleep deprivation, fatigue, constant cough, rash, gastrointestinal upset, or esophageal reflux

A Mnemonic Device for Pain Assessment is PQRST:

P: Precipitating events
Q: Quality of pain or discomfort
R: Radiation of pain
S: Severity of pain
T: Timing

Alert adult patients may be able to use specific words to describe their pain. However, even for adults, it can be difficult to describe and tell how much pain is present. Table 31.1 gives some terms that can be used to describe pain. Be aware of any communication blocks that may prevent the patient from adequately describing the pain. For example, patients who speak a foreign language may require a translator to describe their pain adequately.

Table 31.1 Descriptive Terms for Pain

TYPE OF DESCRIPTION	SPECIFIC TERMS
Degree of pain	Absent, minimal, mild, moderate, fairly severe, very or extremely severe, exquisite, or excruciating
Quality of pain	Crushing, throbbing, pulsating, twisting, pulling, burning, searing, stabbing, tearing, biting, blinding, nauseating, or debilitating
Area of pain	Name of affected body area or part (e.g., right foot or right lower abdomen) localized, radiating, or generalized
Frequency of pain	Constant, intermittent, or occasional

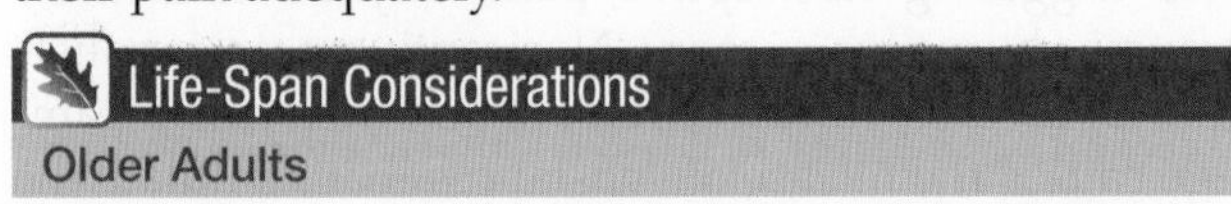
PAIN: Ask patient to rate pain on scale of 0–10
No pain
Worst pain imaginable
0 1 2 3 4 5 6 7 8 9 10

FIGURE 31.4 Numeric pain rating scale.

Life-Span Considerations

Older Adults

The older adult patient may use "aching," "soreness," "stiffness," or "discomfort" rather than "pain" during assessment.

Pain Scales

A variety of pain scales is available to assist patients in communicating their pain level. A numeric scale is often used to help the patient rate the level of pain, with 0 being pain free and 10 being the worst pain imaginable (Fig. 31.4). When requesting pain medication and when assessing the degree of relief following the dose, the patient can refer to the numeric scale. For example, a patient who had an appendectomy this morning may describe his incisional pain as being 8 on a scale of 0 to 10, or very bad, but not the worst possible pain; 1 hour after receiving his medication, he may describe his pain as being a 3, not gone but greatly reduced, allowing him to move about and rest in reasonable comfort.

Children, as well as some adults, may find a numeric scale difficult to use. A picture scale showing faces in varying degrees of pain can also help assess pain (Fig. 31.5). The *Face, Legs, Activity, Cry,* and *Consolability* (FLACC) scale is used for preverbal

0
No hurt
1
Hurts
little bit
2
Hurts
little more
3
Hurts
even more
4
Hurts
whole lot
5
Hurts
worst

FIGURE 31.5 Wong-Baker FACES pain rating scale. (From Hockenberry, M. J., & Wilson, D. [2013]. *Wong's Essentials of Pediatric Nursing* [9th ed.]. St. Louis: Mosby. Used with permission. Copyright Mosby. *Wong's Essentials of Pediatric Nursing* [6th ed.]. St. Louis: Mosby.)

children or noncommunicative patients (Rahu, et al., 2015). For infants, one of several scales is used: the Neonatal Infant Pain Scale (NIPS), Crying, Requires oxygen to maintain saturation, Increased vital signs, Expression, and Sleeplessness (CRIES), or Premature Infant Pain Profile (PIPP). For patients with moderate to severe cognitive deficits or those who have difficulty communicating verbally, the pain thermometer scale, a discomfort scale, or the Pain Assessment Checklist for Seniors with Limited Ability to Communicate (PACSLAC) scale may be used (Cong & McGrath, et al., 2013).

For the confused patient, nonverbal cues that pain is being experienced may include restlessness, rocking, pacing, rigidity, guarding, wincing, crying, grimacing with movement, new inability to sleep, hypersensitivity to touch, withdrawal from usual contact with others, moaning, and grunting. Family or close friends may be able to provide input on how the individual has expressed pain in the past.

Clinical Cues

Management of acute pain, such as postsurgical pain, may be more difficult for patients who have been on opioid medications to control chronic pain. Because they already have an underlying degree of constant pain being controlled by routine medication, they often require higher and/or more frequent doses of analgesia than other patients do. This is not a sign of addiction but rather a legitimate need for a greater degree of analgesia to relieve the additional acute pain.

QSEN Considerations: Teamwork and Collaboration

Memory Jogger

The scale selected to assist in determining the presence and intensity of pain must be indicated on the patient care plan so that it is used consistently by staff.

Assignment Considerations

Reporting Signs of Pain

Remind assistive personnel to report nonverbal signs of pain in patients, such as wincing when being turned, rigid posture, grimacing with movement, or crying with repositioning. Refusal to participate in ordered therapy may also indicate increasing pain, and it should be reported.

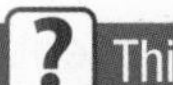

Think Critically

How would you assess pain in a nonverbal patient? How would you assess pain relief?

◆ NURSING DIAGNOSIS

Accurate nursing diagnosis for the patient with pain is based on the patient assessment. Because pain is an individual experience, the reported pain may vary from patient to patient, even though they share a similar medical diagnosis. Nursing diagnoses may include:

- Readiness for enhanced comfort
- Acute pain
- Chronic pain
- Fatigue
- Self-care deficit
- Deficient knowledge
- Sleep deprivation
- Anxiety
- Fear

◆ PLANNING

The plan of care must include pain assessment and management. This should include realistic goals with specific time frames for achieving results. A possible goal might be "patient will report pain at a level of less than 3 on a 0-to-10 scale within 2 days." The patient should assist with setting goals. Goals should be realistic; a patient with a chronic condition may not be pain free, even with the use of analgesics.

◆ IMPLEMENTATION

Pain is an individual experience. **Medications or treatments that prove effective for one patient may not relieve symptoms as well for another patient.** Different methods may need to be tried, alone or in combination, before the patient has effective pain relief (Nursing Care Plan 31.1). Monitor respirations closely in patients receiving opioids.

Nonmedicinal Methods of Pain Control

Just like medications, nonmedicinal pain control methods provide varying degrees of relief, depending on the patient. Use of nonmedicinal methods of pain control may greatly reduce the amount of medication needed. As patients gain pain control and as changes in their condition reduce overall pain, they will voluntarily reduce the use of medications.

Transcutaneous electrical nerve stimulation. **Transcutaneous electrical nerve stimulation (TENS)** uses a small electrical stimulator attached to electrodes to block pain. This therapy is available in high-frequency and low-frequency stimulation. Acute pain may be treated with conventional high-frequency TENS therapy, whereas low-frequency TENS therapy is more effective in the treatment of chronic pain. The electrodes

Nursing Care Plan 31.1 Care of the Patient in Pain

SCENARIO Sara Reynolds, a 48-year-old patient with a history of rheumatoid arthritis, has been admitted to the unit following a right total hip replacement performed this morning. Orders include morphine sulfate via PCA pump, which has just been started. Ms. Reynolds has complained of pain at 8 on a 0-to-10 scale. Her blood pressure and pulse are slightly elevated, but her temperature and respirations are normal. She has been restless and grimaces frequently. You implement the following portion of her plan of care.

PROBLEM/NURSING DIAGNOSIS *Hip replacement*/Pain related to surgical procedure.

Supporting Assessment Data *Subjective:* Patient reports pain at 8 on a 0-to-10 scale. *Objective:* Hip replacement today. Blood pressure and pulse slightly elevated; grimacing and restless.

Goals/Expected Outcomes	Nursing Interventions	Selected Rationale	Evaluation
Patient will report pain at 0 to 4 on a 0-to-10 scale within 2 h.	Teach patient to use the PCA pump.	Knowledge of how to use the pump allows the patient to use it correctly.	*Is pain at 0 to 4?* Yes. Using pump correctly.
	Encourage relaxation techniques; provide diversionary activities such as television, reading, or computer.	Relaxation and diversion are known to lessen pain by focusing the mind elsewhere.	Taught relaxation exercise. Does not wish to watch TV at present.
	Encourage use of PCA before ambulation or exercise.	Medicating before activity reduces pain related to the activity.	Medicated before physical therapist visit.
	Teach patient to splint abdomen and hip area with pillow when coughing or using spirometer.	Splinting reduces pain associated with movement of the abdomen.	Taught splinting technique.
	Observe frequently for pain relief and side effects of medication.	If pain is inadequately relieved, other measures to relieve it can be employed. Knowing whether side effects are occurring allows measures to be taken to alleviate or prevent them.	No side effects noted other than drowsiness. Pain at 3. Progressing toward expected outcomes.

PCA, Patient-controlled analgesia.

CRITICAL THINKING QUESTIONS

1. What factors might influence a child's report of pain?
2. What factors might lead to undertreatment of pain in the older adult population?

are placed on the skin around the area of pain. Low-level current running between the electrodes acts to block the pain sensation. The patient can control the intensity and interval of the current with the dials on the stimulator (Fig. 31.6). A health care professional trained in its use should initiate the application of the TENS unit. This may be a physical therapist, but may also be a nurse or a primary care provider.

The use of TENS requires a medical order. TENS for the relief of postoperative pain is generally most effective when the patient has received instructions on the use of the device before surgery. Postoperative pain and analgesic medications make patient education more difficult than it would have been before surgery for most patients. TENS may also be ordered after traumatic injuries. Occasionally a patient will not tolerate TENS stimulation well. If this is the case, discontinue treatment and notify the primary care provider (Skill 31.1).

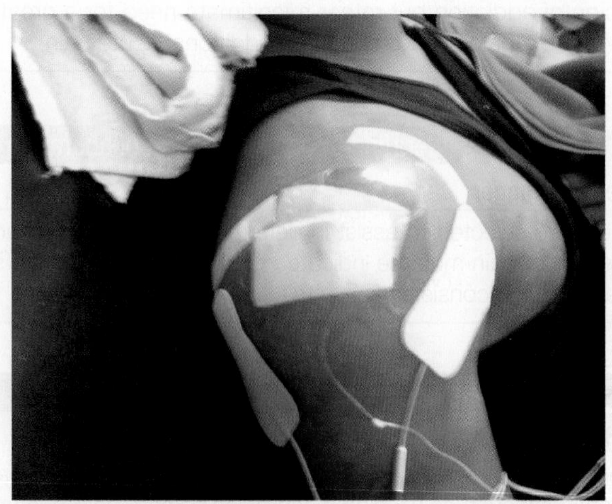

FIGURE 31.6 TENS unit being used after shoulder surgery. (From DeLee, J. C., Drez, D., & Miller M. D. [2009] *DeLee and Drez's Orthopaedic Sports Medicine: Principles and Practices* [3rd ed.]. Philadelphia: Saunders.)

Skill 31.1 Operating a Transcutaneous Electrical Nerve Stimulation Unit

 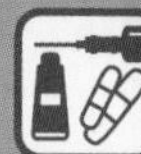 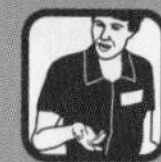 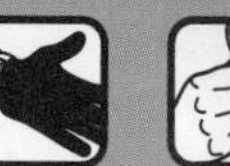 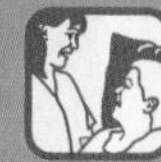 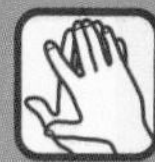 

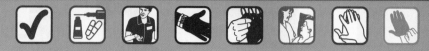

TENS uses low-level electric current via electrodes to block pain sensation. Patients need to be properly instructed in the use of the TENS unit.

SUPPLIES

- TENS unit
- Electrodes
- Conductive jelly (if electrodes are not precoated)
- Tape (if electrodes are not self-adhesive)

Review and carry out the Standard Steps in Appendix A.

ACTION (*RATIONALE*)

Assessment

1. Check the primary care provider's orders. Check to see where electrodes are to be placed. (*Ensures proper placement of electrodes and appropriate TENS settings.*)

Planning

2. Assemble equipment. (*Avoids interruptions and provides for good time management.*)
3. Identify the patient. (*Ensures correct patient receives the TENS.*)
4. Explain the procedure to the patient. (*Decreases patient anxiety and increases cooperation.*)

Implementation

5. Make certain TENS unit is turned off; check to see that the electrodes are properly connected to the unit. (*Avoids premature stimulation of the site.*)
6. Spread conductive jelly on the electrode pads, if electrodes are not precoated. (*Provides for correct electrical conduction.*)
7. Place electrode pads against the patient's skin in the designated places. Use tape to secure if necessary. (*Ensures good conduction; provides stimulation in prescribed places.*)
8. Position patient comfortably. (*Comfort enhances effectiveness of the TENS treatment.*)
9. Explain to the patient that he will feel a tingling sensation. (*Explanations decrease patient anxiety.*)
10. Turn TENS unit on. (*This begins the treatment.*)
11. Increase the amplitude of TENS unit according to patient's response. Check frequently to see how patient is tolerating the procedure. (*Patients should not receive TENS stimulation to the point of discomfort.*)
12. Turn off TENS unit and remove electrodes at the end of the prescribed treatment time. (*Follows the prescribed treatment.*)
13. Assist patient in cleaning the jelly off the skin and rearrange clothing. (*Provides for comfort and good hygiene.*)

Evaluation

14. Assess how patient tolerated the procedure. Assess level of discomfort. (*Evaluates effectiveness of procedure.*)

Documentation

15. Document the date, time, amplitude, and length of time of the procedure; patient tolerance of procedure; and current level of pain. (*Documents use of TENS unit and response to treatment.*)

Documentation Example

TENS unit applied to right shoulder at amplitude of 5 for 20 minutes, tolerated well. Patient states pain at a level of 1 on a 0-to-10 scale following the procedure. (Nurse's time-stamped electronic signature)

Critical Thinking Questions

1. In what patient population might TENS therapy be contraindicated?
2. What safety precautions should be considered for the patient receiving TENS therapy?

Percutaneous electrical nerve stimulation. A treatment showing promise for relief of lower back pain, such as that caused by sciatica, and for relief of some severe headaches, is percutaneous electrical nerve stimulation (PENS). An electric current is sent through thin needle probes positioned in the soft tissues and muscles of the back. A series of intermittent treatments using the electric current are given.

Binders and braces. Binders are cloths wrapped around a limb or body part. They are effective in relieving pain associated with strains, sprains, and surgical incisions. They support the surface and internal tissues during movement, coughing, and other activities. For example, an abdominal binder may be ordered to give additional support and provide comfort after abdominal surgery (see Chapter 38). A brace is a device to immobilize joints. It is stiffer than a binder, and it promotes healing by limiting movement of the joint.

Application of heat and cold. The application of heat or cold, or the alternate application of first one and

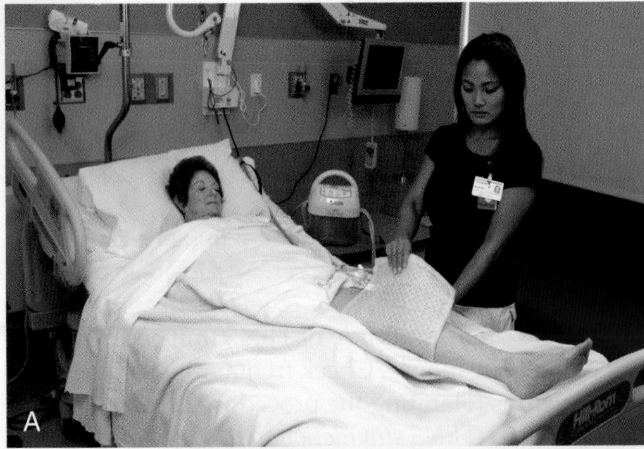

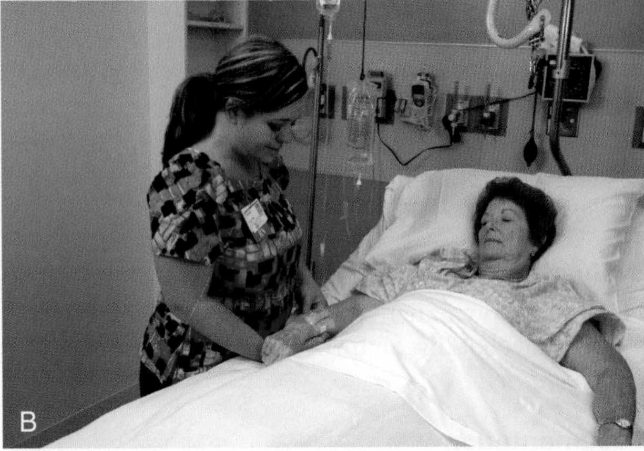

FIGURE 31.7 (A) An Aquathermia K-Pad is used to help relieve pain in the knee. (B) A warm compress is applied to an inflamed IV site.

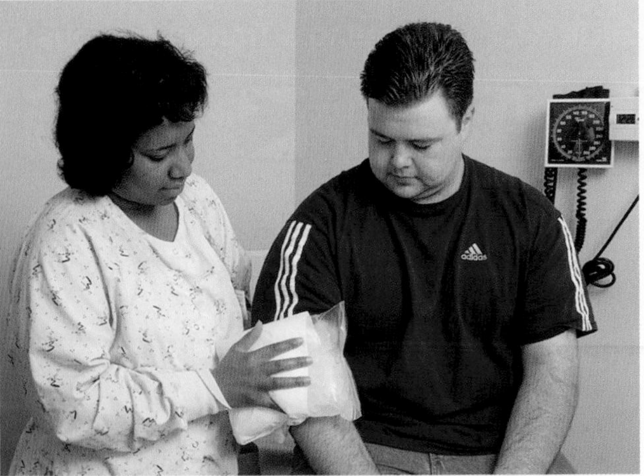

FIGURE 31.8 A cold pack reduces pain and swelling.

then the other, can often soothe or relieve pain from muscular strain or overwork. It is also effective in reducing pain associated with healing tissues.

Sources of warmth include warm water compresses, warm blankets, Aquathermia K-Pads, tub and whirlpool baths, and chemical self-heating packs (Fig. 31.7). The use of heat-producing equipment may require a medical order. When applying heat, check the temperature carefully to avoid burning the patient. Remember that very young and very old patients have skin that is more sensitive to heat damage. In addition, patients with altered levels of consciousness, impaired movement and feeling, or poor circulation may not be aware when something is too hot. These patients can suffer severe burns in a short period. All patients should be closely monitored if heat applications are being used.

Cold is particularly helpful in reducing swelling and can be effective in calming muscle spasms and reducing the pain in joints and muscles from a variety of causes (Fig. 31.8). Gentle ice massage of painful muscles can be done with ice that has been frozen in a paper cup. Tear the edge of the cup away to expose the ice, use the remaining cup as a handle, and massage the area with the ice surface. A bag of frozen peas can be used as an ice pack. Cold is most frequently applied in the form of cold or iced compresses. Some patients have a poor tolerance for cold treatment, so be alert to the patient's response when using cold applications. Occasionally, patients have an increase rather than a decrease in pain when ice is applied. To prevent skin damage, ice should be in contact with the skin for only a few minutes at a time, under direct supervision. Ice packs should be applied with a towel or other barrier between the pack and the skin and not left in place for more than 15 to 20 minutes.

Relaxation. **Relaxation,** or tension release, is helpful in reducing pain, and it allows the patient to obtain greater relief from pain medications. Relaxation is a physical technique that involves conscious relaxation of muscle groups. Before beginning, make the patient comfortable in a quiet, darkened environment. Instruct the patient to first tighten and then release the muscles. Initially, encourage the patient to pay close attention to the difference in the feeling of tension versus relaxation. Frequently, relaxation is done progressively. Have the patient begin by tensing and relaxing (or just relaxing) the toes and feet and then the ankles, calves, knees, thighs, lower abdomen (or stomach), upper abdomen (or chest), shoulders, arms, hands and fingers, neck, face, and head. Give these directions slowly, one body area at a time, with a short space of quiet between each directed relaxation. After a session or two, most patients can do this technique for themselves. Some people with chronic tension-related pain go to sleep this way every night. A variety of relaxation compact disks or audio files are available to assist patients who find this technique helpful.

Biofeedback. **Biofeedback** is a specialized relaxation technique using a machine that measures the degree of muscular tension with skin electrodes. The machine has colored lights that change (usually red to yellow to green) and a tone that changes in pitch from higher to lower as the patient relaxes muscular tension. With this immediate feedback, the patient learns to use relaxation techniques or imagery effectively to decrease tension.

Distraction. **Distraction** assists the patient in focusing on something other than the pain. Patients frequently do this inadvertently, such as when they enjoy visitors and for the moment forget their pain. Unfortunately, nurses sometimes take this as proof that the patient is not in pain at all and see the patient's request for medication as drug-seeking behavior. In fact, the patient still hurts but is just focusing elsewhere.

Watching television, listening to the radio, playing cards or a game, conversing with a friend or volunteer, reading, using a computer, or even thinking about something else may all act as distractions. However, remember that the distraction does not make the pain go away; it merely diverts the attention elsewhere for a time. After the distraction is over, such as at the end of the television program or a visit, the patient may be more aware than ever of the pain. Distraction may be particularly helpful while waiting for an administered dose of medication to take effect. By the time the distraction ends, the pain has begun to be relieved by the analgesic.

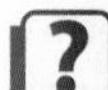

Think Critically

What methods could you use to distract a patient in the following settings: the hospital, a long-term care facility, and at home?

Guided imagery and meditation. These methods differ from relaxation in that they are mental rather than physical techniques. In **guided imagery** (verbally guiding the patient to imagine something) as it is used for pain control, patients are assisted in forming mental images of a pleasant environment where they are comfortable and happy, such as a favorite vacation place. Patients undergoing painful procedures, such as bone marrow aspiration, can learn to use imagery to "leave" the procedure and mentally go somewhere else while it is occurring. Some people have great difficulty seeing things in their minds and need verbal direction to hear or feel pleasant sensations, such as the rustle of leaves or the feel of a breeze as it brushes across their cheeks. Many people who do not visualize well can still get great relief from the technique when it calls on their auditory and kinesthetic abilities.

Patient Education

PAIN CONTROL THROUGH GUIDED IMAGERY

Preparation

- Assist the patient to a comfortable position.
- Lower the lights to a comfortable level, but not completely dark.
- Eliminate any distractions, such as television or radio.
- Close the door. Post a note asking not to be disturbed.

Read the Imagery Script

- Read slowly, in a soft but easily heard voice. Pause frequently to allow the patient to form mental images. The script may be changed to incorporate a place or sensations specific to the patient.
- **Imagery script:**
  - Relax, and gently close your eyes.
  - Take a deep, slow breath in through your nose. *(Pause)* Now slowly exhale through your mouth. Let your tension leave your body as you exhale. *(Pause)* Continue this with each breath. *(Pause)*
  - Imagine you are walking along a forest path. *(Pause)* Smell the fresh air. *(Pause)* Feel the breeze against your face. *(Pause)* Hear the crunch of leaves under your feet.
  - The path leads to your favorite place. It may be a beach, the mountains, or a favorite room in your home. *(Pause)* This is a special place, one where you feel relaxed and secure. *(Pause)*
  - Listen to the sounds around you. *(Pause)* Smell the air. *(Pause)* Take in the comforting sensations of your special place. *(Pause)*
  - Relax even more as you enjoy your surroundings. A feeling of peace and security wraps around you. *(Pause)* Tension leaves as you take in the sensations of this place. *(Pause)*
  - It is now time to leave this place. Get ready to leave, and head back to the forest path. *(Pause)*
  - You feel relaxed and at peace as you return to this room. *(Pause)* You know that you can return to your special place any time. *(Pause)*
  - When you are ready, open your eyes.

After the Imagery Experience

- Allow the patient to share with you if desired. Accept that some patients will not want to share.

Meditation (focusing on an image, thought, the breath, or awareness) can provide the same relief from a painful situation, but it relies on the use of a focus point rather than the mental creation of an alternate environment. During meditation, individuals focus on a visual point, a sound, a repeated phrase, or just the pattern of their own breathing. This focuses attention away from the pain or a painful situation and, for many people, induces profound physical relaxation and reduction in blood pressure and respiratory rate.

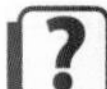

Think Critically

What could you suggest to a patient to use as a visual point for meditation?

Music. Music can be used alone as a source of distraction from pain. It is frequently used effectively in conjunction with other methods. Meditation and relaxation techniques can be done to restful music, and massage can be greatly enhanced by the presence of soft, soothing sounds. Also effective is the use of nature sounds, such as tapes of the ocean, a flowing stream, or the wind and birds in the trees. Listening on headphones allows patients to enjoy their own preferences in music without disturbing others.

Hypnosis. **Hypnosis** is also called therapeutic suggestion. It involves inducing a trance-like state using focusing and relaxation techniques and giving the patient suggestions that may be helpful after the return to an alert state of consciousness. Hypnosis should be done by someone trained in the technique. Hypnosis is only possible and effective when the individual is able to cooperate with the technique; it is pointless to urge it on someone who does not want to be hypnotized.

Massage. **Massage** has long been used to induce relaxation and bring relief from muscle and structural pain. A nightly back rub can bring much comfort to the bedridden patient. Long firm strokes, softer circular strokes, and gentle pounding stimulate circulation, relax muscles, and increase the patient's sense of well-being. This gift of direct comfort from nurse to patient, perhaps more than any other, demonstrates the caring relationship so important to good nursing care. The use of lotion warmed between the hands and then applied to the patient's back refreshes the skin and relieves dryness and itching.

Conditions such as a healing surgical wound or inflammation of the tissues or vessels may preclude direct massage to the area of pain. In such cases, firm massage to another area of the body may allow the patient to focus away from the area of pain. In addition, massage distal or proximal to the point of pain may relieve pain while avoiding direct stimulation to an injured site.

Chiropractic, acupuncture, and acupressure therapies are also used for pain management. These are discussed in Chapter 32.

Medical Methods of Pain Control

Analgesic medications. When pain medications are ordered for patients experiencing pain, you are responsible for monitoring the patient's pain level and administering the medication as ordered. The patient must also be monitored for effectiveness of the medication after administration. The period for reassessment varies depending on the route of administration.

The four basic categories of medications for the relief of pain are (1) nonopioid pain medications, a category that includes **NSAIDs**; (2) cyclooxygenase-2 (COX-2) inhibitors; (3) narcotics or opioids; and (4) adjuvant analgesics. This fourth group includes drugs that are not primarily regarded as analgesics but have been proven effective in the relief of certain types of pain or work with standard analgesics to produce better pain control. COX-2 inhibitors are a type of drug that selectively blocks the COX-2 enzyme, thought to play a role in the cause of arthritis pain. They do not block the COX-1 enzyme, which protects the gastrointestinal system. Therefore, these drugs are not supposed to cause the gastrointestinal side effects, such as gastritis and ulcers, that NSAIDs may cause. Table 31.2 gives examples of the drugs in these four categories. Analgesic treatment is based on the pain assessment.

Clinical Cues

One of the most common side effects of analgesia is constipation. Patients on pain relieving medications should be encouraged to increase their fluid intake if not otherwise contraindicated, and they should be assessed daily regarding bowel function.

Analgesic (pain relieving) medications, whether prescription or nonprescription, are ordered by the primary care provider for the patient. Check the name of the drug, dosage, route, and frequency. If the medication is ordered "as needed" (PRN), the order must include the circumstances under which the drug may be given, such as "PRN for back pain." Analgesics may be given by a numerous routes, including oral, sublingual (SL), topical, intramuscular (IM) injection, intravenous (IV) injection or infusion, PCA, and epidural infusion.

Oral medications. Oral medications have been traditionally used for mild to moderate pain. Recent advances, however, have made available products such as time-released oral morphine, which may be used effectively for severe pain. This dosage form is particularly helpful for patients with chronic severe pain, such as that which occurs with cancer. The use of this type of medication has allowed many individuals with

Table 31.2 Categories of Analgesic Medications

TYPE OF DRUG	PRIMARY MODE OF ACTION	EXAMPLES
Nonopioid analgesics, including NSAIDs	Block pain at the peripheral nervous system level	Over-the-counter: aspirin, acetaminophen, ibuprofen (nonprescription dose), naproxen Prescription: ibuprofen (prescription dose), naproxen, indomethacin
COX-2 inhibitors	Block the COX-2 enzyme, which plays a role in arthritis pain	Anti-inflammatories: celecoxib is currently the only FDA-approved COX-2 inhibitor
Narcotics or opioids	Block pain at the central nervous system level	Narcotic agonists: morphine, oxycodone, hydrocodone, hydromorphone, codeine, levorphanol, oxymorphone, and meperidine (used less frequently because of significant side effects)
Adjuvant analgesics	Various methods of action	Anticonvulsants: phenytoin, carbamazepine Antidepressants: amitriptyline, imipramine, SSRIs Muscle relaxants: baclofen Stimulants: caffeine, dextroamphetamine

COX-2, Cyclooxygenase-2; *FDA*, United States Food and Drug Administration; *NSAIDs*, nonsteroidal anti-inflammatory drugs; *SSRI*, selective serotonin reuptake inhibitors.

severe chronic pain to return to work and a near-normal life for long periods despite serious illness.

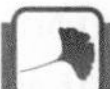 Complementary and Alternative Therapies

Cannabis

When analgesic medications, including opioids, fail to control pain, in some states medical cannabis may be prescribed to help reduce pain. Cannabis (marijuana) can be smoked or mixed into food items and consumed.

Topical medications. Various topical preparations, such as capsaicin, ibuprofen, diclofenac, or menthol cream or gels, may provide relief for muscle or joint pain. Medication patches, such as fentanyl patches, allow the analgesic medicine to be absorbed slowly through the skin. Lidoderm patches are often helpful for neuropathic pain. Fentanyl is approved for relief of severe chronic pain only.

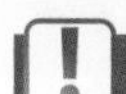 Safety Alert

Fentanyl Patch Overdose

Signs and symptoms of fentanyl overdose are shallow respirations; extreme sleepiness; inability to think, walk, or talk normally; or feelings of faintness, dizziness, or confusion. If symptoms occur, remove the patch and clean the skin, and call the primary care provider immediately.

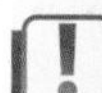 Safety Alert

Safety Education

FENTANYL DANGER FOR CHILDREN

Since patients taking fentanyl have chronic pain, they will be using these patches at home. Several deaths have been reported from children either swallowing the patches or applying them to their skin. Teach the patient to keep the patches away from children; locked up if possible.

A pain medication patch containing metal must be removed before a patient undergoes a magnetic resonance imaging (MRI) scan, otherwise a burn may occur to the skin.

Injected medications. IM or subcutaneous injection of pain medication is usually used for severe pain and only for a relatively short time. Medication given by this method has the advantage of lasting several hours, but administration is painful for the patient, and prolonged use can be detrimental to the tissues. Many individuals, particularly children, fear injections. Small children and older adults also have relatively few sites with adequate muscle tissue; therefore, they can only safely receive medication by this route for a short time. IM injection requires careful technique to avoid nerve injury.

IM injections are used less today than in the past. The dose given is larger than that given intravenously, and the length of time the medication is effective is extended because of the slow absorption from the muscular tissue. Injections are more commonly used for immediate relief of severe pain when an IV line is not in place, although some primary care providers and patients still prefer the IM route.

Intravenous medications. IV pain medication may be given as a **bolus** (concentrated dose given rapidly), as a slow push (over a few minutes), as an intermittent infusion, or by continuous infusion. These techniques are discussed in Chapter 36.

 Assignment Considerations

Monitoring Patients on Narcotic Analgesics

Because many analgesics are constipating, ask assistive personnel to carefully monitor patients who are receiving a narcotic analgesic by any route. Bowel movements need to be tracked, and deviations from the patient's normal pattern reported to the nurse right away. All patients receiving narcotic analgesia should be given mild laxatives, stool softeners, and increased fiber and fluid (unless contraindicated) in the diet.

Administration of pain medication via PCA (discussed in the section "*Patient-controlled analgesia*") has become the preferred route for most patients, although continuous infusion may still be the route of choice for control of severe chronic pain, such as that experienced by some terminally ill cancer patients.

Life-Span Considerations

Older Adults

Because of the decreased kidney and liver function that occurs with aging, an older adult may respond differently to analgesics than a younger adult would. Toxicity with analgesics can occur at normal dosages. Closely monitor the older adult for side effects, such as excessive sedation and constipation (Malec & Shega, 2015).

Patient-controlled analgesia. Currently, the most common method used for injectable opioids in acute care is **PCA** (analgesia doses controlled by the patient). This method uses one of a variety of programmable pumps (Fig. 31.9). The medication comes in special cartridges

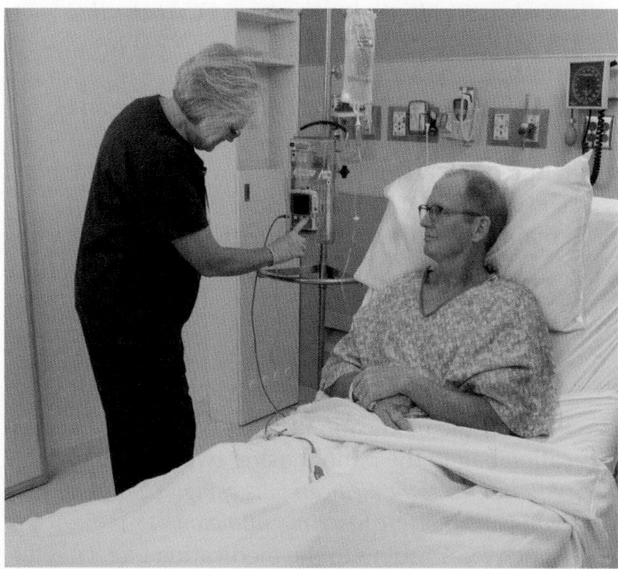

FIGURE 31.9 A portable PCA pump in use by a patient.

or syringes, prediluted to an appropriate strength. The pump is programmed to administer the prescribed dose each time the patient pushes a button, within limitations set by the primary care provider. The primary care provider's order specifies the size of the dose and the minimum time between doses. The pumps are programmed by the registered nurse (RN) or pharmacist. The primary care provider may also order an initial dose or even a continuous infusion dose to be programmed along with the intermittent dose. Within the limits set by the primary care provider's order, the patient can then choose how often to receive the medication.

PCA has proven to greatly reduce patient anxiety about pain by putting the patient in control, and most patients actually use less rather than more medication.

Before caring for a patient with a PCA pump, it is important to understand how it is programmed, how the medication is inserted, and how the machine is locked to prevent anyone from tampering with the medication or the programming (Skill 31.2). PCAs are commonly attached to an IV line, but the medication may also be injected into the subcutaneous tissue on the abdomen for nonhospitalized patients using small, portable pumps.

Skill 31.2 Setting Up (or Monitoring) a Patient-Controlled Analgesia Pump

 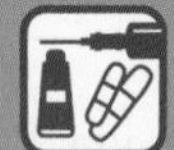 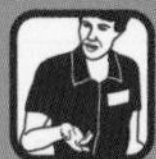  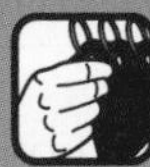 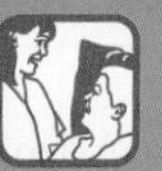 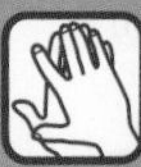 

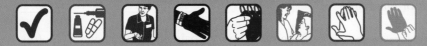

Although the primary responsibility for a PCA pump usually lies with the RN, an LPN/LVN may be required to assist or monitor. Close attention must be paid to both the IV site and side effects of medications.

SUPPLIES

- PCA pump
- IV solution
- PCA medication
- IV administration set
- PCA tubing
- IV starter kit and catheter (if needed)

Review and carry out Standard Steps in Appendix A.

ACTION (*RATIONALE*)

Assessment

1. Check the primary care provider's orders. *(Ensures correct medication dosage and administration.)*
2. Assess patient's knowledge of PCA usage. *(Patients need adequate patient education to use PCA correctly.)*

Planning

3. Assemble the equipment. *(Avoids interruption of procedure; provides for good time management.)*
4. Identify the patient. *(Ensures correct patient receives the PCA.)*
5. Explain procedure to the patient. *(Decreases patient anxiety and increases cooperation.)*

Implementation

6. Start an IV if patient does not have IV access. *(An IV is necessary for standard PCA administration.)*
7. Perform the medication checks of the PCA medication bag to the patient using two identifiers. *(Assures the right medication is being prepared for the right patient before inserting into pump.)*
8. Attach PCA tubing to the medication bag. *(Allows for medication administration.)*
9. Attach, latch, and lock the cassette to the PCA pump. *(Prevents leakage of medication.)*

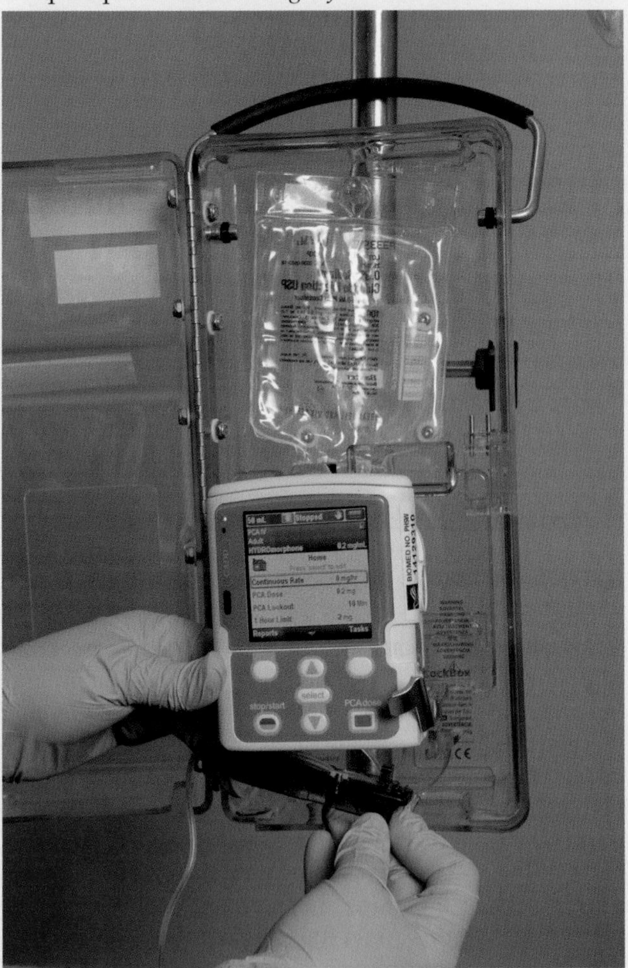

Step 9

10. Secure pump and medication bag in locked medication box. (*Prevents tampering with medication.*)
11. Power on the pump. When "Prime tubing?" displayed, press *Yes* if priming is needed.

(Decreases possibility of air embolism; provides for accurate dosage administration.)

12. Set the PCA pump according to primary care provider's orders. *(This ensures proper drug administration.)*

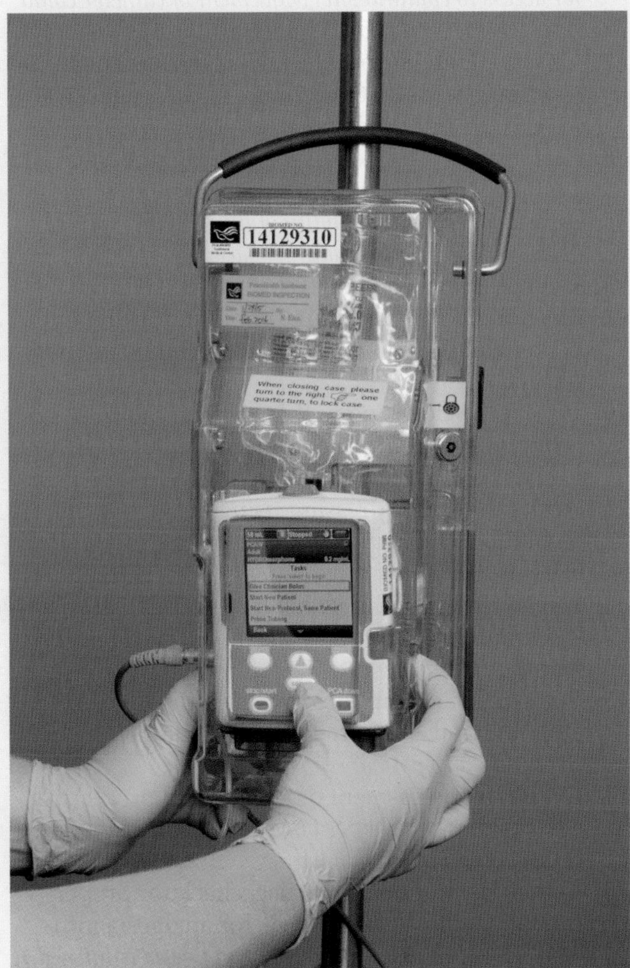

Step **12**

13. Connect the primed IV administration set to the Y adapter of the PCA set. *(Allows for administration of medication through existing IV site.)*
14. Plug the PCA pump into a power source. *(Provides a continuous power source; prevents unnecessary drain on the internal battery.)*
15. Open all slide clamps. *(Allows for PCA administration.)*
16. Review use of PCA with the patient. *(Reinforces previous patient education. Ensures proper use of equipment for pain control.)*

Evaluation

17. Assess patient frequently for ability to use the PCA, effectiveness of medication, and side effects. Assess IV site for redness, drainage, swelling, or tenderness. *(Ensures patient comfort and decreases complications.)*

Documentation

18. Document in the patient's medical record the date and time PCA started, medication, pump settings, observations of the IV site, effectiveness of medication, and patient education. *(Documents use of PCA pump and patient response.)*

Documentation Example

Morphine sulfate via PCA started, 1 mg q 10 min, not to exceed 4 doses/h. No redness, swelling, drainage, tenderness at IV site. Instructions on PCA use given to patient; able to self-administer a dose. States pain at 3 on a 0-to-10 scale. (Nurse's time-stamped electronic signature)

? Critical Thinking Questions

1. How do your beliefs about addiction to pain medication affect the care you provide?
2. What would you teach a patient who expresses a concern about opioid addiction?

? Think Critically

What type of patient education would you perform for a patient using a PCA pump for the first time?

Epidural analgesia. The epidural route has been used for anesthesia for many years. **Epidural analgesia,** however, is a newer form of pain control. An anesthesiologist or nurse anesthetist places a thin catheter in the epidural space near the base of the spine, and then connects the catheter to a small battery-operated programmable pump. The pump administers an opioid analgesic into the epidural space (outside the dural space), either as a bolus followed by a continuous infusion or as repeated bolus doses, as ordered by the primary care provider. **This method is effective in controlling pain while allowing the patient to remain alert.** Its uses include pain relief for obstetric patients in labor, postoperative patients, and patients with cancer. Possible side effects from the opiate component of the infusion include respiratory depression, pruritus, nausea and vomiting, constipation, urinary retention, low pulse rate, and hypotension. Because of rare but potentially dangerous side effects, particularly respiratory depression, patients receiving epidural analgesia are monitored closely. This often includes being placed on an apnea monitor and a pulse oximeter for the first 12 hours. The primary responsibility for caring for the epidural catheter lies with the RN. The licensed practical nurse/licensed vocational nurse (LPN/LVN) monitors the patient's response to the medication (Steps 31.1).

Steps 31.1 Monitoring an Epidural Catheter and Changing the Dressing

A patient may be given an epidural catheter for control of some types of pain. Although an RN or primary care provider starts the administration, other members of the health care team need to monitor the patient closely, both for problems with the catheter and for side effects of medications. The analgesia may be infused by an infusion pump or be given by bolus injection.

Review and carry out the Standard Steps in Appendix A.

ACTION *(RATIONALE)*

1. Assess patient for adequate pain control without signs of oversedation, including decreased level of consciousness or depressed respirations. Be certain that naloxone is immediately available to use in case of an adverse reaction to the analgesia. Monitor vital signs. *(Ensures that pain control is effective and that patient is not experiencing severe central nervous system depression.)*
2. Assess mobility and motor and sensory function before allowing patient out of bed. *(Prevents injury from falling that may occur from sedation, weakness, or postural hypotension.)*
3. Know the facility's policy and procedure for epidural dressing changes. Always change the dressing when soiled, wet, or not intact. Gauze and tape dressings should be changed every 48 to 72 hours, and transparent semipermeable dressings at least weekly. *(A clean, dry, adherent dressing reduces the chances of infection.)*
4. Perform thorough hand hygiene before beginning assessment of the site. *(Prevents spread of microorganisms; infection at the site could travel into the central nervous system.)*
5. Position patient comfortably so that epidural site is exposed. *(Allows for access to epidural site; provides for patient comfort.)*
6. Don gloves. Remove old dressing and discard, being careful not to dislodge catheter. *(Provides for access to epidural site. Movement of catheter could result in the need for reinsertion.)*
7. Observe for signs of infection such as redness, swelling, warmth, tenderness, or drainage. *(Allows for prompt intervention.)*
8. Perform hand hygiene. Open sterile dressings and prepare sterile field. Don sterile gloves. *(Sterile technique reduces possibility of introducing microorganisms into skin or epidural space.)*
9. Using aseptic technique, cleanse the site with alcohol ×3, using a circular motion, starting in the center and working out. *(Alcohol removes dirt and body oils.)*
10. Repeat the cleansing with povidone-iodine (Betadine) ×3. Allow solution to air dry. *(Destroys microorganisms on skin surface.)*
11. Apply the sterile dressing using proper aseptic technique. *(Prevents contamination of epidural site, and prevents infection.)*
12. Anchor the epidural catheter securely to the skin. *(Securing the catheter prevents it from becoming dislodged or migrating into the subarachnoid space.)*
13. Remove soiled supplies and dressings, and restore the unit. Perform hand hygiene. *(Preserves a clean, sanitary patient environment.)*
14. Document assessment of the site and procedure. *(Verifies dressing change and condition of epidural catheter site.)*
15. If an infusion pump is in use, check for proper function and correct settings for analgesia infusion. *(Ensures ordered dosage of analgesia is infused.)*

? Think Critically

How does monitoring a patient with an epidural catheter for pain differ from monitoring a patient with a PCA?

Implantable pumps. Patients with chronic severe pain may have a small pump implanted and attached to an intraspinal catheter to provide long-term pain relief. The pump is placed in a pocket in the subcutaneous tissue of the abdomen, and the attached catheter is threaded intrathecally. The pump is refilled with the ordered medication every 30 to 90 days, depending on flow rate and reservoir size.

◆ EVALUATION

Frequent evaluation of pain control measures is important. As the patient's condition changes, so may the need for pain control. A patient's perception of pain may increase with anxiety, which can be caused in part by ineffective pain control measures. As the patient's condition improves, various interventions, such as medication, may need to be tapered or discontinued.

SLEEP

Proper rest and sleep are important for patients and may be interrupted because of pain, fear, stress, or side effects of medications and necessary treatments. An important nursing action is to assist the patient in obtaining enough sleep to aid in healing and maintaining health. Adults need 7 hours of sleep a night. *Healthy People 2020* set a new goal for sleep: "Increase public knowledge of how adequate sleep and treatment of sleep disorders improve health, productivity, wellness,

BOX 31.1 Healthy People 2020 Goals for Sleep Health

SH-1 Increase the proportion of persons with symptoms of obstructive sleep apnea who seek medical evaluation
SH-2 Reduce the rate of vehicular crashes per 100 million miles traveled that are due to drowsy driving
SH-3 Increase the proportion of students in grades 9 through 12 who get sufficient sleep
SH-4 Increase the proportion of adults who get sufficient sleep

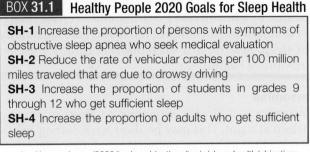

www.healthypeople.gov/2020/topics-objectives/topic/sleep-health/objectives

quality of life, and safety on roads and in the workplace" (*Healthy People 2020*, 2015). The objectives for this goal are presented in Box 31.1.

FUNCTIONS OF SLEEP

Sleep influences memory, mood, cognitive function, secretion of various hormones, immune function, body temperature, and renal function. Adequate rest and sleep are important factors in general health and recovery from illness. Adequate sleep also plays a major role in pain control. Being rested increases pain tolerance and allows an improved response to analgesia.

People who do not get adequate rest often suffer from daytime drowsiness and fatigue. Irritability, depression, and impaired concentration and memory are also common. Both accidents and illness increase in frequency.

STAGES OF SLEEP

Normal sleep follows a course through two states: **non-rapid eye movement (NREM) sleep** and **rapid eye movement (REM) sleep**. REM sleep is the time in which you dream and a period of a high level of activity. Heart rate, blood pressure, and respirations are similar to the levels when awake. NREM sleep is believed to be the time when the body receives the most rest. During this stage, heart rate, blood pressure, and respirations decline. During the course of the night, a person goes through these two states in 90-minute cycles, repeating the cycles five or six times.

NREM sleep is divided into four stages. The first is a transition stage. As a person falls into a light sleep, the muscles relax. This stage usually lasts a few minutes, followed by stage 2, when the person falls into a deeper sleep. Brain wave activity becomes larger, with bursts of electrical activity. This stage lasts 10 to 20 minutes.

As stage 3 begins, the person enters a period called delta sleep, or slow-wave sleep, named for the high-voltage slow brain waves that occur. Respirations and heart rate slow in this stage, and the body becomes immobile. This deep sleep stage lasts 20 to 40 minutes, and dreaming is common. Stage 3 sleep is followed by the deepest stage of sleep, stage 4. During this stage, it is difficult to arouse the sleeping person. This stage lasts approximately 30 minutes.

This is followed by a period of REM sleep. Brain waves become active, almost the same as when awake. This is the stage in which vivid dreams occur, and it lasts approximately 20 minutes. About 25% of the night is spent in REM sleep, and the proportion increases with each sleep cycle during the night.

NORMAL SLEEP REQUIREMENTS

The amount of sleep an individual needs varies from person to person, and the amount of sleep needed changes as a person passes through the life cycle.

Newborns require at least 16 hours of sleep per day, but this is distributed throughout the 24 hours, rather than a being a true sleep cycle. They also spend about 80% of the time in REM sleep. It is speculated that the neural activity occurring during REM sleep is necessary for brain maturation. By 2 to 3 months of age, they begin to develop a true sleep cycle, and REM sleep falls to about 50%. By age 1 year, the child is sleeping 12 to 14 hours per day; he continues to need this amount of sleep until reaching the preschool age, when the amount needed drops to 11 to 13 hours.

School-age children require 10 to 11 hours of sleep per night. REM sleep decreases and deep sleep increases, allowing for repair of damaged cells and the growth of new cells. Insufficient sleep can hamper normal growth and daytime learning.

Growth hormone is secreted during deep sleep in both children and adolescents. Adolescents, however, have different sleep patterns from younger children and adults. Although they need to get 9 to 10 hours of sleep a night, their internal clock does not trigger feelings of sleepiness until late at night because of a natural shift in circadian rhythms that occurs at this period in development. Because school hours demand that they waken by 6:30 or 7 am, many teens are chronically sleep deprived, which affects temperament, academic performance, and their ability to stay awake at critical times, such as when driving a car.

Most adults require approximately 7 to 7½ hours sleep a night, but many get less. Deep sleep time decreases, and REM sleep occurs for about 20% of the night. Many adults are plagued by mild to severe sleep disorders, including varying degrees of insomnia and waking multiple times during the night. Sleep difficulties increase during middle age and can be particularly problematic for menopausal women.

It is a common misconception that older adults need less sleep than younger people do. However, physical conditions such as nocturia and joint pain may interrupt the sleep cycle with increasing frequency. Older adults also tend to have what is called advanced sleep onset—they go to bed earlier and get up earlier than during their younger years. They may also nap during the day. This again represents a shift in the circadian rhythm.

FACTORS AFFECTING SLEEP

Many factors can disrupt the normal sleep cycle. People who work evening and night shifts often have difficulty sleeping during the day. Workers who change shifts during the month have even more difficulty adjusting in order to get enough rest. Students often spend nights studying and find that getting enough sleep can be a problem. Travelers may suffer from jet lag as they go through different time zones. Several hours of sunlight exposure helps reset one's internal clock. People who snore, or have partners who snore, may find that they are awakened frequently. People who snore also have an increased incidence of sleep apnea, which is linked to an increased frequency of cardiac ailments.

Lifestyle can affect the ability to sleep. Caffeine, nicotine, and alcohol consumption can interrupt normal sleep patterns. Caffeine and nicotine can delay sleep, and alcohol may cause nocturnal awakenings.

Clinical Cues

If a patient reports sleeping difficulties, ask if he often drinks something with caffeine after 3 pm. Many drinks contain caffeine, including many carbonated beverages, and it is important to check ingredient labels.

Regular exercise can help a person sleep, but exercise too close to bedtime may be overstimulating and keep a person awake. Taking a nap late in the day may also disrupt nighttime sleep and should be avoided if the individual suffers from insomnia.

Stress and illness also affect sleep. Nighttime worry may keep a person awake or cause awakening in the middle of the night. Illness or discomfort may prevent a person from resting well. An old mattress may contribute to sleeplessness because it is lumpy or no longer supportive.

Environmental factors, such as a room that is too hot or too cold, is too noisy, or has ambient light, can also affect sleep. Patients in the hospital have increased interruptions of regular sleep because of hospital routines that cause noise or require lights, because of the need to be awakened for medications or treatments. Postoperative pain can also be a source of sleep disturbance in the hospital (Dolan, et al., 2016).

Think Critically

What type of stressors might keep a patient awake? Would the stressors be different in the hospital than in a long-term care facility? How can you help to reduce these stressors?

SLEEP DISORDERS

Disorders of sleep can interfere with a person's quality of life and affect health. Accidents may occur due to a lack of sleep. **People with sleep disorders should be treated by a health care practitioner if lifestyle changes or relaxation techniques fail to increase the quality of sleep.** Referral to a sleep disorder clinic for testing may prove helpful.

Insomnia

Insomnia is difficulty in getting to sleep or staying asleep at night. This may be short term, lasting only a few nights, or chronic, lasting a month or longer.

Transient insomnia may be caused by stress, excitement, or a change in sleeping arrangements, as occurs when traveling. Restless leg syndrome may awaken the patient frequently, with a persistent need to move the legs. The sleep pattern usually normalizes as the life situation settles back to routine.

Chronic insomnia may be the result of an underlying medical, behavioral, or psychiatric problem. Depression can often cause insomnia. People suffering from chronic insomnia may require treatment from a health care provider specializing in sleep disorders.

Sleep Apnea

Sleep apnea is a condition in which the person stops breathing for brief periods during sleep. There are three types of sleep apnea: obstructive, central, and mixed complex. They can be further classified as mild, moderate, and severe.

Obstructive apnea is the most common type. It is caused by a relaxation of the soft tissues, which allows partial to total obstruction of the airway. The condition may be further complicated by tissue or bony structure abnormalities. A person with obstructive apnea has visible respiratory effort, but may not be able to move air past the obstruction, causing him to arouse sufficiently to draw breath before falling back into sleep. These individuals often do not remember waking, even though it occurs multiple times through the night, even multiple times per hour.

Central apnea is caused by a failure of the brain to communicate with the respiratory muscles. This results in cessation of breathing with no observable respiratory effort. As the oxygen saturation decreases, the individual resumes breathing. This is much less common than obstructive apnea. Mixed complex sleep apnea is, as the name implies, a combination of obstructive and central sleep apnea.

Obstructive apnea may be treated with a **continuous positive airway pressure (CPAP)** device or a bi-level positive airway pressure (BiPap) device. The devices use a small compressor to maintain airflow via a mask or nasal prongs while the patient sleeps. A dental appliance may be prescribed to reposition the tongue or jaw at night. If a device cannot be tolerated, surgical procedures can be performed to correct the obstruction. Central apnea does not respond to CPAP, but other treatments are available. Apnea is a problem that should be treated by a specialist.

Snoring

Snoring, or harsh sounds that accompany breathing during sleep, is caused by vibration and/or obstruction of the air passages at the back of the mouth and nose. This may result from poor muscle tone, excessive tissue, or deformities such as a deviated septum. Obstructed airways related to colds or allergies can also cause snoring. Snoring may be simple, but can also be a symptom of sleep apnea. Heavy snorers may disrupt their own sleep, as well as the sleep of others.

The mild snorer should exercise to develop good muscle tone and lose weight if needed. Sleeping on the side instead of on the back may help. Remember that snoring can be a symptom of airway obstruction and should be taken seriously. Referral to a primary care provider or a sleep disorder specialist may be necessary.

Narcolepsy

Narcolepsy is sudden-onset, recurrent, uncontrollable, brief episodes of sleep during normal hours of wakefulness in a well-rested person. These sudden sleep periods may occur at any time and last from a few seconds to more than 30 minutes. For example, patients may fall asleep while reading a book, watching TV, attending a meeting, engaging in conversation, or driving. Symptoms usually begin by the age of 25 and may start as excessive daytime sleepiness. There is currently no cure, but drug and behavioral therapies have proven helpful. Regular exercise and exposure to bright light are recommended. Stimulant medication is often used to prevent daytime sleepiness. Diagnosis of narcolepsy is by clinical evaluation, sleep logs or diaries, and the results of sleep laboratory tests. Narcolepsy is not usually an inherited condition.

? Think Critically

What interventions would be needed for the patient with narcolepsy living or being cared for at home? What concerns would you have for this patient as he travels in the community?

❖ APPLICATION OF THE NURSING PROCESS

◆ ASSESSMENT (DATA COLLECTION)

Adequate assessment of the patient having difficulty sleeping is necessary to provide effective interventions. Conduct a thorough history of any sleep-related problems the patient has had. Discuss any current illness or injury in relation to comfort and disruption of sleep.

Encourage patients with sleep difficulties to keep a sleep diary. They should record the time they went to bed, when they woke up, and any time they awoke during the night; usual diet; and all medications and supplements taken, including sleep aids. They should also include information about where they sleep and anything that disturbs sleep, such as neighborhood noise, a snoring partner, wakeful children, or pets.

◆ NURSING DIAGNOSIS

Assessment of the patient with sleep problems allows identification of various nursing diagnoses. These may be related to both the patient's health and sleep disturbances. Possible nursing diagnoses for the patient with sleep disturbances are:

- Readiness for enhanced sleep
- Sleep deprivation
- Fatigue
- Readiness for enhanced comfort
- Acute pain
- Chronic pain
- Anxiety
- Ineffective breathing pattern
- Impaired spontaneous ventilation

Sleep pattern disturbances may be related to many issues, including environmental factors such as noise, health issues, and the necessity of shift work.

◆ PLANNING

When setting up goals related to sleep disturbances, pay attention to the amount of sleep the individual patient needs. A possible goal might be that the patient will sleep undisturbed for 6 hours each night, or awake in the morning feeling rested.

◆ IMPLEMENTATION

Helping the patient adjust lifestyle and bedtime habits can allow him to obtain a sufficient amount of sleep. Avoiding caffeinated beverages for 6 hours before bedtime eliminates stimulants that may interfere with sleep. Eliminating alcohol or nicotine for at least 2 hours before bedtime can also help the patient get to sleep and stay asleep. Encourage the patient to exercise regularly, but not immediately before bedtime. Patients should try to establish a routine time for going to bed and getting up and avoid taking naps late in the day. Going to bed hungry or overly full can interfere with sleep. Reading, playing video games, watching TV, or using a computer in bed should be avoided.

Sleep experts agree that the bedroom should be a refuge, with the bed reserved for sleep and for sexual relations. Discussing the day's problems in bed is also disruptive to the sleep cycle. Many advise that when sleep does not come within 30 minutes, the individual should get up, go into another room, and read or engage in some restful activity until the feeling of sleepiness returns. It is also important that the room be at a comfortable temperature, and the mattress be comfortable and supportive.

Patients in a health care facility are especially prone to environmental disruptions. The use of earplugs or a "white noise" machine may help block out noise. Listening to soft music helps older patients fall asleep quicker and sleep longer. Music can help both acute and chronic sleep disorders (Wang, et al., 2014). **Many patients sleep better if they have a favorite pillow or**

blanket from home. Do not wake patients unless absolutely necessary. Cluster procedures such as vital signs and dressing changes to avoid waking a patient repeatedly. If possible, close the patient's door and avoid talking in the hallway during the night hours.

Think Critically

What would be the difference between interruptions in sleep for the patient in a health care facility and the patient at home? How can you decrease sleep interruptions for a patient in the hospital?

Medication such as sedatives and hypnotics are sometimes prescribed to promote sleep. These should be used only for short-term relief. Over-the-counter sleep medications often contain antihistamines that induce drowsiness. If using medications, the patient should take the dose early enough to allow time for absorption before bedtime. Instruct patients about potential side effects of any medications.

Complementary and Alternative Therapies

Sleep Aids

Melatonin, a natural supplement, can enhance sleep hours for some people. Melatonin is also used to deter jet lag. Calcium and magnesium may ease leg cramps or restless leg syndrome, allowing better quality of sleep. Valerian is an herb that helps some people sleep. As with any supplements, these should be discussed with the primary care provider to ensure they will not interfere with prescribed medications.

◆ EVALUATION

An ongoing evaluation of the effectiveness of interventions is important to assist the patient adequately in achieving sufficient rest. Record the amount of time the patient slept, number and types of interruptions, and patient assessment of quality of sleep.

Get Ready for the NCLEX Examination!

Key Points

- Pain is a subjective experience; there is no objective way to measure pain.
- The major types of pain are acute, chronic, nociceptive, neuropathic, and phantom.
- Pain is what the patient says it is.
- Observable indicators of pain include moaning, crying, irritability, inability to sleep, grimacing or frowning, restlessness, and a rigid posture in bed.
- Pain assessment should include the use of a pain scale.
- Pain is the "fifth vital sign" and is assessed whenever vital signs are measured.
- Pain management can include analgesic medications, TENS, binders, braces, heat and cold application, relaxation, biofeedback, distraction, guided imagery and meditation, music, hypnosis, and massage.
- Adequate rest is necessary for good general health and recovery from illness.
- The two states of sleep are NREM sleep, which is divided into four stages, and REM sleep, which is when we dream.
- Factors affecting sleep include shift work; jet lag; caffeine, nicotine, and alcohol consumption; exercise; environmental factors; stress; and illness.
- Sleep disorders include insomnia, sleep apnea, and narcolepsy.
- Keeping a sleep diary or journal can help in assessing the patient experiencing sleep difficulties.
- Medications should be used only for short-term relief of sleeping problems.

Additional Learning Resources

SG Go to your Study Guide for additional learning activities to help you master this chapter content.

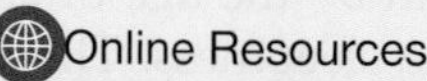 Go to your Evolve website at http://evolve.elsevier.com/Williams/fundamental for additional online resources.

Online Resources
- *American Chronic Pain Association,* www.theacpa.org
- *American Pain Foundation,* www.painfoundation.org
- *American Society for Pain Management Nursing,* www.aspmn.org
- *Cancer pain,* www.cancer-pain.org
- City of Hope Pain & Palliative Care Resource Center, http://prc.coh.org/
- *Best Practices Toolkit,* www.ltctoolkit.rnao.ca/resources/pain#Best-PracticesStandards
- *Pain management resources,* www.pain.com

Review Questions for the NCLEX Examination

*Choose the **best** answer for each question.*

1. When applying the principles of pain treatment, the nurse's **first** consideration should be:
   1. All team members contribute to the plan of care.
   2. The patient's goals must be considered.
   3. The patient's perception of level of pain must be accepted.
   4. Medication side effects must be prevented or managed.
2. A patient, 1 day postoperative, is receiving an analgesic via PCA pump. He reports that the pain is not being controlled adequately. The **first** action the nurse should take is:
   1. Contact the surgeon to increase the dose.
   2. Try nonpharmacologic comfort measures.
   3. Deliver the bolus dose per standing orders.
   4. Assess the pain for location, quality, and intensity.

3. In caring for a patient receiving an opioid, it is most important to monitor for:
   1. Nausea and vomiting.
   2. Respiratory depression.
   3. Hypotension.
   4. Constipation.
4. IM injections of pain medication may be contraindicated for patients who:
   1. Have multiple drug allergies.
   2. Need short-term pain management.
   3. Have poor cognitive abilities.
   4. Have small, poorly developed muscles.
5. Neuropathic pain is most likely to occur in the patient who has:
   1. Ribs fractured in an accident.
   2. A severe ankle sprain.
   3. Bacterial pneumonia.
   4. Diabetes mellitus.
6. Factors that can adversely affect sleep include: *(Select all that apply.)*
   1. Alcohol consumption near bedtime.
   2. A rotating shift schedule.
   3. A very quiet environment.
   4. Watching television in bed.
   5. Reading a book in bed.
   6. A cool bedroom.
7. When a sleep medication is prescribed, the nurse teaches the patient to:
   1. Take the medication 2 hours before bedtime.
   2. Use the medication for short periods.
   3. Use the medication every night.
   4. Take the medication upon retiring for the night.

Critical Thinking Activities

Read each clinical scenario and discuss the questions with your classmates.

Scenario A

Mrs. Thompson, who lives in a long-term care facility, frequently awakens in the middle of the night and finds it difficult to go back to sleep.

1. What interventions could you use to assist her in returning to sleep?
2. What interventions during the day and evening might help prevent the nighttime awakening?

Scenario B

Mr. Rosario, age 48, is an executive with a major company. He works long hours and has little free time. He has had difficulty sleeping for the past 3 months.

1. What factors may be interfering with his sleep?
2. What techniques could you teach him to help him obtain adequate rest?

Scenario C

Ms. Rashad is complaining of postoperative pain after her colectomy surgery yesterday.

1. What type of pain would this be considered?
2. What questions would you ask to assess her pain?

Scenario D

Mr. Chen has been receiving an opioid for his cancer pain.

1. What assessments would you make to identify side effects of the medication?
2. What would you do if Mr. Chen is not able to remain comfortable despite receiving analgesic medication as ordered by the primary care provider?

chapter

32 Complementary and Alternative Therapies

http://evolve.elsevier.com/Williams/fundamental

Objectives

Upon completing this chapter, you should be able to do the following:

Theory

1. Discuss the use of complementary and alternative medicine (CAM) in integrative medicine.
2. Consider each therapy that is considered a part of CAM.
3. Examine five commonly used complementary and alternative therapies.
4. Contrast four mind and body interventions.
5. Direct patients to information needed to make a decision on whether to use an herbal remedy.
6. Describe the desired outcome of spinal manipulation during chiropractic treatment.

Clinical Practice

1. Assist patients in using relaxation and imagery.
2. Assess the use of complementary and alternative therapies by assigned patients.
3. Direct patients to information about complementary and alternative therapies.

Key Terms

acupuncture (ĂK-ū-pŭnk-chŭr, p. 615)
alternative therapies (p. 614)
aromatherapy (ă-RŌ-mă thĕr-ă-pē, p. 619)
chiropractic (kī-rō-PRĂK-tĭk, p. 616)
complementary therapies (p. 614)
herbal (ĔR-băl, p. 618)
imagery (Ĭ-măj-rē, p. 616)
integrative medicine (in-tə-ˌgrā-tiv, p. 615)
phytotherapy (FĪ-tō-thĕr-ă-pē, p. 617)
qi (chē, p. 619)
qi gong (chē gŏng, p. 617)
reiki (RĀ-kē, p. 617)
shaman (ˈSHämən, p. 619)
yoga (p. 614)

 Concepts Covered in This Chapter

- Culture
- Infection
- Pain
- Stress

COMPLEMENTARY AND ALTERNATIVE MEDICINE

Complementary and alternative medicine (CAM) consists of those therapies that are not currently considered part of conventional medical practice. The term **complementary therapies** is used when these practices are employed *in conjunction with* conventional medical treatment. An example would be the use of relaxation therapy along with pain medication to increase a patient's comfort. They become **alternative therapies** when they are used *in place of* mainstream medicine. An example would be eating a special diet to treat cancer rather than undergoing the surgery, radiation, or chemotherapy that has been recommended by one's primary care provider.

In recent decades, the use of complementary and alternative therapies has increased significantly. There are many reasons for this transition. For some, it is related to an overall effort to live a healthier lifestyle, which includes alterations in diet and the adoption of specific practices such as **yoga** (ancient Hindu discipline for harmonizing the body, mind, and spirit) or daily meditation. Other concerns that lead individuals to investigate or begin alternative practices include a desire to decrease or eliminate the use of standard pharmaceuticals, or the failure of conventional medicine to address their health issues, such as chronic pain. Many people cite the impersonal approach and the focus on cure rather than prevention found in standard Western medicine as the primary reason they sought an alternative or integrative practitioner.

Many of the alternatives can be expensive and frequently are not covered by insurance. For a variety of reasons, many people make the decision to invest some or all of the money they have for health maintenance into alternative rather than conventional care.

 QSEN Considerations: Patient-Centered Care

Integrative Medicine

A growing number of conventional medical providers practice integrative medicine. This means they are providing complementary and alternative care along with conventional medicine and providing a holistic approach with more personalized care and easy access to alternative therapies.

The National Institute of Health's National Center for Complementary and Integrative Health (NCCIH) was established to undertake evidence-based research regarding the efficacy of the various complementary and integrative health therapies, and to provide information for the public (see the NCCIH website, https://nccih.nih.gov). **Integrative medicine** focuses on combining conventional and complementary interventions in a collaborated way. NCCIH classifies complementary therapies into two main categories:

- **Mind and Body Interventions:** A variety of techniques designed to enhance the mind's capacity to affect bodily functions and symptoms.
- **Natural Products:** This group contains several different products, such as herbs, vitamins and minerals, and probiotics. These are often referred to as dietary supplements. These substances are commonly found in nature.
- **Other Complementary Interventions**: Many of the complementary therapies fit in one of the two groups of mind and body interventions and natural products. However, some therapies do not fit in either of these groups. These therapies include traditional healers, Ayurvedic medicine, traditional Chinese medicine, homeopathy, and naturopathy.

Examples of these therapies are discussed in this chapter.

MIND AND BODY INTERVENTIONS

Mind-body therapies use a variety of techniques aimed at enhancing the mind's ability to affect the body. These therapies include acupuncture, yoga, chiropractic and osteopathic manipulation, and biofield therapies. Relaxation therapy; therapies that use creative outlets, such as imagery, music, art, or dance; and meditation and prayer are considered mind-body interventions.

ACUPUNCTURE

Acupuncture is a branch of traditional Chinese medicine. Very fine needles are used to stimulate certain points on the body along lines called meridians, to increase or disperse the flow of energy (Fig. 32.1). Studies by the National Institutes of Health have found that acupuncture can be an effective method to treat pain. Acupuncture is also used to increase immunity.

 QSEN Considerations: Safety

Memory Jogger

It is important that only sterile needles be used for acupuncture because of the danger of infection and transmission of human immunodeficiency virus (HIV) or hepatitis.

Acupressure is similar to acupuncture, except it uses pressure points rather than needles, making it lower risk. Acupressure can be effective in treating nausea and lower back or neck pain, as well as menstrual and labor pain (Wagner, 2015).

YOGA

Yoga, a word derived from the Sanskrit meaning "union," is a spiritual practice that combines exercise, controlled breathing, posture, and mental focus to bring about positive effects on the body and mind (Fig. 32.2). It began as part of the ancient medicine system of India, Ayurveda. Yoga has been effective for regulating blood pressure and heart rate, increasing

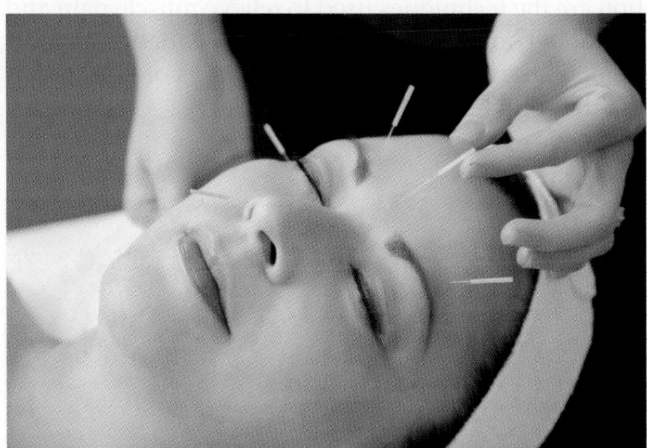

FIGURE 32.1 A patient undergoing acupuncture for relief of pain. (Photo copyright istock.com)

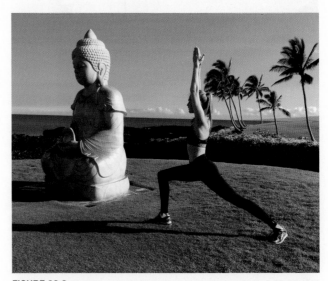

FIGURE 32.2 Yoga is a complementary therapy that focuses on posture, muscles, breathing, and focused consciousness.

circulation, aiding digestion, healing chronic back pain, and helping with other disorders. Yoga may also be practiced for exercise and stress reduction without a spiritual connotation.

CHIROPRACTIC

Chiropractic uses manipulation of the spine for symptomatic relief and improved body functioning by bringing the spinal components back into correct alignment, thereby decreasing or eliminating pain (Fig. 32.3). Exercise, ice, heat, electrical stimulation, and massage may be used in conjunction with spinal manipulation. The treatment does not usually include the use of drugs. Health care providers often refer patients to a doctor of chiropractic medicine, and health insurance often pays for this therapy. Reflexology uses pressure points on the feet and sometimes the palms and ears to relieve symptoms.

MASSAGE THERAPY

Massage therapy uses soft tissue manipulation to improve health. Stroking, kneading, friction, and vibration are the techniques used to relieve muscle pain and promote comfort. There are several varieties of massage, with each using specialized ways of manipulating the soft tissue.

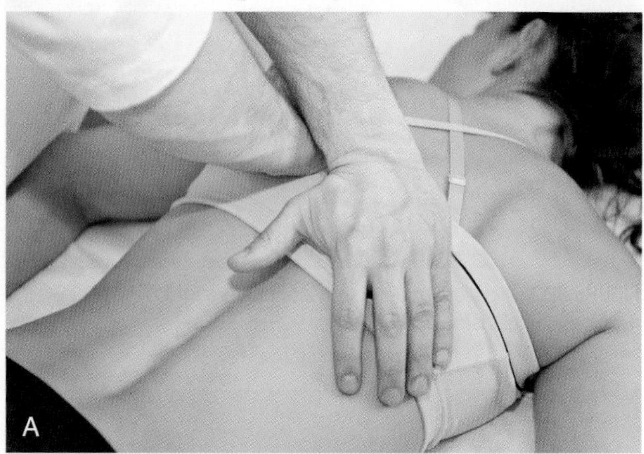

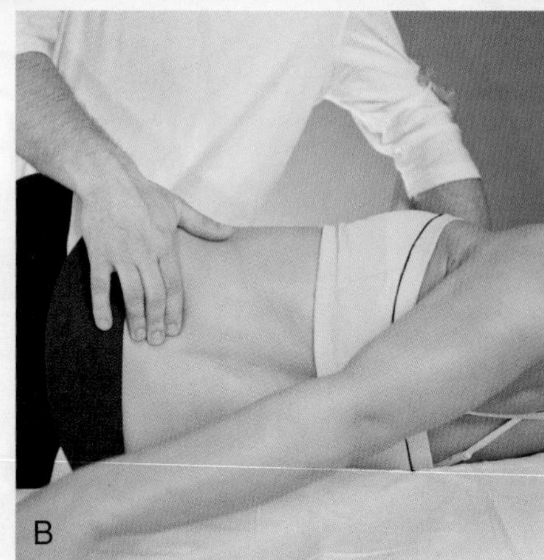

FIGURE 32.3 Chiropractic manipulations. (A) Toggle drop; (B) Lumbar roll. (Photos copyright istock.com)

RELAXATION THERAPY

Relaxation techniques are used to ease stress and are helpful for a variety of chronic illnesses, including headache, irritable bowel syndrome, hypertension, arrhythmias, inflammatory bowel disease, and musculoskeletal pain. Relaxation induces a light state of altered consciousness through refocusing, conscious breathing, and body awareness. Chapter 31 describes some specific relaxation techniques.

IMAGERY

Imagery uses a visual stimulus to produce a particular physiologic change that can decrease stress or promote healing. It is useful in decreasing pain and anxiety, particularly for patients undergoing painful procedures such as bone marrow aspiration. Imagery may produce a physiologic effect on all of the major body systems. Chapter 31 contains an imagery scenario.

MEDITATION

Meditation involves focusing attention on a single repetitive stimulus, thereby decreasing awareness of all other stimuli. It alters consciousness and can bring a beneficial mind–body response. Meditation induces a restful state and lowers heart and respiratory rates, and it may reduce anxiety and depression. It has been helpful for people with asthma, hypertension, diabetes, chronic pain, and other disorders such as sleep disturbances. Meditation can also improve productivity and mood and reduce irritability.

BIOFEEDBACK

Biofeedback is a technique that trains the patient to lessen symptoms by learning to control particular internal physiologic processes that normally occur involuntarily, such as heart rate or blood pressure. It has also been successful in managing pain and controlling panic attacks. The internal activity is measured with electrodes and shown either visually on a screen or as a sound, giving the patient and the practitioner feedback about the internal workings of the body. The person, with practice, can use this information to gain control over the "involuntary" activity. Biofeedback is used effectively for many conditions such as anxiety, hypertension, and seizure disorders, but is particularly successful in treating tension or migraine headaches and chronic pain.

BIOFIELD THERAPIES

Mind and body interventions also include those therapies that use energy fields that are at the core of energy therapies. Biofield therapies are supposed to affect energy fields that surround and penetrate the human body. Such energy fields have not yet been scientifically proven to exist. Examples of energy therapies include qi gong, Reiki, and therapeutic touch. Bioelectromagnetic therapies are based on the use of electromagnetic fields. A therapy may use pulsed fields, magnetic fields, or alternating or direct current. The use of magnets on a body part to relieve pain is an example of a bioelectromagnetic therapy. The research showing the effectiveness of the therapy is largely historical or anecdotal, but some studies validate the notion that magnets reduce pain for some people. Although energy therapies seem to help some individuals, there is a lack of controlled scientific studies validating that the techniques work.

Qi Gong

Qi gong is a form of Chinese exercise-stimulation therapy that seeks to improve health by redirecting mental focus, controlling breathing, improving coordination, and promoting relaxation. Activation of the natural electric currents that flow along meridians in the body helps to rebalance the body's own healing capability. Qi gong has been effective for many people for the management of chronic disease. Recent studies have suggested it might be useful in treating fibromyalgia pain (Sawynok & Lynch, 2014).

Reiki

Reiki stems from the Japanese word meaning "universal life force energy." A practitioner acts as a conduit for healing energy that is directed into the person's energy field or body. The practitioner channels energy to the person, and the person's body does the healing. Energy flows through receptors in the crown, the forehead, the throat, the heart, the stomach, the abdomen, and the groin.

Therapeutic Touch

Therapeutic touch is a technique used to alter body energy fields to restore natural healing powers. The practitioner's hands are passed over the patient to ascertain where tensions or excessive energies exist. Touch may be used to redirect energies and reestablish energy balance.

HYPNOTHERAPY

Hypnotherapy is used to alter behavior, retrieve memories, and induce anesthesia. A hypnotic state is created in which suggestions are implanted that remain during the posthypnotic period. Many physiologic responses have been observed with patients under hypnosis. Hypnotherapy has had moderate success in helping people quit smoking or lose weight. On occasion, people who were not good candidates for general anesthesia have been hypnotized into a deep trance state and were thereby able to undergo a necessary surgical procedure. Hypnosis does not work on all people.

MUSIC, ART, AND DANCE THERAPY

An artistic medium is used to help the individual neutralize conflict or work through a problem. Art therapy has proven helpful when the person has difficulty expressing feelings verbally. Music therapy is beneficial for expression of feelings, reduction of stress and anxiety, enhancement of relaxation, or distraction to aid in pain management. Dance therapy promotes recognition of feelings and awareness of the body. Its goal is to integrate body and mind and promote self-esteem.

HUMOR

Humor has proven to be helpful as a complementary treatment. It can speed the course of healing and decrease pain. Watching movies or comedy sketches or reading humorous literature is distracting, and laughter seems to have a positive effect on the body. Humor generally raises spirits and helps bring about a more positive outlook.

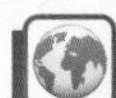

Cultural Considerations

Humor

Nurses should be cautious about using humor because some humor may be considered disrespectful. It is important to understand how humor is viewed within the patient's culture before trying to be funny.

PRAYER

Offering prayers to a higher power helps reduce stress, promotes healing, and may arrest disease. Prayer or spiritual healing may be practiced individually or in groups as intercessory prayer. Prayer chains, in which different people pray for a set time for an individual's recovery over a period of hours or days, are considered beneficial by many people. Research has shown that prayer can be effective in healing for some people. Chapter 14 presents further information on the spiritual aspects of healing.

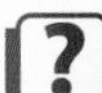

Think Critically

Which complementary or alternative therapies do you think might help an older adult man who is experiencing considerable stress and a consequent rise in his blood pressure?

NATURAL PRODUCTS

Natural products use natural substances, such as foods and herbs. Dietary supplements and vitamins also fall into this category. Many of these therapies have not yet been medically proven. Various clinical trials and research projects are under way at the National Institutes of Health to verify the effectiveness of various herbs and supplements. Many patients use vitamins, supplements, and herb therapies.

HERBAL THERAPY AND DIETARY SUPPLEMENTS

Herbal therapy, or **phytotherapy** (plant therapy), is used by more than 70% of the world's population as a major form of treatment for disorders of the mind and body. **Herbal** medicines contain plant material as their active ingredients and are used to treat a wide variety of health conditions. There are far too many herbs to discuss here; for more information, refer to handbooks and texts about herbs or the Internet (being mindful to search reputable sources).

Many herbs are safe and effective, but others can be dangerous. Herbs may interact with various prescription drugs. **Contraindications to taking an herb should be checked with the primary care provider and pharmacist before using it.** Table 32.1 lists some

Table 32.1 Commonly Used Herbs[a]

COMMON NAME	USES BASED ON SCIENTIFIC EVIDENCE	COMMENTS
Aloe	Constipation	Short-term use only. May cause electrolyte imbalances. May lower blood glucose.
Cranberry	Prevention of urinary tract infection	Drinking cranberry juice appears to be safe. Excessive amounts can lead to gastrointestinal upset or diarrhea.
Echinacea	May reduce incidence and duration of upper respiratory tract infections	Short-term use is recommended. Use with caution in patients with conditions affecting immune system.
Evening primrose	Eczema, skin irritation	Contraindicated in individuals with seizure disorders.
Feverfew	migraine headache prevention	May increase the risk of bleeding. Long-term users may experience withdrawal symptoms.
Garlic	May decrease cholesterol and low-density lipoproteins (studies have been inconsistent)	May increase the risk of bleeding. May lower blood glucose.
Ginger	Nausea and vomiting of pregnancy	May increase the risk of bleeding. May lower blood glucose. Use in pregnancy should not exceed 1 g/day. Supervision by a health care provider is recommended for pregnant women considering the use of ginger.
Ginkgo biloba	Symptoms of claudication	Generally well tolerated in recommended dosages for up to 6 months. May increase the risk of stroke. May increase the risk of bleeding. May affect blood glucose levels.
Ginseng (*Panax* species)	May improve mental performance, may enhance the immune system, and may lower blood glucose	May increase or decrease blood pressure. May increase the risk of bleeding. Avoid use in patients with hormone-sensitive conditions such as breast cancer.
Hawthorn	Mild to moderate heart failure	May add to the effects of cardiac glycosides, antihypertensives, and cholesterol-lowering agents.
Kava	Anxiety	The FDA has issued a warning of severe liver damage linked to its use. Avoid use in patients with liver problems and patients taking medications that affect the liver. May increase drowsiness. Use cautiously with herbs or supplements that are metabolized by the kidneys.
St. John's wort	Short-term treatment of depression (studies on benefits of use are contradictory)	Well tolerated in recommended dosages for 1-3 months. May lead to serious interactions with herbs, supplements, OTC drugs, or prescription drugs. Interferes with the metabolism of drugs that use cytochrome P450 enzyme system. May lead to increased side effects when taken with other antidepressants. Advise the patients to consult a health care professional before self-medicating with St. John's wort.
Zinc	Upper respiratory tract infections	Relatively safe. Should not be taken with dairy products or caffeine, which will reduce its absorption.

FDA, Food and Drug Administration; *OTC*, over-the-counter.
[a]Advise patients who are pregnant or lactating to consult a health care practitioner before using any herbs. There is limited scientific evidence for the use of most herbs during pregnancy or lactation.
(From Lewis, S. L., Dirksen, S. R., Heitkemper, M. M., & Bucher L. [2014]. *Medical-surgical nursing: Assessment and management of clinical problems* [9th ed.]. St. Louis, MO: Mosby.)

commonly used herbs and their scientifically based uses. Herbal preparations are not regulated by the US Food and Drug Administration (FDA), but are regarded as food supplements and subject to those regulations. Not all herbs have been scientifically researched in the United States as to efficacy and safety.

Increasing concerns about both the cost of prescription drugs and their toxic side effects are causing many patients to turn to herbal remedies to treat their maladies. Echinacea is used to combat cold symptoms, and ginkgo biloba is taken to improve memory. Some older men take saw palmetto or pumpkin seeds to shrink the hypertrophy of the prostate gland that comes with age. St. John's wort is used to combat mild to moderate depression. Many women rely on black cohosh rather than hormone therapy to treat the hot flashes and mood swings of menopause.

 QSEN Considerations: Safety

Ephedra Warning

Ephedra, or ma huang, once a common ingredient in weight loss preparations, is a cardiac stimulant that can cause a variety of adverse side effects, including death. The FDA has banned the sale of weight loss products that contain ephedra, and patients should be counseled to stay away from this herb.

In addition to herbs, various dietary supplements are commonly used. Vitamin D_3 is a supplement that may prevent a variety of health problems.

Information on various herbs and supplements can be found on the Internet. One database is at www.herbmed.org. Supplement information is available from the Food & Nutrition Information Center at http://fnic.nal.usda.gov/dietary-supplements.

AROMATHERAPY

Aromatherapy uses oils from plants that are either absorbed through the skin during massage or inhaled. The aromatic properties of certain herbs are thought to act on the brain to evoke pleasant feelings related to past experiences and emotions. Aromatherapy may be combined with a body-based therapy.

 Think Critically

What type of complementary therapy might be effective for the teenager who is experiencing a lot of pain after an automobile accident?

OTHER COMPLEMENTARY INTERVENTIONS

Homeopathy, naturopathy, traditional Chinese medicine, traditional healers, and Ayurveda (traditional medicine from India) are examples of other complementary interventions. Each of these is briefly described next.

HOMEOPATHIC MEDICINE

Homeopathy teaches that symptoms are signs of the body's effort to get rid of disease and that disease can be cured by giving small doses of substances that produce symptoms of the disease or disorder in a healthy person. This process stimulates the person's natural defenses, alleviating the problem. Homeopathy is based on three principles: (1) like cures like; (2) the greater the dilution of the remedy, the greater its potency; and (3) illness is specific to the individual. Homeopathic remedies are derived from plants, animals, or minerals.

NATUROPATHIC MEDICINE

Naturopathic medicine is a philosophy directed at the prevention of disease. Its basis is the use of natural means to promote health. Lifestyle management; natural foods; massage; and substances such as botanicals, light, and fresh air are used along with regular exercise to maintain the body at a high level of wellness through use of the body's inherent healing ability.

TRADITIONAL CHINESE MEDICINE

Traditional Chinese medicine is a comprehensive system based on the opposition of polarities (yin and yang); the elements of wood, fire, earth, metal, and water; and the flow of energy (or **qi**) in the body. It looks for underlying causes of imbalances and patterns of disharmony in the body. Chinese medicine uses more than 50,000 medicinal plants, acupuncture, and massage. Tai chi, a form of stretching exercise that promotes relaxation and increased circulation, and qi gong, another type of exercise and stimulation therapy emphasizing breathing, coordination, and relaxation, are also recommended.

AYURVEDA

Ayurveda is the traditional Indian system of medicine dating from before the first century AD. It uses combinations of herbs, minerals, purgatives, massage, meditation, and special diets. The focus of Ayurveda is on restoring and strengthening the person's body, mind, and spirit. Its healing focus is on maintenance of balance and wholeness to prevent illness. Ayurveda is more than medical treatment, it is a way of life, and it may incorporate a variety of other practices.

SHAMANISM

Many ancient cultures practice shamanism. A trained practitioner, the **shaman**, uses techniques to achieve a nonordinary reality, or a "shamanic" state of consciousness.

With the patient present, the practitioner journeys to other planes of existence to retrieve information that is necessary for the healing process. The patient and the shamanic practitioner work together to make use of the information obtained. The shaman may perform various ceremonies, including the burning of particular plants and herbs, to rebalance the individual with nature.

FOLK MEDICINE

Folk medicine practices are seen in many cultures. In Mexico, it is called *curanderismo.* In this practice, illness is seen as an imbalance. This may be between hot and cold in the body, between the patient and the environment, between parts of the body, or between the patient and the spiritual realm. Folk medicine combines many healing practices and is prevalent throughout Latin America. Biologic compounds, foods, and herbs are used to treat the physical components of the illness. The *curandero* also treats the supernatural components. *Susto* (fear) is thought to cause the soul to separate from the body, resulting in illness. *Mal de ojo* (evil eye) generally is thought to affect children and causes fever, irritability, headache, and weeping. *Empacho* is a gastrointestinal disorder thought to be caused by a blockage in the stomach or intestine. Practitioners are believed to have a *don,* or God-given talent for specific healing, and usually specialize in treating those areas of illness related to their *don.*

AMERICAN INDIAN MEDICINE

In American Indian medicine, healing herbs and ceremonies with a spiritual emphasis are used to treat ailing patients. The therapies are based on the belief that spirit, mind, and emotions all interact with the environment. A patient's disease or disorder is believed to be caused by a disharmony in the patient's connection to nature, Mother Earth, and the spirit world. The focus of treatment is bringing the patient back into harmony.

There are many forms of therapy, including the sweat lodge ceremony; the sacred pipe; and sacred sage, sweet grass, cedar, and other herbs burned and wafted over the patient with the use of a feather. Herbs may also be used in tea or in a bath or burned with the smoke inhaled. Shaking rattles help break up blocks of dead or jammed energy, and drums align the heartbeat of Mother Earth with the patient's spirit. All therapies are performed by highly trained medicine people. Specific treatments, ceremonies, and beliefs vary throughout the many tribal cultures that are contained within the designation of American Indian Medicine. The patient may use mainstream medical therapies as well.

THE NURSE'S ROLE IN COMPLEMENTARY AND ALTERNATIVE THERAPIES

The nurse should be knowledgeable about the various types of complementary and alternative therapies so that basic information can be given to patients if they ask. **It is vital for health care providers to know whether patients are taking over-the-counter herbal or homeopathic substances** because these may interact with prescription medications, even leading to organ transplant rejection. One example includes ginkgo biloba, which prolongs bleeding time and interacts with warfarin. Mixing fluoxetine with St. John's wort can cause toxicity, and there are many others. The University Health Network (UHN) in Canada requests its patients who are either waiting for an organ transplant or have received one to avoid essentially all herbal or natural health products (UHN Multi-Organ Transplant Program, 2015).

Patients may request a referral to a CAM practitioner. **Referrals to a specific practitioner are not part of the nurse's role**. You can and should explain the necessity for determining the educational background, qualifications, and certification of any practitioner before seeking services. Whenever a patient is using any of these therapies, the health care provider should be informed.

Question patients about the use of a CAM therapy in a nonjudgmental manner. It is not your place to encourage or discourage the patient's use of alternative or complementary therapy. Only guide the patient on where to find information about the therapy and how to choose a practitioner. The patient should find out how many treatments will be required, the cost of treatment, and the possible benefits. Strongly encourage a pretransplant patient to self-educate and discuss with the primary care provider and pharmacist prior to consuming any herbal or natural products.

Clinical Cues

Patients often do not discuss their use of CAM with their primary care providers. Some think that, because what they are doing or taking is natural, it does not interfere with prescribed medicine. Others are afraid their primary care provider will disapprove and insist they cease the alternative practice or that they use prescription medications instead of other supplements and herbs. It is important that the nurse assist patients in understanding why it is necessary for the primary care provider to know what supplements and alternative treatments they are using.

Get Ready for the NCLEX Examination!

Key Points

- Complementary therapies are used along with conventional medical treatments.
- Alternative therapies are those used instead of conventional medical treatment.
- NCCIH is researching the efficacy of various therapies.
- There are two main categories of complementary therapies: mind and body interventions and natural products.
- Homeopathic medicine, naturopathic medicine, traditional Chinese medicine, traditional healers, and Ayurveda are examples of complementary therapies that are not part of mind and body interventions or natural products.
- Herbs and other supplements may interact with prescription medications.
- Many herbs may be safely taken (see Table 32.1).
- Be prepared to direct patients to information about complementary and alternative therapies.
- Encourage the patient to check the qualifications and certification of a CAM practitioner.

Additional Learning Resources

SG Go to your Study Guide for additional learning activities to help you master this chapter content.

evolve Go to your Evolve website at http://evolve.elsevier.com/Williams/fundamental for additional online resources.

Online Resources

- *Alternative Medicine Wellness Community,* www.alternativedr.com
- *American Botanical Council*, http://www.herbmed.org/
- *Bandolier* (evidence-based thinking about health care), www.medicine.ox.ac.uk/bandolier
- *Cochrane CAM Field,* www.compmed.umm.edu/cochrane.asp
- *Evidence-Based Complementary and Alternative Medicine,* http://www.hindawi.com/journals/ecam/
- *National Cancer Institute's Office of Cancer Complementary and Alternative Medicine,* http://cam.cancer.gov/
- *National Center for Complementary and Integrative Medicine,* https://nccih.nih.gov/

Review Questions for the NCLEX Examination

*Choose the **best** answer for each question.*

1. Your patient asks you what phytotherapy means. You respond that it refers to:
   1. Plant, animal, or mineral substances given in small amounts to diminish symptoms.
   2. Plant-based prescription drugs used to treat allergies.
   3. Homemade remedies handed down from generation to generation.
   4. Herbs compounded into medicines.
2. It is important to know whether a patient is using herbal therapies because:
   1. Certain herbs can interact adversely with prescription drugs.
   2. Herbs block the action of most prescription drugs.
   3. Herbs often cause odd side effects that may mimic disease.
   4. No one should take herbs while ill.
3. Chiropractic therapy: *(Select all that apply.)*
   1. Is rarely covered by insurance.
   2. Is usually used in combination with pain relieving medications.
   3. Uses spinal manipulation to relieve pain and restore function.
   4. May be combined with exercise, ice, heat, and electrical stimulation massage.
   5. Is typically combined with medications to enhance its effectiveness.
4. A patient who takes several herbs and supplements is scheduled for surgery in 2 weeks. The nurse should advise discontinuing: (*Select all that apply.)*
   1. Kava.
   2. Garlic.
   3. Ginseng.
   4. Omega-3 fatty acids.
   5. Ibuprofen.
5. A logical choice of a complementary therapy for a person who has difficulty expressing her feelings might be:
   1. Acupuncture.
   2. Reiki therapy.
   3. Relaxation therapy.
   4. Art therapy.
6. An herb once commonly used in weight loss preparations and now banned by the FDA is:
   1. Valerian.
   2. Ginseng.
   3. Ginger.
   4. Ephedra.

Critical Thinking Activities

Read each clinical scenario and discuss the questions with your classmates.

Scenario A

What would you say to a patient who has been suffering with back pain who wants to try a Reiki practitioner?

Scenario B

A woman who wants to stop taking hormone therapy for menopausal symptoms is seeking alternative therapies. What alternative therapies would you suggest she find out more about?

Scenario C

Your patient is a young adult who is experiencing chronic pain and does not like to take pain medication. What complementary therapies might you suggest he explore?

chapter 33

Pharmacology and Preparation for Drug Administration

http://evolve.elsevier.com/Williams/fundamental

Objectives

Upon completing this chapter, you should be able to do the following:

Theory

1. Summarize the different classifications of drugs based on their specific actions.
2. Explain the legal implications of administration of drugs by nurses.
3. Summarize the general actions of drugs in the body.
4. Discuss areas of concern regarding medication administration to children or older adults.
5. Analyze issues of medication administration in home care.
6. Identify measures used to prevent medication errors.
7. Evaluate reasons why patients may be nonadherent with drug treatment.

Clinical Practice

1. Locate information about a drug, including action, use, usual dosage, side effects, interactions, recommended routes of administration, and nursing implications.
2. Identify information the patient must be taught to use a drug safely.
3. Accurately calculate various drug dosages.
4. Demonstrate safe practices in administration of medications.
5. Correctly document medications that you administer.

Key Terms

adverse drug reaction (ADR) (or adverse drug event [ADE]) (p. 631)
adverse effects (p. 627)
agonists (ĂG-ŏ-nĭsts, p. 628)
anaphylaxis (ă-nă-fă-LĂK-sĭs, p. 628)
antagonists (ăn-TĂG-ŏ-nĭsts, p. 628)
"black box" warnings (p. 628)
contraindications (kŏn-tră-ĭn-dĭ-KĀ-shŭns, p. 634)
degrade (dĭ-GRĀD, p. 627)
drug interactions (p. 622)
electronic medication administration record (eMAR) (p. 634)
generic name (jĕ-NĔR-ĭk, p. 623)
half-life (p. 627)
Institute for Safe Medication Practices (ISMP) (p. 625)
medication administration record (MAR) (p. 634)
medication reconciliation (p. 634)
nonadherence (nŏn-kŏm-HER-ăns, p. 633)
noncompliance (nŏn-kŏm-PLĪ-ăns, p. 633)
nursing implications (p. 623)
peak action (p. 627)
peak and trough levels (p. 628)
pharmacodynamics (făr-mă-kō-dī-NĂM-ĭks, p. 627)
pharmacokinetics (făr-mă-kō-kĭ-NĔT-ĭks, p. 626)
side effects (p. 627)
synergistic effect (sĭn-ĕr-JĬS-tĭk, p. 628)
therapeutic range (thĕr-ă-PŪ-tĭk, p. 628)
toxic effects (p. 628)
trade name (p. 623)

Concepts Covered in This Chapter

- Adherence
- Pain
- Palliation
- Patient education
- Safety

PHARMACOLOGY

Because of the vast increase in pharmaceutical agents used for medical treatment, and the multiple drugs that many patients take, nurses must be knowledgeable about possible drug effects, side effects, and **drug interactions** (where one drug modifies the action of another). For the patient to receive the full benefit of the drug, nurses must also be aware of foods that interfere with the desired uptake or action of the medication. Issues of cost containment demand that nurses be aware of how drugs affect diagnostic testing. If a drug causes a false-positive result, then unnecessary and expensive treatment may be erroneously ordered. Likewise, a drug that causes a false-negative result may lead a primary care provider to overlook a disease condition.

Along with physicians and pharmacists, nurses are held legally responsible for the safe and therapeutic effects of the drugs.

 QSEN Considerations: Teamwork and Collaboration

Error Prevention Is Teamwork

A multidisciplinary effort to prevent error is necessary because it is estimated that as many as 98,000 people die from errors in the hospital setting alone (US Food and Drug Administration, 2013).

To prepare for medication administration, you need to (1) be able to locate the information about each drug, (2) consistently calculate drug dosages accurately, (3) devise a method for consistently using the Six Rights of medication administration, and (4) recognize the nursing implications (points you need to remember about the drug or teach to the patient) for each drug administered.

CLASSIFICATION OF DRUGS

Although drugs may have three names—a chemical name, a **generic name** (name not protected by trademark), and a **trade name** (name protected by a trademark)—knowing the generic and trade names is sufficient for the nurse. The chemical name describes the chemical composition of the drug. Some drugs have many different trade names because they are manufactured by several different companies. For example, ibuprofen (generic name) may be marketed under the trade names Advil, Motrin, and others.

Learn to categorize medications with similar characteristics by their class. Classifications may be defined by the effect of the drug on a body system (e.g., anticonvulsants), the symptoms the drug relieves (e.g., antihypertensives), or the drug's desired effect (e.g., analgesics). Similar types of problems are treated by the same class of drug, although the class may be broken into subgroups depending on how the drug works in the body to produce the desired overall effect. A drug may also have a variety of properties and effects and therefore may belong to more than one class. A common example is aspirin, which has antipyretic, anti-inflammatory, analgesic, and anticlotting effects.

Another way to learn the drugs is according to groups categorized by their generic drug name endings. Drugs with the same name ending often have similar characteristics and are used for the same type of problem (Table 33.1).

It is extremely important to learn the general characteristics of each drug classification and the **nursing implications, which are your guide to safe and effective medication administration** (Table 33.2). For a complete list of drug classifications, consult a drug handbook or pharmacology textbook. *Mosby's Drug Reference* or comprehensive drug websites such as pdr.net or drugs.com are also convenient references. An easy-to-use medication interaction checker can be found at http://reference.medscape.com/drug-interactionchecker.

The nurse's role in drug therapy is to administer an individual dose of a medication at a specified time.

Table 33.1 Examples of Drug Categories by Generic Name Endings

GENERIC NAME ENDING	TYPE OF DRUG	COMMON ACTION
"Prils" (e.g., lisinopril)	ACE inhibitors	Antihypertensive that relaxes arterial vessels
"Sartans" (e.g., losartan)	Angiotensin receptor blockers	Antihypertensive that blocks action of vasoconstriction effects of angiotensin II
"Olols, alols, and ilols"(e.g., atenolol, labetalol, metoprolol)	Beta blockers	Antihypertensives/antianginals that block beta adrenergic receptors in vascular smooth muscle
"Statins" (e.g., atorvastatin)	Antilipemics	Inhibit HMG-CoA reductase enzyme, reducing cholesterol synthesis
"Dipines" (e.g., amlopidipine)	Peripheral vessel calcium channel blockers	Antihypertensives/antianginals that produce relaxation of coronary smooth muscle and vascular smooth muscle; dilate coronary arteries
"Afils" (e.g., sildenafil)	Erectile agents	Peripheral vasodilator that promotes a penile erection
"Floxacins" (e.g., ciprofloxacin)	Broad-spectrum anti-infectives	Inhibit bacteria by interfering with DNA
"Prazoles" (e.g., esomeprazole)	Proton pump inhibitors	Suppress gastric secretions, preventing gastric reflux and gastric and duodenal ulcers
"Tidines" (e.g., famotidine, ranitidine)	Block histamine-2 receptors	Inhibits histamine at H_2 receptor sites, decreasing gastric secretions
"Azoles" (e.g., fluconazole)	Antifungals	Cause direct damage to the fungal membrane
"Cyclovirs" (e.g., acyclovir)	Antiherpetic	Interferes with DNA synthesis, causing decreased viral replication

Adapted from a presentation by Barb Bancroft at the California Vocational Nurse Educators Conference in Burlingame, California, April 17, 2015.

Table 33.2 Selected Groups of Drugs Classified by Action

CLASSIFICATION	ACTION	EXAMPLES
Circulatory System and Heart		
Anticoagulants	Inhibit clotting of blood	Sodium warfarin heparin
Antianginals	Increase blood flow to the heart	Nitroglycerin, isosorbide dinitrate, diltiazem
Antiarrhythmics	Regulate the heart rate	Lidocaine, atropine, amiodarone
Antihypertensives	Control high blood pressure	Atenolol, enalapril maleate, captopril, clonidine
Antilipidemics	Lower abnormal blood lipid levels	Lovastatin atorvastatin
Antiplatelets	Inhibit platelet aggregation	Clopidogrel bisulfate
Cardiotonics	Strengthen the contraction of the heart	Digoxin digitalis
Diuretics	Reduce edema and increase urine output	Furosemide, chlorothiazide, bumetanide
Hemostatics	Promote clotting of blood	Vitamin K_5, absorbable gelatin sponge (Gelfoam)
Emotional and Mental States		
Hypnotics, sedatives	Relieve anxiety, reduce activity, and promote sleep	Chloral hydrate, secobarbital, flurazepam, zolpidem tartrate
Stimulants	Increase mental alertness and function	Caffeine, methylphenidate, dextroamphetamine, modafinil
Tricyclic antidepressants	Relieve depression	Amitriptyline doxepin
Selective serotonin reuptake inhibitors (SSRIs)	Relieve depression	Paroxetine, fluoxetine, citalopram, sertraline
Anxiolytics	Relieve anxiety	Lorazepam, buspirone, diazepam
Antipsychotics	Relieve psychotic symptoms	Aripiprazole, haloperidol, olanzapine, ziprasidone
Muscular System and Integument		
Antihistamines	Reduce congestion and allergic reactions	Diphenhydramine chlorpheniramine
Muscle relaxants	Control muscle spasms and tension	Baclofen carisoprodol
Neurologic System		
Narcotics (opioids)	Relieve moderate to severe pain	Morphine, codeine, meperidine, hydromorphone, fentanyl, oxycodone
Non-narcotics (nonopioids)	Relieve mild pain	Aspirin acetaminophen
NSAIDs	Reduce inflammation and pain	Ibuprofen, naproxen, sulindac
Alzheimer disease drugs	Slow progression of disease	Donepezil rivastigmine
Antiepiliptics	Control epileptic seizures and tremors	Phenytoin, paramethadione, phenobarbital
Respiratory System		
Antitussives	Relieve cough	Codeine, dextromethorphan, guaifenesin
Bronchodilators and expectorants	Relieve obstruction of air passages	Terbutaline, albuterol, metaproterenol
Endocrine System		
Adrenal hormones	All hormones act to regulate body growth, function, and metabolism	Corticotropin, aldosterone, epinephrine, cortisone
Female hormones	—	Estrogen, estrone, progestin, ethinyl estradiol
Male hormone	—	Testosterone
Pancreatic hormone	Reduces blood glucose	Regular insulin, isophane insulin, Humalog, Humulin (NPH), lente insulin
Hypoglycemics	Reduce blood glucose	Glyburide, metformin, chlorpropamide
Gastrointestinal System		
Antacids	Neutralize stomach acids	Aluminum hydroxide, magaldrate, aluminum carbonate
Antisecretories	Decrease gastric acid secretion	Ranitidine, omeprazole, pantoprazole, lansoprazole
Anticholinergics	Reduce spasms and secretions of stomach	Propantheline

Table 33.2 Selected Groups of Drugs Classified by Action—cont'd

CLASSIFICATION	ACTION	EXAMPLES
Antidiarrheals	Reduce bowel irritability and movements	Diphenoxylate, kaolin and pectin, loperamide, octreotide
Antiemetics	Relieve nausea and control vomiting	Promethazine, metoclopramide, dolasetron mesylate, ondansetron
Cathartics, laxatives	Promote bowel movements	Bisacodyl, magnesium hydroxide, senna
Stool softeners	Add water or bulk to stool and aid defecation	Docusate calcium docusate sodium
Antibiotics	Inhibit the growth of or kill microorganisms	Erythromycin, cephalosporin, penicillin, vancomycin, ciprofloxacin, clarithromycin

NSAIDs, Nonsteroidal anti-inflammatory drugs; *SSRIs*, selective serotonin reuptake inhibitors.

Table 33.3 Schedule of Controlled Drugs

CLASSIFICATION	CRITERIA AND EXAMPLES OF CONTROLLED DRUGS
Schedule I	Drugs with no currently accepted medical use in the United States, a high potential for abuse, and lacking accepted safety measures. The group includes some opioids, psychedelics, cannabis derivatives, methaqualone, and phencyclidine. *Examples: heroin, lysergic acid diethylamide (LSD), phenolsulfonphthalein (PSP), peyote, and 3,4-methylenedioxymethamphetamine ("Ecstasy").*
Schedule II	Drugs with a medical use, a high potential for abuse, with severe psychological or physical dependence. The group includes many opioids, psychostimulants, barbiturates, and cannabinoids. *Examples: hydromorphone (Dilaudid), methadone (Dolophine), meperidine (Demerol), oxycodone (OxyContin, Percocet), and fentanyl (Sublimaze and Duragesic), codeine, and hydrocodone.*
Schedule III	Drugs that are medically useful but with less potential for abuse that lead to moderate or low physical and high psychological dependence. The group includes lesser opioids, stimulants, some barbiturates, miscellaneous depressants, anabolic steroids, and products containing not more than 90 mg of codeine per dosage unit. *Examples: paregoric, butabarbital, acetaminophen with codeine, and buprenorphine*
Schedule IV	Drugs that are medically useful, but with less potential for abuse than the Schedule III drugs, their abuse causing limited physical or psychological dependence. The group includes some lesser opioids, stimulants that suppress appetite, some barbiturates, benzodiazepines, and miscellaneous depressants. *Examples: tranquilizers such as chlordiazepoxide (Librium), diazepam (Valium), fenfluramine, temazepam, and chloral hydrate*
Schedule V	Drugs with medical use, low potential for abuse, and producing less physical dependence than the Schedule IV drugs, and cough preparations containing not more than 200 mg of codeine per 100 milliliters or per 100 g. *Examples: mixtures with small amounts of narcotics (e.g., cough syrup containing codeine such as Robitussin AC, Phenergan with Codeine, and ezogabine.*

Safety Alert

Appropriate Form of the Drug

You must administer the appropriate form of each drug. For example, if the prescriber orders two 325 mg tablets of acetaminophen, you cannot substitute the liquid form without a change in the order. In addition, be vigilant in reading the labels of drugs. For example, the **Institute for Safe Medication Practices (ISMP),** an organization devoted to safe medication practices and the prevention of errors, reported that numerous mistakes have been made when nurses did not notice the warning on the label for methylprednisolone acetate (Depo-Medrol), which is *not* for intravenous (IV) use, compared to methylprednisolone sodium succinate (Solu-Medrol), which can be used for IV administration.

Statutes regulating the type and forms of drugs and nurse practice laws vary from state to state; thus, you are responsible for knowing and adhering to state statutes.

The form of a drug determines its route of administration. The composition of a particular form is designed to enhance its absorption and metabolism in the body. In other words a medication given by a different route may not work (a liquid injectable medication may not be absorbed properly if given orally) or could even be dangerous (an oral medication injected). Many drugs come in several forms, such as tablets, capsules, ointments, solutions, suspensions, and suppositories.

LEGAL CONTROL OF DRUGS

Physicians, dentists, osteopaths, and veterinarians prescribe medications; physicians' assistants, nurse practitioners, and advanced practice nurses (APNs) prescribe medications in collaboration with physicians. Drugs may be dispensed and administered by pharmacists and by those prescribing them.

Federal laws have been passed that extend and refine controls on drug distribution, sales, testing, naming, and labeling. The Comprehensive Drug Abuse Prevention and Control Act of 1970 further regulates dispensing and handling of all controlled substances (Table 33.3). It classifies drugs according to their medical usefulness and their potential for abuse. Many controlled substances are used daily in health care agencies, and you must comply with regulations and agency policies to prevent misuse of these drugs.

In the hospital, the responsibility for the security of controlled drugs is shared by the pharmacists and the nurses. Stock supplies of controlled drugs are stored in the pharmacy and dispensed as needed to the nursing units. In a majority of hospitals, Schedule II and III drugs are dispensed in limited amounts to the nursing units, where they are stored in a locked narcotics drawer, compartment, or automated dispensing unit. **The licensed nurse is responsible for the security of these medications and must account for each dose that is used.** Although the method of accounting varies among hospitals, a record is kept on which the nurse notes each dose that is given, to whom, and when. Other information may be included, such as the patient's room and hospital number or the name of the primary care provider. A proof-of-use record accounts for each dose dispensed to the nursing unit. Information is recorded when the dose is administered to the patient. When the contents of the locked narcotics drawer are counted at the change of shift, there should be a record of each dose given, a dose of the drug remaining for each unrecorded line, and the total remaining. It is common practice for two nurses from consecutive shifts to count the drugs together. The completed proof-of-use records are eventually returned to the pharmacy and must be kept for a specified time. Automated dispensing units track doses removed by each nurse by computer. An end-of-shift printout is run to identify any discrepancies, and each week an inventory is taken of all narcotics.

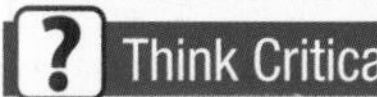

Think Critically

What would you do if you noticed frequent discrepancies in the proof-of-use record whenever Nurse A is working?

Drug Standards

Standards for drug quality, purity, packaging, safety, labeling, and dose form were set by the Pure Food and Drug Act of 1906. For a drug to pass US Food and Drug Administration (FDA) approval and be marketed, it must meet standards in five areas: purity, potency, bioavailability, efficacy, and safety (Table 33.4).

Table 33.4 Drug Standards Manufacturers Must Meet

STANDARD	DESCRIPTION
Purity	Types and concentrations of substances other than the drug that can be in the tablet, capsule, suspension, or other form of drug
Potency	The amount of active drug in the preparation contributing to its strength
Bioavailability	The drug's ability to dissolve, be absorbed, and be transported in the body to its desired site of action
Efficacy	Laboratory studies providing proof that the drug is effective for its intended use
Safety	Sufficient studies completed to indicate potential side effects, adverse effects, and toxic reactions; safety is determined from the data

BASIC CONCEPTS OF PHARMACOLOGY

Drug Action and Pharmacokinetics

Drugs or medications are substances used in the treatment, palliation, diagnosis, cure, and prevention of disease. Any drug can be either beneficial or harmful, depending on the cellular reaction. Essentially, cell functions are either stimulated or depressed in various ways. Digoxin, for example, stimulates heart muscle fibers to contract more powerfully, and its effect on the heart's electrical properties causes changes in rate and rhythm. Barbiturates depress the function of cell groups in the central nervous system, causing drowsiness. Antineoplastic drugs, such as vincristine, have the ability to block cell division.

The study of how drugs enter the body and reach their site of action, and how they are metabolized and excreted, is called **pharmacokinetics.** Knowledge of pharmacokinetics is used by nurses in timing drug administration. Nurses judge the patient's risk for alterations in drug action considering physiologic condition and other drugs the patient is taking.

Absorption. To reach the cellular level, solid drugs in the form of capsules, pills, or powders must be dissolved within the body before the medication is absorbed into the bloodstream and distributed to the tissues. Drugs already in solution, such as oral liquids or injections, are generally absorbed more rapidly. The rate of absorption is determined by many factors. Body weight, age, sex, disease conditions, genetic factors, immune mechanisms, and physiologic and emotional factors modify reactions to a given drug. Even such factors as hot or cold weather affect the absorption rate. Infants display a lower tolerance for drugs than children do; this relates to the immaturity of organs needed to detoxify and excrete the drugs. Differences in absorption by route are shown in Table 33.5.

Other Factors Affecting Drug Action. Distribution to tissues and the cellular site of action depends on the drug's chemical and physical properties and the patient's physical status. A direct relationship exists between the amount of drug administered and the amount of body tissue in which it is distributed. An increase in body fat tends to delay drug distribution. **The less a patient weighs, the more concentrated the drug will be in the tissues, and, consequently, the more powerful the effect.**

The rapidity with which concentration at a target site occurs depends on the blood supply to the site.

Table 33.5 Differences in Absorption by Route

ROUTE	RATE OF ABSORPTION
Skin (transdermal)	Slow absorption
Mucous membranes	Quick absorption
Respiratory tract	Quick absorption
Oral	Slow absorption (liquids are faster than pills, tablets, or capsules)
Intramuscular	Depends on the form of the drug: aqueous is quicker compared with oil, which slows absorption
Subcutaneous	Slow absorption
Intravenous	Most rapid absorption

Local vasodilation or vasoconstriction affects the rate of blood flow. Biologic membranes also affect drug distribution. The blood-brain barrier is permeable only to fat-soluble drugs, and only these drugs can reach the brain and cerebrospinal fluid. **Most drugs cross the placental barrier and affect the fetus.**

Most drugs bind to the protein albumin to some extent. Only the unbound portion of the drug in the bloodstream is then distributed to the target tissue. If a patient is taking two drugs that are protein bound, one or the other drug may have a higher concentration in the unbound state than it would if it had been given alone. This is because the drug with the lower unbound concentration has a greater ability to bind to available protein, leaving less protein to bind to the other drug.

At the site of action, the drug is soon metabolized into an inactive form that can be more easily excreted. This occurs when enzymes detoxify, **degrade** (break down), and remove the active drug chemicals. Most drugs are metabolized in the liver, but the lungs, blood, the intestines, and the kidneys contribute to metabolism. **When liver function is decreased because of disease or aging, a drug may be eliminated more slowly than usual, resulting in an accumulation of the drug that could lead to toxic levels.**

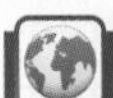 **Cultural Considerations**

Ethnopharmacology

Ethnopharmacologic research shows that different ethnic groups may metabolize drugs differently. Generic forms of drugs are frequently prescribed by providers or requested by patients because of lower cost; however, generic drugs often contain a filler such as lactose, and people of African, Hispanic, and Asian descent, as well as Native Americans, frequently are lactose intolerant (Mayo Clinic Staff, 2015). The symptoms caused by lactose intolerance, such as abdominal distention or bloating, could potentially contribute to nonadherence.

Drugs are mainly excreted by the kidneys, but some excretion occurs via the bowel, the liver, the lungs, and the exocrine glands. Alcohol and gaseous and volatile compounds such as anesthetics are excreted through the lungs. Deep breathing and coughing help the postsurgery patient rid the body of anesthetic more rapidly. Drugs metabolized in the liver may be excreted into the intestine in the bile. The chemicals may be reabsorbed through the intestines. Therefore, an increase in peristalsis accelerates drug excretion, and factors that slow peristalsis may prolong the drug's effect. Some drugs are excreted by the kidney unchanged, but most drugs are metabolized and then excreted by the kidney. If kidney function declines, drug excretion drops, placing the patient at risk for drug toxicity. **Adequate fluid intake (50 mL/kg per day) is essential for the patient to eliminate drugs properly.**

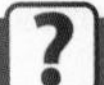 **Did You Know?**

Dialysis and Medications

When your patient is on hemodialysis, many medications are "dialyzed out" of the system during dialysis and rendered ineffective for the patient. Always check the primary care provider's preference if a medication should be held or delayed until after dialysis.

Drug Response and Pharmacodynamics

The study of a drug's effect on cellular physiology and biochemistry and its mechanism of action is known as **pharmacodynamics.** Response to a drug can cause a primary or secondary physiologic effect, or both. The primary effect is the desired effect; the secondary effect may be desirable or undesirable, causing **side effects** (unintended actions) or **adverse effects** (undesirable effects with more serious consequences). For example, antihistamines such as diphenhydramine hydrochloride compete with histamine at receptor sites, producing a primary antihistamine effect. A secondary effect is the inhibition of central acetylcholine, which produces a sedative effect. The secondary effect is undesirable when driving a car, but might be desirable at bedtime.

 **QSEN Considerations: Teamwork and Collaboration**

Alert UAPs about Possible Medication Side Effects

When your patient is taking a medication that may cause secondary effects such as dizziness, inform unlicensed assistive personnel (UAP) that the patient may need assistance with ambulation or hygiene.

Onset, peak, and duration of action differ for each drug. **Peak action** occurs when the highest blood or plasma concentration of the drug is achieved. **The length of time the drug exerts a pharmacologic effect is the duration of action.** The onset of drug action begins when the drug reaches a minimum effective concentration level. Each drug has a serum **half-life**, or the time it takes excretion to lower the drug concentration by half. The next dose of a drug is scheduled at the time the previous dose should reach its half-life, thus sustaining a therapeutic level of the drug. The provider orders **peak (highest concentration) and trough (lowest concentration) levels** for certain drugs to ensure an effective concentration level.

When giving sequential doses of a drug, it is important to time the doses so that the drug's concentration level in the blood never drops below the minimum effective level. However, if doses of a drug are given too close together, the peak may be exceeded, causing a toxic concentration of the drug in the body.

Drugs work by attaching to receptor sites on cells or preventing other substances from attaching to those sites. The action of many drugs depends on their ability to attach to specific receptor sites. The better the drug fits the receptor site, the better the drug's intended action will be. Most cell receptors are protein in structure. Drugs that produce a response are **agonists,** and drugs that block a response are **antagonists.**

Most drugs do not bind only to specific or selective sites. They produce multiple side effects because of binding to other sites in addition to the intended ones. For example, a drug that binds to and, therefore, blocks cholinergic receptors will produce anticholinergic responses. The drug may be intended to dry up secretions by blocking gland secretion before surgery, but it may also cause urinary retention because of effects on the bladder. An anticholinergic drug also affects the heart, the lungs, and the eyes. For this reason, **if you know how a drug works, you can usually figure out what its side effects will be.** Those side effects depend on which receptor sites the drug is stimulating or blocking. Some drugs work nonselectively and affect multiple types of receptor sites. Epinephrine is such a drug; it acts on $alpha_1$, $beta_1$, and $beta_2$ receptors. Other drugs produce a response by stimulating or inhibiting enzymes or hormones and do not act on receptor sites at all.

Drugs have four types of action:

1. **Stimulation or depression** (direct action on a receptor site), such as when the rate of cell activity is stimulated or secretion from a gland is increased, or cell activity is depressed and the function of a specific organ is reduced
2. **Replacement,** such as injected insulin for people who do not produce their own
3. **Inhibition** or **killing** of organisms, such as the action of an antibiotic when it blocks synthesis of the bacterial cell wall
4. **Irritation,** such as that produced by a laxative on the colon wall, resulting in peristalsis and defecation

The less specific the drug's action, the more side effects the drug may have. Most drugs have some side effects. Sometimes side effects include adverse effects. An example of an adverse reaction is nausea produced by an antibiotic when its desired action is to kill pathogenic organisms. Another type of adverse effect is an allergic reaction, such as developing a rash or hives after taking penicillin. When an allergic adverse reaction occurs, the patient is cautioned never to take the drug again because an allergic response will become more

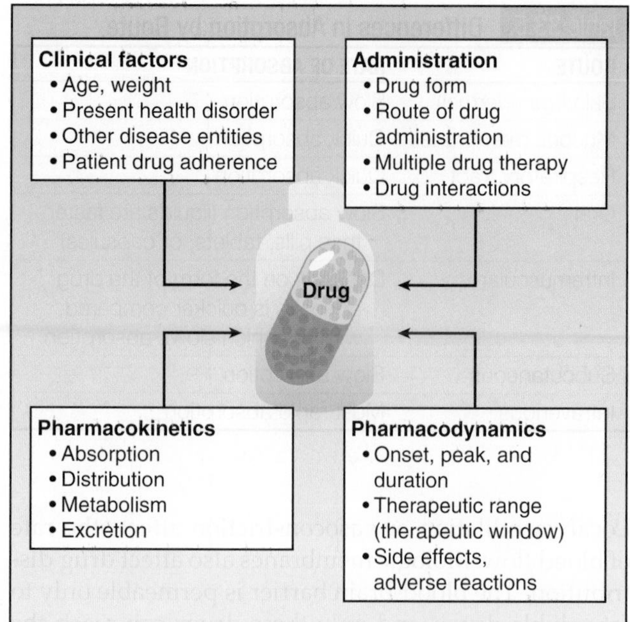

FIGURE 33.1 Factors affecting drug therapy. (Modified from Kee, J. L., Hayes, E. R., & McCuistion, L. E. [2015]. *Pharmacology: A patient-centered nursing process approach* Figure 1.13 [8th ed.]. St. Louis: Elsevier Saunders)

severe the next time a drug is encountered and could cause **anaphylaxis** (severe allergic reaction), which could lead to death. **The possibility of adverse drug effects, side effects, allergic reactions, and undesirable interactions with other drugs and foods increases with the number of drugs administered.**

The **therapeutic range** is the range of levels of the drug in the blood that will produce the desired effect without causing toxic effects. **Toxic effects** (harmful effects) occur when the blood level of a drug rises above the therapeutic range and causes unintended damage to normal cells. For drugs that have a narrow therapeutic range, blood levels are monitored to prevent toxicity. For example, the therapeutic range of phenytoin, an anticonvulsant, is 10 to 20 mcg/mL of blood serum. Toxic effects occur if the blood level rises above 30 mcg/mL. Figure 33.1 reviews the factors that affect drug therapy. Nurses should also be aware that some drugs have **"black box" warnings. A black box warning is the strongest warning by the Food and Drug Administration (FDA) that a medication can carry and remain on the market in the United States.** The prescription medication must have a warning in a "black box" to alert the patient and health care provider about important safety concerns, such as serious side effects or life-threatening risks (US Food and Drug Administration, 2012).

A drug interaction may result in an increase or a decrease in the action of the other drug, or may alter the way in which the drug is absorbed, metabolized, or eliminated from the body. A **synergistic effect** (combined interaction) occurs when the action of the two drugs combined is increased or greater than the effect of the drugs given separately. Alcohol has a synergistic effect when

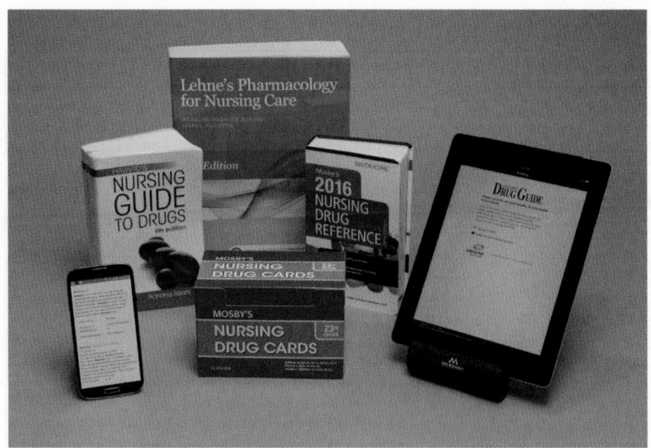

FIGURE 33.2 Drug reference books and resources.

combined with any drug that depresses the central nervous system (CNS) because it is also a CNS depressant.

Drug and Food Incompatibilities

The presence of food in the stomach can affect the drug in many ways. It can speed up, reduce, or even prevent the absorption of the drug into the bloodstream. Food delays the emptying of the stomach and so may delay the onset of the therapeutic effects of the drug. The acidic gastric juices may affect the rate of breakdown of tablets and may prevent the drug from reaching the intestinal wall, where it can be absorbed.

In addition, some drugs are incompatible with others. When such drugs are given at the same time, their effects are changed. Some drug actions are accentuated by other drugs, others have an additive effect, and still other drugs may be inactivated by the other medication. For example, antacids change the pH of the stomach and may inactivate many medications that require an acidic environment for absorption. The nurse is responsible for knowing the factors affecting the use of each medication given. For updated information on food and drug incompatibilities, consult drug handbooks, pharmacology books, professional journals, drug package inserts, computerized drug databases, or check with the pharmacist (Fig. 33.2). Many prescription drugs include precautions on how the drug is to be taken in relation to food and liquids as part of the label for the patient's information.

Clinical Cues

A patient may be using over-the-counter (OTC) medications, herbal remedies, or illicit substances. He may not report these because "they are not drugs from a doctor." However, these substances can cause drug-drug interactions. So question your patients specifically about OTC drugs, herbals, and illicit substances, in a nonjudgmental manner, when taking a drug history.

MEDICATION ADMINISTRATION AND SAFETY

When a prescription or order is created for a drug to be dispensed or administered to a patient, the drug name, the amount of the drug per dose, the number of doses (e.g., tablets or capsules), the route by which to administer the drug, and the frequency or number of times a day the drug is to be taken is written by the physician or qualified person. **You must analyze the order and determine whether the drug, the dose, and the timing of the drug are appropriate for the patient.** For this reason, you must be aware of the usual dosages for an adult or for a child for each drug. Sometimes the route ordered is not appropriate; this might happen when a patient is experiencing nausea and vomiting but has a medication order for an oral route. If the drug comes in a rectal suppository form or an injectable form, you can consult with the prescribing provider and have the order changed. See Table 33.6 for routes.

The nurse is also responsible for monitoring laboratory results related to drug administration. For

Table 33.6 Routes for Drug Administration

Route	Description
Oral Routes	
PO	Medication is given by mouth and swallowed with fluid.
SL	Medication is placed under the tongue, where it readily dissolves and it should not be swallowed.
Buccal	Solid medication is placed in the mouth against the mucous membrane of the cheek until it dissolves. It should not be chewed or swallowed.
Parenteral Routes	
Intradermal	Medication is injected into the dermis just under the epidermis.
Subcutaneous	Medication is injected into the tissues just below the dermis.
IM	Medication is injected into a muscle.
IV	Medication is injected into a vein.
Epidural	Medication is injected into the epidural space of spinal column.[a]
Intrathecal	Medication is injected into the intrathecal space of spinal column.[a]
Skin	
Topical	Medication is applied to the skin, eye, or ear for local effect.
Transdermal	Medication is applied in a small area for slow systemic absorption.
Mucous Membranes	
Vaginal	Medication is inserted into the vagina for local treatment.
Rectal	Medication is inserted into the rectum for local or systemic effect.
Inhalation	Medication is inhaled into the nose or lungs for local and systemic effect.

IM, intramuscular; *IV*, intravenous; *PO*, Oral; *SL*, sublingual.
[a]Medication administration via these routes is beyond the scope of LPN/LVN practice, but you may see this type of order.

Table 33.7 **Abbreviations, Acronyms, and Symbols Not to Be Used in Documentation**

ABBREVIATION	POTENTIAL PROBLEM	PREFERRED TERM
U ("unit")	Mistaken for 0 (zero), 4 (four), or "cc."	Write "unit."
IU ("international unit")	Mistaken for "IV" (intravenous) or "10" (ten).	Write "international unit."
q am, q pm	Mistaken for "9" am or "9" pm	Write "morning, daily," "evening, daily," or "every morning" or "every evening."
ss (sliding scale)	Mistaken for "55"	Write "sliding scale."
Q.D., QD, q.d., qd, Q.O.D., QOD, q.o.d., qod (Latin abbreviations for "once daily" and "every other day")	Mistaken for each other. The period after the Q can be mistaken for an "I," and the "O" can be mistaken for "I."	Write "daily" and "every other day."
Trailing zero (*X*.0 mg) Lack of leading zero (.*X* mg)	Decimal point is missed.	Never write a zero by itself after a decimal point (*X* mg), and always use a zero before a decimal point (0.*X* mg).
MS (for "morphine sulfate") MSO_4, $MgSO_4$ ("magnesium sulfate")	Confused for one another.	Write "morphine sulfate" or "magnesium sulfate."
μg ("microgram")	Mistaken for mg (milligrams), resulting in 1000-fold dosing overdose.	Write "mcg" or "micrograms."
H.S. (for "half-strength" or as Latin abbreviation for "bedtime")	Mistaken for either "half-strength" or "hour of sleep" (at bedtime); q. H.S. mistaken for "every hour." All can result in a dosing error.	Write out "half-strength" or "at bedtime."
T.I.W. ("three times a week")	Mistaken for "three times a day" or "twice weekly," resulting in an overdose.	Write "three times weekly" or "three times weekly."
S.C. or S.Q. ("subcutaneous")	Mistaken as SL for "sublingual," or "5 every."	Write "Sub-Q," "subQ," "subcut.," or "subcutaneously."
D/C ("discharge")	Interpreted as "discontinue" whatever medications follow (typically discharge meds).	Write "discharge."
c.c. ("cubic centimeter")	Mistaken for U ("units") when poorly written.	Write "mL" or "ml" or "milliliters" (mL is preferred).
A.S., A.D., A.U. (Latin abbreviations for "left ear," "right ear," or "both ears")	Mistaken for each other (e.g., AS for OS, AD for OD, AU for OU).	Write: "left ear," "right ear," or "both ears"; "left eye," "right eye," or "both eyes."
O.S., O.D., O.U. (Latin abbreviation for "left eye," "right eye," or "both eyes")	—	—
> (greater than), < (less than)	Misinterpreted as the number 7 (seven) or the letter L. Confused for one another.	Write "greater than" and "less than."
Abbreviations for drug names	Misinterpreted because of similar abbreviations for many drugs.	Write drug names in full.
Apothecary units	Unfamiliar to many practitioners. Confused with metric units.	Use metric units.
@	Mistaken for the number 2 (two).	Write "at."
×3d ("for 3 days")	Mistaken as "for 3 doses."	Write "for 3 days."

Data from Official "Do Not Use" List @ The Joint Commission, 2012. http://www.jointcommission.org/topics/patient_safety.aspx.
Institute for Safe Medication Practices. (2012). *List of Error Prone Abbreviations, Symbols, and Dose Designations*. www.ismp.org/tools/errorproneabbreviations.pdf.

example, if a patient is taking furosemide, an appropriate nursing action is to check the potassium level before administering the drug. In addition, the ISMP suggests that laboratory values be reported directly to licensed personnel.

According to The Joint Commission's National Patient Safety Goals, health care facilities should incorporate the evidence-based practice of a "standardized list of abbreviations, acronyms, symbols, and dose designations that are not to be used" (Table 33.7). The Joint Commission's Do Not Use List does not apply to pre-programmed electronic medical records but this may change in the future (The Joint Commission, 2015a). It is possible you will see one of these abbreviations; if that occurs, consider the order in relation to the patient's condition to be certain you understand its meaning.

Develop a routine for safely giving medications and stick to it each time you do the procedure to avoid

Box 33.1 Safety Guidelines to Prevent Medication Errors

WHEN PREPARING TO ADMINISTER MEDICATIONS

- Plan ahead and do not rush when preparing medications for administration.
- Prepare medications for administration in as distraction-free an environment as possible.
- Follow the "Six Rights" every time you prepare and give medications.
- Clarify with the prescriber any illegible writing in a handwritten drug order.
- Do not administer a drug that is not labeled clearly and correctly with name and amount.
- Check any questionable order or unfamiliar drug or dosage with the pharmacist.
- If an ordered drug dosage seems odd, question it and check the order with the pharmacist or prescribing provider.
- Have another nurse independently recalculate your calculations and then compare results.
- Review the patient's MAR or eMAR for any possible drug interactions.
- Determine whether the patient is receiving more than one drug with the same action. If so, question the orders.
- Ask another nurse to perform an *independent* (meaning without input from you) double-check (IDC) for the order and dose you are going to give for any high-alert drug such as IV potassium, anticoagulants, IV cardiac drugs, opioids, and insulin.
- Keep the drug in its original container. Discard leftover portions of unused medication from single-dose packages.
- Question the pharmacist whenever multiple tablets or vials are needed to prepare a single dose of medication.
- Become aware of drugs with similar names and carefully check the original order and the reason why the patient is receiving the drug before administering it.
- Question an excessive dosage increase in a patient's medication.
- Be familiar with every drug you administer. Look it up if you cannot remember the information you need to administer it safely.
- Check each medication with the order thoroughly three times before administration.

AT THE TIME OF MEDICATION ADMINISTRATION TO THE PATIENT

- Always have the patient state his full name. Verify the name and number on the patient's wristband with the information on the MAR or eMAR. Ask about allergies each time you administer medications to the patient.
- Check each drug at the bedside with the patient's MAR or eMAR before administration.
- Sign that a medication has been given only after the patient has received it.
- Do not leave a medication dose at the patient's bedside.

WORKING WITH THE PATIENT FOR ERROR PREVENTION

- Encourage the patient to be an active partner to prevent errors.
- Teach the patient about the necessity of proper patient identification.
- Familiarize the patient with the color, the shape, and the purpose of each medication.
- Obtain a complete drug history from the patient.
- If the patient questions the appearance or dosage, double-check the order and purpose before administering the drug.

If a medication error does occur, always report it.

making a medication error. **Medication errors can result in an adverse drug reaction (ADR) (also referred to as an adverse drug event [ADE]), which is the fourth leading cause of death in the United States (US Food and Drug Administration, 2014). If an error is made, it must be reported immediately to your clinical instructor and/or charge nurse. A medication error can be a life-threatening event, and patient safety must come first.**

! Safety Alert

Look-Alike, Sound-Alike Drugs

Look-alike drugs and packaging and sound-alike names increase the likelihood of mistakenly giving the wrong medication. The ISMP recommends that institutions minimize their stock of these types of drugs. If you identify this problem on your unit, notify the unit manager.

The ISMP publishes a newsletter that provides educational information for health care providers related to safe medication administration (www.ismp.org/newsletters/nursing/backissues.asp). There is a telephone number to report medication errors to the ISMP ([800]-FAIL-SAF[E]), a website on which you may report (https://www.ismp.org/errorReporting/reportErrortoISMP.aspx), or it may be done via e-mail (ismpinfo@ismp.org). The reporter's identity and location are confidential and never published. Anonymous reports are also accepted. Many nurses fear the negative consequences and individual blame associated with reporting, but reporting errors is an opportunity to improve individual practice and health system policies. Box 33.1 and Concept Map 33.1 include information you need to administer medications safely.

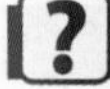
Did You Know?

Computerized Provider Order Entry Helps Prevent Errors

In a study by the Agency for Healthcare Research and Quality (2013a), computerized provider order entry (CPOE) was shown to cut the number of medication errors in half.

CONSIDERATIONS FOR INFANTS AND CHILDREN

Differences in size, age, weight, surface area, and organ maturity all affect the ability to absorb, metabolize, and excrete drugs. Drug dosages are lower for infants and children than for adults and must be carefully calculated and administered. **Doses are based on**

Compare to name on MAR
Check ID band
Drug in-date
Document after drug is given
Ask name
Right patient
Right drug
Right time
Right route
Follow 6 Rights
Right dose
Right documentation
Medication error prevention
Is drug effective?
Is patient receiving more than one drug with the same action?
Are there adverse effects evident?
Is patient allergic to any medication?
Questions to ask yourself
Why is patient receiving the drug?
Should lab values be checked?
Is drug order legible?
Is dosage OK for this patient?
Are there possible drug interactions?

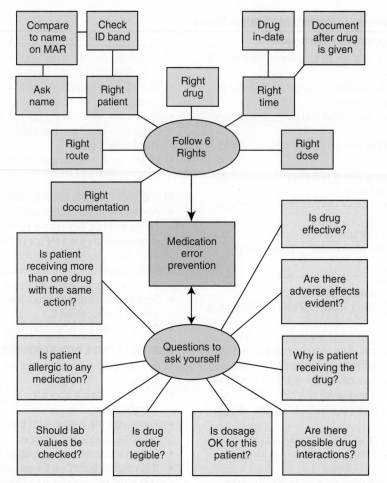

CONCEPT MAP 33.1 Steps to medication error prevention. *ID*, Identification; *MAR*, medication administration record.

the child's age and body weight, and are not given in a standardized amount. Pediatric nurses routinely double-check and recalculate all doses that are ordered by prescribers.

Check with the child's parents for the most effective, least traumatic way to give the child a medication. Sometimes it is best to let the parent administer the oral medication while you supervise. Explain in short sentences, with simple language at the child's level of understanding, what the drug is for, and how it is to be given. Be supportive, and approach the child with confidence and an attitude of expecting cooperation.

Clinical Cues

When giving medication to young children, do not say the medication is like "candy"; simply say that it will help him or her get well. After the medication has been given, praise the child and offer a simple reward such as a sticker.

CONSIDERATIONS FOR THE OLDER ADULT

The following points are related to administering medications to an older adult:

- Older adults may have chronic medical conditions and take multiple medications; check drug interactions carefully.
- Changes in the neurologic system, metabolic rate, and kidney and liver function of the older adult indicate a need for smaller doses of a drug than for the middle-aged patient.
- Older adults often have a decreased level of albumin. This causes a greater potential for unbound drug in the system and a risk for increased drug activity and toxicity.
- Metabolism of drugs is slowed in the older adult, and normal doses may build to toxic levels when liver or kidney function is decreased. Older adults experience twice as many adverse reactions as younger people.
- Older adults on long-term anti-inflammatory therapy for arthritis should be monitored for gastrointestinal bleeding and anemia.
- Older adults may need a pill organizer or alarm to help them remember which drugs to take and to remind them whether they have taken a dose of medication.
- Older adults are likely to have greater blood pressure fluctuations with position changes and are more susceptible to falls when taking drugs that can cause orthostatic hypotension.
- Older adults may become quickly dehydrated and experience electrolyte imbalances when taking

diuretics; these drugs may increase the uric acid level, which contributes to gout.

- Older adults with decreased kidney function are susceptible to digoxin toxicity. Watch for early signs of toxicity: appetite loss, confusion, fatigue, and depression.
- Patients with limited financial resources may not be able to afford needed medications; a tactful inquiry is sometimes necessary.
- Some older adults have limited vision and can misread the label on medication containers; suggest that another person verify or color-code medications.
- With age, swallowing muscles weaken, and the patient is more susceptible to choking; position the patient upright and have him take a sip of water and then the oral medication with additional water.
- If the patient has had a stroke, causing weakness on one side, be certain that the medication is placed on the strongest side of the mouth (always assess swallowing ability before giving anything by mouth to a patient who has had a stroke or neurologic problem causing weakness).
- Many older adults have difficulty opening "childproof" caps on medication bottles; the pharmacy can dispense medication in bottles with caps that are easy to remove.
- Approximately one-third of older adults are nonadherent with their medication regimens because of confusion, forgetfulness, poor vision, and other socioeconomic reasons. In such cases, help is needed to provide a method of adhering to the regimen.

Clinical Cues

When assessing your patient's ability to swallow, put him in a high Fowler position. Ask him to swallow as you observe movements in his throat and his ability to follow instructions. Gently place your thumb and finger over the larynx and ask him to swallow again as you feel the swallow movement. Next, try giving him 1 teaspoon of water and observe as he swallows.

CONSIDERATIONS FOR HOME CARE

Provide the patient and caregiver with written instructions about what to report to the primary care provider. If possible, observe the caregiver or patient as he prepares the medication(s) to validate the process of administration that is being used. Verify that the patient can obtain the needed medications; if not, notify the provider. Caution patients about keeping medications out of reach of children. Check medicine cabinets for out-of-date medications and discard them. Obtain feedback that indicates the caregiver understands what each medication is for, when it is to be given, side effects to monitor, and adverse effects to report to the primary care provider. In accordance with *Healthy People 2020*, pharmacists and prescribers should counsel patients and families about the risks and uses of medications. Nurses must support this by reinforcing patient education and encouraging patients and caregivers to ask questions.

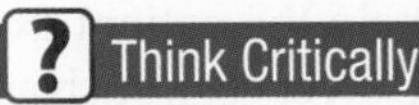

Think Critically

You are providing home care for an older adult who is taking multiple medications prescribed by several different providers. You notice that some of the medications could have drug-drug interactions. Why might this occur? What would you do about this situation?

PROBLEMS OF NONADHERENCE

There are many reasons why patients do not take the drugs that are prescribed for them on the schedule that is indicated by the prescription. Almost half of medications prescribed for chronic conditions are not taken according to directions; 20% to 30% of them are never even filled at the pharmacy (Agency for Healthcare Research and Quality, 2013b).

QSEN Considerations: Patient-Centered Care

Noncompliance versus Nonadherence

Traditionally the behavior of not following medical advice and recommendations was labeled ***noncompliance***, such as the noncompliant ("difficult") patient who refuses to comply with a medical order or treatment. Many people believe this term is a stereotypical and negative label, so the term ***nonadherence*** was introduced, implying that patients are partners with shared decision making about their care. There are many reasons why someone does not or *cannot* follow medical recommendations that have nothing to do with the desire to act contrary to medical advice. Although this author prefers the term *nonadherent*, NANDA terminology still uses the term *noncompliant*, so both terms will be used.

One reason patients might be nonadherent is because they do not comprehend the drug's action or why it is being taken. Patients might not understand that a steady blood level is needed for it to work effectively. Evidence-based practice suggests that adherence increases when patients are knowledgeable about the medication. It is your responsibility to teach patients about the purpose, benefits, and side effects of the medication; how to use the medication; and what to do if a dose is missed. In addition, some patients need information on how to obtain future supplies (National Institute for Health and Care Excellence, 2015).

Another reason for stopping a drug is that the patient cannot tolerate one of its side effects. In the male, urinary retention and sexual dysfunction are common reasons for nonadherence. Often a dosage adjustment or change in the drug prescribed will alleviate these problems. Otherwise, if the drug is vital to the patient's health, another medication may be used to counteract the undesirable side effect.

Listen to your patient's concerns about their ability to follow the medication regimen. Patients often stop taking medication because they cannot afford to buy more and, after taking the first round of the prescription, state, "I feel fine." Once the patient understands what can happen without medication, it may receive higher priority in the budget. You can also help the patient explore ways to obtain medications at a lower cost, such as asking about availability of generic medications or consulting social services about eligibility for prescription assistance programs. Community pharmacists may be aware of local resources used by patients.

Other evidence-based interventions to increase adherence include suggesting that patients record their medications, encouraging self-monitoring of the condition, simplifying the regimen, providing alternative packaging, discussing how the patient would like to deal with side effects, possibly switching medications or dosage, and helping patients weigh the benefits against the side effects (National Institute for Health and Care Excellence, 2015).

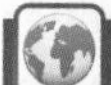

Cultural Considerations

Adherence and Age

Do not assume that a younger and well-educated patient will be more adherent taking medications compared with older patients. No one wants to be perceived as unhealthy and having to rely on medications; thus, a younger patient may be inclined to discontinue medications as symptoms improve.

❖ APPLICATION OF THE NURSING PROCESS

◆ ASSESSMENT (DATA COLLECTION)

Assessment of the patient's condition and medication history is essential before administering a medication. One method is to ask the patient to bring all medications from home, including OTC medications and supplements so that the health care team can review each medication. **Medication reconciliation** is the process of reviewing the patient's complete medication regimen at admission, transfer, and discharge, and comparing it with the new regimen proposed for the new care setting (Agency for Healthcare Research and Quality, 2015).

QSEN Considerations: Teamwork and Collaboration

Medication Reconciliation is Teamwork

The Joint Commission requires all health care staff to participate in medication reconciliation, and some countries recommend patient involvement as well (National Institute for Health and Care Excellence, 2015).

According to The Joint Commission (2015b), the recommended steps of medication reconciliation are:

1. Obtain information on the current medications being taken when the patient is admitted to the hospital or seen in the outpatient setting.
2. Define the types of information to be collected in non–24-hour settings and different patient circumstances (e.g., name, dose, frequency, route, and purpose).
3. Compare the information from the patient with medications being ordered for the patient to identify and resolve discrepancies.
4. Provide the patient with written medication instructions after hospital discharge or completion of outpatient encounter.
5. Explain to the patient the importance of managing medication information after hospital discharge or completion of outpatient encounter.

When you know about the patient's medical problems, you can correlate the reason for the prescribed drug. When assessing for allergies, check all locations where allergies are listed in your facility's medical record; **also, ask the patient.** You must know whether there are any **contraindications** (reasons not to administer) for giving the drug ordered by the route ordered. **If giving a medication that affects vital signs, know the current readings before administration to determine whether it will be safe to give the drug.** If the drug has a narrow therapeutic range, it is important to assess the serum blood level of the drug. Check laboratory results for a serum drug level and determine whether it is within safe and therapeutic limits. Additionally, check laboratory results, such as serum potassium or blood glucose, that will influence the decision to administer or hold certain medications.

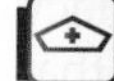

Clinical Cues

Get in the habit of asking about allergies to medication **every time** you give a drug, even if you have already asked the patient about allergies earlier in the day. Later in your career, this habit will be in place when you are caring for multiple patients at a very fast pace.

Assess information about each drug, noting how the drug works, its purpose, usual dosages, routes of administration, side effects, and the nursing implications for administration and monitoring of the patient. Look at the other drugs listed on the **medication administration record (MAR)** or **electronic medication administration record (eMAR)** (record listing medications prescribed and times to be given), and determine whether there are any possible drug interactions with the drug you are about to give. Assess for any food interactions and counsel the patient appropriately.

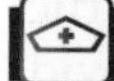

Clinical Cues

Make an effort to develop a strong professional relationship with the pharmacist and memorize that telephone number. Pharmacists provide a wealth of clinical information, including drug interactions and compatibilities.

Other factors to assess include whether the patient can swallow an oral medication or has sufficient muscle tissue to absorb an intramuscular injection, and what site will be best to use for such an injection. Assess for side or adverse effects from previous doses of the drug. Determine the patient's attitude about drugs because this may suggest whether the patient is likely to adhere to the medication regimen (Nursing Care Plan 33.1).

Nursing Care Plan 33.1 Care of the Patient Who Is Nonadherent

SCENARIO Richard Paloni was diagnosed with hypertension and started on metoprolol 50 mg PO bid and hydrochlorothiazide 10 mg PO bid. When he came into the clinic for a follow-up visit, his blood pressure was 166/96 mm Hg. It is determined that Mr. Paloni does not understand his disease or the need for continuous medication. He had not been taking the medication since his prescription ran out. When asked why he had quit taking his medication, he stated he thought the medicine had cured his blood pressure problem because he feels fine.

PROBLEM/NURSING DIAGNOSIS *Does not understand disease or need for medication*/Deficient knowledge related to effects and control of hypertension.

Supporting Assessment Data ***Subjective:*** States, "thought the medicine had cured my blood pressure problem, since I feel fine." Has not been taking medication since his prescription ran out. ***Objective:*** Blood pressure 166/96 mm Hg.

Goals/Expected Outcomes	Nursing Interventions	Selected Rationale	Evaluation
Patient will verbalize possible outcomes of uncontrolled hypertension during next visit.	Assess patient's knowledge of how hypertension affects the body.	Establishes knowledge base about his disease process.	*What does patient know about his hypertension?* States, "My doctor told me I had high blood pressure."
	Instruct regarding effects of hypertension on the body. Advise of potential complications of uncontrolled hypertension.	Promotes understanding of damage uncontrolled hypertension can do.	*What information was given to patient?* Pamphlet regarding high blood pressure control and complications reviewed with patient. Agrees to read material and ask questions tomorrow.
Patient will verbalize action of antihypertensive medication and importance of taking it as scheduled by next visit.	Discuss how metoprolol and hydrochlorothiazide work in the body to lower the blood pressure.	Knowledge of how a drug works and an understanding of what it is expected to do promote adherence.	*What was the patient able to recall about medication teaching?* Knows to take metoprolol and hydrochlorothiazide two times a day. States, "Hydrochlorothiazide will increase urine output, and metoprolol slows my heart rate and decreases my blood pressure." Outcomes partially met. Continue with plan.

PROBLEM/NURSING DIAGNOSIS *Not taking medication*/Noncompliance related to lack of understanding about his disease and medication.

Supporting Assessment Data ***Subjective:*** "I didn't see the need to refill the prescription." Quit taking medication after prescription ran out. ***Objective:*** Blood pressure 166/96 mm Hg.

Goals/Expected Outcomes	Nursing Interventions	Selected Rationale	Evaluation
Patient will take antihypertensive as it is prescribed on a continuing basis.	Explain that blood pressure is lowered by appropriate medication adherence.	Understanding of how medication works promotes adherence.	*Is the patient taking his medication as ordered?* States, "I should take my medicine every day."
	Explain that the medication must be taken every day for it to remain in the bloodstream, where it can work to lower the blood pressure.	Taking the drug on a set daily schedule keeps a steady amount in the bloodstream, which will maintain the blood pressure at a lower level.	Discussed maintaining blood level of the drug by taking it regularly. Reports, "I'm sure that I will be proud of myself for remembering to take care of myself."
Patient will take antihypertensive as prescribed on a continuing basis.	Explore whether patient can afford to buy the medication. Establish how patient will routinely take the medication.	Must be able to obtain the drug in order to take it to lower the blood pressure.	States, "I understand the need for regular doses of the medication." States, "Insurance will cover most of the cost," and "I will take it each morning when I brush my teeth." Progressing toward expected outcome. Continue with plan.

CRITICAL THINKING QUESTIONS

1. What specifically would you teach Mr. Paloni about the possible consequences of uncontrolled hypertension?
2. What feelings would you (the nurse) experience if Mr. Paloni continues with nonadherence despite your best efforts to teach him about the importance of taking his blood pressure medication?

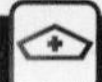 Clinical Cues

When you are at the bedside doing your third and final medication check, ask the patient if he is noticing any ill effects that he associates with taking his medications: for example, "Sir, this is your antibiotic medication. Does this medication seem to be causing any problems for you?" (e.g., diarrhea or nausea). This is one method of assessing the patient's subjective response to the medication. Of course, you are also responsible for evaluating relevant laboratory values and observing for effects that the patient may not associate with the medication.

When working in a home care or clinic situation, assess for any patient limitations that might make self-administration difficult, such as poor eyesight, weakness or paralysis, or confusion and forgetfulness. If such limitations exist, try to identify ways that the patient might receive the medications in a safe manner. Assess the patient's knowledge about the drug therapy to determine areas of needed instruction.

◆ NURSING DIAGNOSIS

Possible nursing diagnoses for patients receiving drug therapy include:

- Deficient knowledge related to use and adverse effects of prescribed drugs
- Noncompliance with medication regimen

◆ PLANNING

Examples of expected outcomes are:

- Patient will verbalize reason he is taking the drug.
- Before discharge, patient will list signs of adverse effects to report to the primary care provider.
- Patient will take medications as prescribed.

Safely and accurately administering drugs requires planning. Unfamiliar drugs should be verified by using reference drug books, computerized drug databases, or package inserts, before the scheduled time to give them. A medication administration schedule should be incorporated into the daily work organization plan. Specific planning is required to evaluate properly whether the patient has any signs or symptoms of adverse effects. Plan time for patient education about the information needed to take each drug prescribed safely.

Before administering a drug, check the **Six Rights** of medication administration. Be certain you have:

1. **The right drug**
2. **The right dose**
3. **The right route**
4. **The right time**
5. **The right patient**
6. **The right documentation**

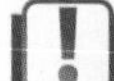 Safety Alert

Patient Identifiers

In accordance with National Patient Safety Goals, at least two patient identifiers must be used to ensure the medication is administered to the correct patient. Say to the patient, "State your name for me, please." (Do not call the patient by name; some patients who do not hear well will say "yes"; confused patients may answer to any name.) Look at the patient's identification wristband or number. Some facilities may also require validation of the birth date.

 Legal and Ethical Considerations

How Many Rights are "Right?"

Deep in nursing tradition is the "Five Rights" of medication administration (drug, dose, route, time, patient). Nurses have historically performed these safety checks while preparing and administering medication, on three separate occasions: "*the three checks of the five rights*." These three checks are performed (a) when retrieving the medication, (b) while preparing the medication, and (c) immediately before giving the medication. A sixth right has been added, the documentation piece, since documentation takes place immediately following (or concurrently with) medication administration. A quick literature search, however, demonstrates that there now exist other various expansions on the traditional Five Rights: six, seven, nine, ten, even *fourteen* rights of medication administration! The information in the more expansive versions of the rights is included in this chapter (see following section: Implementation) and will, of course, be an important part of your assessment prior to medication administration. Fourteen pieces of information, however, is cumbersome to keep in your mind while performing medication administration at the bedside. This textbook, therefore, will emphasize the traditional Five Rights plus documentation, making a total of Six Rights for Medication Administration.

 Legal and Ethical Considerations

Nurses' Rights Related to Medication Administration

If inadequate supplies, insufficient information, insufficient time, or other systemic problems are occurring that negatively affect your ability to administer medications safely, report the issues to the charge nurse, using a constructive problem-solving approach.

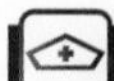 Clinical Cues

Plan to give routinely scheduled medications to those needing extra help last. Always give the most important medication first (e.g., give digoxin first and a multivitamin last).

Before preparing medications for your assigned patients, verify which patients are to have nothing by mouth (NPO) before surgery or tests and have an order to "hold breakfast." Check with the charge nurse about giving these patients their medications when tests are completed. Dialysis patients also may need to have medications held, especially blood pressure medications, but this may vary by primary care provider preference.

Clinical Cues

Although most facilities have drug information books or computerized drug information, consider buying and carrying your own drug handbook. Mark frequently used drugs with sticky notes, and highlight points that you want to remember. The advantage of consistently using your own book is that you can find information more quickly. You will also find that drugs that you highlighted as a beginning student will reappear throughout your career.

Plan. Check whether you need to take juice or milk and crackers to the patient for a particular drug to be taken. If a patient needs a drug crushed and mixed in applesauce or pudding, take the supplies to the bedside with you. This saves a trip back to the workroom. If a patient needs help to sit upright or has difficulty taking medications, extra time is needed.

◆ IMPLEMENTATION

When giving medications, the nurse is guided by many principles. Facility policies vary, but you will safely and accurately give medications if you follow these principles:

- Medications are given by the person who prepared them. If not given, the drug should not be returned to the drug cabinet or cart unless it is still in the unopened, labeled unit-dose package.
- Medications are never to be left at the bedside because they may be forgotten, lost, or taken by another patient. Exceptions include drugs such as antacids, nitroglycerin, or birth control pills; written order by the primary care provider is required. You must monitor for side effects and document the doses taken.
- Narcotics and other controlled drugs are kept in locked cabinets. You are legally responsible for the security of these cabinets and must account for each dose used.
- Check medication orders before giving drugs. Routinely compare medication records with those drugs listed on the MAR or eMAR to see that there are no errors or omissions. If you have a question about the accuracy, refer to the original order in the medical record.
- Avoid distractions or interruptions when preparing or administering medications.
- Research information on unfamiliar drugs: action, dosage, and nursing implications.
- **Observe the Six Rights when administering drugs.**
- Observe the principles of aseptic technique. Perform hand hygiene before beginning to dispense medications and after patient contact. Avoid touching the inside of medication containers or cups. Dispose of pills dropped on the floor. Do not handle or touch medications; pour the pills or tablets into the bottle cover and then transfer them into the medication cup (Fig. 33.3).
- Obtain a complete medication history from the patient and look for possible drug interactions among the medications the patient is taking.
- Is the medication order consistent with the patient's diagnosis and plan of treatment? If the answer is no, or if there is doubt, check with the charge nurse or the primary care provider.
- Is the medication similar in action to another medication the patient has been receiving? Is he still getting the other drug? If so, question both orders.

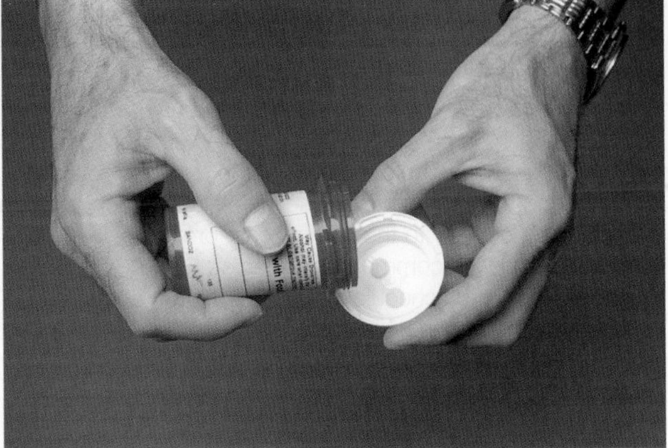

FIGURE 33.3 Pour pills from the patient's own supply into the vial cover.

- Check the medical record and MAR or eMAR for listed patient allergies and ask the patient about allergies whenever you administer medications; look for the allergy identification band.
- Perform patient education about the drug: what it looks like, its intended action, possible side effects, and how to take it. Explain why it should be taken with food or on an empty stomach and why it is important to take it on schedule.
- Check all MAR or eMAR entries with the original order for accuracy.
- Check pertinent laboratory values and assess for side effects of the drug before giving the next dose of a medication.
- Avoid contamination of your own skin or inhalation to minimize the chance of allergy or development of drug sensitivity.
- Document after the drug is given. Note the route, time, and site (if pertinent). In addition, document information about assessment for side effects from previous doses of the drug. Include any patient education that was done about the medication, the dosage schedule, or precautions.

QSEN Considerations: Safety

Evidence-Based Medication Safety Practices

- Staff nurse education
- Use of "no-interruption wear" (vest or sash) that a nurse wears while preparing medications
- Delineation of a "no-interruption zone" where medications are prepared, and if a nurse is standing in this zone, nobody should speak with the nurse unless it is an emergency
- Signage placed indicating medication preparation is in progress; some facilities are implementing a "med pass time" twice daily at 9 am and 9 pm, where all nonurgent questions and calls for nurses are held temporarily
- A printed card with guidelines for responding to interruptions

Sources: Williams et al. (2014), Institute for Healthcare Improvement (2015), and Cleveland Clinic (2015).

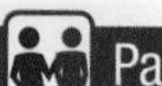

Patient Education

DRUG INFORMATION

Teach patients the following points about each prescribed drug:

- Why the drug is prescribed and what it is supposed to do
- How long it will be before results of the drug will be evident
- Signs and symptoms of adverse effects and which ones to report immediately to the primary care provider
- How to deal with common side effects
- The dosage and schedule for taking the drug and the rationale for the schedule
- The amount of fluid and types of food that should or should not be consumed
- Any special instructions pertinent to the drug, such as weighing daily, eating high-potassium foods, or avoiding salt
- What to do if a dose is accidentally forgotten
- Activities that may be affected, such as driving or exercise
- Reasons for not keeping medications at the bedside (except for medications such as nitroglycerin)
- The need to keep medications in their labeled containers
- The need to consult with the primary care provider before taking any OTC medications or supplements
- The importance of any needed periodic laboratory tests
- The need to keep a list of all current medications

Evolving technologies contribute to safe and accurate medication administration. For example, Accu-flo (formerly known as eMedPass) is a user-friendly system used in assisted living, long-term care, and rehabilitation facilities that incorporates a touch screen of patient photos and medication icons. The system has integrated bar code medication administration features and eMAR documentation. Studies report up to 80% fewer medication administration errors after implementation of bar code medication administration systems (Leung et al., 2015).

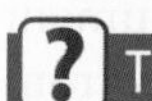

Think Critically

Another nurse asks you to obtain a drug for her patient from the medication cart while you are getting medications for your patients. Discuss some of the problems that could occur.

Calculating the Drug Dosage to Be Given

Several methods can be used to calculate accurately the dosage for a particular drug order. A few examples are given here as a refresher. Use a math workbook to practice and improve your ability to make accurate calculations.

Examples of Conversion Problems. Sometimes it is necessary to perform mathematical conversions to obtain the correct dose. The equivalents must be memorized first or you must use a conversion table (Box 33.2).

To set up a conversion problem, let us assume that grams need to be converted to milligrams (mg). The order reads:

1.5 g of sulfisoxazole orally stat

Box 33.2 Approximate Measurement Equivalents

VOLUME EQUIVALENTS

METRIC (ML)		APOTHECARY		HOUSEHOLD
1	=	—	—	15-16 drops (gtt)
5	=	—	—	1 tsp
15	=	—	—	1 Tbsp
30	=	1 fl oz	—	—
500	=	16 fl oz	=	1 pint
1000	=	32 fl oz	=	1 quart

WEIGHT EQUIVALENTS

METRIC				APOTHECARY
1 mg	=	1000 mcg	—	—
60-65 mg	=	—	—	1 grain
1000 mg	=	1 g	—	—
30 g	=	—	—	1 oz
500 g	=	—	—	1.1 lb
1000 g	=	1 kg	=	2.2 lb

fl oz, Fluid ounce; *g,* gram; *kg,* kilogram; *lb,* pound; *mcg,* microgram; *mg,* milligram; *oz,* ounce; *Tbsp,* tablespoon; *tsp,* teaspoon.

[a]Current recommendations for safety in medication administration state not to use the apothecary system, but some prescribing providers may still use the apothecary system in medication orders. There is variation of measurement conversion to the metric system. For example, one grain varies from 60 to 65 mg. The conversion should not vary by more than 10%. (Data from American Society of Health-System Pharmacists [2015]. Drug products, labeling, and packaging: ASHP policy positions. http://www.ashp.org/DocLibrary/BestPractices/ProductsPositions.aspx)

The order calls for 1.5 g of medication *(amount desired).* First, convert the 1.5 g to mg. The conversion problem is:

$$1.5\text{ g} = x\text{ mg}\ (\textit{amount desired})$$

Cross-multiply:

$$\frac{1000\text{ mg}}{x\text{ mg}} \times \frac{1\text{ g}}{1.5\text{ g}}$$

$$x = 1500\text{ mg}\ (\textit{amount desired})$$

On hand are 500-mg tablets. The dosage problem then would be:

$$1500\text{ mg} = x\text{ tablets}$$

Cross-multiply:

$$\frac{1500\text{ mg}}{500\text{ mg}} \times \frac{x}{1\text{ tablet}}$$

$$500x = 1500$$

Divide both sides by 500:

$$\frac{500x}{500} = \frac{1500}{500}$$

$$x = 3\text{ tablets}$$

One tablet contains 500 mg (amount on hand); 3 tablets = 1500 mg, or 1.5 g.

Let us try another problem that requires converting milligrams to micrograms (mcg). The primary care provider orders an oral dose of digoxin 0.25 mg (desired dose). The pharmacy delivers digoxin tablets that contain 125 mcg per tablet.

The order calls for 0.25 mg of medication *(amount desired)*. First, convert the 0.25 mg to micrograms. The conversion problem is:

$$0.25\text{ mg} = x\text{ mcg}\ (\textit{amount desired})$$

Cross-multiply:

$$\frac{1000\text{ micrograms}}{x\text{ micrograms}} \times \frac{1\text{ milligram}}{0.25\text{ milligrams}}$$

$$x = 250\text{ micrograms}\ (\textit{amount desired})$$

On hand are 125-mcg tablets. The dosage problem then would be:

$$250\text{ mcg} = x\text{ tablets}$$

Cross-multiply:

$$\frac{250\text{ micrograms}}{125\text{ micrograms}} \times \frac{x}{1\text{ tablet}}$$

$$125x = 2$$

Divide both sides by 125:

$$\frac{125x}{125} = \frac{250}{125}$$

$$x = 2\text{ tablets}$$

One tablet contains 125 mcg (amount on hand); 2 tablets = 250 mcg or 0.25 mg.

Drug Problem Formula. You have an order for glipizide, 2.5 mg PO (D = dose desired). On hand you have glipizide, 5 mg/tablet (H = amount on hand). Set up the problem putting the unknown factor on top. D and H need to be measured in like units, so do the conversion problem first.

$$D/H = x$$

Now cross-multiply, ignoring the units until the end.

$$\frac{2.5\text{ mg}}{5\text{ mg}} \times \frac{x\text{ tablets}}{1\text{ tablet}}$$

$$5x = 2.5$$

Divide both sides by 5:

$$\frac{5x}{5} = \frac{2.5}{5}$$

$$x = 0.5\text{ tablets}$$

(Because the x was in front of tablets, then x = 0.5 tablets.) Give ½ tablet.

For liquid medications, follow the same formula. The order specifies guaifenesin, 75 mg PO tid. On hand is guaifenesin syrup, 100 mg/5 mL.

The problem is set up as follows:

$$D/H = \text{Volume}$$

Cross-multiply:

$$\frac{75\text{ mg}}{100\text{ mg}} \times \frac{x}{5\text{ mL}}$$

$$100x = 375$$

Divide both sides by 100:

$$\frac{100x}{100} = \frac{375}{100}$$

$$x = 3.75$$

Give 3.75 mL of guaifenesin syrup.

For an injection, use the same formula. The order reads chlorpromazine, 40 mg for agitation. On hand is chlorpromazine, 25 mg/mL.

Cross-multiply:

$$\frac{40\text{ mg}}{25\text{ mg}} \times \frac{x}{1\text{ mL}}$$

$$25x = 40$$

Divide both sides by 25:

$$\frac{25x}{25} = \frac{40}{25}$$

$$x = 1.6$$

Give 1.6 mL.

Practicing the Six Rights

Give the Right Drug. Check MARs against the prescriber's original orders in the medical record to make certain that the order was transcribed correctly. This transcription is usually performed or verified by a registered nurse on admission and as the prescriber enters new orders. Each time a drug dose is administered, check the order against the drug label for the correct name of drug. **Check the expiration date of the drug at this time.** If the spelling in the computer or in the paper medical record is different from the name on the drug label, check the original order. If there is a discrepancy, consult the prescriber. Tell the patient the name of the drug and show the medication to him before administering it.

Give the Right Dose. Many medication errors occur because the dosage given to the patient is not the dosage ordered. Carefully compare the dose you are about to give with the dose indicated, as ordered in the medical record. Oral doses are supplied in standard amounts per pill or capsule. When the dose is ordered by capsules, tablets, or suppositories, make sure that the ordered dose does not exceed the maximum recommendation. When the dose ordered is in milligrams rather than in capsules, tablets, or milliliters, a mathematical calculation is needed to ensure accuracy. Evidence-based practice indicates that 

older adults in particular should receive the lowest dose possible (Rochon, 2015). Although it is the prescribing provider's responsibility to prescribe the dose, it is your responsibility to question an order if the dosage seems incorrect for the patient or the condition.

Give the Right Drug by the Right Route. The fact that the patient does not feel the need for pain medication by injection anymore does not mean that the nurse can give it in oral form. The order must be changed for the drug to be legally given orally. In some cases, the order is to give the drug orally, but the patient cannot swallow the capsule or tablet. Look for how the drug is supplied to determine the safety of crushing. **For example, sublingual, buccal, enteric-coated, and extended-release products and products with carcinogenic potential should not be crushed.** The ISMP has a "do not crush" list (www.ismp.org/Tools/DoNotCrush.pdf), and the pharmacist can help with this information. Certainly, when a liquid form of the drug is available, a more exact dosage is achieved than with a crushed pill; a liquid dose is also more time-efficient for the nurse. When a liquid form is available, ask the primary care provider to change the order.

Give the Right Drug at the Right Time. The times at which patients are to receive medications should be written down on the work organization sheet. Day shift medications are most commonly given at 9:00 am and 1:00 pm; medications ordered for 7:30, 8:00, 9:30, or 11:00 am, or any other nonroutine time, should be highlighted on the computer printout so that they are not forgotten. The agency protocol may state that a drug may be given within 30 minutes of the time ordered simply because it is not possible to give all the drugs ordered to all patients exactly at the appointed time. In some acute care agencies, this flexibility means that the drug may be given from 30 minutes before the ordered time to 30 minutes after that time. Other agencies require that the drug be given within a 30-minute window from 15 minutes before to 15 minutes after the ordered time.

! Safety Alert

Some eMAR fields change to a red color when a medication administration goes beyond the 30 minute window. Do not let the fear of the color change hurry you into making a medication error! It is better to give the correct dose of a medication 5 minutes late than an incorrect dosage on time.

Nurses must remember that the purpose of drug scheduling is to maintain a consistent level of the drug in the blood. For that reason, drugs should be given as close to the ordered time as possible. Antiarrhythmic heart medications in particular should be given very close to the appointed time.

Give the right drug to the right patient. You must identify the patient correctly using two identifiers. Check the wristband information for both name and identification number, and verify that these match the imprint on the MAR or eMAR. Also, ask the patient, "state your name," and birthday if required.

The FDA has formally recommended that all hospitals adopt bar code medication administration systems. The patient is issued a bracelet with an individual bar code on it. The same bar code is placed on the patient's MAR or eMAR and on each unit-dose medication dispensed by the pharmacy. The nurse scans the patient's bracelet when administering medications. The scanner verifies that the same code is on the patient's bracelet and on the medication packet (Fig. 33.4). In some systems, the nurse may also scan the bar code on her own identification tag, and the system then documents that this particular nurse gave the medication.

Document at the right time. Record the drug given, the dose, the time, the route, and your initials when documenting on a MAR. Sign with your first initial, last name, and designation (student vocational nurse [SVN], or student practical nurse [SPN]). This information is automatically recorded when documented in an eMAR. When documenting a PRN (as needed) medication, be sure to include the reason the medication was given, the dose and route, and the location if it was given by injection. Some nurses develop the habit of documenting medications when they are taken from the medication cart drawer or bin. If the patient is not available to take the drug when the nurse reaches the room, and if things become hectic on the unit, the dose is forgotten. **Never document that a dose was given until after the patient receives it.** When an ordered dose is *not* administered, this should also be noted on the MAR. On an eMAR it will automatically show as not administered; make a note in the record as to why it was not administered.

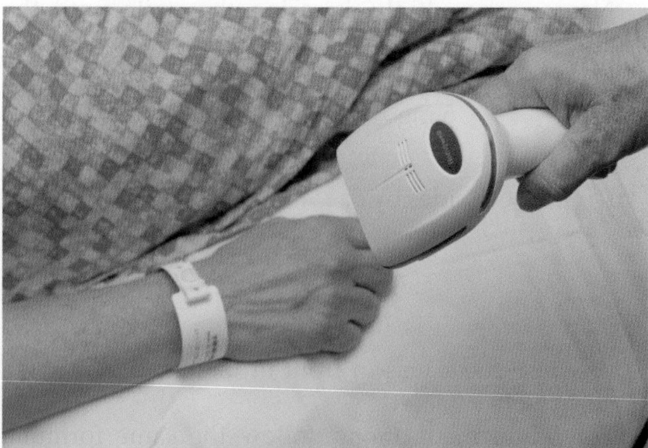

FIGURE 33.4 The nurse checks the bar code on the patient's bracelet and on the medication packet.

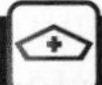

Clinical Cues

Always double-check if the patient tells you the pill looks different or makes any other comment that causes doubt that this medication is correct. A medication order can be written in the wrong medical record, or you might have made an error when preparing the medication.

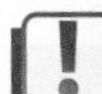

Safety Alert

Watch That Decimal Point!

A common dosage error is a mistaken decimal point or a floating zero. For example, the primary care provider writes ".030 mL of medication." One nurse says use 3/100 mL; one nurse says use 3/10 mL; one nurse says use 3 mL; and one nurse says use 30 mL. Who is correct? Where is the error? Another provider writes "5.0 mg" of medication." One nurse says use 5 mg and another nurse says 50 mg. Who is correct? Where is the error?

Documentation also includes noting the patient's response to the medication. Obviously adverse effects or allergic reactions must be included, but a positive response, such as pain relief, is also important. Any patient concerns about the drug therapy should also be mentioned. In addition, remember to document any patient education that is performed while you are administering the medications.

The right drug, dose, route, time, and patient should be checked three times. The third check should be done at the bedside before opening the unit-dose package. Because unit-dose systems have become the standard, nurses do not seem to check medications as carefully as they did when they used a stock drug supply. One method for instituting three checks using the Six Rights for each medication is listed in Box 33.3.

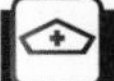

Clinical Cues

The prudent nurse will ask another nurse to check the prepared doses of certain drugs before administering them. All insulin is **always** double-checked in this manner; anticoagulants, injectable digoxin, and other drugs that have a potentially toxic or lethal effect on the patient are double-checked. Many agencies have a list of drugs that require a check by two different nurses before the drug is given.

Safety Alert

"Inattentional" Blindness

Mental fatigue or overload may contribute to failure to attend to the obvious and result in "inattentional blindness," the phenomenon of seeing what we *expect* to see. This sometimes happens when medication labels for different concentrations of the same medication have similar packaging, and numerous medication errors have been committed because of this. Even the most conscientious and experienced nurse who knows what to do and how to do it may find herself saying, "I am not sure why I made that stupid mistake." Use of colors, shapes, and visual displays might help the brain regain focus and see what is being overlooked, although some studies question this logic (Kreitz et al., 2015a) and only found the personality trait of "openness" to reduce inattentional blindness (Kreitz et al., 2015b).

Box 33.3 Performing the Six Rights

For safety, check *three* times: Take out the patient's medication drawer or bin and place it alongside the MAR or eMAR containing the drug orders. Count the number of medications to be administered at this particular time: for example, there are 15 drugs scheduled to be administered at 0900.

1. **The right drug:** Locate the first drug on the MAR or eMAR list that is to be given at 0900. Remove it from the drawer and carefully compare the drug name on the label with the drug name on the MAR or eMAR. Check the expiration date. If outdated, discard and obtain another dose. Why is the patient receiving this medication? If the answer is not apparent, stop and check.
2. **The right dose:** Check the dose on the MAR or eMAR and compare it with the dose you have in your hand. Verify the correct dose by calculation if needed. Determine whether the dosage is within normal recommendations. Place the correct dose unopened in a medication cup or on a medication tray (or in a plastic baggy if there is a large number of medications).
3. **The right route:** Check the route ordered with the type of medication you have prepared.
4. **The right time:** Verify that the time the drug is scheduled is this date and this hour (e.g., 0900). Remember that some drugs are ordered on an every-other-day or every-third-day schedule. **Perform the second check of the medications.** Put the drawer or bin away and then, for each drug, meticulously check the drug, dose, time, and route against the MAR or eMAR again.
5. **The right patient:** Check the patient's identity by comparing the name and hospital number on the patient's identification band with the imprint on the MAR or eMAR. Ask the patient to state his or her name. Verify that the patient has no allergy to the medication before administration. Assess for adverse effects the patient might be experiencing from previous doses of each medication. **Perform the third check** by checking the drug, dose, time, and route one more time before opening the medication package and administering the dose. If you cannot take the MAR or eMAR into the room (e.g., patient is in contact isolation), make or obtain a label to ensure proper patient identification.
6. **The right documentation:** The administration of the medication, dose, time, and route are documented on the MAR or eMAR *after* the patient receives the medication. Additional notes about the patient's response to medication, side effects, or notification of the primary care provider for medication issues should be documented in the nurses' notes.

◆ EVALUATION

Evaluation of drug therapy is related to whether the desired therapeutic effect is occurring. For example, when antibiotics are given, the temperature, the white blood cell count, and perhaps other laboratory values are assessed along with an evaluation of the patient's general condition (e.g., how the patient feels). Evaluation is also necessary regarding the side effects of medications. Each patient is assessed for the signs and symptoms of side effects for every drug being administered. Evaluate whether the expected outcomes listed on the nursing care plan are being met. If they are not, revise the plan of care.

Get Ready for the NCLEX Examination!

Key Points

- Nurses are legally responsible for the safe and therapeutic effects of drugs they administer.
- Drug therapy is used for treatment, palliation, cure, prevention, or diagnosis of disease.
- It is important to understand the general characteristics for different classes of drugs and the nursing implications.
- Controlled drugs are kept in locked compartments, and each dose must be accounted for at all times.
- Drugs are absorbed at different rates depending on their form and physical factors within the body.
- Distribution of a drug is affected by the drug's chemical and physical properties and the patient's physical status. A greater percentage of body fat results in slower drug distribution; the less a patient weighs, the more concentrated the drug is and the more powerful its effect.
- Older adults often have decreased albumin, causing an increase in unbound drug in circulation; this causes increased drug activity and possible toxicity.
- Most drugs are metabolized in the liver and excreted by the kidneys.
- Most drugs produce a primary and a secondary effect. The primary effect is the intended effect; the secondary effect may be desirable or undesirable. Secondary effects are often the side effects of the drug.
- Drug doses must be given on schedule to maintain a therapeutic level of the drug in the patient's blood serum. The therapeutic range of a drug is that which produces the desired effect without causing toxic effects.
- Drugs have four types of action: stimulation or depression, replacement, inhibition or killing, and irritation.
- Drugs tend to interact, altering the way a drug is absorbed, metabolized, or eliminated from the body.
- Alcohol has a synergistic effect when combined with drugs that depress the CNS.
- Foods can affect the absorption or action of drugs.
- The Six Rights must be followed when administering drugs.
- When medication is given to children, the dose is based on age and body weight.
- Nonadherence can be related to lack of information, financial problems, health beliefs, unpleasant side effects, or cognitive issues.
- Evaluation of drug therapy requires data about the patient's response to the drug. Side effects are also evaluated.

Additional Learning Resources

SG Go to your Study Guide for additional learning activities to help you master this chapter content.

evolve Go to your Evolve website at http://evolve.elsevier.com/Williams/fundamental for additional online resources.

Review Questions for the NCLEX Examination

*Choose the **best** answer for each question.*

1. The primary care provider orders a medication blood level after making an adjustment in a patient's prescribed dose of antiseizure medication. What is the purpose of monitoring the drug level after dose adjustment?
   1. There are synergistic effects with other drugs.
   2. The patient is suspected of nonadherence.
   3. The drug has a narrow therapeutic range.
   4. There is danger of anaphylaxis and allergic reaction.
2. An older adult is taking a nonsteroidal anti-inflammatory drug (NSAID) for arthritis on a continuing basis. Which assessment question is the most relevant?
   1. Are you having problems with constipation?
   2. Are you remembering to wear sunscreen and a hat?
   3. Have you had any recent changes in appetite?
   4. Have you noticed any dark discoloration of the stool?
3. Which actions demonstrate the nurse's application of the Six Rights to ensure the safe administration of medication? *(Select all that apply.)*
   1. Carefully checks the original order in the MAR or eMAR
   2. Selects a quiet time to administer medication without interruption
   3. Evaluates the prescribed medication in context of the patient's condition
   4. Asks another nurse to double-check dosage and to obtain it from the medication cart
   5. Places name alert labels on individual medication drawers for similar surnames
4. The surgeon orders 500 mg PO tablets q 8 hours. The pharmacy delivers the medication in tablet form, but the patient tells the nurse that he cannot swallow the tablets and that his family doctor always gives him liquid medications. What is the most appropriate nursing action?
   1. Gently encourage the patient to take the medication that the surgeon has ordered.
   2. Call the pharmacy and ask them to send the liquid form of the medication.
   3. Call the patient's primary care provider to verify what the patient usually takes.
   4. Call the surgeon, explain the situation, and ask for the order to be changed.
5. The nurse is caring for a patient who was admitted for a serious bacterial infection. In addition, the patient also has a history of high blood pressure, high cholesterol, and an ulcer. Which medication is the nurse most likely to question if it is included in the admission orders?
   1. metoprolol
   2. acyclovir

3. esomeprazole
4. ciprofloxacin

6. The nurse is caring for several patients. Which patients are most likely to require a lower than normal dosage of their medications? *(Select all that apply.)*
   1. A healthy woman who is 3 months' pregnant
   2. An older man with several chronic health problems
   3. A middle-aged woman who is mildly obese for height and age
   4. A middle-aged man with chronic alcoholism
   5. An infant girl with normal weight for height and age
7. The nurse has administered morning medications, and several patients are experiencing effects related to the medications. Which patient should the nurse attend to first?
   1. The patient who received an antihypertensive and complains of dizziness when attempting to stand
   2. The patient who received an antihistamine and reports feeling drowsy and sleepy
   3. The patient who received an antibiotic and now has hives and welts all over the trunk, face, and lips
   4. The patient who received an anticholinergic and now has a dry mouth and feels thirsty

Critical Thinking Activities

Read each clinical scenario and discuss the questions with your classmates.

Scenario A

George Hamarabi, age 72, is receiving cefuroxime 250 mg bid for his pneumonia.

1. What would you need to teach Mr. Hamarabi about this antibiotic?
2. He has been on the medication for 4 days. How would you evaluate whether the medication treatment is effective?

Scenario B

Florence Simoneski, age 78, is receiving enteric-coated aspirin for her arthritis. She is hospitalized with dehydration and is very weak. She cannot swallow the enteric-coated aspirin tablets. What would you do?

Scenario C

You are assigned to care for an older adult who is somewhat confused and who rejects your overtures. She refuses to tell you her name when you ask her to state her name before administering her medication. What should you do?

Scenario D

Calculate the necessary drug dosages.

1. Potassium chloride 10 mEq is ordered; 40 mEq/10 mL is the preparation available. How many milliliters will you give?
2. The order reads 400 mg IM. The vial reads 1 g/2 mL. How many milliliters will you give?

chapter 34

Administering Oral, Topical, and Inhalant Medications

http://evolve.elsevier.com/Williams/fundamental

Objectives

Upon completing this chapter, you should be able to do the following:

Theory

1. Describe the legal and professional responsibilities of the licensed practical nurse/licensed vocational nurse (LPN/LVN) related to medication administration.
2. Identify all of the parts of a complete medication order.
3. Compare and contrast the hard copy medication administration record (MAR) and the electronic medication administration record (eMAR).
4. Discuss the types of technology used in hospitals and their effect on medication errors.
5. Identify the advantages and disadvantages of the unit-dose system and the prescription system.
6. Summarize four principles to be followed when giving a medication through a feeding tube.
7. Analyze special considerations when administering oral and topical medications to an older adult.
8. Evaluate your responsibilities in the event of a medication error.

Clinical Practice

1. Recognize the different types of medication orders (e.g., scheduled or routine, PRN, stat, and one time).
2. According to the facilities policy, identify the times used for scheduled medications (i.e., daily, BID, TID, and QID).
3. Demonstrate the accounting for doses of controlled medications that must be withdrawn from the locked narcotics cabinet or dispensed from an automatic dispensing unit.
4. Prepare and apply topical medications such as eye ointments, eardrops, nasal medications, transdermal patches, and topical ointments.
5. Write a care plan for a patient who is receiving medication that includes patient-specific data, an identified nursing diagnosis, and interventions that you would use.
6. Give oral and topical medications using the Six Rights of Medication Administration.
7. Teach a patient to use a metered-dose inhaler.
8. Instill a vaginal and a rectal suppository safely and effectively.
9. Document medication administration and your patient's response to the therapy.

Skills & Steps

Skills

Steps

Key Terms

buccal (BŬK-ăl, p. 658)
douche (DŪSH, p. 662)
meniscus (mĕ-NĬS-kŭs, p. 658)
metered-dose inhalers (MDIs) (p. 661)
ophthalmic (ŏf-THĂL-mĭk, p. 658)
otic (Ō-tĭk, p. 660)
PO (p. 647)
PRN (p. 646)
root cause analysis (p. 669)
spansule (SPĂN-syūl, p. 653)
stat (STĂT, p. 646)
sublingual (sŭb-LĬNG-wăl, p. 658)
topical (TŎP-ĭ-kăl, p. 647)
transdermal (trănz-DĔR-măl, p. 666)
unit dose (p. 649)

Concepts Covered in This Chapter

- Adherence
- Communication
- Pain
- Patient education
- Safety

NURSING RESPONSIBILITIES IN MEDICATION ADMINISTRATION

A recent study showed that about one-third of the medication errors that caused harm to patients occurred in the medication preparation and administration phase (Smeulers et al., 2015). Medication administration requires the nurse to interpret the medication order correctly and then give the correct medication to the patient. Nurses are legally responsible for being knowledgeable about each medication they administer to patients: the correct dose, the route by which it should be given, desired effects, side effects, interactions with other medications, and any  contraindications. Assessment of the patient after medication administration provides data for evaluating the medication's effectiveness and guiding patient education. On discharge from the health care facility, patients need to know how often to take each drug, whether the medication should be taken before or after meals, whether certain foods or fluids should be avoided, the expected effect, what to do about side effects if they occur, and what to do if they forget to take a dose at the prescribed time. In accordance with National Patient Safety Goals, involving and educating patients and families in care and treatment is a safety measure.

All procedures related to medication administration should be followed exactly to promote safety and avoid making a medication error. If the wrong medication is given to a patient, it could have serious consequences. Should an error be made, report it promptly in accordance with agency policy and take appropriate action to promote patient safety and well-being. Medication errors should be reported even if there is no harm to the patient. **Medication orders that are unclear, incomplete, or ambiguous should be questioned to avoid errors** (Institute for Safe Medication Practices, 2011).

Think Critically

You are a new nurse. The primary care provider has written a medication order, but it is difficult to read. You call for clarification, but the provider abruptly states, "It's my standard order," and hangs up. What would you do in this situation?

The Six Rights of medication administration provide a framework for safe delivery of drugs to patients (see Chapter 33). Box 34.1 presents pertinent National Patient Safety Goals of The Joint Commission as they relate to medication administration. Practice in the clinical setting helps establish a consistent, efficient routine for giving drugs. Concept Map 34.1 depicts the nurse's responsibilities when administering medications.

Box 34.1 Safe Medication Administration Guidelines

- Ask yourself why this drug is prescribed for this patient. Know the drug, the patient, and all of the patient's medical conditions.
- Always record a verbal order clearly in its entirety and "read back" for verification that you heard the order correctly.
- Become familiar with the "high-alert drug list" from your facility's pharmacy and know the nursing implications.
- Become familiar with the list of abbreviations that are no longer to be used and ask for verification of any questionable abbreviations in a provider's order.
- Review special precautions concerning medications for children and older adults.
- If you need to administer more than three tablets or capsules, check with the pharmacist to verify that the ordered amount is within safe dosage range.
- Check drug references before crushing a medication or opening a capsule.
- Do not unwrap a unit-dose drug before you are at the patient's bedside and ready to administer the medication.
- Check two patient identifiers every time before administering drugs to a patient.
- Report every medication error so that medication safety can be improved.
- Be alert for look-alike or sound-alike medications, and advocate that these be kept to a minimum and stored in a fashion that reduces error.
- Label all medications if removed from original container (e.g., syringe or medication cup).
- Be especially alert to prevent complications for patients taking anticoagulant medications.

MEDICATION ORDERS

The primary care provider prescribes the type of treatment in a series of instructions written in the medical record. The written prescription for a drug is called the **medication order** or the **drug order.** Provider's orders are part of the patient record.

Medication orders must meet certain standards specified by state law and by regulations established by inspecting agencies. A complete drug order must include the patient's full name, the name of the drug, the dosage to be given, the route of administration, how often it is to be given, the date and time written, and the prescriber's signature. Some orders also specify the total number of doses that are to be given. Examples of medication orders are given in Table 34.1.

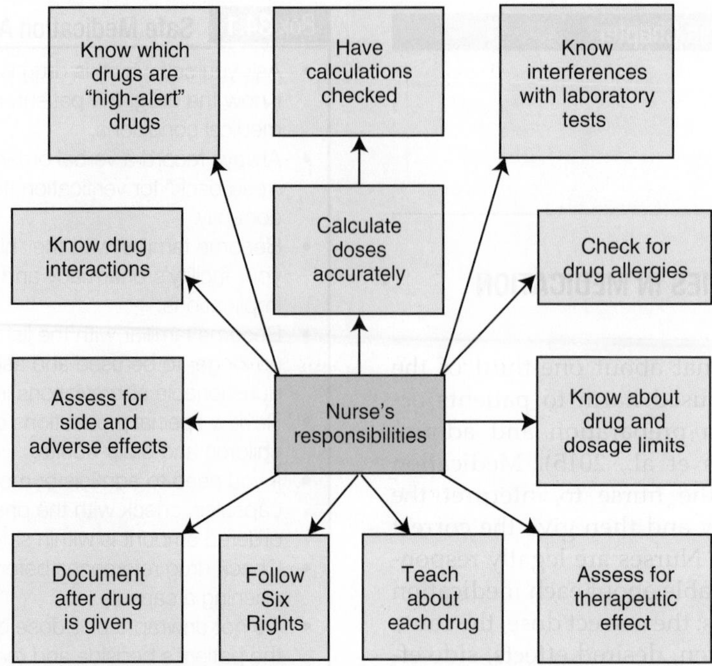

CONCEPT MAP 34.1 Nurse's responsibilities in medication administration.

Table 34.1 Examples of Drug Orders

ORDER	MEANING
Digoxin 0.25 mg PO daily	Digoxin (a drug that strengthens the heart) in a dose of 0.25 mg to be given orally every day
Methylpredniso-lone 4 mg PO qid	Methylprednisolone (a type of corti-sone) in a dose of 4 mg to be given orally four times a day
Acyclovir 200 mg PO q 4 h (five times daily) when awake	Acyclovir (an antiviral medication) in a dose of 200 mg to be given orally every 4 hours during waking hours for a total of 5 doses each day

Table 34.2 Examples of PRN Orders

ORDER	MEANING
Oxycodone HCl 5 mg PO q 6 h PRN pain	Oxycodone (an analgesic) 5 mg given by mouth every 6 hours as needed for pain
Magnesium hydroxide (Milk of magnesia) 30 mL PO at bed-time PRN	Magnesium hydroxide (a laxative) 30 mL by mouth given at bed-time as needed for constipation

PO, Per os; *PRN*, pro re nata.

TYPES OF ORDERS

In your practice, you will encounter several common types of medication orders:

- A routine or scheduled medication order is carried out until it is canceled by the health care provider or until the prescribed number of doses has been given. "Cefuroxime 250 mg PO bid for 10 days" is an example of a routine order.
- A **PRN (Latin for *pro re nata*)** order is written to treat specific symptoms experienced by the patient on an as needed ("PRN") basis. Examples of these medications include analgesics (to control pain), tranquilizers or sedatives (for restlessness), and laxatives (for constipation). Some PRN medication orders specify when or how often the medication can be given (e.g., at bedtime PRN, meaning "at bedtime as needed," or q 4 h PRN, meaning "as often as every 4 hours as needed"). Table 34.2 shows two examples of PRN orders. Every PRN order must indicate frequency of administration and symptom or condition with which to treat.
- A one-time (single) order is written for a drug to be given once. Such orders are common before surgery or a diagnostic procedure. An example is "Valium 10 mg IM on call to G.I. lab." Once administered, the order is discontinued.
- A **stat** (immediate) order is for a single dose of a medication to be given right away. The nurse should administer the medication within 15 minutes of the order being written. A stat order is used in emergencies when the patient's condition has suddenly changed. An example is "diphenhydramine 50 mg IM stat" to help counteract an allergic reaction.
- The primary care provider must give or write a renewal order to continue certain medications. Opiate analgesics generally have a 48- or 72-hour limit; sedatives and antibiotics may have a 5- or 7-day limit; and some agencies may impose a 30-day limit on all medications. At the end of the specified period, the order is no longer valid, and no additional doses of the drug may be given. If you think the medication will need to be continued, contact the provider and obtain a new order rather than just holding the drug.

- Orders by protocol may exist in specialty units such as the emergency department, labor and delivery, or intensive care units. The general medical-surgical unit may have a protocol for an emergency situation, such as administering intravenous (IV) dextrose for dangerously low blood glucose levels. This would be an example of a hypoglycemic protocol. These protocols are in place for experienced nurses who are capable of interpreting findings, making accurate assessments, and using clinical judgment to treat according to the protocol. As a student, you are not responsible for carrying out protocol orders, but you must be able to recognize an emergency situation and immediately report it to your instructor or charge nurse.

Many abbreviations and symbols are used in medication orders that you must know. The most common ones are given in Table 34.3.

Table 34.3 Abbreviations and Symbols Used in Medication Orders

ABBREVIATION	MEANING
ac	Before meals
ad lib	Freely
BID or bid	Twice a day
g or gm	Gram
gtt	Drops
H or hr	Hour
I.D.	Intradermal
IM	Intramuscular
IV	Intravenous
IVPB	Intravenous piggyback
Kg	Kilogram
KVO	Keep vein open
L	Liter
Mcg	Microgram
mEq	Milliequivalent
mL	Milliliter
MDI	Metered-dose inhaler
NGT	Nasogastric tube
PCA	Patient-controlled analgesia
pc	After meals
PR	Per rectum
PRN or prn	As needed
Q	Every
QID or qid	four times a day
Rx	Take
STAT or stat	Immediately
Subling or SL	Sublingual
Sub-Q or subcut	Subcutaneous
SR	Sustained release
TID or tid	three times a day

REGULARLY SCHEDULED OR ROUTINE MEDICATION ORDERS

To maintain the desired level of medication in the bloodstream, the drug may be given several times a day. The primary care provider's order specifies how often the medication is to be given, such as three times a day (tid), every 4 hours (q 4 h), and so forth.

Each health care agency has policies that designate the time of day corresponding to the frequency ordered by the primary care provider. It is imperative that the agency policy be followed. For example, on some nursing units the schedule of times might be:

ORDER	SCHEDULE
Daily	0900
bid	0900 and 1700
tid	0900, 1300, and 1700
qid	0900, 1300, 1700, and 2100
q 4 h	0100, 0500, 0900, 1300 (and so on)

? Think Critically

Can you correctly interpret the following medication orders?

- cefprozil 500 mg PO q 12 h × 10 days
- ferrous sulfate 300 mg tabs PO bid
- digoxin 0.125 mg PO daily

DOSAGE OF MEDICATIONS

Use of the apothecary system is discouraged for measuring medication dosage in the United States. If you do encounter an order that uses it, consult the pharmacist for the proper conversion. A conversion table may also be available in the unit's medication room. **Checking calculations for a divided dose with another colleague is recommended at all times as a medication safety measure.** Consult pediatric textbooks for additional information on confirming dosages and preparing divided doses of medications for infants and children.

ROUTES OF ORAL AND TOPICAL MEDICATION ADMINISTRATION

The selected route of administration depends on several factors: the patient's condition, the nature of the drug (taste, stability, and so on), and the rate of absorption via one route versus another. Oral and topical medications come in many different forms. The oral route (**PO**, or per os, which means "by mouth") is used for many solid and liquid medications because it is the simplest, most convenient, and least expensive (Table 34.4). Those patients who have difficulty swallowing pills must have them crushed and given mixed in some food or juice. Some pills cannot be crushed because this changes their effect on the body. In this case, ask the primary care provider to order the medication in liquid form.

Topical medications are instilled in the form of eye drops or ear drops, or applied as ointments, pastes, or lotions to the skin or mucous membrane. The rectal route is often used to give medications to children or for patients who are vomiting. (Skills detailing the procedures for giving solutions as enemas can be reviewed in Chapter 30.) Many medications affecting the respiratory system are given as inhalants.

MEDICATION ADMINISTRATION AND TECHNOLOGY

The use of technology has contributed to an increase in medication safety. Systems such as computerized provider order entry (CPOE), bar coding, and smartphones, mobile devices, and personal digital assistants (PDAs) are a few examples of technology being used by health care providers today. CPOE allows the provider to enter all patients' medication orders directly into the hospital's computer system. The order is automatically transmitted to the pharmacy, and the nurse's electronic medication administration record (eMAR) is automatically updated. This significantly decreases the potential for transcription errors, one of the many causes of

Table 34.4 Oral and Topical Medications

FORM OF DRUG	CHARACTERISTICS	PRESCRIPTION ABBREVIATION	ROUTE
	ORAL MEDICATIONS		
Tablet	Powder compressed into a tablet with a binding substance	Tab	Given by mouth
Capsule	Powder placed in a capsule	Cap	Given by mouth
Spansule	Time-release pellets placed in a capsule shell	Span	Given by mouth (do not open)
Enteric coated	Tablet with a coating that does not dissolve until it is in the intestine	EC	Given by mouth (do not crush)
Elixir	Sweetened flavoring substance with an active medicinal ingredient	Elix	Given by mouth or feeding tube
Lozenge	Medicated tablet or disk		Given by mouth; to be sucked on until it totally dissolves
Sublingual	Tablet formulated to quickly dissolve under the tongue	Subling	Given by mouth by placing under the tongue (not to be swallowed)
Buccal	Tablet formulated to dissolve when placed in the inner cheek of the mouth	Bucc	Given by mouth by placing in the inner cheek pocket (not to be swallowed)
Syrup	A thick sugar solution combined with a medicinal ingredient	Syr	Given by mouth or by feeding tube; often used for children's medication preparations and cough medicines
Suspension	Medication particles suspended rather than dissolved in a liquid substance	Susp	Given by mouth or by feeding tube; antibiotics are often prepared this way for children
	TOPICAL MEDICATIONS		
Lotion	A liquid suspension		Applied to the skin
Ointment	A semisolid, thick preparation containing a medicinal agent	Oint	Applied to the skin or mucous membrane
Cream	A semisolid, thin preparation containing a medicinal agent		Applied to the skin or mucous membrane
Tincture	Medication dissolved in alcohol	Tinct, tr	Applied to the skin
Drops	Liquid medication provided in a dropper bottle or a bottle with a detachable dropper	gt, gtt	Usually formulated for the nose, eye, or ear, although infant vitamins and other medications are made as drops
Patch	An adhesive substance with medication bonded to it that is slowly absorbed into the skin		Applied to the skin for up to 7 days for transdermal absorption
Inhalant	A liquid placed in a pressurized container or a squeeze bottle so that it will form an aerosol when activated		Inhaled through the mouth or the nose
Suppository	Solid medication mixed with a viscous substance that dissolves at body temperature	Supp	Placed in the vagina, rectum, or urethra, depending on the type of suppository

medication errors. Other features of the CPOE system include alerts about adverse reactions, drug and food incompatibilities, nursing implications for administration, and updates on new drug information. CPOE also has the potential to incorporate patient-specific information such as allergies, laboratory results, and vital signs, to ensure the nurse is aware of contraindications to the prescribed medications. A survey released in 2014 showed an all-time record of 1339 hospitals using CPOE in at least one inpatient unit, compared with 384 in 2010 (Leapfrog, 2014).

Bar code scanners are used to scan the medication package and the patient identification (ID) bands. When scanning is combined with a patient-specific profile, an electronic cross check of the Six Rights is ensured. When bar code scanning is used properly, it decreases the likelihood of administering the wrong drug to the wrong patient. Bar coding can also be set up with alerts for the nurse if a pill must be split in half, if a medication should be held because of a slow heart rate, or if the provider needs to be notified before or after administering a specific medication.

Mobile devices, smartphones, and PDAs are being used to download patient information such as diagnostic test results, lab findings, and treatment plans so the nurse can have access to patient information instantly. These devices also allow the nurse to document findings, which can be shared with providers immediately. This use of technology has increased the quality of data collection, and has improved the appropriateness of diagnosis and treatment decisions made by practitioners. When combined with the use of CPOE, nurses are able to perform treatments and administer medications in a timelier manner. The use of mobile devices, smartphones, and PDAs benefit the nurse, as well as the patients.

Clinical Cues

Computerized systems promote safety by cross checking information. For example, if you are administering the medication at the wrong time, the computer will query if you want to proceed. As a nursing student, you are likely to observe nurses who readily override these queries. Be aware that they may be performing an override because they have information that you do not have. Alternatively, they could be inappropriately overriding a safety feature to save time. Consult your instructor on how to handle such situations.

QSEN Considerations: Informatics

Using Technology to Improve Safety

Health care providers should value technologies that support clinical decision making, error prevention, and care coordination.

MEDICATION ADMINISTRATION RECORD

The medication administration record (MAR) is a part of the patient's medical record that the nurse refers to when administering medications to the patient. The medications are transcribed onto the MAR after the nurse receives the written order from the provider (Fig. 34.1). For convenience, the forms may be in binders kept in the medication area, and they may be referred to when giving regularly scheduled and PRN medications.

If CPOE is used, the medication order is automatically transcribed onto the eMAR. On both the MAR and eMAR, the nurse must document all medications that are administered or held, as well as any other data required by the facility. With computer systems, the eMAR is easier to retrieve and update; however, this also means that the nurse (or student nurse) is responsible for using the most current version of the eMAR. **Nurses and students should never rely on a hard copy of the MAR that was printed out at the beginning of the shift, as the information contained on it can change at any time.**

Think Critically

What are the advantages and disadvantages of the MAR? What are the advantages and disadvantages of the eMAR?

MEDICATION ADMINISTRATION SYSTEMS

There are three types of medication administration systems: the stock supply of medicines, the individual prescription system, and the unit-dose method. The unit-dose system is the most commonly used medication administration system. The advantages of the unit-dose system and the individual prescription system have made the stock supply system less popular. The unit-dose system can be modified in various ways and can be operated from a stationary (fixed) or a mobile center.

The fixed site is generally a small medication room that contains an automated dispensing machine (ADM) (e.g., Pyxis, Omnicell, and Cerner) individualized patient drawers, and medication administration supplies that are easily accessible for the nurse. The mobile method requires a cart that can be pushed from room to room as the medications are prepared and administered. These carts contain individualized patient drawers, as well as supplies commonly needed by the nurse to administer medications.

UNIT-DOSE SYSTEM

Unit dose refers to drugs packaged in single, individual doses. The unit-dose system provides a premeasured, prepackaged, and prelabeled dose of a medication for each patient (Fig. 34.2). Almost all oral medications, liquids, suppositories, and lotions are now available in unit doses and in prefilled cartridges or syringes for injection. This system is considered safest. With the mobile method, the pharmacy delivers a 24-hour supply of drugs for each patient, and then the nurse has access to each individually prescribed dose for that

24-hour period. In the long-term care facility, a week's or month's supply of each medication is often provided in a bubble pack. Each day's dose is pushed out of a bubble on the pack and is administered as ordered. When using an ADM, the pharmacy can enter a patient-specific profile, allowing the nurse to access medications only within that patient's profile. In some hospitals where the CPOE system communicates directly to the ADM, medications are added to the profile immediately so that nurses can administer medications as long as that medication is available in the ADM.

Clinical Cues

The unit-dose packaging can help you avoid drug dosage errors. For example, 1 g is ordered, but the drug comes in a unit-dose package of 0.25 mg per tablet; you would need 4000 tablets! Whenever you are preparing medications, **if three or more unit-dose packages are required to achieve the dose, recheck the order and your calculations.** Call the prescriber for clarification as needed.

The unit-dose system provides many benefits. The pharmacy supplies the exact dose of medication ordered, and each dose is opened and administered at the bedside, enhancing patient safety and reducing medication errors. The system also saves time for the nurse. Another benefit is that the patient is charged only for medications that are used. Finally, this system allows nursing units to keep a minimum amount of drugs on hand.

PRESCRIPTION SYSTEM

The prescription system is similar to the unit-dose system except that the pharmacy supplies enough doses for several days. This system is used in community pharmacies and in outpatient clinics. A prescription is written for each drug ordered and filled by the pharmacist, who then provides individual containers holding doses for several days. Its advantages include that only a limited amount of drugs needs to be kept in the outpatient clinic. Home care patients use prescription system–prepared drugs from the local pharmacy or by-mail pharmacies.

PREPARATION OF ORAL CONTROLLED SUBSTANCES FROM A DISPENSER

A controlled dispensing system is used for distributing opiate analgesics and hypnotics. **Legally controlled**

MEDICATION ADMINISTRATION RECORD PART I

ALLERGIES Penicillin
DIAGNOSIS HF
SIGNATURE L. Henderson, LPN; S. deWit, RN; P. Hall, LVN; D. Thomas, LVN

△ = IVPB TUBING CHANGE
A-RT. DELTOID
B-LT. DELTOID
C-RT. UP. OUT. QUAD.
D-LT. UP. OUT. QUAD.
E-RT. ABDOMEN
F-LT. ABDOMEN
I-RT. THIGH
J-LT. THIGH
K-RT. VENT. GLUTEAL
L-LT. VENT. GLUTEAL

RECOPIED BY:

ADDRESSOGRAPH Smith, John

INITL	DATE ORD.	DATE RNEW	DRUG AND DOSE	DC'D DATE	ROUTE FREQUENCY	SCHEDULE			DATE	DATE	DATE	DATE	DATE
L.H.	4/26/17		Digoxin 0.125 mg		P.O. qd			N					
						9		D	4/27 9 SD	4/28 9 SD			
								E	AP 82	AP 78			
L.H.	4/26/17		Furosemide 20 mg		P.O. bid			N					
						9		D	4/27 9 SD	4/28 9 SD			
						5		E	4/27 5 PH	4/28 5 O.T			
L.H.	4/26/17		SLO-K 500 mg.		P.O. tid			N					
						9	1	D	4/27 9 SD 1 SD	9 SD + SD			
						5		E	4/27 5 PH	5 O.2.			

FIGURE 34.1A Medication administration record (sample paper version).

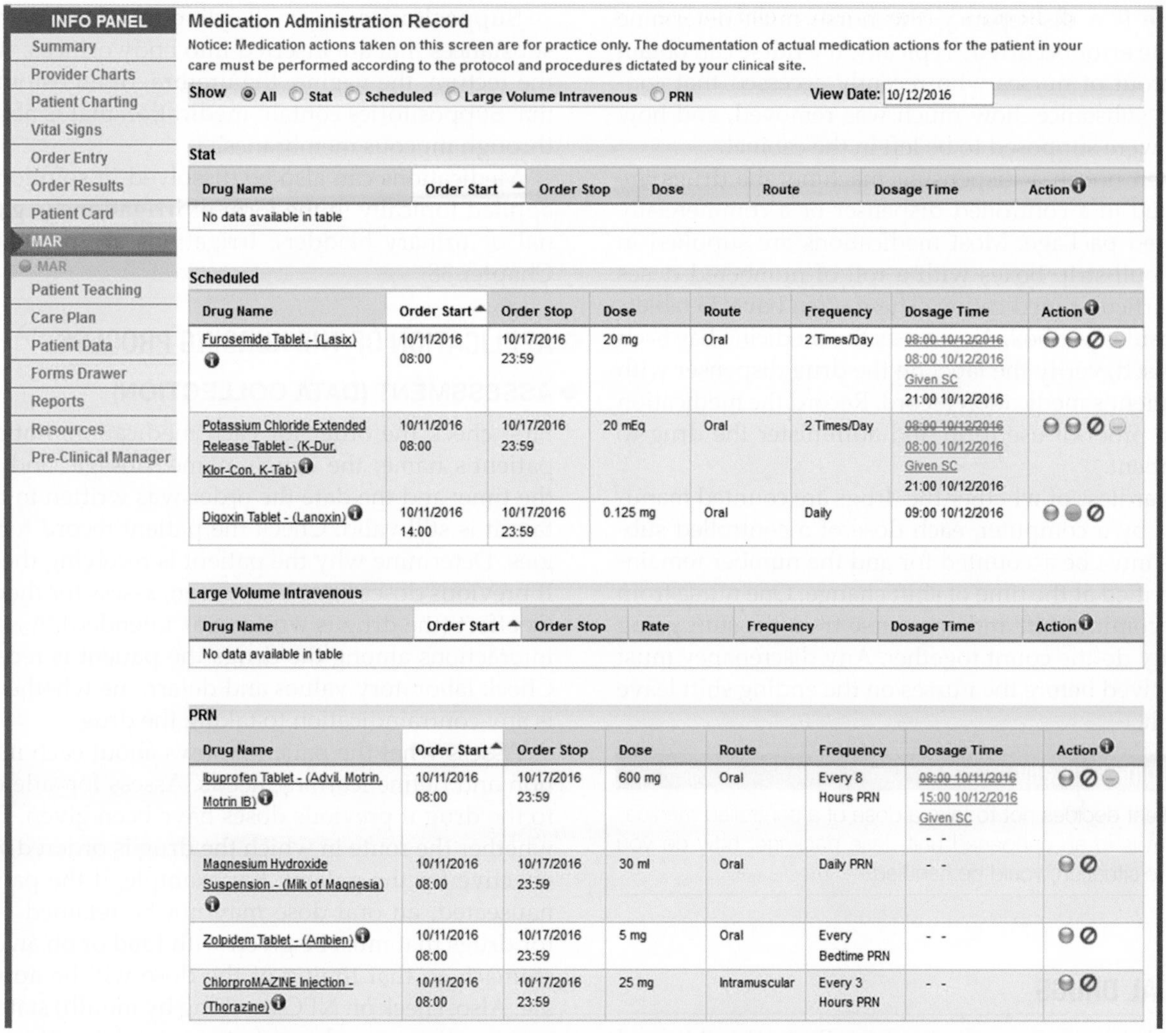

INFO PANEL
Summary
Provider Charts
Patient Charting
Vital Signs
Order Entry
Order Results
Patient Card
MAR
MAR
Patient Teaching
Care Plan
Patient Data
Forms Drawer
Reports
Resources
Pre-Clinical Manager

Medication Administration Record

Notice: Medication actions taken on this screen are for practice only. The documentation of actual medication actions for the patient in your care must be performed according to the protocol and procedures dictated by your clinical site.

Show ◉ All ○ Stat ○ Scheduled ○ Large Volume Intravenous ○ PRN   View Date: 10/12/2016

Stat

Drug Name	Order Start	Order Stop	Dose	Route	Dosage Time	Action
No data available in table						

Scheduled

Drug Name	Order Start	Order Stop	Dose	Route	Frequency	Dosage Time	Action
Furosemide Tablet - (Lasix)	10/11/2016 08:00	10/17/2016 23:59	20 mg	Oral	2 Times/Day	~~08:00 10/12/2016~~ 08:00 10/12/2016 Given SC 21:00 10/12/2016	
Potassium Chloride Extended Release Tablet - (K-Dur, Klor-Con, K-Tab)	10/11/2016 08:00	10/17/2016 23:59	20 mEq	Oral	2 Times/Day	~~08:00 10/12/2016~~ 08:00 10/12/2016 Given SC 21:00 10/12/2016	
Digoxin Tablet - (Lanoxin)	10/11/2016 14:00	10/17/2016 23:59	0.125 mg	Oral	Daily	09:00 10/12/2016	

Large Volume Intravenous

Drug Name	Order Start	Order Stop	Rate	Frequency	Dosage Time	Action
No data available in table						

PRN

Drug Name	Order Start	Order Stop	Dose	Route	Frequency	Dosage Time	Action
Ibuprofen Tablet - (Advil, Motrin, Motrin IB)	10/11/2016 08:00	10/17/2016 23:59	600 mg	Oral	Every 8 Hours PRN	~~08:00 10/11/2016~~ 15:00 10/12/2016 Given SC - -	
Magnesium Hydroxide Suspension - (Milk of Magnesia)	10/11/2016 08:00	10/17/2016 23:59	30 ml	Oral	Daily PRN	- -	
Zolpidem Tablet - (Ambien)	10/11/2016 08:00	10/17/2016 23:59	5 mg	Oral	Every Bedtime PRN	- -	
ChlorproMAZINE Injection - (Thorazine)	10/11/2016 08:00	10/17/2016 23:59	25 mg	Intramuscular	Every 3 Hours PRN	- -	

FIGURE 34.1B Medication administration record (sample electronic version).

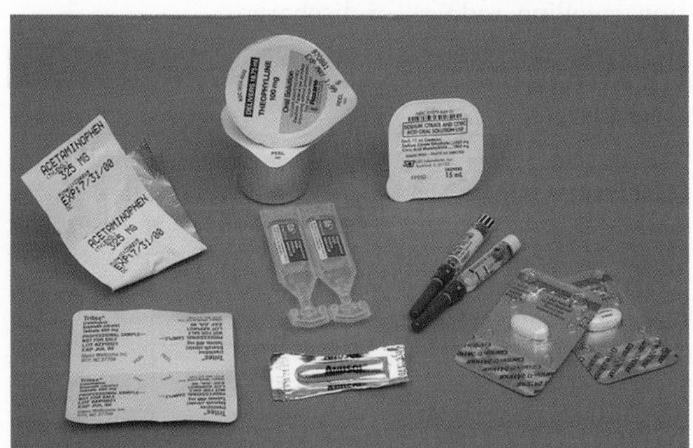

FIGURE 34.2 Unit-dose medications.

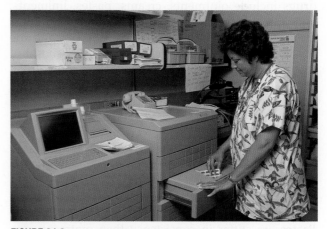

FIGURE 34.3 Nurse obtaining medication from an automated dispensing unit.

substances must be locked away safely at all times. ADMs are often used in the clinical setting to monitor and control narcotic use (Fig. 34.3). A significant advantage of this type of system is that a username and password or biometric identification system (fingerprint) is used to enter the system. This eliminates the problem of having to find the nurse who has the keys to the locked cabinet, and increases efficiency. Each nurse has a username and password for gaining entry to the system. Biometric identification ensures unauthorized users do not gain access. Once the nurse removes the controlled substance, s/he is required to count the remaining medications left in the drawer or cabinet. This count must match the computer count.

If there is a discrepancy, the nurse must determine how the error occurred. Typically, the nurse can obtain a printout of nurses who recently accessed that controlled substance, how much was removed, and how many were supposed to be left in the cabinet.

When not in a dispensing machine, the drugs are supplied in a controlled dispenser or a commercially prepared package. Most medications are supplied in small pull-strip boxes with a roll of numbered doses of a particular medication. These often have 25 tablets or capsules per box. As soon as the medicine has been dispensed, verify the label on the drug dispenser with the patient's medication record. Record the medication on the proof-of-use form and administer the drug to the patient.

Regardless of whether the drugs are counted manually or by a computer, each dose of a controlled substance must be accounted for and the number remaining verified at the time of shift change. One nurse from the oncoming shift and one nurse from the shift going off duty do the count together. Any discrepancy must be resolved before the nurses on the ending shift leave the unit.

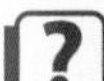 Think Critically

If a patient decides not to take a dose of a controlled medication that is in an unopened unit-dose package, how do you think the situation would be handled?

TOPICAL DRUGS

Topical drugs are applied externally to the skin and the mucous membranes. Common forms of topical drugs include ointments, creams, pastes, liniments, and lotions that are used to treat local conditions. Drug solutions instilled in the eye, the ear, and the nose are topical and act locally on these tissues, but they may also have a systemic effect on the patient. Drops and ointments for the eye must be sterile and nonirritating to the tissues. Solutions to be instilled in the eye, the ear, or the nose are generally prepared in dropper bottles.

Ointments are medicines manufactured in an oily base, such as petrolatum or lanolin, which keeps the drug in prolonged contact with the skin surface to obtain a soothing and anti-inflammatory effect. To protect against local infections, many contain antibiotics. **Pastes** are stiffer in consistency than ointments are, and they do not melt at body temperature. Aluminum paste and zinc oxide are examples of pastes that are used to absorb secretions and protect the skin. **Lotions** and **liniments** are topical drugs in liquid form, such as calamine lotion, used to cool, soothe, and reduce inflammation or itching of the skin. Lotions are patted on gently, whereas liniments are rubbed into the skin. Liniments provide temporary relief of pain or soothing warmth by their action, which dilates the superficial blood vessels.

Suppositories are small cylinder-shaped, semisolid substances that are inserted into body orifices, such as the rectum, the vagina, the urethra, or an ostomy stoma. Suppositories contain medication that is absorbed through mucous membranes.

Medications can also be dissolved in solutions and applied topically in the form of **irrigations** (e.g., vaginal or urinary bladder). Irrigations are presented in Chapter 38.

❖ APPLICATION OF THE NURSING PROCESS

◆ ASSESSMENT (DATA COLLECTION)

First check the order for each medication, noting the patient's name; the drug's name, dosage, and route; the time; and the date the order was written to be certain it is still valid. Check the patient record for allergies. Determine why the patient is receiving the drug. If previous doses have been given, assess for therapeutic effect (the drug is working as intended). Assess for interactions among the drugs the patient is receiving. Check laboratory values and determine whether there is any contraindication to taking the drug.

Assess what the patient knows about each medication and define learning needs. Assess for side effects to the drug if previous doses have been given. Decide whether the route in which the drug is ordered will be effective for the patient. For example, if the patient is nauseated, an oral dose may not be retained. Assess for drugs that must be given with food or on an empty stomach so that timing of the dose will be appropriate. Also, check on NPO (nothing by mouth) status and any pending procedures that require delay of administering medication. When topical medications are to be applied, assess for adverse effects such as inflammation, swelling, redness, or discharge.

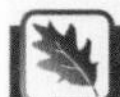 Life-Span Considerations

Older Adults

Assess your patient's manual dexterity. If your patient seems shaky or has trouble with fine motor movements, take a clean towel and spread it across her chest before handing her pills or tablets. If she (or you) drops the pill on the clean towel, it can be retrieved, but if a pill falls on the floor or dirty linens, you will have to stop and obtain a new pill from the pharmacy.

◆ NURSING DIAGNOSIS

Look at the classification of each medication and determine how nursing diagnoses are related to each prescribed medication. A hospitalized patient has acute problems but may be getting medications for other chronic problems. These chronic problems need to be addressed with nursing diagnoses on the care plan. For example, a patient who had a colon resection may also be diabetic and hypertensive. Patient care is often complex. By looking at the medications patients are receiving that are unrelated to the primary condition for which they are hospitalized, you can uncover and address chronic conditions. For example, if the patient is in the hospital for a hip replacement and the major nursing diagnosis on the care plan is Impaired physical mobility related to hip replacement, but the eMAR includes digoxin as a scheduled medication, then the patient may also have the nursing diagnosis of Decreased cardiac output. Digoxin is given to increase contractility of the heart. A few examples of nursing diagnoses for which medications are part of the treatment plan include:

- Acute pain (analgesics)
- Ineffective peripheral tissue perfusion related to increased blood pressure (antihypertensives)
- Risk for decreased cardiac tissue perfusion related to cardiac arrhythmia (antiarrhythmics)
- Impaired tissue integrity related to wound infection (antibiotics)
- Imbalanced nutrition: less than body requirements related to nausea (antiemetics)
- Deficient knowledge related to the action or side effects of prescribed medications

Life-Span Considerations

Older Adults

Over time, the older adult will experience an increasing number of ailments and illnesses. Older adults frequently receive prescriptions from more than one provider, especially if they are being treated for chronic conditions (Rambhade et al., 2012).

◆ PLANNING

Plan and incorporate times for medication administration into the daily shift work schedule. A grid on the daily worksheet for assigned patients and the times of their medications is useful. Plan to take juice or crackers to the room when a patient's medication is scheduled between meals and needs to be taken with food. If a patient has difficulty swallowing, allow time to sit the patient upright and coach her in the swallowing process. Plan to assess for side effects of the medication before giving the next scheduled dose. The overall goals of medication administration are:

- All medications ordered will be safely administered to each patient on time.
- Serious side effects of medication will be identified quickly.
- The medication will be effective.
- No allergic reaction to the medication will occur.
- The patient will understand why the drug is prescribed, adhere to the medication schedule, and report serious side effects.

Expected outcomes for the previous nursing diagnoses might be:

- Pain will be relieved for 3 hours after administration of analgesic.
- Blood pressure will be controlled within normal limits by antihypertensive medication within 1 week.
- Heart rate will be regular and strong while taking antiarrhythmic medication.
- Wound culture will be negative at end of antibiotic therapy.
- The patient will eat a meal without nausea with antiemetic 30 minutes before the meal.
- The patient will verbalize the reason for medication and side effects that might occur.

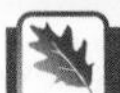
Life-Span Considerations

Older Adults

Older adults (or psychiatric patients) sometimes hold oral medication in the buccal (inner cheek) area rather than swallowing it; check the mouth to be certain that the medication has been swallowed if in doubt.

Think Critically

One of your patients requires 15 different morning medications. One of the medications must be cut in half to achieve the correct dose. What could you do to remind yourself that the tablet must be cut in half at the bedside?

◆ IMPLEMENTATION

When preparing any medication, remember to check the label three times and follow the Six Rights of medication administration. Always check for patient allergy to the medication before giving it, and document *after* administering the drug. Patient education is an integral part of medication administration (Nursing Care Plan 34.1).

Life-Span Considerations

Older Adults

For older adults with visual acuity deficits, make a chart using large dark letters on a white background. Include the drug's name, dose, time, and purpose. If the patient cannot read, tape a sample pill to the chart.

Oral Medication

Oral drugs may be supplied in many different forms. Examples include tablets, capsules, **spansules** (time-released pellets put into a capsule), lozenges, gelcaps, caplets, oral powders, tinctures, emulsions, and liquids in the form of a syrup, an elixir, or a suspension. Occasionally, you will have to cut a tablet in half to achieve the correct dose. Evidence-based practice indicates that you should use a tablet splitter (also called pill cutter) for this purpose because attempting to split the medication with scissors or to break it by hand will result in large dose deviations (Habib et al., 2014). When giving a drug in tablet or capsule form, be certain to offer sufficient water with which to swallow the medication. Some people want to take all of their pills at once; others want to take them one at a time. **Remember: Any water that is used must be entered on the intake sheet if the patient is on intake and output recording** (Skill 34.1). It is important to assess for side effects of the drug before giving another dose of the medication.

Nursing Care Plan 34.1 Care of the Patient Discharged With a New Medication

SCENARIO Phillip Hertog suffered a myocardial infarction and is being discharged home tomorrow. He has nitroglycerin ordered and has never used this medication and doesn't "understand the directions."

PROBLEM/NURSING DIAGNOSIS *Never used this medication; doesn't understand how to use it*/Deficient knowledge related to prescription for nitroglycerin sublingual tablets.

Supporting Assessment Data *Subjective:* States has never used nitroglycerin and does not "understand the directions." *Objective:* Has an anxious expression and is picking at the bedcovers.

Goals/Expected Outcomes	Nursing Interventions	Selected Rationale	Evaluation
Patient will verbalize correct way to take nitroglycerin by discharge.	Teach: • When chest pain occurs, he should sit down.	A resting position decreases the work of the heart.	*What was the patient able to recall about taking nitroglycerin?*
	• Place a sublingual tablet under the tongue.	Sublingual means under the tongue.	States, "Place a tablet under the tongue."
	• If pain has not eased within 5 min, place another sublingual tablet under the tongue.	A larger dose of nitroglycerin may be needed.	
Patient will state how many tablets he can use when he has chest pain.	• Repeat two times at 5-min intervals if the pain has not eased.		*Does the patient know how many tablets to use for chest pain?*
Patient will state what to do if medication does not relieve pain.	• Do not swallow pill.	Stomach acid may inactivate the medication, and it will not be absorbed as rapidly.	States, "Maximum of three tablets should be taken." Agrees not to swallow.
	• Call 911 if the pain continues after three tablets have been used.	Chest pain may indicate a myocardial infarction is occurring.	Chest pain symptoms reviewed.
	• Tablets are to be kept in an airtight, lightproof container.	Light makes tablets deteriorate and become ineffective.	Will keep tablets out of the light.
	• Tablets should be carried with him at all times and should be by the bedside at night.	Tablets must be at hand when chest pain occurs.	Agrees to have a bottle in his pocket or on the nightstand.
	• Headache is an expected side effect.	Patient must know this is an expected side effect.	Verbalizes awareness of possible headache.
	Answer any questions. Leave printed instructions with him.	Printed instructions reinforce verbal instructions and are at home for later referral.	Verbal and written instructions provided.
	Obtain verbal feedback from him regarding the instructions before discharge.	Verbal feedback, when correct, indicates understanding of the procedure to follow.	Correctly verbalized all points covered. Meeting expected outcomes.

CRITICAL THINKING QUESTIONS

1. What would you say to Mr. Hertog if he complains that the nitroglycerin tablets give him a terrible headache?
2. What instructions would you give Mr. Hertog about the side effects of nitroglycerin?

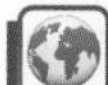

Cultural Considerations

Color, Size, and Milligrams of Pills

Some of your patients may believe that the size or color of a pill, or the dose, is related to efficacy. For example, your patient may voice a preference for a red pill, or your Cambodian patient may believe that a large pill contains a large dose. A comparative Western belief would be that your American patient believes that a large number of milligrams is related to therapeutic effect.

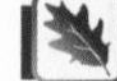

Life-Span Considerations

Older Adults

If an older adult patient has difficulty swallowing a pill, instruct him to take a sip of water and swallow it; then place the pill toward the back of the tongue. Have him take a large sip of water, place the tongue on the roof of the mouth, and with the chin tilted slightly downward, swallow; follow with more water. Consider crushing or cutting the pill unless contraindicated, or ask the provider for a liquid form of the drug.

Skill 34.1 Administering Oral Medications

 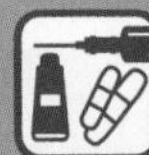 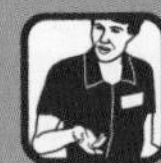 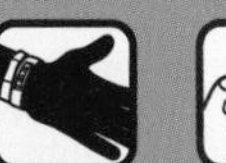 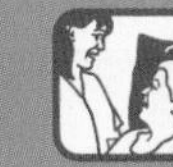 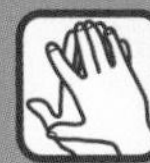 

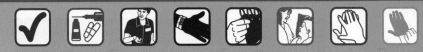

Most oral medications come in unit-dose packaging. You must locate where the medications are stored: the unit-dose cart, the individual patient medication drawer, or the central medication room. (The location varies by facility.) Patients are identified by at least two identifiers. Follow the principles of medication administration and consistently use the eMAR when checking and giving medications.

Supplies

- Unit-dose cart or patient drawer stocked with medications
- Medication cups (or a plastic baggy if there are many medications)
- Disposable gloves
- Straws
- Drinking cups
- Tongue blades
- Water or juice

Review and carry out the Standard Steps in Appendix A.

ACTION *(RATIONALE)*

Assessment (Data Collection)

1. Verify that the medication record has been compared with the provider's orders. Check each patient's allergies. *(Mistakes are sometimes made when transcribing orders onto the MAR, even in computerized systems. Allergic reactions can be fatal.)*
2. Determine that MARs are current for all patients to receive medications. *(The provider may write new orders at any time of the day.)*
3. Assess for side effects of previously given doses of the drug(s). Question the patient or assess the area where a topical medication was applied and is to be given. *(Prevents potential adverse effect of the drug.)*

Planning

4. Assess supplies on the cart and restock as necessary. *(Drinking cups, disposable gloves, and medication cups for liquid medication are needed. A pill cutter should be used if tablets need to be split.)*

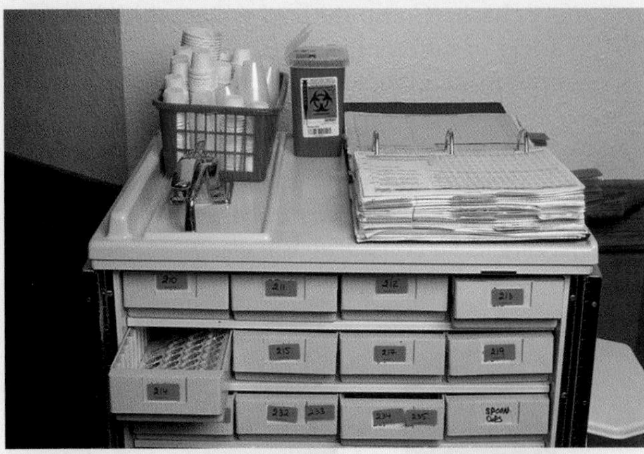

Step 4

5. Determine which patients are NPO (including those who are scheduled to have dialysis) and which are off the floor for procedures or surgery. *(Patients who are NPO must not receive oral medications; sometimes a medication can be taken with one sip of water. Some medications, such as antihypertensives, are held before dialysis. You must organize your work around procedures or surgery.)*
6. Calculate doses as needed. *(Ensures that the correct amount of drug will be administered.)*
7. Check to see whether narcotics or PRN medications are needed. *(These are stored in locked cabinets.)*

Implementation

8. Perform hand hygiene. *(Medications must be administered using aseptic technique.)*
9. Take the medication cart or individual patient's drawer to the patient's room. *(Administer medications to one patient at a time.)*
10. Verify that the patient is present to receive medications. *(If the patient is not available, medications will be delayed.)*
11. Remove the patient drawer containing the medications, and place it on the work space on top of the cart. Position the MAR sheet beside the drawer. If you are using an electronic MAR, position the screen so that you can easily compare each medication label to the MAR order. Perform the first check of each medication due at this hour by removing the medication from the drawer and checking the package label with the MAR order. Note the following:
    a. Drug name
    b. Dosage
    c. Date and time to be given
    d. Expiration date of the drug and the order

    Place the package beside the information on the MAR and proceed to the next medication ordered for this time. If you have many medications, make a small pencil mark beside the medication name so that you will know that you have checked it and place the package in a plastic baggy. If you are using an eMAR, the system may have a check box that allows you to note the first medication safety check. (Computerized systems will have a variety of different features.) Review signs and symptoms of adverse effects for which you must assess; look up any medication with which you are unfamiliar. *(This completes the first check of the Six Rights. Legally, you must know the action, normal dosage, adverse effects, interactions, and nursing implications for every drug you give.)*

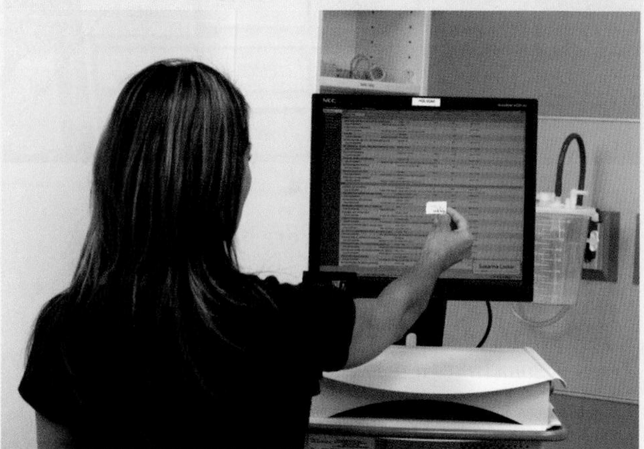

Step **11**

12. Return the drawer to its place in the cart, and then carefully check each medication a second time with the MAR or eMAR, verifying the following:
    a. Drug name
    b. Dosage
    c. Route ordered
    d. Date and time to be given

    Place each package into the medicine cup (or plastic baggy), unopened, as the second check is finished. *(Counting the number of medications on the MAR or eMAR to be given at the designated time [e.g., 0900] and then counting the medications you have out can prevent overlooking a dose. All MAR entries must be checked; some patients need many medications. Unit-dose packages are not to be opened until after the third medication check, when you are with the patient.)*
13. Pour the liquid medication dose into a medication cup unless it is in a dose-measured cup already; carefully check the dosage amount. To pour a liquid medication from a multidose bottle, read the dose from the bottom of the meniscus, the lowest point. Label the cup. When liquid medications are supplied in a premeasured cup, remove the lid carefully at the bedside so as not to spill the contents. If a multidose bottle is supplied, measure the dose accurately. *(Liquids must be accurately measured, but excess should not be poured back into the multidose bottle. Labeling the cup helps to prevent error.)*

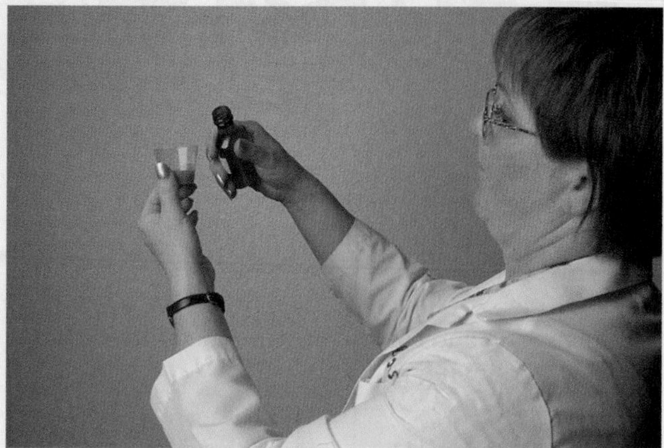

Step **13**

14. Take the medications and the MAR sheet to the patient. If using an eMAR and bar code scanner, take the workstation on wheels (WOW) into the patient's room. Identify the patient by comparing the information on the wristband with the information imprinted on the MAR, and by asking the patient to state his or her name; scan the patient's wristband if using bar code scanning; explain the procedure, thereby completing the Six Rights check. *(Identification of the patient's full name and hospital number is the best method. Some patients respond to any name.)*

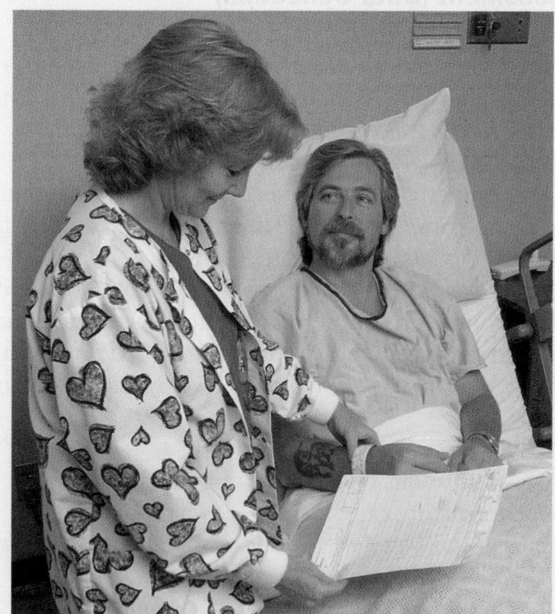

Step **14**

15. Check each medication for the third time as you prepare to open it to give to the patient. Tell the patient what the medication is (e.g., "your heart medication"). Check the following:
    a. Drug name
    b. Dosage
    c. Route ordered
    d. Date and time

If the patient does not recognize the medication or indicates that no "heart medication" has ever been taken, for example, stop and recheck the original order. If there is no question, open the medication and place it in the medicine cup. *(When the drug is kept in its wrapper, it can be returned to the drawer if the patient refuses it or if it is not the correct medication. The third check of the medicine provides added safety in following the Six Rights. Many medication errors are made because the date and time were not also checked along with the drug name and dosage. Even though drugs are dispensed in unit-dose packages, more than one package or part of a tablet may be required for the ordered dose.)*

16. Pour water for the patient to take the pills; perform any assessment necessary before the patient takes the medication (e.g., take an apical pulse rate before administering digitalis preparations, assess the blood pressure before giving an antihypertensive medication; record the data). Assess for adverse effects from previous doses of the medications you are about to give. Assess to see whether any PRN medications are needed at this time. *(Liquid is necessary for swallowing pills. The heart rate and rhythm must be known before digitalis is administered; certain antihypertensive medications are withheld if the blood pressure is below a specified level. You must assess for adverse effects of a drug before giving another dose. Giving PRN medications while in the room saves time.)*
17. Give the medications to the patient with water or other acceptable liquid. Adhere to fluid restriction requirements for patients whose intake of fluid is restricted. *(Patients whose intake of fluid is restricted must space their fluid intake over 24 hours and are not allowed unlimited fluid for taking medications.)*
18. Observe the patient take the medications, and for those patients who have difficulty swallowing, check the inside of the mouth to see that the pills were actually swallowed. For patients who have difficulty swallowing, placing the pill as far back on the tongue as possible before the patient takes a sip of water helps. *(Sometimes pills fall onto the bed or floor when the patient places the medicine cup to the mouth. A pill may remain in the mouth if the patient has difficulty swallowing.)*
19. Initial the doses given and sign your name on the MAR (or document in the eMAR) according to agency policy. If the medicine is not given, circle the time of the dose and follow agency policy regarding further documentation. *(Documentation of an administered dose is done after the patient has taken the medication. Typically, you must document the reason for holding the medication [e.g., surgery or vomiting]).*
20. Proceed to prepare and administer medications to the next patient. *(The patient should receive medications within 30 to 60 minutes of the scheduled time, depending on the type of drug and agency requirements.)*
21. Return common equipment and supplies to the central area. *(You may delay the work of others if you do not return common equipment in a timely fashion.)*

Evaluation

22. Evaluate whether the patient had any signs or symptoms of adverse effects and whether the medication appears to be effective in treating the condition. Recheck each MAR or eMAR for the time you are giving medications to ensure that every medication scheduled for that time has been signed off. (After the medication has been documented in the eMAR, the appearance of the medication typeface will change from bold to faded, depending on the system, indicating that the medication administration has been recorded.) *(If there are adverse or ineffective results, the provider should be notified before other doses are administered. Rechecking ensures no dose has been overlooked.)*

Special Considerations

- If medications are prepared for administration in the medication room, complete the two checks for each drug ordered before going to the patient's room; perform the third check at the bedside.
- Patients should be sitting up as high as possible to swallow medications. Instruct not to hyperextend the neck when swallowing, but to tuck in the chin slightly instead. Offer a straw if the patient has difficulty drinking from a cup.
- When a patient is on intake and output (I & O) recording, the amount of water used to take medications must be noted on the I & O sheet.
- Consider possible drug interactions among the drugs ordered for the patient.
- If indicated, check the swallowing reflex by offering a sip of water.
- Sublingual or buccal medications are left under the tongue or in the cheek pocket to allow for absorption via the oral mucosa.
- If an agency uses computerized systems for dispensing, administering, or documenting, you will need computer training, but the basic safety principles and the Six Rights still apply.

? Critical Thinking Questions

1. What would you check to verify that the patient is not allergic to a medication?
2. What will you do if the patient looks at the pill you are administering and says, "I don't recognize this pill. Is it really ordered for me?"

When preparing liquid medications, pour the dose into a graduated medicine cup. The exact level of the dose is read at the lowest point of the **meniscus** (curved upper surface) of the liquid in the cup when held at eye level (Fig. 34.4). Always pour the liquid out the side of the bottle, away from the label, so that any residual liquid will not run down the label and distort the words on it.

Clinical Cues

For infants, measure oral liquid medication with an oral syringe. The mother or nurse cuddles the infant in an upright position on the lap. Insert the tip of the oral syringe on the side of mouth and give it slowly. An alternative method for infants who can bottle feed is to use a Medibottle, which allows the attachment of a medication syringe to a nipple.

Sublingual medications are placed under the tongue. They should never be swallowed. The drug dissolves in the sublingual pocket and is quickly absorbed by the vessels in the oral mucosa. **Buccal** medications are placed in the pocket between the teeth and the cheek. Swallowing these medications alters their absorption and may make them ineffective.

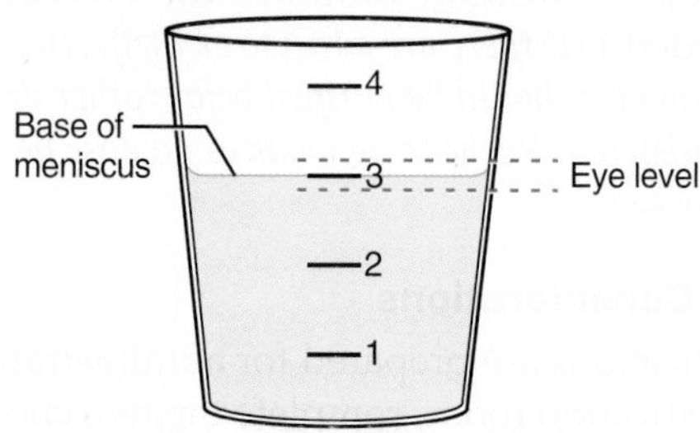

FIGURE 34.4 Reading the dose prepared at the meniscus of the liquid.

Eye and Ear Medications

Ophthalmic (eye) medications may be in the form of drops, ointment, or an eye disk. An error with an eye medication can cause significant damage, and it is imperative to check each medication carefully before instilling it. The word *ophthalmic* must be clearly visible on the medication container, and the medication must be in date. Skill 34.2 shows the steps for instilling eye drops and eye ointment. Eye medications must be kept sterile. Careful hand hygiene is necessary before beginning the procedure. If the patient is wearing contact lenses, they must be removed. Some medications will stain the lenses; ointments will coat and may destroy them.

Safety Alert

Oral Syringes for Safety

Small amounts (less than 30 mL) of oral medications can be measured with a syringe. To increase safety, use an **oral syringe** to prevent accidental intramuscular (IM), IV, or subcutaneous administration of oral medications. If the facility does not carry oral syringes, discuss this with the charge nurse because errors occur when nurses are forced to use "what's available" (Grissinger, 2013).

Skill 34.2 Instilling Eye Medication

 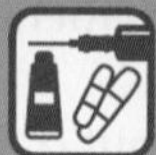 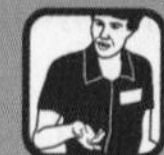  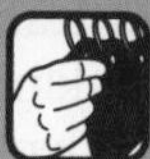 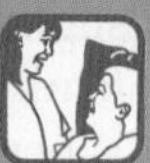 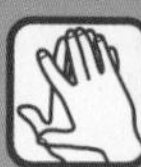 

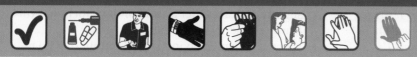

Eye medications are used to control glaucoma, treat eye infections, decrease inflammation, provide moisture to the eye, dilate the eye, and cleanse the eye. Each medication bottle is ordered only for an individual patient.

Supplies

- Ophthalmic solution or ointment (as ordered)
- Disposable gloves
- Medication administration record (MAR or eMAR)
- Tissues or cotton balls

Review and carry out the Standard Steps in Appendix A.

ACTION *(RATIONALE)*

Assessment (Data Collection)

1. Determine that the ordered eye medications are on hand. If the patient has contact lenses or glasses, assist the patient in removing and storing lenses or glasses. *(Contact lenses could be damaged.)*
2. Check the eye medication with the MAR or eMAR, following the Six Rights of medication administration, twice before performing hand hygiene and once after identifying the patient. Double check whether the instillation is for the right eye, the left eye, or both eyes. *(Prevents medication errors.)*
3. Assess the eye(s) for inflammation, swelling, discharge, and change in vision. *(May be an adverse effect of medication.)*

Planning

4. Consider the order in which the eye medications are to be instilled if there is more than one. *(Some types of medications must be instilled before other types.)*
5. You may need to remove a dressing, clean the eye, or instill drops over a set time period. *(Instilling eye medication often takes longer than giving an oral medication.)*

Intervention

6. Check the patient's identification band, comparing it with the MAR or eMAR. Ask the patient to state her name. Scan the patient's wristband if using bar code scanning. Perform hand hygiene and don gloves. *(Give medication to the right patient. Aseptic technique is required.)*

Eye Drop Application

7. Remove the cap from the bottle of medication; place it upside down on the table. *(The cap must be sterile.)*
8. Place the patient in a sitting or reclining position. Ask the patient to look at the ceiling and tilt the head slightly to the side of the affected eye. With a tissue beneath the fingers, retract the lower lid over the bony orbit by pulling it downward to expose the conjunctival sac. If the patient is sitting in a chair, stand beside the chair. *(Looking upward inhibits the desire to blink.)*
9. Stabilize the container above the eye over the conjunctival sac and drop the designated number of drops directly into the conjunctival sac without touching the surface of the eye. Do not place drops on the cornea. Block the entrance to the lacrimal gland by placing a finger over it. *(Drops on the cornea cause discomfort and/or damage. Medication can enter systemic circulation through lacrimal gland.)*

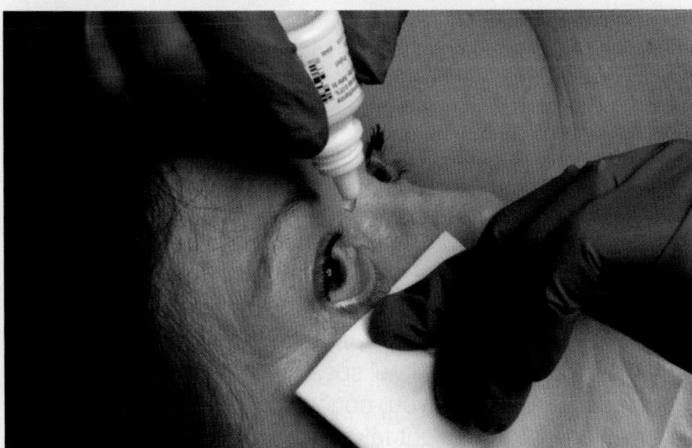

Step 9

10. Replace the cap on the bottle without contaminating the dropper tip or the rim of the top. If the dropper tip becomes contaminated, replace the medication with a new bottle. *(Medication is contaminated if the tip becomes contaminated.)*

Eye Ointment Application

11. For eye ointment, remove the cap from the tube and set it down on a table upside down. Expose the conjunctival sac, and apply a thin ribbon of ointment along the entire length of the visible conjunctival sac. To end the ribbon, simply twist the tube with a lateral movement of the wrist without touching the eye or the lid. Recap the tube and return it to storage. *(Tip will be contaminated if it touches the eye. Medication placed in the conjunctival sac will spread over the eye.)*

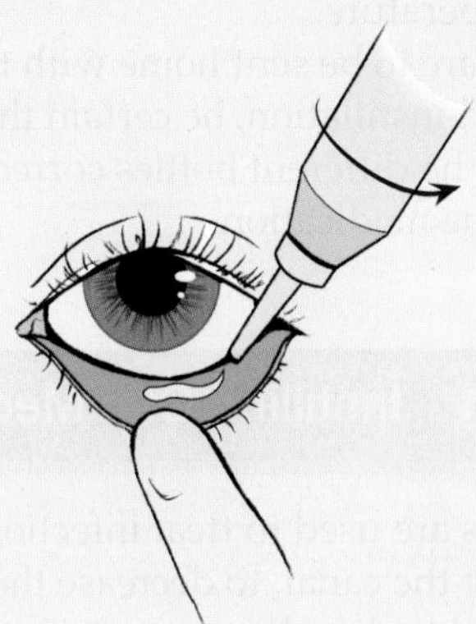

Step 11

12. Ask the patient to close the eyelid gently and move the eyes side to side and up and down with eyelids closed to distribute the medication. *(Closing the eyelid tightly causes medication to be pushed out. Rolling the eyeball around distributes ointment over the entire eyeball.)*
13. With a tissue or a cotton ball, gently remove excess medication from the outside of the lid and discard into a designated container. *(Removes excess medication from the face.)*

For Eye Drops and Ointment

14. Remove gloves and perform hand hygiene. Return the medications to their storage location. *(Reduces transfer of microorganisms. Prepares medications for the next use.)*

Evaluation

15. Assess for the desired effect of the eye medication and for adverse effects. *(If adverse effects occur, the medication may need to be changed.)*
16. Evaluate your own technique and consider any changes to be made for the next instillation. *(Provides feedback on technical skill.)*

Documentation

17. Document the doses given on the MAR or eMAR. *(The right documentation verifies that medication was given.)*

Special Considerations

- If a dressing was removed, reapply a dressing using aseptic technique.
- If eye crusting or debris is present, clean the lids and lashes with sterile normal saline and sterile

cotton balls before instilling the medication. Wipe from the inner canthus at the nose to the outer canthus near the temple. Use a clean cotton ball for each wiping stroke.

- Eye medications should be at room temperature for administration; eye ointment will flow more easily at room temperature.
- If eye drops are to be sent home with the patient for continued instillation, be certain that the patient can identify the different bottles correctly, if there is more than one medication.
- Assess the area for inflammation, swelling, pain, and discharge; determine whether vision has changed.

Critical Thinking Questions

1. How can you mark multiple eye drop bottles that the patient will be using at home, so that there is no mistake about when to use them and in what order?
2. Why would you avoid dropping the eye drops directly on the cornea?

Steps 34.1 Instilling Otic Medication

Ear medications are used to treat infection or inflammation of the canal, to decrease the pain of otitis media, and to dissolve cerumen (earwax). A cotton ball is placed in the ear after the drops have been instilled to prevent medication from dripping out and soiling clothes.

Review and carry out the Standard Steps in Appendix A.

ACTION *(RATIONALE)*

1. Position the patient supine and in the lateral position so that the affected ear is uppermost. *(Drops will flow into the ear by gravity.)*
2. Draw medication into the dropper by depressing the bulb and letting it go. *(Suction draws medication into dropper.)*
3. Straighten the ear canal by drawing the pinna upward and toward the back of the head. For children younger than 3 years, draw the earlobe slightly down and back. Insert the tip of the medicine dropper into the external ear canal; instill the medication and withdraw the dropper (see Fig. 34.5). *(Places medication in the intended location.)*
4. Place cotton in the external meatus to prevent the medication from escaping. Have patient remain in the lateral position for 5 to 10 minutes. *(Allows medicine to penetrate the length of the ear canal.)*

Communication

Patient Education to Increase Adherence

Rita Sanchez is being discharged after hospitalization for a bacterial pneumonia. Her primary care provider has prescribed clarithromycin tablets for her to take at home. You go to instruct her about this medication and find she has taken it before and did not like the side effects.

Ms. Sanchez: "Clarithromycin makes my mouth taste terrible, and I lost my appetite the last time I took it."

Nurse: "Why was it prescribed for you the last time?"

Ms. Sanchez: "I had bronchitis."

Nurse: "I'm sorry it caused such an unpleasant side effect. Did it cause stomach pain or diarrhea?"

Ms. Sanchez: "No, I didn't have those problems with it."

Nurse: "Your doctor has prescribed clarithromycin because it is the best one to treat the infection."

Ms. Sanchez: "But I'm not going to get my strength back if I can't eat."

Nurse: "I understand your concern. You might try brushing your teeth several times a day and using a mild mouthwash every 2 hours while you are awake to get rid of the taste in your mouth."

Ms. Sanchez: "Do you really think that will help?"

Nurse: "There is a good chance that it will help. Chewing gum between meals may also decrease the bad taste. Try eating six small meals a day until the medication is gone."

Ms. Sanchez: "Are you sure there isn't another medication that I can take instead of this one?"

Nurse: "Well, your sputum culture showed that this medication is the most effective at treating the bacteria responsible for the infection. I will speak with your primary care provider and tell him your concerns and see if there is anything else you might take."

Ms. Sanchez: "Why, thank you very much."

Otic (ear) medication is primarily used in children to decrease the pain of otitis media, but may also be used to treat external otitis and to soften cerumen (earwax) so that it can be removed more easily. Otic medication administration is presented in Steps 34.1. For the child younger than 3 years, pull the earlobe downward to straighten the canal; in the adult, pull the top of the pinna out and upward (Fig. 34.5).

Nasal Medications

Nasal medications come in soft plastic atomizer or dropper bottles. An atomizer bottle contains

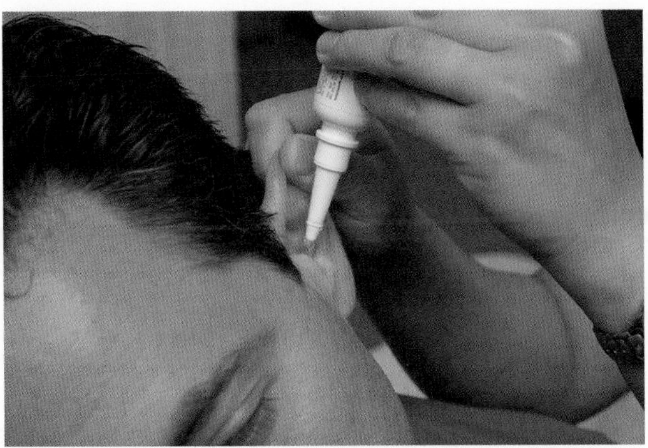

FIGURE 34.5 Straightening the ear canal for otic drops.

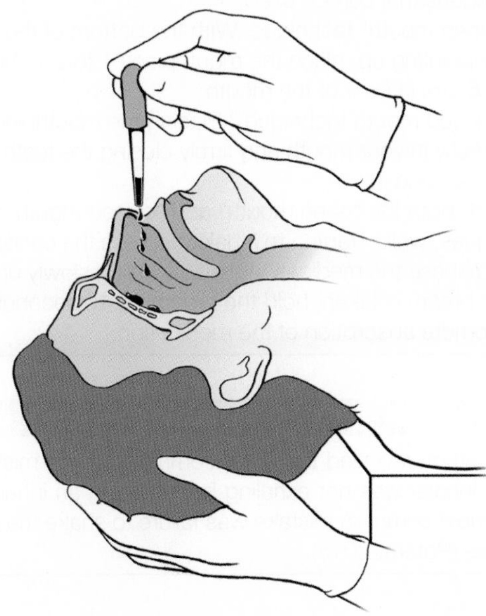

FIGURE 34.6 Instilling nose drops (Proetz position).

decongestant, antihistamine, antibiotic, or steroid, depending on the patient's need. To use an atomizer bottle, have the patient clear the nose as much as possible. While holding one nostril shut, the patient inserts the top of the atomizer into the other nostril. The patient squeezes the bottle while breathing in and repeats the process on the other side. One or two squirts per nostril is the usual dose. The top of the bottle should be wiped clean before the cap is replaced.

When nose drops are prescribed, the patient should lie down face up, with the head off the bed and the neck hyperextended. The drops are pulled into the dropper by depressing the rubber top of the dropper while the stem is in the liquid and letting go. The tip of the dropper is held just above the nostril, and the correct number of drops is gently expelled into the nostril by lightly squeezing the rubber top (Fig. 34.6). The patient should remain in the head-back position for a few minutes.

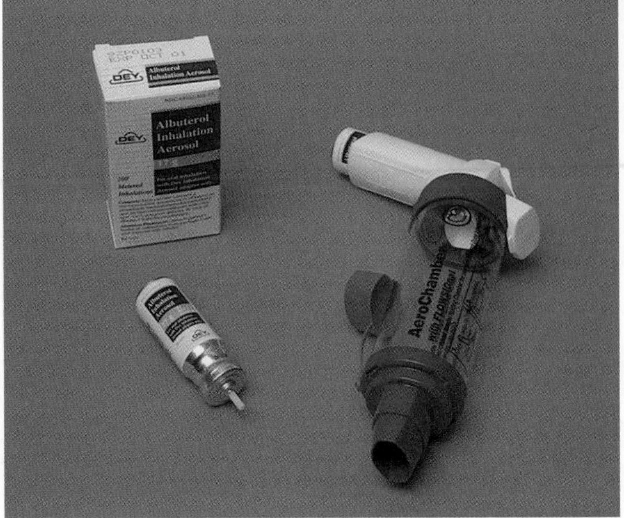

FIGURE 34.7 Metered-dose inhaler, medication canister, and spacer.

Safety Alert

One or Both Nostrils?

Nasal medications that are intended for local effect on the nasal mucosa, such as saline nose drops or drops for seasonal allergies, are administered in both nostrils. Nasal medications that are intended for systemic effects, such as sumatriptan (Imitrex), should be given in one nostril only.

Inhalation Medications

Inhalation therapy is used for patients with respiratory conditions, which can originate in any area from the nasal passageways to the deep lung tissues. Drugs used for inhalation therapy are always water soluble to ensure quick absorption into the respiratory system without creating tissue inflammation. Various mechanical devices, such as atomizers, sprays, and hand-held metered-dose inhalers (MDIs), are designed for aerosol treatment (Fig. 34.7).

Metered-dose inhalers (MDIs) and nasal sprays come in containers labeled with directions for use. The MDI is held in front of the mouth; the cylinder for the inhalant is depressed; and a spray of medication is released into the chamber (spacer) to be inhaled. Many medications are available in MDI form: antispasmodics, bronchodilators, mucolytic agents, proteolytic enzymes, and anti-inflammatory medications. Using a spacer with the device enhances delivery of the medication deeper into the bronchioles. Patients must be taught how to use an MDI properly (Fig. 34.8). Five groups of drugs are commonly dispensed in inhalers for treatment of the lungs (Table 34.5). The patient should not take more than one drug from any one of the groups.

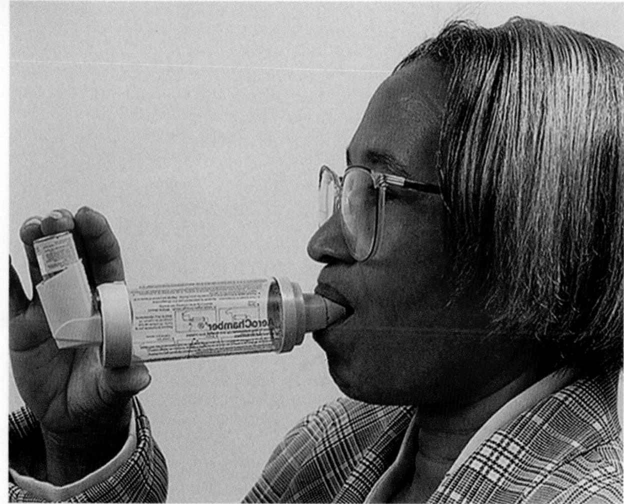

FIGURE 34.8 Using a metered-dose inhaler with a spacer. (From Taussig, L. M., & Landau, L. I. [Eds.], [2008]. *Pediatric respiratory medicine* [2nd ed.]. St. Louis, MO: Mosby. From Potter, P. A., & Perry, A. G. [2008]. *Fundamentals of nursing* [7th ed.]. St. Louis, MO: Mosby.)

Table 34.5 Inhalant Drugs for Respiratory Problems

DRUG	EXAMPLE
Beta-agonist drugs (stimulants) that open the small airways	Metaproterenol (Alupent), albuterol (Proventil, Ventolin), terbutaline (Brethaire), levalbuterol (Xopenex)
Anticholinergics used to decrease bronchospasm and open the large airways	Atropine ipratropium (Atrovent)
Corticosteroids used to decrease inflammation	Beclomethasone (Beclovent and Vanceril), triamcinolone (Azmacort), flunisolide (AeroBid)
Leukotriene modifiers for maintenance therapy of chronic asthma	Montelukast (Singulair)
Antiallergic medications used to decrease mucosal response to allergens	Cromolyn sodium (Intal)

Patient Education

How to Use a Metered-Dose Inhaler With a Spacer

When a patient is taking both a corticosteroid and a bronchodilator, teach her to take the bronchodilator first to open the airways so that the corticosteroid will be absorbed. Using a spacer with the MDI is the preferred method (Cleveland Clinic, 2015). Instruct the patient to use the following steps:

- Always sit or stand to use the MDI.
- Attach the medication canister by holding the long end of the mouthpiece and inserting the stemmed top of the canister into it.
- Shake the canister for 5 seconds to mix medication with propellant, and remove the mouthpiece cap.
- Insert the MDI into the open end of the spacer (opposite the mouthpiece).
- Place the mouthpiece of the chamber in the mouth between the teeth and seal the lips around it. Completely exhale from the nose.
- Depress the canister once to release the medication into the spacer.
- Breathe in slowly. If you hear a "horn-like" sound while inhaling, slow your inhalation down. After inhalation, hold the breath for 10 seconds and try not to cough. This allows the medication to penetrate the lung mucosa.
- Exhale through the nose and take two or three short breaths to obtain the remaining medication in the spacer.
- If a second puff is ordered, wait at least 1 minute before repeating the procedure. This allows the first dose to be fully absorbed before the second is given.
- If using a MDI without a spacer, there are two possible techniques that can be used:
  - "Open mouth" technique: With the bottom of the canister pointing up, place the mouthpiece 1 to 2 inches (2.5 to 5 cm) in front of the mouth.
  - "Closed mouth technique:" Placing the mouthpiece directly in your mouth and firmly closing the teeth and lips around it.
  - With both the "open mouth" and "closed mouth" techniques, while starting to inhale, depress the canister to release the medication. Keep inhaling slowly until a full breath is taken; hold the breath for 10 seconds to promote absorption of the medication.

Memory Jogger

A recent study revealed the most common patient mistake in using an inhaler was not exhaling before using an inhaler; the second most common mistake was failure to shake the inhaler before use (Potera, 2015).

Vaginal Medications

A vaginal irrigation is also called a **douche.** Topical solution is introduced into the vaginal cavity for the following purposes:

- To cleanse the vagina in preparation for surgery
- To supply antiseptics to reduce bacterial growth
- To remove odors or foul discharge
- To apply heat or cold to soothe inflamed tissues or reduce oozing of blood

The normal secretions of the vaginal tissues are naturally acidic, which helps protect against vaginal infection. Vaginal irrigations are considered a clean procedure, except when given after surgery or childbirth; then principles of surgical asepsis are followed. Medicated solutions used for vaginal irrigations are 2% sodium bicarbonate solution, diluted hydrogen peroxide, povidone-iodine solution, a weak solution of acetic acid (1 tablespoon vinegar to 1000 mL of fluid), or a medication that is diluted in water. The amount of solution ranges from 1500 to 2000 mL, given slowly over a period of 10 to 15 minutes at body temperature unless the purpose is

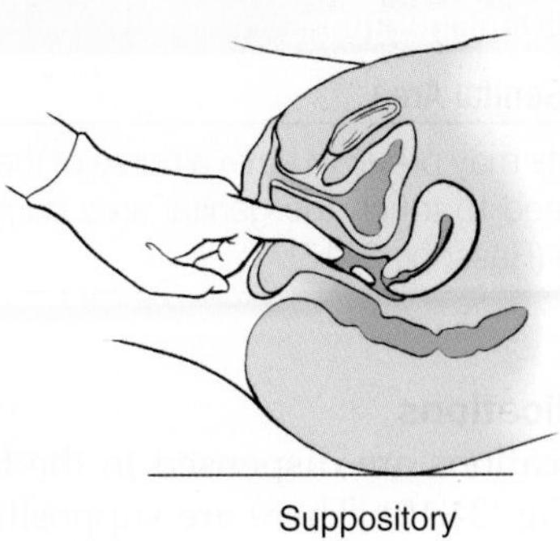

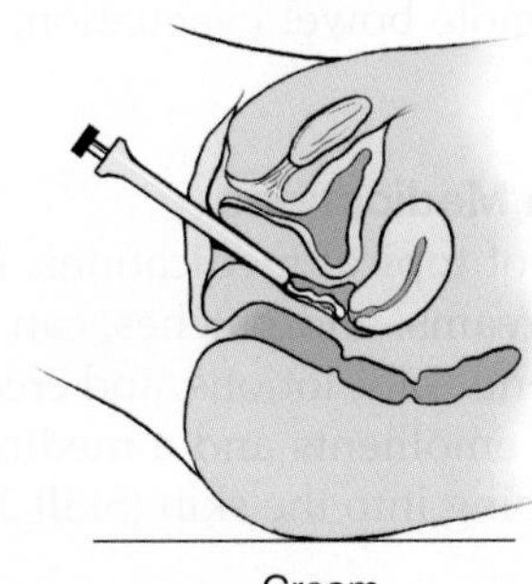

FIGURE 34.9 Inserting vaginal medications.

to apply heat; then it should be 110°F (43.3°C). The patient should receive instruction in the correct way to perform the irrigation.

Other topical medications applied to the vagina are suppositories, ointments, and creams prescribed to treat infections and inflammation. Applicators are used for inserting the smaller vaginal suppositories at the distal end of the vagina. An applicator is also required for vaginal ointments. The applicator fits the top of the tube, and enough medication is squeezed into the barrel to fill it, after which the applicator is inserted into the vagina and the plunger is depressed to deposit the ointment (Fig. 34.9). After use, the applicator is washed with soap and water and stored for the patient's future use, or it is discarded. The patient may be instructed on how to insert the medication herself. After medication has been inserted, a small pad or panty shield may be worn to keep from soiling clothing or bedding.

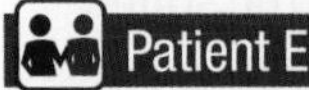 Patient Education

How to Perform Vaginal Irrigations and Instill Vaginal Medications

A vaginal douche works best when done in a dorsal recumbent position in the tub, but it can be done when sitting on a commode. The bladder should be emptied first. Medication is best instilled at bedtime to enhance retention of the medication for a prolonged time.

Instruct the patient to do the following:

FOR IRRIGATION WITH A VAGINAL DOUCHE

- Perform hand hygiene. Prepare the douche solution per the directions with the medication.
- Fill the douche bag, run a small amount of fluid through the tubing to clear the air in the tube, and close the clamp.
- Hang the douche container no more than 18 inches above the level of the hips. Otherwise, the pressure of the fluid will be too great. A coat hanger placed on a towel rack may work for hanging the bag.
- Gently insert the irrigating nozzle, directing it downward or backward to the back of the vagina.
- Holding the labia closed around the nozzle, unclamp the clamp, allowing the solution to flow slowly into the vagina. When the pressure becomes slightly uncomfortable, ease your grip, allowing the solution to flow out of the vagina. Hold the labia closed again until the vagina fills; repeat the process until all the irrigating solution has been used. *With the labia closed, the solution will distend the folds of the vagina, reaching all areas.*
- The nozzle may be rotated during the irrigation.
- Close the clamp and remove the nozzle. Dry the perineum.
- Rinse the equipment, wash the nozzle with soap and warm water, and rinse it well. Hang the bag upside down to drain and dry.

FOR INSERTION OF A VAGINAL SUPPOSITORY

- Wait at least an hour after a vaginal irrigation before inserting medication so that residual irrigation fluid does not wash the medication away.
- Perform hand hygiene.
- Remove the wrapper from the suppository. Lubricate the rounded end of the suppository with a small amount of water-soluble lubricant for easier insertion.
- Lie down, bend the legs, and spread the knees, or bend a leg and prop a foot on a chair seat or the commode.
- Gently open the labial folds with the nondominant hand.
- Insert the rounded end of the suppository into the vagina with the dominant hand and direct it toward the posterior wall, placing it the full finger's length into the vaginal vault so it will not be easily expelled. Use a vaginal applicator according to package directions if one was supplied with the medication.
- Withdraw the finger or applicator and wash hands and applicator thoroughly.
- Use a panty liner or sanitary pad to collect drainage from the medication to avoid staining clothing.

FOR INSTILLATION OF VAGINAL CREAM OR FOAM

- Perform hand hygiene.
- Fill the cream or foam applicator according to the directions on the package insert.
- Lie down, bend the knees, and spread the legs.
- Gently separate the labial folds with the nondominant hand.
- With the dominant hand, gently insert the applicator about 2 to 4 inches and press the plunger to deposit the medication into the vagina.
- Remove the applicator and wipe excess cream from the labia.
- Remain recumbent for at least 10 minutes to allow medication to disperse.
- Clean the applicator and wash hands thoroughly.
- Use a panty liner or sanitary napkin to catch medication drainage to avoid staining clothing.
- Report any persistent burning or irritation to the primary care provider because this may indicate an adverse reaction.

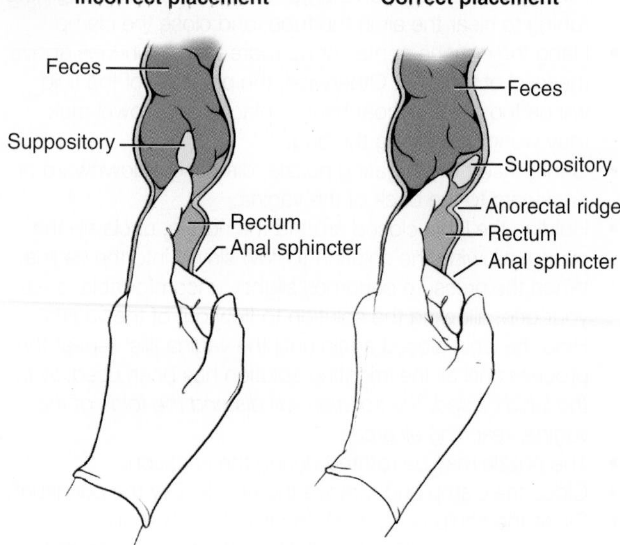

FIGURE 34.10 Inserting a rectal suppository to promote bowel evacuation.

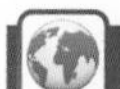

Cultural Considerations

Touching the Genital Area

Muslim patients may prefer to have a nurse of the same gender if there is a need to touch the genital area during medication administration (Rassool, 2015).

Rectal Medications

Rectal medications are dispensed in the form of suppositories (Fig. 34.10). There are suppositories to prevent vomiting, soothe hemorrhoids, prevent bladder spasms, promote bowel evacuation, and reduce fever (Steps 34.2).

Topical Skin Medications

Many types of topical medications, including lotions, ointments, creams, and patches, can be applied to the skin. Ointments, oils, lotions, and creams are combinations of skin emollients and a medication and are applied by rubbing into the skin (Skill 34.3).

Steps 34.2 Inserting a Rectal Suppository

A rectal suppository may be inserted to stimulate a bowel movement, to deliver a medication when the patient cannot take it another way, or to treat hemorrhoids.

Review and carry out the Standard Steps in Appendix A.

ACTION *(RATIONALE)*

1. After checking the order, obtain the suppository, gloves, and water-soluble lubricant. *(Suppositories are frequently stored in the refrigerator.)*
2. Perform hand hygiene, identify the patient, provide privacy, explain the procedure, raise the bed to working height, and lower the near side rail if up. *(Ensures the correct patient receives suppository. Teaches patient the purpose of suppository. Allows easy access to the patient.)*
3. Place the patient in the left Sims' position and fold the top bedding obliquely back over the hips to expose the buttocks. Lower the pajama pants or fold the gown out of the way; turn on a light so that the anus will be easily visualized. *(Provides for easier insertion of suppository into rectum.)*
4. Put on gloves and open lubricant, squeezing it onto a paper towel. Remove the foil wrapper from suppository and dip the point into the lubricant, being careful not to get it on your gloved fingers. *(A suppository will soften with prolonged handling and become more difficult to insert.)*
5. With the other hand, draw the top gluteal fold upward to expose the anus. Ask the patient to take a deep breath through the mouth as you place the suppository into the anus (directed toward the umbilicus) with a slight twisting motion. Gently push the suppository along the wall of the anus up into the rectum with your index finger as far as you can reach. Withdraw your finger and hold both buttocks tightly together for a few seconds while the patient breathes deeply until the urge to expel the suppository has passed. *(Positions suppository above the sphincter so it will not be immediately expelled.)*
6. Wipe excess lubricant from anus. Instruct the patient to try to hold the suppository in place for at least 20 minutes. *(The suppository will melt and deposit medication or stimulate the bowel within this time frame.)*
7. Remove the gloves and wrap them in the soiled paper towel; discard in the proper waste container. Perform hand hygiene. *(Reduces transfer of microorganisms.)*
8. Document administration of the suppository and the outcome of its use. *(Provides data on the success or failure of treatment.)*

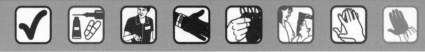

Skill 34.3 Administering Topical Skin Medications

 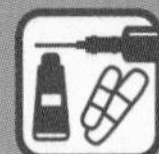 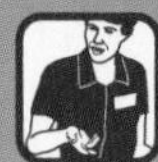 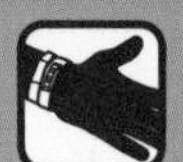 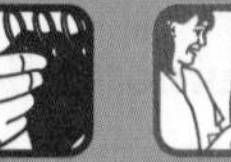 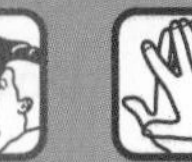 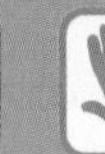 

Many types of topical medications can be applied to the skin. Lotions, ointments, creams, and patches are all used on the skin. The steps for medication administration must be followed when applying any topical medication.

Supplies

- Medication
- Disposable gloves
- Medication administration record (MAR or eMAR)
- Tongue blade
- Waste container

Review and carry out the Standard Steps in Appendix A.

ACTION *(RATIONALE)*

Assessment (Data Collection)

1. Determine that ordered medication is on hand and that patient is available for the application and has already bathed. *(Saves time; prevents medication from being washed off.)*
2. Assess for any side or adverse effects of the medication. *(If there is an adverse reaction, notify the provider before giving additional doses.)*

Planning

3. Gather any dressing materials that may be needed. *(Promotes work efficiency.)*
4. Plan sufficient time to perform the application without interruption. *(Dressings and large areas require more time.)*

Implementation

5. Check the medication against the MAR or eMAR twice, following the Six Rights of medication administration. *(Ensures giving the right drug in the right dose and applying it on the right location.)*
6. Identify the patient by checking the identification band with the MAR (and using the bar code scanner if using eMAR). Ask the patient to state her name. *(Ensures the right patient receives the medication.)*
7. Perform hand hygiene and don gloves. *(Gloves protect you from absorbing medication through the hands. For example, nitroglycerin ointment could give you a headache if it gets on your hands.)*

To Apply Lotion

8. Place the medication bottle and supply of gauze dressings or cotton balls on a convenient working surface. Shake the bottle well; perform the third drug check with the MAR or eMAR; remove the cap and place it upside down on the working surface. *(Third check of the drug helps to prevent medication error.)*
9. Pick up a gauze dressing or cotton ball. With the bottle in your nondominant hand with the label facing upward, carefully pour the lotion onto the applicator. Catch excess solution in a basin, paper wrapper, or waste container. *(Prevents soiling the label if some of the medicine drips down the side of the bottle while pouring. Applying the lotion to the gauze or cotton ball prevents spills.)*
10. Apply the lotion to the affected area by patting it on lightly. Do not rub. Repeat steps 9 and 10 until the area is covered, using a new applicator each time. Observe the skin for change in color, swelling, rash, and so on. *(Rubbing makes pruritus [itching] worse. Friction irritates lesions.)*
11. Discard the gauze or cotton balls in the designated container; remove gloves and replace the cap on the lotion. *(Disposes of potentially infectious waste; preserves the medication.)*

To Apply Cream or Ointment

12. Apply the medication with a gloved finger or tongue blade to dry skin. Apply a thin film in the direction of hair growth. *(A tongue blade spreads an even layer of ointment.)*
13. Apply a dressing if ordered. *(A dressing helps keep the cream or ointment on the skin.)*

To Apply Antianginal Ointment

14. Measure out the correct amount of ointment on a paper measuring guide. *(The dose must be exact.)*

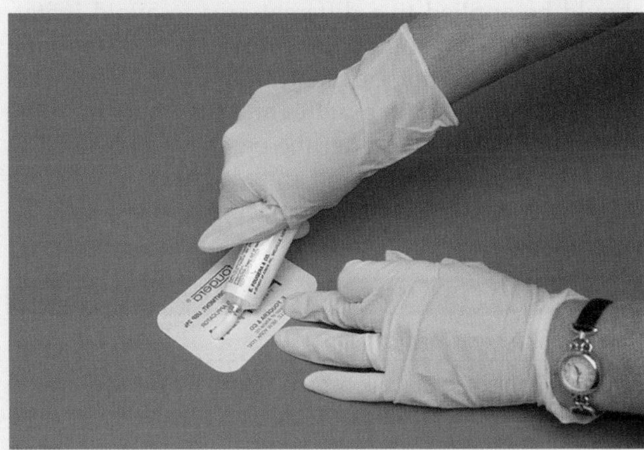

Step 14

15. Wash off any remaining ointment from a previous application. *(Remaining ointment would increase the dose the patient is receiving.)*
16. Gently apply the paper to the patient's skin, distributing the ointment over about a 2-inch area, but not rubbing it into the skin. Rotate the site with each application; use the chest and upper arms to apply over as hairless an area as possible. Tape the paper in place around the edges, or place a piece of plastic wrap over the paper and tape it into place. *(Medication slowly disperses into the skin and bloodstream. Hair may prevent contact of the ointment with the skin, decreasing absorption. Taping and/or covering the paper with plastic wrap protects patient's clothing.)*
17. Remove gloves and perform hand hygiene; return medication to the storage area. *(Reduces transfer of microorganisms; prepares medication for the next use.)*

Evaluation

18. Evaluate the skin for tolerance of the medication; assess for adverse effects. Assess for systemic therapeutic effect of antianginal ointment. *(If ineffective or adverse effects occur, consult the provider.)*

Documentation

19. Document the medication dose on the MAR or eMAR. Document the condition of the skin in the patient's medical record. *(Data about skin are compared with baseline.)*

Documentation Example

Old nitroglycerin ointment removed from right anterior chest. Skin cleansed. No redness or irritation noted. Patient advised that sites should be rotated and condition of the skin should be noted at each medication application change. (Nurse's time-stamped electronic signature)

Critical Thinking Questions

1. Why is it important to check the previous skin site where the medication patch was applied?
2. If the chest is covered with hair, where else can you apply the paste? Why should the previous area of application be wiped clean before applying the paste to a new spot?

Transdermal (through the skin) medications are supplied in a sustained-release patch that is applied to clean, dry, hairless skin and left in place, or as a paste that is spread on a small area of skin. The drug is slowly absorbed through the skin and into the bloodstream. Examples of drugs that are available in skin patch form include nitroglycerin to dilate coronary arteries; scopolamine to relieve motion sickness; nicotine to assist in smoking cessation; and fentanyl, an opioid analgesic, for severe chronic pain. Skin patches should be applied to areas where there is adequate circulation, such as the chest, shoulders, or upper arm. Scopolamine patches are placed behind the ear. Each new patch should be applied to a different area to avoid irritating the skin. Hair should be removed before applying a patch. The effect of the medication from a skin patch will begin in about 30 minutes and may remain in the system for 30 minutes after the patch is removed. The patch should be dated and initialed so it is evident when it was applied. Before placing a new patch, be sure the old one has been removed.

Safety Alert

Dangers of Topical Medications

Because topical medications are applied externally, many people do not view them as "medicine"; however, this can be a deadly mistake. Serious adverse reactions and even deaths have been reported following topical medication administration. Chemical burns have occurred following use of products containing menthol, methyl salicylate, or capsaicin. One 17-year-old cross-country runner died following using too much cream containing methyl salicylate for muscle pain, which was absorbed systemically. Topical anesthetics used before cosmetic procedures have also resulted in patients dying (Cohen, 2013). Topical steroids also come in a variety of strengths; be vigilant and carefully check the dosage before you apply the medication.

Assignment Considerations

COORDINATING HYGIENIC CARE AND TOPICAL MEDICATION ADMINISTRATION

When your patient must receive a topical medication such as ointment or a transdermal patch, try to coordinate with the unlicensed assistive personnel (UAP) so that showering or bathing does not interfere with the medication absorption. Remove the old patch, assess the area, and then have the UAP assist the patient with showering or bathing before applying the new medication. If the new medication has been applied before hygiene, instruct the UAP to cover the area with a plastic protector.

Nitroglycerin is also dispensed as a paste. It is applied to the skin, but not rubbed in. A ribbon of the ointment in the amount prescribed is applied to the measuring applicator, and the paper is folded to distribute the paste or a wooden applicator is used to spread the paste over a 2¼- × 3½-inch (5.6- × 8.8-cm) area of the paper. The paper is placed paste side down on a clean, hairless area of skin and taped into place. Be sure to write the date and time on the paper.

For patients administering this medication at home, instruct them to cover the applicator with a piece of plastic kitchen wrap to prevent the ointment from staining their clothes. When one applicator is removed, cleanse the skin and apply the next applicator in a different, clean area.

Administering Medications via Feeding Tube

Many oral medications can be given through a feeding tube. It is best to use liquid medications to prevent clogging of the feeding tube, but not all medications are available in liquid form. The nurse may crush tablets or pills, open a capsule and remove the contents, or aspirate liquid from a capsule. The contents are then dissolved in water and administered through the feeding tube. **Medications that should not be crushed and administered through the tube are sublingual or buccal, enteric coated, sustained-release, or potentially carcinogenic** (e.g., antineoplastic) **products**. Be sure to check with the pharmacy before crushing any medications. For a small bore tube, medications must be well dissolved in the liquid before administration. Do not mix the medication with a tube feeding because many things can interrupt delivery of the entire dose of medication (Skill 34.4).

Skill 34.4 Administering Medications Through a Feeding Tube

 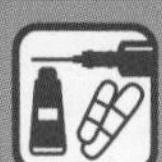 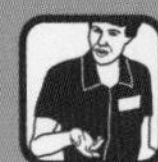  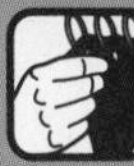 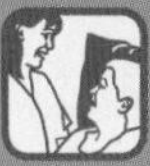  

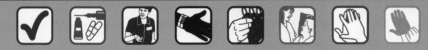

When the patient cannot take anything by mouth but has a feeding tube in place, oral medications can be administered through the tube. The medication dose must be followed by more water to irrigate the tube so that it does not clog. Each medication is mixed with water individually; medications are not combined, to prevent clumping. Seek help if the patient is a child or infant, is on fluid restriction, has multiple medications, or is having problems with gastric residual; the volume of water for mixing medications or flushing the tube may have to be adapted to meet these conditions.

Supplies

- Medicine cup
- Pill crusher
- Warm water
- Syringe and needle
- Large irrigation syringe
- Disposable gloves
- Medication administration record (MAR or eMAR)
- Medication(s)

Review and carry out the Standard Steps in Appendix A.

ACTION *(RATIONALE)*

Assessment (Data Collection)

1. Check the order and assess for allergies and adverse effects. Check the medications with the MAR or eMAR, performing two checks before preparing each medication and one check after preparing each one. Check that crushing tablets or opening capsules is acceptable for prescribed medications. *(Follows the principles of the Six Rights of medication administration. If medication cannot be crushed or if capsules cannot be opened, notify the provider so that the form can be changed to liquid.)*
2. Assess for patency and the position of feeding tube. *(Follow the correct procedure for verifying placement and patency of the feeding tube [see Chapter 27].)*

Planning

3. Verify that needed supplies are on hand. Fill a container with warm water. *(Warm water works better than cold to dissolve medications.)*
4. Perform hand hygiene. *(Medicines are prepared with aseptic technique.)*
5. Crush each medication that comes in a tablet, if it can safely be crushed and administered. If medication is a liquid in a gel capsule, the liquid may be aspirated with a syringe and needle. For capsules containing powder, open the capsule and pour the powder into a medicine cup. *(Medications must be dissolved or clogging will occur.)*

Implementation

6. Mix each medication with 30 mL of warm water. Gelatin capsules may be dissolved by dropping the capsule into warm water and allowing it to sit for 15 minutes. *(If medications clog the tube, the tube may have to be replaced.)*
7. Correctly identify the patient by checking the identification band with the name and hospital number on the MAR or eMAR. Ask the patient to state his name. Scan the patient's wristband if using bar code scanning. *(Prevents giving a medication to the wrong patient.)*
8. Place the patient in a high Fowler position, unless contraindicated. *(Gravity helps medication pass through the tube. Elevating the head at least 30-degrees helps prevent aspiration.)*
9. Put on gloves and attach the irrigation syringe to the tube while keeping the tube pinched off. *(Readies the syringe to receive the water and medication. Prevents air from entering tube.)*

10. Firmly hold the tube where it connects with the syringe and flush the tube with 30 mL of water. Next, add the dissolved medication just as the water is about to finish entering the tube. If necessary, apply gentle pressure with the syringe plunger or bulb to instill the liquid. *(Syringe can disconnect when the plunger is engaged, and fluid will spill onto bed linens. Water flushes tube feeding from the tube and decreases viscosity of fluid within the tube. Adding the medication before the syringe is empty prevents air from entering tube. Pressure may be needed to initiate the flow.)*

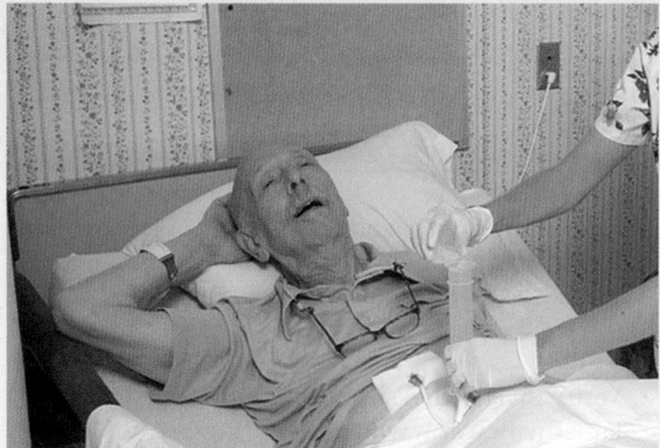

Step **10**

11. Follow the first medication with at least 15 to 30 mL of water before administering the next one. Add the next medication each time before the syringe is empty. *(Ensures the various medications do not interact in tube and clog it. Prevents air from entering tube.)*
12. Follow the last medication with 30 to 60 mL of water. Pinch off the tube as the syringe empties. *(Water flushes the tube of all medication and ensures patency of tube. Pinching off the tube prevents air from entering tube.)*

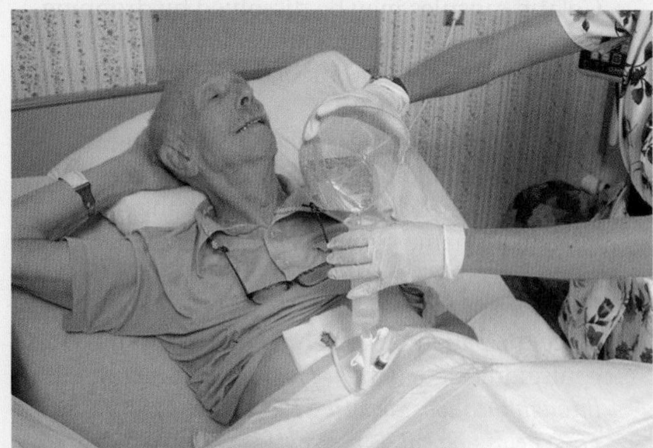

Step **12**

13. Clamp or plug the tube for 30 minutes before reconnecting a decompression tube to suction. For a feeding tube, clamp it only if the medications cannot be mixed with food. Otherwise, the tube may be reconnected to the tube feeding. If tube feedings are intermittent, the tube is simply left clamped. *(Prevents suctioning out the medication before it is absorbed. Prevents drug and food interactions. Reinitiates tube feeding.)*

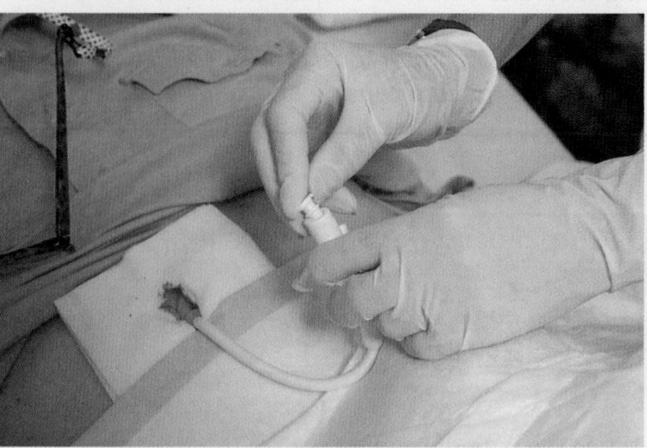

Step **13**

14. Leave the head of the bed elevated for at least 30 minutes, preferably for 60 minutes. *(Decreases risk of aspiration.)*
15. Clean up equipment, remove gloves, and perform hand hygiene. *(Reduces transfer of microorganisms.)*

Evaluation

16. Evaluate patency of tube by visualizing the free flow of liquid into it. *(If liquid does not flow smoothly, the tube may be becoming clogged and may require further irrigation.)*
17. Assess for adverse effects of the medication(s). *(If adverse effects occur, notify the provider.)*
18. Evaluate for abdominal distention or nausea. *(Medications may irritate the stomach; if so, consult the provider.)*

Documentation

19. Document the doses given on the MAR or eMAR. *(The right documentation is essential for continuity of care.)*
20. Enter the amount of fluid given on the intake portion of the intake and output sheet or on the appropriate computer screen. *(Tracks the patient's intake.)*
21. Document any problems encountered and corrective actions. *(When a problem is identified, always document steps that were taken to address or correct the problem.)*

? Critical Thinking Questions

1. Your patient has a feeding tube and is to receive an enteric coated medication. What should you do?
2. What would you do if the tube becomes clogged and you cannot get it to clear with water irrigation?

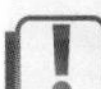 Clinical Cues

Potassium crystals may look small, but they do not dissolve readily and should not be administered through small bore feeding tubes because the crystals will clog the tube.

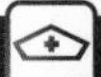 Safety Alert

Preventing Aspiration

Evidence-based practice to prevent aspiration includes checking the placement of the feeding tube, elevating the head of the bed, and allowing the patient to remain in an upright position for at least 30 minutes after instilling medications and fluids through a nasogastric tube (American Association of Critical Care Nurses, 2011).

Clinical Cues

Although the "beads" inside a spansule appear small, they can readily clog a small bore feeding tube. Generally, these beads are designed for sustained release and should not be crushed or diluted; therefore, the spansule should not be opened. If your patient has a feeding tube and needs a sustained-release medication, consult with the pharmacist and the primary care provider for a possible alternative form or dosing options.

◆ EVALUATION

Evaluate for therapeutic effectiveness or signs of adverse effects before administration of the next dose. Sometimes signs and symptoms do not appear until after the prescription has been finished. Evaluation statements might be as follows:

- Experienced nausea within 30 minutes of taking antibiotic.
- Refused antihistamine; itching has subsided.
- White blood cell count is 7000/mm^3; temperature 99°F (37.2°C); states, "I feel better."
- Red rash on chest possibly from antibiotic; primary care provider notified.
- Verbalizes that she will take antihypertensive even if she feels well.

Sample evaluation statements related to expected outcomes stated earlier in the chapter include:

- Pain is relieved for 3½ hours by analgesic.
- Blood pressure 120/80 to 130/80 mm Hg while patient is taking antihypertensive medication.
- Heart rate regular and 70 to 85/min while patient is taking antiarrhythmic medication.
- Wound culture negative after 5 days of antibiotic therapy.
- No nausea when antiemetic taken 30 minutes before eating a meal.
- Patient verbalizes medication "controls my blood pressure."

 Think Critically

What would you do if your patient had been receiving an antibiotic for 6 days, but all your evaluation data indicated that the patient's condition had not improved?

 Life-Span Considerations

Older Adults

Older adults who see more than one provider sometimes have the same drug prescription with two different trade-name drugs. They then end up taking twice as much of the drug as they should be taking and suffer adverse effects or toxicity. Always ask to check all of the patient's prescription bottles; this contributes to the evidence-based process of medication reconciliation (Siu, 2015).

Documentation

Documentation of medication administration is largely done on the eMAR. PRN medications, one-time doses, and preoperative medications may also be documented in the nurse's notes (according to agency policy). Data to be documented include:

- Medication name, dosage, route, and time administered.
- Blood pressure and pulse before administration of antihypertensives and beta-blocker drugs.
- The reason for administration of a PRN medication.
- Assessment data regarding side effects of the medication.
- Patient education regarding the medication (see Home Care Considerations).
- Evaluation data indicative of medication effectiveness.

MEDICATION ERRORS

Preventable medication errors are prominent cost and quality issues in the United States. It is estimated that they affect more than 7 million patients, contribute to 7000 deaths, and cost almost $21 billion in direct medical costs across all care settings annually (Lahue et al., 2012).

All medication errors must be reported as soon as they are discovered, regardless of whether or not the patient was harmed or injured. An incident or occurrence form is filled out for the medication error, and the agency policy for reporting medication errors is followed. After notifying the provider, carry out orders to safeguard the patient. The goal is to prevent harm to the patient from the error and to prevent similar errors from happening again. The nurse who discovers the error is the one to report it and fill out the report. Therefore, the nurse who made the error may not be the same nurse who reports it and fills out the occurrence form. In accordance with National Patient Safety Goals, health facilities and all health care workers should support efforts to track and monitor adverse events to improve health care delivery systems. The Joint Commission requires that a process called **root cause analysis** be used to investigate a sentinel event, which is an occurrence that causes a patient's death or serious injury. The purpose of the root cause analysis is to help a health care system understand why the event occurred and how to prevent it in the future (Agency for Healthcare Research and Quality, 2014).

 QSEN Considerations: Quality Improvement

Improving Processes

Performing a root cause analysis when medication errors occur is necessary to improve processes that are already in place. Even with safeguards provided by the use of technology, errors still occur.

 QSEN Considerations: Safety

Improving Practice

Engage in root cause analysis rather than blaming when errors or near misses occur.

 Home Care Considerations

Medication Administration for the Home Care Patient

- A 7-day medication planner container is helpful for the patient who is unreliable in taking medications or for one who has difficulty removing the tops from medication vials (Fig. 34.11). The patient can easily see whether a medication has been taken. A friend or neighbor can be enlisted to help set up the medications once a week if the patient lives alone.
- All medication must be kept out of reach of children. Even if children are not living in the home, this is a concern if any children visit.

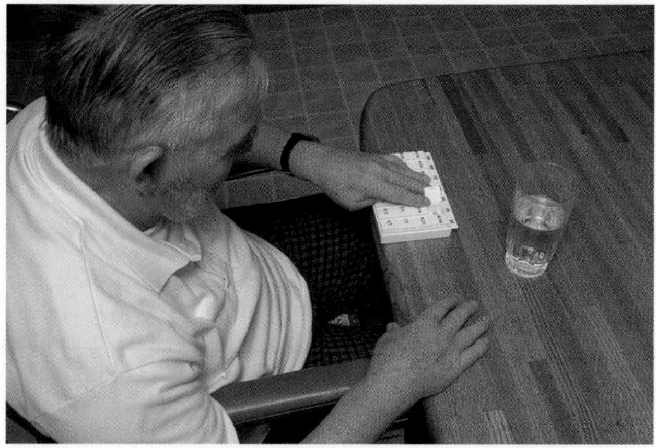

FIGURE 34.11 A 7-day medication planner helps the patient remember to take his medication.

- Check expiration dates for all prescription and nonprescription medications in the home. Discard expired medications.
- Assess use of over-the-counter medications when performing a medication history.
- Advise patients that if they are ordering prescriptions by mail, they need to inform the local pharmacist of these medications. The local pharmacy should have a complete list of everything the patient is taking so that duplicates, drug interactions, or overdosage can be prevented.
- If possible, assess the patient's (or caregiver's) preparation of the medication to observe the methods and techniques being used.

Get Ready for the NCLEX Examination!

Key Points

- All medications must be administered carefully following the Six Rights: the right drug, the right dose, the right route, the right time, and the right patient, with the right documentation.
- Medications should be administered only if the order is legally complete.
- You must give only the medication ordered, and it must be given by the route ordered.
- Most medications are given at routine scheduled times, one, two, three, or four times a day.
- PRN medications are given at ordered intervals if the patient needs or wants them; you may not give a lesser amount than that ordered.
- Stat orders are to be carried out immediately.
- Most narcotic orders are good for only 3 days and then must be renewed.
- All medication orders are stopped when a patient goes to surgery or undergoes general anesthesia for a procedure.
- Doses of medication administered are recorded on the eMAR after the patient takes the medication.
- Medication orders are transcribed onto the eMAR or the computer-generated nursing care plan.
- The unit-dose system is the most commonly used medication administration system. ADMs use this system on nursing units.
- The prescription system is used in pharmacies in the community and in outpatient clinics.
- Controlled substances are kept in double-locked cabinets or drawers and are carefully counted and recorded when administered. ADMs require accurate count of controlled substances; otherwise, a discrepancy exists in the computer.
- Checked each medication three times before administering it.
- Topical medications come in the form of lotions, ointments, creams, pastes, liniments, suppositories, drops, patches, and aerosols.
- Place sublingual medications under the tongue; place buccal medications in the inner cheek pocket. These medications should not be swallowed.
- Administer ophthalmic medications in one or both eyes using surgical asepsis.
- Transdermal medications are administered in a sustained-release patch. Remove the old patch before applying a new one.
- Irrigate feeding tubes with 15 to 30 mL of water between each medication and with 30 to 60 mL after the last medication is given. Clamp decompression tubes for 30 to 60 minutes before returning to suction after medications have been given.
- Report medication errors promptly and take action to ensure patient safety and to improve individual performance and agency policy.

Additional Learning Resources

SG Go to your Study Guide for additional learning activities to help you master this chapter content.

evolve Go to your Evolve website at http://evolve.elsevier.com/Williams/fundamental for additional online resources.

Suggested viewing: *Chasing Zero: Winning the War on Healthcare Harm* **(documentary featuring Dennis Quaid).** www.safetyleaders.org/pages/chasingZeroDocumentary.jsp

Review Questions for the NCLEX Examination

*Choose the **best** answer for each question.*

1. The primary care provider has just written several medication orders for several different patients. Which order has the highest priority?
   1. Hydrocodone and acetaminophen 5 mg PO q 4 to 6 hr PRN pain
   2. Lorazepam 2 mg IV bolus stat
   3. Gentamicin 200 mg IV q 8 hr
   4. Cefazolin 250 mg IVP on call to OR
2. A nursing student is administering medication to a patient via a nasogastric tube. The supervising nurse would intervene if the student:
   1. Crushes an ordered tablet and mixes it with 30 mL of warm water.
   2. Reconnects the tube to low suction as soon as the medication is administered.
   3. Flushes the tube with 50 mL of water after giving the last medication.
   4. Places the patient in a high Fowler position before administering medications.
3. The use of eMAR and barcoding in inpatient facilities has the following benefits *(Select all that apply)*:
   1. The potential to check the medications list against the patient's drug allergies.
   2. Eliminates medication errors as long as both systems are used correctly.
   3. Guarantees timely administration of medications by the nurse.
   4. Informs the nurse of drug-drug incompatibilities
   5. Performs a root cause analysis in the event of a medication error.
4. A nurse is instructing a patient on how to use an MDI. Which statements by the patient indicate that she understands the correct way to use the MDI? *(Select all that apply.)*
   1. "I should wait 1 minute between puffs."
   2. "I must close one nostril before depressing the canister."
   3. "I take a deep breath and hold it before placing the mouthpiece."
   4. "I need to inhale the medication and hold it for at least 10 seconds."
   5. "I should inhale quickly and deeply until the spacer makes a horn-like sound."
5. After preparation of a liquid medication, the patient refuses it. What is the most appropriate nursing action?
   1. Record the medication as "not taken" and discard it.
   2. Record the dose as taken because it must be charged.
   3. Insist the patient take the medication.
   4. Return the medication to the container.
6. A nurse is preparing to give a PRN pain medication when he realizes that, in the shift report, the day shift nurse said she gave it just before the end of her shift. It is not documented on the eMAR. Which action should the nurse take?
   1. Give the medication according to the eMAR.
   2. Call the day shift nurse's cell phone to ask for clarification.
   3. Ask the patient and family member if they remember if the day shift nurse gave the medication. If they say it wasn't given, go ahead and give it.
   4. Compare the eMAR with the CPOE. As long as they are both correct, it is okay to give the medication.
7. A surgery patient is to be discharged home and needs six doses of analgesic tablets for discomfort. What is the most appropriate nursing action?
   1. Dispense six tablets from the controlled-substance dispenser.
   2. Obtain a written prescription for the medication.
   3. Call the hospital pharmacist to fill the order.
   4. Ask the patient to call the primary care provider's office for the prescription.
8. A patient reports that he is taking an aspirin every day "to prevent heart attack," as well as enteric coated aspirin. Which nursing action is the priority?
   1. Tell him to stop taking either the aspirin or the enteric coated aspirin.
   2. Tell him to call his primary care provider or his pharmacist for clarification.
   3. Collect additional data about his health and medication history.
   4. Give him a pamphlet about enteric coated aspirin and explain drug-drug interactions.

Critical Thinking Activities

Read each clinical scenario and discuss the questions with your classmates.

Scenario A

You are in the medication room preparing medications for your patients when a nurse who is standing next to you is called to take a patient to another nursing unit. She shows you the medications she has prepared for one of her patients and asks you to please administer them so they will not be given late. What do you say? How can this situation be handled so that the patient receives needed medications on time?

Scenario B

Dan Hartford is receiving ampicillin for a respiratory tract infection. You notice that his face seems to have a red rash on it. When you question him, he states he has been itching a little across his chest and on his legs. As you are assessing his skin, you notice that his allergy band indicates that he has a penicillin allergy.

1. What, specifically, would you do?
2. If you had administered the ampicillin without noticing the penicillin allergy band, how would you feel?

Scenario C

Connie Simonelli is to receive 15 mL of magnesium hydroxide/aluminum hydroxide/simethicone (Mylanta II), a liquid antacid medication. How would you measure the correct amount of liquid medication?

Scenario D

You go into a room to give Florence Tolstoy her medication. When you ask to check her armband, you find that she does not have one on. What do you do? How can you properly identify the patient?

Scenario E

You enter Mr. King's room so that you can administer his morning medications: blood pressure medication, a daily vitamin, a pain medication, and a cholesterol medication. The nursing assistant had informed you that Mr. King's blood pressure was high, so you want to check the blood pressure yourself. However, Mr. King is angry and he tells you that he asked the night shift nurse for pain medication 2 hours ago. He is packing his clothes and says he is leaving the hospital. Discuss what you could do to help Mr. King at this point.

chapter 35

Administering Intradermal, Subcutaneous, and Intramuscular Injections

http://evolve.elsevier.com/Williams/fundamental

Objectives

Upon completing this chapter, you should be able to do the following:

Theory

1. Identify the principles for safe and effective administration of intradermal, subcutaneous, and intramuscular injections.
2. List the routes used for administering parenteral medications and the advantages and disadvantages of each route for pediatric, adult, and older adults.
3. Summarize the signs and symptoms of anaphylactic shock.

Clinical Practice

1. Using clinical judgment, choose the appropriate syringe and needle for the type of injection ordered.
2. Follow Standard Precautions when administering injections and disposing of used equipment.
3. Aseptically and accurately withdraw and measure the ordered dose of a medication from a vial or an ampule.
4. Demonstrate reconstitution of a medication from a powder.
5. Demonstrate the correct method for drawing up two types of medications, including insulin, in one syringe.
6. Use the Six Rights of medication administration, including checking for patient drug allergies.
7. Prepare and administer an intradermal injection, using the Six Rights and aseptic technique.
8. Correctly prepare and administer a subcutaneous injection with 100% accuracy.
9. Correctly prepare and administer an intramuscular injection with 100% accuracy.
10. Locate the appropriate site on a patient to give an intradermal, subcutaneous, or intramuscular injection by identifying correct anatomic landmarks.
11. Evaluate your documentation of injections after administration.

Skills & Steps

Key Terms

ampules (ĂM-pūlz, p. 678)
anaphylactic shock (ăn-ă-fī-LĂK-tĭk, p. 695)
bevel (BĔV-ĕl, p. 676)
bleb (BLĔB, p. 675)
core (KŌR, p. 680)
diluent (DĬL-ū-ĕnt, p. 681)
fibrosis (fī-BRŌ-sĭs, p. 683)
gauge (GĀJ, p. 675)
gluteal (GLŪ-tē-ăl, p. 691)
induration (ĭn-dŭr-Ā-shŭn, p. 686)
injection (ĭn-JĔK-shŭn, p. 674)
intradermal (ID) (ĭn-tră-DĔR-măl, p. 674)
intramuscular (IM) (ĭn-tră-MŬS-kū-lăr, p. 674)
lumen (LŪ-mĕn, p. 676)
parenteral (pĕ-RĔN-tĕr-ăl, p. 674)
solute (SŎL-ūt, p. 681)
subcutaneous (sŭb-kū-TĀ-nē-ĕs, p. 674)
tuberculin syringe (too-BĔR-kū-lĭn sĭ-RĬNJ, p. 675)
urticaria (ŭr-tĭ-KĀ-rē-ă, p. 695)
vials (VĪ-ălz, p. 678)
viscous (VĬS-kŭs, p. 677)
Z-track technique (p. 695)

Concepts Covered in This Chapter

- Anxiety
- Clinical judgment
- Evidence
- Safety
- Tissue integrity

Being asked to give an **injection** (forcing fluid into a part of the body) to another person makes many student nurses apprehensive. Giving an injection means the possibility of causing pain. Ways to decrease your anxiety include (1) focusing on the beneficial effects of medications, (2) developing dexterity in administering injections, and (3) practice, practice, practice in the skills lab! Learning the sites for injections is necessary for safety. **Intramuscular (IM)** (into the muscle), **subcutaneous** (beneath the skin layers), and **intradermal (ID)** (into the dermis) routes of administration are specific to the type and purpose of the medication.

PRINCIPLES OF PARENTERAL INJECTIONS

Parenteral (not delivered via the gastrointestinal tract) routes require the use of (1) a syringe and needle or (2) an intravenous (IV) catheter, to introduce medications into the body tissues or fluids. Medications that are given parenterally must be sterile, nonallergenic to the patient, and readily absorbable. Injections are given for the following purposes:

- When the patient cannot take medication by mouth.
- To hasten the action of the drug.
- When a continuous infusion of medication is necessary.
- When digestive juices would counteract the effects of the drug if given by the oral route.

Injectable drugs have a potential for rapid effects, so observe the following precautions:

- Ensure that the dose is accurate.
- Select the correct site to prevent damage to the tissue.
- Use sterile equipment and aseptic technique to prevent infection and sepsis.

The parenteral routes involve injecting medications into various layers of the skin or into veins. The skin's outer layer, or epidermis, is continually sloughing off dying cells. Below the epidermis is the dermis, or true skin, which contains hair follicles, sweat glands, sebaceous glands, blood vessels, and nerve endings (Fig. 35.1). Combined, these layers of the skin are 1 to 2 mm in thickness. Directly below the dermis is the subcutaneous, or hypodermal, layer of connective tissue (also known as superficial fascia), which contains varying amounts of fat cells. In some parts of the body, the subcutaneous layer may be more than 3 cm thick. It anchors the skin to the underlying organs. Although not often considered a part of the integument, the subcutaneous layer has considerable interconnectivity with the dermis. The skin has an extensive lymphatic and capillary system; the latter plays a major role in the absorption of medications. **The more vascular the tissue, the quicker the medication is absorbed.**

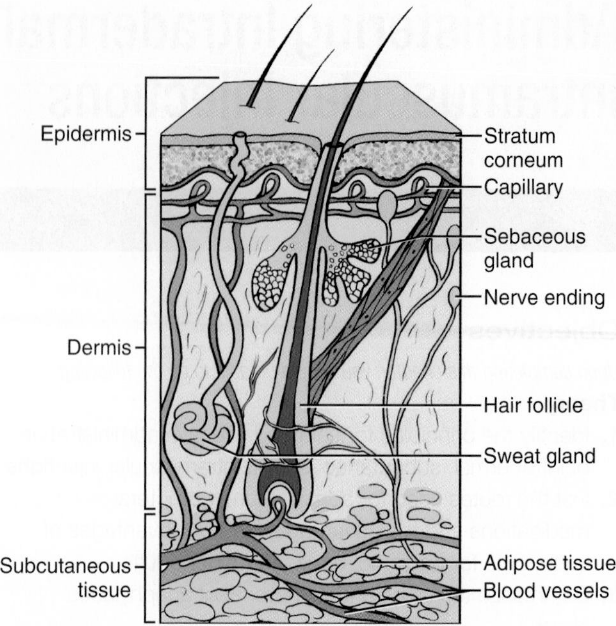

FIGURE 35.1 Structure of the skin.

Box 35.1 Principles for Safe, Effective Administration of Parenteral Medications

- Know the medication you will administer and observe for side effects and therapeutic action.
- Check for drug allergies before administration of injection.
- Use only sterile needles and syringes.
- Select the appropriate length of needle to deposit the medication in the proper tissue layer.
- Label the syringe with the patient's name, the name of the drug, and the dose.
- Obtain assistance as needed when the patient is a frightened child or an uncooperative adult.
- Rotate injection sites for patients receiving repeated injections by establishing a predetermined plan.
- Select an injection site that is relatively free of hair, lesions, inflammation, rashes, moles, and freckles.
- Select the injection site carefully to avoid major nerves, blood vessels, and underlying organs.

The wrong site or route may cause damage to a major nerve or blood vessel or even death. Contamination of the equipment or the medication may cause infection or abscess formation. Box 35.1 presents the principles that must be observed for safe and effective administration of parenteral medications.

ROUTES FOR PARENTERAL MEDICATION

The intradermal (ID), subcutaneous (Subcut.), intramuscular (IM), and intravascular (IV) routes are used for parenteral medication administration (Fig. 35.2). The IV route is presented in Chapter 36.

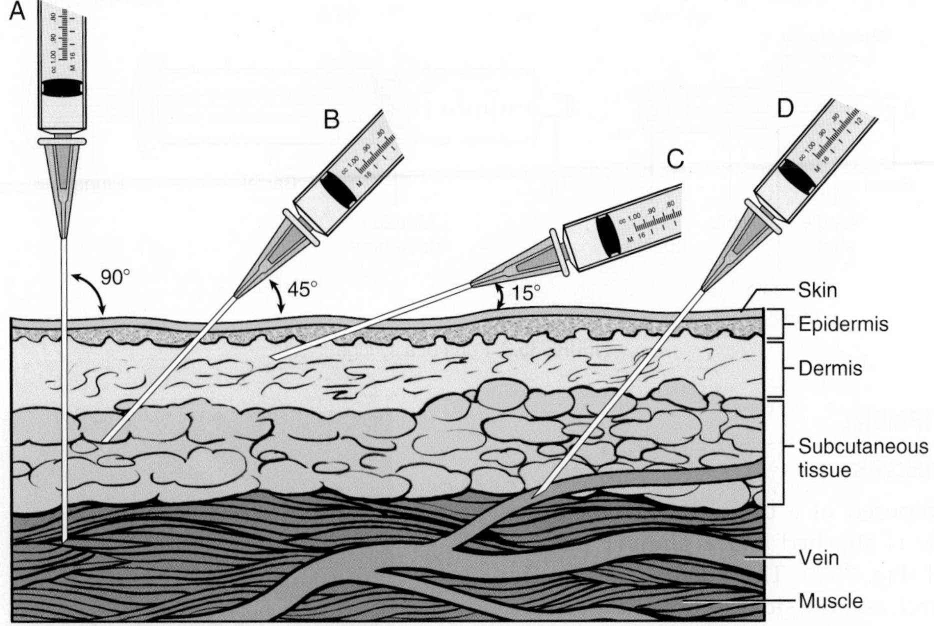

FIGURE 35.2 Injection routes. (A) Intramuscular. (B) Subcutaneous. (C) Intradermal. (D) Intravenous.

Cultural Considerations

Belief in Needles

Patients from certain cultures may believe that a medication is more effective if it is given as a "shot" rather than a pill or capsule.

INTRADERMAL ROUTE

The ID route, which deposits small amounts of drug solution into the dermal layer, is used extensively for skin testing, such as tuberculin testing, generally on the inner surface of the forearm. The **tuberculin syringe** (syringe with graduated measurements to 1 mL) is used to measure these small dosages. A fine 25-, 27-, or 29-**gauge** (scale of measurement) needle is used at a 5- to 15-degree angle of insertion. This 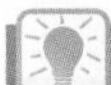 creates a pool of medication under the thin layer of skin that forms a **bleb** (bump; visible elevation of the epidermis).

SUBCUTANEOUS ROUTE

The subcutaneous route is used for injecting medication into the tissues below the dermal layer of the skin, usually in the upper portion of the upper outer arm, the anterior surface of the thigh, or the abdomen where there are no major vessels or nerves. Small amounts of solution (0.05 to 1.0 mL in volume; see agency policy) are injected subcutaneously with either a tuberculin or 3-mL syringe. A 27-gauge, ⅜- to ½-inch, or a 25-gauge, ⅝-inch needle is used. The needle is inserted at a 45- or 90-degree angle, depending on needle length and the patient's size.

Absorption time is slower than with an IM injection because of the lack of blood vessels in this area compared with muscle. These sites are used for medications that require slow absorption for sustained action.

INTRAMUSCULAR ROUTE

Using the IM route means medication is injected in the muscular layer. The absorption time for IM medications varies; aqueous solutions are absorbed more rapidly than those in an oil suspension are. **The most frequently used IM sites are the deltoid, ventrogluteal, vastus lateralis, and rectus femoris of the thigh.** The angle of injection is 90 degrees, and, depending on the patient's size, a needle from 1 to 3 inches in length is used.

QSEN Considerations: Evidence-Based Practice

Aspiration is not Evidence Based

Historically, nurses have aspirated (pulled back on the syringe plunger to create suction) to check for blood before injecting when administering intramuscular medications, to avoid injecting directly into a blood vessel. However, the evidence does not support this practice, with the exception of injections into the dorsogluteal muscle (Sisson, 2015). Because injection into the dorsogluteal is no longer recommended (because it is located near major blood vessels and nerves) nor described in this text, the step of aspirating for blood is no longer included in the skill "administering an intramuscular injection" (Skill 35.3).

Clinical Cues

Up to 3 mL can be safely injected in the ventrogluteal, vastus lateralis, and rectus femoris sites in most adult patients; however, the muscle mass of older or thin patients may only accommodate 2 mL in a single injection (Perry, et al, 2016). Larger amounts may be given in one injection in a large adult muscle in some instances (see agency policy).

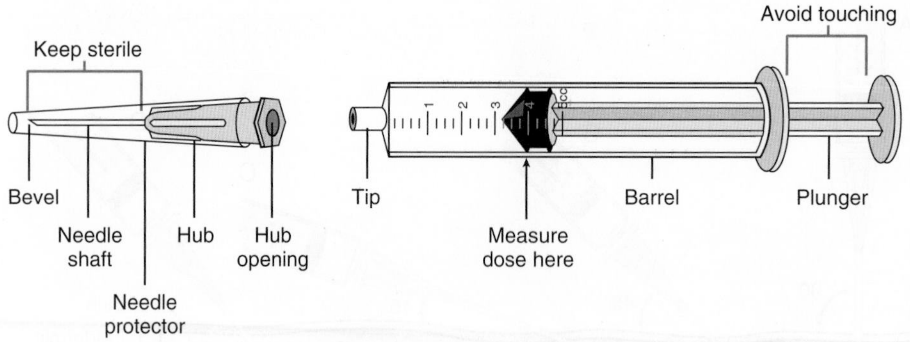

Avoid touching

Keep sterile

Bevel

Needle shaft

Hub

Hub opening

Needle protector

Tip

Measure dose here

Barrel

Plunger

FIGURE 35.3 Parts of a syringe.

INJECTION EQUIPMENT

TYPES OF SYRINGES

Syringes are composed of a barrel that has a tip to which the needle is attached and a plunger that fits inside the barrel (Fig. 35.3). **The needle, the tip, the inside of the barrel, and the sides of the plunger must be kept sterile.**

Disposable syringes are used almost exclusively in North America because they are convenient, safe, and economical (Fig. 35.4). The 3-mL syringe is popular because it is large enough for subcutaneous and most IM injections. The U-100 insulin syringe is calibrated to measure 100 units of insulin. For lower doses, the U-50 insulin syringe is calibrated for 50 units (Fig. 35.5). The insulin needle is part of the syringe and is not removable. The insulin syringe sometimes has a milliliter scale on it as well. Tuberculin syringes are 1 mL in size and are calibrated to measure drug doses as small as 0.01 mL (Fig. 35.6).

? Think Critically

You have to inject 3 mL of medication. What size of syringe will you select? State your rationale.

Clinical Cues

Small gauge syringes such as the tuberculin syringe and the insulin syringe are easily confused and misread. Carefully examine the medication order and the scale on the syringe to ensure that you are interpreting the order correctly and using the right syringe and the right scale.

Syringe tips are also a consideration. For example, a Luer-Lok tip would be the choice for an intramuscular injection because the locking mechanism prevents a sudden separation of the needle and syringe when pressure is applied to inject medication into the muscle mass. The non–Luer-Lok or slip tip is acceptable for an ID injection because little pressure is needed to inject the medications into the dermal layer.

A few injectable medications are supplied in the form of unit-dose cartridges. These require a special holder for the cartridge and needle, such as the Carpuject system, to administer the injection.

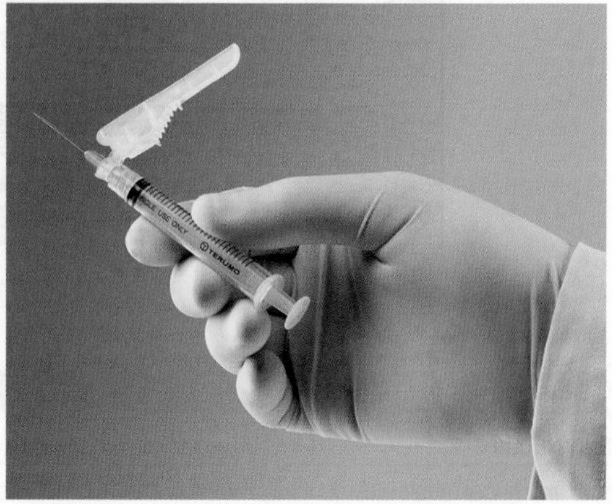

FIGURE 35.4 Disposable syringe. (Copyright 2012, Terumo Medical Corp., Somerset, NJ.)

MEASUREMENT SCALES

Each syringe is calibrated, and the measurements are marked on the barrel for accurate medication measurement. The syringe chosen for the injection must have a measurement scale that is appropriate for the required dose of medication. **The 3-mL syringe measures tenths of a milliliter (0.1 mL)** (Fig. 35.7). Although the 0.1-mL scale is accurate for tenths of a milliliter, it is not appropriate or accurate enough to measure doses in hundredths, such as 0.25 mL. A tuberculin syringe easily measures this amount; it is best to use a tuberculin syringe for such small doses.

NEEDLE GAUGE AND LENGTH

A needle is a metal tube through which liquid medication flows. It consists of a hub fitting onto the end of a syringe, a hollow shaft (also called a **cannula**), and a **bevel** (the slanted part of the needle tip) ending in a sharp point. The inner part of the cannula is the **lumen** (opening or interior diameter). Needles are generally disposable and are discarded **immediately** after use.

Needles are available in standard sizes measured in gauge from 13 to 30, although an agency may not buy all sizes; Figure 35.8 shows the most commonly used sizes. **The larger the number of the gauge, the smaller the needle.** Because an ID injection goes under the epidermis (the outer layer of skin), a 25-, 27-, or 29-gauge

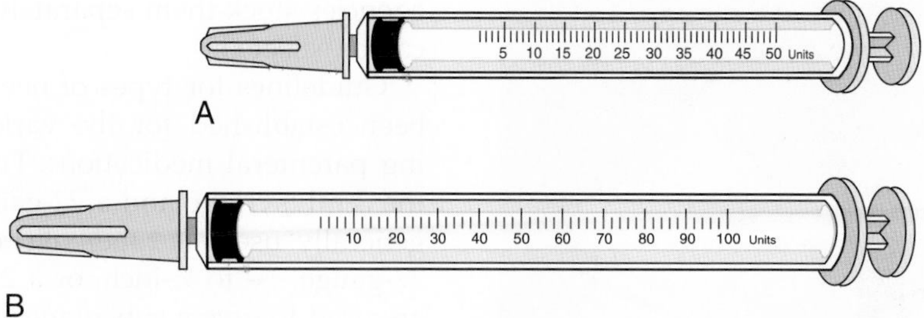

FIGURE 35.5 Insulin syringes. (A) A 50-unit syringe. (B) A 100-unit syringe.

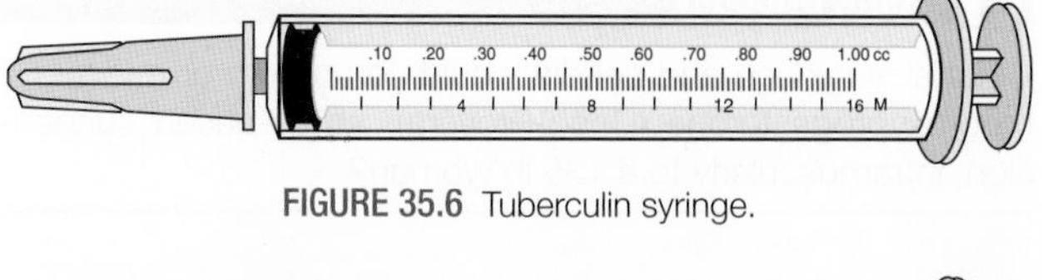

FIGURE 35.6 Tuberculin syringe.

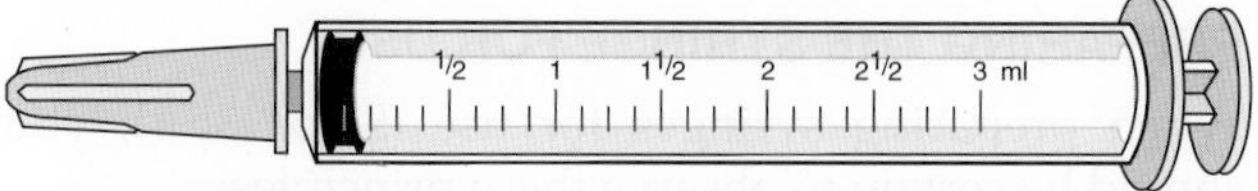

FIGURE 35.7 Measurement scale on a 3-mL syringe.

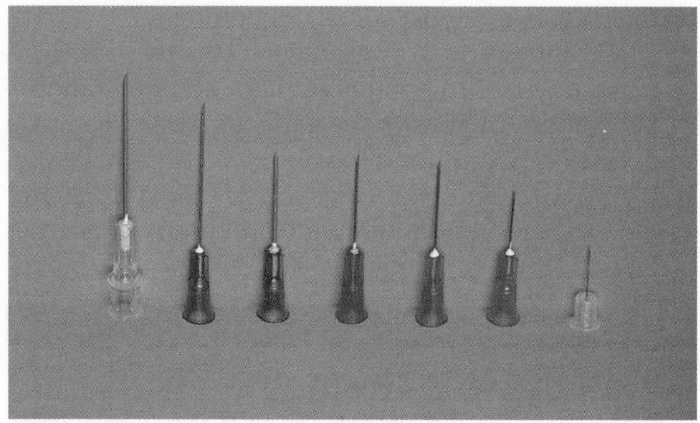

FIGURE 35.8 Various needle sizes. (Display is shown without protector covers for comparison of needle sizes.)

needle works best. The 25-gauge needle is strong enough to puncture the skin and reach below the dermis for subcutaneous injections. Heavier-duty 20-, 21-, 22-, and 23-gauge needles are needed to penetrate the large muscle layers when IM injections are given in those sites. The length of the needle is measured from its beveled tip to the junction of the shaft and the hub. Most often 1- or 1½-inch needles are used for adult parenteral injections. Adult IM injections frequently use 22- and 23-gauge needles, although 20- and 21-gauge needles are preferred for **viscous** (thick and sticky) solutions or medications in oil suspensions.

Clinical Cues

An obese person requires a longer needle than one who is normal weight; a very thin person requires a shorter needle. Health professionals may use shorter needles in the mistaken belief that is it kinder to the patient; however, too short of a needle will deposit the medication into the fat or subcutaneous tissue. This can also occur if the needle is not fully advanced into the skin (Hopkins & Arias, 2013).

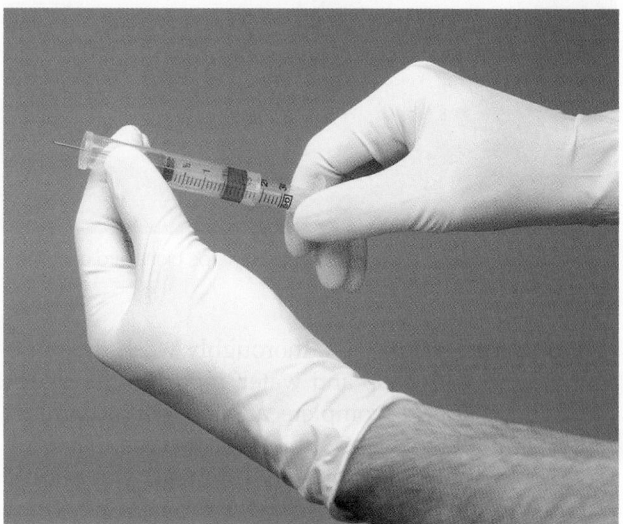

FIGURE 35.9 Needle with a protective sheath.

PREVENTING NEEDLE STICKS

A needle stick occurs any time a needle accidentally pricks the skin. The danger of the spread of HIV, hepatitis B virus, and hepatitis C virus has created much concern about needle safety. A variety of safety devices have been developed to dispose of used needles safely. A protective cover may snap over the needle, or activation of the safety device may cause the needle to retract into a protective plastic sheath (Fig. 35.9). The Occupational Safety and Health Administration (OSHA) requires that safety equipment be used in most situations in all states. **Always use the needleless option to draw up medications whenever it is available.** Learning to use these safety features should precede preparing medications or practicing injections.

If you must use a needle to draw up potentially irritating medications, the needle is then changed to a new safety needle before injection to eliminate the possibility of depositing medication in surface tissue.

Clinical Cues

If you must recap a **CLEAN** needle, use a one-hand scoop technique. Place the needle cap on a flat, firm surface, preferably with the closed end of the needle cover against an object. With one hand holding the syringe barrel, slide the needle into the needle cap. Secure the cap by pushing it against a vertical surface (e.g., the drawer front on the bedside table, the wall, or a door)—never the other hand.

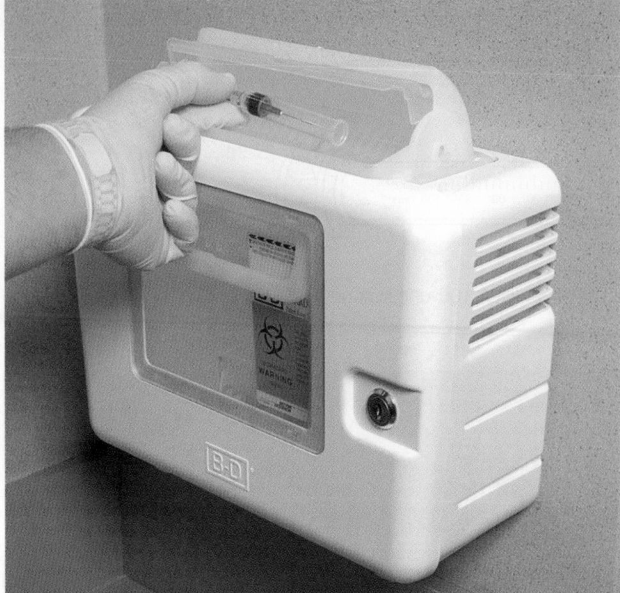

FIGURE 35.10 Drop a used syringe into a sharps biohazard container immediately.

If a needle stick occurs, thoroughly wash the puncture wound with soap and water, report to the charge nurse immediately, complete an incident/occurrence report, and follow agency policy for treatment and follow-up. **In the immediate environment, you should attempt to develop a conscious awareness of where contaminated needles might be left or carried by other health care workers to prevent needle stick injuries.**

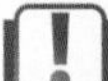 Safety Alert

Reducing Needle Stick Injuries

Recapping is not recommended for used needles. All syringes and needles are **dropped, not pushed,** into a sharps container immediately after use (Fig. 35.10). If a sharps container is not available in each patient's room, notify the nurse manager.

 Assignment Considerations

Preventing Needle Sticks Among Health Care Team Members

If you ask the unlicensed assistive personnel (UAP) to clean up or remove equipment after the health care provider has performed a procedure, remind her to look for sharps first rather than picking up used equipment in a bundle. Each person who uses sharps is responsible for placing them in the appropriate container; however, the UAP should be advised to protect herself from an accidental needle stick if a sharp has been overlooked and left on the equipment tray.

SYRINGE AND NEEDLE SELECTION

In preparing to give an injection, the first step is to select the appropriate size and type of needle and syringe for the medication to be given and for the patient's age and size. Today the needle and syringe are usually supplied in a preassembled safety unit, although some agencies stock them separately, and the desired types can be selected.

Guidelines for types of needles and syringes have been established for the various methods of injecting parenteral medications. For giving IM injections, the 3-mL syringe and a 22-gauge, 1½-inch needle are generally used. A tuberculin or 3-mL syringe and a 27-gauge, ⅜- to ½-inch, or a 25-gauge, ⅝-inch needle are used to give a subcutaneous injection. These sizes are modified as necessary to accommodate different medications, doses, and patient needs.

? Think Critically

What size syringe and needle would you use to give 2 mL of medroxyprogesterone (Depo-Provera), an oil-based suspension, intramuscularly to a 135 lb woman?

PREPARING THE SYRINGE FOR USE

When preparing syringes for use (Steps 35.1), you should be certain to observe these principles:

- Use aseptic technique in handling the syringe and needle. Protect the surfaces that must remain sterile: the needle, tip, inner barrel, and plunger.
- Discard the syringe or needle if it becomes contaminated during drug preparation for administration.
- Label the syringe with the patient's name, the name of the medication, and the dose.
- Do not prepare the medication in one syringe and then transfer the solution into another syringe (McNew, 2013).

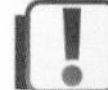 Safety Alert

Label Syringes and Other Containers

In accordance with the National Patient Safety Goals, when medication is removed from the original container and placed in a syringe or medication cup, it should be clearly labeled. Use a piece of tape or obtain a label stamped with the patient's name and identification number; write the name of the drug and the dosage on it; and attach it to the syringe or medication cup to ensure right drug, right dose, and right patient.

PARENTERAL SOLUTIONS

Medications for injection are dispensed in various kinds of units: glass **ampules** (all-glass containers containing medication) containing a single dose, single-dose **vials** (small bottles), mix-o-vials, and multiple-dose vials (Fig. 35.11). The mix-o-vial contains powder in the base and solution in the top, which are mixed together for use. The unit-dose cartridge consists of a vial with an attached needle for use with the Carpuject holder (Fig. 35.12). Parenteral medications must be kept sterile.

USING A MEDICATION AMPULE

Ampules are made entirely of glass or polyurethane and contain a single standard dose of the medication.

Steps 35.1 Preparing a Syringe for Use

Disposable syringes are packaged in a paper wrapper or are encased in plastic to protect their sterility. The Carpuject cartridge is inserted and fastened into a syringe mechanism.

ACTION *(RATIONALE)*

Removing Protective Wrapping

1. Perform hand hygiene and select the desired size and type of syringe. *(Maintains asepsis; ensures that appropriate syringe will be used.)*
2. For a paper-wrapped syringe, peel open the wrapper while maintaining asepsis. *(The inside of syringe and needle must be kept sterile.)*
3. For a rigid plastic casing, twist the plastic cap counterclockwise and remove it; slide the cover down off the barrel of the syringe. When ready, remove the protective cover from the needle by pulling it straight off. *(The barrel of the syringe and the protected needle slip out of the top of the plastic sheath.)*
4. Pull out the plunger on the holder mechanism. Insert the cartridge into the holder from the side, sliding the needle through the bottom opening. *(Positions the cartridge in the holder mechanism.)*
5. Twist the cartridge to lock it at the needle end. *(Stabilizes the cartridge in the holder mechanism.)*
6. Place the end of the plunger against the screw end of the cartridge and turn the plunger clockwise until fastened. *(Fastens the plunger to the cartridge for further stabilization.)*
7. Remove unwanted excess medication or air from the unit. *(The order may not call for a full dose of the medication; excess air may be present in the cartridge.)*

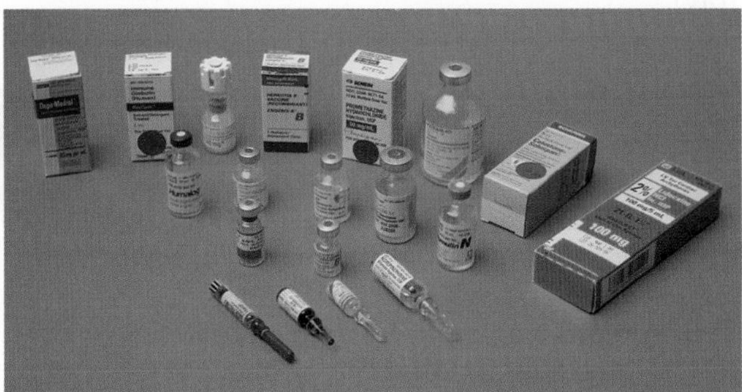

FIGURE 35.11 Containers of parenteral medication.

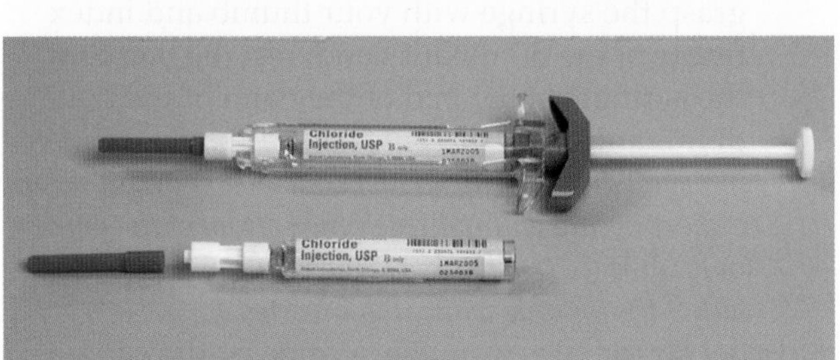

FIGURE 35.12 Carpuject cartridge and holder.

Most ampules are prescored on the neck so that the glass will break more evenly with slight pressure at that portion.

Before opening an ampule, remove the medication from the neck or stem of the ampule, or some will be wasted when the ampule is opened. To move the medication, tap or flick the stem several times with a finger to free the trapped solution (Fig. 35.13).

Clinical Cues

Before breaking open the ampule, you should wrap the neck with the rubber ampule guard, an alcohol swab, or a gauze pad to avoid accidental cuts. Press the thumbs outward against the neck so the ampule will break outward away from you.

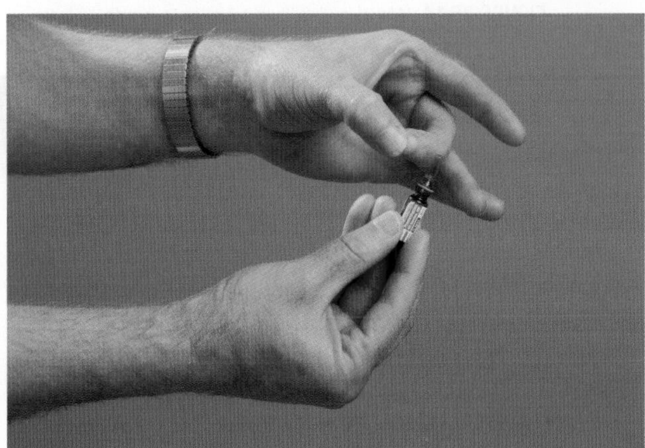

FIGURE 35.13 Moving fluid from the neck of the ampule.

Use a filter needle to withdraw medication from an ampule because small particles of glass may fall into the medication when the ampule neck is removed (Fig. 35.14). The open ampule may be stabilized on a flat surface for withdrawal of the drug when a long needle is used. If a short needle is used, the ampule may be inverted to withdraw the correct dose. The tip must be beneath the surface of the solution to withdraw it. Do not inject air into the ampule, or the medication will bubble up and out of the ampule (Steps 35.2).

Clinical Cues

Medication in an ampule is packaged in a specific amount per milliliter; however, usually the ampule contains more than the total amount indicated in the event of spillage. **Carefully verify that the exact amount ordered is in the syringe before giving the injection.**

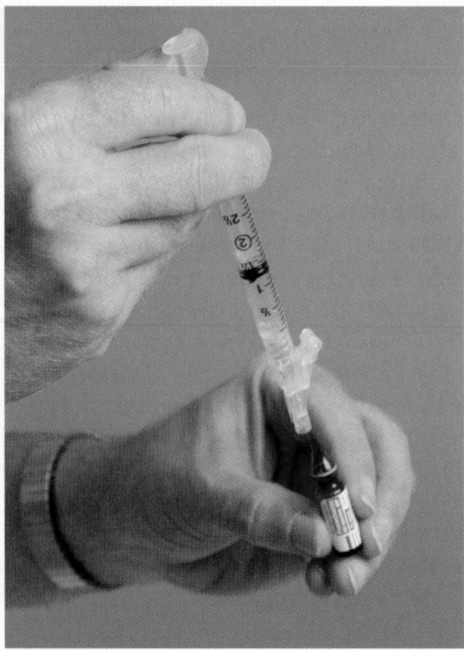

FIGURE 35.14 Withdrawing fluid from an ampule.

USING A MEDICATION VIAL

A vial is a small bottle with a rubber stopper attached with a metal band. A vial may contain one or more doses of medication. Single-dose vials are small, usually 1 or 2 mL; multiple-dose vials are 5, 10, 20, or 30 mL or larger. Use of single-dose vials is always preferred when possible (Boyle, 2014). The desired amount of medication is removed by inserting a sterile needleless device or the needle of a syringe through the rubber stopper into the liquid with the vial inverted and drawing up the solution (Fig. 35.15).

If you are using a needle, take care to avoid coring the stopper by using a slight lateral pressure to pierce the core and inserting the needle bevel up. The sharp edges of the needle can create a small **core** (circular cutout piece) that can be pushed into the bottle and become a source of contamination (Hanan & Durgin, 2015) (Steps 35.3). Do not put a medication vial into your pocket, and discard any vial that may have been contaminated (e.g., a vial that is left on a procedure tray).

Steps 35.2 Withdrawing Medication From an Ampule

Ampules contain a single dose. The glass ampule neck must be broken to extract the medication.

ACTION *(RATIONALE)*

1. After checking the medication order and performing any calculation necessary for the correct dose, perform hand hygiene. *(Checking and calculating dosage prevents medication error.)*
2. Dislodge any fluid from the stem of the ampule by tapping the stem or by holding the ampule upside down and then quickly inverting it. *(Fluid from the stem must be moved into the ampule to obtain the dose.)*
3. Break the neck of the ampule with an ampule breaker, or wrap the neck with gauze or an alcohol swab, place both your thumbs together at the neck, and apply outward pressure to snap the neck away from you. *(Breaking the neck outward prevents glass splinters from flying into the eyes or skin.)*
4. Remove the needle from the syringe and replace it with a sterile filter needle. Keep the regular needle sterile for later replacement on the syringe. *(Filter needle traps any glass particles and keeps them out of the syringe. The filter needle is replaced by the regular needle after medication is drawn up.)*
5. Place the needle into the solution without touching the neck of the ampule. Keeping the bevel of the needle below the surface of the solution, pull back on the syringe plunger with your dominant hand to the correct line on the measuring scale.
   a. Place the ampule on a flat surface, insert the needle into the ampule close to the bottom of the medication, and withdraw the desired dose of medication. *(This method requires a steady hand so as not to tip the ampule while drawing up the medication.)*
   b. Alternatively, hold the ampule between your thumb and middle or index finger of the nondominant hand and, with the needle inserted into the solution, invert the ampule while you grasp the syringe with your thumb and index finger of the dominant hand; rest the barrel of the syringe on the pad of the palm of the nondominant hand. *(Keeping the bevel in the solution prevents drawing up air. This method is useful when a short needle will not reach the bottom of the ampule. Surface tension keeps the solution from leaking out of the ampule while it is inverted.)*
6. Expel air bubbles from the syringe by drawing more air into the syringe to make a larger bubble; then, holding the syringe with the needle upright, tap with your finger to move the air bubble toward the needle, and push the plunger to expel the air. Stop when one drop of liquid appears in the bevel of the needle. Ascertain that the dose is correct. *(Air must be removed to measure the exact dose ordered.)*
7. Change back to the sterile needle that was removed from the syringe. *(Prevents glass particles caught in the filter needle from entering the patient.)*
8. Label the syringe with the patient's name, the name of the drug, and the dosage. *(When a medication is removed from the original container or vial, labeling the new container [e.g., syringe or medication cup] prevents accidentally giving the wrong drug to the wrong patient.)*

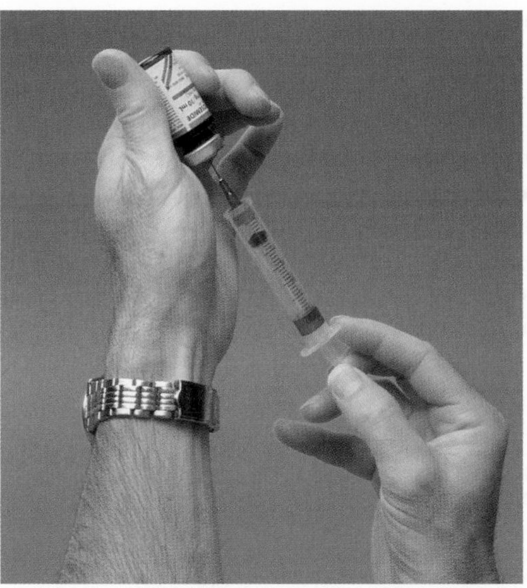

FIGURE 35.15 Drawing medication from a vial.

RECONSTITUTION OF A DRUG

Drugs that are unstable in solution are prepared in a powdered or solid form. The **solute** (solid material) in the vial is mixed with a **diluent** (specified fluid to dissolve the solute) before the drug is drawn up into a syringe. Sterile water and sterile normal saline are typical diluents. The label or the drug insert packaged with the vial provides instructions about the type and amount of diluent to use. **The solute must be thoroughly mixed with the diluent before use.** The label on the vial indicates the amount of medication per volume after correct dilution (e.g., 250 mg/mL).

Follow the directions that accompany the vial for storage of the medication after reconstitution.

COMPATIBILITY OF MEDICATIONS

Not all drugs are compatible with others when mixed together. The reaction of incompatibilities can range

Steps 35.3 Withdrawing Medication From a Vial

Medication may be supplied in a single-dose or a multiple-dose vial. When withdrawing from a multiple-dose vial and mixing drugs, be careful not to allow any other medication to enter the vial.

ACTION *(RATIONALE)*

1. After checking the medication with the order for the correct drug and dose, select an appropriate-size syringe and needle; perform hand hygiene. *(Ensures that you are preparing the correct dose of the drug ordered; maintains asepsis.)*
2. Remove the plastic tab covering the vial rubber stopper, and rub the stopper with an antiseptic swab. Discard the swab. *(This removes residue that may have condensed on the stopper during manufacture.)*
3. Pull the plunger of the syringe back to the exact mark on the barrel of the syringe for the prescribed amount of the medication. *(Air equal to the amount of medication to be drawn up is drawn into the syringe.)*
4. Place the vial on a flat countertop and hold the vial between your thumb and your index and third finger of your nondominant hand. Insert the needleless device (or needle) into the vial at a slight angle with lateral pressure. *(Inserting the needleless device into the vial at an angle with lateral pressure prevents coring of the stopper.)* (Note to student: A needle will work in this circumstance, but use of a needleless device is recommended whenever available.)
5. Keep the needle tip above the solution surface and push the plunger into the barrel to inject the air. *(The air is injected into the vial to prevent a vacuum in the vial, which may inhibit withdrawal of solution, especially in multiple-dose vials.)*
6. Invert the vial and, while holding it at eye level, pull the needleless device back so the tip is below the solution surface. Pull the plunger down until slightly more than the required amount of medication is in the syringe (see Fig. 35.15). Tap any air bubbles to the top near the needle and readjust the plunger, expelling air and excess medication, so that the exact amount of the dose is in the syringe. *(Keeping the bevel of the needleless device below the solution surface prevents air bubbles in the syringe. Expelling the air allows correct visualization of the dose in the syringe.)*
7. Verify the dose and remove the needleless device from the vial and replace it with the appropriate size sterile needle. *(Rechecking the calculation helps prevent medication errors.)*
8. Label the syringe with the patient's name, the name of the drug, and the dose. *(When a medication is removed from the original container or vial, labeling the new container [e.g., syringe or medication cup] prevents accidentally giving the wrong drug to the wrong patient.)*
9. For multiple-dose vials, label with the date, the time, and your initials after opening the vial; use agency protocol. Refrigerate the remainder of the vial if necessary. *(Open medication has a specific time that it will remain usable; the amount of time varies from one medication to another. Many medications need to be refrigerated after reconstitution or opening.)*

from color change, precipitation, and clouding to invisible chemical changes rendering the drug inactive.

When medications are compatible, as with different types of insulin, you inject an amount of air equal to the desired dose of each drug into their respective vials. This reduces the vacuum inside the multidose vial and makes it easier to withdraw the medication. Air is placed in the longer-acting insulin vial first (Fig. 35.16). After injecting air into the second vial, withdraw the desired dose. Insert the needle again into the first vial, into which air has already been injected, and withdraw the exact desired dose of this drug. If too much is drawn up, the contents of the syringe must be discarded, and the medications redrawn because, once the drugs are mixed in the syringe, there is no way to separate the drugs to discard the excess. When mixing medications in the same syringe, take care not to inject any of the medication already drawn up from the first vial into the second multidose vial (Steps 35.4).

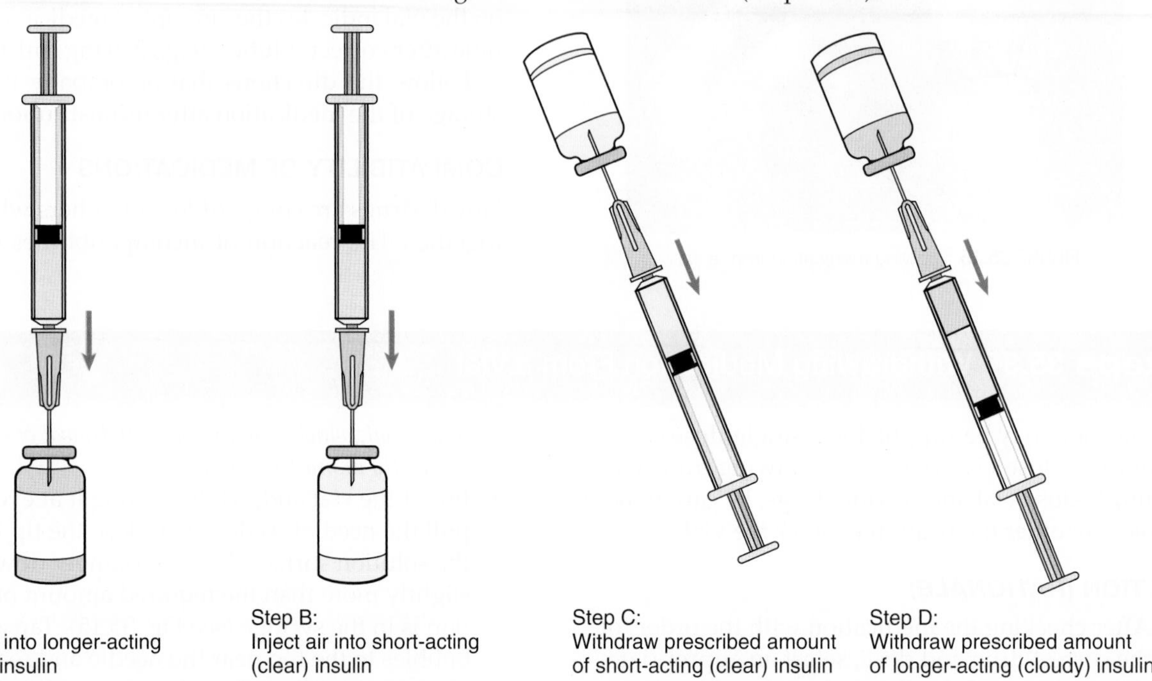
Step A:
Inject air into longer-acting (cloudy) insulin
Step B:
Inject air into short-acting (clear) insulin
Step C:
Withdraw prescribed amount of short-acting (clear) insulin
Step D:
Withdraw prescribed amount of longer-acting (cloudy) insulin

FIGURE 35.16 Mixing doses of insulin from multidose vials.

Steps 35.4 Combining Insulins

Often short-acting insulin is ordered to be mixed with longer-acting insulin. These steps are used to mix the two insulins. An insulin syringe is used to draw up the insulins. (Insulin syringes are usually packaged with a needle in place that cannot be detached.)

ACTION *(RATIONALE)*

1. Check expiration dates on both bottles of insulin. *(Outdated insulin is not reliable and should not be used.)*
2. Check for change in color, clumping, or granular appearance of insulin and discard if such has occurred. *(Insulin that has been contaminated or exposed to heat is no longer good.)*
3. To mix an insulin suspension, swirl the vial gently, rotate between palms. *(Mixes the insulin evenly without causing air bubbles, which would interfere with accurate dose.)*
4. Roll the vial of the long-acting (cloudy) insulin to distribute the insulin evenly in the suspension. *(Dosage will be inaccurate unless the insulin is evenly mixed.)*
5. Swab the tops of both vials of insulin with alcohol swabs. *(Cleans the top of the stopper, removing debris and microorganisms.)*
6. Use an insulin syringe calibrated in units. *(Primary care provider orders the insulin in units. Use of an insulin syringe facilitates measuring the exact dose.)*
7. Pull the plunger of the syringe, drawing in air, to the amount needed from the first bottle, the long-acting insulin. *(Prepares air to be injected into vial.)*
8. Insert the needle into the first vial with the long-acting insulin, and inject the air into the vial. Withdraw the needle. *(Air injected into the vial reduces the vacuum and makes it easier to withdraw the medication [see Fig. 35.16].)*
9. Pull the plunger of the syringe, drawing in air, to the amount of insulin needed from the second vial, the short-acting (clear) insulin. *(Prepares air to be injected into vial.)*
10. Insert the needle into the second vial with the short-acting insulin, and inject the air into the vial with the needle above the surface of the medication.

(Air injected into the vial prevents a vacuum, which will pull regular insulin into the long-acting insulin vial; makes it easier to withdraw medication.)

11. Invert the vial and, keeping the bevel of the needle beneath the surface of the insulin, withdraw the exact amount of short-acting insulin needed from this vial; tap out any air bubbles. Remove the needle. *(The bevel must be below the surface of the liquid to draw up the medication. Air bubbles interfere with measuring exact correct dose.)*
12. Keeping the plunger at the exact place, insert the needle into the first bottle with the long-acting insulin and withdraw exactly the amount ordered. Do not let any of the medication in the syringe enter the vial. *(Mixes the two insulins within the syringe in the exact amounts ordered. If fluid from the syringe enters the vial, the doses of both insulins will be incorrect, and the vial will be contaminated with the short-acting insulin.)*
13. Recap the needle, using the scoop technique, if you are not with the patient, and proceed to the patient to administer the insulin. *(Protects the needle sterility and protects others from needle sticks.)*

Clinical Cues

Occasionally the patient may need several injectable medications. If the medications can be combined, the patient will have to endure only one injection; however, before combining two or more drugs in a syringe, check with the pharmacist or consult a drug reference for compatibilities.

APPLICATION OF THE NURSING PROCESS

Administering an injection is considered an implementation of the nursing process; the other steps of the process are also followed.

ASSESSMENT (DATA COLLECTION)

Check the primary care provider's order for the medication. Note the patient's name, generic and trade medication name, dosage, route, and time. Verify the identity of the patient who is to receive the injection, using two identifiers, to prevent medication errors and harm to the patient. Check the medical record for indication of drug allergies, and question the patient about allergies each time a parenteral medication is given. **An allergy to an injectable medication that goes into the tissue or bloodstream could result in anaphylaxis.** Check the expiration date on the label of the medication container before drawing it up. Out-of-date medication should not be administered because it may have changed chemically. Determine the reason the patient is receiving this medication. If the reason is not evident, the medication order may have been written on the wrong medical record.

Therapeutic effects of previous doses need to be assessed. This may include reviewing the patient's symptomatic response and checking laboratory data, such as white blood cell (WBC) count. Determine the medication's desired action, potential side effects, precautions, and recommended nursing interventions. **It is imperative to know both what the medication is supposed to do (therapeutic action) and what adverse or side effects may occur to assess the patient for their presence properly.** Assess the patient for signs of side effects to previous doses of the medication. If harmful side effects have occurred, the medication must be discontinued and the primary care provider consulted.

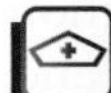
Clinical Cues

Apply your knowledge of pathophysiology and pharmacology; question a medication order that does not match your patient's condition, medical diagnosis, or symptoms.

Determine previous injection sites by consulting the medication administration record (MAR) or electronic medication administration record (eMAR) and the patient. It is best to rotate injection sites to promote the best absorption of the medication and to decrease tissue irritation or **fibrosis** (formation of fibrous tissue) (Lee, 2012). Assess the patient's size and anatomy, and locate the appropriate landmarks at the chosen injection site. Determine whether blood circulation is adequate. The needle size and length are determined by the type of injection to be given, as well as the size of muscle tissue and the amount of fat at the patient's injection site. Adequate circulation is essential for drug absorption.

NURSING DIAGNOSIS

The nursing diagnosis that covers the administration of a particular medication depends on the purpose of the drug. A few possible nursing diagnoses are:

- Acute pain related to inflammation or surgery (analgesic)
- Risk for infection related to surgical procedure (antibiotic)
- Imbalanced nutrition, less than body requirements, related to inability to use glucose (insulin)
- Activity intolerance related to postoperative discomfort (pain medication)
- Deficient fluid volume related to vomiting (antie metic)

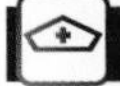
Clinical Cues

In planning for medication administration, it is important to check that patients' medications are on the unit before the time they are to be administered. Perform any calculations needed to reconstitute a drug ahead of administration time.

◆ **PLANNING**

Sample goals/expected outcomes for the previous nursing diagnoses might be:

- Pain will be relieved for 3 hours by medication.
- No signs of infection will be present at discharge.
- Blood glucose level will be maintained within normal limits.
- Patient will demonstrate willingness to ambulate, cough, and deep breathe within 30 minutes after an injection of pain medication.
- Nausea and vomiting will be controlled by antiemetic medication.

◆ **IMPLEMENTATION**

Giving injections involves correctly checking and preparing the medication and administering it skillfully. It is necessary to use clinical judgment to choose the correct needle size and syringe for the type of injection to be given. Maintaining asepsis while drawing up and giving injections is mandatory. **Always follow the Six Rights when administering a parenteral medication (right drug, right route, right dose, right time, right patient, and right documentation).**

Once disposable needles and syringes have been used, they must be discarded in such a way that they cannot pose a danger to others.

 **Home Care Considerations**

Disposing of Sharps in the Home Care Setting

In the home care setting, the patient may be giving himself heparin or insulin injections. Regulations for sharps disposal from home vary according to state and local jurisdiction, so it is important to know the local laws. For example, some counties require home "sharps containers" to be rigid and no larger than 2 L. Most communities offer drop boxes outside of hospitals or pharmacies for used sharps. Tips on getting rid of sharps can be found at: <http://www.fda.gov/MedicalDevices/ProductsandMedicalProcedures/HomeHealthandConsumer/ConsumerProducts/Sharps/default.htm>.

Intradermal Injections

ID injections are most frequently used for tuberculosis or allergy testing. **For the ID route, a small amount of solution is injected.** Extreme care must be taken to measure the dose accurately because the solutions are capable of producing severe reactions. A tuberculin syringe and a short needle, ¼ to ½ inch in length, are used. The ventral aspect of the forearm is the customary injection site, but when this site is not available for use, the dorsal and lateral sides of the upper arm can also be used because they are readily observable. The needle is inserted at an angle of about 5 to 15 degrees between the upper layers of the skin. The injected solution will raise the epidermis to form a bleb. It is then slowly absorbed from the site because the blood vessels are deeper.

Tuberculin is a biologic product used for skin testing for exposure to tuberculosis. The basis of the test is that a person infected with *Mycobacterium tuberculosis* develops sensitivity to certain products of this organism, which are contained in the culture extracts called tuberculins.

Tuberculin testing is the first step in a series to confirm that a patient is infected with the tubercle bacillus and may have clinical tuberculosis. The tuberculin skin test (TST) is the preferred method (Skill 35.1). Box 35.2 provides guidelines for reading the results of a TST. A positive tuberculin

Skill 35.1 Administering an Intradermal Injection

 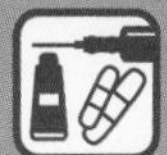 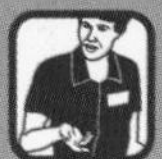 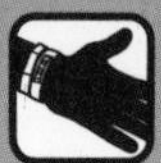 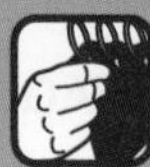 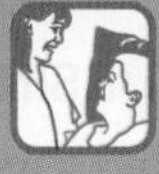 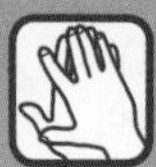 

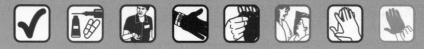

Intradermal injections are used for various skin tests, such as the tuberculin skin test. The object is to inject an antigen to determine whether the patient has an inflammatory reaction, indicating that previous exposure to the antigen has caused antibodies to be manufactured by the body.

SUPPLIES

- Tuberculin syringe with ¼- to ½-inch needle
- Medication to be injected
- Gloves
- Medication administration record (MAR or eMAR) or order
- Alcohol swabs

Review and carry out the Standard Steps in Appendix A.

ACTION *(RATIONALE)*

Assessment (Data Collection)

1. Assess whether the patient understands the procedure for the ID injection and its purpose. Assess for previous reaction to the agent to be injected. *(Determines whether patient education is needed. Identifies possible contraindication to injection.)*

Planning

2. Determine when 48 to 72 hours after the injection will occur (or the proper time for reading the result) and whether someone will be available to read the result. *(The injection may need to be delayed on the weekend or because of the patient's personal schedule, which will interfere with proper reading of the result.)*

Implementation

3. Check the medication label against the MAR or eMAR. *(This is the first check to prevent medication errors.)*
4. Perform hand hygiene and draw up the medication. Perform the second check per the Six Rights at this time. *(Prepares medication for injection. Helps prevent a medication error.)*
5. Clean the preparation area and take the injection and the MAR or workstation on wheels (WOW) to the patient. Perform the third check of the medication with the MAR or eMAR. *(The third check is always done at the bedside.)*
6. Properly identify the patient using two identifiers. Select a relatively hairless site, usually on the inside of the forearm. (Agency policy may specify right or left.) Have the patient extend the elbow and support the forearm on a flat surface. Cleanse the site well with an antiseptic swab using firm, gentle circular motions, or use soap and water. Clean an area approximately 2 inches in diameter. Allow the skin to dry. *(The inside of the forearm is used for intradermal injections. If the skin is still wet with alcohol when the injection is given, the patient will experience more stinging.)*
7. Hold the syringe vertically and verify that the exact dose is present in the syringe. *(Intradermal doses are usually very small. The scale may be difficult to read. Ask your instructor to check your dose.)*
8. Don gloves; stand or sit in front of the patient and turn the patient's forearm palm upward, facing you. With the index finger and thumb, pull the skin taut at the selected site on the forearm. Insert the needle, with the **bevel up**, at a 5- to 15-degree angle for approximately ⅛ inch (3 mm). You should be able to see the outline of the point of the needle. If you are in the dermis, you will feel resistance to the needle; if you can move the needle freely, you are in the subcutaneous tissue and must start over. *(Positioning the needle bevel up minimizes resistance of the skin when the needle is inserted, decreasing discomfort. The needle must be in the dermis at a 5- to 15-degree angle for the medication to form a bleb.)*

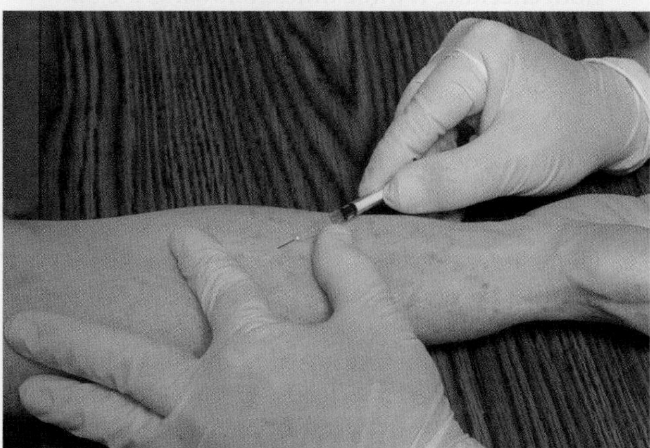

Step 8

9. Lift up the needle's point slightly and inject the solution slowly; a bleb, or bump, of 6 to 10 mm in diameter should form. *(If a bleb is not formed, the medication has been deposited into the subcutaneous tissue and the test will not be valid.)*

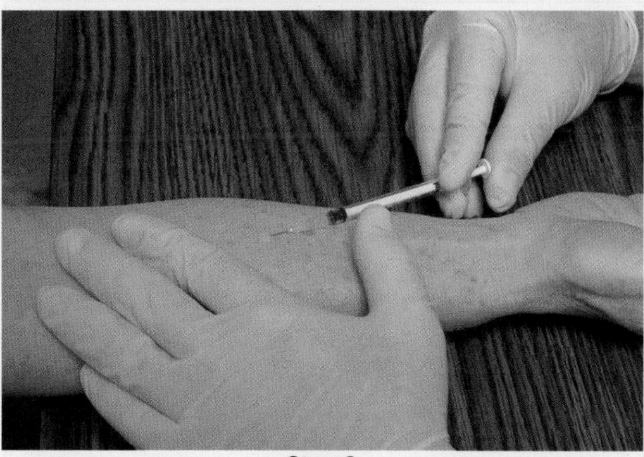

Step 9

10. Carefully withdraw the needle and wipe the skin very gently with the antiseptic swab **after** you remove the needle; **do not apply pressure. Activate the safety guard over the used needle; do not recap.** *(Move your fingers to prevent accidental needle sticks. Applying pressure will disperse the bleb. Activating the needle guard prevents needle sticks.)*
11. Dispose of the syringe and needle by dropping them into the sharps container; remove and dispose of gloves; perform hand hygiene. *(Prevents needle sticks to self or others.)*
12. Circle the injection site with a skin pencil. *(Facilitates locating the site when it is time to read the reaction.)*

Evaluation

13. Verify that the bleb remains. *(The procedure is repeated if a bleb is not visible or is less than 6 mm. If a repeat injection is needed, select a site at least 2 inches from the original site and document.)*
14. Read the result of the skin test at the proper interval. *(Different antigens used for testing require different intervals before reading the result.)*

Documentation

15. Document the dose on the MAR or eMAR and record the exact site of the injection. *(Documenting the exact site shows where to read the result in 48 to 72 hours.)*
16. When the result is read, document the findings in the medical record. *(The right documentation records information for future reference.)*

Documentation Example

TST 0.1 mL on left inner forearm; to return in 48 to 72 hours for reading. (Nurse's time-stamped electronic signature)

Critical Thinking Questions

1. What would you do if a large portion of the solution for the TST leaked out of the bleb after you removed the needle from the skin?
2. How would you handle the situation if the patient states he has had a positive reaction in the past to a tuberculosis test?

Box 35.2 Reading the Tuberculin Skin Test Results

Locate the injection site indicated on the patient record and marked with a skin pencil. Inspect the injection site under a good light, noting any erythema. Palpate the margin of the induration. With a millimeter ruler, measure the transverse diameter of the indurated area across the point at which the needle entered. The reading is recorded in millimeters of **induration** (quality of being hard). Induration, not erythema, is the key to the positive reaction. The result is read between 48 and 72 h after injection.

POSITIVE REACTION

The test is positive when the swelling at the site of injection is more than 5 mm in diameter in people who have a history of contact with infectious tuberculosis or in immunocompromised patients.

Induration of more than 10 mm in diameter is positive in recent immigrants from countries where tuberculosis is prevalent, in medically underserved groups, and in the homeless.

For those people at low risk, induration of more than 15 mm is considered positive (deWit & Kumagai, 2012).

NEGATIVE REACTION

The induration measures less than 5 mm.

test result denotes that exposure has occurred, but it does not signify the presence of active disease. Follow-up of a positive tuberculin test result involves a chest x-ray examination and possibly other blood tests.

Subcutaneous Injections

Medications administered by the subcutaneous route are absorbed more slowly by the body than those are via the IM route (Skill 35.2). The subcutaneous route is used for a variety of medications, including insulin, heparin, and some preoperative medications and narcotics to relieve pain. Sites that can be used for subcutaneous injections are shown in Figure 35.17. For most patients the preferred sites are the lateral surfaces of the upper arm or the anterior and lateral aspects of the thigh. Heparin is given in the abdominal subcutaneous sites (Box 35.3; Nursing Care Plan 35.1); the best site for insulin is also the abdomen because it provides the most reliable, steady absorption (Morris, 2014). In accordance with National Patient Safety Goals, you should encourage your patients to be actively involved with medication administration. For example, teach your diabetic patients to rotate sites for insulin administration and, if ordered, how to use an insulin pen.

Skill 35.2 Administering a Subcutaneous Injection

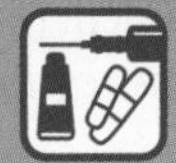
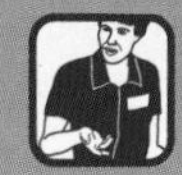

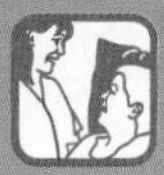
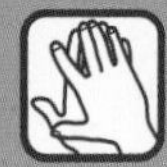
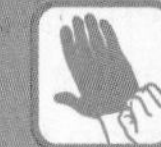

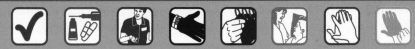

Certain drugs must be injected subcutaneously rather than intramuscularly to be absorbed properly and at the desired speed. Heparin, insulin, allergy extract, and certain types of immunizations, as well as some other medications, are given subcutaneously.

SUPPLIES

- Medication
- Gloves
- Medication administration record (MAR or eMAR)
- Alcohol swabs
- Syringe and needle (preferably ⅜ to ⅝ inch in length)

Review and carry out the Standard Steps in Appendix A.

ACTION *(RATIONALE)*

Assessment (Data Collection)

1. Check the medication order and determine that the medication is available on the unit. Check for presence of drug allergies. *(Ensures that time is not lost acquiring the medication. Indicates whether patient might be allergic to the medication.)*
2. Determine that patient is in the room and ready to receive the injection. *(Prevents having to wait to give injection once it is drawn up. Some drugs deteriorate in plastic syringes.)*

Planning

3. Plan the site at which to place the injection. Using your clinical judgment, choose an appropriate syringe and needle. *(Consider the patient's size and weight, as well as the condition of the various sites in which a subcutaneous injection may be given.)*

Implementation

4. Perform hand hygiene and prepare the medication, checking it three times following the Six Rights. *(Checking the medication three times using the Six Rights helps prevent medication errors.)*
5. Identify patient by checking wristband with MAR and having patient state his name. Alternatively, use a bar code device to check bar code on the name band and eMAR. *(Prevents medication errors and injury to patients.)*
6. Don gloves, select site for injection, and expose the area for good visibility. Open the alcohol swab package and cleanse selected site gently by using a circular motion until an area approximately 2 inches in diameter is cleansed. Place the swab between index and middle fingers of your nondominant hand. Allow the skin to dry. *(Cleanses the area; positions swab for use after injection. Vigorous rubbing increases blood flow and increases rapidity of absorption.)*

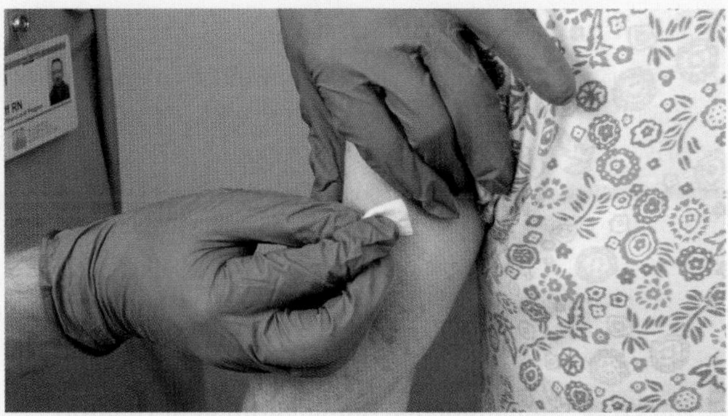

Step 6

7. Pick up the prepared syringe in one hand and remove the needle guard by pulling it straight off the needle with the other hand to avoid contaminating the needle, dulling it, or suffering a needle stick. *(Asepsis and safety must be maintained.)*
8. Support the skin at the site by gently bunching up the tissue between your thumb and index finger. *(Picking up the tissue helps you assess thickness of subcutaneous layer into which you will inject the drug and prevents medication from being injected into the muscle.)*

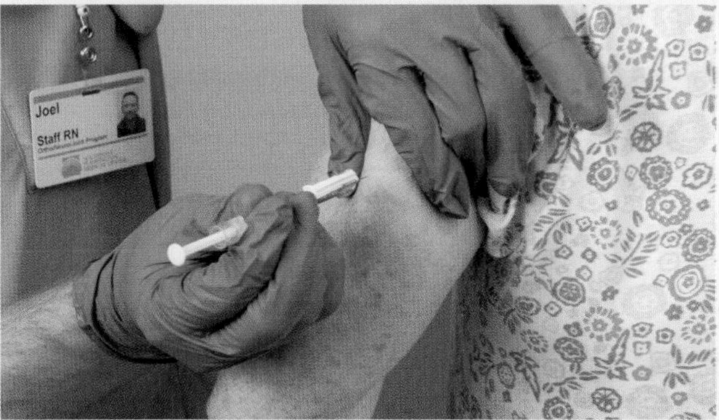

Step 8

9. Hold the barrel of the syringe in your hand between the thumb and index finger, bracing with the remaining three fingers. Insert needle into the skin at a 45- or 90-degree angle depending on length of the needle, with a firm, quick forward thrust; release the pinched-up skin. *(Stabilizes tissue so that needle will pierce cleanly. A shorter needle uses a 90-degree angle; a longer needle uses a 45-degree angle to stay in subcutaneous tissue.)*

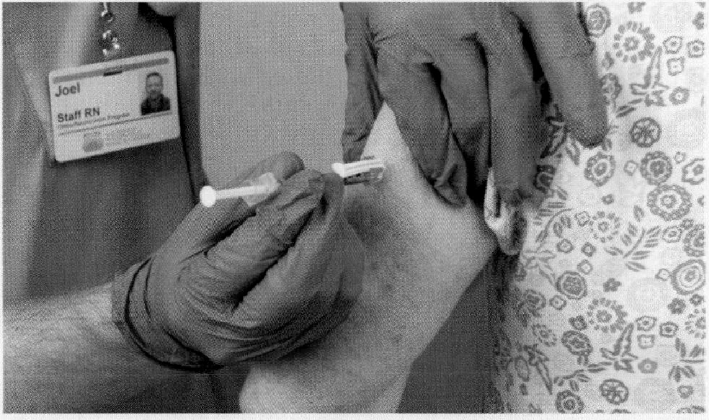

Step 9

10. Press the plunger with a smooth, slow motion until all medication is injected. *(Places medication in the tissue.)*
11. Remove needle by pulling it out on the angle of insertion while stabilizing skin with the other hand. Activate safety guard on the needle. *(Pulling the needle out quickly while stabilizing skin causes the least discomfort for patient. Activating needle guard prevents needle sticks.)*
12. Wipe injection site with an alcohol swab to remove any blood that may appear at the puncture. Do not rub or massage an allergy extract, heparin, or insulin injections. *(Massaging can alter rate of absorption.)*
13. Drop needle and syringe in the sharps container. Remove gloves; perform hand hygiene. *(Pushing used equipment into sharps container increases risk of needle sticks. Reduces transfer of microorganisms.)*

Evaluation

14. Check with patient in 30 minutes to evaluate the therapeutic effect of the medication if it was an analgesic. *(Analgesics should be working within 30 minutes. Allergy injection sites are checked at 30 minutes for local reaction. Immunizations cannot be visually evaluated for therapeutic effect; however, patients should be observed for untoward effects.)*

Documentation

15. Document the injection on the MAR, eMAR, or patient clinic record, noting the location in which the injection was given. *(Verifies that injection was given as ordered.)*

Documentation Example

Allergy injection 0.5 mL of trees and grasses mixture, 50,000 mcg/mL in left upper outer arm subcutaneously. (Nurse's time-stamped electronic signature)

Special Considerations

- The needle angle used depends on the length of the needle and the amount of subcutaneous tissue at the site. If 2 inches (5 cm) of tissue can be grasped, insert the needle at a 90-degree angle; if only 1 inch of tissue can be grasped, use a 45-degree angle for the injection.
- Allergy injection sites should be rotated from one side of the body to the other.
- Heparin injections are given in the abdomen on both sides of and below the umbilicus outside of a 2-inch radius around the umbilicus from the lower costal margins to the iliac crests. Wait at least 15 to 30 seconds before removing the needle from the injection site.
- If bruising occurs after a heparin injection, ice the area chosen for the next injection.

- Keep a record of where each insulin injection is given. Insulin is absorbed more quickly and uniformly when injected into the abdominal sites.

Critical Thinking Questions

1. Your patient states he never rotates his insulin injections at home and asks why you are doing it now. What would you tell him?
2. Why would you avoid rubbing or massaging allergy extract, heparin, or insulin injections?

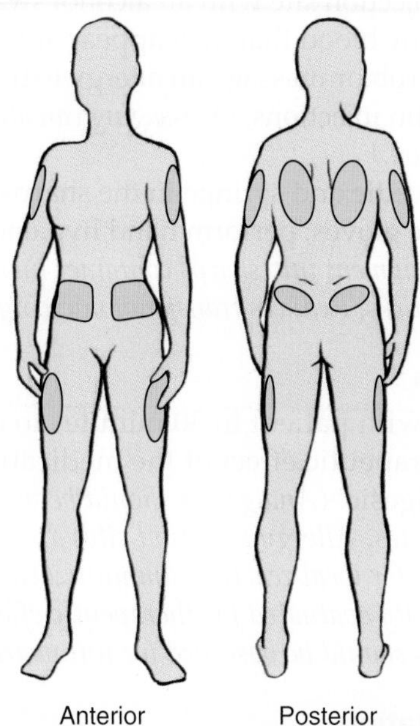

FIGURE 35.17 Subcutaneous injection sites.

Box 35.3 Subcutaneous Administration of Heparin

When heparin is administered subcutaneously, it requires additional precautions during administration. Because of its anticoagulant properties, it can stimulate bleeding into the tissues. Always have another nurse double-check your syringe for the correct amount and the vial for the correct strength and dose.

- Sites on the abdomen from below the costal margins to the iliac crests are used because this area is not involved in muscular activity, whereas the arms and legs are.
- Sites should be rotated within the abdominal area, alternating from one side to another; avoid giving a subsequent injection too close to a previous one.
- Do not massage the site after the drug has been injected because this may cause bruising of the tissue, bleeding, and severe **ecchymosis** (purplish area under the skin caused by bleeding).

Nursing Care Plan 35.1 Care of the Patient Receiving Heparin Injections

SCENARIO Lena Thomas, age 56, was admitted with a deep vein thrombosis (DVT) of the right leg. She has been receiving intravenous heparin but is to be discharged today. She was started on warfarin sodium by mouth yesterday. Because it takes 3 days for the warfarin levels to be effective for maintenance of anticoagulation, she will receive heparin injections twice a day for 2 days. The home health nurse will give the injections.

PROBLEM/NURSING DIAGNOSIS *Has a blood clot in right leg*/Risk for injury related to potential for thrombus formation.

Supporting Assessment Data *Subjective:* Injured leg. Developed swelling, redness, and pain in right leg. *Objective:* Swelling decreasing, redness diminished, pain lessened.

Goals/Expected Outcomes	Nursing Interventions	Selected Rationale	Evaluation
Patient will not display signs of emboli during the recovery period.	Apply antithrombotic elastic stockings to both legs.	Elastic stockings apply pressure to tissue and vessels to encourage venous return and prevent pooling of blood in the leg.	*Did the patient have any signs of emboli?* No signs of emboli (i.e., no change of mental status and denies SOB or chest pain).
	Discourage rubbing of the legs.	Rubbing an area where a thrombus is located may dislodge it, and it then would become an embolus.	The patient agrees not to rub his legs.

Nursing Care Plan 35.1 Care of the Patient Receiving Heparin Injections—cont'd

Goals/Expected Outcomes	Nursing Interventions	Selected Rationale	Evaluation
	Check APTT before administering heparin. Call the primary care provider if APTT is less than 50 seconds or greater than 100 seconds.	Normal APTT is 30-40 seconds. Desired therapeutic range is 1.5 to 2.5 times normal. Dosage adjustment is needed if not in the therapeutic range.	APTT is 70 seconds.
	Administer 5000 units sodium heparin subcutaneously in the abdomen q 12 h.	Heparin prevents DVT formation. Heparin is absorbed best from abdominal sites.	5000 units of heparin administered Subcut in Rt. abdomen at 0900; no adverse effects.
	If bruising occurs, ice the area for 3 to 5 min before the next injection; stabilize the needle well so as not to cause bleeding in the tissues from needle movement.	Cold causes vessel constriction and helps prevent bleeding that causes bruising. Stabilizing the needle prevents tissue damage that could cause bruising.	No signs of bruising.
Swelling and pain will be gone within 2 weeks.	Keep the leg elevated when sitting.	Elevation prevents pooling of blood and edema.	*Did the swelling and pain resolve?* Leg is elevated on a pillow; encouraged to change position q 2 h. Swelling and pain decreased.
	Do not stand for long periods.	Standing allows blood to pool in legs.	Patient is aware of the need to rest and elevate legs.
Patient will verbalize symptoms of emboli to report to the primary care provider.	Assess for signs of pulmonary crackles or SOB indicating possible pulmonary emboli; assess for neurologic changes that might indicate a brain embolus; instruct to call 911 if she experiences chest pain with SOB because this might indicate a coronary embolus.	Pulmonary emboli cause SOB and anxiety; neurologic changes may indicate a brain embolus and stroke. A coronary embolus may cause a myocardial infarction requiring emergency treatment.	*Was the patient able to verbalize symptoms to watch for?* Patient and family verbalize signs of emboli correctly (i.e., SOB, anxiety, chest pain, change in mental status).
	Teach family how to recognize signs of emboli.	If family has knowledge of signs and symptoms of emboli, they can obtain emergency services quickly.	Family participated in a patient education session and is able to state how to call 911 services. Outcomes met.

CRITICAL THINKING QUESTIONS

1. Explain how you would evaluate the effectiveness of the heparin.
2. Explain the process of preparing and administering a heparin injection.
3. Explain how you would select the syringe and needle size for a heparin injection.

APTT, Activated partial thromboplastin time; *SOB*, shortness of breath.

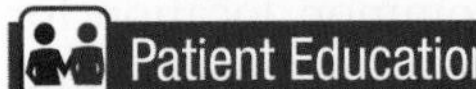

Patient Education

How to Use the Insulin Pen (Humulin or Humalog)

The insulin pen is a convenient, safe way to administer insulin. It is lightweight and can be carried in a pocket or a purse. The insulin pen is usually dispensed with 300 units of the prescribed insulin.

To use a pen:

- Be certain the needle is firmly attached to the pen. Use a new needle every time you use the pen for an injection.

PRIMING THE PEN

- Pull out the dose knob and turn it clockwise until a "0" appears in the dose window.
- Now turn the dose knob clockwise until a "2" appears.
- Remove the cover from the needle and point the pen upward.
- Tap the plastic barrel lightly, then push the injection button down all the way, until a click is heard and you see a drop of insulin at the needle tip.
- Turn the dose knob clockwise until the arrow appears in the dose window. Pull out the dose knob. A "0" will appear in the window.
- Dial the correct number of units for your dose of insulin (Fig. 35.18).
- If you dial up too large a dose, turn the dose knob backward until the correct dose appears in the dose window.

INJECTION, DISPOSAL, AND STORAGE

- Using clinical judgment, choose the injection site and insert the needle straight into the skin; press the injection button.

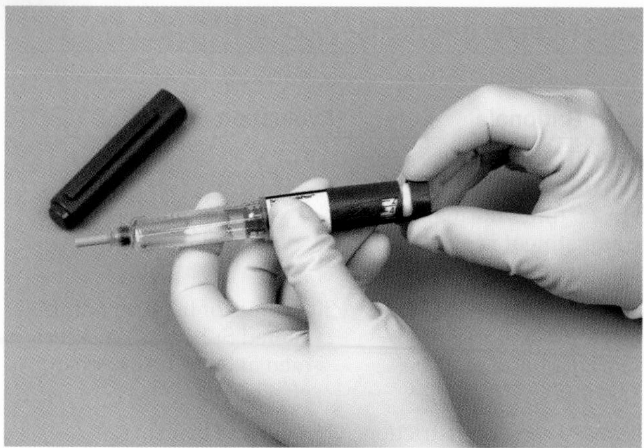

FIGURE 35.18 Dialing an insulin pen.

Count to five slowly before you remove the needle. A click will be heard when the injection is complete.

- Replace the outer needle shield. Unscrew the capped needle and appropriately dispose of it as instructed. (Used needles are a biohazard.)
- Place the cap on the pen for storage. Store the pen at room temperature, below 86°F.
- Protect the pen from direct heat and light.
- The pen should not be refrigerated once it has been used (Holland, 2014).
- Discard the pen 28 days after initial use, even if there is insulin remaining.

Home Care Considerations

Monitoring Injections Given in the Home Care Setting

- When family members or patients in the home care setting are giving injections, periodically assess whether the injection is being given with correct technique by observing the injection preparation and administration.
- Be certain that used syringes and needles are being disposed of safely. Remind patients and families that reusing needles is not recommended even in home settings because of the risk of infection and increased pain, bleeding, or even breakage of reused needles.
- From time to time, thoroughly review the principles of asepsis for the home care patient receiving injections.

Safety Alert

Double-Check Insulin, Heparin, and Other High-Alert Medication Doses With Another Nurse

There are many medications on the Institute for Safe Medication Practice's (ISMP) high-alert list; these medications can have devastating consequences when medication errors occur. The ISMP encourages agencies to develop strategies to minimize the chances of high-alert medication errors. One such strategy is the independent double-checking of medication and dose; many facilities have had the requirement to double-check insulin and heparin for years (ISMP, 2014). When you are giving insulin, heparin, injectable heart medications, or parenteral chemotherapy drugs to a patient, always have another nurse *independently* double-check for correct medication and correct dose. Show the other nurse the medication vial and ask her to read the amount in the syringe. This evidence-based practice should continue even after you have graduated and have many years of experience. For the full list of high-alert medications for acute care settings, see: <www.ismp.org/tools/institutionalhighAlert.asp>.

Think Critically

Although the abdomen is the best site for insulin, why might the nurse elect to administer the insulin in the patient's upper arm while the patient is in the hospital?

Intramuscular Injections

IM injections are used if the patient cannot take medicine orally, the medication is not prepared in an oral form, or a faster action is desired. IM injections can provide onset of action within 15 minutes because muscle tissue is highly vascular, and, thus, drug absorption is faster than by the subcutaneous route.

Selection of the injection site is a critical decision. **Improper site selection can result in damaged nerves, abscesses, necrosis, sloughing of skin, and pain.** Therefore, consider the individual's stage of development, body build, and physical condition, along with the viscosity and amount of the drug to be administered. If more than 3 mL of medication must be given at one time to an adult, the dose should be divided in half and given in two different large muscle sites.

QSEN Considerations: Evidence-Based Practice

Injection Skin Preparation and Disinfection

IM injection sites have traditionally been disinfected with alcohol; however, according to the most recent World Health Organization (WHO) guidelines (2010), washing skin with soap and water before subcutaneous, intradermal, and intramuscular (for immunizations) is the recommended skin preparation. Therapeutic intramuscular administration (other medications) is stated by the WHO as an "unresolved" issue, recommending skin be disinfected with alcohol, although noting there is "insufficient evidence" for doing so and that further studies are warranted (WHO, 2010).

The mid-deltoid muscle is a common location for IM injection; however, the actual area involved is limited because of its proximity to major vessels, nerves, and bones. The area for the mid-deltoid injection is triangular, with the base of the triangle beginning 1 to 2 inches below the acromion process and extending down to just above the axilla fold (Fig. 35.19). The correct site for injection can be located by placing four fingers across the deltoid muscle, with the little finger on the acromion process; the site is three finger widths below the acromion process (Perry et al., 2016). This site is convenient because it is usually easily accessible; it is not used in infants or children with underdeveloped muscles.

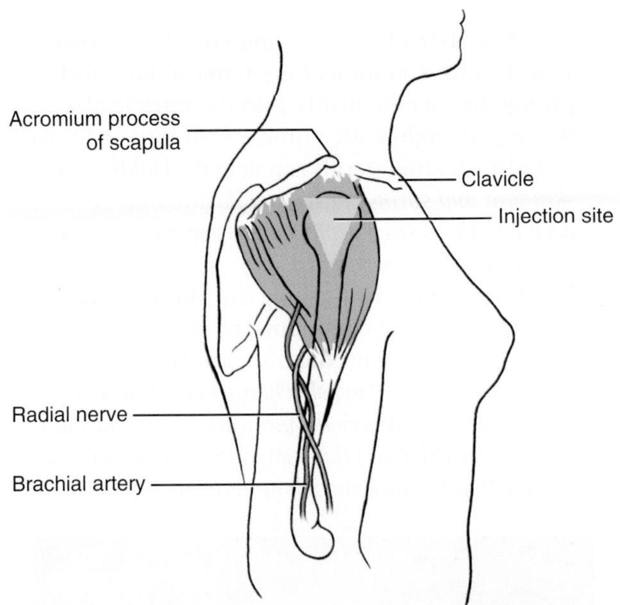

FIGURE 35.19 Locating the site for a mid-deltoid IM injection. *IM*, Intramuscular.

In the past the dorsogluteal (**gluteal:** pertaining to the buttocks) site was used; however, evidence-based practice indicates that it is **no longer recommended** because of the high potential for injury to the sciatic nerve and the blood vessels.

The ventrogluteal area is the preferred IM injection site (Hopkins & Arias, 2013) involving the gluteus medius and minimus muscles (see Skill 35.3). The muscle layer is thick, and this site has a very small fatty layer. The site can be used for both adults and children and is especially helpful if patients are only able to lie on their back or turn to one side or the other. To locate the injection site, place the palm over the greater trochanter, put the index finger on the anterior iliac spine, and spread the middle finger as far as possible toward the posterior iliac crest (Fig. 35.20). **The center of the "V" bounded by the index and middle fingers is the precise injection site to be used.**

Skill 35.3 Administering an Intramuscular Injection

 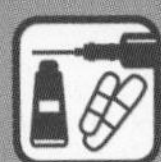 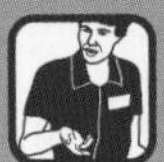 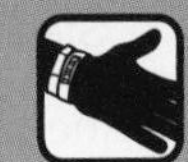 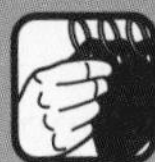 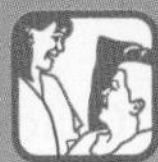 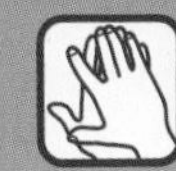 

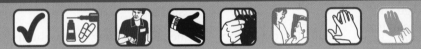

Many drugs are given only by intramuscular injection. The site must be carefully selected to prevent injury to the patient. Intramuscular injection sites are shown in Figures 35.19 to 35.22.

SUPPLIES

- Syringe and needle 1 to 3 inches in length
- Medication
- Gloves
- Medication administration record (MAR or eMAR)
- Alcohol swabs or soap and water for cleansing
- Adhesive bandage (optional)

Review and carry out the Standard Steps in Appendix A.

ACTION *(RATIONALE)*

Assessment (Data Collection)

1. Determine that patient is in the room and ready for the injection. Assess for allergy to the drug. *(Medication should be given immediately after preparation. Allergic reactions must be avoided.)*

Planning

2. Plan the site at which the injection is to be given. *(Deltoid, ventrogluteal, vastus lateralis, or rectus femoris sites may be used.)*

Implementation

3. Verify the medication label with the MAR, checking the medication three times, using the Six Rights. Alternatively, check the bar code on the patient's bracelet and the code on the eMAR. *(Adhering to the Six Rights of medication administration and checking each medication three times for drug, dose, route, date, and time prevents medication errors.)*
4. Perform hand hygiene and don gloves. Select and expose the injection site so that the view is unobstructed. For the ventrogluteal site, the patient may be supine or turned to the side. *(Ventrogluteal site is the safest site for adults. IM site chosen must be within defined landmarks; a good view is necessary to inject at the correct location.)*

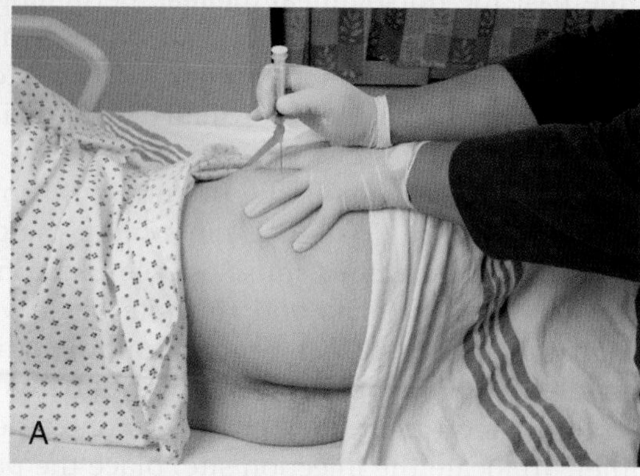

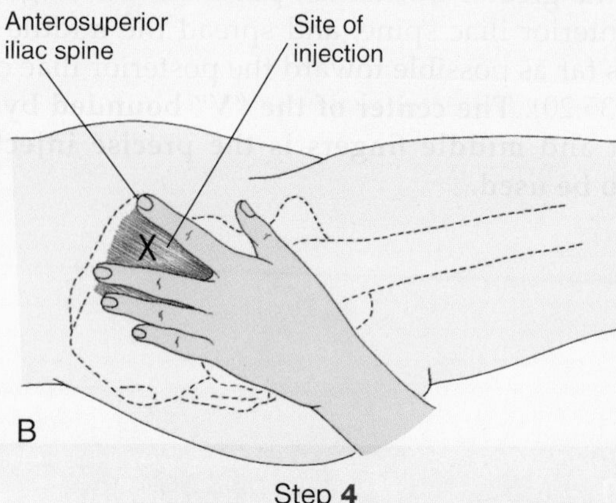

Step 4

5. Remove an alcohol swab from the package and cleanse a space 2 inches in diameter using a firm circular motion. Place the swab between fingers of the nondominant hand for later use, or place it just lateral to the site. Allow area to dry. *(Prevents transfer of microorganisms. Cleanses the site. Makes swab available after the injection. Wet alcohol on the skin may cause stinging on injection.)*
6. Pick up the syringe and verify it contains correct dose. *(Ensures correct dose according to the Six Rights.)*
7. Spread the skin at the site with nondominant hand, pressing firmly around the site to compress the subcutaneous and muscle tissues. *(Taut skin reduces resistance to the needle when it enters tissues and causes less pain.)*

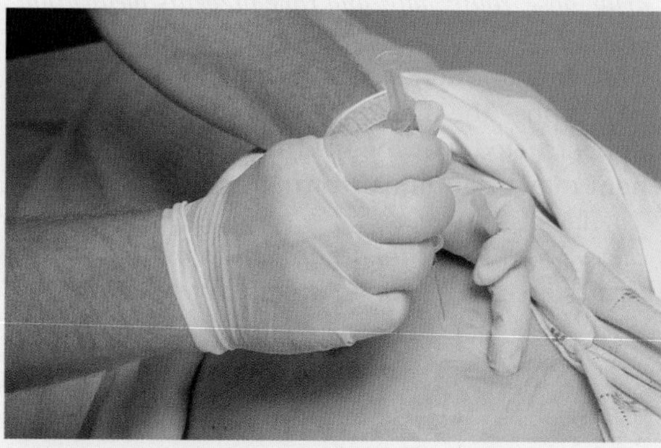

Step 7

8. Grasp the barrel of the syringe firmly between your thumb and index finger, like a dart, and plunge the needle firmly into the muscle at a 90-degree angle with a quick, firm forward thrust until the desired depth is reached. *(Holding the skin taut and syringe steady while introducing the needle to the desired depth in one stroke causes the least discomfort to patient.)*
9. Inject medication by pushing the plunger into the barrel with a slow, continuous motion. Be careful not to displace the needle from its original position as you inject. *(Injecting slowly is less painful because tissue has time to absorb the medication. A medication prepared for IM absorption may cause local tissue reaction if left in the fatty subcutaneous or ID tissue.)*

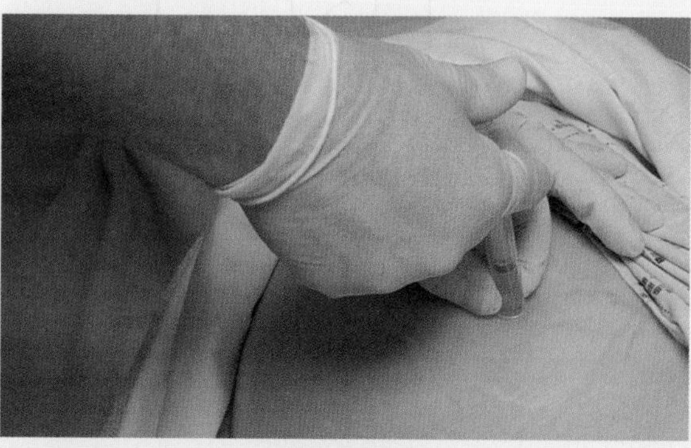

Step 9

10. Quickly remove the needle, drawing it straight up with a quick motion. Activate the needle guard. Using a gauze pad, apply light pressure to the site. Apply an adhesive bandage if there is superficial bleeding. Do not massage. *(Removing the needle with a quick motion is less painful than removing it slowly. Enclosing the needle in a guard prevents needle sticks. A gauze pad is usually sufficient to contain any bleeding; apply an adhesive bandage if needed.)*

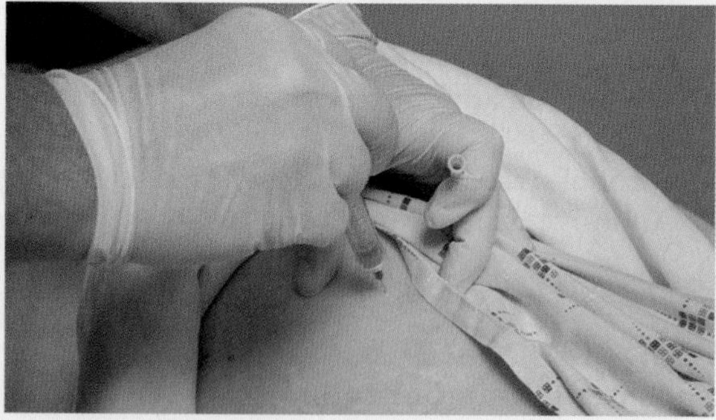

Step 10

11. Dispose of the syringe, remove gloves, and perform hand hygiene. *(Prevents needle sticks and decreases transfer of microorganisms.)*

Evaluation

12. Assess patient tolerance of injection. Depending on the medication injected, check for therapeutic

effect of the injection at a proper interval. *(If adverse effects of medication occur, document them and inform the primary care provider promptly. If the medication appears to be ineffective, consult primary care provider.)*

Documentation

13. Document the dose and the site on the MAR or eMAR. If the medication is PRN, document in the nurse's notes. *(The reason for injection and patient's response are documented for all PRN medications.)*

Documentation Examples

Morphine 8 mg IM RVG (right ventrogluteal) for complaints of pain of 7 on a scale of 0 to 10 at incision. (Nurse's time-stamped electronic signature)

States pain has lessened considerably; now a 4 on a scale of 0 to 10. (Nurse's time-stamped electronic signature)

Special Considerations

- Use clinical judgment to carefully consider the size of muscle mass in the older adult and choose a safe injection site. Many older adults have muscle wasting (atrophy). A shorter needle may be necessary. The vastus lateralis and ventrogluteal sites are the preferred sites in older adults.
- Apply pressure to the injection site in the older adult for longer than for a younger person, to prevent bleeding and hematoma formation. Clotting time is often decreased in older adults.
- When the patient is receiving a series of injections, check the former sites for induration at the time of choosing a site for the next injection.
- If a medication causes excessive discomfort when injected, place ice over the site for 3 to 5 minutes before injecting.

? Critical Thinking Questions

1. You are working with an experienced nurse who encourages you to use the dorsogluteal site to give an IM injection. What would you say to the nurse?
2. You are working with the same experienced nurse who insists you vigorously massage the injection site after withdrawing the needle. What would you say this time?

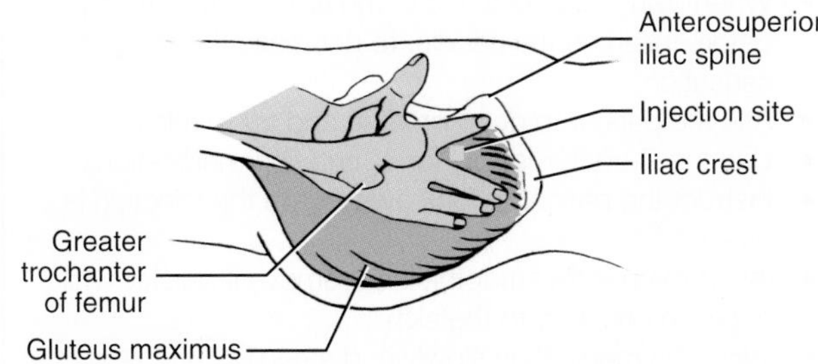

FIGURE 35.20 Locating the site for a ventrogluteal IM injection. *IM*, Intramuscular.

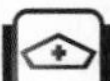 **Clinical Cues**

One milliliter of medication can be safely injected into the middeltoid site for adults (Hopkins & Arias, 2013). Check agency policy before injecting a larger amount.

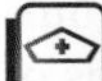 **Clinical Cues**

The ventrogluteal area is considered the safest intramuscular injection site in adults to avoid damage to nerves or blood vessels. However, rather than leaving your hand in the "V" position, after identifying the correct injection site, place an alcohol swab on the patient's skin to mark the site (e.g., develop a routine of always placing an alcohol swab directly adjacent to the injection site, "pointing" toward it). This is especially important if you suspect that the patient might move during the procedure (e.g., if the patient is confused or unable to follow instructions).

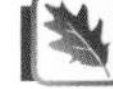 **Life-Span Considerations**

OLDER ADULTS

Older adults may have decreased muscle mass. The body of the muscle may have to be palpated and then grasped to ensure injection into the muscle mass. A shorter needle than average may need to be used.

The vastus lateralis muscle is also a preferred IM injection site for adults, children, and infants (Immunize.org, 2015) because it is easily accessible and free of major nerves and blood vessels (Hopkins & Arias, 2013). The area extends from the anterolateral aspect of the thigh to the midlateral thigh, a hand's width below the proximal end of the greater trochanter and a hand's width above the upper knee (Fig. 35.21). The middle third of the muscle is the best site for injection. This muscle can be used when the patient is recumbent with the knee slightly flexed in the Sims position or is sitting upright.

The rectus femoris muscle can also be used as an IM site in the adult, as well as when other sites are contraindicated in children. It is located on the anterior aspect of the thigh (Fig. 35.22) and is used by people who give their own IM injections because it is easy to reach. The disadvantage of this site is that the injection may cause considerable discomfort.

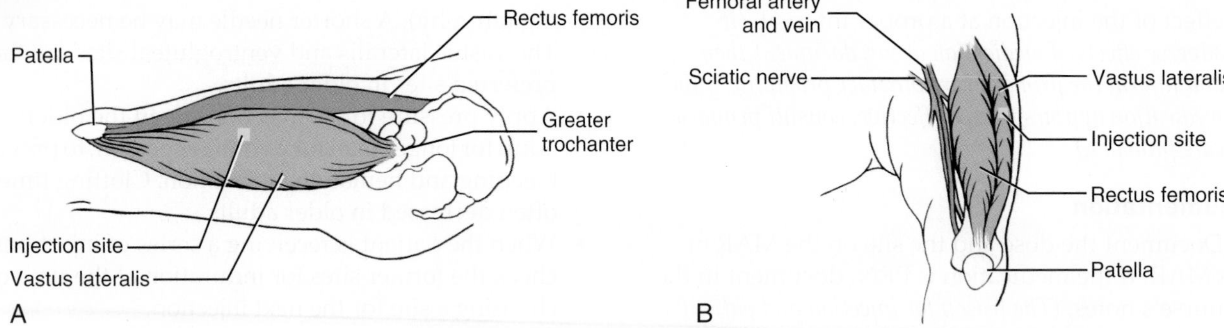

FIGURE 35.21 Locating the vastus lateralis IM injection site. (A) Side view. (B) Front view. *IM,* Intramuscular.

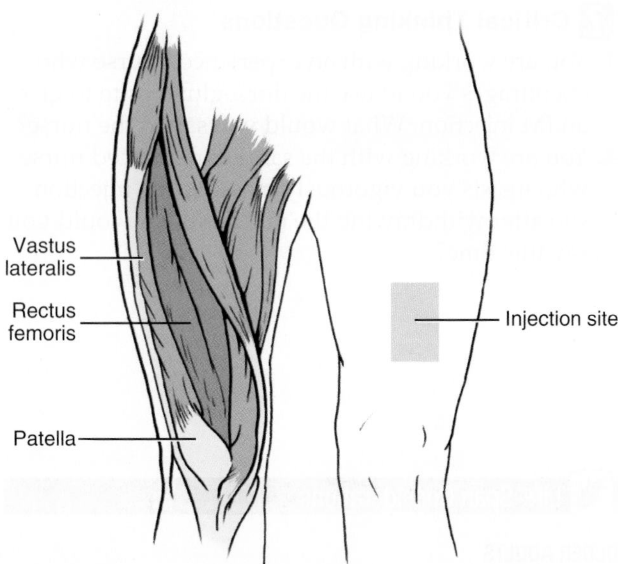

FIGURE 35.22 Locating the rectus femoris IM injection site. *IM,* Intramuscular.

Clinical Cues

IM injections are less painful when the muscle is relaxed. Because the gluteal muscles are tense when the hip is extended or the leg is externally rotated, ask the patient to lie in a prone position with the toes turned inward or to lie in the Sims position.

Intramuscular injections in children. It is preferable to find another way to give medication to children because IM injections are painful and traumatic for the child. Unfortunately, some pediatric immunizations must be given IM. Ways to decrease injection discomfort are listed in Box 35.4.

The needle size and the angle of the injection depend on the size of the infant or child. For infants a ⅝-inch needle is used, whereas for older children a ⅝- or 1-inch needle may be used. The angle is varied depending on the child's size and anatomy; the needle's point must reach the desired area in the muscle. An adult may take a 90-degree angle; a child or smaller person may need a 45-degree angle for the injection.

Box 35.4 Ways to Decrease Injection Discomfort

- For a child, EMLA cream (a mixture of lidocaine and prilocaine, available by prescription) can be applied to the site where the injection will be administered to numb the area. The cream is applied 1 hour before injection time.
- Apply an ice pack for 3 to 5 minutes to numb the skin.
- Use the smallest gauge needle that is appropriate.
- Select a site without signs of inflammation, lesions, or bony prominences and without large underlying vessels or nerves.
- Ask the patient to assume a prone position with the feet turned inward, or the Sims position, to relax the muscles.
- Press down with your thumb over the injection site for 10 seconds to numb it.
- When using alcohol to clean the area, allow it to dry before inserting the needle, to decrease the stinging sensation.
- Ask the patient to deep breathe and try to relax.
- Use the Z-track method for all irritating medications.
- Instruct the patient to look away while the injection is given.
- Insert the needle smoothly and remove it quickly while applying pressure to the skin.
- Inject the medication slowly and steadily.
- Apply light pressure to the site with a gauze pad after withdrawing the needle. Never massage an injection given via Z-track method.
- Encourage active use of the muscle after the injection.

When giving a deltoid injection to a child, give the injection in the thickest part of the muscle; the needle should point at a slight angle toward the shoulder. IM immunizations for children over 13 months of age can be given in the deltoid site, unless the muscle appears poorly developed.

Clinical Cues

The vastus lateralis is the site of choice for infants younger than 12 months, as well as children older than 13 months of age for intramuscular injections. For children older than 13 months of age, you can also use deltoid muscle if it is well developed (Centers for Disease Control and Prevention, 2015).

When giving injections to children, you must assess and understand their level of biophysical and psychosocial development. Knowledge of the various stages of child growth and development enables you to give an appropriate explanation to the child and to provide emotional support before, during, and after the injection. When it is necessary to restrain a child to give the injection safely, you should have someone hold the child. Your manner can help to reassure the child. If the child is old enough to understand, be honest and say, "It will just hurt for a minute." After the injection, talk in a soothing way and cuddle the child to reestablish trust.

Clinical Cues

Playacting is a helpful way of explaining procedures to children in the preschoolage group. You can demonstrate the entire procedure on a doll, indicating the reasons for the injection and the way the doll responds to it, so that the child has an idea of what will happen and how to behave. Give the child an opportunity to look at or handle empty vials or syringes. Explain that the medicine will help him get well and that then he will be able to play.

School-age children want to know how and why things work. Give a clear and simple explanation of why the injection is needed and how it is done. Compliment the child for being good about the discomfort; children thrive on praise and rewards.

Teenagers may avoid expressing their real feelings of anxiety and fear because they are coping with many physical and emotional changes. Many adolescents are extremely modest and self-conscious, so take care to avoid unnecessary exposure of their bodies.

Communication

Communicating With Your Pediatric Patient

Jin Tang is a 5-year-old who has been brought to the clinic by his mother to have immunizations before entering school. He is crying as you enter the room.

Jin: "I don't want a shot! I don't want a shot!"

Nurse: "Jin, hi. My name is Sally and I am a nurse. Sit on your mom's lap and let's talk for a minute."

Jin: "Are you going to give me a shot?"

Nurse: "Right now we are just talking. Can you count numbers?"

Jin: "Yes. I can count really fast. I learned that in preschool."

Nurse: "Can you show me?"

Jin: "1, 2, 3, 4, 5...."

Nurse: "Wow, that was great!" If you count really fast while I give you the medicine, it would help me."

Jin: "I don't want a shot. It hurts."

Nurse: "It does hurt, just a little, but it will be quick if you'll help me. Nurse Janie will help us too. She is going to give you a big hug and you count really fast and then when we are done, your mom will come and give you a bigger hug."

The Z-track technique. With IM injections, medication can leak upward into the subcutaneous tissues, causing staining, bruising, and significant pain for several weeks or longer with some medications. Nurses are encouraged to use the **Z-track technique** (causing a needle track, or pathway, in the shape of a "Z") any time an IM injection is given (Fig. 35.23) (Steps 35.5) to prevent this leakage and associated pain (Hopkins & Arias, 2013). The Z-track technique *must* be used whenever a deep IM injection of iron dextran and other irritating solutions such as hydroxyzine hydrochloride and several antipsychotic agents are given (check the drug insert that comes with the medication).

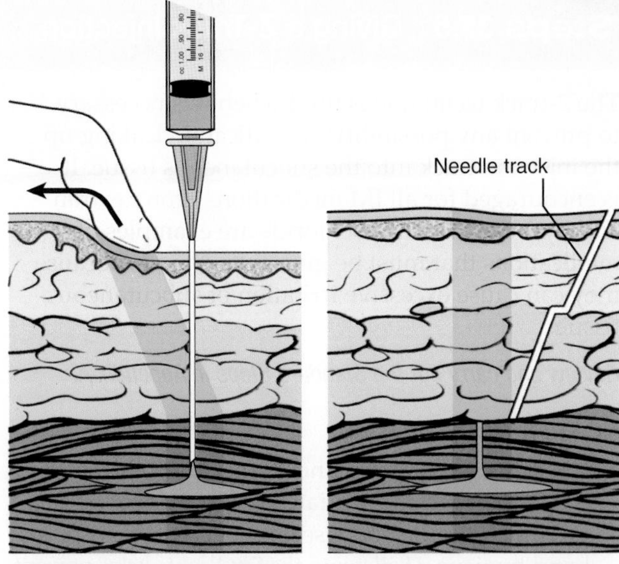

FIGURE 35.23 Z-track technique for IM injection. *IM,* Intramuscular.

Anaphylactic Shock

When an allergen is taken in by a sensitized person, the reaction can range from mild to severe; in fact, death can occur within minutes. Many medications may cause this **anaphylactic** reaction, but parenteral medications present a greater risk because they are absorbed quickly. Symptoms of **anaphylactic shock** (circulatory failure from an allergic reaction) include **urticaria** (a reaction characterized by reddened, slightly elevated patches known as wheals); bronchiolar constriction that manifests as wheezing or difficulty breathing; edema; and, finally, circulatory collapse. Circulatory collapse may occur as the initial symptom. In accordance with National Patient Safety Goals, nurses should be vigilant for changes in patient condition. Oxygen supplementation, cardiopulmonary resuscitation, or the administration of emergency drugs may be necessary.

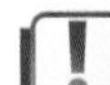

Safety Alert

Watch for Allergic Reactions

Critical nursing responsibilities when administering a parenteral drug are to check for allergy to the drug before administration and to observe the patient for 30 minutes after the drug has been given for the first time.

Steps 35.5 Giving a Z-Track Injection

The Z-track technique is used when it is necessary to prevent any possibility of medication leaking up the injection track into the subcutaneous tissue. It is encouraged for all IM medications. Iron dextran and hydroxyzine hydrochloride are examples of medications that must be given via Z-track, because they can cause excessive irritation of subcutaneous tissue.

Review and carry out the Standard Steps in Appendix A.

ACTION *(RATIONALE)*

1. Check the medication and dosage with the order; obtain the appropriate syringe with at least a 1½-inch needle and a second needle. Perform hand hygiene. *(Following the Six Rights helps prevent medication errors. A 3-inch or longer needle is needed for iron dextran preparations.)*
2. Draw up the correct amount of medication. *(Right dose and right drug.)*
3. Change the needle. *(Medication can adhere to the outside of the shaft and cause irritation to the overlying tissue during the injection.)*
4. Follow the Six Rights, perform hand hygiene, and don gloves. Assess the patient for drug allergy. Using clinical judgment, choose a large muscle injection site. *(Gloves reduce the transfer of microorganisms. Prevention of dangerous allergic reactions is always necessary. A large muscle is better for absorbing medication.)*
5. With the nondominant hand, press the side of the hand down and retract the skin and tissue laterally. Cleanse the site. Insert needle at a 90-degree angle. Maintain this hand position, with traction on the skin until after medication is injected. *(Retracting skin and tissue provides a slanted needle track when the needle enters the tissue; layers of tissue block the needle track after the needle is removed and tissue returns to normal position.)*
6. Slowly inject medication. Wait for 10 seconds before withdrawing needle. *(Injecting medication slowly allows tissue to absorb the medication and prevents untoward bruising. Waiting allows time for the medication to disperse into tissue; this helps prevent medication from traveling back up the needle track.)*
7. Withdraw the needle with a slow movement while releasing the tissue. Gently wipe injection site with alcohol swab. Do not massage site. Use alternate sites for subsequent injections. *(Releasing tissue while withdrawing the needle disrupts the needle track, preventing medication from traveling to skin surface. Massage might force the medication out into the subcutaneous tissue.)*
8. Document the injection was given, including site used and technique. *(The right documentation verifies that the patient received the medication and notes site in case of local reaction.)*

Some allergic reactions may occur for up to 2 weeks after the medication was administered. Allergic reactions are more common the second or successive times the medication is received.

! Safety Alert

Dispose of the Cap; Do Not Contribute to Pressure Sores

As a student nurse, you will be nervous as you give your first several injections. You will feel flush with success and relief after you give the medication and withdraw the needle! Before you walk away to celebrate, double-check that you have not left the cap, a piece of the syringe, or other debris on the bed linens. This foreign material can accidentally work its way underneath the patient and create skin irritation and breakdown.

◆ EVALUATION

Administration of an injection is evaluated in terms of whether it was given properly and whether it achieved its purpose (Table 35.1). For drugs such as antibiotics, if no improvement is seen within 2 to 3 days, notify the primary care provider. Assess for any adverse reaction to the medication, check the injection site for signs of inflammation. Always leave the patient in a safe and comfortable position.

Documentation

Injection documentation should include the medication, the dosage, the route, and the site at which the injection was given. The testing substance is noted for ID injections. Routine injections are recorded on the MAR or eMAR only. The PRN (as needed) and stat doses may also be recorded in the nurse's notes, along with the reason the medication was given and the result and duration of effect of the injection.

Table 35.1 Evaluating the Effectiveness of Injections

The main way to determine the effectiveness of injections is to assess for signs that the desired effect is taking place. This means checking to see whether the signs and symptoms of the problem for which the medication is being given are subsiding, and looking at laboratory test results. Here are some specific examples.

TYPE OF DRUG	EVALUATION CRITERIA
Antibiotic	Temperature is returning to normal. Signs of infection are subsiding: decreased redness, swelling, pain, or tenderness. WBCs are returning to normal.
Antiemetic	Nausea subsides within 30-60 minutes; vomiting is controlled for 3 hours.
Narcotic	Pain subsides within 30-60 minutes and stays under control for 3-4 hours.
Heparin	No signs of new clots are found (e.g., no calf pain or swelling). APTT laboratory values are within therapeutic limits.
Allergy extracts	Allergy symptoms subside: decreased sneezing, stuffy head, and runny nose.
Iron dextran	RBC count, hemoglobin, and hematocrit rise toward normal levels.
Preoperative sedatives	Patient becomes drowsy and more relaxed.

APTT, Activated partial thromboplastin time; *RBC,* red blood cell; *WBC,* white blood cell.

Get Ready for the NCLEX Examination!

Key Points

- Parenteral routes are used when medication cannot be taken by mouth or quick drug action is desired.
- Once injected, medication cannot be retrieved; extreme care regarding dosage and route is essential.
- Improper selection of site may cause nerve, blood vessel, or tissue damage.
- Injections must be prepared and given using aseptic technique to prevent infection.
- The routes for parenteral medication include ID, subcutaneous, and IM.
- The ID route deposits medication into the dermal layer of the skin. A tuberculin syringe is used for ID injections.
- Subcutaneous injections are placed beneath the dermis and above muscle; 0.05 to 1 mL of solution may be injected subcutaneously.
- The angle of injection for a subcutaneous medication depends on the patient's size and the length of the needle used.
- Sites for IM injections include the ventrogluteal, the deltoid, the vastus lateralis, and the rectus femoris. The angle of injection is 90 degrees; the needle length varies depending on the site chosen and the patient's size.
- Three milliliters of solution may be safely injected into the ventrogluteal, the vastus lateralis, and the rectus femoris IM sites in an adult.
- A 2- to 3-mL syringe is usually used for an IM injection with a 1- to 1½-inch needle that is 23 to 20 gauge.
- Medications for injection come packaged in ampules, vials, or individual unit-dose cartridges.
- A filter needle is used to draw medication from an ampule; the needle is changed before administering the injection.
- The larger the number of the needle gauge, the smaller the needle and the finer the cannula.
- The selection of a gauge of needle depends on the viscosity of the fluid to be injected and the route of administration.
- A needle stick from a used needle may transmit HIV or hepatitis B or C virus. Needles are not recapped after use, but are immediately dropped into a sharps biohazard container.
- Use safety needle devices.
- For two medications to be mixed, they must be compatible. Consult drug inserts, drug handbooks, or the pharmacist regarding the route and compatibility of drugs being administered concurrently.
- Assessment before administering an injection includes (1) checking for allergies to the medication; (2) verifying the drug, the dose, the route, the time, the expiration date, and patient identification; (3) determining why the patient is receiving the drug; and (4) checking for possible drug interactions with other prescribed and over-the-counter drugs. Use the Six Rights of medication administration.
- When a repeat injection of a drug is given, assess for side effects of the drug, previous site condition, and evidence of therapeutic effect before administration of the dose.
- ID injections are used for allergy testing and the administration of the TST.
- Rotation of sites for medications, such as heparin and insulin, prevents fibrosis of the tissue.
- The vastus lateralis site is the preferred site for IM injection in infants under the age of 12 months.
- The ventrogluteal IM injection site is the safest site to use in the adult.
- A Z-track technique is encouraged with all IM injections, but must be used with particularly irritating medications to decrease pain and bruising by sealing the drug in the muscle tissue.
- Injected medications are capable of causing anaphylactic shock. Symptoms of an anaphylactic reaction are urticaria, bronchiolar constriction, edema, and circulatory collapse. Cardiopulmonary resuscitation and the administration of emergency drugs may be necessary.
- Each injection is documented on the MAR or eMAR; PRN medications and their effect may also be documented in the nurse's notes.

Additional Learning Resources

SG Go to your Study Guide for additional learning activities to help you master this chapter content.

evolve Go to your Evolve website at http://evolve.elsevier.com/Williams/fundamental for additional online resources.

Review Questions for the NCLEX Examination

*Choose the **best** answer for each question.*

1. The nurse is preparing to give an average-size adult patient an IM injection of 3 mL of viscous medication. Which equipment should the nurse use?
   1. A 3-mL syringe with a 25-gauge 1-inch needle
   2. A 5-mL syringe with a 20-gauge 1½-inch needle
   3. A 10-mL syringe with a 25-gauge 1½-inch needle
   4. A 3-mL syringe with an 18-gauge 2-inch needle
2. During an IM injection, the patient moves as the nurse is withdrawing the needle and the nurse accidentally sustains a needle stick injury. What is the priority action?
   1. Check the patient's medical record for a diagnosis of HIV or hepatitis.
   2. Call the infection control nurse and ask for advice.
   3. Scrub the needle stick site with warm water and soap.
   4. Report immediately to the emergency department for treatment.
3. The nurse is supervising a nursing student who is trying to withdraw 2 mL of medication from an ampule. The nurse would intervene if the student performed which action?
   1. Wraps the neck of the ampule with an alcohol swab
   2. Draws up 2 mL of air into the syringe to insert in the ampule
   3. Taps the stem of ampule to dislodge medication that is trapped in the stem
   4. Inserts a filter needle into the ampule below the surface of the fluid
4. A patient needs an ID injection for a TST, but he currently has bilateral forearm casts in place. What is the best alternative site?
   1. Abdomen
   2. Lateral upper arm
   3. Medial upper thigh
   4. Antecubital space
5. The nurse must give an injection to a 7-year-old. What actions should the nurse use to prepare the child? *(Select all that apply.)*
   1. Obtain a helper and swaddle the child in a snug blanket.
   2. Allow the child to hold and examine a demonstration syringe.
   3. Give a brief explanation of what will happen.
   4. Instruct the child on a distraction task that he can do during the procedure.
   5. Promise a reward for good behavior.
6. When the nurse is preparing a parenteral injection, medical asepsis is permissible for handling the:
   1. Shaft of the plunger.
   2. Needle shaft and tip.
   3. Barrel of the syringe.
   4. Solution in the vial.
7. The nurse must give an IM injection to an 8-month-old. Which injection site is the best choice for this patient?
   1. Dorsogluteal
   2. Vastus lateralis
   3. Deltoid
   4. Ventrogluteal

Critical Thinking Activities

Read each clinical scenario and discuss the questions with your classmates.

Scenario A
You have an order to administer an IM injection to Mrs. Sorenson, who is a petite older adult. Discuss special considerations when giving IM injections to older adults.

Scenario B
You administer an antibiotic as ordered via IM injection. Within 10 minutes, the patient complains of feeling peculiar and short of breath. What would you do?

Scenario C
Jacob Giovanni, age 5, has come to the clinic with his mother to get the immunizations he will need to enter kindergarten. He is calm but appears scared. You must give him four injections. How would you handle the situation and interact with Jacob?

Scenario D
You must administer a morning dose of insulin to a patient, but this is the first time you have had the opportunity to give an injection to an actual patient.

1. What strategies can you use to overcome your own anxieties about performing this procedure for the first time?
2. What information will you seek before telling your instructor that you are ready to prepare the dose?

chapter 36

Administering Intravenous Solutions and Medications

http://evolve.elsevier.com/Williams/fundamental

Objectives

Upon completing this chapter, you should be able to do the following:

Theory

1. Identify four purposes for administering intravenous (IV) therapy.
2. Evaluate the advantages and disadvantages of using an infusion pump to deliver fluids or medications.
3. List three possible complications that can arise from the use of the IV route and the corrective actions you should take for each one.
4. State at least seven guidelines related to IV therapy of fluids or medications.
5. Summarize special considerations for older adults who need IV therapy.
6. Recognize the signs and symptoms of a blood transfusion reaction, and describe the steps you should take if one occurs.

Clinical Practice

1. Prepare to give medications using each of the following methods:
   a. Using an infusion pump to deliver a primary infusion.
   b. Using an infusion pump to deliver an IV piggyback.
   c. Using a controlled-volume device.
   d. Using an intermittent IV or a PRN (as needed) lock.
   e. Giving the medication as a bolus.
2. Devise a care plan with patient-specific data for a patient who needs IV fluid therapy.
3. Calculate the IV fluid flow rate from various IV orders.
4. Initiate IV therapy by performing venipuncture with an IV cannula (catheter over the stylet), using aseptic technique, and starting the ordered infusion.
5. Add a new bag of fluid to replace one from which the solution has infused.
6. Discontinue an IV infusion and evaluate the site and surrounding tissue.
7. Safely monitor a patient receiving a blood transfusion; document your actions and the patient's response to therapy.
8. Collect data on a patient who is receiving total parenteral nutrition; document your findings and the patient's response to therapy.

Skills & Steps

Skills

Steps

Key Terms

autologous (ăw-TŎL-ŏ-gŭs, p. 728)
bolus (p. 704)
bore (p. 712)
burette (bŭ-RĔT, p. 705)
catheter embolus (KĂ-thĕ-tĕr ĔM-bō-lŭs, p. 709)
epidural (p. 709)
extravasation (p. 709)
hypertonic (hī-pĕr-TŎN-ĭk, p. 702)
hypotonic (hī-pō-TŎN-ĭk, p. 702)
infiltrated (ĬN-fĭl-trā-tĭd, p. 706)
infusion (p. 700)
infusion pump (p. 704)
insulin pump (p. 707)
intrathecal (p. 709)
intravenous (IV) (p. 700)
isotonic (ī-sō-TŎN-ĭk, p. 700)

Key Terms—Cont'd

macrodrops (p. 703)
microdrops (p. 703)
"scrub the hub" (p. 704)
total parenteral nutrition (TPN) (p. 705)
transfusion (trănz-FŪ-shŭn, p. 704)
vascular access devices (VĂS-kū-lăr, p. 708)
vesicant (p. 709)
viscous (VĬS-kŭs, p. 703)

Concepts Covered in This Chapter

- Clinical judgment
- Evidence
- Patient education
- Safety
- Tissue integrity

INTRAVENOUS THERAPY

The **intravenous (IV)** route is the primary method of supplying the patient with fluids and medications via the veins when the patient cannot take them orally. The IV route has the advantage of making drugs or fluid instantly available for circulation to all tissues. The disadvantage is that, if an error is made, adverse effects will occur more rapidly. IV **infusion** (slow introduction of fluid into a vein) can be used to maintain hydration. IV bolus can be used to treat dehydration rapidly.

IVs are given to supply the body with fluids, electrolytes, nutritional components, or drugs. Examples of substances delivered by the IV route include:

- Fluids and electrolytes that the patient is unable to take orally in sufficient amounts.
- Medications that are more effective when given by this route or cannot be given any other way.
- Blood, plasma, or other blood components.
- Nutritional formulas containing glucose, amino acids, and lipids.

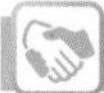

Community Considerations

Intravenous Vitamin Fad

A recent health fad is taking vitamin supplements via the IV route, and specialized health clinics and health spas are offering this rather expensive treatment (Kirkey, 2015). However, it has not been proven more effective than taking oral vitamins or eating fruits and veggies.

The average adult needs 1500 to 2000 mL of fluids in a 24-hour period to replace fluids eliminated by the body. Some patients have decreased fluid intake. Others experience fluid loss through hemorrhage, severe or prolonged vomiting or diarrhea (Nursing Care Plan 36.1), profuse perspiration, and moderate to excessive drainage from wounds, especially from burn wounds. Fluid balance is also affected by increased metabolic processes, for example, during a fever. Accurate recording of the patient's intake and output (I & O) is needed to determine the amount of fluids necessary for daily replacement. The primary care provider considers laboratory tests related to electrolytes when ordering replacements such as sodium, potassium, and chloride.

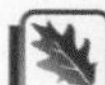

Life-Span Considerations

Older Adults

Monitor electrolyte levels closely; fluid therapy can rapidly change the fluid and electrolyte balance.

LICENSED PRACTICAL NURSE/LICENSED VOCATIONAL NURSE'S ROLE IN INTRAVENOUS THERAPY

All nurses must monitor IV therapy. Patients who require fluids by the IV method are placed on I & O recording to monitor for fluid overload. In some states the nurse practice act and facility policy allow practical nurses to hang IV piggyback medications, add medications to IV solutions, calculate IV infusion rates, insert peripheral catheters, and teach patients about IV therapy. Often an extra course is required for certification for the licensed practical nurse/licensed vocational nurse (LPN/LVN) to perform IV therapy and to start IVs.

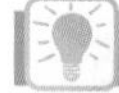

QSEN Considerations: Safety

Can I Administer IV Medications?

Check your state's nurse practice act to determine whether an IV certification is necessary to administer IV medications. In some states, LPN/LVNs are not allowed to perform IV therapy.

Think Critically

In accordance with *Healthy People 2020*, all health care professionals should be educating patients about their medications. What might cause a nurse to neglect or forget to educate the patient about IV medications?

TYPES OF INTRAVENOUS SOLUTION

The primary care provider orders the type of solution to be given, the amount to be infused, and the rate of infusion (as either the number of hours for the solution to infuse or the volume per hour). Many types of solutions are available, and still others can be prepared to meet a patient's specific needs. The solutions most frequently used are those containing glucose, saline, electrolytes, vitamins, and amino acids. Blood and blood products are also given intravenously. Table 36.1 lists common IV solutions.

IV solutions are isotonic, hypotonic, or hypertonic. **Isotonic** solutions have the same concentration, or osmolality, as blood and are used to expand the body's fluid volume (see Table 36.1). When exposed to isotonic

Nursing Care Plan 36.1 Care of the Patient With Deficient Fluid Volume and Hyponatremia

SCENARIO Jane Weston, age 78, is transferred from a local long-term care facility. She reports "flu" with nausea and vomiting and poor intake. Dehydration is noted. There is a question as to whether she has suffered a small stroke or is just dehydrated and has consequent electrolyte imbalance. She is receiving D_5 ½NS IV solution and is being encouraged to eat and drink. (Dehydration may increase the viscosity of the blood, which can lead to clotting in susceptible individuals.)

PROBLEM/NURSING DIAGNOSIS *Vomiting, not eating, dehydrated*/Deficient fluid volume related to nausea, vomiting, and lack of oral intake.

Supporting Assessment Data *Subjective:* "I've been so nauseated. I don't want to eat." *Objective:* Tongue dry and furrowed; 4-lb weight loss; poor skin turgor, scanty urine output.

Goals/Expected Outcomes	Nursing Interventions	Selected Rationale	Evaluation
Patient will be adequately hydrated within 2 days as evidenced by weight gain, normal condition of mucous membranes, and normal urine output.	Give IV solution at 125 mL/h as ordered.	IV solution will rehydrate patient.	*How is the patient responding to therapy?* IV fluids infusing at 125 mL/h. No redness, swelling or pain at the site. Membranes moist.
	Check laboratory values of electrolytes.	Provides data as to whether imbalances are improving.	Laboratory results pending.
	Assess the lungs for signs of crackles indicating fluid overload.	Crackles in lungs may indicate fluid overload from IV infusions.	Lung sounds clear. No crackles auscultated.
	Perform neurologic assessment q 4 h.	Imbalance of fluids and electrolytes will affect mental status. Additionally, possible cerebral edema from fluid overload or stroke in progress is relevant for this patient.	Oriented to person and place, unsure about date. Able to follow commands. Speech clear and appropriate.
	Encourage oral fluids, including sodas containing sodium.	Fluids with sodium help return the sodium level to normal and rehydrate.	Likes soda and asks for chicken broth.
	Give small amounts of fluids q 30 to 60 min. Assist to drink fluids.	Encourages gradual return to oral intake; helps with rehydration.	Taking 7 to 10 small sips of soda q 30 to 60 min.
	Encourage oral intake as nausea subsides.	The patient is more likely to resume oral intake once nausea is relieved.	Currently denies nausea. Will take fluid with coaching; needs reminders.
	Determine what the patient would like to eat.	Preferred foods may appeal to flagging appetite.	Continues to refuse offers of food.
	Initiate I & O recording.	Comparison of input versus output provides information to assess fluid balance.	Intake this shift 1230 mL.
	Watch urine output closely. Report greater than 30 mL/h output to primary care provider.	Decreasing urine flow may indicate or contribute to kidney failure.	Output: 600 mL of clear, dark yellow urine.
	Turn at least q 2 h. Assess pressure areas each time patient is turned.	Dehydration makes skin more vulnerable to pressure areas and pressure injuries. Turning relieves pressure over bony prominences.	Skin intact. Coached and assisted to turn q 2 h. Progressing toward expected outcomes. Continue plan.

CRITICAL THINKING QUESTIONS

1. What are some issues that you must consider when older adult patients need IV therapy?
2. Ms. Weston complains about the IV. What assessments should you perform?

I & O, Intake and output; *IV*, intravenous.

Table 36.1 Common Intravenous Therapy Solutions, Tonicity, and Examples of Clinical Use

SOLUTION	TONICITY	EXAMPLES OF CLINICAL USE
0.9% Saline	Isotonic	Trauma, diabetic ketoacidosis, blood transfusions, and hyponatremia
0.45% Saline	Hypotonic	Supplies normal daily salt and water requirements
5% Dextrose in water	Isotonic	Vehicle for some IV piggyback medications; hyperkalemia
10% Dextrose in water	Hypertonic	if TPN is abruptly discontinued
5% Dextrose in 0.9% saline	Hypertonic	Early treatment of burns
5% Dextrose in 0.45% saline	Hypertonic	Postoperative; common maintenance fluid
5% Dextrose in 0.225% saline	Isotonic	Postoperative; common maintenance fluid
Ringer lactate	Isotonic	Trauma, dehydration from severe diarrhea or vomiting
5% Dextrose in Ringer lactate	Hypertonic	Burns; dehydration from severe diarrhea or vomiting

IV, Intravenous; *TPN*, total parenteral nutrition.

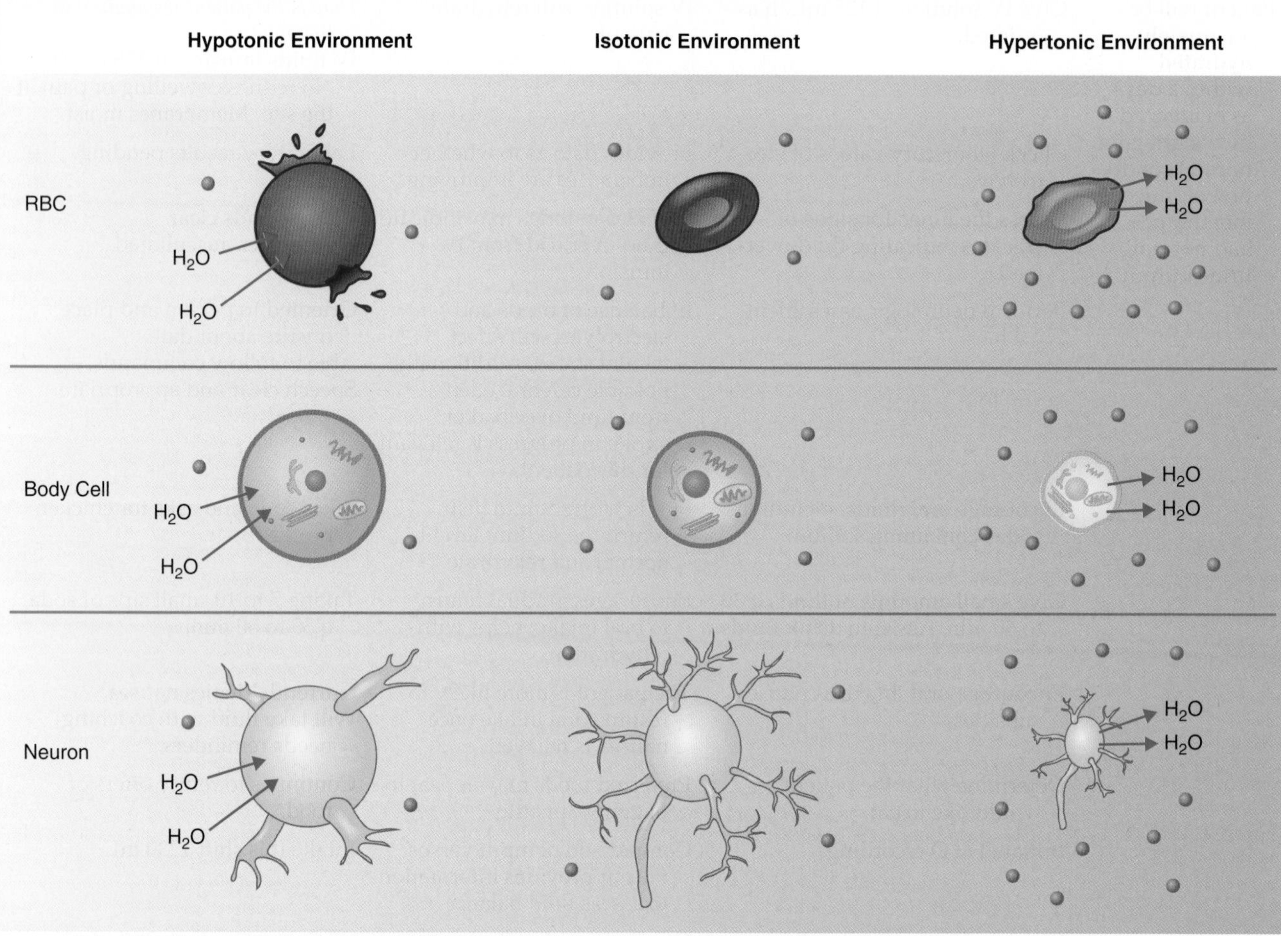

FIGURE 36.1 Hypotonic, isotonic, and hypertonic solutions.

solutions body cells stay approximately the same size. **Hypotonic** solutions contain less solute than extravascular fluid and may cause fluid to shift out of the vascular compartment and into the cells. This can cause a dangerous situation, as cells can rupture (Fig. 36.1). Hypotonic solutions are generally considered unsafe to administer to children (Beck et al., 2013). **Hypertonic** solutions have a greater tonicity compared with blood. They are used to replace electrolytes and, when given as concentrated dextrose solutions, produce a shift in fluid from the intracellular compartment to the extracellular compartment, causing shrinkage of cells (see Fig. 36.1). Concentrated solutions of glucose, mannitol, or sucrose are given to reduce cerebral edema in patients with head injury because the osmotic pressure draws water out of the cells, whereas hypotonic solutions would not be given because the potential fluid shifting could exacerbate cerebral edema (Rangel-Castilla, 2014).

? Think Critically

You are caring for a postoperative patient who had a routine and uncomplicated surgery. Which type of IV solution (isotonic, hypotonic, or hypertonic) is the primary care provider most likely to order for this patient? Why?

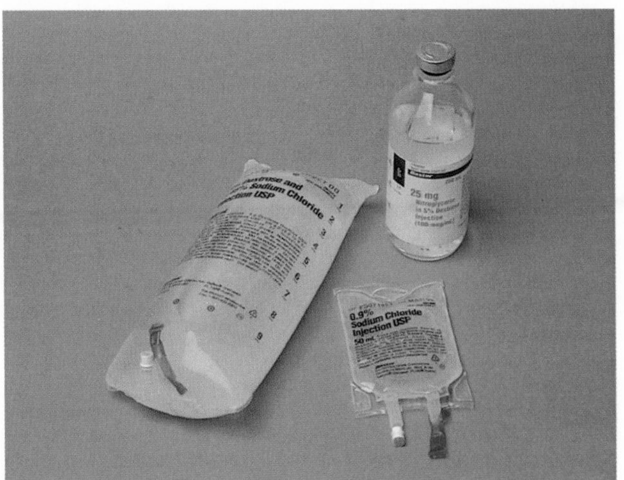

FIGURE 36.2 Intravenous solution containers.

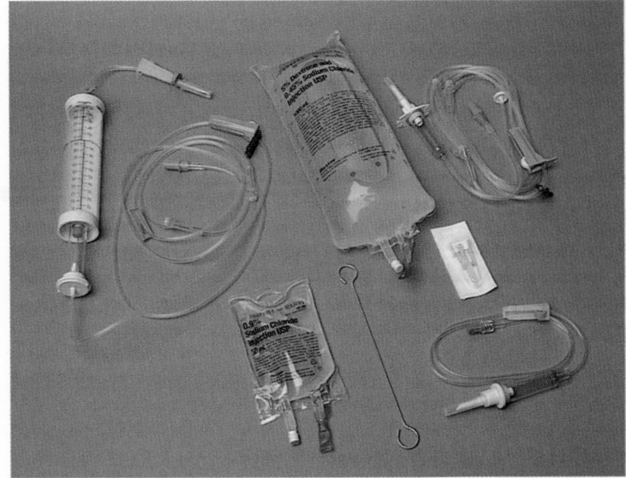

FIGURE 36.3 Intravenous fluid and medication administration sets.

Solutions that are given intravenously must be sterile. They are supplied in plastic bags of 250-, 500-, and 1000-mL amounts. Smaller bags of sterile water, dextrose in water, and normal saline are used to dissolve or dilute various drugs for parenteral use. Glass bottles are occasionally used for a few solutions and some IV drugs. Check the expiration date and inspect the container for clarity of solution; the solution should be clear.

The typical IV bag (Fig. 36.2) has calibrations along the sides for approximating the amount of fluid left in the bag. A plastic cover on the tubing port is pulled off for insertion of the tubing spike. A plastic or foil tab is removed to access the medication port. The top of the bag has a tab for hanging on an IV pole.

The IV bottle is also marked with calibrations on the side. The flat metal or plastic cover on the top of the bottle is pulled off to expose a rubber stopper or diaphragm held in place by a metal rim. The diaphragm is removed, revealing a rubber stopper with an outlet vent for insertion of the IV tubing, and an inlet for adding medications. Some IV bottles contain a tube that acts automatically as an air vent; for others, a vented tubing set must be used to let air in.

EQUIPMENT FOR INTRAVENOUS ADMINISTRATION

ADMINISTRATION SETS

Many different types of administration sets are available, some of which are specific for the type of IV solution, container, or IV pump (Fig. 36.3). Administration sets can be classified as (1) primary IV sets; (2) secondary, or piggyback, IV sets; (3) parallel, or Y, IV sets; and (4) controlled-volume IV sets. As long as the patient is not receiving blood, blood products, fat emulsions, or propofol infusion, change IV tubing no more frequently than every 96 hours but at least every 7 days for infection control purposes. Check agency policy for frequency of tubing change, and properly label tubing with the date and time (Centers for Disease Control and Prevention, 2011).

Solutions can also be given intermittently through an intermittent IV device. Filters are recommended for the infusion of many solutions (check agency policy on filter use).

Primary Intravenous Set

The primary IV infusion setup consists of a bag of solution, a regular tubing set, a needleless connector, and an IV stand. A filter may be added. The IV tubing set consists of the spike end, which is inserted into the bag; the drip chamber; the tubing; a flow regulator or clamp; and a Luer-Lok connector. The spike and the connector at the ends of the tubing are covered with plastic protectors to maintain sterility. The primary line usually has one or two injection ports. The primary IV infusion setup is used for any type of IV therapy except the administration of blood products, which requires a special set with a filter in the drip chamber. Several different brands of IV administration tubing sets are on the market; check the directions for the type used in your agency.

? Think Critically

How would the diameter and length of IV equipment, such as tubing and catheters, affect the flow of fluid?

The primary IV tubing set, used in gravity delivery, is sized by the number of drops per milliliter (gtt/mL) to be delivered into the drip chamber. There are three major sizes:

1. Regular drops (10 to 20 gtt/mL of fluid as specified by the manufacturer), used for administering IV therapy to most adult patients.
2. **Macrodrops** (10 to 15 gtt/mL), used for **viscous** (sticky or thick) fluids, such as blood; may be used for regular fluids.
3. **Microdrops** (60 gtt/mL), used when small amounts of fluid are required or when extreme care must be used to measure the exact amount; most often used for giving IV fluids to infants and children; recommended for older adults with fragile veins.

If you are using an infusion pump, you must use primary tubing that is designed to fit the pump. Manufacturer design varies greatly, and the tubing is not interchangeable among different equipment; however, all types of tubing have the familiar roller clamp, which allows for manual control in the event of equipment or power failure.

Think Critically

Why is the microdrop set safer for pediatric patients? Can you identify other types of patients or health conditions for which a microdrop set would be a good choice?

Secondary, or Piggyback, Intravenous Set

Medications to be given intravenously are often added to an existing IV line by using the piggyback method. When this is used, the primary infusion is interrupted to infuse medications such as antibiotics and antineoplastic drugs at regularly scheduled times. These drugs are diluted in 50 to 150 mL of solution and given by infusion, not by **bolus** (small dose of medication administered IV). The secondary bag containing the medication, also known as the piggyback, is hung higher than the level of fluid in the primary IV so that gravity forces it to empty first. Do not clamp or alter the flow of the primary bag. **If the secondary bag is positioned correctly, the primary IV will begin to flow as soon as the secondary bag is finished.**

Clinical Cues

"Scrub the hub" is a slogan that was developed to emphasize the importance of using a sterile alcohol pad to scrub the injection port with friction for at least 15 seconds when accessing a central line injection port or IV connection. Exceed the standard of care by scrubbing the hub when accessing a peripheral IV line.

The prevention of needle sticks, which may transmit HIV, hepatitis B virus, hepatitis C virus, or other infectious diseases, is important for your safety and that of your patients and co-workers. Use of needleless devices for attaching secondary tubing for the infusion of medication is highly recommended to prevent injury and exposure to these diseases (Fig. 36.4).

Parallel, or Y, Intravenous Set

A Y-type administration set is used to infuse certain blood products (Fig. 36.5). The blood product is placed on one side, and a bag of normal saline is placed on the other side. The saline is started first, and then the blood administration is begun. The saline is stopped while the blood is running. **Blood products are never infused into the same IV line as medications or other fluids.** When the **transfusion** (introduction of blood components into the bloodstream) is complete, the tubing is flushed with the normal saline solution.

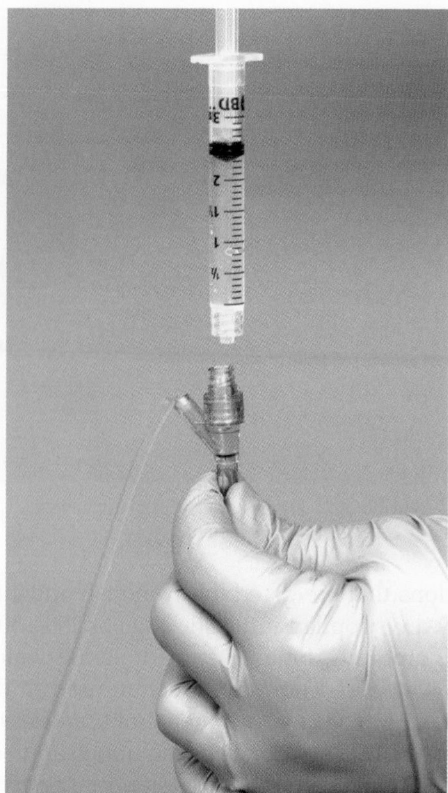

FIGURE 36.4 Luer-Lok needleless intravenous syringe and port.

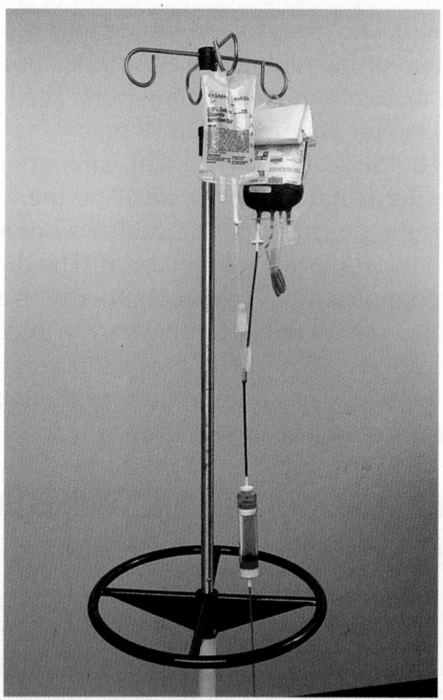

FIGURE 36.5 Y-type blood administration setup.

Controlled-Volume Intravenous Set

A dose of diluted medication can also be given through a controlled-volume administration set. In most cases, an **infusion pump** (a machine that delivers IV fluids at a rate that is set by the nurse) is used to administer fluid or medication. However, the controlled-volume system is sometimes used as a safety

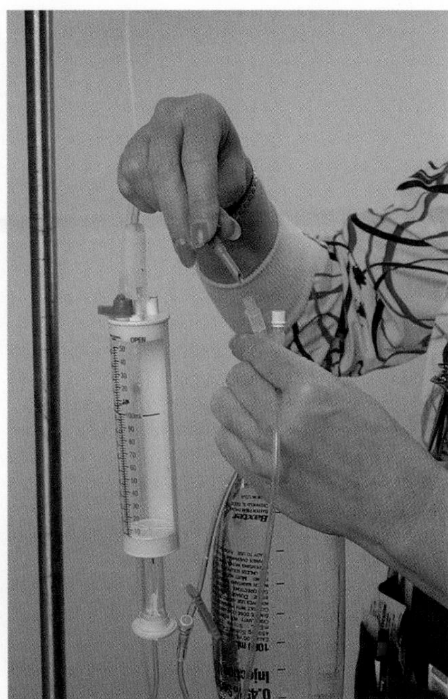

FIGURE 36.6 Controlled-volume set.

backup between the primary IV bag and the entry to the infusion pump to prevent free flow of fluid. The set contains a **burette** (tube-like chamber that holds 150 mL of fluid) (Fig. 36.6) into which the medication is injected along with a specified volume of fluid from the primary bag, which is then clamped off. When an IV infusion pump is not used, the medication from the burette goes into the drip chamber, and the roller clamp on the IV tubing is used to regulate the flow. This set can also be used when a small amount of fluid is to be infused over a long period. It can be used for administration of fluids to infants, children, and older adults. Using a controlled-volume set decreases likelihood of fluid overload because only a specified amount of fluid (e.g., 50 to 100 mL) is available to be infused at any one time.

Clinical Cues

Patients who receive IV fluids must be observed for signs of fluid overload, such as sudden weight gain, crackles in lungs on auscultation, and peripheral edema. The LPN/LVN must accurately record I & O and report changes, observe for subtle changes in urinary patterns, and monitor laboratory results, including: electrolytes, BUN, and serum creatinine.

Intermittent Intravenous Device (Saline or PRN Lock)

Some patients do not require fluid by the IV route but may need to receive IV medications at intervals or have an IV access in case emergency medications are needed. An intermittent access device is preferred for patients who receive intermittent antibiotics, heparin, corticosteroids, antimetabolites, and other IV push drugs. One advantage of the saline lock is the freedom of movement for the patient. Because no solution is continuously infusing through the lock, saline or dilute heparin is used to flush the device to maintain patency by keeping a clot from forming at the tip of the catheter. Follow the facility's policy as to the type, amount, and frequency used to flush the device. The device is established by applying a Luer-Lok cap or an extension set, which is a short piece of tubing, to the IV cannula. The peripheral device is referred to as a saline lock, PRN lock, or intermittent lock (Fig. 36.7).

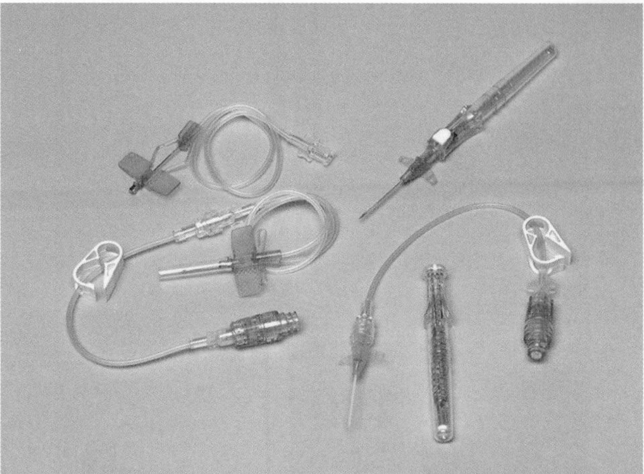

FIGURE 36.7 Intermittent intravenous device (i.e., PRN lock).

Safety Alert

Flushing the Lock

Most locks are flushed with saline, but rarely the lock will be flushed with a dilute heparin solution, NOT the higher concentration used as a medication. This heparin solution may be in multiple-dose vials (not recommended for neonates to whom the preservative can be toxic) or prefilled syringes. It is critically important to be sure you are using the correct concentration of heparin, because a mistake can result in patient death. For this reason, most units "lock" the locks with saline rather than heparin.

Filters

Filters trap small particles such as undissolved medication or salts that have precipitated from solution. They prevent such particles from entering the vein. A 0.22-micron filter is used for most solutions. For solutions containing lipids or albumin, a 1.2-micron filter is used. A special filter is needed for blood components.

INFUSION PUMPS AND CONTROLLERS

Use of infusion pumps is an added safety measure. Many facilities require use of pumps to regulate the flow of routine IV fluids, especially those containing potassium. The latest infusion pumps are also referred to as Smart Pumps because they contain robust and sophisticated drug libraries that nurses are able to use to prevent medication errors from occurring.

Use of pumps is mandatory when patients are receiving **total parenteral nutrition (TPN)** (technique of providing needed nutrition intravenously) or for medications

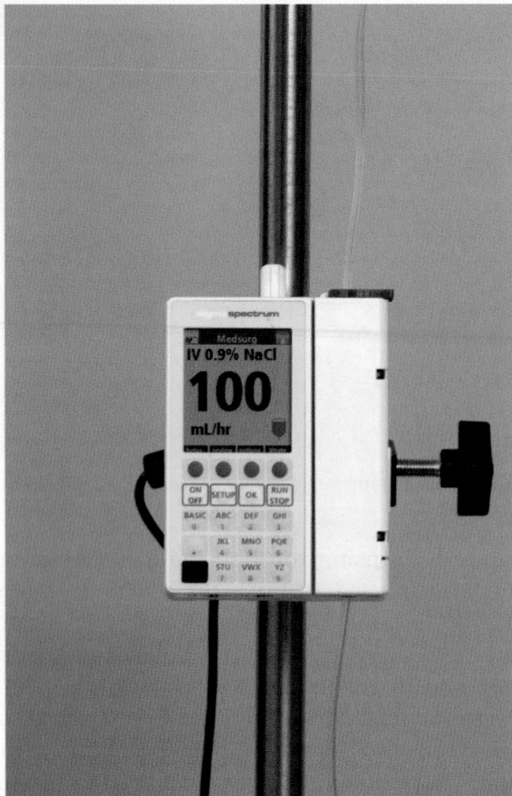

FIGURE 36.8 Intravenous infusion pump.

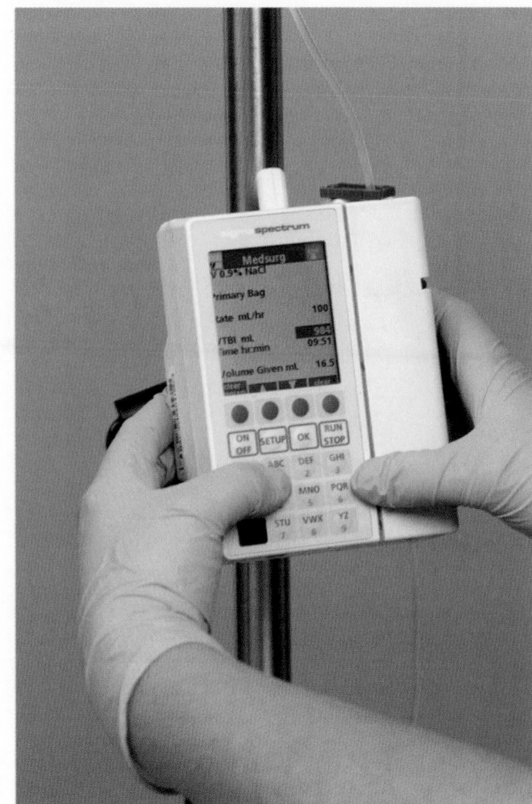

FIGURE 36.9 Setting the rate and volume on the infusion pump.

that require critical accuracy, such as heparin, insulin, cardiovascular medications, chemotherapy drugs, or medications that are used to induce labor (Fig. 36.8).

Clinical Cues

Potassium is always diluted in fluid and given as a carefully controlled infusion. **Potassium is never given as a bolus because it can cause cardiac arrest.**

Programmed infusion pumps are more accurate and provide better control over the amount of solution being infused. These pumps deliver IV fluids automatically at a rate that is programmed by the nurse (Fig. 36.9). They have alarms that warn when the IV container is empty, when air is present in the tubing, or when there is an occlusion. They also alarm when the site is **infiltrated** (solution is deposited in tissue outside the vein); however, the infiltration can be extensive before the machine detects an obstruction of flow. You must have additional training before you attempt to use infusion pump equipment, and remember a pump is never a substitute for good nursing observation.

Patient Education

SILENCE ALARM BUTTON

The patient or family may observe the nursing staff using the silence alarm button, and they may push the button in an attempt "to help the nurse." Teach them to call for assistance. Reassure them that you will quickly respond to the alarms.

Disadvantages of pumps include expense and special administration sets. There have also been incidents of pump failure. Health care facilities should purchase infusion pumps that have administration sets with set-based anti–free-flow mechanisms that prevent gravity free flow by closing off the tubing when the administration set is removed from the pump. Other pumps must have a free-flow safety device attached to the tubing before it enters the pump. The US Food and Drug Administration (FDA, 2015) advises clinicians to consider the following strategies to help reduce risk to patients.

- Plan: have a backup plan in the event of pump failure; participate in educational opportunities relating to the facility's smart pump; use a secondary device to check the expected volume infused.
- Label: clearly label tubing and pump channels with the name of the medication infusing, especially if multiple lines are running.
- Check: verify pump settings; have another nurse double-check your settings when infusing high-risk medications. Monitor: carefully watch patients for signs of overinfusion or underinfusion.
- Use: consult with super-users for additional assistance and training, use available resources to prevent and respond to pump problems, and follow the Six Rights for medication administration.
- Report: promptly report adverse events to the FDA; remove any equipment that is not working properly.

Box 36.1 Intravenous Pumps: Tips for Use and Troubleshooting

- IV pumps vary greatly by manufacturer; obtain assistance as needed to learn the specific features.
- Check the medication, calculate the correct dosage, and determine the pump setting before entering the patient's room (see Box 36.2).
- For adult usage, most pumps measure delivery rate in milliliters per hour. Set the pump for the correct rate in milliliters per hour.
- Pumps usually allow you to set a total volume; the machine will alarm when it reaches that volume. (Use this feature to call you back at the end of the infusion, or sooner as needed.)
- Before you leave the room, check to ensure that the patient is comfortable, there is no swelling at the insertion site, appropriate clamps are open, and intermittent dripping (not continuous) is occurring in the drip chamber.
- Pumps can malfunction; assessing the site and equipment every 1 to 2 hours is a typical policy.
- **If the IV pump is continually alarming:** Check the IV site for infiltration, pain, and other signs of infiltration. Check tubing for kinks or air in the line. Check clamps and flow regulators. Check IV bag to see whether there is fluid for infusion. Make certain the pump is plugged into an electrical source. Recheck settings on the pump. Change the position of the patient's extremity. Try turning the pump off and resetting it. Try another pump.

IV, intravenous.

Some pumps can handle multiple infusion lines and can be programmed separately for each line. Box 36.1 includes tips for using an IV pump.

Think Critically

Your patient needs an IV infusion and you are unable to find an IV pump. You have called central supply and several other units and were told that no pumps are available at this time. It is the facility policy that an IV pump should always be used. What will you do?

Patient-controlled analgesia (PCA) pumps are commonly used in both hospitals and home settings. This pump is used for pain control, and it has a remote-control button by which the patient can administer a controlled bolus of pain medication. The pump is programmed to allow a set amount at specified intervals.

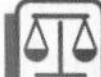

Legal and Ethical Considerations

The American Society for Pain Management Nursing supports the use of authorized agent-controlled analgesia, where a nurse or caregiver is authorized (under specific guidelines) to activate delivery of analgesic medication for a patient who is unable to self-administer pain medication via the PCA pump. This is based on the ethical principle of beneficence, to provide comfort to those who are unable to act on their own behalf.

A mini-infusion pump (also known as syringe pump) uses an ordinary syringe to deliver very small amounts of medication or fluid in a controlled time. These are used more frequently on pediatric units.

The **insulin pump** is another small, self-contained pump device used to deliver doses of the hormone insulin. The insulin pump is a small portable device that can be programmed to deliver a continuous infusion of regular insulin that mimics normal physiology. The patient must be highly motivated and capable of changing the insertion site every 2 or 3 days, refilling the pump with insulin, reprogramming the device, checking blood glucose four to six times per day, and monitoring for signs of infection.

VENOUS ACCESS DEVICES

Intravenous Needles and Catheters

Safety venous access devices decrease the risk of accidental needle sticks. These devices have either a stylet that retracts into a closed sleeve or a plastic sleeve that advances over the stylet as it is removed from the skin. Venous access devices come in many different sizes called gauges; the smaller the size needed, the larger the gauge number. For instance, a 24-gauge needle is very small, and would be used for an older adult with very small veins. An 18-gauge needle delivers larger volumes of fluid, and would be placed in a trauma patient upon arrival to the ED for rapid transfusion of blood or fluids. When using the scalp veins of infants, finer-gauge needles must be used. The nurse must determine the appropriate gauge needed based on both how it will be used and the size of a suitable vein. For clear aqueous solutions, a 20- to 22-gauge needle is used, but for viscous fluids, blood products, or rapid administration of large amounts of fluid, a larger (18- or 19-gauge) needle or catheter is needed.

Two basic types of IV needles and catheters are used for peripheral IV fluid administration. The winged-tip or butterfly needle is meant for short-term therapy, such as to give single-dose IV medication or to obtain blood samples. After insertion, the wings are taped to the skin. These needles are supplied in odd-numbered gauges (17, 19, 23, and 25). The butterfly needle is also frequently used for pediatric or older adult patients (because of the smaller gauges for use in smaller vessels). These needles are rigid and may cause more discomfort than other needles. Mobility must be restricted to prevent dislodgement of the needle.

Over-the-needle catheters consist of a needle with a catheter sheath over it. After the device is placed into the vein and the cannula (catheter sheath) is threaded, the needle is removed, leaving the flexible catheter in the vein. Catheters of this type are thought to cause less irritation, thereby decreasing the incidence of infection and phlebitis.

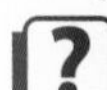 Clinical Cues

Peripheral catheters are typically replaced every 72 hours (Centers for Disease Control and Prevention, 2011). Facility policy may dictate that catheters that are inserted in the emergency department or in the field by paramedics be replaced sooner.

Although an arm board may be used to support and immobilize the arm during IV therapy, this is not desirable because the patient's elbow or wrist movement may be severely restricted, causing discomfort. Newer ergonomic armboards can be safer and potentially reduce risks of injury (IV House, 2016).

? Think Critically

What special care do you think is needed when the patient's IV site is secured with an arm board?

Central Venous Catheters and Peripherally Inserted Central Catheters

When a peripheral vein is difficult to locate in the adult or the veins are not suitable for IV therapy, a catheter is inserted into the large subclavian vein and positioned in the superior vena cava or the right atrium. This type of catheter can be left in place for 6 to 8 weeks. The nurse assists the physician during the subclavian catheter insertion by providing the sterile catheter tray, draping the patient, opening sterile packages, and preparing the IV administration set for use. If the patient needs a central line for more than 6 to 8 weeks, a long-term catheter such as a tunneled Broviac, Hickman, or Groshong is inserted. This procedure is done in the operating room.

Peripherally inserted central catheters (PICCs) or midline catheters (MLs) are often used in children or in adults who need peripheral IV therapy that requires placement where there is high blood flow. They are also a first choice in home care IV therapy of 6 to 8 weeks. These catheters are long and are inserted in the larger basilic or cephalic vein of the upper arm. The ML ideally sits just inside the subclavian vein; the PICC may be advanced as far as the superior vena cava (Fig. 36.10). Other **vascular access devices** (devices such as a needle or catheter that allow direct access to the circulatory system) in the form of central venous catheters or implanted infusion ports are used for patients who need long-term drug therapy, fluid therapy, or chemotherapy. These catheters are inserted by the physician or a specially trained nurse.

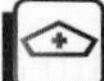 Clinical Cues

Remember not to take the blood pressure on the arm that has a PICC or ML catheter in place.

Short-term central venous catheters are inserted into a large vein, usually the subclavian or jugular, by the physician. Long-term central venous catheters that are threaded to the tip of the right atrium of the heart are placed by surgical tunneling through subcutaneous tissue and then through the subclavian vein into the superior vena cava (Fig. 36.11). The surgeon first enters the vein and then makes the subcutaneous tunnel or pocket. Central venous catheters range from 15 to 30 cm in length. Several types are available. Some have a single lumen; others have two, three, or more lumens.

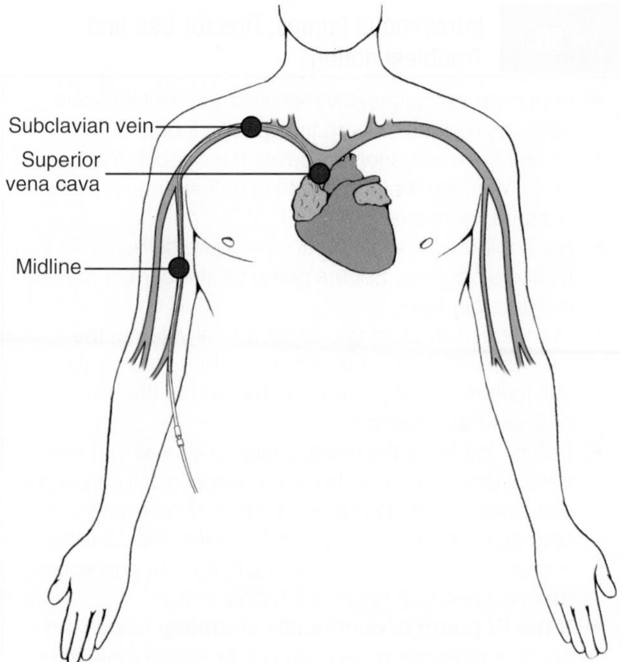

FIGURE 36.10 Placement of a PICC line.

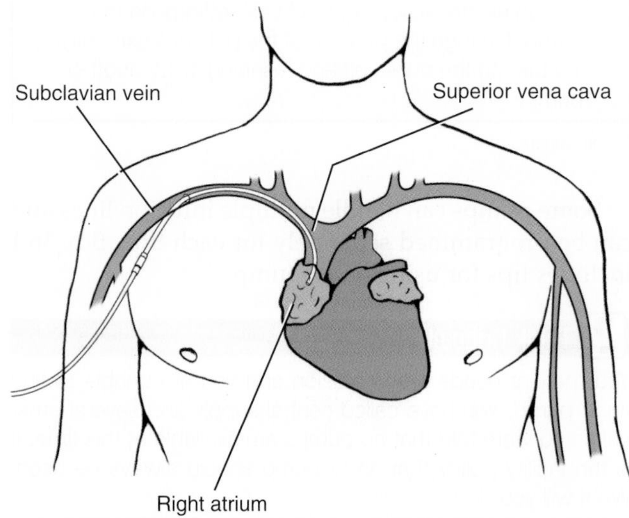

FIGURE 36.11 Placement of a subclavian central line.

These catheters are periodically flushed, much the same as for a PRN lock, to keep the lumens patent. Agency policy dictates specific amount and type of flush solution (i.e., saline or heparin), frequency, size of the syringe, and guidelines for when to obtain an order for special declotting solutions. Agency policy also indicates whether central line management is a responsibility only of registered nurses (RNs). **Correct placement of**

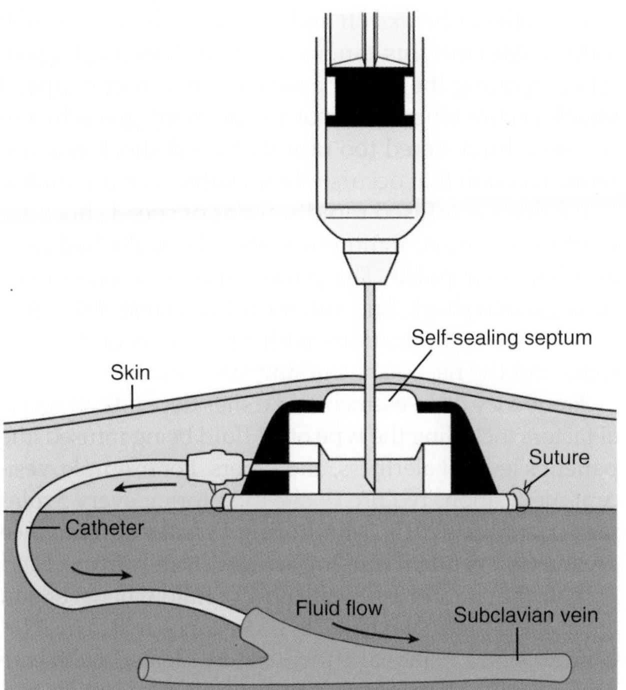

FIGURE 36.12 Implanted infusion port and Huber needle.

subclavian catheters must be verified by radiographic studies before any fluid is infused through them.

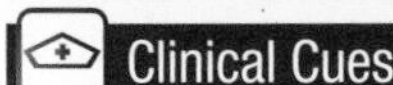

Clinical Cues

Never use a syringe that is smaller than 10 mL for flushing a central IV line (Institute for Safe Medical Practices, 2015). Although it may seem illogical at first, small diameter syringes generate more pressure than larger syringes do, thereby presenting an increased risk of damage to the catheter.

Infusion Port

An infusion port with a single- or dual-lumen catheter can be implanted (Fig. 36.12). Most ports are placed subcutaneously on the chest beneath the right clavicle, and the catheter is threaded through a large vein and into the superior vena cava. Sometimes these ports are implanted in other areas for intraspinal or intraperitoneal infusion. Specially designed Huber noncoring needles are used to infuse solutions and medications through the port. Other types of needles cause damage to the port.

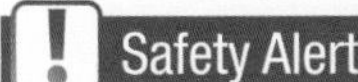

Safety Alert

A Lethal Error: Medication Routes Are Not Interchangeable

The physician may order medication to be given by the **epidural** (epidural space of the spinal column) or **intrathecal** (intrathecal space of the spinal column) route. These routes of administration are beyond the scope of practice for LPN/LVNs; however, be aware that medication vials can be labeled specifically for IV, epidural, or intrathecal administration. Fatalities have occurred when epidural medications have been connected to the patient's peripheral IV line. **Read the labels and immediately alert the charge nurse if you find these medications are being stored together.**

COMPLICATIONS OF INTRAVENOUS THERAPY

Complications of IV therapy are potentially serious and costly. Potential complications include infiltration, extravasation, phlebitis, systemic infection, and **catheter embolus** (piece of the catheter obstructing blood flow). Medicare and Medicaid do not reimburse for infections or complications related to poor care of catheters (Kornbau et al., 2015).

QSEN Considerations: Patient-Centered Care

Patient and Family Participation

One of the most effective ways to prevent complications is to teach the patient to immediately report any changes or discomfort at the IV site. National Patient Safety Goals advocate the active participation of the patient and the family to increase safety.

INFILTRATION

Infiltration is the most common problem encountered with IV therapy. Infiltration occurs when a nonvesicant fluid or medication leaks out of the vein into the tissue. Signs and symptoms include local edema, skin blanching, skin coolness, leakage at the puncture site, pain, and feelings of tightness, and sometimes numbness. Flow can be slow and sluggish; however, this is not a definitive sign, particularly in the early phase of infiltration when the fluid can be progressively leaking into the surrounding tissue. If infiltration occurs, discontinue the infusion, remove the catheter, and reestablish another IV line at a different site. Fluid that is in the tissue will usually reabsorb within 24 hours. Follow agency policy for treatment.

EXTRAVASATION

Extravasation is the infiltration of a **vesicant** (chemical irritant that causes tissue destruction) drug from an IV line. The appearance of the site and the patient's subjective complaints may initially be similar to those with an infiltration, but damage may go unnoticed for 48 to 72 hours, leading to severe tissue damage (Chiu et al., 2015). The results can be infection, disfigurement, or loss of function. Be aware of drugs that may have vesicant properties, for example, some antibiotics, or certain antineoplastic drugs (there are many others). Assess the site before administering the dose, dilute the drug as directed, avoid vein sites such as the dorsum of the hand or the antecubital fossa, and be aware of available antidotes so that an order can be obtained for prompt administration as needed (Reynolds et al., 2014). If extravasation does occur, do not discontinue the IV, because the antidote must be delivered directly to the problem area (Kreidieh et al., 2016). Extravasation of a vesicant is reported to the primary care provider; additional documentation, such as an incident report, will be required.

PHLEBITIS

Phlebitis is caused by irritation of the vein by the needle, the catheter, medications, or additives in the IV solution. The typical signs of phlebitis are erythema, warmth, swelling, and tenderness. The IV must be discontinued and another site found for reinitiating therapy. Application of warm compresses to the inflamed site decreases discomfort.

BLOODSTREAM INFECTION

Bloodstream infection **(septicemia)** occurs when infectious pathogens are introduced into the bloodstream. Central line-associated bloodstream infections (CLABSIs) are the cause of thousands of deaths in the United States each year, and cost billions of dollars (Centers for Disease Control and Prevention, 2016). There is a risk for infection during breaks in sterile technique during cannula insertion or any time the system is opened to change the bag or tubing. Signs and symptoms are fever, chills, pain, headache, nausea, vomiting, and extreme fatigue. Blood cultures are ordered, and aggressive antibiotic therapy is started. The IV site is immediately discontinued. Evidence-based care to prevent central line infection includes implementing a central line bundle and using maximum barrier precautions during insertion, ultrasound-guided placement, a saline-only flush protocol, and chlorhexidine disks at the insertion site. Other suggested interventions are rigorous hand hygiene, tubing and "scrub the hub" for at least 15 seconds with alcohol whenever a port or IV connector is accessed (Fig. 36.13) (Harnage, 2012). Additionally, daily review of the necessity for leaving the catheter in place, along with prompt removal of an unneeded line is needed. Caps are to be changed no more often than every 72 hours (The Joint Commission, 2013). Antibiotic-impregnated central venous catheters are another proven method of reducing infections in adults and are presently being studied in children (Gilbert et al., 2016) and neonates (Lai et al., 2016).

OTHER COMPLICATIONS

There are several additional serious complications of IV therapy. Catheter embolus can occur when a piece of the catheter breaks off and travels in the vein until it lodges. **Air embolus** can occur when changing bags or when opening the line of a subclavian catheter. **Speed shock** occurs when fluids or medications given by bolus are administered too rapidly. Speed shock is a systemic reaction that occurs when a substance unfamiliar to the body is infused rapidly. Signs of speed shock are light-headedness, tightness in the chest, flushed face, and irregular pulse. The patient may lose consciousness, go into shock, and suffer cardiac arrest. Table 36.2 lists all the complications with their signs and symptoms and the necessary nursing interventions.

Frequency of assessment of IV sites depends on several factors including the type of IV fluid being infused, the patient's level of alertness, and others. For example, vesicant medications require IV site monitoring every 5 minutes (Hadaway, 2015). **Monitoring IV sites at least once an hour is a prudent nursing action.** Visually inspect and palpate the site and assess the flow of fluid whenever you are at the patient's bedside. In accordance with The Joint Commission's National Patient Safety Goals, health care professionals are expected "to improve recognition and response to changes in the patient's condition."

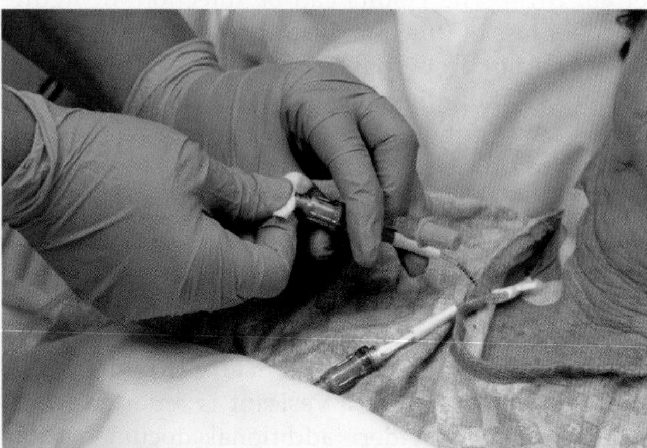

FIGURE 36.13 "Scrub the hub" before accessing ports or connectors to inject medication or attach intravenous tubing.

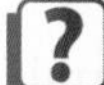 **Think Critically**

Your documentation demonstrates that you observed and noted signs of phlebitis related to your patient's IV site. You corrected the problem but forgot to document your actions. Several years later, the patient retains a lawyer and attempts to sue the hospital for a variety of issues. What are the implications of your missing documentation?

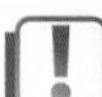 **Safety Alert**

Where Does That Line Go?

Evidence-based practice indicates that, when working with IV tubing connections, you must trace the tube all the way from its point of origin to the patient's body to ensure you are making the correct connection. There have been incidents in which IV tubing was inadvertently attached to the cuff of a tracheostomy tube, or other tubes (feeding tubes, automatic blood pressure tubing, or urinary catheter irrigation tubing) were inadvertently connected to IV tubing. Most mistakes of this magnitude result in patient death.

❖ APPLICATION OF THE NURSING PROCESS

◆ ASSESSMENT (DATA COLLECTION)

Each nurse is responsible for determining that the correct IV solution is hanging. The IV site must be assessed every 1 to 2 hours during a shift to ensure patency and absence of complications. The flow rate is checked to make certain that the fluid is running at the prescribed rate.

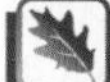 **Life-Span Considerations**

Older Adults

Older adults who have IV fluid infusing are at risk for fluid overload. Auscultate the lungs at least once each shift for sounds of crackles. Rapid pulse, shortness of breath, and distended neck veins are other possible signs of fluid overload.

When giving IV medications, review the drug's action, possible side effects, correct dosage, and nursing implications and the patient's drug allergies before preparing the drug. Check for possible drug-solution incompatibilities. If incompatibilities exist, the IV line must be flushed with sterile saline before the other drug or solution is started and flushed again when the infusion or injection is finished (Bentley et al., 2015). Assess for potential drug interactions when more than one drug is being administered. **Always assess for adverse or side effects of previously administered doses of IV or piggyback medications before administering the next dose.** Assess the existing IV site and catheter size before beginning an infusion of a blood product. The site must be free of any signs of infection or infiltration.

◆ NURSING DIAGNOSIS

Common nursing diagnoses for patients who are undergoing IV therapy might include:

- Deficient fluid volume related to inability to take fluids by mouth (fluid replacement).
- Risk for infection related to invasive procedure (IV insertion).
- Imbalanced nutrition, less than body requirements, related to an inability to take oral foods or fluids (TPN).

◆ PLANNING

Allow time to provide care for the IV site (see Assignment Considerations), hang solutions, change tubing or IV sites, and perform needed assessments. Allow extra time if you have to monitor a blood transfusion.

Table 36.2 Complications of Intravenous Therapy and Nursing Interventions

COMPLICATION	MANIFESTATIONS	NURSING CARE
Local		
Infiltration	Arm swollen, tender, cool to touch; may or may not have blood return	Remove IV catheter and restart IV in the other extremity. (Consult agency policy for certain IV solutions or drugs.)
Extravasation	Initial symptoms often similar to infiltration, but damage can result in infection, disfigurement, or loss of function	Be aware of which drugs have vesicant properties. Stop infusion. Do not remove the catheter. Notify the primary care provider for order for appropriate antidote.
Phlebitis	Vein hard with skin red, swollen, tender, warm; blood return present; IV infusion may or may not be sluggish	Remove IV catheter, notify the primary care provider, and apply warm packs to the IV site.
Thrombophlebitis	Site red, tender, warm; IV infusion sluggish	Never irrigate the IV catheter; remove the IV catheter, notify the primary care provider, and restart IV in opposite extremity.
IV site infection	Site hot, red, painful but not hard or swollen; IV infusion sluggish	Remove IV catheter; restart in opposite extremity; use new tubing and solution.
Systemic		
Catheter embolus	Decrease in BP; weak, rapid pulse; cyanosis of nail beds; loss of consciousness (could also have a local effect only: pain along a vein)	Remove the IV catheter and inspect, place a tourniquet high on the limb of the IV site, notify the primary care provider, obtain x-ray film, and prepare for surgery to remove the catheter pieces.
Infection	Fever, chills, and general malaise	Change the infusion system, notify the primary care provider, and obtain cultures as ordered.
Speed shock	Flushed face, severe headache, chest pain, irregular pulse, decreased BP, loss of consciousness, and cardiac arrest	Stop the infusion, notify the primary care provider, and monitor vital signs frequently.
Circulatory overload	Increased BP, distended neck veins, rapid breathing, dyspnea, moist cough, and crackles	Elevate the head of the bed, keep the patient warm, assess for edema, slow the infusion rate, and notify the primary care provider.
Air embolus	Sudden drop in BP and increase in pulse	Place the patient on the left side and lower the head of the bed; inspect the IV infusion system for disconnection or leak; notify the primary care provider.
Allergic reaction	Catheter: red streak along the vein and pain at the IV site Medication: site red, itching, rash	Remove the IV catheter, restart the IV using a different type of IV catheter, and notify the primary care provider; discontinue the medication.

IV, Intravenous.
Modified from Leahy, J. M., & Kizilay, P. E. (1998). *Foundations of nursing practice: A nursing process approach* (pp. 822). Philadelphia, PA: W. B. Saunders.

Sample goals/expected outcomes for the previous nursing diagnoses include:

- No signs of dehydration will be displayed.
- The patient will display no signs of infection at IV site.
- The patient's nutritional status will improve as evidenced by a weight gain of 0.5 lb/week.

Assignment Considerations

Protecting IV Sites During Showering and Bathing

When caring for a patient with a peripheral IV, plan additional time for bathing and assisting with daily activities. Alert the unlicensed assistive personnel (UAPs) to which patients have IVs. Commercial plastic sheaths can be used to cover an IV site on an extremity, or a clean plastic bag can be taped to protect the site.

Calculation of Flow Rates

The factors that influence the rate of flow of an IV solution are catheter size, height of the solution container, and viscosity of the fluid. Fluids flow less rapidly through a catheter with a small **bore** (internal diameter) than through a catheter with a larger bore. In the gravity method, the higher the container, the faster the fluid will flow.

The use of infusion pumps is increasingly common, and typically, the device calculates the flow rate; however, the pump relies on the user to enter the correct data. For example, the order may read normal saline to infuse at 125 mL/hour; therefore, the nurse must enter the "volume" to be delivered (125 mL) and "the amount of time" (60 minutes) required for the volume to infuse. Pumps offer a variety of programmable functions. The device may do the math, but you are responsible for correct use of the equipment and correct entry of the required parameters.

To calculate the flow rate using the gravity method, you must know how many drops are contained in each milliliter (drop factor) as it passes through the drip chamber of the tubing. The standard set produces 10 to 20 gtt/mL, and the pediatric or microdrop chamber produces 60 gtt/mL. There are charts with precalculated rates for the various drip chambers and standard volumes and times. The basic formula for calculating the rate of flow is given in Box 36.2. When IV therapy is administered, the fluid enters the circulation immediately. The adult adapts best to fluids at a steady rate of 80 to 250 mL/hour. Rapid infusion can lead to fluid overload and heart failure.

◆ IMPLEMENTATION

The patient who has a peripheral IV will be a bit more limited in performing usual tasks. Help may be needed to open containers on the dietary tray, and if the IV is in the dominant hand, assistance may be required for many of the tasks of daily living. Nursing guidelines for IV therapy are presented in Box 36.3.

Box 36.2 Calculating the Intravenous Flow Rate

- Formula for flow rate calculation:

$$\frac{\text{Amount of solution (in mL)} \times \text{No drops/mL}}{\text{Time (in min)}} = \text{Drops/min}$$

- When the order reads "1000 mL of D_5W over 10 hours," use a regular drip set (15 gtt/mL):

$$\frac{1000\text{ mL} \times 15\text{ gtt/mL}}{10\text{ h} \times 60\text{ min}} = \frac{15,000}{600} = 25\text{ gtt/min}$$

- When the order reads "D5 ½NS at 125 mL/h," use:

$$\frac{125\text{ mL} \times 15\text{ gtt/mL}}{60\text{ min}} = \frac{1875}{60} = 31.25\text{ or }31\text{ gtt/min}$$

- Formula for using a standard adult pump (mL/h):

$$\frac{\text{Amount of solution (in mL)} \times 60\text{ min/h}}{\text{Time (in min)}} = \text{mL/h}$$

- When the order reads "250 mg of medication in 100 mL, deliver over 30 minutes," use:

$$\frac{100\text{ mL of solution} \times 60\text{ min/h}}{30\text{ min}} = 200\text{ mL/h}$$

Box 36.3 Intravenous Therapy Guidelines

- **Keep IV fluid sterile.** Everything coming into contact with the solution must be sterile, including the inside surface of the catheter hub and all connecting points between the bag and drip chamber and between the tubing and the needleless connector.
- Protect the catheter site from contamination to avoid possible infection. An airtight, transparent dressing is used over the catheter site. Keep tubing free of air. Clear tubing of air before connecting to the catheter. Do not allow the current bag to run dry before changing to the next one.
- **Hang fluids at the correct height.** Keep the bag of fluid sufficiently above the level of the catheter site to maintain flow; avoid having it too high because this significantly increases the effect of gravity.
- **Carefully regulate the rate of flow.** If the IV is behind schedule, do not run in a large amount of fluid to catch up. Rather, recalculate either (1) the span of time for the infusion or (2) the rate of drops per minute for the fluid to run at the ordered rate. (For an infusion pump, access the function of the pump.)
- **Monitor intake and output when a patient is receiving IV fluids or blood.** Keep accurate intake and output records and compare intake with output over 24 hours.
- **Hang the solution that should run in first in a higher position.** Attach the piggyback tubing to a port beneath the roller clamp on the primary tubing. Lower the primary bag without clamping the tubing so it will begin to flow when the piggyback has run in.
- **Assess the site frequently for signs of complications.** Monitor for infiltration, extravasation, swelling at the IV site, irritation of the vein, formation of a clot stopping the flow, or systemic reaction. Take vital signs several times a day to detect early signs of infection or adverse reaction.

I & O, Intake and output; *IV*, intravenous.

Initiating Intravenous Therapy

Students must have supervision when performing a venipuncture. Before venipuncture is performed, gather the equipment, obtain or prepare the IV infusion (with or without medication), select the most appropriate vein, and prepare the site (Skill 36.1). Whenever an IV site is initiated or changed or an IV solution is hung, document this on the parenteral infusion record (Fig. 36.14).

Selection of the intravenous site. Selection of a vein for IV use depends on several factors, including the vein's accessibility and general condition, the type of fluid or medication to be given, and the duration of IV therapy. The veins preferred for infusions and intermittent doses of medications are those distal to the antecubital area; a new site cannot be placed distal to an old site. The cephalic, basilic, and antebrachial veins of the lower arm and the veins on the back of the hand are sites for most adult patients (Fig. 36.15). It is necessary to be able to feel or see the vein. If there is difficulty detecting the vein, a device called the venoscope can be used to illuminate the tissue and outline the vein.

Skill 36.1 Starting the Primary Intravenous Infusion

 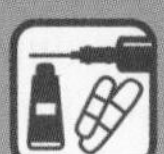 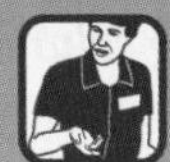 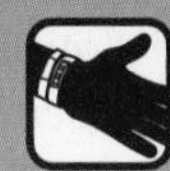 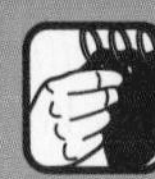 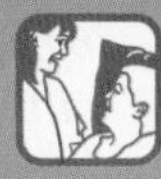 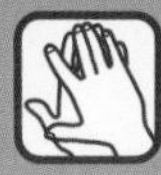 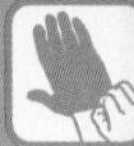

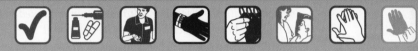

Use strict aseptic technique when handling IV fluids and tubing because an IV site provides access for bacteria to enter the bloodstream. Agency policy will provide guidelines for IV catheter insertion.

Supplies

- IV solution as ordered
- IV administration set
- IV cannula
- Scissors
- IV infusion pump (according to agency policy)
- IV stand or pole
- IV start kit (chlorhexidine swabs, alcohol swabs, label, tape, transparent dressing, and tourniquet)
- Gloves
- Commercial device to secure the site
- Towel or underpad
- Arm board (optional)
- Medication administration record (MAR) or workstation on wheels (WOW)

Review and carry out the Standard Steps in Appendix A.

ACTION *(RATIONALE)*

Assessment (Data Collection)

1. Inspect the patient's hands and forearms, and select the site for venipuncture. Choose the most distal site possible. *(Start the IV in the most distal vein, and progress proximally with each successive site.)*

Planning

2. Verify that the patient is ready for the procedure and gather all equipment. Explain what you will do. *(Prepares the patient and prevents time loss.)*

Implementation

Preparing the IV Infusion

3. Obtain the correct IV solution; check the solution against the order. *(The Six Rights of medication administration applies to IV fluids and to additives.)*
4. Remove the covering from the IV bag, and check the solution for clarity, leaks, and particulate matter. Note the expiration date. *(Do not use out-of-date or contaminated solutions.)*
5. Open the administration set, and position the roller clamp where it will be easy to reach and regulate while watching the drops in the drip chamber. Close the roller clamp, and remove the pull tab from the IV bag spike port. Maintain sterility while removing the cap on the tubing spike. Insert the spike; do not touch the spike to anything but the inside of the spike port. *(If the clamp is not closed, the fluid will run quickly through the tubing when the bag is inverted. Contaminated equipment must be discarded.)*
6. Squeeze the drip chamber while raising the bag, and then place the container on a hook or IV stand. Allow the drip chamber to fill partially. *(This method reduces air bubbles that enter the IV tubing.)*

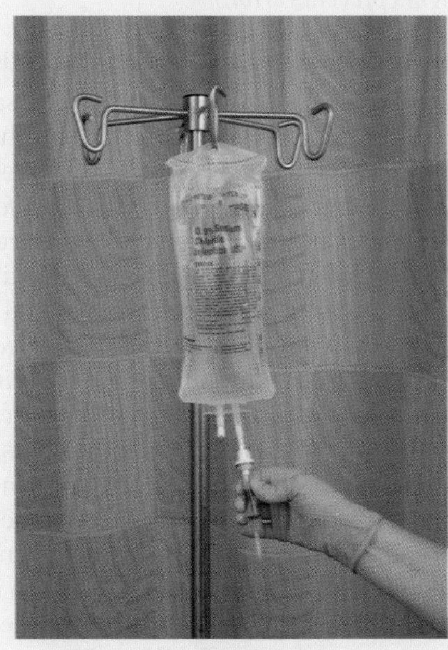

Step 6

7. Remove the air from the tubing by slowly opening the roller clamp after loosening the protector cap over the needle adapter to allow the air to escape; allow a small amount of fluid to escape from the tubing, verifying that all air is removed. *(Patients are conscious of air in the tubing. In addition, pumps sense small amounts of air and continuously alarm until the air is removed.)*

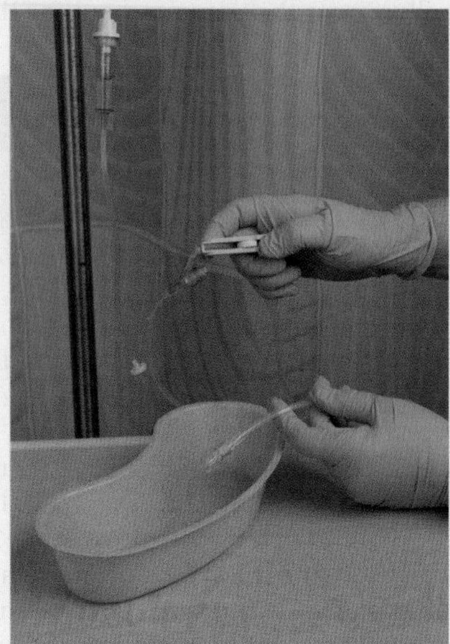

Step 7

8. Close the roller clamp and retighten the cap. *(The roller clamp is used to manually stop or regulate flow.)*
9. Verify the IV solution and additives, if any, with the MAR or eMAR. Take the IV solution and the MAR or WOW to the patient's bedside. *(The MAR or eMAR is used to identify the patient and to perform the third medication check.)*
10. Verify the patient's identification. *(Following the Six Rights prevents error.)*

Placing the IV Catheter and Starting the Infusion

11. Remove excess hair from the site if necessary by clipping (do not shave) the area around the chosen site and where the adhesive will be applied. *(Hair harbors microorganisms that contribute to infection.)*
12. Turn on the examination light, allow the extremity to hang down off the bed for a short time, or wrap it in a warm, moist pack for several minutes to distend the vein. Prepare the IV start equipment and perform hand hygiene. *(The vein must be visualized and distended to introduce the cannula.)*
13. Apply the tourniquet and check the veins. The tourniquet should be positioned on the midforearm if the dorsum of the hand is to be used. If the forearm area is to be used, the tourniquet is placed on the upper arm or at least 4 to 6 inches above the site. Do not place the tourniquet so tightly as to restrict arterial flow. Release the tourniquet and prepare equipment. *(The venous flow must be restricted in the vein for it to distend enough to introduce the cannula. Leaving the tourniquet causes discomfort.)*
14. Put down a protective pad under the extremity, and cleanse the site with antiseptic solution according to agency policy. This may be 70% alcohol, tincture of iodine, or chlorhexidine gluconate solution (Centers for Disease Control and Prevention, 2011). Clean an area of about 2 inches, starting at the center, and working in a circular motion outward. Allow the area to dry. Do not wave your hands or blow on the area to dry it. *(A protective pad prevents bedding and other surfaces from becoming soiled with the cleansing solution or contaminated with blood. Waving over the area or blowing on it deposits microorganisms on the newly cleansed skin.)*
15. Don gloves, and reapply the tourniquet; ask the patient to open and close the fist a few times, and then hold it closed. Stabilize the skin below the IV site by placing your thumb about 2 inches directly below the insertion site. A local anesthetic at the insertion site is sometimes allowed by agency policy. *(Gloves are required when contact with blood is possible. Using a tourniquet and pumping the fist distend the vein. For the cannula to enter the vein smoothly and with less discomfort, the skin must be taut. Use of a local anesthetic is controversial; an order or protocol is necessary before using an anesthetic.)*

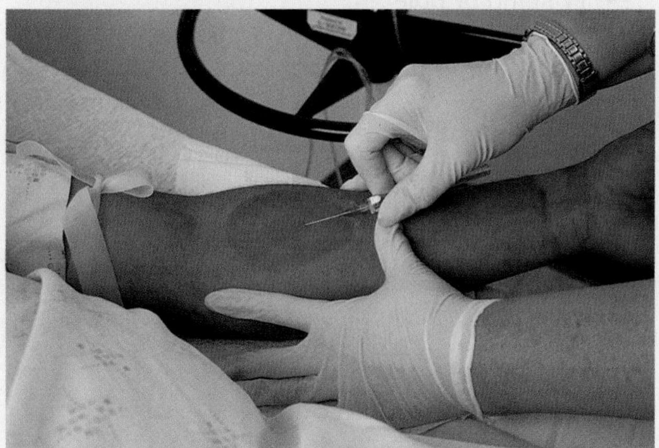

Step 15

16. Insert the IV cannula into the vein by either the indirect or the direct method. Using the indirect method, first insert the cannula into the subcutaneous space directly parallel to the side of the vein. Then move the tip toward the vein, and gently ease the cannula into the vein. Using the direct method, hold the cannula with the bevel upright and at a 15- to 25-degree angle to pierce the skin, and then lower the cannula until it is nearly parallel to the skin when piercing the vein. Enter the skin and vein in one quick, steady, forward thrust. Decreased resistance or a "pop" will be felt as the needle enters the vein. When the cannula punctures the vein, you will see blood

(flashback) return into the hub of the unit. *(The indirect method of cannula insertion has less chance of pushing completely through the vein. The direct method is best when the vein is large and stable.)*

17. After you see the flashback, insert the cannula an additional ⅛ inch and then slide the catheter off the stylet into the vein for its full length while keeping the stylet steady. Remove the tourniquet and ask the patient to open the fist. If you go through the vein wall, remove the tourniquet, withdraw the whole unit, and apply pressure. *(Advancing the cannula when it is not in the vein causes pain and tissue damage. If you continue to push the stylet after the flashback, you will go through vein wall, and fluid will infiltrate into the surrounding tissues. A tight tourniquet impedes solution. Pressure applied to the vein prevents bleeding while you are attaching the tubing.)*

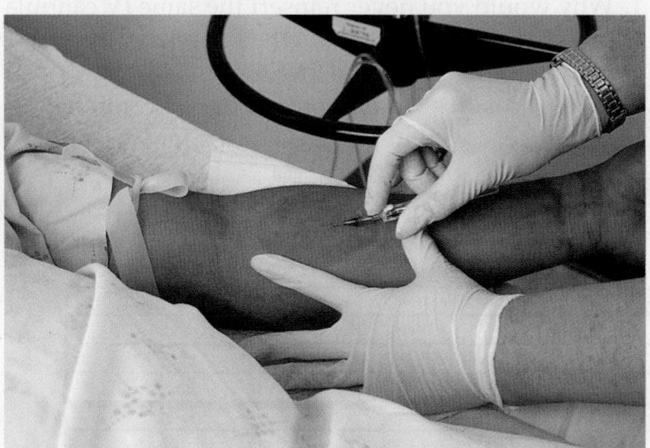

Step **17**

18. Remove the protective cap over the needle adapter on the IV tubing, attach the tubing to the catheter hub, and open the clamp to begin the infusion slowly. Observe the site for swelling or leaking, indicating that the site is infiltrating. *(Observe a slow flow to establish the patency of the IV before setting the rate. If the IV is not patent, remove the catheter.)*

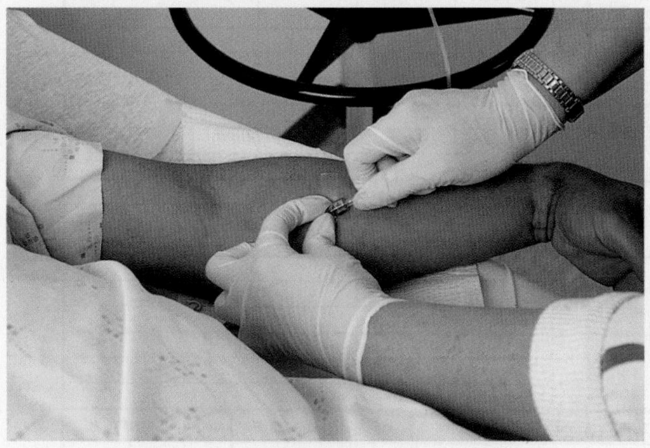

Step **18**

19. If the site is patent, secure the catheter with a manufactured catheter stabilization device. Apply a transparent dressing. Loop the IV tubing on the extremity, and secure it again with tape. Supply an arm board if needed to immobilize or support the IV area. Label the dressing with the date and your initials. *(A transparent dressing protects the site from microorganisms while allowing visualization of the site. Do not apply nonsterile tape near the insertion site or underneath the transparent dressing. Taping the IV tubing prevents possible dislodgement when the patient moves around.)*

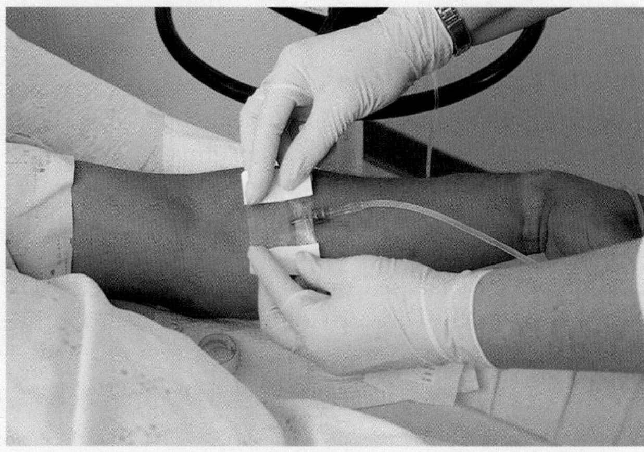

Step **19**

20. Regulate the solution flow according to the order by adjusting the roller clamp and counting the drops per minute (or set the infusion pump to infuse at the correct rate). *(The position of the arm, movement, and securing the catheter to stabilize it in the vein can alter the rate of flow.)*

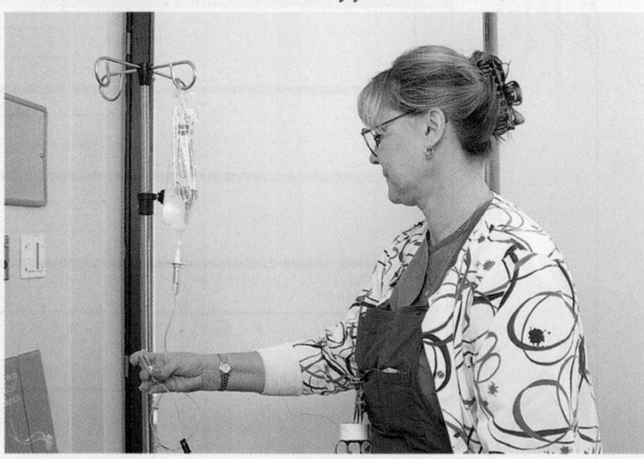

Step **20**

Evaluation

21. Verify that the solution is running at the correct rate into the vein without pain and that the IV catheter is held securely in place. *(Ensures that the IV is patent and secure.)*
22. Clean up used supplies and make the patient comfortable. Remove gloves and perform hand hygiene. *(Prevents spread of microorganisms and fosters patient well-being.)*

Documentation

23. Documentation should include the location of the site, the type of catheter inserted, and the solution started. In some agencies, this information is documented on an IV flow sheet. *(The right documentation includes when the catheter was inserted so that it can be changed at the appropriate time.)*

Documentation Example

#18 Angiocath × 1 inch inserted in L interior forearm with aseptic technique. IV 1000 mL of D_5W infusing at 125 mL/h per infusion pump. Transparent dressing applied. (Nurse's time-stamped electronic signature)

Special Considerations

- Verify patient allergies before cleansing the skin or touching the patient with a latex glove.
- Antibiotic ointment at the insertion site is not recommended because it can contribute to the growth of fungal infections and antimicrobial resistance (Centers for Disease Control and Prevention, 2011).
- The Centers for Disease Control and Prevention (2011) recommends that catheters be secured with either sterile gauze and tape or a transparent, semipermeable dressing. The site should be assessed daily, either visually (through the transparent dressing) or via palpation if gauze and tape are used. If the site is tender to palpation or the patient has a fever without known cause, remove the dressing and inspect the site visually.
- If you cannot initiate a patent IV in two attempts, ask another nurse to perform the task.
- A peripheral IV site is changed every 72 to 96 hours or according to agency policy.
- Never perform venipuncture in an extremity where there is a hemodialysis access shunt or on the side of a mastectomy or paralysis.
- If the solution is running slowly, check for infiltration, adjust the securing device or dressing, or try slightly rotating the catheter tip away from the vein wall.

Critical Thinking Questions

1. Why would you never reinsert the same IV cannula in a slightly different spot when you have missed getting into the vein the first time?
2. What measures would you take if you could not see or feel a vein in the area chosen for IV cannula insertion?

IV, Intravenous; *MAR*, medication administration record; *WOW*, workstation on wheels.

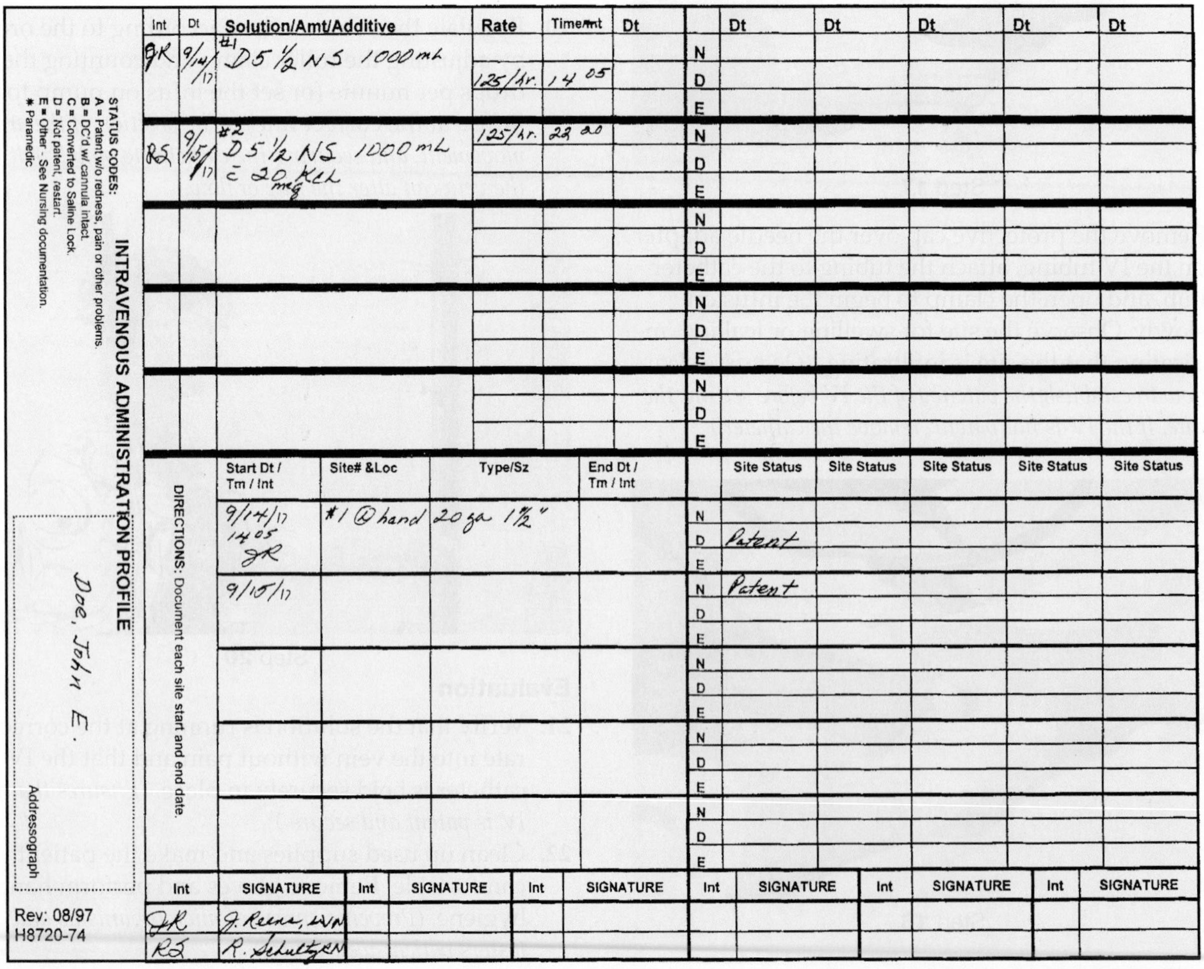

INTRAVENOUS ADMINISTRATION PROFILE

STATUS CODES:
A = Patent w/o redness, pain or other problems.
B = DC'd w/ cannula intact.
C = Converted to Saline Lock.
D = Not patent, restart.
E = Other - See Nursing documentation.
* Paramedic.

Int	Dt	Solution/Amt/Additive	Rate	Time/Amt	Dt		Dt	Dt	Dt	Dt	Dt
JR	9/14/17	#1 D5 ½ NS 1000 mL	125/hr.	14 05		N D E					
RS	9/15/17	#2 D5 ½ NS 1000 mL ē 20 KCL mEq	125/hr.	22 00		N D E					
						N D E					
						N D E					
						N D E					

DIRECTIONS: Document each site start and end date.

Start Dt / Tm / Int	Site# &Loc	Type/Sz	End Dt / Tm / Int		Site Status	Site Status	Site Status	Site Status	Site Status
9/14/17 1405 JR	#1 Ⓡ hand	20 ga 1½"		N D E	Patent (D)				
9/15/17				N D E	Patent (N)				
				N D E					
				N D E					
				N D E					

Int	SIGNATURE	Int	SIGNATURE	Int	SIGNATURE	Int	SIGNATURE	Int	SIGNATURE	Int	SIGNATURE
JR	J. Reena, WN										
RS	R. Schultz RN										

Doe, John E.

Addressograph

Rev: 08/97
H8720-74

FIGURE 36.14 Parenteral infusion record.

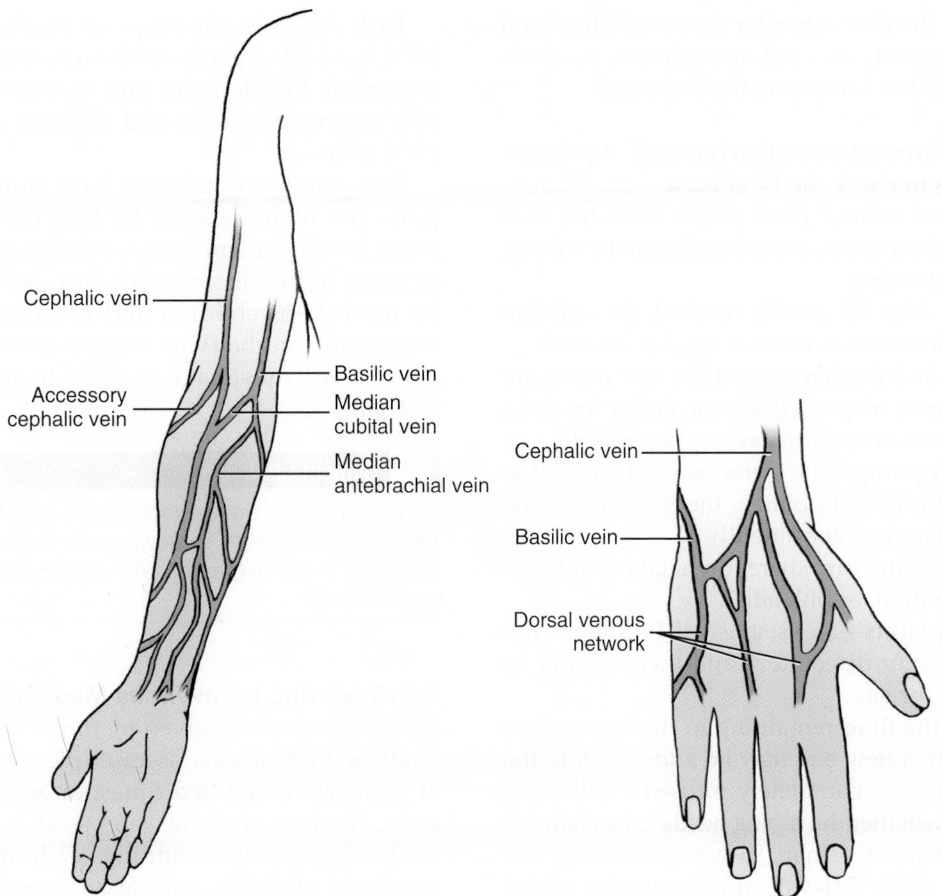

FIGURE 36.15 Sites for insertion of the intravenous cannula.

The veins in the antecubital space are not used extensively for IV infusions because movement causes irritation or damage to the vein, and keeping the arm extended may cause muscle or nerve damage. Veins of the foot are rarely used for adults, but could be used in an emergency if no other sites are available. The scalp veins are frequently used in infants because they are easily accessible, the needle is less likely to be dislodged from this site, and the veins of the arms are too small.

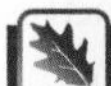

Life-Span Considerations

Older Adults

Using a blood pressure cuff rather than a tourniquet is sometimes better for the fragile veins of older adults. Place the cuff about 6 inches above the selected site. Inflate the cuff to about 10 mm Hg above the diastolic pressure to dilate the vein. If the patient is fluid depleted, inflate to 20 mm Hg over the diastolic pressure.

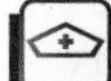

Clinical Cues

For pediatric patients (or confused older adults) who are pulling at the tubing and catheter, a sleeve or roller gauze can be used to cover the site and equipment. Alternatively, a commercial shield shape can be taped over the catheter site (Fig. 36.16). These devices can prevent accidental dislodgement, but obscure quick visualization of the site. You must weigh benefits against the inconvenience.

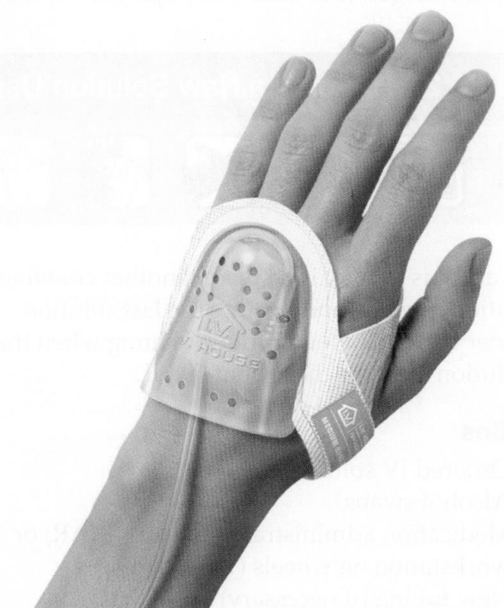

FIGURE 36.16 IV house protective device. (Courtesy IV House, St. Louis, MO.)

Managing Intravenous Therapy

When your patient has an IV, you are responsible for ensuring that the correct solution is infusing at the prescribed rate. **Movement of the patient can alter**

the rate. Check the flow rate after the patient has been ambulating, returns from a test or treatment, has been turned in bed, or has been up to the bathroom.

Keeping the intravenous solution running. A primary responsibility is to check the IV at least every 60 minutes and observe each of these points with the eyes traveling from the solution container, down the tubing, and to the catheter site:

- **The IV flow**—for the gravity method, the solution should drip into the chamber at regular intervals.
- **The rate of the infusion**—count the rate if you are using the gravity method. If it is too fast or too slow, adjust it to the correct infusion rate per minute.
- **The infusion pump**—if a pump is used, check the programmed rate and volume; the dripping in the chamber will occur intermittently.
- **The insertion site**—are there any signs of infiltration, extravasation, or phlebitis?
- **Patient complaints**—an established IV should not cause any pain or discomfort, and there should be no leaking at the site.
- **The level of the fluid remaining in the bag**—when 50 mL are left, a new bag may be added before the current solution is completely infused (Skill 36.2). Check to see whether the tubing needs to be changed (no more frequently than 96-hour intervals, but at least once every 7 days), and change the tubing when a new bag is hung (Steps 36.1) (O'Grady et al., 2011). Check your facility's policy for frequency of tubing changes. (For additional tips, see Table 36.3).

Each state sets the scope of practice for the LPN/LVN, but each organization can narrow the scope. It is important, therefore, for you to know what your specific organization does and does not allow the LPN/LVN to do.

The solution container is hung from an IV stand or pole. The tubing should be long enough to provide room for the patient to move about in bed, turn over, or carry out necessary activities. Soft restraints may be needed for children and confused patients who might pull out the IV or cause it to infiltrate. Remember that you must have an order to apply any kind of restraint.

Clinical Cues

As a courtesy to the oncoming shift, and to ensure that the patient's IV continues to flow, check the amount of solution remaining in the bag at the end of your shift and hang a new bag if needed.

Administering Intravenous Medications

Medications can be given by the IV route as one-time (stat) or PRN doses, as multiple doses to be given at regularly scheduled times, or as continuous infusions. Various methods are used to administer IV medications, such as adding medications to the primary bag of fluids, adding a secondary line or piggyback to the primary line, using controlled-volume burettes, or directly injecting the medication into the vein (Skill 36.3).

Skill 36.2 Hanging a New Solution Using an Existing Intravenous Infusion Setup

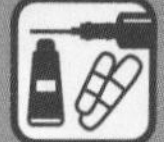
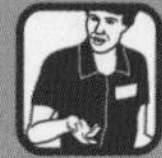

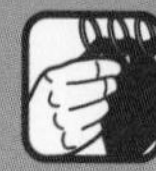
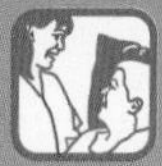
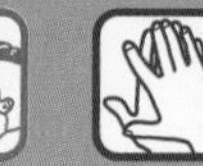

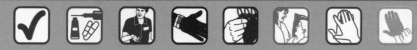

When an IV is to remain in place, another container of solution must be hung before the last solution container runs dry. New solution is hung when the old solution level reaches about 50 mL.

Supplies

- Ordered IV solution
- Alcohol swabs
- Medication administration record (MAR) or workstation on wheels (WOW)
- New tubing (if necessary)

Review and carry out the Standard Steps in Appendix A.

ACTION *(RATIONALE)*

Assessment (Data Collection)

1. Check orders for type of solution. *(IV solutions require a medical order.)*
2. Select the correct solution and inspect it for cloudiness, particles, and other signs of contamination. *(Contaminated solution must not be used.)*

Planning

3. Check the expiration date on existing tubing; obtain the correct new tubing if needed. *(Tubing should be changed no more frequently than every 96 hours but at least every 7 days depending on agency policy.)*

Implementation

4. Go to the patient's bedside, and properly identify the patient using two identifiers. Inspect the IV site for signs of complications. *(If infection or infiltration is present, the site should be changed.)*
5. Hang the IV container on the IV pole. Remove the container that is almost empty, crimp the tubing close to the drip chamber or close the

Skill 36.2 Hanging a New Solution Using an Existing Intravenous Infusion Setup—cont'd

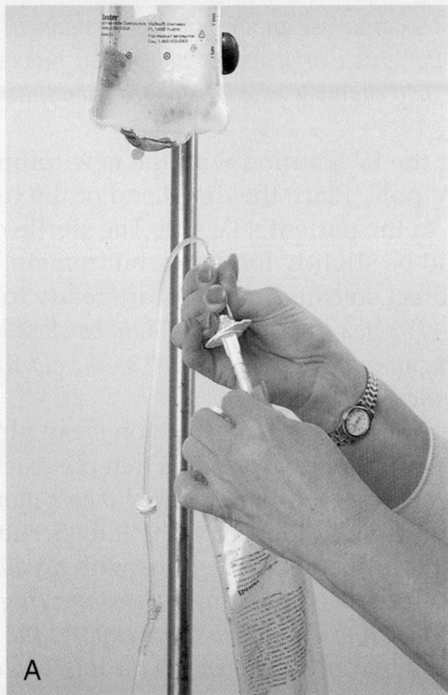
A

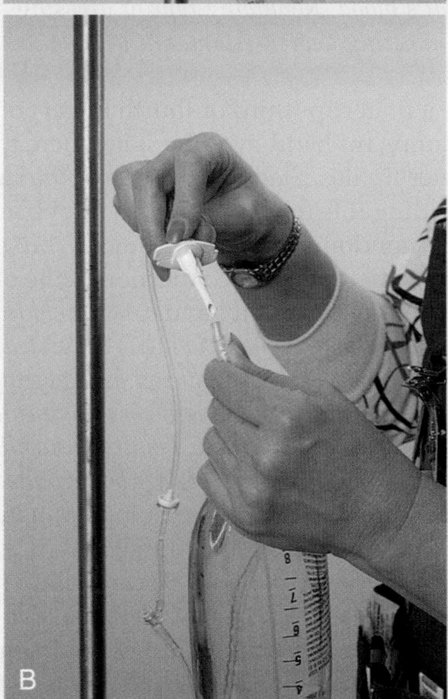
B

Step 5

roller clamp, and remove the spike from the used container. Keep the spike from becoming contaminated. Remove the tab from the IV tubing port on the new container, and insert the tubing spike while stabilizing the container with your other hand. *(The tubing must be occluded while you change IV containers to prevent air from entering tubing. If the spike becomes contaminated, obtain new tubing.)*

6. Remove any air bubbles that entered the tubing by tapping the tube with your finger or a pencil as you stretch it taut. Squeezing the tubing below the bubbles will sometimes encourage them to move up to the drip chamber. *(Air bubbles can cause an air embolus if sufficient air collects. Air moves upward to the drip chamber when dislodged from the side of the tubing.)*
7. Check the flow rate and readjust it as needed to the prescribed rate. *(If using the gravity method, the greater quantity of fluid in the new container causes a larger pressure gradient, and the new solution may flow more rapidly. For a pump, verify the settings and function before leaving the room.)*
8. Dispose of the empty container in the proper receptacle. Remove and destroy any labels that include the patient's name. *(Some agencies require that the container be drained dry before it is discarded. In accordance with HIPAA, protect your patient's identity.)*

Evaluation

9. Before leaving the room, check the solution label with the order again, assess the site for signs of infiltration, and make certain that the fluid is infusing at the correct rate. *(Verifies that correct solution is infusing through a patent site.)*

Documentation

10. Record the added fluid on the IV flow sheet. *(The amount and type of fluid added and the infusion rate are documented along with an assessment of the IV site.)*

Critical Thinking Questions

1. You are performing the initial morning assessment for your patient. You find that the bag that is infusing is not the correct solution according to the report that you received at shift change. What would you do?
2. At what point would you switch out an old IV solution for a new bag of solution? (How much is left in the bag?) Why would you choose to change the solution at this point?

HIPAA, Health Insurance Portability and Accountability Act; *IV*, intravenous; *MAR*, medication administration record; *WOW*, workstation on wheels.

Steps 36.1 Changing Intravenous Tubing

Change primary tubing every 96 hours (or according to agency policy). For intermittent infusion sets (without a primary infusion), change every 24 hours. Blood tubing should be changed after every unit. Change the tubing more frequently if contamination occurs or if sterility is in question.

Review and carry out the Standard Steps in Appendix A.

ACTION *(RATIONALE)*

1. Check the IV order to see whether continued therapy is necessary. *(If the patient is being discharged or if the therapy is completed, the tubing change is an unnecessary cost to the patient.)*
2. Obtain the correct tubing; a needleless connector (if necessary); an alcohol pad; and a label with the date, the time, and your initials. *(There are a variety of IV tubing types and connectors. Obtaining the correct equipment saves time and money. A label indicates when the next tubing change is due.)*
3. Close the roller clamp on the existing IV. Open the new tubing, stretch it slightly, and move the roller clamp to approximately 4 to 6 inches from the drip chamber; then shut the roller clamp. Place the label on the new tube. *(Closing the clamp prevents an air bolus from being delivered during the tubing change. Closing the roller clamp prevents turbulence during flushing and decreases air bubble formation. Failure to place the label results in added expense to the patient because other nurses must change the tubing if it is not dated.)*
4. Remove the IV container from the IV pole and hold it so that the access is facing slightly upward. This access site must be kept sterile, so it should not be touched or allowed to come into contact with nonsterile surfaces. Remove the spike of the old tubing from the container and hand the old tubing to an assistant or drape the tubing over the IV pole. Remove the protective cap from the spike of the new IV tubing, and insert the spike while stabilizing the container with your other hand. *(The port of the IV container and the spike of the new IV tubing must be kept sterile at all times. If the port or spike is accidentally contaminated, obtain a new IV fluid bag and new tubing.)*
5. Flush the IV tubing with the IV fluid and remove any air bubbles by tapping the tube with a finger or a pencil as the tube is stretched taut. Squeezing the tubing below the bubbles will sometimes encourage them to move up to the drip chamber. *(Bubbles can cause an air embolus if sufficient air collects. Patients worry about bubbles. Air moves upward to the drip chamber when dislodged from the side of tubing.)*
6. Hang the IV solution with the new tubing on the IV pole. Place the distal end of the tubing close to the patient's IV site. The sterile cap should be slightly loosened, but remain in place to protect sterility until you are ready to reconnect. *(The new tubing unit should be close by so that it can quickly be connected as the old tubing is disconnected.)*
7. Perform hand hygiene and don clean gloves. Undo any tape or dressings that obstruct access to the IV catheter hub. Place a sterile gauze pad underneath the hub. Scrub the catheter hub and connections with an alcohol pad before disconnecting. *(Disconnecting the old IV tubing from the catheter hub exposes the patient to risk of infection and exposes the nurse to the patient's blood. Removing tape or dressings before disconnecting decreases amount of time the hub is exposed.)*
8. Place a fingertip (third or fourth finger) of the nondominant hand over the skin where the catheter tip lies. Stabilize the hub of the catheter by holding it firmly between the thumb and index finger (nondominant hand). Quickly, but gently, unscrew the Luer-Lok connection of the old tubing with the dominant hand. *(As the old tubing is disconnected and the new tubing is connected, blood will flow or ooze from the catheter hub. Placing some pressure over the tip of the catheter underneath the skin decreases the blood flow. Failure to stabilize the catheter will result in the catheter being pulled out.)*
9. Hold the new tubing in the dominant hand and remove the cap using the thumb and index finger of the nondominant hand. Be careful not to contaminate the end of the new tubing as the cap is removed. Quickly screw the new tubing into the Luer-Lok connection. *(The sterility of the end of the new tubing and the hub must be maintained to prevent hospital-acquired infection.)*
10. Clean the patient's skin with alcohol or chlorhexidine and apply a new dressing and tape. *(Blood that remains on the skin provides a medium for bacterial growth.)*
11. Regulate the solution flow according to the order by adjusting the roller clamp and counting the drops per minute (or set the infusion pump to infuse at the correct rate). *(The position of the arm, movement, and securing the catheter to stabilize it in the vein can alter the rate of flow.)*

IV, Intravenous.

Table 36.3 Troubleshooting: Intravenous Flow

CHECK	RATIONALE
Height of infusion container (infusion pumps may be somewhat less sensitive to the height of the container)	The patient may have changed position. The container should be at least 36 inches above the heart.
System vent	Air vent occlusion will prevent the flow.
Position of tubing	Tubing may be kinked, obstructing the flow. Tubing hanging below the bed interferes with gravity flow.
Position of the extremity where the site is located	Flexion of the extremity may compress the vein, slowing the flow.
Any possible obstruction to the flow	A protective device on the limb may be too tight. Tape may be compressing the extremity.
When the filter was changed	The filter may be occluded.
Position of the catheter within the vein	The catheter may be lying against the vein wall. Turning the catheter slightly may reposition the tip.
If other measures are unsuccessful, try to aspirate blood from the catheter	A small clot may be obstructing the catheter. Aspiration may withdraw the clot.
Never force flush an IV catheter	Forcefully flushing a catheter sends the clot into the bloodstream. This creates an embolus that could lodge anywhere, including the brain, heart, or lungs.

IV, Intravenous.

Skill 36.3 Administering Intravenous Piggyback Medication

 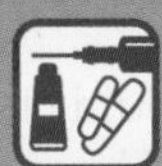 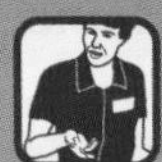 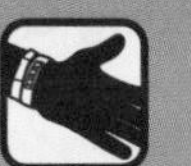 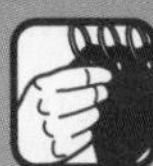 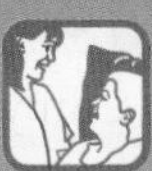 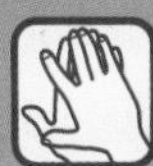 

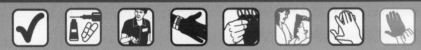

Various types of medications are administered intermittently by piggyback, or secondary line, infusion. The drug solution is generally prepared by the pharmacy. Some drugs in solution must be refrigerated. If this is the case, remove the medication from the refrigerator 30 minutes before administration.

Supplies

- Ordered medication in solution
- IV piggyback administration set
- Needleless connector
- Alcohol swabs
- Medication administration record (MAR) or workstation on wheels (WOW)

Review and carry out the Standard Steps in Appendix A.

ACTION *(RATIONALE)*

Assessment (Data Collection)

1. Check the medication against the MAR or eMAR. Assess for allergies. *(Use the Six Rights when administering IV medications. An allergy to IV medication can be life threatening.)*

Planning

2. Calculate the flow rate. Check with the pharmacy or consult a drug handbook for the specific drug you will administer. *(Most IV piggyback drugs are given over 20 to 90 minutes.)*

Implementation

3. Open the secondary (piggyback) administration set, close the clamp, and insert the spike end of the tubing into the tubing port, using aseptic technique. *(The process of preparing secondary tubing is similar to preparing primary tubing.)*
4. Squeeze the drip chamber while inverting the IV piggyback container, and hang it from an IV hook. *(This maneuver partially fills the drip chamber so that air will not flow into the tubing.)*
5. Loosen the connector cover; slowly open the clamp, and clear the air by running fluid through the tubing into the trash or a sink. *(Allows fluid to run through the tubing without allowing more air to bubble into the tubing.)*
6. Verify the drug and dosage again, and go to the patient's room. Properly identify the patient, using two identifiers. If infusing an antibiotic, re-verify any allergies the patient might have. *(The third check is performed at the bedside. Medication allergies can be life threatening.)*
7. Hang the piggyback container on the IV pole. "Scrub the hub" of the injection port of the primary site with an alcohol swab for 15 seconds. *(Scrubbing the hub is recommended to prevent catheter-related bloodstream infections.)*

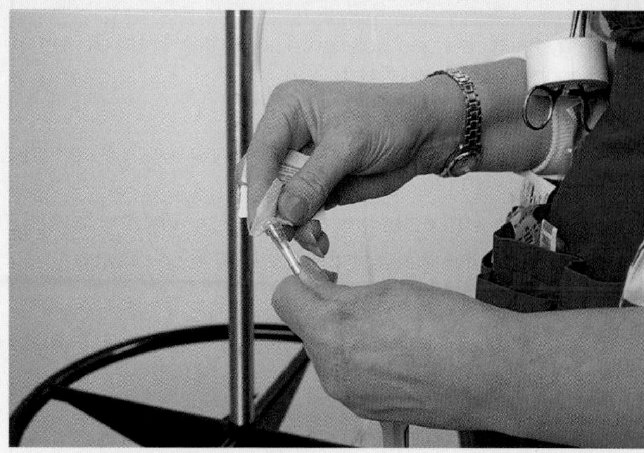

Step **7**

8. Attach the IV piggyback tubing to the port with a needleless adaptor or a snap lock device; open the clamp of the secondary set, and adjust the rate of flow. If the piggyback will not flow, lower the primary IV container using an IV hanger. If you are using an infusion pump, make certain that all the clamps are open and troubleshoot the pump. *(Fluid in a higher container will flow before the fluid in the lower container. See Box 36.1 for troubleshooting an infusion pump.)*

Evaluation

9. Evaluate whether the medication is effective by assessing for signs of improvement. Evaluate the vein and surrounding tissue for irritation or inflammation. *(Monitoring blood counts, other laboratory values, vital signs, and the patient's subjective report indicates the effectiveness of the therapy.)*
10. Assess for adverse or side effects to the medication administered. *(If adverse effects occur, discontinue the medication and notify the primary care provider.)*

Documentation

11. Document the IV medication on the MAR or eMAR. *(The right documentation promotes continuity of care.)*

Special Considerations

- Always assess for allergies and adverse effects before infusing each dose of medication.
- "Scrub the hub" for 15 seconds when accessing an injection port of IV tubing.
- Use a needleless connector with a securing clamp to attach the piggyback to the primary tubing, to prevent disconnection with patient movement.
- Always assess the IV site before infusing any IV medication to make certain that the IV site is patent.

Critical Thinking Questions

1. Can you identify everything you would check before starting to infuse an IV piggyback medication for a patient?
2. What would you need to do if the IV piggyback ordered is incompatible with one of the additives in the main IV solution infusing at the time you are to administer the IV piggyback?

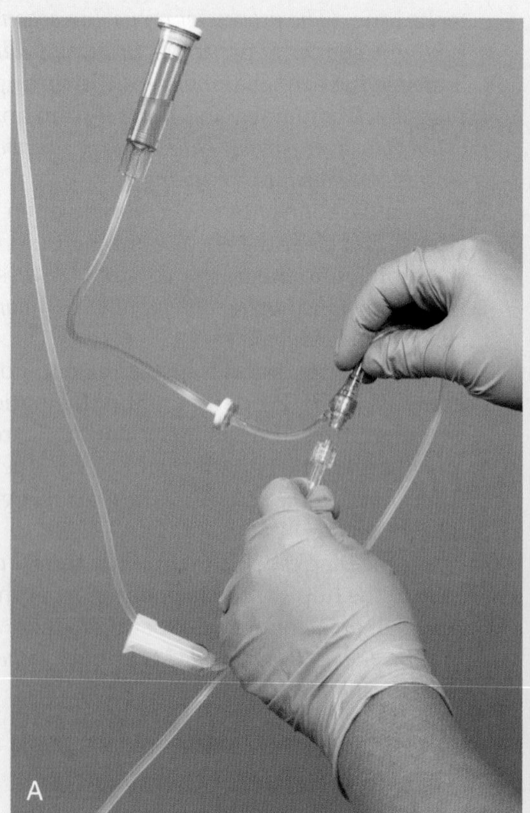

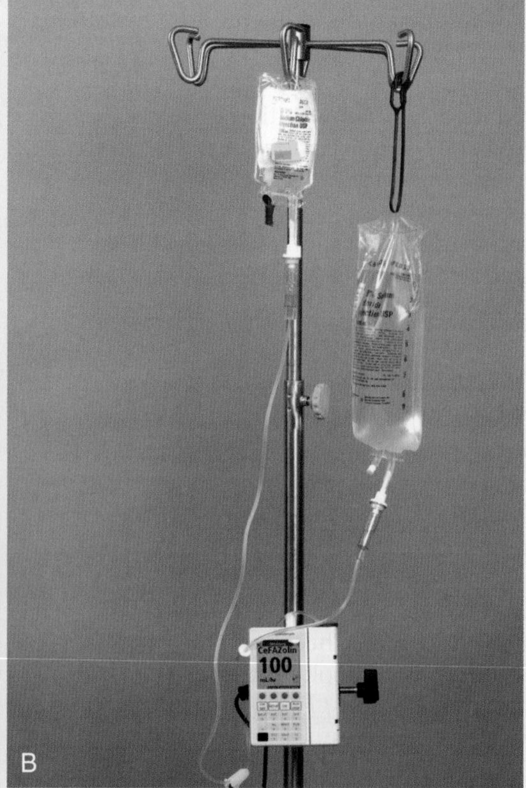

Step **8**

IV, Intravenous; *MAR*, medication administration record; *WOW*, workstation on wheels.

Steps 36.2 Adding Medication to an Intravenous Solution

Adding a medication to an IV solution is frequently done by the pharmacy; however, on occasion nurses would perform this task.

Review and carry out the Standard Steps in Appendix A.

ACTION *(RATIONALE)*

1. Check the medication and IV solution against the order; calculate the medication dosage if necessary. *(Observing the Six Rights prevents medication errors. Ask another nurse to check your calculations.)*
2. Prepare an additive label to be placed on the IV container after the medication is added. The label should include the patient's name, the room number, the name of the drug, the dosage, the date and time, and your initials. *(A label indicates what has been added to the solution.)*
3. Prepare the medication, and draw it up in a syringe using aseptic technique. *(Prevents contamination of the medication and the IV solution.)*
4. Remove the tab from the medication injection port on the IV container, swab it with an antiseptic swab to remove any residue that may have been deposited during manufacture, and inject the medication into the container. *(Deposits the medication into the solution.)*
5. Place the additive label on the container. Mix the solution with the medication by inverting the container or rotating it several times. *(The medication and solution must be thoroughly mixed to provide the right dilution and distribution of the medication.)*

IV, Intravenous.

Some potent drugs and those causing irritation in concentrated strengths are diluted in 1000 mL of fluids. Typical drugs used in this way are potassium, insulin, sodium bicarbonate, calcium, magnesium sulfate, vitamin B complex, and vitamin C. Usually these medications are added by the pharmacist. If you have to add medication to IV fluids or dilute medications, you must follow package directions for type and amount of diluent, use strict aseptic technique, and use a needleless device (Steps 36.2).

Medications can be given intermittently at timed intervals and administered by the piggyback method. The medication is added to a small bag of fluid, usually 50 to 150 mL. When the patient has a PRN lock rather than a continuous IV infusion, the method of hanging an intermittent infusion differs slightly (Skill 36.4).

Another method of administering IV medications is to mix them in a small amount of solution in a controlled-volume burette (Skill 36.5). Medications given in this manner interrupt the primary infusion of fluids. Monitor the medication closely, and open the clamp to restart the flow of the primary solution when the medication has infused. **The tubing is reused for subsequent fluids and additional doses of medication, thus increasing the possibility of contamination.**

Giving the medication directly into the vein over a few minutes is termed giving a *bolus,* or *IV push, injection* (Steps 36.3). The medication can be instilled via the injection port on the IV tubing, through a PRN lock, or directly into the vein. Many state nurse practice acts do not allow LPN/LVNs to give a bolus injection.

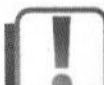 **Safety Alert**

Intravenous Push Promethazine

IV push promethazine has been associated with serious tissue damage leading to loss of circulation and amputation. The Institute for Safe Medication Practices set forth guidelines for nurses administering IV push promethazine that include the following measures to reduce the risk of tissue damage: dilute the drug, limit the concentration and the initial dose, provide an alert on the paper or electronic medication administration record (MAR or eMAR), inject the drug into a running IV, use the port that is farthest from the patient's veins, **never use a hand, wrist, or foot vein**, and advise the patient to report discomfort immediately (Pharmacy & Therapeutics Committee, Marquette General Hospital, 2014). If the patient complains of discomfort at the injection site, stop the infusion immediately and notify the RN/MD.

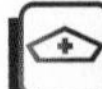 **Clinical Cues**

Most facilities have guidelines for IV antibiotic administration for community-acquired pneumonia (CAP), usually with the goal of first dose of antibiotic to be given within 4 hours of patient arrival, often in the emergency department (Kamangar, 2015).

Administering Heparin Infusions

One of the National Patient Safety Goals is to "reduce the likelihood of patient harm associated with the use of anticoagulation therapy." Nursing measures to meet this goal include scrupulous attention to dosage and adjustment of IV infusions such as a heparin drip; use of an IV pump is mandatory for safe delivery. Agency protocol may allow RNs to adjust the IV dose of heparin based on laboratory values such as partial

Skill 36.4 Administering Medication via Saline or PRN Lock

 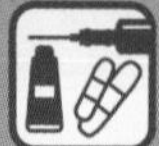 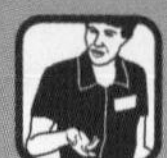  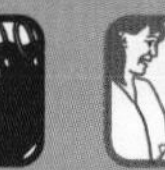 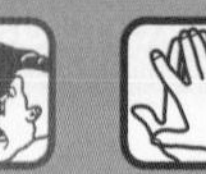 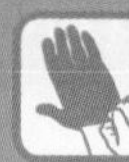

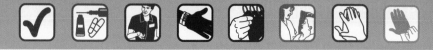

When the patient does not need large quantities of IV fluid but does need IV medications intermittently, a saline or PRN lock is inserted. If an IV is already infusing, it can be changed to an intermittent IV by removing the tubing and attaching an injection cap or a short extension set to the catheter.

Supplies

- Gloves
- IV cannula and injection cap (or an extension set with an injection cap)
- Normal saline
- IV start kit (usually includes chlorhexidine or alcohol swabs, label, tape, transparent dressing, and tourniquet)
- Underpad
- Syringe and needleless connector or snap connector
- Medication administration record (MAR) or workstation on wheels (WOW)
- Commercial device for securing the site

Review and carry out the Standard Steps in Appendix A.

ACTION *(RATIONALE)*

Assessment (Data Collection)

1. Determine need for saline or PRN lock rather than continuous IV; check the primary care provider's orders. *(Intermittent infusion is more comfortable for the patient.)*

Planning

2. Look at the patient's veins and choose the best site for the saline or PRN lock. *(Unless the lock will be used long-term, a site on the forearm will be most comfortable for the patient.)*

Implementation

Flushing the Saline or PRN Lock

3. Perform hand hygiene and flush injection cap (or extension set with cap) with saline. *(Prepares cap or extension set so that it will be ready as soon as IV catheter is inserted.)*
4. Perform hand hygiene, prepare the skin, don gloves; insert the IV cannula (see Skill 36.1) and attach the injection cap (or extension set) to the catheter; flush with 2 mL of normal saline. *(Checks patency of catheter.)*
5. Secure the lock with the commercial securement device. Label the site with the date and your initials. *(Prevents the lock from dislodging. Shows when lock was started.)*

Administering Medications via the Saline or PRN Lock

6. Prepare the medication following the Six Rights. The medication may be mixed as an IV piggyback or drawn up in a syringe. *(Six Rights are always followed to prevent medication errors.)*
7. Prepare a syringe containing normal saline. *(Flushing with saline is used to check patency, to clear the lock of medication, and to leave fluid in the lock to prevent clotting.)*
8. "Scrub the hub" of the cap with an alcohol swab for 15 seconds. Insert the needleless connector into the bull's eye on the lock or connect the syringe to the lock, and aspirate for blood return to determine the patency of the lock. *(If you cannot aspirate blood, the lock is not necessarily blocked because the catheter may just be against the side wall of the vein.)* Slowly inject the saline. If resistance occurs, stop and replace the lock. *(Verifies that the lock is patent before the medication is injected.)*

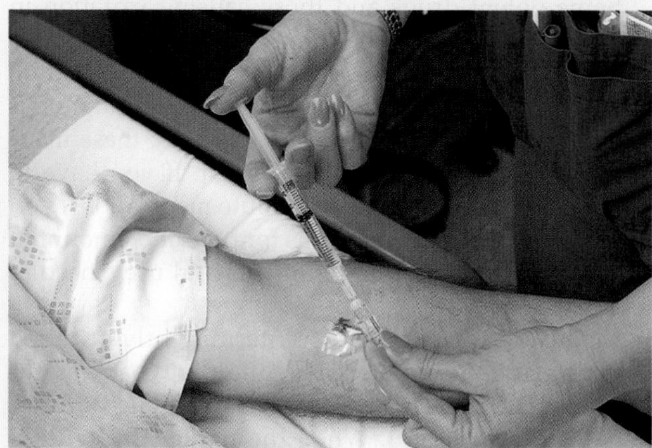

Step 8

9. Verify the drug, the dosage, and patient identification one more time, and then hook up the IV piggyback or inject the medication over the recommended period. *(The third check is done to prevent error.)*

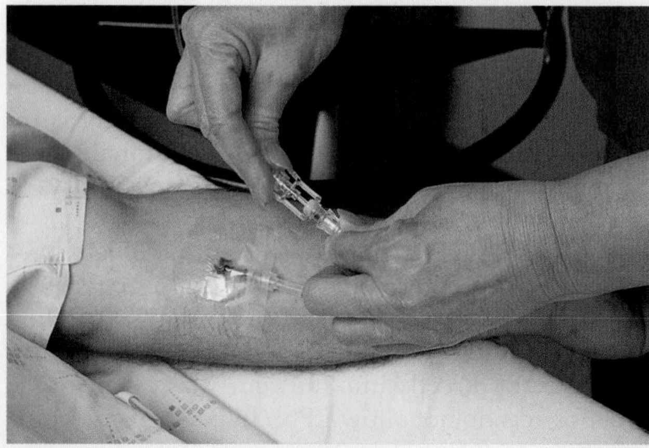

Step 9

Skill 36.4 Administering Medication via Saline or PRN Lock—cont'd

10. After the medication administration is completed, "scrub the hub" for 15 seconds and flush the lock with 2 mL of normal saline. Some agencies follow the flush with a heparin solution; check agency policy. *(Prevents a blood clot from forming and occluding catheter.)*
11. Clean up used equipment and make the patient comfortable. Remove gloves. *(Restores order in the unit. Prevents transfer of microorganisms.)*

Evaluation

12. Observe for blood flow on aspiration of the lock to evaluate patency. *(If no blood flow is seen, injecting 2 mL of saline without pain or swelling at the site indicates that lock is patent.)*

Documentation

13. Document insertion of the saline or PRN lock on the IV flow sheet. Document each medication administered on the MAR or eMAR. *(Right documentation includes site, size of catheter, date, amount and type of flush solution, and medication given.)*

? Critical Thinking Questions

1. You cannot always obtain a blood return from a PRN or intermittent lock. How would you verify that it is patent before you infuse a medication into the lock?
2. How often should a PRN or intermittent lock be changed to another site?

IV, intravenous; *MAR*, medication administration record; *WOW*, workstation on wheels.

Skill 36.5 Administering Medication With a Controlled-Volume Set

 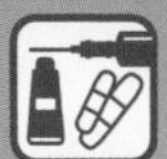 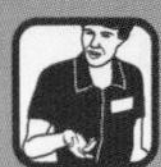 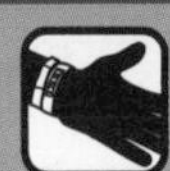 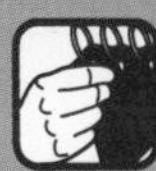 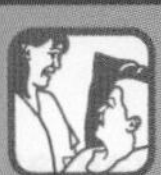 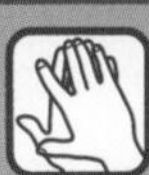 

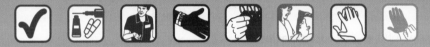

A controlled-volume set is still sometimes used when small amounts of fluid are required just to keep a vein open, for pediatric or older adult patients, or when backup safety for a pump is needed. It could also be used for diluting doses of medication in place of the IV piggyback container or when a pump is not available.

Supplies

- Ordered medication
- Alcohol swabs
- Medication administration record (MAR) or workstation on wheels (WOW)
- Medication label
- Syringe and needleless device
- In-line burette
- IV solution

Review and carry out the Standard Steps in Appendix A.

ACTION *(RATIONALE)*

Assessment (Data Collection)

1. Check the medication with the order; calculate the dosage if needed. Verify compatibility of drug with primary IV solution. Assess for adverse effects of previous doses. *(Following the Six Rights helps prevent medication errors. Incompatibility may cause the drug to precipitate or may inactivate it. Assessment for adverse effects should precede administration of successive doses.)*

Planning

2. Calculate the drop rate (or the pump setting) to instill the medication in the correct amount of time. Note the ending time on your daily work sheet. *(The medication must be administered over a set period of time. The primary IV must be opened again as soon as the medication finishes.)*

Implementation

3. Prepare the medication, and draw it up in a syringe. *(Medication must be added to the burette.)*
4. Take the syringe and the MAR or WOW to the patient's bedside. Properly identify the patient using two identifiers, and recheck the medication. *(The third check is performed at the bedside.)*
5. Fill the burette by opening the upper clamp on the tubing to the primary bag and running 50 to 150 mL of fluid, as specified in the order. Close the clamp on the upper tubing to the solution bag. *(If the upper clamp is not closed, fluid from the primary bag will continue to flow into the burette.)*
6. Lower the burette, locate the injection port on the top of it, "scrub the hub" of the injection port with an alcohol swab for 15 seconds, and inject the medication. Mix the medication with the solution by gently tilting the burette back and forth. *(Dilutes medication for ordered dosage.)*

Skill 36.5 Administering Medication With a Controlled-Volume Set—cont'd

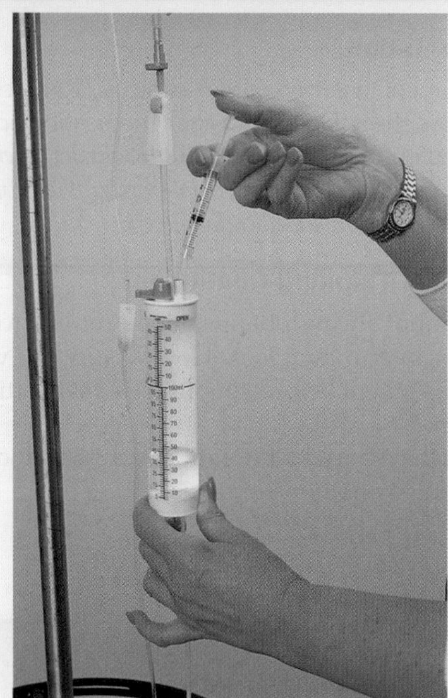

Step 6

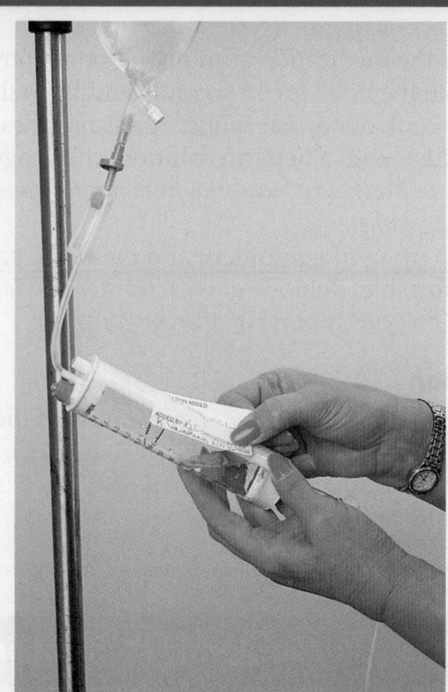

Step 8

7. Open the lower clamp, and adjust the rate of flow from the burette. *(The lower clamp controls the flow to the patient. You may have to increase the height of the burette.)*
8. Label the burette with the name of the drug, the dose, the time, the rate, and your initials. *(Identifies the contents of the burette; if it is not labeled, the contents may be mistaken for ordinary IV solution.)*
9. When the burette is empty, restart the flow from the primary bag by opening the clamp on the upper tubing. Adjust the flow rate. *(Once the burette is empty, the primary bag must be regulated for flow.)*

Evaluation

10. Evaluate the IV site to see whether the medication is causing irritation of the vein. Evaluate the patient for signs that the medication is effective. *(Some medications are irritating to the vein.)*

Documentation

11. Document the medication given on the MAR or eMAR. *(The right documentation verifies that the medication was given.)*

Critical Thinking Question

1. Can you explain what will happen if you forget to clamp off the line from the IV container to the burette when using this controlled-volume device?

IV, Intravenous; *MAR*, medication administration record; *WOW*, workstation on wheels.

thromboplastin time (PTT), or policy may dictate that the primary care provider be notified about each laboratory value and then the provider would order specific dosage adjustments. Nursing students should not adjust the dosage or change the pump settings of heparin infusions; however, you are responsible for monitoring for bleeding signs such as bruising, bleeding of the gums, or blood in the stool.

Administering Antineoplastic Medications

Antineoplastic medications (also called *chemotherapy*) are used to destroy or alter the growth of malignant cells and are toxic to both normal and abnormal cells. Many are irritating to tissue. Toxic antineoplastic drugs usually have a special label attached with a caution warning.

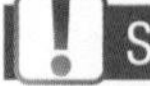 Safety Alert

Administration of Antineoplastic Medications

Most agencies require special training and certification before a nurse is allowed to prepare or administer chemotherapy drugs. Antineoplastic medications can be absorbed through the skin, by inhalation of droplets, or by oral contamination from residue on the nurse's hands. Frequent or long-term exposure to these drugs can lead to alterations in the cells of ova, sperm, or fetal tissue.

Discontinuing an Intravenous Infusion

When an infusion is to be discontinued, the flow is stopped, and the catheter is removed (Steps 36.4). Discontinuation is documented on the IV flow sheet.

Steps 36.3 Administering an Intravenous Bolus Medication (Intravenous Push)

The primary care provider may order medication to be given by the IV push route; although most LPN/LVNs cannot do this under their state nurse practice act, some locales may allow this with additional training.

Review and carry out the Standard Steps in Appendix A.

ACTION *(RATIONALE)*

1. Gather equipment and perform hand hygiene. *(Readies equipment. Prevents transfer of microorganisms.)*
2. Follow the Six Rights when preparing the medication. *(Prevents medication errors.)*
3. Check to see that the medication and any IV solution flowing are compatible. *(Prevents precipitation or inactivation of medication.)*
4. Perform hand hygiene and don gloves; flush the intermittent lock as instructed in Skill 36.4 or scrub the injection port on the primary tubing closest to the patient (the farthest port should be used for some medications) with an alcohol swab. *(Prepares the access for injection of the medication. Some medications should be given in the most distal port because they are irritating to the veins. Check drug handbooks or computer drug databases and consult the pharmacist as needed.)*
5. Connect the syringe or needleless device to the port. *(Allows the medication to flow into the vein.)*
6. Occlude the IV tubing above the port while injecting the medication if injecting into a port on the primary tubing. *(Prevents backflow into the tubing.)*
7. Hold your watch within view as you inject the medication over the recommended time period; inject evenly over the entire time period. *(No medication should ever be injected in less than 1 minute; some require 5 minutes or more.)*
8. Disconnect the syringe from the intermittent lock or the IV injection port; slowly open the IV tubing to flush and then reestablish correct rate. *(Slowly flushing prevents a rapid bolus of medication that is contained within the section of tubing; reestablishes the correct infusion rate after interruption for bolus delivery.)*
9. Flush the intermittent lock, if used. *(Clears medication from the lock and protects it from clotting.)*
10. Dispose of equipment in biohazard container; remove gloves and perform hand hygiene. *(Reduces transfer of microorganisms.)*
11. Document the medication administered on the MAR and patient response on the nurse's notes. *(Include the patient's response because effects usually occur within seconds to minutes after the injection.)*

IV, intravenous.

Steps 36.4 Discontinuing an Intravenous Infusion or PRN Lock

When the patient no longer needs IV fluids, IV medications, or access for emergency drugs, the catheter is removed. Follow Standard Precautions when removing an IV catheter because a slight amount of bleeding almost always occurs.

Review and carry out the Standard Steps in Appendix A.

ACTION *(RATIONALE)*

1. Check the primary care provider's order for discontinuing the IV. *(Prevents inadvertently discontinuing the IV and having to restart it.)*
2. Identify the patient using two identifiers and remove the IV dressing carefully. *(Gentle removal of the dressing prevents moving the IV catheter, which might cause tissue irritation.)*
3. Perform hand hygiene and don gloves; stop the IV flow by clamping the tubing. Hold a sterile gauze pad over the insertion site lightly. Withdraw the catheter. Examine it to verify it is intact. Immediately apply pressure to the site to stop bleeding. *(If tubing is not clamped, the fluid will continue to drip after the catheter is removed. Dry sterile gauze will stop the bleeding quicker. If the catheter is torn or broken, there is risk for catheter emboli. Applying pressure helps prevent hematoma formation.)*
4. When the bleeding has stopped, gently clean blood off the skin around the site, and apply an adhesive bandage. *(A bandage protects the insertion site from microorganisms while it heals.)*
5. Document removal of the catheter and appearance of the site. *(Examples of documentation might include phrases such as "catheter intact and absence of infection" or "tissue damage at the time of removal.")*

IV, Intravenous.

Some acute care units require IV access while patients are hospitalized, so for those patients, their IV is converted to a saline lock.

Administering Blood and Blood Products

A transfusion is the IV administration of whole blood, or one or more of its components. Components frequently transfused include fresh or frozen plasma, packed red blood cells (RBCs), and platelets. Normal saline is the only solution used in conjunction with a blood transfusion. **Autologous** (from the patient's own body) infusions are common during and after surgery. In this instance, the patient's own blood is reinfused. Blood is either collected during surgery (e.g., from chest drainage) or donated by the patient during the weeks before surgery for later reinfusion. Packed RBCs are commonly given for acute or chronic anemia; platelets and fresh frozen plasma are transfused to replenish platelets and provide clotting factors. **The patient must sign a consent to receive blood,** generally no more than 48 to 72 hours before the transfusion. Obtain baseline vital signs before starting the infusion of blood products. All facilities have strict policies regarding frequency of monitoring the patient's condition and response to the blood product.

Observe closely for transfusion reactions. Reactions to blood transfusion usually occur shortly after the start of the transfusion (within 5 to 15 minutes). Reactions are most common when packed RBCs or whole blood is given. Signs of reaction include hives, itching, facial flushing, chills, back pain, apprehension, and fever. If a reaction to the blood occurs, the blood should be instantly shut off. Start the normal saline (with fresh tubing) to keep the IV access open in case emergency drugs are needed. Notify the primary care provider immediately (Skill 36.6).

Legal & Ethical Considerations

Right to Refuse Blood Transfusions

An adult Jehovah's Witness patient may refuse to have a blood transfusion; however, according to US law, if the patient is a minor and the treatment would be lifesaving, legal precedent allows physicians and/or hospitals to take protective custody of the child to do what they view as medically necessary, which may include blood transfusions (Talati, 2012). The family should be treated with respect and empathy. Blood substitutes or alternative treatments may be used in certain cases.

Skill 36.6 Administering Blood Products

 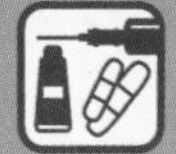 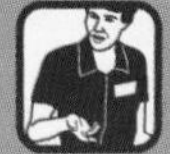 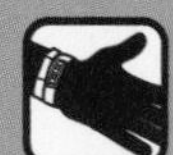 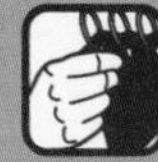 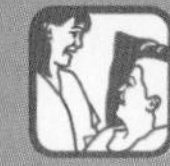 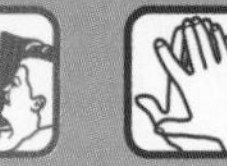 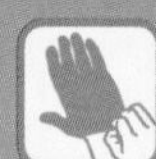

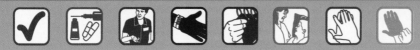

There is no margin for error when administering blood products because adverse reactions can be life threatening. In accordance with National Patient Safety Goals, the nurse must use two identifiers: the patient's name and number on the identification bracelet, or the patient verbally stating name and birth date, are suitable identifiers. Most agencies require that two nurses verify the blood component, the patient number, and blood component unit numbers. Some state laws may prohibit the LPN/LVN from initiating blood products but allow monitoring of a stable patient.

Supplies

- Blood product administration set (Y tubing and filter)
- Alcohol swabs
- Normal saline 0.9% IV solution
- Blood bank slip
- Ordered blood component
- Tape
- Gloves
- Infusion pump

Review and carry out the Standard Steps in Appendix A.

ACTION *(RATIONALE)*

Assessment (Data Collection)

1. The patient must have a patent IV of at least 20-gauge (Stupnytskyi et al., 2014). Plasma products may be infused via a 22-gauge catheter. *(A catheter with a bore smaller than 20 gauge may break up red cells.)*

Planning

2. Gather the equipment, verify that the patient is ready, and obtain the blood product from the blood bank. (Packed red cells are the component used for this example.) *(Administration of blood product must begin within 30 minutes after the product leaves the blood bank.)*

Implementation

3. With another nurse, verify the blood component, and compare the donor numbers and the ABO group and Rh type on the request slip with the label and numbers on the blood component bag. One nurse should read the numbers from the blood bank transfusion record slip while the other checks the numbers on the blood component bag. Verify the expiration date on the blood component bag; check the bag for clots. *(Verification process may differ*

Skill 36.6 Administering Blood Products—cont'd

slightly by agency. Both nurses must sign the transfusion verification form. Expired blood components or bags with clots must be returned to the blood bank.)

4. Close all clamps on the Y administration set. Spike a normal saline container. Prime the filter and tubing with normal saline by opening the slide clamp below the drip chamber of the normal saline and the lower roller clamp. Spike the blood component bag. For packed red cells, invert and lower the packed red cell bag, open the clamp to the bag, and open the slide clamp to the normal saline while keeping the roller clamp closed. Allow about 50 mL of saline to run into the packed red cells. Close the clamps. *(A Y set is always used for blood component infusion. Priming the filter and tubing with normal saline removes air. Combining a small amount of saline with packed red cells decreases the viscosity and facilitates flow; check agency policy. Close clamps to prevent loss of blood product.)*

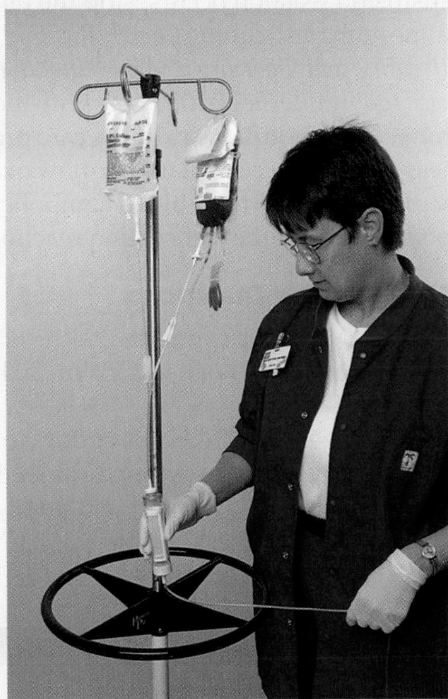

Step 4

5. Take the administration set to the patient's room; properly identify the patient using two identifiers, comparing the full name and hospital identification number on the patient's wristband with the transfusion record information. Compare the blood bracelet identification number with the number on the blood component. *(All identifying information and numbers must match exactly. If discrepancies occur, notify the blood bank. Transfusions are not begun until the discrepancy is resolved.)*
6. Don gloves, and connect the Y administration set to the indwelling catheter. Start the normal saline to clear the catheter, and verify the patency of the site. *(Gloves must be used when contact with blood is likely. The patency of the site must be verified before beginning the transfusion.)*
7. Obtain baseline vital signs. If the patient's temperature is over 100°F, consult the primary care provider. Assess the patient's physical status, particularly looking for signs or symptoms that mimic a transfusion reaction. *(Knowing baseline status helps determine later if a transfusion reaction is occurring.)*
8. Clamp off the saline, and open the clamp to the blood. Set the flow rate at 2 mL/min for the first 15 minutes. Remain with the patient for at least the first 5 minutes. Reassess the patient and take vital signs at the end of 15 minutes. If there are no signs of an adverse reaction, the infusion rate may be increased to the calculated flow rate. Take vital signs at the end of 30 minutes and then every 30 minutes (or according to agency policy) until the transfusion is complete. Ask the patient to tell you if she feels "funny" or has chills, back pain, itching, or shortness of breath. Watch for flushing. **Blood must be infused within 4 hours of release from the blood bank.** Monitor the drip rate continually, and use normal saline to dilute the blood product as needed. Use of an infusion pump is recommended to control the rate. *(Adverse reactions occur most frequently during the first 5 minutes, although delayed reactions can occur. The patient must be monitored throughout the transfusion for any signs of an adverse reaction. It is essential that the patient understand the importance of reporting any symptoms. Average infusion time is 2 hours per unit. Blood is viscous, and the filters will clog and the flow will eventually stop; use of saline dilutes the blood product and decreases viscosity. New tubing may be needed.)*

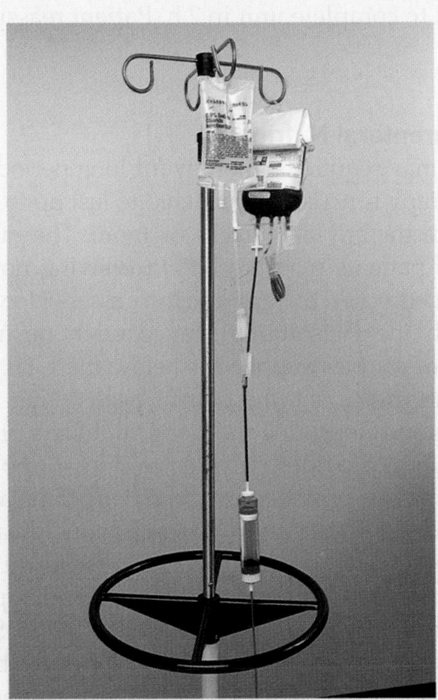

Step 8

Skill 36.6 Administering Blood Products—cont'd

9. When the blood component has been infused, flush the line with normal saline. Reinstitute IV fluid orders with a new solution and tubing, or maintain saline at a "keep vein open" rate (30 to 50 mL/h) until you are certain that the patient is stable and has had no reaction. Then convert to a PRN lock or discontinue the IV site per orders. *(Previously hanging IV solution and tubing are considered contaminated and must be discarded.)*

Evaluation

10. Monitor vital signs and assess for shortness of breath, rash, back pain, apprehension, fever, tachycardia, nausea and vomiting, and other signs of transfusion reaction. *(A transfusion reaction requires immediate intervention.)*

Documentation

11. Document the infusion on the IV flow sheet. Add the amount infused to the IV intake record. Save the label from the blood bag with numbers of the unit and crossmatch identification numbers with the donor type and Rh type; note volume infused, date and time, any reaction signs and symptoms, and your signature. Adverse reactions must be documented in the nurse's notes. *(Documents the transfusion and patient response. Typically, labels and blood forms are returned to the blood bank; consult agency policy.)*

Documentation Example

Vital signs: T 98.4°F; BP 132/86; P 74; R 16. First unit of packed RBCs via 18 angiocath in rt. forearm. Begun at 2 mL/min. No signs of adverse effects in 15 min. Vital signs: T 98.4°F, BP 136/86; P 76, R 16. Flow rate adjusted to complete unit in 2 h. Patient reassured that someone will check on her every 15 to 30 min, but also instructed to call for symptoms such as chills, shortness of breath, apprehension, or discomfort. (Nurse's time-stamped electronic signature)

Special Considerations

- A blood product infusion should begin within 30 minutes of leaving the blood bank.
- A blood warmer may be used if the patient is in critical condition.
- The patient and the blood transfusion should be checked every 15 to 30 minutes to ensure patient safety and continuance of ordered rate.
- Blood components that are still hanging after 4 hours without refrigeration must be discontinued.
- In the post infusion period, the patient's urine is observed for signs of hematuria, indicating a transfusion reaction.
- If a transfusion reaction occurs, stop the blood, start saline with fresh tubing *(merely flushing the Y tubing with saline will flush any blood product that remains in the used tubing into the patient)*, stay with the patient, and immediately notify the primary care provider. If shortness of breath occurs, start low-flow oxygen per agency protocol. Return the blood component bag to the blood bank with the transfusion reaction form.

Critical Thinking Questions

1. What type of IV fluid is connected to the Y tubing when RBCs are given to patients? Why is this IV fluid selected?
2. You are infusing packed red cells and the patient calls you to the room and says that she is feeling short of breath and itchy. What would you do?

IV, Intravenous; *RBCs*, red blood cells.

Total Parenteral Nutrition

Patients may require IV therapy for long periods. Short-term therapy is usually considered to last up to 2 weeks; long-term therapy is 6 weeks or more. The nutritional status of patients who are NPO (receiving nothing by mouth) and on IV therapy must be assessed every day. Although the IV solution may contain dextrose, the amount of calories supplied is below the total daily requirement; moreover, the patient needs other essential nutrients and fiber. One thousand milliliters of 5% glucose solution provides only 200 calories. Supplemental calories may be provided by the use of amino acids and fat emulsions. Dextrose in concentrations greater than 10% is best given through central lines because it is irritating to peripheral veins and can lead to thrombophlebitis. TPN is primarily given through a central line. Specially prepared solutions can be given peripherally, but these may provide fewer calories if the dextrose content is less. Additional information on TPN is found in Chapter 27.

Home Care Considerations

Using Intravenous Medications in the Home

- When there is a long-term need for IV therapy, the patient or family may be instructed on how to administer the solutions safely. The solutions and medications are prepared and delivered by a home infusion company. For safety, an infusion pump is often used.
- The patient should have an emergency telephone number for problems with therapy or equipment.
- Clearly written instructions in the appropriate language regarding dosage schedules for IV medications, preparation of IV piggyback bags and tubing, PRN lock flushes, how to change the primary IV tubing, and so forth must be available for the patient or family member responsible for IV care.
- The patient or family member should give a return demonstration before giving unsupervised IV care.
- Coordinate IV patient education with the IV infusion company to avoid conflicting instructions for the patient.

◆ EVALUATION

Evaluation requires constant patient assessment. Evaluation of the effect of IV therapy relates to the reason it was given. If fluids are being given for hydration, check for good skin turgor, adequate urine output, and moist mucous membranes. If TPN is being given, assess the patient's weight gain and monitor the blood glucose level. When IV antibiotics are administered, check the leukocyte count, temperature, and any wound to see if signs of infection are clearing; also check for signs or symptoms of allergic reaction. When antibiotics are given to prevent infection after surgery, monitor the incision for signs of inflammation and track the body temperature to see whether the medication is effective. When a blood product is administered, monitor the blood count to see if values improve. Monitor for signs and symptoms of transfusion reaction.

Documentation

Documentation of IV medication is done on the MAR or eMAR. Data included in the documentation are similar to those for other types of medications. In addition, the IV site is assessed every 1 to 2 hours according to agency policy, and observations are entered on a flow sheet or in the nurse's notes. IV fluid is counted as intake and recorded on the I & O sheet. Your documentation should reflect an absence of complications. **If you identify a problem, document your observations and include your follow-up actions to address the problem.**

Get Ready for the NCLEX Examination!

Key Points

- IV solutions supply the body with fluids, electrolytes, nutritional components, or medications that cannot be supplied as rapidly or efficiently by other means.
- The average adult needs 1500 to 2000 mL of fluid per 24 hours to replace fluids eliminated by the body.
- Medications may be given as IV solution additives, as piggyback medications, by controlled-volume burette, or by bolus.
- All medications are administered following the Six Rights and are documented on the MAR or eMAR.
- All IV solutions must be sterile; interior surfaces of connectors, adapters, and equipment that comes in contact with the solution must also be kept sterile.
- The three most common infusion tubing sets are the primary, the secondary, and the Y-type tubing.
- Regular drop sets deliver 10 to 20 gtt/mL, macrodrip sets deliver 10 to 15 gtt/mL, and microdrip sets deliver 60 gtt/mL.
- Infusion pumps are programmed by the nurse to deliver a set volume in a specified period.
- Piggyback (intermittent) IV medications are commonly mixed in 50 to 250 mL of solution.
- The most frequently used peripheral IV sites are the veins of the forearm and hand. Scalp veins may be used in infants.
- PICC and ML catheters are used for IV therapy when high blood flow is needed; they are also used for long-term IV therapy.
- Central venous catheters are inserted into the subclavian or jugular vein by a physician.
- All IV catheters must be periodically flushed using a 10-mL syringe with sterile saline (or dilute heparin) to maintain patency if continuous fluid is not infusing.
- Longer-term IV therapy requires a tunneled catheter, PICC line, ML catheter, or implanted infusion port.
- Infiltration is the most common complication of IV therapy; other complications are listed in Table 36.2.
- Assess the site and the patient every 1 to 2 hours when administering IV fluids or medications.
- You are responsible for correctly calculating the ordered flow rate, regulating the infusion, ensuring that the correct fluid is infusing, and watching for complications.
- Always "scrub the hub" with an alcohol swab for 15 seconds before flushing or before interrupting the system to attach new connectors, adapters, or IV tubing.
- All IV sites and solutions infused are recorded on the IV flow sheet. IV medications are recorded on the MAR or eMAR.
- Always use normal saline to flush the line when blood products are administered.
- If a transfusion reaction occurs, immediately stop the blood and start normal saline with fresh tubing.
- Clearly written instructions and demonstrations are given to home care patients who are undergoing IV therapy.

Additional Learning Resources

SG Go to your Study Guide for additional learning activities to help you master this chapter content.

evolve Go to your Evolve website at http://evolve.elsevier.com/Williams/fundamental for additional online resources.

Review Questions for the NCLEX Examination

*Choose the **best** answer for each question.*

1. Because of a communication error, the pharmacy says that there is a long delay for a replacement bag of TPN to be mixed and delivered to the unit for the patient. While awaiting the replacement bag of TPN, the nurse recognizes that a medical order is needed for which type of IV fluid?
   1. 0.45% Saline
   2. 5% Dextrose in water
   3. 10% Dextrose in water
   4. Lactated Ringer

2. What is the nurse's primary responsibility in the daily care of a patient with a central line?
   1. Use sterile technique during insertion.
   2. Flush the line according to agency policy.
   3. Verify catheter placement with an x-ray examination.
   4. Rotate the insertion site every 72 hours.
3. A patient is receiving heparin intravenously. What signs and symptoms would alert you to the patient having adverse effects of heparin? *(Select all that apply.)*
   1. Sleeplessness
   2. Bleeding gums
   3. Blood in urine
   4. Coughing
   5. Bruising
4. A nurse is adding a secondary piggyback to the patient's existing IV. To use the gravity system, the nurse should hang:
   1. The piggyback bag higher than the maintenance IV bag.
   2. The maintenance IV bag at the same height as the piggyback bag.
   3. The piggyback bag and the maintenance IV bag using Y tubing.
   4. The maintenance IV bag after the piggyback bag is completed.
5. In which circumstance would the use of a burette be advised as a safety device?
   1. A trauma patient needs several units of packed red blood cells.
   2. The patient needs IV fluids, but no infusion pump is available.
   3. An infant is at risk for IV fluid volume overload.
   4. A confused patient keeps trying to unplug the infusion pump.
6. The nurse must assess for complications of IV therapy. Signs of common complications include: *(Select all that apply.)*
   1. Swelling and coolness at the site.
   2. Redness along the vein.
   3. Pale skin at the insertion site.
   4. Immobility of the extremity.
   5. Erythema and tenderness.
7. The patient is receiving a blood transfusion and develops a fever, shortness of breath, and a diffuse rash within 10 minutes after the start of the transfusion. What is the priority action?
   1. Take vital signs and call the primary care provider.
   2. Place the patient in a supine position and start oxygen.
   3. Stop the blood and change the IV tubing.
   4. Slow the blood and check the vital signs.
8. A patient returns from physical therapy, and her IV has a very sluggish flow, but it was functioning well before going to physical therapy. What is the priority nursing action?
   1. Call the physical therapist and ask if anything happened to the IV during the treatment session.
   2. Discontinue the IV and restart the IV at a new site.
   3. Assess the IV insertion site and tubing and try repositioning the extremity.
   4. Use a heparin flush to clear the line.

Critical Thinking Activities

Read each clinical scenario and discuss the questions with your classmates.

Scenario A

Daris Hostetler has lost a lot of blood from injuries sustained in an automobile accident. The primary care provider orders three units of packed RBCs for him.

1. Describe the procedure used to prepare to infuse the first unit of packed RBCs.
2. What points are essential to check with another nurse for each unit of packed RBCs?
3. After the second unit is begun, Mr. Hostetler complains of shortness of breath and is apprehensive. Identify the steps you would take in order of priority.

Scenario B

Sherida Patel, age 82, is receiving IV therapy after surgery for her fractured hip.

1. What areas of assessment (related to the IV therapy) would you pay especially close attention to for this older adult patient?
2. Mrs. Patel becomes confused and develops crackles in the base of the lungs. What would you do?

Scenario C

The patient has a potassium level of 3.2 mEq/L. The primary care provider orders 20 mEq of potassium added to 250 mL of 5% dextrose in 0.45% saline to infuse over 2 hours.

1. What is the purpose of diluting potassium in the 5% dextrose in 0.45% saline solution?
2. List at least three nursing actions that you would use to prevent the complications or adverse reactions related to the potassium infusion.

Scenario D

You are assigned to care for a patient who requires IV therapy. You have the opportunity to insert a peripheral IV, but you have never done this procedure before on a real patient.

1. Discuss some of the feelings you might have regarding this first time opportunity.
2. What are some things you should do before you attempt the procedure?
3. You have tried twice to hit the vein. Your instructor tells you that although you were not successful, you still used the correct sterile technique. Later that day, the patient seems a little hesitant to allow you to perform other care. What could you do?

chapter 37

Care of the Surgical Patient

http://evolve.elsevier.com/Williams/fundamental

Objectives

Upon completing this chapter, you should be able to do the following:

Theory

1. Discuss reasons for performing surgery.
2. Identify potential risk factors for complications of surgery.
3. Explain the nurse's role in the various phases of perioperative nursing.
4. Illustrate how robotic surgery has shortened recovery time.
5. Compare the types of anesthesia used for surgery.
6. Verify the safety measures in place to prevent errors regarding the surgical site.
7. Assist the patient with psychological preparation for surgery.
8. State the nurse's role during the signing of a surgical consent form.
9. Compare the roles of the scrub person and the circulating nurse.
10. Select interventions to prevent each of the potential postoperative complications.

Clinical Practice

1. Perform preoperative patient education for the patient and the family.
2. Implement physical preparation of the patient before surgery.
3. Prepare to perform an immediate postoperative assessment when a patient returns to the nursing unit.
4. Promote adequate ventilation of the lungs during recovery from anesthesia.
5. Assess for postoperative pain and provide comfort measures and pain relief.
6. Promote early ambulation and return to independence in activities of daily living.
7. Perform discharge patient education necessary for postoperative home self-care.

Skills

Skill 37.1 Applying Antiembolism Stockings 753

Key Terms

anesthesia (ăn-ĕs-THĒ-zē-ă, p. 736)
atelectasis (ă-tē-LĔK-tă-sĭs, p. 751)
autologous transfusion (ăw-tō-lŏ-gŭs trănz-FYŪ-shŭn, p. 739)
conscious (KŎN-shŭs, p. 736)
curative surgery (KYŪR-ă-tĭv, p. 734)
dehiscence (dĕ-HĬS-ĕns, p. 755)
elective (ē-LĔK-tĭv, p. 734)
embolus (ĔM-bō-lŭs, p. 755)
evisceration (ĕ-vĭs-ĕr-Ā-shŭn, p. 755)
laser (LĀ-sĕr, p. 735)
palliative surgery (PĂL-ē-ă-tĭv, p. 734)
paralytic ileus (păr-ă-LĬT-ĭk ĬL-ē-ŭs, p. 754)
perioperative (pĕr-ē-ŎP-ĕr-ă-tĭv, p. 735)
pneumonia (nū-MŌ-nē-ă, p. 755)
prosthesis (prŏs-THĒ-sĭs, p. 738)
stasis (STĀ-sĭs, p. 739)
thrombophlebitis (thrŏm-bō-flĕ-BĪ-tĭs, p. 739)
thrombosis (thrŏm-BŌ-sĭs, p. 752)
unconscious (ŭn-KŎN-shŭs, p. 736)

Concepts Covered in This Chapter

- Anxiety
- Communication
- Coping
- Culture
- Elimination
- Gas exchange
- Infection
- Inflammation
- Mobility
- Nutrition
- Pain
- Patient education
- Perfusion
- Safety
- Sensory perception
- Stress

REASONS FOR SURGERY

A procedure may be **elective** (voluntary), such as when a hernia repair is scheduled a week away. **Emergency surgery** is often necessary in trauma cases in which serious consequences will occur if surgery is not done immediately. **Palliative surgery** (to relieve pain or complications) is performed to make a patient more comfortable. Removing a metastatic tumor from the abdomen that is causing considerable pain is an example. **Diagnostic surgery,** such as a biopsy of a mass, is done to provide data for a diagnosis of the problem. **Reconstructive surgery,** such as mammoplasty after a mastectomy, is done to restore appearance or function. **Curative surgery** alleviates (cures) a problem, as when a gallbladder full of stones causing blockage or pain is removed.

PATIENTS AT HIGHER RISK FOR SURGICAL COMPLICATIONS

The infant and the older adult are at higher risk for surgical complications because of either immature body systems or a decline in function of various body systems. Maintaining core body temperature is one concern for these patients. Both age groups are at risk for dehydration or overhydration. Aging causes changes in the cardiovascular, respiratory, renal, integumentary, neurologic, and metabolic systems. Other types of patients who are at higher risk during and after surgery are those with bleeding disorders, cancer, heart disease, chronic respiratory disease, diabetes, liver disease, immune disorders, chronic pain, upper respiratory tract infection, fever, or drug abuse issues (Table 37.1). **These patients are subject to a variety of complications and should be carefully assessed during the postoperative period.**

All patients are at risk for surgical site infection. By adhering to the guidelines established in the Surgical Care Improvement Project (SCIP), an estimated 40% to 60% of surgical site infections can be prevented (Phillips et al., 2015) (Box 37.1). SCIP was created in collaboration with The Centers for Medicare & Medicaid Services, The Joint Commission, The Centers for Disease Control and Prevention, American College of

Table 37.1 Surgical Risk Factors

FACTOR	KEY POINTS
Diabetes mellitus and other chronic diseases	Stress of surgery may cause swings in blood glucose levels that are difficult to control, even for patients without diabetes. Patient may receive intravenous insulin during and after surgery. Wound healing tends to be delayed in the diabetic patient, making the risk of dehiscence greater. There is a higher incidence of infection in the surgical wounds of diabetic patients. Liver and kidney disease makes it more difficult to metabolize and eliminate anesthesia and waste products.
Advanced age with inactivity	Healing is slower in older adults. The risk of disuse syndrome, hypostatic pneumonia, and thrombus formation is higher in an inactive older adult.
Very young age	Infants have difficulty controlling temperature and maintaining normal circulatory blood volume; they are at risk of dehydration.
Malnutrition	Inadequate nutritional stores lead to poor wound healing and skin breakdown.
Dehydration	Reduced circulating volume reduces kidney perfusion and predisposes to a reduced urine output and thrombus formation. Dehydration also alters electrolyte values. The dehydrated patient is at increased risk for problems with pressure areas during surgery.
Obesity	The extremely heavy patient does not breathe as deeply and is at risk of hypostatic pneumonia. Excessive fatty tissue also is a factor in poor wound healing.
Cardiovascular problems	Patients with hypertension, left ventricular hypertrophy, cardiac arrhythmias, or history of heart failure are at a high risk for myocardial infarction from the stresses of surgery and anesthesia.
Peripheral vascular disease	Poor circulation in the extremities predisposes the patient to possible thrombus formation and pressure sores on the lower legs and feet. Antiembolism stockings or devices are generally prescribed for use during and after surgery.
Substance abuse or alcohol dependence	Substance abuse may alter reaction to anesthetic agents. Alcohol dependence may cause withdrawal symptoms if the use of alcohol is discontinued abruptly.
Smoking	Causes increased lung secretions from anesthesia and predisposes the patient to atelectasis and pneumonia postoperatively. Smokers are prone to thrombus formation.
Regular use of certain drugs	Aspirin and anticoagulants make the patient prone to excessive bleeding. Corticosteroids reduce the body's response to infection and delay the healing process.
Excessive fear	Stimulates the sympathetic nervous system and causes the release of hormones, causing swings in the body's chemistry and vital signs. Increased muscle tension makes surgery more difficult. Physical manifestations of fear can interfere with achieving the desired state of anesthesia.

Box 37.1 Recommended Measures to Prevent Surgical Site Infections

- Administer prophylactic antibiotics just before incision time.
- Do not remove hair at the surgical site. If removal of hair is essential, remove hair with clippers or a depilatory.
- Hair is to be removed, when essential, immediately before surgery.
- A razor should not be used to remove hair because it causes nicks and abrasions in the skin.
- Glycemic control should be maintained with blood glucose below 200 mg/dL in the first 48 hours postoperatively.
- Body temperature during and after surgery should be maintained at 96.8 to 100.4°F (36 to 38°C), particularly for those patients having colorectal surgery.

Adapted from Phillips, N., Chettle, C. C., & Barzoloski-O'Connor, B. (2015). Reducing the risk of surgical site infections with the surgical care improvement project (SCIP). Nurse.com West, 28(5), 78–83.

Surgeons and American Hospital Association. This improvement project is designed to monitor and increase patient safety.

PERIOPERATIVE NURSING

Perioperative nursing refers to care of the patient from the time of the decision to have surgery through recovery from the procedure. Learning the terminology for surgical procedures will help in identifying what the surgeon is going to do (Box 37.2). Surgery may be performed as a same-day, or outpatient, procedure, or an inpatient procedure in a hospital or surgery center. Minor surgery is often performed in a physician's office. Patients having same-day surgery are admitted and discharged the same day. Preparation for surgery begins before admission. Diagnostic tests are done in the days just before the scheduled surgery. Patient education for postoperative care must be done efficiently because length of stay is short to reduce hospitalization costs. Your ability to deliver and reinforce patient education for postoperative and home care is crucial to the patient's well-being and quick recovery.

Home Care Considerations

Home Care for Discharged Postsurgical Patients

Discharge planning begins at the time of admission. Whether the patient is a same-day surgery patient or an inpatient, the same general points need to be covered as part of patient education before discharge.

- The patient must know about each medication to be taken, including when to take it.
- Discuss the diet, any restrictions, and guidelines for fluid intake. Alcohol must be avoided for 24 hours after surgery.
- List any restrictions on activity, and provide instructions for use of any special equipment, such as crutches, a splint, or a walker.
- Patients should not drive or make important decisions for 24 hours after anesthesia.
- Explain the type of bath or shower permitted and any special needs (such as shower chair or dressing cover) that may be required during this activity.
- Discuss cleansing and dressing of the wound, along with where to obtain supplies.
- Provide a list of signs and symptoms to report to the surgeon, such as temperature above 100°F, increasing malaise, severe pain or swelling, bleeding through the bandage, decreased sensation below the surgical site, or severe nausea and vomiting.
- Provide written instructions on when to make a follow-up appointment with the provider.
- Send written instructions home with the patient for all essential points of care.

Box 37.2 Terminology for Surgical Procedures

Suffixes are often attached to a stem word to describe a surgical procedure. For example, *appendectomy* means cutting out the appendix.

Lysis: removal or destruction of (lysis of adhesions: removal of adhesions)
Anastomosis: joining of two parts, ducts, or blood vessels
-ectomy: cutting out or off (colectomy: cutting out a part of the colon)
-ostomy: furnishing with a mouth or an outlet (colostomy: creating an outlet from the body for the colon)
-otomy: cutting into (thoracotomy: cutting into the chest cavity)
-plasty: revision, molding, or repair of tissue (mammoplasty: revision of the breast)
-pexy: fixation, anchoring in place (orchiopexy: fixation of an undescended testicle in the scrotum)

ENHANCEMENTS TO SURGICAL TECHNIQUE

LASER SURGERY

Laser (*L*ight *A*mplification by the *S*timulated *E*mission of *R*adiation) surgery is common and is often combined with microscopic, endoscopic, and robotic-enhanced procedures. A laser is a tube that contains a medium such as carbon dioxide or another active gas, which is energized by electricity. Mirrors reflect the energized molecules back and forth, generating a bright light in the form of a beam. The light beam is converted to heat as tissue absorbs it. There are several varieties of lasers for different uses, and they may require a dedicated surgical area or room.

FIBEROPTIC SURGERY

Fiberoptics allow the use of endoscopes with high-resolution video cameras passed through a very small incision for an ever-increasing variety of surgical procedures. Operating microscopes can be combined with an endoscope for microscopic surgery. Small growths and organs can be removed without making a traditional surgical incision. However, two or three other puncture holes are made for the instruments and video camera attachment that provide access and a visual field for the procedure.

ROBOTIC SURGERY

More surgeons are using remote controlled robots to perform surgeries. Robotics is seen as a key to less invasive, less traumatic surgeries in the future. The robot is operated from a nearby computer while the surgeon views magnified three-dimensional images of the surgical field on the computer's screen. This equipment often requires a specially trained surgeon or surgical team and a special area or room. The robot's tiny camera has multiple lenses that allow magnification up to 12 times that of normal vision. Assistants and a second surgeon are next to the patient, but the main surgeon performs the surgery at the computer. For heart surgery the robot's needle-like "fingers" are introduced through pencil-sized holes in the chest to perform certain techniques. Remote controlled instruments are inserted through small incisions. Some types of robotics are voice activated by the surgeon.

A big advantage of using the robot is that it has "rock steady" hands, providing precision that is beyond human dexterity. Because only small incisions are needed, the patient has less pain postoperatively and requires less time to heal. There is less scarring, and fewer infections seem to develop with this evolving surgical technique.

ANESTHESIA

Anesthesia (the loss of sensory perception) has been in use for surgical procedures since the 1840s. Newer anesthetics and techniques make anesthesia safer than ever, but **there is still a risk any time a patient is anesthetized.** The goals of anesthesia are (1) to prevent pain; (2) to achieve adequate muscle relaxation; and (3) to calm fear, ease anxiety, and induce forgetfulness of an unpleasant experience. Anesthetics are administered in a number of ways to achieve these goals. The choice of anesthetic rests with the anesthesiologist or nurse anesthetist, considering the type of surgery to be performed and the patient's age and physical condition.

GENERAL ANESTHESIA

General anesthesia is induced by the administration of an inhalant gas or an intravenous (IV) medication. During general anesthesia the patient is in a deep sleep state with muscle relaxation and is not aware of anything going on in the operating room (OR). General anesthesia has four stages (Box 37.3). When the patient awakens from anesthesia, progression through the stages occurs in reverse. Quiet must be maintained while the patient is in stage II because noise may excite the patient, resulting in instability of vital signs.

Box 37.3 The Four Stages of Anesthesia

Stage I: The stage of analgesia. Begins with the administration of the anesthetic agent and ends when the patient becomes **unconscious** (incapable of responding to sensory stimuli). Hearing is amplified at the end of this stage.

Stage II: The excitement phase. Muscles become tense, but swallowing and vomiting reflexes are still present. Breathing may become irregular or the breath may be held. The environment should be kept quiet during this period.

Stage III: Surgical anesthesia state. Begins with the return of regular breathing. Vital functions are depressed; eyes are fixed; and reflexes are lost or temporarily depressed. The surgical procedure is begun during this stage.

Stage IV: Complete respiratory depression. Spontaneous respirations are absent. The patient is maintained by the anesthesia machine, which supplies oxygen and a set rate of breaths.

Life Span Considerations

Older Adult

- An accurate height and weight of the older adult are important for calculation of anesthetic agents and medication dosages.
- Kidney function declines in the older adult, and drugs are not eliminated from the body as quickly. Reduced dosages are often needed.

REGIONAL ANESTHESIA

Regional anesthesia is accomplished by administering a nerve block. It is often more economical than general anesthesia. This may be accomplished by injecting the spinal, epidural, caudal, or peripheral nerve area. The block anesthetizes the local area or the area distal to the block. Spinal or epidural blocks are frequently used for high-risk patients undergoing pelvic or lower extremity surgery; epidural blocks are widely used in obstetric procedures.

PROCEDURAL (MODERATE) SEDATION ANESTHESIA

A local anesthetic agent at the surgical site plus IV sedation is used to provide systemic analgesia, **conscious** (awareness of one's surroundings) sedation, and depression of the autonomic nervous system. The technique can be used for any surgery or procedure that can be done with local anesthesia and is being used more and more frequently. The patient is monitored closely for blood pressure changes, oxygen saturation levels, and heart activity.

LOCAL ANESTHESIA

Local anesthesia is used for minor procedures, such as superficial tissue biopsies, surface cyst excision, insertion of a pacemaker, and insertion of vascular access devices. The patient who has had local anesthesia is transferred directly to the nursing unit and does not need care in the postanesthesia care recovery unit (PACU, also called PAR or PARU).

PREOPERATIVE PROCEDURES

Care of the surgical patient is divided into four phases: preoperative, intraoperative, postanesthesia immediate care, and postoperative care. During the preoperative phase, nonanemic patients may donate their own blood 2 to 4 weeks before surgery to be banked in case of postoperative autologous (related to self) transfusion need. This eliminates any possibility of transfusion with blood contaminated with a blood-borne virus, such as human immunodeficiency virus (HIV) or hepatitis B or C.

SURGICAL CONSENT

A surgical consent form must be signed before surgery and before preoperative medications are given (i.e., before the patient's mind is affected by the medications). This is a legal form; it must be completed in ink with the correct spelling of procedures to be done. **The surgeon is responsible for obtaining an informed surgical consent.** The need for the procedure, a description of the procedure to be performed, its risks and benefits, and alternative treatments available and their possible consequences must be explained to the patient in understandable terms, and the explanation (not just the patient's signature) should be witnessed by at least one health care professional. Any questions must be answered. The surgeon often explains the procedure with the nurse present, answers questions, and then asks the nurse to obtain the patient's signature on the form. **If the patient does not understand the procedure or has further questions for the surgeon, refer the matter back to the surgeon.** If the patient is a minor, is confused, or is mentally incompetent, another responsible party such as a parent, spouse, or guardian must be present for the explanation and may need to sign the consent form. The signature of the patient or the responsible party is witnessed by another party, often a staff member. The consent form must show the procedure to be performed and the risks involved, must include the time and date, and must be signed in ink. A witnessed "X" is acceptable if the patient cannot sign with a signature, if allowed by institutional policy.

If emergency surgery is needed and the patient is not conscious or able to give consent, immediate family is contacted. Telephone permission may be given as long as there are two witnesses on extension lines. If no family can be found, the opinion of a second surgeon regarding the need for surgery is sought, and then the surgery may take place.

All responsible adults are asked to complete advance directives when admitted to the hospital if they do not already have such a document on file; these are discussed in Chapter 3. Advance directives indicate the patient's desires regarding lifesaving or life-preserving measures in the event of a cardiac arrest or other complication that threatens basic function.

 **Think Critically**

You are taking preoperative vital signs and preparing the patient for surgery when he says, "I've changed my mind. I don't want to have this surgery after all." What would you do?

SURGICAL SITE IDENTIFICATION

One of the 2016 National Patient Safety Goals continues to recommend procedures to **"Eliminate wrong-site, wrong-patient, wrong-procedure surgery."** A preoperative checklist verification process is used to ensure that appropriate medical records and imaging studies are available. A process must also be implemented to mark the surgical site and involve the patient in the marking process. This should be done before preoperative medications are given so that the patient is alert to participate in this procedure.

 **QSEN Considerations: Safety**

Time-Out

Before surgery commences, a "time-out" is called, and the correct patient, correct site, and correct body part are verified by the operating team via the medical orders, operative permit, and imaging studies.

PHYSICAL EXAMINATION

The referring provider, the surgeon, or a surgical resident takes a medical history, performs a physical examination, and orders necessary tests (Box 37.4). This may be done in the provider's office. The dictated report must be in the record before the patient goes to surgery. The patient should be in the best possible physical condition, unless it is an emergency procedure. Most surgeons postpone surgery if the patient's hemoglobin level is too low.

Box 37.4 Recommended Diagnostic Tests Before Surgery

- Complete blood count (CBC)
- Urinalysis
- Chest x-ray examination
- Electrocardiogram (older than age 40)
- Pregnancy test for women of childbearing age
- Electrolytes, blood glucose, liver function, and kidney function tests (SMA-12)
- Prothrombin time (PT) and activated partial thromboplastin time (APTT)
- Blood type and crossmatch

❖ APPLICATION OF THE NURSING PROCESS

PREOPERATIVE CARE

During the preoperative period, the patient is prepared physically and psychologically for surgery. If the patient is very ill, a significant other may join in the interview process. Focus completely on the patient in an unhurried manner. Ask open-ended questions and listen attentively.

◆ ASSESSMENT (DATA COLLECTION)

The nursing history and assessment focus on possible factors that indicate the patient is at higher risk for complications from surgery (see Table 37.1). An important part of your assessment is determining what supplements and herbs a patient consumes (Table 37.2). The surgeon and anesthesiologist must be aware of what substances are in the patient's body in addition to his regular medications. Besides checking for drug allergies, it is important to determine if the patient has a latex allergy.

Clinical Cues

Indications of latex allergy may be reactions to avocados, kiwifruit, bananas, chestnuts, potatoes, peaches, or apricots.

Communication

Preoperative Interaction

Carolyn Silva, age 67, is scheduled for a partial colectomy. She has had several bouts of diverticulitis with considerable pain and malaise. She seems apprehensive about the surgery.

Nurse: "Mrs. Silva, do you understand what the surgeon is going to do on Wednesday?"

Mrs. Silva: "Yes, but I'm nervous about having this done."

Nurse: "The thought of surgery makes you nervous?"

Mrs. Silva: "Well, it's more than that. I have several family members who have had colon cancer and I can't help thinking that cancer is what will be found."

Nurse: "You are scared you have cancer. As I recall you had a colonoscopy a few weeks ago and it didn't show any lesion suspicious of cancer in the colon."

Mrs. Silva: "That's right, but what if the doctor just didn't see it?"

Nurse: "There are no guarantees until you get a clean pathology report, but the colonoscopy showed that you had severe inflammation in this one part of the colon and that is what is to be taken out."

Mrs. Silva: "Oh, I know. I'm just a worrywart."

Nurse: "Perhaps holding positive thoughts about the outcome of this surgery would help reduce your fears. Try to visualize yourself with a healthy colon, with the diseased piece gone, and no more episodes of severe pain and illness."

Mrs. Silva: "I'll try it. It does seem foolish to spend energy worrying until I know something more is wrong."

Nurse: "I'll be at the desk completing documentation for my patients. If you need me, press the call button."

Psychosocial assessment includes fears, attitudes, and concerns about any changes in body image and lifestyle that the surgery may cause (Box 37.5).

Table 37.2 Herbs and Supplements Affecting Surgical Outcomes

SUBSTANCE	POSSIBLE EFFECT
Arnica	May be useful in soft tissue healing
Astragalus and ginseng	May cause increased blood pressure before and during surgery
Garlic, vitamin E, ginkgo, and fish oils	May increase bleeding tendency
Ginger	Can be useful for the prevention of postoperative nausea
Kava and valerian	May cause excess sedation

Adapted from Lewis, S. L., Dirksen, S. R., Heitkemper, M. M., & Bucher L. (2014). *Medical-surgical nursing: Assessment and management of clinical problems* (9th ed., p. 320). St. Louis, MO: Elsevier Mosby.

Box 37.5 Preoperative Psychosocial Data Collection

Inquire regarding feelings and concerns about:

- Body image—scars or loss of a body part
- Possible change in role or relationships after surgery
- Specific anxieties or fears about surgery or anesthesia
- Concerns about care after discharge
- Financial concerns
- The effect on lifestyle that surgery may have
- Past experience of surgery or anesthesia and perceived impressions from others
- Knowledge of surgery, recovery, the patient's role, and the effect on life
- Expectation of surgery results

The OR is notified if the patient is hard of hearing, has impaired vision when glasses are not in place, or has a **prosthesis** (an artificial body part).

 **Life Span Considerations**

Older Adult

One of the greatest fears of the older adult facing surgery is a loss of independence. It is important to stress the measures that will be taken to return the patient to independence after surgery.

Cultural beliefs and values regarding surgery must be considered. If the patient does not speak the same language as the surgical team, an interpreter should be enlisted to assist with communication. A patient's family member should not be used as an interpreter because of confidentiality and possible errors in translation. If a female patient's culture has strict rules for female attire, she needs assurance of sufficient privacy and protection of modesty to ease any fears she might have; such issues and interventions must be conveyed to the OR. Some cultures require a female care provider to perform pelvic examinations. If the patient's culture has certain taboos regarding an aspect of the surgery, the surgical team needs to know about them and plan a way to achieve a good outcome without violating such a taboo. It is especially important to know whether the patient will accept a blood transfusion.

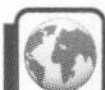

Cultural Considerations

Prohibition of a Non-Self Blood Transfusion

Jehovah's Witnesses refuse a blood transfusion because it is prohibited by their religion. In years past, many surgeries could not be performed on these individuals because the chance of death was too great. New bloodless medicine strategies have allowed many surgeries to occur safely that were denied before; therefore the use of alternative blood products and procedures should be discussed.

- **Autologous transfusion** (transfusion of one's own blood) is one method, using a cell-saver gathering system for blood lost during surgery or in the 2 days after surgery. These cells are washed and then reinfused. This procedure is acceptable to Jehovah's Witnesses as long as there is a continuously closed circuit for collection and reinfusion.
- Hemodilution during surgery may be used, in which up to seven units of the patient's blood are removed and replaced with crystalloids or colloids. The cells are usually reinfused later, again via a closed system. The replacement fluids decrease blood viscosity, increase blood flow in tissues, and help to maintain oxygen transport and blood pressure.
- The use of lasers, electrocautery, argon beam coagulators, and harmonic scalpels, which cause blood to coagulate after tissue is cut, decreases blood loss.
- If the patient is anemic before surgery, epoetin alfa is used along with vitamins B_{12} and C to stimulate red blood cell production.

Think Critically

The patient has told you during your assessment that she drinks a glass of wine with dinner each night. Later her husband informs you that she tends to drink three or four glasses of wine each evening. What should you do with this information?

◆ NURSING DIAGNOSIS

Nursing diagnoses in the preoperative stage include actual and potential problems identified by your data collection and the registered nurse (RN) assessment. Examples of common nursing diagnoses include:

- Anxiety related to the surgical experience and outcome.
- Fear related to risk for death, effects of impending surgery, or loss of control due to anesthesia.
- Grieving related to impending loss of body function or body part.
- Deficient knowledge related to preoperative and postoperative routines.
- Sleep deprivation related to stress or unfamiliar environment.
- Ineffective coping related to lack of problem-solving skills or adequate support.
- Ineffective role performance related to inability to care for children during hospitalization.

◆ PLANNING

Expected outcomes are written for the individual nursing diagnoses assigned to each patient. However, **general goals** for all preoperative patients are the same in that the patient will be:

- Prepared for surgery physically and emotionally.
- Able to demonstrate deep breathing, coughing, and leg exercises.
- Able to verbalize understanding of the procedure and the expectations of him in the postoperative period.
- Able to maintain fluid and electrolyte balance throughout the perioperative period.

When preoperative patients are assigned, plan the work for the shift carefully to have the patients ready without neglecting the needs of other assigned patients. At the beginning of the shift, check to see that any ordered preoperative medications are on hand. Check the surgery schedule and estimate the time that the patient will need to be prepared for surgery.

◆ IMPLEMENTATION

Preoperatively, divide your time between preparing the patient for surgery and patient education about what will happen and how to assist in the recovery period. The same-day surgery patient receives teaching from the medical office nurse or a surgical intake nurse. Patient education sessions may be scheduled when the patient comes for diagnostic testing. Sending written instructions home with the patient reinforces what has been taught. Give the patient a telephone number to call for answers to questions that arise before entering the facility for surgery.

Patient Education for Postoperative Exercises

Teaching the patient breathing, coughing, turning, and leg exercises is a high priority during the preoperative period. Venous return is often hampered during the surgical procedure because of the position assumed on the operating table and pooling of blood in the lower extremities. The **stasis** (stoppage of flow) of blood places the patient at risk for **thrombophlebitis** (a blood clot causing inflammation of a vessel). Specific leg exercises help to prevent this complication (Fig. 37.1). Explain the importance of doing the exercises and show the patient how to do each one; ask for a return demonstration.

Patient Education

Postoperative Foot and Leg Exercises

- Flex and extend the right foot, moving the toes upward and downward, four or five times.
- Repeat with the left foot.
- With the right foot, trace circles to the right five times; repeat with circles to the left.
- Repeat with the left foot.
- Bend the right leg at the knee, sliding the foot back toward the buttocks as far as possible; raise the bent leg off the

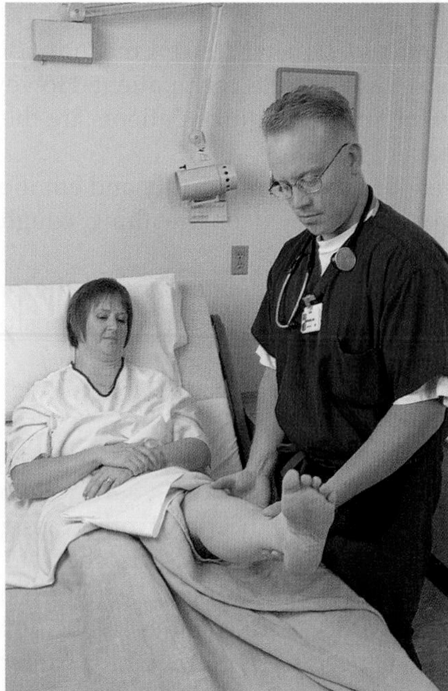

FIGURE 37.1 Performing patient education: postoperative leg exercises. (Courtesy Southwest Washington Medical Center, Vancouver, WA.)

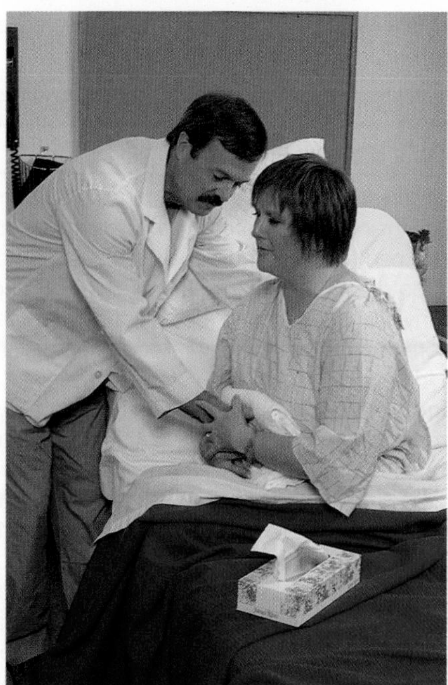

FIGURE 37.2 Performing patient education: deep breathing and coughing.

bed, extend the leg and dorsiflex the foot; extend the foot and lower the leg to the bed.
- Repeat with the left leg and foot.
- Tighten the buttocks muscles for a count of 10 and release to exercise the quadriceps muscles.
- Repeat each exercise four more times.

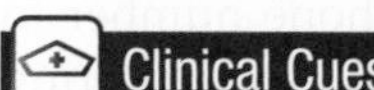

Clinical Cues

One way for patients to remember to do the exercises is to perform them whenever a commercial comes on TV. The exercises should be done at least 5 to 10 times every hour while awake after surgery until the patient is up and about normally.

For deep breathing and coughing, it is preferable for the patient to sit up with the back away from the mattress or chair. This allows for full lung expansion. The surgical incision should be splinted with a pillow (Fig. 37.2).

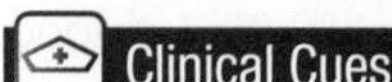

Clinical Cues

A small, firm, coughing pillow can be made by folding a bath towel, putting it in a pillowcase, and folding the pillowcase over and taping it. It is helpful to have a significant other present for these patient education sessions so that coaching and encouragement can later be given to the patient.

Deep breathing and coughing should be performed every 2 hours for 72 hours after general anesthesia. The surgeon may order use of an incentive spirometer. Instruct the patient in its use and supervise until the patient has mastered the technique. Help the same-day surgery patient devise a schedule for doing the exercises.

Show the patient how to turn in bed by flexing the legs to relax the abdominal muscles, grabbing on to the side rail, and slowly turning to the side. This maneuver is also used for getting up out of bed. Instruct the patient about what to expect before, during, and after surgery.

Patient Education

Lung Exercises

Postoperatively, the patient will be asked to deep breathe and cough to open the lungs and clear secretions. When doing these exercises, the patient will sit up away from the mattress. The exercises should be performed every 2 hours during waking hours.

DEEP BREATHING
- Take a deep breath in through the nose, hold for a few seconds, and slowly exhale.
- Repeat twice more.

FORCED EXHALATION COUGHING

Splint the abdominal or chest incision and:
- Take a deep breath through the nose, and cough as you exhale with the mouth open but covered with a tissue.
- If you cannot move secretions with your cough, use a forced exhalation cough.
- Take a deep breath through the nose and forcibly and quickly exhale, producing a huff-cough.
- Repeat the process.
- Repeat again, using three short "huffs" as you exhale to bring the secretions to the mouth where they can be expectorated.

USING AN INCENTIVE SPIROMETER
- Insert the mouthpiece, covering it completely with the lips.
- Take a slow deep breath and hold it for at least 3 seconds.
- Exhale slowly, keeping the lips puckered.
- Breathe normally for a few breaths.
- Try to increase the inspired volume by at least 100 mL with each breath on the spirometer.
- Once maximal volume is achieved, attempt to inspire this volume 10 times, resting a few breaths in between each attempt.
- Clean the mouthpiece of the spirometer when finished.

NPO Status

Food and fluids are restricted before surgery, and the patient is placed on NPO (nothing by mouth) status. A light meal such as toast and clear fluids may be allowed up to 6 hours before surgery and a heavier meal 8 hours before surgery. For elective surgery, the American Society of Anesthesiologists updated the practice guideline in 2011 for preoperative fasting in healthy patients (Johnstone, 2013). Clear liquids, such as black coffee, tea, apple juice, or carbonated beverages, may be consumed up to 2 hours before surgery in some elective cases. Sometimes the surgeon allows an oral blood pressure or heart medication to be given with a sip of water the morning of surgery. **Always check the medical order before giving anything by mouth in the immediate preoperative period.** The purpose of the restriction is to prevent vomiting and aspiration, which can occur, but is rarely seen with modern anesthesia.

Elimination

If the patient is having colon surgery, enemas may be ordered, to be given "until clear." The patient may be on a special soft or liquid diet for 3 days before surgery to decrease the content of the bowel.

Clinical Cues

Ask the patient to empty the bladder, unless a catheter is in place, as you finish the preoperative checklist. Relaxation induced by medications and anesthesia causes the urge to urinate if the bladder is not empty.

Expected Tubes and Equipment

If a nasogastric (NG) tube will be inserted during surgery for postoperative use, explain its purpose, its care, and what it will feel like to the patient. Give an estimate of how long the tube will remain in the stomach. Explain the function, care, and probable duration of use of other expected tubes, such as drains, an IV line, oxygen delivery and monitoring devices, a chest tube, and a urinary catheter.

Rest and Sedation

It is desirable for the patient to be as well rested as possible before surgery so the body is not compromised in meeting the stresses of anesthesia and the procedure. A sedative is usually ordered for the night before surgery, but, if in the hospital, the patient often must ask for it. Same-day surgery patients need to be told how early to take the sedative and retire the night before surgery because they will need to arise early to enter the facility.

Pain Control

Many surgeons order a patient-controlled analgesia (PCA) pump for their patients postoperatively. Patients should receive instruction about the pump and how to operate it before surgery. If patients will be receiving injections for pain control, explain that this type of medication is ordered on an as needed basis every 3 to 4 hours, and they must ask for it.

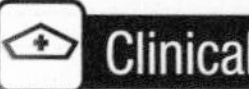
Clinical Cues

Explain that requesting pain medication before the pain becomes severe makes the pain easier to control. The patient will be much more comfortable if pain medication is administered regularly for the first 48 hours postoperatively. Assess the effectiveness of medication delivered by the PCA pump and notify the surgeon if pain is not being well controlled with use of the pump.

Skin Preparation

The patient may be asked to shower with a special antibacterial cleanser the night or morning before surgery to remove as many microorganisms from the skin as possible. Removing hair from the operative site may be done just before surgery but is not generally recommended (see Box 37.1). Explain the process, the area to be prepared, and timing of the prep to the patient. Although this is often done in the OR, it may be part of your job to clip hair or use a depilatory before the patient goes to surgery. If a depilatory is used, perform a skin test for sensitivity close to the surgical site many hours before its use.

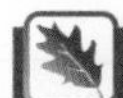
Life Span Considerations

Older Adult

- Perform patient education with the older adult patient in short segments to prevent confusion and to increase the patient's comprehension.
- Provide written reminders of the instructions to the patient.

Immediate Preoperative Care

Dress the patient in a clean hospital gown, with underwear removed, for the OR. Cover the hair with a surgical paper cap. Arrange long hair so that it will tangle minimally; remove all hairpins and barrettes. Remove jewelry, money, and credit cards and give them to a significant other to keep or secure them in a valuables envelope and place it in a locked environment, according to facility policy. If a wedding band is to be worn to surgery, tape it to the finger without restricting circulation. If dentures are removed, place them in a labeled cup and keep them in a designated place according to facility policy. Sometimes the anesthesiologist orders the dentures left in place to facilitate the administration of anesthesia by mask.

Check the patient's identification bracelet against the medical record for accuracy to avoid any error or mix-up of patients in the OR.

Attend to all items on the preoperative checklist that can be handled ahead of time early in the morning (Fig. 37.3). This prevents hurrying, mistakes, and delays in the departure for the OR. If the facility wants the surgical area marked before the patient leaves the room, confer with the patient and appropriately mark or have patient appropriately mark the site according

PREOP/PREPROCEDURE CHECKLIST/REPORT FORM

PATIENT LABEL

1SURG

		YES	N/A
Date	Time		
Surgery/procedure			
Correct patient ID band on		☐	
	In medical record	☐	
	Dictated	☐	

History and Physical
H&P 24 hours to 30 days: update with "No Pertinent Change in History & Physical" stamp
H&P 31-180 days: H&P update form #2396
OB H&P Update for Surgery/Procedures form #2543

	YES	N/A
Initiate Anesthesia Preop order 101.S09. As appropriate initiate OB Anesthesia Order 144.P11	☐	
Include at least one page of patient ID stickers	☐	
Procedural consent: Signed/In medical record	☐	
Procedural site verified with patient/guardian	☐	
Procedural site marked when laterality (including internal laterality), multiple structures (fingers, toes, lesions) or multiple levels (spine). Specify site: ______	☐	☐
Preop antibiotic given	☐	☐
Interpreter if needed	☐	☐
HBOC transfer report in medical record (when applicable)	☐	☐
Acuscan MAR-LOS custom report in medical record (when applicable)	☐	☐

OB ☐ The Department of Social and Health Services consent for sterilization completed and in medical record dated ≥ 30 days prior to procedure (*unless meets exception criteria, listed in Standards of Care Notebook)
☐ Notify anesthesia provider

Diagnostic ☐ Labs in medical record ☐ X-rays with patient (when appropriate) ☐ When applicable Glucose: ______/time ______
☐ Type and screen ☐ ECG (when applicable) Blood units available: # ______

Medications/IV ☐ MAR in medical record ☐ IV/Saline lock in place ☐ If TPN running, start second peripheral IV site

Belongings	Labeled	With Patient/Family	To OR
Contacts			
Glasses			
Hearing aids R L Both			
Dentures ☐ Upper ☐ Lower ☐ Partial			

Prep ☐ Personal clothing removed ☐ Prep completed
☐ Snap gown ☐ Voided, time: ______ ☐ Foley
☐ Jewelry/body piercings: ☐ None ☐ Taped ☐ Family ☐ Patient registration safe
☐ Prep education done Last oral/fluid intake: ______ Time:

Unit based or bedside procedures: FINAL VERIFICATION
☐ Correct patient ☐ Correct side/site ☐ Correct position
☐ Correct procedure ☐ Correct equipment/trays

REPORT USING ISBAR-R: Provide an opportunity to ask and answer questions. Include significant history/special needs.

INITIALS/OR SIGNATURE IF SIGNATURE PAGE NOT USED

FIGURE 37.3 Preoperative communication record to be filled in as the patient is prepared for surgery.

4/10/13 0730 Preop checklist
complete. Surgical site &
knee verified with patient
and marked. - S. Crebs, LPN
0800 transported via gurney. Handoff report to OR team. S. Crebs, LPN

FIGURE 37.4 Entry in nurse's notes.

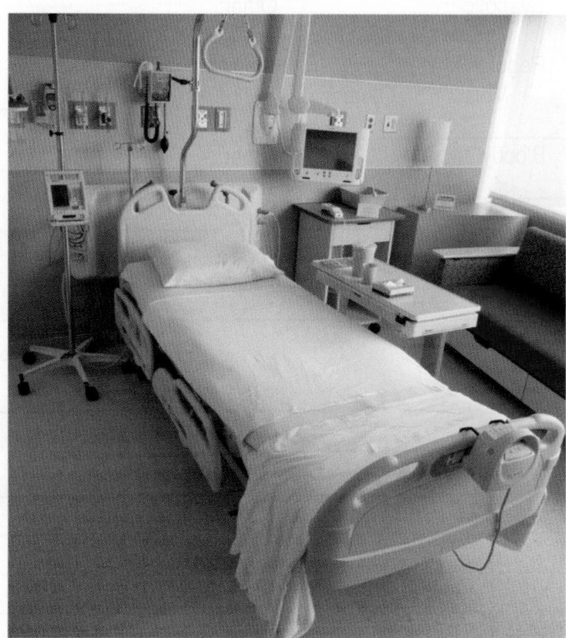

FIGURE 37.5 Postoperative unit prepared for the patient. (Courtesy Southwest Washington Medical Center, Vancouver, WA.)

to agency policy. Seek feedback from the patient and document that the site is marked properly.

Assist in transferring the patient to the stretcher when the transport person comes to take the patient to surgery. Compare the patient's identification bracelet name and numbers with the transport request sheet. Check the medical record to make certain that everything ordered has been done, and make a final entry in the nurse's notes (Fig. 37.4).

Preoperative medications. Most preoperative medications are given intravenously in the surgical holding area rather than on the nursing unit. Preoperative medications are given:

- To reduce anxiety and promote a restful state.
- To decrease secretion of mucus and other body fluids.
- To counteract nausea and reduce emesis.
- To enhance the effects of the anesthetic.

Complementary and Alternative Therapies

Use of Acupuncture to Prevent Postoperative Nausea

An acupuncturist may treat the patient in the holding area to prevent postoperative nausea and vomiting. Such treatment has been shown effective and is helpful for patients who have difficulty with anesthetics and pain medication side effects (Glickman-Simon & Tessier, 2014).

Preparation of the Patient Unit

While patients are in surgery, prepare the patient unit for their return. Make the bed with fresh linen, including a draw sheet placed at shoulder height. Place an underpad at the hip area. Fanfold the top covers to the far side of the bed or to the bottom of the bed. Have the bed in a raised position at the height of the gurney that will return the patient, and arrange furniture so that the gurney can be pulled up alongside the bed (Fig. 37.5).

Gather an emesis basin, tissues, a workstation on wheels (WOW), frequent vital signs sheet or postoperative record (if paper documentation is used), an intake and output sheet, a small towel and washcloth, and a pencil, and place them on the bedside table or console (Fig. 37.6). Place an IV pole at the head of the bed. Connect oxygen and suction equipment if their need is anticipated. A thermometer, sphygmomanometer and stethoscope, and pulse oximeter should be nearby on the patient's return to the unit. If a PCA pump, sequential pneumatic compression devices, or a passive range-of-motion machine will be needed, see that they are obtained and ready.

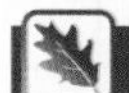

Life Span Considerations

Older Adult

- Kidney function is decreased in the older adult, which makes them less tolerant of normal adult dosages of medications. Monitor for medication toxicity.
- Meperidine may cause confusion if used continuously.

◆ EVALUATION

Evaluation is accomplished by determining whether the expected outcomes and goals have been met. If the patient is properly prepared for surgery, is kept NPO, is reasonably calm, and is knowledgeable about the procedure and what is expected of him, then the general goals have been met. If the patient was not ready for transport at the appointed time, then you need to review your steps to see where improvement can occur. Other areas to evaluate are whether the patient's valuables were safely returned after surgery,

POSTOPERATIVE RECORD

Department: ____________

Date: ____________ Time Received on Unit ____________

Type of Surgery: ____________

INITIAL POST-OP ASSESSMENT (Circle Appropriate Response)

CONSCIOUSNESS: .... Awake Arousable Unconscious Other: ______

AIRWAY: .... None Oral Nasal Endotracheal

RESPIRATION: .... Deep Shallow Regular Irregular

OXYGEN THERAPY: .... ______ liter. None Cannula mask Vent Tent Other: ______

COLOR: .... WNL Pale Cyanotic Other: ______

PULSES: .... Location: ______
Strong Weak Regular Irregular

SKIN: .... Warm Dry Cool Moist Other: ______

DRESSINGS: .... None Location: ______
Dry Serous Bloody Other: ______

DRAINS: .... None Location: ______ Type: ______
Location: ______ Type: ______

ORTHOPEDIC: .... None Cost: Location: ______ Dry Moist
Splint: Location: ______
Traction: Type: ______ # of weight: ______
PAS TEDS

GI: .... Nausea Emesis

GU: .... Foley Suprapubic Other: ______

RECEIVED BY: ______ R.N.

(See 24 Hours Patient Care Flow Sheet and Nurses Documentation Notes for Ongoing Assessment Date)

	Initial*	15"	30"	1 Hr.	1.5 Hrs.	2.5 Hrs.	3.5 Hrs.			
Actual Time										
Temp.										
B.P.										
Pulse										
Resp. *										
C.M.S.										
TCDB										
Dressing										
Voided/Amt.										
Fluids										
Fundus/Lochia										
Initials										

** Received from PAR*

Initials	Signature

Addressograph

H8720-59 (05/02/94) G.e65

FIGURE 37.6 Postoperative record used when the patient returns to the unit.

and whether dentures, glasses, or hearing aids were found and reinserted. If any of these items was misplaced, then procedures need to be changed. Expected outcomes written for individual nursing diagnoses must also be addressed during evaluation (Nursing Care Plan 37.1).

Nursing Care Plan 37.1 Care of the Patient Undergoing a Colon Resection

SCENARIO Helen Walters, age 67, has just had a colon resection. She was admitted early this morning, but will stay in the hospital for a couple of days. She has a history of diverticulitis (inflammation of pockets in the colon). She is a widow. Her daughter will care for her when she goes home.

PROBLEM/NURSING DIAGNOSIS *Fresh surgical incision*/Pain related to surgical incision.

Supporting Assessment Data: *Subjective:* Moaning and asking for pain medication on return from PACU. *Objective:* Abdominal incision for colon resection.

Goals/Expected Outcomes	Nursing Interventions	Selected Rationale	Evaluation
Pain will be controlled by analgesia 30 min after administration as reported by the patient.	Set up and begin administration of the PCA pump immediately after the initial assessment and give a bolus dose of morphine as ordered if no contraindication is found.	The ability to self-medicate for pain decreases anxiety, and the patient usually needs less medication.	*Is pain controlled within 30 min?* States is more comfortable.
	Remind patient how to work PCA pump.	Patient must know how to work the pump to receive pain medication.	
	Note response to PCA medication and closely monitor respiratory rate.	Morphine can depress the respiratory rate.	Relaxed body posture.
Pain will be controlled by oral analgesia, by discharge.			*Is pain controlled by oral analgesia?* Not yet.

PROBLEM/NURSING DIAGNOSIS *Skin incision*/Impaired skin integrity related to surgical incision.

Supporting Assessment Data: *Objective:* Abdominal incision with dressing intact and dry.

Goals/Expected Outcomes	Nursing Interventions	Selected Rationale	Evaluation
Wound will be free of signs of infection.	Keep Hemovac suction functioning properly. Note the character and amount of drainage; document.	The Hemovac must be compressed to exert suction.	*Are there signs of infection present?* The wound is without signs of infection.
	Assess for signs of infection with dressing changes.	Redness, warmth, swelling, and draining purulent exudate indicate infection.	
	Monitor temperature and WBC count.	WBC will rise in the presence of infection.	
	Reinforce dressing as needed. Assess for bleeding q h × 4 h, then q 2 h × 24 h.	Bleeding indicates a complication.	
	Use aseptic technique for dressing changes.	Asepsis prevents wound infection.	
Wound will heal completely.	Assess for signs of proper healing.	Good approximation of wound edges and decreasing redness indicate proper healing.	*Is the wound completely healed?* No, but progressing toward outcomes; continue plan.

Continued

Nursing Care Plan 37.1 Care of the Patient Undergoing a Colon Resection—cont'd

PROBLEM/NURSING DIAGNOSIS *Recovering from anesthesia*/Risk for ineffective airway clearance related to effects of anesthesia, immobility, and incisional pain.

Supporting Assessment Data: *Subjective:* States has discomfort taking a deep breath or coughing. *Objective:* Under anesthesia for 3 hours; abdominal incision. Resp. 18.

Goals/Expected Outcomes	Nursing Interventions	Selected Rationale	Evaluation
Patient will not develop atelectasis.	Remind how to splint the incision to cough.	Splinting when coughing reduces pressure on the incision during coughing and helps prevent pain and dehiscence.	*Does patient have atelectasis?* No signs of atelectasis. Splinting adequately. Using incentive spirometer q 2 h effectively.
	Have patient breathe deeply and cough while sitting on side of bed q 2 h after fully alert.	Sitting to cough aids in lung expansion and expulsion of secretions.	
	Remind to use incentive spirometer at least q 2 h.	Sustained inspiration opens alveoli.	
Lung sounds will be clear.	Auscultate lungs initially and during each shift.	Lung sound changes may indicate complications.	*Are lung sounds clear?* Lung sounds are clear with decreased sound in the bases.
	Encourage ambulation after 8 h.	Ambulation promotes greater lung expansion and deeper breathing.	
	Monitor temperature and respirations.	Rising temperature and increased respirations may indicate a complication.	Progressing toward outcomes. Continue plan.

PROBLEM/NURSING DIAGNOSIS *NPO status*/Risk for deficient fluid volume related to surgery and NG suction.

Supporting Assessment Data: *Objective:* Bowel resection; NPO status.

Goals/Expected Outcomes	Nursing Interventions	Selected Rationale	Evaluation
Fluid balance will be within normal limits.	Maintain low intermittent suction on the NG tube.	Suction must be set as ordered.	*Is fluid balance within normal limits?* Not yet.
	Irrigate with 30 mL normal saline q 2 h.	Normal saline will not alter electrolyte imbalance.	Suction maintained. Irrigated q 2 h.
	Monitor the character of drainage.	Bleeding in drainage could indicate a complication.	Secretions are clear to light brown.
	Check for signs of dehydration. Maintain IV fluids at the correct flow rate.	Removing stomach secretions without replacing fluids sufficiently can cause dehydration.	Skin turgor is elastic with moist mucous membranes.
	Monitor for signs of overhydration: auscultate the lungs for crackles.	Crackles in the lungs indicate moisture, which can indicate overhydration.	No signs or symptoms of edema.
	Auscultate for return of bowel sounds each shift.	The NG tube cannot be removed until bowel sounds return.	No bowel sounds detected.

Nursing Care Plan 37.1 Care of the Patient Undergoing a Colon Resection—cont'd

Goals/Expected Outcomes	Nursing Interventions	Selected Rationale	Evaluation
	Monitor I & O.	I & O records help monitor for fluid imbalance.	Intake 660 mL; output 485 mL. Progressing toward outcomes. Continue plan.

PROBLEM/NURSING DIAGNOSIS *Afraid might have cancer*/Anxiety related to outcome of surgery.

Supporting Assessment Data: *Subjective:* "I hope there wasn't any cancer." *Objective:* Concerned expression on face.

Goals/Expected Outcomes	Nursing Interventions	Selected Rationale	Evaluation
Anxiety will decrease as evidenced by patient's statements.	Reassure patient that surgeon said there was no sign of a mass in the excised portion of colon.	Reassuring information helps dispel anxiety.	*Do patient's statements indicate anxiety has dissipated?* No signs of anxiety.
	Remind patient that her diagnosis was diverticulitis, not cancer.	Helps patient focus on the positive.	Progressing toward outcomes. Continue plan.

PROBLEM/NURSING DIAGNOSIS *Just had abdominal surgery*/Self-care deficit, bathing/hygiene and grooming, related to surgical incision and discomfort.

Supporting Assessment Data: *Subjective:* States it is difficult to move or bend. *Objective:* Abdominal incision.

Goals/Expected Outcomes	Nursing Interventions	Selected Rationale	Evaluation
Patient will bathe daily, receiving assistance as needed.	Bathing promotes cleanliness and decreases microorganisms on the skin that might lead to wound infection.	Assist patient with bathing and washing the feet and back.	*Is the patient being bathed daily?* Yes. Meeting outcomes.
Patient will receive assistance with hygiene and grooming.	Provide dental care equipment and assist as needed with cleansing of the teeth. Apply skin lotion. Assist into a clean gown.	Assisting with hygiene and grooming conserves energy needed for healing. Prevents patient from overtiring.	*Is the patient assisted with hygiene and grooming?* Yes.

CRITICAL THINKING QUESTIONS

1. What actions would you take if the patient does not seem to be getting sufficient pain relief when using the PCA pump?
2. Would you expect the I & O to be essentially balanced for the first 24 hours on the day of surgery? What about the day after surgery?

I & O, Intake and output; *IV*, intravenous; *NG*, nasogastric; *NPO*, nothing by mouth; *PACU*, postanesthesia care unit; *PCA*, patient-controlled analgesia; *q*, every; *WBC*, white blood cell.

INTRAOPERATIVE CARE

The patient is transported to a holding room where the circulating nurse verifies the patient's identification and that all preoperative orders have been accomplished. The anesthesiologist or nurse anesthetist starts an IV if one is not already in place. The surgical consent form is checked to ensure that the patient is being prepared for the correct surgery on the correct body part. The surgical site is verified with the patient and marked, if not already done, before medications are given. Any ordered preoperative medications are administered. When the OR is ready, the patient is transferred to the operating table (Fig. 37.7). Patient identification is verified again by the circulating nurse. The patient is positioned with padding to prevent injury to nerves and to minimize pressure over bony prominences. Safety straps are secured over the patient.

All personnel who will be entering the OR wear clean scrub outfits, hair covers, shoe covers, and masks; the surgical team, including the surgeon, assistant surgeon, and scrub person, perform a surgical

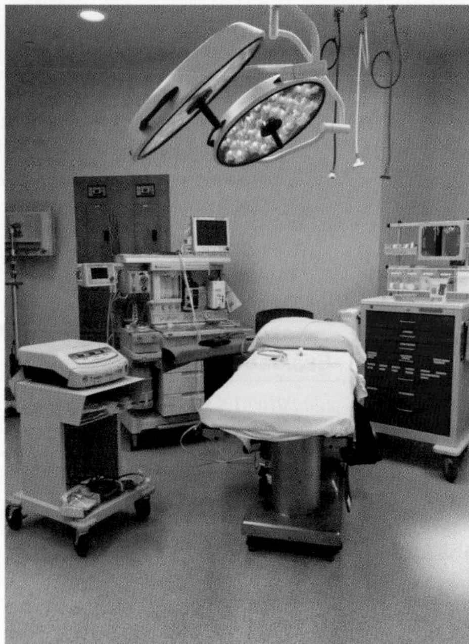

FIGURE 37.7 Traditional operating room.

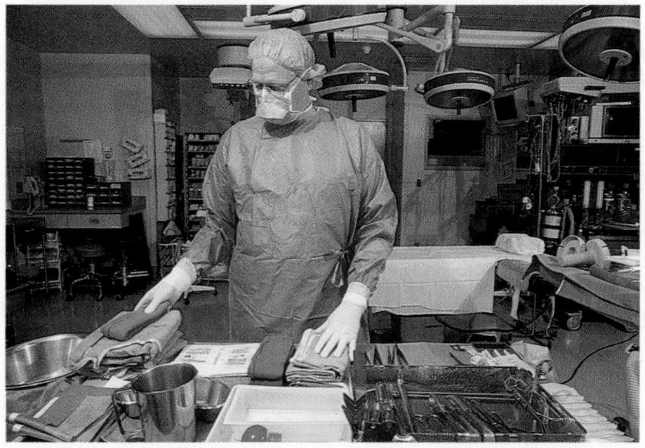

FIGURE 37.8 Preparing the surgical instruments and supplies.

scrub before entering the room. After the surgical scrub, the team is sterile gowned and gloved. **Strict surgical asepsis is mandatory throughout the surgical area.** The circulating nurse or scrub person and OR technician prepare the instruments and sterile supplies (Fig. 37.8). As the patient is draped, anesthesia is begun. Further skin preparation is done at this time.

Maintaining a normal body temperature in surgery is important in the prevention of surgical infections. Hypothermia during the perioperative period increases the risk of surgical site infection and delays recovery (Steelman & Graling, 2013). Prevention of hypothermia can be done by active warming during the surgery with a forced-air warming blanket and prewarmed IV fluids.

◆ ROLE OF THE SCRUB PERSON AND CIRCULATING NURSE

A surgical technician or a specially trained nurse (licensed practical nurse/licensed vocational nurse [LPN/LVN] or RN) may be the scrub person. A licensed nurse usually fulfills the duties of the circulating nurse (Box 37.6).

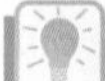 QSEN Considerations: Teamwork and Collaboration

Maintaining Sterility in the Operating Room

It is important to work as a team and report breaks in sterile technique to the person who breaks sterility. Maintaining the sterile OR environment is everyone's responsibility.

◆ POSTANESTHESIA IMMEDIATE CARE

Postanesthesia Care Unit

The period immediately after surgery with general anesthesia or after a major procedure performed with spinal anesthesia is a critical time and requires constant observation by specially trained nurses. The PACU provides care for all basic needs (Fig. 37.9). The patient is positioned to prevent aspiration and promote lung expansion. The patient is kept warm by covering with warmed blankets and is reassured that the surgery is over. Vital signs are taken every 5 to 15 minutes until stable. Emergency equipment is on hand (Fig. 37.10). The anesthesia recovery period usually takes 2 to 6 hours. The patient remains in the PACU until the vital signs are stable and he is awake and able to respond to stimuli. Many facilities use the Aldrete scoring system to determine readiness for transfer. This scoring system rates a patient's activity, respiration, circulation, consciousness, and skin color on a scale of 1 to 3. A total score of 9 or 10 usually indicates the patient is ready for transfer. Because patients are coming out of anesthesia through the various stages and are unstable, the environment is kept as quiet as possible. Communication among the staff is kept to a minimum and is done in hushed tones. Once the patient is awake, family is sometimes allowed to visit for a few minutes so that they are assured that their loved one is alive and recovering.

◆ POSTANESTHESIA CARE IN THE SAME-DAY SURGERY UNIT

For many procedures, the patient may be transferred from the OR directly back to the same-day surgery unit. Monitor the patient's respiration, circulation, vital signs, neurologic status, fluid balance, wound drainage and dressings, and comfort level. When the vital signs are stable, the patient is allowed to sit up and then begins to ambulate. When able to ambulate unassisted, the patient may be discharged if vital signs are stable. Recovery time in the same-day surgery unit takes about 1 to 4 hours. Discharge patient education is begun before the surgery and continues, once the patient is again alert. Written instructions are always sent home with the patient.

BOX 37.6 Functions of the Circulating Nurse and the Scrub Person

MAJOR FUNCTIONS OF THE CIRCULATING NURSE

- Coordinates care, oversees the environment, and cares for the patient in the operating room
- Verifies that consent is signed and accurate and that surgical site is marked
- Greets patient and performs patient assessment
- Checks medical record and preoperative forms for completeness
- Sets up the operating room; adjusts lights, stools, and discard buckets; and ensures supplies and diagnostic support are available
- Gathers and checks all equipment anticipated to be used, ensuring its safe function
- Opens sterile supplies for scrub nurse
- Provides needed padding and warming or cooling devices for the operating table
- Assists with ties of surgical team's gowns
- Assists with the transfer of the patient to the operating table and positions the patient
- Places an electrocautery ground pad under the patient if electrocautery is to be used
- Assists the anesthesia induction provider with anesthesia
- May prep the patient's skin before sterile draping occurs
- May insert a urinary catheter
- Handles labeling and disposition of specimens
- Coordinates activities with the radiology and pathology departments
- Monitors urine and blood loss during surgery and reports findings to the surgeon
- Observes for breaks in sterile technique and announces them to the team
- Monitors traffic and noise within the operating room
- Communicates information on the surgery's progress to family during long procedures
- Documents care, events, interventions, and findings
- Helps transfer patient to a gurney and accompanies patient to the recovery area, providing handoff report of the surgery and patient condition to recovery nurse

MAJOR FUNCTIONS OF THE SCRUB PERSON

- Gathers all equipment for the procedure
- Prepares all sterile supplies and instruments using sterile technique
- Gowns and gloves surgeons on entry to the operating room
- Assists with sterile draping of the patient
- Maintains sterility within the sterile field during surgery
- Hands instruments and supplies to the operating team during surgery
- Maintains a neat instrument table
- Labels and handles surgical specimens correctly
- Maintains an accurate count of sponges, sharps, and instruments on the sterile field; verifies counts with the circulating nurse before and after surgery
- Monitors for breaks in sterile technique and points them out
- Cleans up after the surgery is over

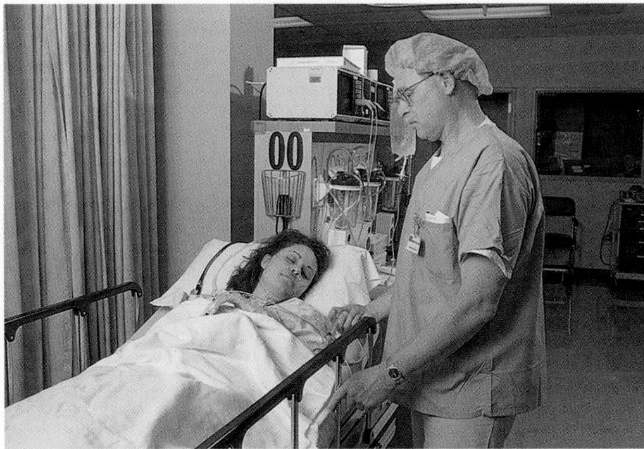

FIGURE 37.9 Postanesthesia recovery unit.

? Think Critically

What is the number one priority of care for the patient in the PACU?

POSTOPERATIVE CARE

◆ ASSESSMENT (DATA COLLECTION)

On receiving the patient from the PACU nurse, check his identity, settle him in bed, and perform an initial postoperative assessment. This provides a baseline for frequent postoperative assessments to prevent or quickly catch signs of complications. Initial postoperative assessment is outlined in Table 37.3. **Vital signs and careful assessment are performed every 15 minutes for the first hour, every 30 minutes for the next 2 hours, every hour for the next 4 hours, and then every 4 hours until the patient is completely recovered from anesthesia and vital signs have returned to normal.** Vital signs are taken more frequently if they are unstable according to nursing judgment.

◆ NURSING DIAGNOSIS

Nursing diagnoses commonly used for postoperative patients who had general anesthesia include:

- Pain related to disruption of tissue
- Risk for infection related to surgical wound
- Impaired gas exchange related to the effect of anesthesia on the lungs
- Ineffective airway clearance related to inability to breathe deeply and cough without discomfort
- Self-care deficit, bathing, related to decreased mobility, tubes, and dressings
- Risk for injury related to sedation, decreased level of consciousness, or excessive blood loss
- Ineffective peripheral tissue perfusion related to surgery, anesthesia, and positioning on the operating table
- Ineffective coping related to loss of body part or change in body image

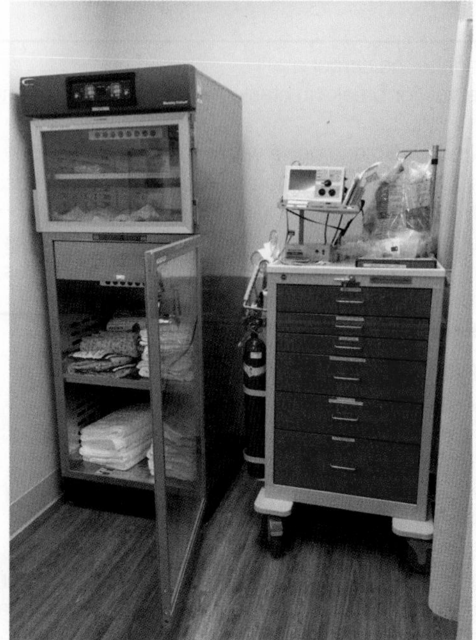
FIGURE 37.10 PACU blanket warmer and crash cart.

For patients who have undergone spinal anesthesia, include the first two diagnoses on the list above, plus the following:

- Impaired physical mobility related to effects of spinal anesthesia
- Risk for injury related to decreased sensation and movement in lower extremities

◆ PLANNING

The expected outcomes depend on the individual specific nursing diagnoses. General nursing goals are:

- Maintain patent airway and adequate respiratory exchange.
- Maintain adequate tissue perfusion.
- Promote comfort and rest.
- Promote wound healing.
- Promote psychological adjustment to lifestyle or body image changes.
- Prevent complications.

When planning the shift work, allow time for frequent postoperative assessments. Careful planning is essential to care for the early postoperative patient properly and not neglect the needs of other assigned patients.

Table 37.3 Postoperative Assessment

AREA	ASSESSMENT	SCHEDULE
Airway	Lung sounds, depth and quality of air movement, and respiratory rate.	Auscultate the lungs initially; respiratory rate q 15 min until fully aroused from anesthesia, and then assess the quality of respirations with vital signs assessment.
Oxygenation	Oxygen saturation; oxygen delivery at the rate ordered and patent system.	Note per vital signs schedule and whenever in the room. Check the oxygen delivery system with the initial assessment.
Circulation	Auscultate the heart; check peripheral pulses and sensation, especially distal to the surgical site. Assess skin color.	Initially, q 4 h × 2 and then with vital signs. If surgery was on an extremity, assess each time vital signs are measured.
Mental status	Level of consciousness and orientation.	Initially and then with full vital signs.
Vital signs	Temperature, BP, pulse, and respirations.	Check temperature initially and then q 8 h once stable. Check vital signs q 15 min × 1 h; q 30 min × 2 h; q 1 h × 4; q 4 h × 24-48 h; or per agency protocol.
Fluid status and hydration	IV site and flow rate; I & O; skin turgor; oral membranes.	Check the IV initially and when in the room; I & O each shift; skin turgor and oral membranes initially and each shift.
Surgical site	Check for bleeding; mark drainage on dressing; check wound drainage in containers.	Initially and q 1 h × 4; then with vital signs.
Gastrointestinal	Auscultate bowel sounds; assess the abdomen; check NG drainage color, character, and amount.	Initially, then q 8 h. Check drainage whenever in the room.
Tubes	Check for patency and function of each.	Initially; then with vital signs after 1 h.
Kidney function	Assess urine output from the urinary catheter; must void within 8 h if no catheter is in place.	Initially and q 1 h × 4; then if greater than 30 mL/h, q 4 h.
Pain	Use a pain scale and observation of nonverbal behaviors.	Initially and with vital signs; assess at least q 2 h.
Skin	Pressure areas over bony prominences.	Initially and q 2 h.

BP, blood pressure; *h*, hour; *I & O*, Intake and output; *IV*, intravenous; *min*, minute; *NG*, nasogastric; *NPO*, nothing by mouth; *q*, every.

◆ IMPLEMENTATION

Protect the Patient from Injury

Maintaining an open airway is a priority measure. The patient must be positioned on the side or with the head turned to the side to prevent aspiration, if not contraindicated, until fully recovered, alert, and with the swallowing reflex intact.

Side rails are kept raised for safety until patients are fully recovered from anesthesia. Reassure the patient who has had spinal anesthesia that it is normal for the legs to feel numb and heavy and that feeling will soon return to normal. Sense of position will return to the legs first; then sensation to deep pressure; then voluntary movement; and finally feeling of superficial pain and temperature. A feeling of "pins and needles" in the legs is common. The patient is prone to hypotension until all effects of the spinal anesthesia are resolved. Monitor the patient for a spinal headache, but it is not necessary to stay completely flat for the first 12 hours because this has proven ineffective. If a headache develops, staying flat reduces the pain.

Clinical Cues

Encourage the patient to drink plenty of fluids, including those containing caffeine. The fluids and caffeine raise the vascular pressure at the spinal puncture site and help to seal the hole.

Check the surgical site when the patient returns to the unit. The dressing should be dry. If it is stained, outline the area with pen and note the time so that further bleeding can be assessed later. If the bleeding has saturated the dressing, reinforce with more dressing supplies; the dressing is not changed without an order to do so. Check the surgical site each hour for the first 4 hours, and then every 2 hours if bleeding has not occurred. Report excessive bleeding to the surgeon. Check the bed linens under the patient as well because sometimes blood runs under the dressing and pools under the patient.

Assess drains for patency when checking the wound, and empty and recompress drainage devices as needed. Record the amount of drainage on the intake and output record (Table 37.4). Position the drainage devices so that there is no pulling on the entry sites. During assessment, check the tubes for kinking and ensure that the patient is not lying on them. Common types of drains left in to help remove fluid from the surgical site are Penrose, Hemovac, and Jackson-Pratt (J-P) bulb drains, chest tubes, and a T-tube to the common bile duct.

Promote Respiratory Function

The postoperative patient is at risk for respiratory problems from the effects of anesthesia on the lungs, from being in one position on the OR table for the duration of surgery, and from limited mobility in the immediate postoperative period. The patient may have oxygen per nasal cannula ordered for 24 hours after surgery. Some

Table 37.4 Expected Drainage From Tubes and Catheters Postoperatively

TYPE OF DRAINAGE	AMOUNT OF DRAINAGE IN 24 HOURS
Urine	800-1500 mL for first 24 h Minimum expected output: 0.5 mL/kg per h
Gastric contents	Up to 1500 mL/day
Wound drainage	Variable with procedure and type of drain; may decrease over hours or days
T-tube and bile	Up to 500 mL

Adapted from Lewis, S. L., Dirksen, S. R., Heitkemper, M. M., Bucher, L., & Camera, I. M. (2014). *Medical-surgical nursing: Assessment and management of clinical problems* (9th ed., p. 361). St. Louis, MO: Elsevier Mosby.

degree of **atelectasis** (collapse of alveoli in the lungs) exists after anesthesia. A mild hypoxia is usually present for about 48 hours postoperatively. Auscultate the lungs carefully for absence of sound or for crackles, indicating retained secretions. Assess the rate and depth of breathing and encourage the patient to deep breathe and cough every 2 hours. This is essential to prevent pneumonia and relieve atelectasis. Hypostatic pneumonia occurs when lack of movement or of position change causes stasis of secretions, which become a breeding ground for bacteria. **Coughing may be contraindicated for patients who have had hernia repair or eye, ear, or brain surgery.** Check the surgeon's orders.

Coughing mobilizes secretions for expectoration. If the patient cannot cough effectively, instruct him to take a deep breath and forcibly exhale with the mouth open; have him repeat the "huff" maneuver again; then ask him to take a deep breath and cough strongly as he exhales to move the secretions out of the airways. Little coughs just clear the throat. Be certain the patient turns every 2 hours, as well, because this changes the distribution of gas and blood flow in the lungs and helps move secretions.

Signs of complications are complaints of shortness of breath, pain on inspiration, and extreme fatigue (which is related to hypoxemia). The use of an incentive spirometer is especially helpful to prevent atelectasis and hypoventilation. The older adult patient may need extra coaching to master the technique.

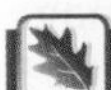

Life Span Considerations

Older Adult

The risk of hypoventilation is greater in the older adult because lung expansion may be hampered by calcification of costal cartilage and weakened respiratory muscles.

A pulse oximeter may be used to determine blood oxygenation. Monitor the readings periodically, and report arterial oxygen saturation (SaO_2) readings below 92% to the provider. Pulse oximetry is covered in Chapter 28.

Promote Circulation

When considerable blood is lost during surgery, transfusion may be ordered. Autologous transfusion may be done if the patient donated blood several weeks before surgery or if the patient's blood was collected as it was lost. This blood is filtered and returned to the patient.

When the procedure involved an extremity or the pelvic area, check the distal or peripheral pulse during each full assessment. Swelling at the surgical site can compress vessels and decrease blood flow distal to the area. The skin should be warm to the touch, and there should be good capillary refill in the fingers or toes.

 **Life Span Considerations**

Older Adult

- Because older adults have fragile skin and less subcutaneous tissue, check bony prominences carefully for signs of breakdown.
- Joint strains can occur from the positioning necessary for certain types of surgery; perform position changes slowly and gently.

Blood pressure and pulse should be compared with preoperative values to determine significant changes. An increase in pulse may indicate that internal bleeding is occurring, but it can also signify incomplete pain control. Blood pressure falling below the normal baseline level may indicate major bleeding.

The use of antiembolism (elastic) stockings increases venous return from the legs and helps to prevent stasis of blood in the lower extremities (Skill 37.1). If the patient is at risk of venous **thrombosis** (blood clot), the surgeon will order sequential pneumatic compression devices to be applied to the legs and/or an anticoagulant. These devices alternately compress and release, squeezing the vessels and propelling blood along them (Fig. 37.11).

Maintain Fluid Balance

The urine output is monitored after surgery. **If the patient has an indwelling catheter, the urine in the bag is observed every hour in the early postoperative period.** There should be a urinometer on the drainage bag for this purpose. If the urine flow is less than 5 mL/kg per hour, report it to the charge nurse. If flow is less than 60 mL over a two hour period, notify the surgeon. Check the catheter to ensure it is not kinked and that the connecting tubing is not lying beneath the patient. If no catheter is present, the patient must void within 8 hours of surgery. If the patient is unable to empty the bladder spontaneously, obtain an order for catheterization.

The patient usually has an IV infusion running when he returns from surgery. Depending on the type of surgery, IV fluids may be continued for a few days or may be discontinued after the fluid has infused. Check to make certain that the fluid running is the one that the surgeon ordered. **No potassium additive should be given until the urine flow is at least 5 mL/kg per hour.** Potassium may cause hyperkalemia if kidney function is not adequate. Assess the IV site for patency and lack of complications when vital signs are taken. Recheck the IV flow rate as well. Record all IV fluid administered as intake on the intake and output record.

As soon as the patient is conscious and the swallowing reflex has returned, offer the patient a few ice chips or sips of water unless there is an order to maintain NPO status. Record all intake on the intake and output record. At the end of each shift, note the difference between the intake and output. Check the surgical and PACU records for intake and output including blood loss during the intraoperative and immediate postoperative periods. The body initially retains fluid because of the stress reaction from surgery. Postoperatively, the output slowly rises until it is more than the intake; after 2 or 3 days, a balance should be reached.

Anesthesia may make the patient nauseated, and vomiting may occur. Keep the emesis basin nearby, and position the patient on the side to prevent aspiration. The surgeon usually writes an order for medication in the event of excessive nausea or vomiting. It is best to medicate the patient before actual vomiting occurs. After emesis, provide mouth care. If vomiting is uncontrolled with medication, a NG tube may have to be inserted to suction stomach contents and prevent further fluid and electrolyte loss.

Surgeons often leave in a NG tube after most abdominal procedures because handling of the gastrointestinal tract and general anesthesia cause peristalsis to halt, and secretions will not flow through the system properly. When a NG tube is in place, check that the suction is set according to orders and is working properly. Assess the amount of drainage produced every 1 to 2 hours. **If the tubing is kept above the level of the stomach, drainage will occur more easily.** If the drainage turns dark brown and grainy, it should be checked for blood with a special reagent. Report the presence of blood to the surgeon.

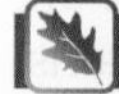 **Life Span Considerations**

Older Adult

- Fluid and electrolyte shifts may cause confusion in the older adult postoperatively.
- The skin and vessels are fragile in the older adult; assess the IV site frequently for signs of infiltration.
- Adjustment of the body to fluid shifts is difficult, and the older adult is prone to postural hypotension when changing to a standing position. Be certain to support the patient adequately.

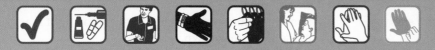

Skill 37.1 Applying Antiembolism Stockings

 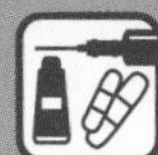 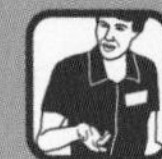 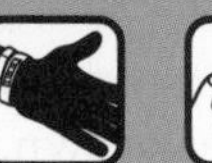 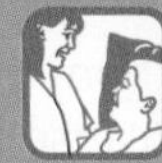 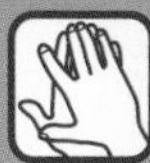 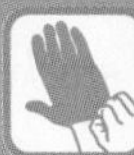

Many surgeons order some type of antiembolism stockings after major surgery. Patients frequently return from the postanesthesia care unit (PACU) with the stockings already in place. In such cases, the preoperative orders include fitting the patient for antiembolism stockings, which are then sent with the patient to the operating room.

Supplies

- Antiembolism stockings
- Measuring tape

Review and carry out the Standard Steps in Appendix A.

ACTION *(RATIONALE)*

Assessment (Data Collection)

1. Check the orders for the type of stocking to be applied. *(Stockings come in three lengths: knee high, thigh high, and full length.)*

Planning

2. Measure the patient's leg length and circumference for the length of stocking ordered. Obtain the correct size stocking. *(Ensures stockings will fit properly.)*

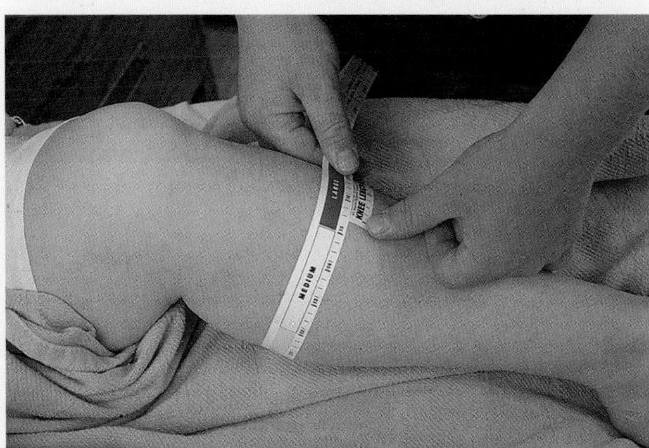

Step 2

Implementation

3. Be certain patient's legs are clean and dry. *(Dry skin makes stocking application easier and smoother.)*
4. Place your hand in one stocking and turn it inside out, down to the heel. *(This makes it easier to slip the stocking onto the foot without discomfort to the patient.)*
5. Stretch open the stocking at the heel, and fit it over the patient's foot. *(The stockings must fit smoothly without wrinkles that might damage the skin's surface.)*

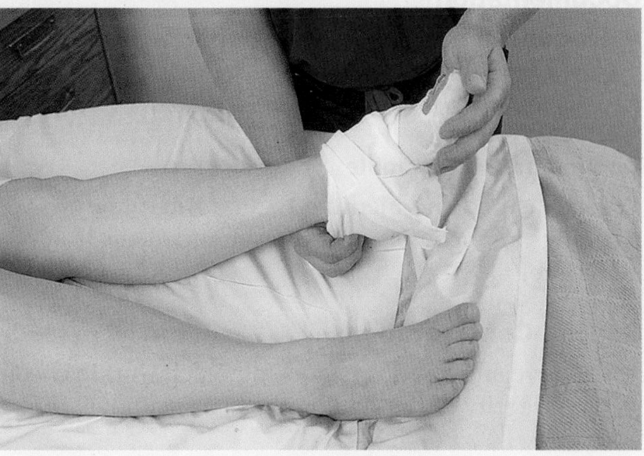

Step 5

6. Grasp the top of the stocking, and fit it over the ankle and calf. *(If knee-high stockings are being used, do not pull them over knee or fold the top of the stocking down. The stockings must be the correct length or they can impair circulation or damage the skin's surface.)*
7. If using thigh high, fit the top of the stocking over the knee and thigh. Smooth the entire surface to eliminate any wrinkles. Repeat steps 4 through 7 for the second stocking. Instruct patient not to cross the legs or ankles when sitting in a bed or chair. *(Crossing the limbs causes pressure points that can hinder circulation.)*

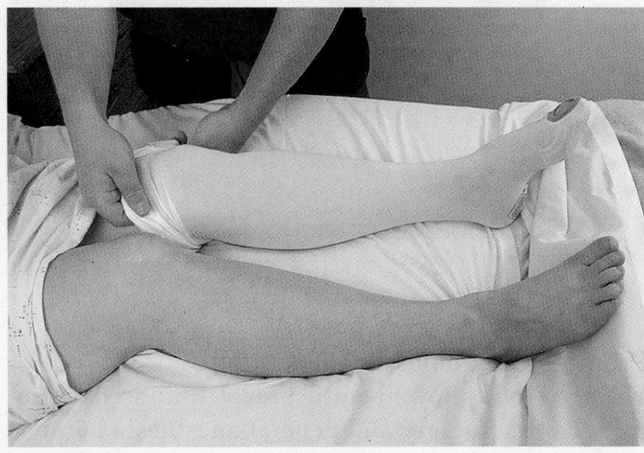

Step 7

Evaluation

8. Are the stockings at the right height for what was ordered? Are the stockings on smoothly, without any wrinkles? Do the stockings fit properly—not too tight or too loose at any point? *(Answers to these*

Skill 37.1 Applying Antiembolism Stockings—cont'd

questions indicate whether the correctly fitted stocking is applied properly.)

Documentation

9. Document the size, type, and application of the stockings. (*Verifies that ordered stockings are in place and supports charges for the stockings.)*

Documentation Example

Legs measured and medium regular thigh-high stockings applied. (Nurse's time-stamped electronic signature)

Special Considerations

- Remove antiembolism stockings each shift to check the integrity of the skin on the heels and over the bony prominences. Stockings that are too tight may cause skin breakdown.
- Wash stockings when soiled. Obtain a second pair for use while stockings are drying. To wash, use mild soap and warm, not hot, water. Rinse thoroughly, squeeze out excess water, and roll up in a towel to remove further moisture; allow to air dry.
- Do not have stockings off the patient for more than 30 minutes at any one time.

Critical Thinking Questions

1. What would you do if you measured a patient for thigh-high elastic stockings and the supply room did not have a size available that you need?
2. How does drying the legs thoroughly make applying elastic stockings easier?

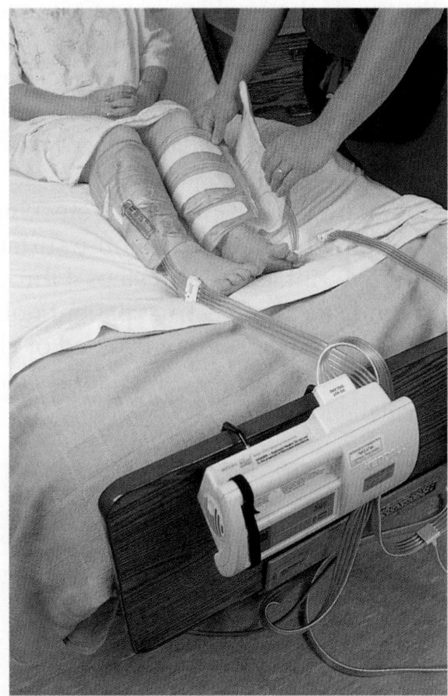

FIGURE 37.11 Applying leg sequential compression devices.

Promote Gastrointestinal Function

Eating is not allowed until bowel sounds have returned after surgery and general anesthesia because of the risk of development of **paralytic ileus** (failure of forward movement of bowel contents). Listen for bowel sounds and document at least once per shift. When eating is resumed, clear liquids are usually ordered, followed by full liquids, then a regular diet if the preceding diets have been tolerated. After spinal anesthesia, the patient may be allowed to eat right away.

After the patient is eating again, he should have a bowel movement within 2 or 3 days. If one does not occur, an order for a suppository may be needed to stimulate a bowel movement. Patients receiving narcotic analgesics may become constipated and require stool softeners or laxatives to produce normal bowel movements.

Promote Comfort

If the patient is complaining of pain on return to the unit, check through the notes from the PACU and see if any pain medication was given. Note what preoperative medications were administered and when they were given.

Clinical Cues

When droperidol plus fentanyl is given as a preoperative medication, narcotic pain medication is reduced by half for the 8 hours after the preoperative medication, or the narcotic analgesic will gravely depress respirations.

If respirations are within normal limits and there is no contraindication to doing so, medicate promptly with the ordered analgesic. If it is too soon to give more analgesia, reposition the patient, be certain the bladder is not distended and causing discomfort, check that the patient is warm enough, and use other comfort measures such as distraction and imagery to relieve the pain. Note when analgesia is due and have it ready to administer at the appointed time.

The patient may feel cold and should be kept warm with extra blankets or warmed bath blankets applied under the top covers. Placing socks on the feet may help. Some anesthetic agents may cause tremors as they wear off. If uncontrollable shivering occurs, contact the care provider for medication orders.

Check dressings on extremities to be certain that they are not so tight that circulation is impaired. Monitor the distal pulse and skin temperature. Check with the surgeon or charge nurse before loosening a dressing.

Abdominal distention and considerable flatus may occur after general anesthesia because the gastrointestinal tract action ceases. This may cause discomfort. Ambulating is helpful in moving and evacuating gas. Taking only small amounts of liquid or food at a time, drinking liquids that are neither very hot nor very cold, and refraining from drinking with a straw helps to keep flatus to a minimum. If permitted, the patient can try resting in a slight Trendelenburg position, with the legs and rectum higher than the stomach; this may assist in the evacuation of flatus. Chewing gum, if permitted, may also aid the return of proper gastrointestinal function.

Occasionally continuous hiccups occur after surgery, making the patient quite uncomfortable. Having the patient breathe into a paper bag often relieves the hiccups, but persistent hiccups require more vigorous treatment to be prescribed by the provider.

Rest and Activity

The patient needs to sleep after surgery. Keep the room quiet and group nursing activities to avoid waking the patient more than necessary. Every 2 hours the patient must do leg exercises and change position. Orders for ambulation may begin 8 hours postoperatively. Raise the head of the bed first, and let the body adjust to the position change. Then sit the patient on the side of the bed, allowing the legs to dangle over the side with the feet on the floor. After a few minutes, slowly help the patient to stand. Have the patient walk around the room using a gait belt, or for at least a few steps. Have someone assist you if the patient is very weak. Pain medication can be timed so that it is effective but the patient is not too groggy. Emphasize to the patient that exercise is vital to prevent circulatory problems. **Do not rub the legs to promote circulation. Such an action may disrupt a clot that has formed and cause an embolus** (a clot that travels and lodges in a vessel) to the lung, heart, or brain. Praise the patient for any efforts. Continue to ambulate on a set schedule until the patient is out of bed independently.

If the patient is on bed rest, range-of-motion exercises must be performed at least four times a day. The patient may do active range of motion on most joints, but passive range of motion on joints the patient is unable to exercise must be done unless physical therapy visits have been ordered. See Chapter 18 for directions for range-of-motion exercises.

Prevent Infection

Aseptic technique must be used when caring for the postoperative patient. Good handwashing is the primary means of preventing infection. Perform dressing changes with strict aseptic technique while the patient is in the hospital; the patient may use clean technique at home. Encouraging fluids to flush the bladder helps to prevent a bladder infection for the patient who was catheterized or has an indwelling catheter. Turning, coughing, and deep breathing, plus ambulation, assist in preventing **pneumonia** (inflammation and consolidation of the lung with exudate) from retained secretions and lack of movement.

Inspect the surgical wound site each shift and assess for signs of infection: local pain, increased tenderness, warmth, redness, or purulent drainage. Monitor the blood count for increasing leukocytes (white blood cells), and monitor the temperature for unexpected increase.

Complications of Surgery

A major nursing responsibility is continuous monitoring for signs of the various complications that may occur because of surgery. Table 37.5 summarizes postoperative complications and nursing actions to prevent them. **Dehiscence** (separation of the layers of the surgical wound) and **evisceration** (extrusion of the viscera through the surgical incision) may occur when the patient is coughing, particularly if the abdominal incision is not properly splinted.

◆ EVALUATION

Evaluation is based on whether goals and expected outcomes have been met. Evaluative statements regarding previously stated general goals might be:

- Lungs clear to auscultation; respirations 18
- Pulse 82, BP 136/86, peripheral pulses present
- Pain controlled for 4 hours with analgesia; states pain medication controls pain for approximately 4 hours
- Incision clean, dry, and without redness
- States is glad he will not have periods of pain and malaise anymore
- No signs of thrombophlebitis or infection

Each nursing care plan is evaluated on whether the individual specific outcomes have been met. Further examples of evaluation are in the nursing care plans for this chapter.

Table 37.5 Postoperative Complications

PROBLEM	SIGNS AND SYMPTOMS	PREVENTIVE INTERVENTIONS
Atelectasis	Decreased breath sounds over areas not aerating; dyspnea	Deep breathing and coughing; use of incentive spirometer; early ambulation; teaching to cough properly.
Pneumonia: hypostatic, aspiration, or bacterial	Fever, malaise, increased sputum, purulent sputum, cough, flushed skin, dyspnea, pain on inspiration, and abnormal breath sounds, crackles, and gurgles (low-pitched wheezes)	Deep breathing, coughing, and frequent turning; early ambulation; incentive spirometer; range-of-motion exercises if unable to ambulate; medication if bacterial.
Paralytic (adynamic) ileus	No bowel sounds 24-36 hours post operatively or fewer than 5 sounds per minute	Monitor bowel sounds; encourage early ambulation; NPO as ordered. Do not feed until bowel sounds return.
Thrombophlebitis	Pain or warmth in the calf of the leg, swollen leg, warm area to touch on the leg; possible temperature elevation	Encourage leg exercises; keep the patient well hydrated; encourage ambulation; antiembolism stockings or devices.
Urinary retention	Distended bladder; inability to void spontaneously	Palpate the bladder; encourage voiding; catheterize if unable to void within 8 hours per order; medicate to increase urinary sphincter tone as ordered.
Urinary tract infection	Dysuria, frequency, and foul-smelling urine	Force fluids when allowed; encourage frequent voiding; keep the catheter clean and patent; use aseptic technique to empty the drainage bag.
Wound infection	Redness, swelling, pain, warmth, drainage, fever, increased leukocytes, and rapid pulse and respirations (Fever 72 hours postoperatively indicates infection in some system or in the wound.)	Assess wound characteristics and drainage. Monitor WBC levels and temperature. Use aseptic technique for wound care; encourage adequate nutrition and fluids; encourage activity.
Pulmonary embolus	Shortness of breath, anxiety, chest pain, rapid pulse and respirations, cyanosis, cough, and bloody sputum	Use antiembolism stockings; ensure adequate fluid intake; assist with frequent turning or ambulation; administer preventive anticoagulant if ordered.
Hemorrhage and shock	Evidence of copious bleeding; decreased blood pressure, elevated pulse, cold clammy skin, and decreased urine output	Administer blood or volume expander; stop bleeding. Place in shock position with feet and legs elevated and head flat; administer ordered medications to raise blood pressure; administer oxygen; measure vital signs frequently.
Wound dehiscence or evisceration	Discharge of serosanguinous drainage from the wound and sensation that "something gave"; separation of wound edges with intestines visible through the abdominal incision	Teach to splint properly for coughing. Place the patient supine; cover the wound with sterile saline-soaked gauze or towels; return to the OR for repair; monitor for shock.
Fluid imbalance	**Signs of overhydration:** crackles in lungs, edema, and weight gain **Signs of dehydration:** weight loss, diminished pulse, dry mucous membranes, and decreased tissue turgor	Control the IV flow rate. Monitor I&O and correct imbalances. Output will be less than intake in the first 72 hours postoperatively with general anesthesia. Auscultate the lungs each shift. Monitor weight; check for edema.

h, hour; *I & O*, Intake and output; *IV*, intravenous; *min*, minute; *NPO*, nothing by mouth; *WBC*, white blood cells.

Get Ready for the NCLEX Examination!

Key Points

- Surgical procedures may be elective, emergency, palliative, diagnostic, curative, or reconstructive.
- The use of lasers, fiberoptic endoscopes with high-resolution video cameras, operating microscopes, and robotic technology has revolutionized surgery.
- Anesthesia is used to prevent pain, achieve adequate muscle relaxation, calm fear, allay anxiety, and induce forgetfulness of an unpleasant experience.
- Inhalant gases and IV medications are used to induce general anesthesia, and the patient progresses through four stages to total anesthesia.
- Regional anesthesia, moderate sedation, or local anesthesia is used for many surgical procedures.
- The surgeon must obtain informed consent from the patient before surgery is performed.
- A thorough assessment is performed by the nurse, and any risk factors for surgery are identified.
- The nursing care plan is amended as the patient progresses through preoperative, intraoperative, and postoperative periods.
- Preoperative patient education of exercises to be performed postoperatively is important; the patient is taught leg, breathing, and coughing exercises.
- The scrub person and the circulating nurse provide care for the patient while in the OR.
- The PACU monitors patients closely until they are fully aroused from anesthesia.
- Nursing interventions are aimed at providing pain control, comfort, and fluid balance; protecting the patient from injury; maintaining vital functions; and preventing infection.
- The nurse tries to prevent or intervene in the many potential complications of surgery.
- Discharge planning begins at admission and covers all areas of basic needs, wound care, and activity restrictions.
- Written instructions regarding all aspects of postoperative care should be sent home with the patient.

Additional Learning Resources

SG Go to your Study Guide for additional learning activities to help you master this chapter content.

evolve Go to your Evolve website at http://evolve.elsevier.com/Williams/fundamental for additional online resources.

Review Questions for the NCLEX Examination

*Choose the **best** answer for each question.*

1. A similarity of roles for the scrub person and the circulating nurse is that they both:
   1. Set up initial sterile instruments and supplies.
   2. Position lights and step stools.
   3. Are communication links with personnel outside the room.
   4. Advise the team of breaks in sterile technique.
2. When a patient arrives in the PACU with a surgical dressing, an intravenous infusion, and a urinary catheter, the **priority** action of the nurse is assessment of:
   1. Urine output.
   2. IV line patency.
   3. Airway patency.
   4. Wound drainage.
3. As part of a patient's immediate care in the PACU, the nurse would: *(Select all that apply.)*
   1. Check vital signs every 15 minutes.
   2. Assess adequacy of respirations.
   3. Monitor the dressing.
   4. Observe the drainage from the NG tube.
   5. Note the amount of urine output.
4. A patient returns to his room after surgery. When he arrives, you notice that he is still groggy from anesthesia and that he has an IV running in one arm. As you help settle him in bed, you: *(Select all that apply.)*
   1. Assess the IV for patency and correct fluid and rate.
   2. Position to prevent aspiration while still groggy.
   3. Quickly medicate for pain.
   4. Take his vital signs every 15 minutes for 1 hour.
   5. Reassure him that the surgery is over.
5. If your fresh postoperative patient has not voided within 8 hours of the end of surgery, you would **first**:
   1. Seek an order to catheterize the patient.
   2. Assist the patient to attempt to void using measures to encourage voiding.
   3. Allow another hour in which the patient might spontaneously void.
   4. Obtain catheterization equipment and bring it to the bedside.
6. The second day postoperatively, the NG tube is removed and an order is written for fluids as tolerated and a liquid diet. The patient is eager to try taking fluids. What should the nurse recommend that he do?
   1. Wait until his liquid diet tray arrives at mealtime.
   2. Start with small sips of water at first to see if they are retained.
   3. Take in a variety of fluids totaling 3000 mL/day.
   4. Go ahead and drink all the water he wants.
7. The patient has a PCA pump to be used for pain control. Should his pain not be adequately controlled with use of the pump, the nurse would **first:** *(Select all that apply.)*
   1. Administer an oral analgesic in addition to the pump medication.
   2. Seek a medication order change from the provider.
   3. Use nonpharmacologic comfort measures.
   4. Be certain that none of the drainage tubes are kinked.
   5. Encourage the use of distraction.

8. On his third postoperative day, a patient states that he does not feel well and that he has a lot more pain in the incision area. You inspect the incision and notice that the lower end of it is very red. From these symptoms, you suspect that this patient has developed:
   1. An embolus.
   2. An ileus.
   3. A wound infection.
   4. An evisceration.

Critical Thinking Activities

Read each clinical scenario and discuss the questions with your classmates.

Scenario A

Theresa Hijazi is scheduled for surgery this morning. You are assigned two other patients to care for, as well as Theresa. One of these patients is stable and will be going home. The other patient is going for a computed tomography (CT) scan at 11 am.

1. Describe in detail how you would plan your morning care for these three patients.
2. Theresa shares with you that she really doesn't understand just what the surgeon is going to do to her. How would you handle the situation?

Scenario B

You have prepared your 16-year-old patient for surgery, given instructions, and left him a clean gown to put on. When you return to assist in transferring him to the gurney for the trip to the OR, you find he has put on underwear and is wearing a St. Christopher's medal around his neck.

1. What would you do about the underwear?
2. How would you handle the situation with the St. Christopher's medal?

Scenario C

You are told to prepare the unit in 404 for the return of a patient from surgery.

1. What supplies do you need?
2. How would you arrange the unit?
3. How often will you need to take vital signs?
4. How often will you do other assessments?
5. What will you assess?

chapter 38

Providing Wound Care and Treating Pressure Injuries

http://evolve.elsevier.com/Williams/fundamental

Objectives

Upon completing this chapter, you should be able to do the following:

Theory

1. Describe the physiologic process by which wounds heal.
2. Discuss factors that affect wound healing.
3. Describe four signs and symptoms of wound infection.
4. Discuss correct nursing actions to be taken if wound dehiscence or evisceration occurs.
5. Explain the major purpose of a wound drain.
6. Identify the advantages of negative pressure wound therapy.
7. Compare and contrast the therapeutic effects of heat and cold.

Clinical Practice

1. Perform wound care, including emptying a drainage device and applying a sterile dressing.
2. Provide appropriate care for a pressure injury.
3. Perform wound irrigation.
4. Remove sutures or staples from a wound and apply thin adhesive strips (Steri-Strips).
5. Give a heat or cold treatment to a patient.

Skills & Steps

Key Terms

abscess (ĂB-sĕs, p. 765)
adhesions (ăd-HĒ-shŭnz, p. 762)
adipose (ĂD-ĭ-pōs, p. 762)
approximate (ă-PRŎX-ĭ-māt, p. 762)
approximation (ă-prŏx-ĭ-MĀ-shŭn, p. 772)
binders (p. 770)
cellulitis (sĕl-ū-LĪ-tĭs, p. 765)
collagen (KŎL-ă-jĕn, p. 762)
débridement (dĕ-BRĒD-măw, p. 767)
erythema (ĕr-ĭ-THĒ-mă, p. 761)
eschar (ĔS-kăr, p. 767)
exudate (ĔKS-ū-dāt, p. 765)
fibrin (p. 761)
first intention (ĭn-TĔN-shŭn, p. 762)
fistula (FĬS-tū-lă, p. 765)
granulation tissue (grăn-ū-LĀ-shŭn, p. 774)
hemostasis (hē-mō-STĀ-sĭs, p. 761)
immunocompromised (ĭm-ū-nō-KŎM-prō-mīzd, p. 765)
integument (ĭn-TĔG-ū-mĕnt, p. 760)
keloid (KĒ-loyd, p. 762)
laceration (lăs-ĕr-Ā-shŭn, p. 762)
lysis (LĪ-sĭs, p. 762)
maceration (măs-ĕr-Ā-shŭn, p. 781)
macrophages (MĂK-rō-fāj-ĕz, p. 762)
necrosis (nē-KRŌ-sĭs, p. 761)
phagocytosis (făg-ō-sī-TŌ-sĭs, p. 761)
platelet aggregation (PLĀT-lĕt ăg-rĕ-GĀ-shŭn, p. 761)
purulent (PŪ-rū-lĕnt, p. 765)
sanguineous (săng-GWĬN-ē-ŭs, p. 765)
second intention (p. 762)
serosanguineous (sĕr-ō-săng-GWĬN-ē-ŭs, p. 766)
sinus (SĪ-nŭs, p. 766)
sloughing (SLŪF-ĭng, p. 767)
suppuration (sŭp-ū-RĀ-shŭn, p. 785)
third intention (p. 762)

Concepts Covered in This Chapter

- Clinical judgment
- Infection
- Nutrition
- Pain
- Patient education
- Professionalism
- Sensory perception
- Tissue integrity

TYPES OF WOUNDS AND THE HEALING PROCESS

Wounds occur in a variety of ways. A surgical incision causes a clean and controlled break in skin integrity, whereas trauma may cause an irregular break in the skin. Pressure can cause tissue breakdown and alter skin integrity. Burns can partially or completely destroy skin. The skin and mucous membranes are protective barriers for the body against infection. Thus, injury to the **integument** (skin) brings risk of infection and may cause permanent damage. When the integument is injured, a complex healing process is initiated. Nurses act to prevent the invasion of microorganisms into wounds and to support and enhance the body's ability to affect wound repair.

Wounds may be **open,** occurring through the skin, or **closed,** without a break in the skin (Table 38.1). Closed wounds are typically caused by blunt trauma, twisting, pulling, straining, or deceleration force against the body.

Wounds may be partial thickness (superficial) or full thickness. **Partial-thickness** wounds heal more quickly because new skin cells are produced by the epithelial cells remaining in the dermal layer of the skin. The fibrin clot that forms after an injury acts as the framework, and regrowth occurs across the open wound area. When a **full-thickness** wound occurs, the dermal layer is no longer present except at the wound margins. To heal, all dead (necrotic) tissue must be

Table 38.1 Wound Types and Characteristics

TYPE	CHARACTERISTICS	DOCUMENTATION DESCRIPTION
	CLOSED	
Contusion (bruise)	Tissue injury without breaking of skin	Purple contusion 5 × 7 cm on left thigh
Hematoma	Tissue injury that damages a blood vessel; pooling of blood under the unbroken skin	4 cm diameter hematoma on right forearm
Sprain	Wrenching or twisting of a joint with partial rupture of its ligaments; causes swelling	Swelling of right foot and around malleolus No bruising noted
	OPEN	
Incision	Surgically made separation of tissues with clean, smooth edges	Approx 7 cm incision on right lower quadrant of abdomen; well approximated; clean and dry with sutures intact
Laceration	Traumatic separation of tissues with irregular, torn edges	5 cm jagged laceration approx 4 cm deep on lateral aspect of left lower leg
Abrasion	Traumatic scraping away of surface layers of skin	Raw appearing abraded area 6 cm diameter beneath left elbow
Puncture	Wound made by sharp, pointed object through skin or mucous membranes and underlying tissue	Small, circular entry wound on bottom of left foot from stepping on nail
Penetrating	Variable-size open wound through skin and underlying tissues made by a bullet or metal or wood fragment; may extend deeply into body	Jagged deep wound on left chest at third intercostal space, 5 cm lateral to sternum
Avulsion	Tearing away of a structure or a part, such as a fingertip, accidentally or surgically	Avulsion of tip of left little finger from accident with knife Attached only by skin
Ulceration	Excavation of skin and/or underlying tissue from injury or necrosis	Ulceration on lateral aspect of left lower leg 4½ × 5¾ × 2 cm deep; yellow drainage present; wound edges reddened
Perforation	Internal organ or body cavity tissue opened, usually because of infection or a penetrating wound	Abdomen pale, hard to palpation with blue-tinged discoloration noted in right upper quadrant
Crush (could cause open or closed wound)	Tissue significantly disrupted or compressed because of high level of force being applied (e.g., person pinned against a wall by a car hitting him at a moderate speed); may or may not be visible lacerations or maceration of surrounding tissue	Both lower extremities with gross deformities; significant hematomas present, left greater than right, below the knees, no pulses palpated in popliteal or pedal regions bilaterally

removed so that granulation tissue can gradually fill in the defect (Fig. 38.1). The wound heals by contraction.

Wounds may be **clean** (free of microorganisms) or **dirty** (containing microorganisms). An infected wound contains a large number of microorganisms that invaded the tissue and released a variety of toxins.

When a wound occurs, the two primary methods of healing are replacement of cells and regeneration. **Replacement** occurs in the form of fibrous connective tissue that does not have the same functional characteristics as the tissue lost when the wound occurred. When cells are not damaged beyond recovery, they restore themselves, with little to no permanent evidence of injury. If the blood supply has been disrupted to the new wound bed and **necrosis** (death or injury to cells) has occurred, the affected tissue must heal by **regeneration.** New cells similar in structure and function to the dead cells are produced if the tissue is a type that will regenerate. Skin, mucous membranes, bone marrow, muscle, bone, liver, kidney, and lung tissue can regenerate with tissue that is structurally similar to that which was lost. Heart muscle and nerve cells are generally unable to regenerate.

PHASES OF WOUND HEALING

No matter what the cause of the wound, healing occurs in three distinct phases: the inflammatory phase; the proliferation or reconstruction phase; and the maturation, or remodeling, phase. **Inflammation** is a localized protective response brought on by injury or destruction of tissues. **The inflammatory phase begins immediately after injury and lasts approximately 3 or 4 days.** It includes constriction of blood vessels, **platelet aggregation** (clumping), and the formation of **fibrin** (protein essential to clotting) from the action of thrombin on fibrinogen and epithelial cell migration. This is the process of **hemostasis** (blood clotting or vessel compression) and clot formation. A scab forms to protect against pathogens. Epithelial cells migrate from the margins of the wound toward the base of the scab, and within about 48 hours a thin layer of epithelial tissue forms over the wound. Chemical reactions releasing histamine and prostaglandin occur. Small blood vessels then dilate and become more permeable, causing serous fluid to leak into the traumatized area. The collection of plasma and electrolytes leaking into the interstitial spaces causes edema. The wound becomes reddened, swollen, and tender. Reactions that are more chemical bring phagocytic neutrophils to cleanse the wound. The phagocytic cells remove debris and protect against bacterial invasion by **phagocytosis** (engulfing of microorganisms or foreign particles).

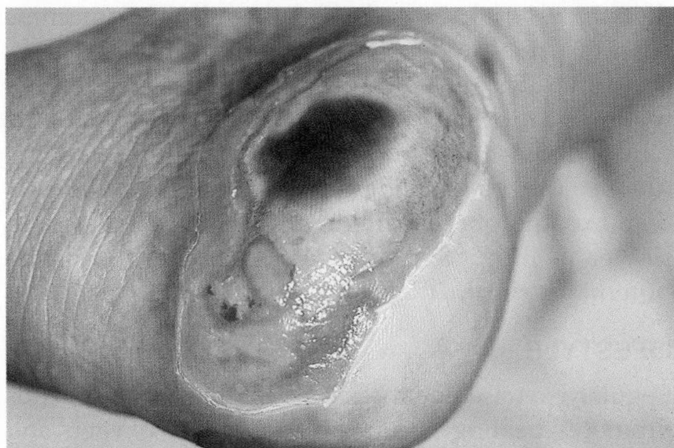

FIGURE 38.1 The brown necrotic tissue must be débrided before healing can take place in this pressure injury. (From Potter, P. A., & Perry, G. A. [2009]. *Fundamentals of Nursing* [7th ed.]. St. Louis: Mosby.)

The clinical signs of the inflammatory process are as follows:

- Swelling or edema of the injured part
- **Erythema** (redness) resulting from the increased blood supply
- Heat or increased temperature at the site
- Pain stemming from pressure on nerve receptors
- A possible loss of function resulting from all these changes

 Communication

Concern About Scarring

Carl Heffner has had open heart surgery and comes to the cardiac rehabilitation center three times a week. The saphenous veins from both legs were used for grafts, so he has three healing incisions from this surgery. He is 64 and divorced.

Mr. Heffner: "When it gets warm this summer, I will hate wearing shorts to work out with these leg scars. They are so ugly. I feel like I have little red snakes going up my legs."

Nurse: "You are worried about the appearance of your legs?"

Mr. Heffner: "Yes, people must find these scars repulsive. I've always looked away when I've seen someone at the gym with all these scars."

Nurse: "Is it difficult to think of yourself looking different than you did before the surgery?"

Mr. Heffner: "Yes, I've always taken a great deal of pride in my appearance. There was a time when women told me I was handsome. Now I'm just a wreck."

Nurse: "How are you feeling now, compared with before your surgery?"

Mr. Heffner: "I feel much better. I am able to do more and am not fatigued all the time. I'm even thinking of playing tennis again."

Nurse: "So before your surgery, you had fairly constant chest pain, were very fatigued, and had to give up playing tennis. Let's look at what the surgery has meant to your life on the whole."

Mr. Heffner: "Well, sure, I'm much better after the surgery and I'm grateful to be alive. My stamina is improving daily and it looks like I will be able to play tennis again. I am really looking forward to that. But I am very self-conscious about getting out on the court in shorts. My buddies will probably tease me."

Nurse: "Have any of the other players had heart surgery?"

Mr. Heffner: "Yes, Charlie has, but he doesn't have these big red scars on his legs."

Nurse: "Did you know him at the time of his surgery?"

Mr. Heffner: "No, I came to the group a couple of years after that."
Nurse: "I think if you look, you will see that Charlie's leg scar has become white and isn't nearly as noticeable now. Yours will mature in that way also. It just takes time for the scar to mature and the red color to fade."
Mr. Heffner: "You think they won't be so prominent later on?"
Nurse: "Yes, they will smooth out and fade."
Mr. Heffner: "I could live with that a lot easier. Plus, players are supposed to keep their eyes on the ball, not on their partner's or opponent's legs!"
Nurse: "That's the spirit, Mr. H.!"

The proliferation stage begins on the third or fourth day after injury and lasts 2 to 3 weeks. In this phase the wound is filled with new connective tissue, and new epithelium will cover the wound. **Macrophages** (monocytes that are phagocytic) continue to clean the wound of debris, stimulating fibroblasts, which synthesize collagen. **Collagen** (fibrous structural protein of all connective tissue) is the main ingredient of scar tissue. New capillary networks provide oxygen and nutrients to support the collagen and further synthesis of granulation tissue. This tissue is deep pink in appearance. A full-thickness wound begins to close by contraction as new tissue is grown. Scarring is influenced by the degree of stress on the wound. In 15 to 20 days the risk of wound separation or rupture is less likely.

The final stage of healing, maturation, begins approximately 3 weeks after injury. Scar maturation, or remodeling, is the process of collagen **lysis** (breakdown) and collagen synthesis by the macrophages to produce the strongest scar tissue possible. Scar tissue slowly thins and becomes paler in color. At the end of this process, the scar is firm and inelastic.

The length of each phase depends on the type of injury and whether the wound heals by first, second, or third intention. The stages of healing are interwoven rather than linear. Different parts of a wound can be in different stages of healing. The process of wound healing is presented in Concept Map 38.1. To ensure adequate and timely wound healing, the nurse should implement the key steps found in Box 38.1.

When a wound occurs around a joint, attention is needed to maintain joint mobility and prevent a **contracture** (abnormal shortening of muscle tissue) that will restrict joint extension. If collagen overgrowth occurs, which is frequent in dark-pigmented skin, a **keloid** (permanent raised, enlarged scar) occurs (Fig. 38.2). In the interior of the body, **adhesions** (fibrous bands that hold together tissues that are normally separated) may grow and interfere with function of the internal organs.

A wound with little tissue loss, such as a surgical incision, heals by **first intention** (closure) (Fig. 38.3). The edges of the wound **approximate** (close together), and there is only a slight chance of infection. A wound with tissue loss, such as a decubitus (pressure) injury or severe **laceration** (a torn, ragged, or mangled wound), typically heals by **second intention.** The edges of the wound do not approximate, and the wound is left open and fills with scar tissue. Because of the longer healing period, the chance of infection is higher. **Third intention** healing, also known as delayed or secondary closure, occurs when there is delayed suturing of a wound. Such wounds are sutured after the granulation tissue has begun to form. An abdominal wound left open for drainage and then later closed is an example of healing by third intention.

? Think Critically

If a patient asks why swelling occurs after an injury, what would you say?

FACTORS AFFECTING WOUND HEALING

AGE

Healthy children and adults heal more quickly than those with chronic health conditions and older adults. Metabolism and regeneration in the chronically ill and older adult are slower. Peripheral vascular disease impairs blood flow, which can impede healing. Atherosclerosis and atrophy reduce skin capillaries and impair blood flow to the wound. A decline in immune function reduces the formation of antibodies and monocytes necessary for wound healing. Reduced liver function impairs the synthesis of blood factors. Decreases in lung function reduce available oxygen needed for synthesis of collagen and the formation of new epithelial cells. Older skin is much thinner, more fragile, and more easily damaged than the skin of younger people; thus, older patients' skin should be handled carefully when performing wound care to avoid further wound formation.

NUTRITION

Added protein and adequate fluid are of great importance when a patient has a chronic wound. A diet that is rich in carbohydrates, lipids, vitamins A and C, thiamine, pyridoxine, and riboflavin, plus the minerals zinc, iron, and copper, is needed for wound healing. Malnourished patients and patients with diabetes are at risk for delayed wound healing. **Adipose** (fatty) tissue has less blood supply and predisposes the obese patient to wound infection and slower healing. (See Chapter 26 for more information on nutrition.)

LIFESTYLE

Regular exercise enhances blood circulation and thus promotes healing because blood brings oxygen and nutrients to the wound. Smoking reduces the functional hemoglobin of the blood, which limits oxygen-carrying capacity. The person who does not smoke and who exercises regularly typically heals more quickly.

Wound

Inflammatory phase

Vascular constriction

Platelet aggression

Fibrin formation

Hemostasis and clot formation

Chemical release

Small vessels dilate

Fluid accumulates, causing edema

Redness, tenderness, and swelling

Phagocytes enter → phagocytosis

Proliferation phase

Phagocytosis continues

Fibroblasts synthesize collagen

New capillary networks

Granulation tissue forms

Contraction

Possible contracture

Epithelialization

Maturation (remodeling) phase

Collagen lysis and production

Scar remodeling

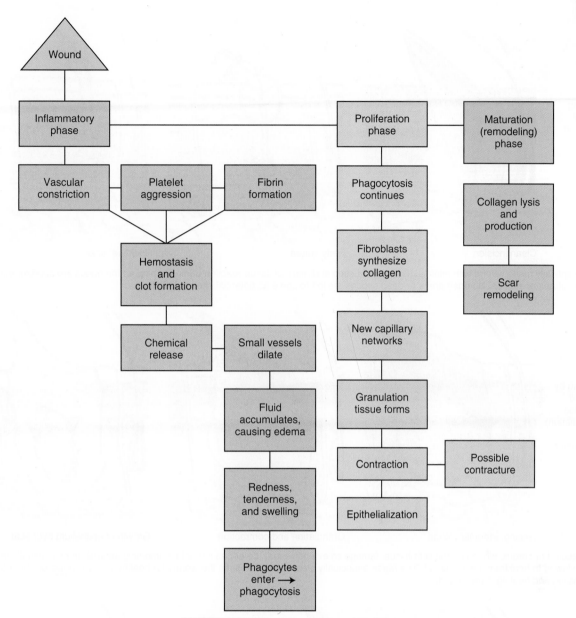

CONCEPT MAP 38.1 Process of wound healing.

Box 38.1 Key Steps to Ensure Appropriate Wound Healing

- Keep surrounding skin and tissue clean and dry.
- Ensure adequate oxygen and nutrient supply to the wound by maintaining appropriate body positioning to prevent undue or prolonged pressure.
- Ensure dressings, compression stockings, NPWT and wound VAC units, and drains are applied and positioned correctly so that circulation is not impaired and the risk of developing lymphedema is minimized.
- Report any signs or symptoms of infection immediately to ensure appropriate therapies are quickly initiated.
- Provide appropriate nutrition and optimize blood glucose levels to aid in the healing process.

NPWT, Negative pressure wound therapy; *VAC,* vacuum-assisted closure.

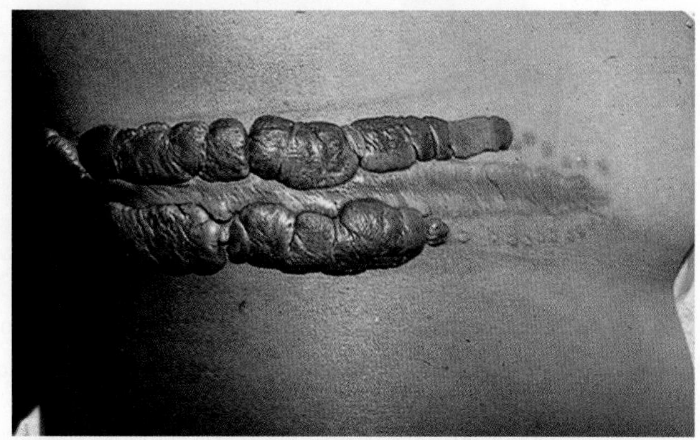

FIGURE 38.2 Keloid along a sutured wound. (From Habif, T. P. [1991]. *Clinical Dermatology: A Color Guide to Diagnosis and Therapy* [2nd ed.]. St. Louis: Mosby.)

Healing by first intention

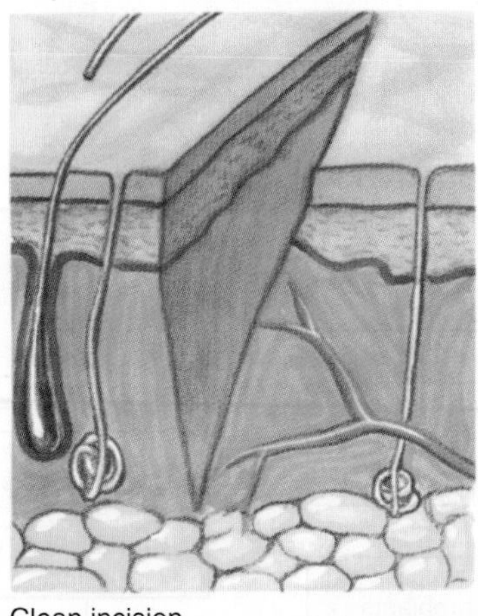

Clean incision

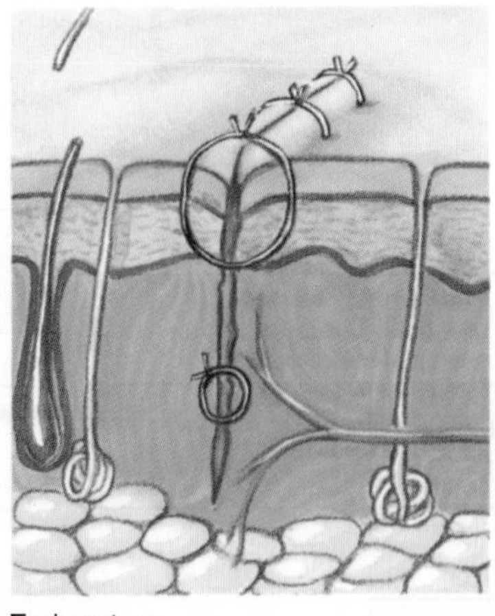

Early suture

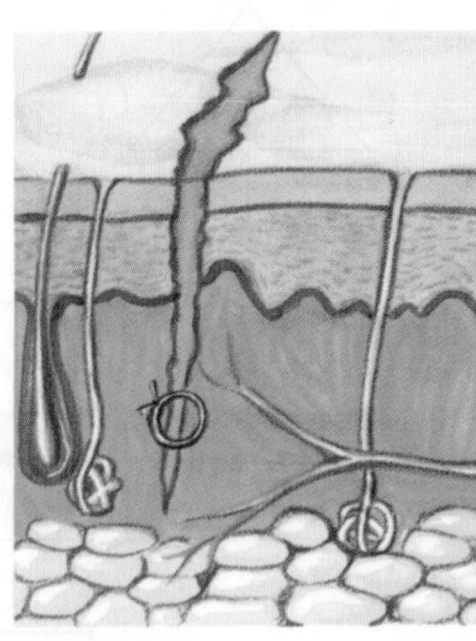

"Hairline" scar

An aseptically made wound with minimal tissue destruction and minimal tissue reaction begins to heal as the edges are approximated by close sutures or staples. No open areas or dead spaces are left to serve as potential sites of infection.

Healing by second intention (granulation) and contraction

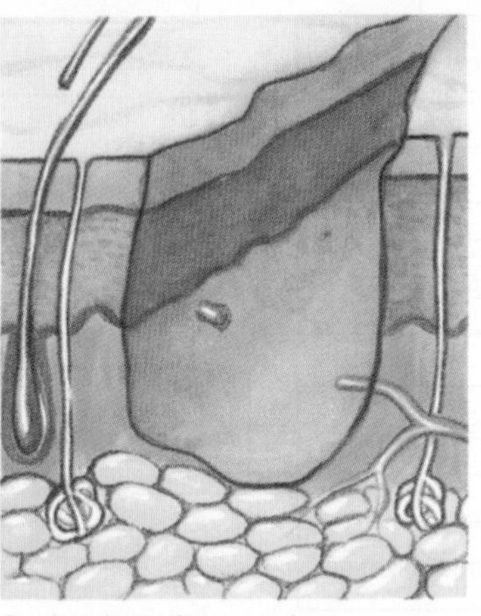

Gaping, irregular wound

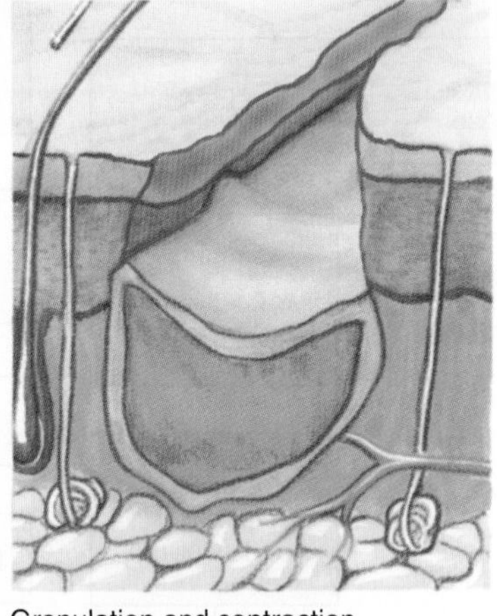

Granulation and contraction

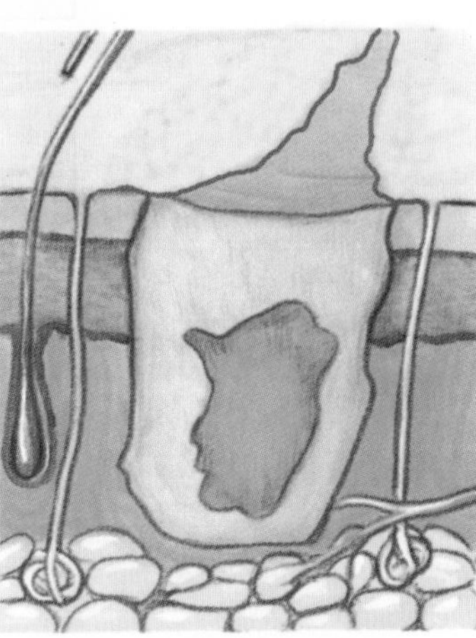

Growth of epithelium over scar

An infected or chronic wound or one with tissue damage so extensive that the edges cannot be smoothly approximated is usually left open and allowed to heal from the inside out. The nurse periodically cleans and assesses the wound for healthy tissue production. Scar tissue is extensive, and healing is prolonged.

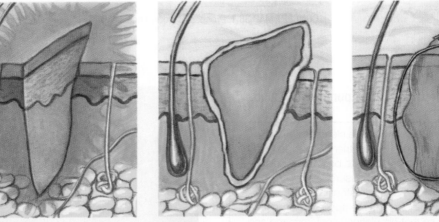

Healing by third intention (delayed closure)

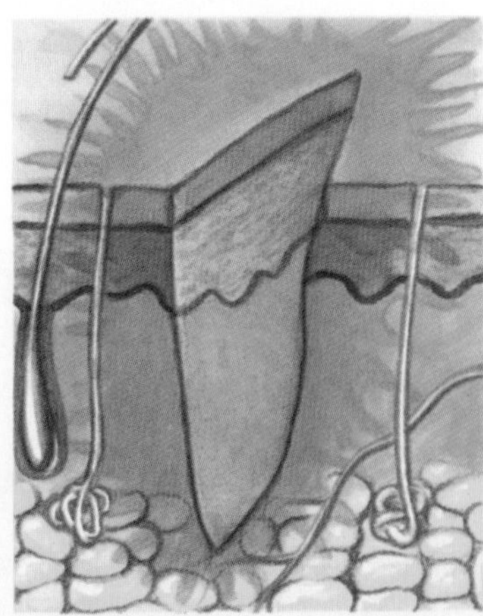

Infected wound

Granulation

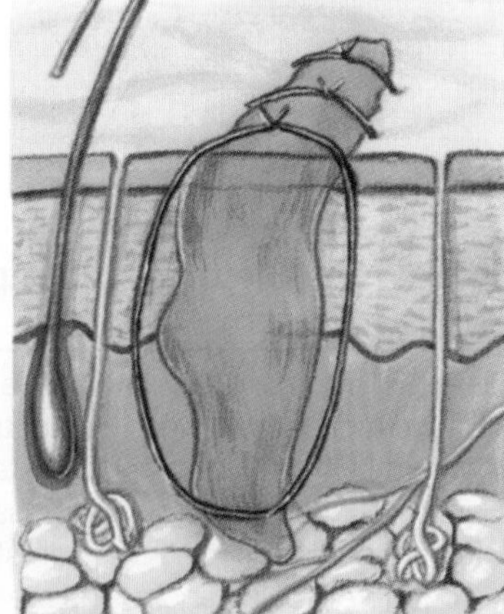

Closure with wide scar

A potentially infected surgical wound may be left open for several days. If no clinical signs of infection occur, the wound is then closed surgically.

FIGURE 38.3 The process of wound healing. (From Ignatavicius, D. D., & Workman, M. L. [2002]. *Medical-Surgical Nursing: Critical Thinking for Collaborative Care* [4th ed.]. Philadelphia: Saunders.)

MEDICATIONS

Use of steroids, immunosuppressants and other anti-inflammatory drugs, anticoagulants such as heparin, and antineoplastic agents interfere with various aspects of the healing process. Steroids may mask the signs of wound infection because they inhibit the inflammatory response. Inflammation is generally a signal of infection, but it may not occur when steroids are present.

INFECTION

A wound infection slows the healing process. The acute phase of an infection is characterized by a sudden onset of symptoms and by the vascular changes of inflammation, especially swelling caused by fluid collecting in tissue. The acute phase is followed by an increase in white blood cells (WBCs), which overwhelm the invading microorganisms and clear away the damaged tissues so that healing can occur. A bacterial infection of the skin or mucous membranes frequently causes fluid drainage from the wound or damaged tissue.

Clinical Cues

Assess drainage for color, consistency, odor, and amount, and document the findings. The color may range from creamy yellow to dark green. **Purulent** (containing purulent exudate) drainage contains dead phagocytes, bacteria, and tissue and is thick in consistency. As the infection disappears, the drainage lessens, has minimal to no odor, is more serous or watery, and lightens in color. All signs of inflammation subside as healing occurs.

CHRONIC ILLNESS

Patients who have a chronic illness, such as diabetes, cardiovascular disease, or a disorder of the immune system, may take longer to heal. Slowed wound healing occurs from decreased oxygen and nutrients at the cellular level, disruptions in the normal metabolism of substances in the body that aid in the healing process, or inability of the body to fight infection.

Patients who are **immunocompromised** (with poorly functioning immune systems) have delayed wound healing because fibroblast function, collagen synthesis, and phagocytosis are affected. These patients are at high risk for health care–associated infection (HAI). This type of infection is one that someone acquires while receiving treatment for another condition in a health care setting.

COMPLICATIONS OF WOUND HEALING

HEMORRHAGE

Some bleeding from a wound is normal, but hemorrhage is abnormal. Internal hemorrhage is evidenced by swelling or distention in the area of the wound and, perhaps, **sanguineous** (bloody) drainage from a surgical drain.

Clinical Cues

Monitor all patients with fresh surgical wounds for signs of hemorrhage. Be certain to check underneath the patient who had abdominal surgery to be certain blood is not seeping from the side of the dressing under the patient.

If internal hemorrhage is extensive, hypovolemic shock may occur with a fall in blood pressure, rapid and thready pulse, increased respiratory rate, restlessness, diaphoresis, and cold clammy skin. Intervene promptly to prevent a potentially life-threatening situation.

In other cases a **hematoma** may occur. A hematoma may appear as a swelling that is bluish red. If a hematoma is large, it may place pressure on blood vessels and obstruct blood flow to the surrounding tissue. A hematoma may also cause the patient to exhibit a slight elevation in temperature.

The risk of hemorrhage is greatest during the first 48 hours after surgery; when it occurs, it requires emergency intervention. If external hemorrhage occurs, apply extra pressure using sterile dressings to the site; closely monitor the patient's vital signs. Notify the surgeon because the patient may need to be immediately returned to the operating room for further intervention.

INFECTION

A wound may be infected with microorganisms at the time of injury, during surgery, or postoperatively. Local signs that a wound is infected include increased pain, redness, warmth in the surrounding tissues, and purulent **exudate** (fluid accumulation containing cellular debris). Traumatic wounds are more likely to become infected than surgical wounds. A localized infection called an **abscess** is an accumulation of purulent exudate made up of debris from phagocytosis when microorganisms have been present. The fluid may be white, yellow, pink, or green, depending on the infecting microorganisms. Surgical wound infection is often an HAI, but can be from microorganisms that are present in the wound bed or on the surface of the skin.

The microorganism most frequently present in wound infections is *Staphylococcus aureus.* Other microorganisms commonly responsible for wound infections include *Escherichia coli, Streptococcus pyogenes,* methicillin-resistant *Staphylococcus aureus* (MRSA), and *Pseudomonas aeruginosa.* When wound infection is suspected, a specimen of wound exudate is obtained and tested. A Culturette tube is used to obtain a specimen for the culture (see Chapter 24), and a sensitivity test is performed to determine which antimicrobial agent is most effective against the offending organism (Fig. 38.4).

Cellulitis is an inflammation of the tissue surrounding the initial wound, with redness and **induration** (skin hardening). A **fistula** is an abnormal passage or

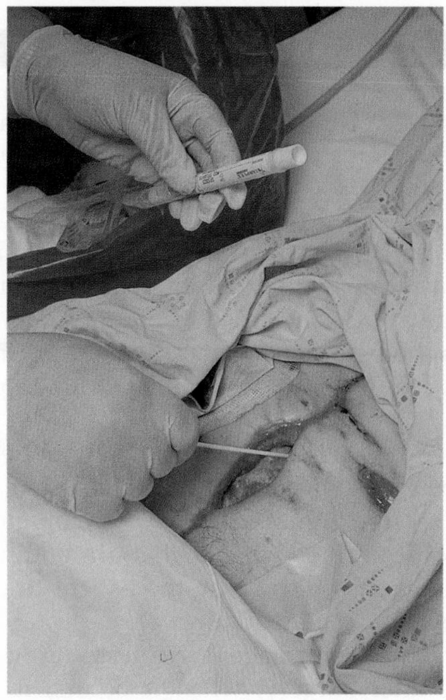

FIGURE 38.4 Take a specimen from the interior of the wound for a culture.

communication usually formed between two internal organs or leading from an internal organ to the surface of the body. A fistula may result from an infection, or it may be present congenitally. Common postoperative fistulas are designated according to the organs or parts with which they communicate, such as a rectovaginal, anal, or biliary fistula. A **sinus** is a fistula leading from a purulent exudate-filled cavity to the outside of the body.

The best way to prevent wound infection is to maintain strict asepsis when performing wound care. Use sterile equipment, meticulous hand hygiene, sterile gloves, and sterile dressings. To prevent shedding of microorganisms into the wound, contain long hair so that it is not swinging over the wound and remove the stethoscope from around the neck. Refrain from talking while dressing a wound to prevent microorganisms in the mouth or saliva from possibly landing in the wound.

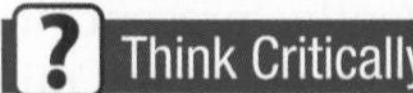

Think Critically

What discharge instructions would you give a patient about assessing for signs of wound infection?

DEHISCENCE AND EVISCERATION

Dehiscence is the spontaneous opening of an incision. Dehiscence of an abdominal wound often involves separation of the layers beneath the skin as well. **Evisceration** is the protrusion of an internal organ through the incision. Risk factors for dehiscence are obesity, poor nutrition, multiple traumas, excessive coughing, vomiting, strong sneezing, suture failure, and dehydration. The greatest risk for wound dehiscence is on the fourth or fifth postoperative day, before extensive collagen has built up. **A sign of impending dehiscence may be an increase in the flow of serosanguineous (serum and blood mixture) drainage into the wound dressing.** When dehiscence occurs, the patient may state that "something has given way." If dehiscence or evisceration occurs, quickly place the patient supine and place large sterile dressings, or towels soaked in normal saline, over the incision and viscera. Notify the surgeon immediately and prepare the patient for return to surgery.

Life Span Considerations

Older Adults

Complications of wound healing, such as dehiscence and evisceration, may occur more frequently in older adults because of the prolonged healing process.

Think Critically

What would you do if you were ambulating in the hall with a patient who has an abdominal incision and he bends forward suddenly and says "something gave way"?

TREATMENT OF WOUNDS

WOUND CLOSURE

Sutures and staples are typically used to hold the edges of a surgical wound together until the wound can heal. Traumatic wounds are usually cleaned, trimmed, and sutured closed. Sutures used to attach tissues beneath the skin are made of absorbable material, are not removed, and are reabsorbed or dissolve within a few days. Skin sutures are made of silk, cotton, linen, wire, nylon, or Dacron. Silver wire clips are also sometimes used. Large retention sutures may be used on a wound when the surgeon believes there is a danger of dehiscence (Fig. 38.5). These are usually wire, and the portion of the suture outside the skin is covered with rubber. Sometimes the wound is small, and Steri-Strips can be used. These are small, reinforced adhesive strips placed over the break in the skin that effectively hold the wound edges together while healing takes place.

Dermabond is synthetic, noninvasive glue that decreases the trauma from removing a dressing, while providing a seal that protects underlying tissue without the need for bandages. This may sometimes be used in place of sutures in small areas. It loosens and comes off in 7 to 10 days. It is not used on mucous membranes.

The recommended method of open wound classification is based on the wound's color rather than its cause or dimensions. There are three basic wound types: red, yellow, and black. The type of wound indicates the type of dressing needed. **Red wounds** are clean and ready to heal. Protection is the best method of treatment. A **yellow wound** has a layer of yellow

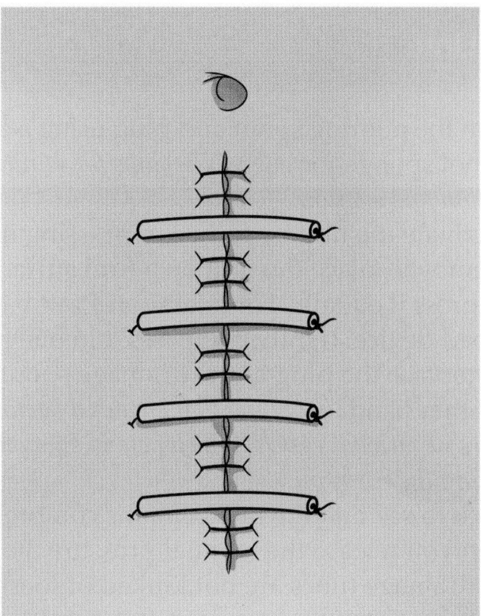

FIGURE 38.5 Retention sutures.

fibrous debris or exudate. Wounds can be yellow if there are a large amount of leukocytes present (Grady, 2014). **Sloughing** (natural shedding of dead tissue) may cause drainage. A yellow wound needs to be frequently cleansed and should have a dressing that will absorb the drainage and débride the surface mechanically. A yellow wound often becomes infected. **Black wounds** need **débridement** (removal of all foreign or unhealthy tissue from a wound) of the **eschar** (sloughing dead tissue, usually caused by a thermal injury or gangrene) to heal. Eschar can be mechanically débrided by a surgeon, softened by soaks or enzyme substances, and gradually removed as it separates. Licensed practical/vocational nurses (LPN/LVNs) can become certified in wound care; they can also perform débridement of wounds if allowed by their state boards of nursing and allowed by the agency's policies and procedures.

DRAINS AND DRAINAGE DEVICES

At surgery, one or more drains may be placed to provide an exit for blood, purulent exudate, fluids, or air that accumulates and could increase the risk of infection. The drain may be active or passive. An active drain is attached to a wound suction device to remove any accumulated exudate or other material. A passive drain has no suction device attachment; it works by the increased pressure inside the wound and depends on gravity and capillary action to pull out any fluid buildup. The drain is placed within the surgical area and exits through a "stab" wound (a puncture or slit made by the surgeon) at a location different from the incision. A Penrose drain is a flat rubber tube. Often a safety pin is placed at the external end of the drain to prevent it from slipping into the wound (Fig. 38.6). Whenever this drain is ordered to be shortened, place a new safety pin proximal to where you will cut the drain tubing to the desired length before cutting the tubing. Catheters of various sizes can also be used as drains.

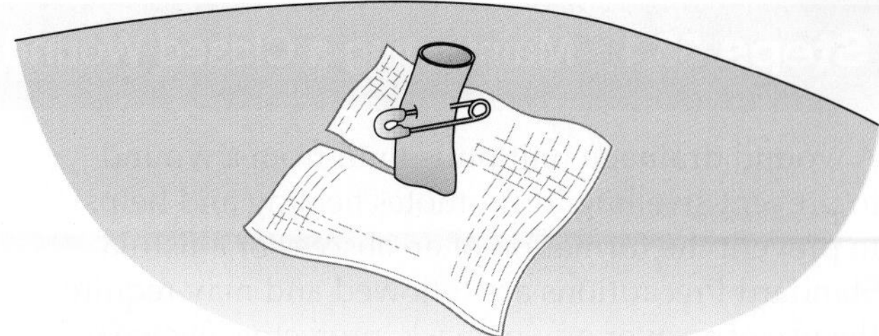

FIGURE 38.6 Penrose drain in a "stab wound" close to an abdominal incision. (Redrawn from Potter, P. A., & Perry, G.A. [2005]. *Fundamentals of Nursing* [6th ed.]. St. Louis: Mosby.)

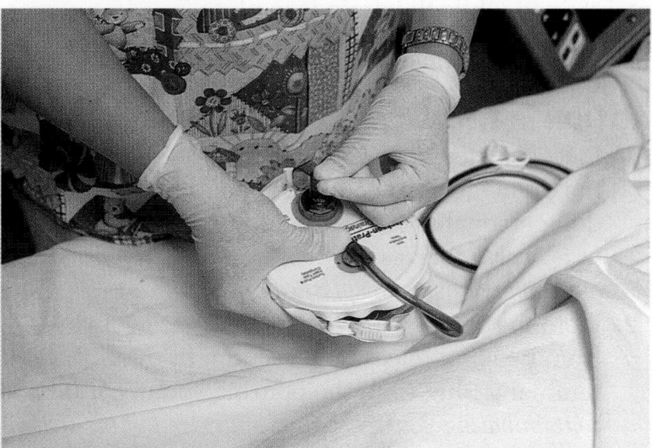

FIGURE 38.7 Compress the Hemovac-type drainage system to activate it.

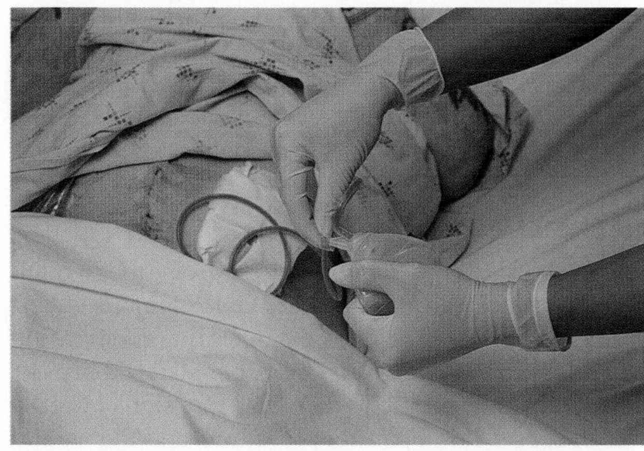

FIGURE 38.8 After emptying drainage, compress the bulb of the Jackson-Pratt–type drainage device to activate it.

Plastic drainage tubes can be connected to a drainage system that is compressed and closed, applying slight suction to the drainage tube to help to evacuate wound fluids (Fig. 38.7). The Hemovac evacuators and Jackson-Pratt drains are examples of this (Fig. 38.8). The fluid in a drainage device is measured and then emptied at the end of each shift, and the amount drained is entered on the intake and output record (Steps 38.1). Draining excess fluid from a wound area helps to prevent the formation of an abscess or a fistula. Drains are sometimes used when traumatic wounds are sutured closed. The skin around the drain is cleansed during each dressing change.

Steps 38.1 Maintaining a Closed Wound Drainage Unit

A wound drainage unit pulls fluid from a wound to prevent swelling. It promotes healing and helps to prevent the formation of an abscess or a fistula. Standard Precautions are followed and may require the use of a cover gown, mask, protective eyewear, and gloves. Jackson-Pratt drainage system bulbs should be drained and recompressed at least once every 4 hours and when they are at least two-thirds full. This ensures that the negative pressure is maintained while the drain is in place.

Review and carry out the Standard Steps in Appendix A.

ACTION *(RATIONALE)*

1. Place a waterproof underpad on the bed under the drainage device. Perform hand hygiene, and don personal protective equipment (PPE). *(Protects the bedding if spill occurs. Protects from transfer of microorganisms in splashed fluids.)*
2. Hold the device with the spout pointing away from you and release the vacuum by gently removing plug from the pouring spout. *(Avoids contaminating yourself if fluid spurts out of the spout.)*
3. Do not touch the drainage spout or plug. *(Touching these areas contaminates these surfaces, increasing risk of infection.)*
4. Empty the contents into a measuring container. Note the amount and appearance of drainage. *(Allows accurate output measurement. Provides data for documentation and evaluation.)*
5. Clean the pouring spout and plug using a separate alcohol sponge for each. *(Prepares for reinitiation of vacuum and suction.)*
6. Reactivate the unit by fully compressing it. For a Hemovac, place the unit on a firm surface and compress it equally. For a Jackson-Pratt balloon-shaped device, tightly compress it in one hand and replace the plug in the drainage spout with the other hand. *(Compression creates a vacuum and causes negative pressure, which acts to suction drainage into the reservoir.)*
7. Check to see that the unit remains compressed when you release the manual pressure. Be certain that drainage tubes are not kinked or loose. *(Reinstitutes suction of the wound and ensures the drain[s] can safely collect fluid as it drains.)*
8. Secure device to patient's gown below the level of the wound. *(Prevents pulling on the drains and wound if device is caught on something and aids in draining fluid from wound.)*
9. Remove and dispose of PPE, and wash your hands. Note the amount of drainage on the shift intake and output record. *(Prevents transfer of microorganisms and tracks the amount of drainage.)*
10. Document amount, color, and odor of drainage and that system is recharged/compressed and drainage tubes are unkinked. *(Provides a record of your actions and findings.)*

DÉBRIDEMENT

Necrotic tissue must be removed from the wound before healing can occur. **Sharp débridement** is performed at the bedside or in the operating room, using sterile scissors, forceps, and a scalpel blade. Sharp débridement is performed when there are signs of cellulitis or sepsis. It is a painful procedure, and the wound bleeds afterward. The surgeon or nurse practitioner usually performs this function, although nurses can perform it under certain conditions (described earlier). Nurses often are directed to perform **enzymatic débridement,** which uses topical substances that break down and liquefy the dead tissue. These substances are placed in the wound, and another dressing is placed over it to hold them in place. This is useful for uninfected wounds.

Chemical débridement using Dakin solution or sterile maggots is occasionally used on a wound with necrotic tissue that is not responding to other treatments. **Autolytic débridement** is a longer process that uses the body's enzymes to break down nonviable tissue in the wound. It is best used on small, uninfected wounds because the type of dressing used provides a warm, moist environment that could encourage growth of bacteria if they are present. Closely monitor the wound for signs of infection during the autolytic process. **Mechanical débridement** is the physical removal of wound debris by irrigation or hydrotherapy with a whirlpool bath or ultrasound mist. The physical therapist performs the whirlpool procedure. With ultrasound mist therapy, microscopic saline bubbles and sound waves clean and débride the wound bed and remove bacteria while stimulating cell growth. Treatments are usually ordered three times a week. The procedure is usually painless but may be followed by tingling and redness of the site.

The mist is delivered in a grid pattern, perpendicular to the wound.

Wet-to-dry dressings are an older form of dressing changes that mechanically débride because tissue sticks to the dressing material, and a layer of cells is pulled off when the dressings are removed. They are no longer recommended because they disrupt newly regenerated tissue.

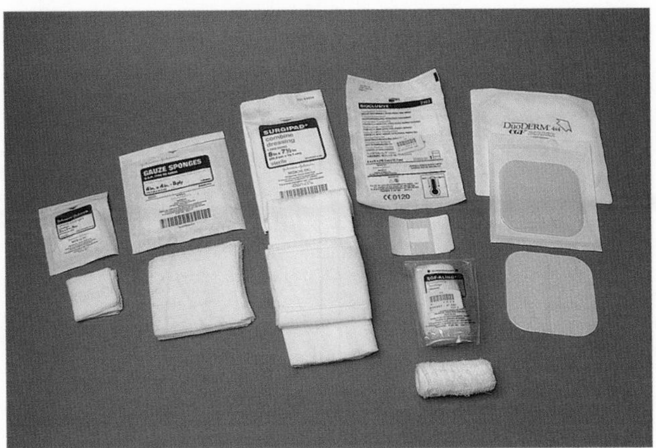

FIGURE 38.9 Various types of dressings.

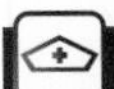 Clinical Cues

The only necrotic wound for which débridement is not recommended is a pressure injury on a heel. According to Agency for Healthcare Research and Quality guidelines (National Pressure Ulcer Advisory Panel, 2015), this type of pressure injury is not débrided if the eschar is dry and if edema, erythema, or drainage is not present.

DRESSINGS

Dressings, which are protective coverings placed over wounds, serve a number of purposes. They prevent microorganisms from freely entering or escaping the wound, and they absorb drainage. Dressings can be used for applying pressure to control bleeding and for improving the adherence of a skin graft to the grafted site. In addition, dressings help to support and stabilize tissues and reduce discomfort from a wound.

A wide variety of dressing materials are available for dressing a wound (Fig. 38.9). Choices are based on the location, size, and type of wound; whether infection is present or débridement is needed; and the frequency with which the dressing will be changed. Several standard sizes of dry sterile gauze are available: 2 × 2 inch (5 × 5 cm), 4 × 4 inch (10 × 10 cm), and 4 × 8 inch (10 × 20 cm). The size and number of gauze pads needed depend on the size of the wound and the amount of exudate. Dressings may be folded or cut with sterile scissors to fit around drains.

Telfa and other nonadherent dressings have a shiny, nonadherent surface on one side that is applied to the wound. Exudate seeps through this surface and collects in the absorbent material on the other side. This dressing causes less wound trauma when it is removed.

Surgi-Pads or abdominal pads (ABDs) are used to cover small gauze dressings. They hold the dressings in place and absorb and collect excess drainage. The more absorbent surface of the Surgi-Pad is placed facing the wound; the less absorbent outward side helps to protect from external contamination. The outer side is usually indicated by a blue stripe or a seam.

Whichever dressings are used, the purpose is to fully cover the wound and supply sufficient absorbent material to contain any exudate produced. The outermost dressing should completely cover the inner dressings.

It has been known for some time that superficial wounds heal faster when kept moist than when kept dry. A variety of air or fluid occlusive and semi-occlusive wound dressings have been developed, including thin films, hydrocolloids, and foams. These dressings keep the wound moist while insulating and protecting it from external contamination. Foam dressings absorb drainage. These dressings are used more frequently than gauze for chronic or hard-to-heal wounds.

Two commonly used dressings are transparent film and hydrocolloid dressings. Many combination varieties and other wound dressings are also available. It is important to determine the desired action for treatment of the wound before choosing the appropriate dressing. Other types of dressings include hydrogels, calcium alginate, composites, collagens, and enzymatic débriders.

Transparent Film Dressings

Clear film dressings, such as OpSite or Tegaderm, allow you to assess the wound without removing the dressing. The transparent dressing does not require the use of tape and is less bulky than a gauze dressing. These dressings are often used to cover intravenous catheter sites and to protect a stage 1 or 2 pressure injury. They are useful for superficial, partial-thickness wounds. They do not absorb drainage. A transparent film dressing should be changed when it no longer adheres to the skin properly. They may remain in place from 3 to 7 days. Do not use a transparent film dressing over an infected wound.

 Assignment Considerations

Pressure Injury and Wound Observation

Remind unlicensed assistive personnel (UAPs) to report any changes, such as drainage, increased reddening, or a loose dressing, to you. Perform your own assessments of wounds and pressure injuries. Assessment is not the UAP's job.

Hydrocolloid Dressing

Hydrocolloid dressings, such as DuoDERM, keep a wound moist and have been shown to reduce wound size (Kirman, 2015). They are water and air occlusive and self-adhesive. You cannot see through a hydrocolloid dressing. This dressing facilitates autolytic débridement and provides thermal insulation, keeping the wound warm. Once applied, this dressing may stay in place for 3 to 5 days, as long as it stays intact with good skin contact on all edges. Hydrocolloids are not recommended for heavily draining wounds.

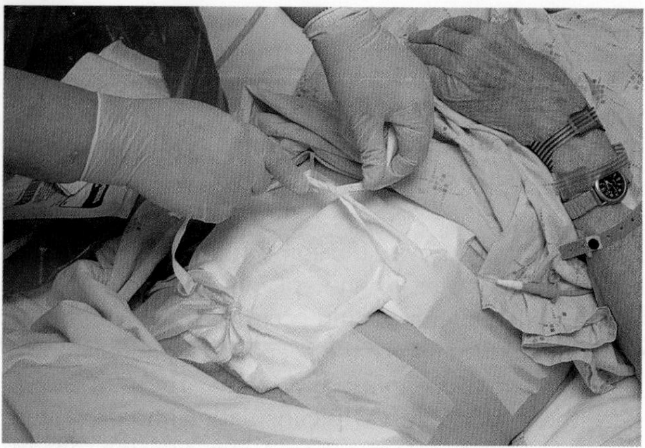

FIGURE 38.10 Montgomery straps may be used to hold a dressing in place.

Box 38.2 Principles for the Application of Tape on a Dressing

- Place the tape so that the wound will stay covered by the dressing and the tape will adhere to intact skin. Place strips of tape at the ends of the dressing, and space tape strips evenly across the middle.
- The tape should be long and wide enough to adhere firmly to intact skin on each side of the dressing but not so long that activity will loosen it.
- Place the tape opposite to body action in the wound location. Tape should go across a joint or crease, not lengthwise along it (see Fig. 38.11).
- Turning under the end of the tape leaves a tab, making removal easier.

Securing Dressings

The dressing is secured to the wound using tape, stretch roller gauze (Conform, Kerlix, Kling), mesh netting, an elastic bandage, or Montgomery straps (tie tapes). The correct product must be selected for the purpose. Elastic tape or bandages provide pressure; stretch gauze and mesh netting allow some movement without dislodging the dressing; and Montgomery straps allow changing of the dressing without removing and reapplying tape, which can cause repeated skin irritation (Fig. 38.10).

Tincture of benzoin may be applied to protect sensitive skin before the dressing is taped (Box 38.2). Strips of hydrocolloid dressing can be placed on either side of the wound edges, the dressing applied, and then tape applied to the hydrocolloid strips for wounds that need frequent dressing changes. Non-allergenic tapes are available for the patient who has an allergy to other types of tape. Ensure that tape adheres to the skin for several inches on both sides of the dressing, and if it is a large dressing, place a length of tape across the middle of the dressing (Fig. 38.11). Do not apply tape over irritated or broken skin. To remove tape, gently loosen the tape ends and gently pull each parallel to the skin surface **toward** the wound while applying light traction to the skin away from the wound as the tape is loosened. If the tape will not loosen, adhesive remover may be used.

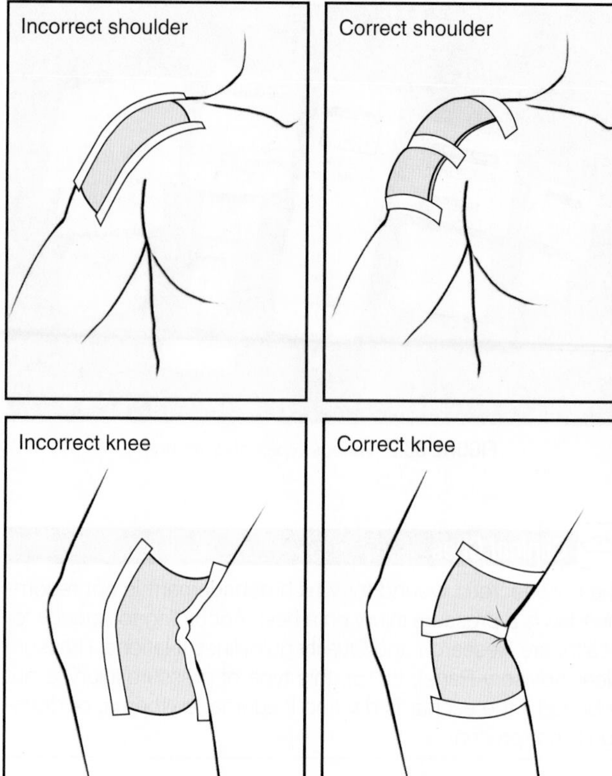

FIGURE 38.11 Tape across a joint or a crease.

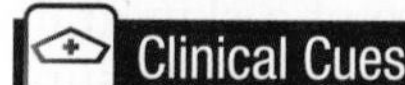

Clinical Cues

In the home setting, self-adherent plastic wrap can be used to secure dressings on patients who have problems with tape. Use the plastic wrap only for securing dressings over uninfected wounds.

BINDERS

Binders (wide elasticized fabric bands) are used to decrease tension around a wound or suture line, increase patient comfort, decrease lactation after childbirth, or hold dressings in place. An abdominal binder provides support and comfort for an abdominal incision when the patient must perform deep breathing and coughing exercises and when getting in and out of bed (Fig. 38.12). An elastic athletic supporter is used to hold dressings in place on the male scrotum and perineum. Elastic mesh panties can be used to hold dressings in place for the female perineum.

Think Critically

Why should you assess the number and type of dressings needed for a particular dressing change before taking dressings to the patient's bedside?

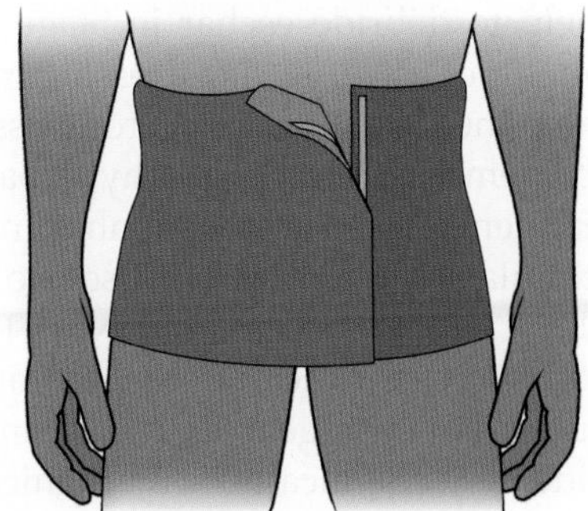

FIGURE 38.12 An abdominal binder provides support.

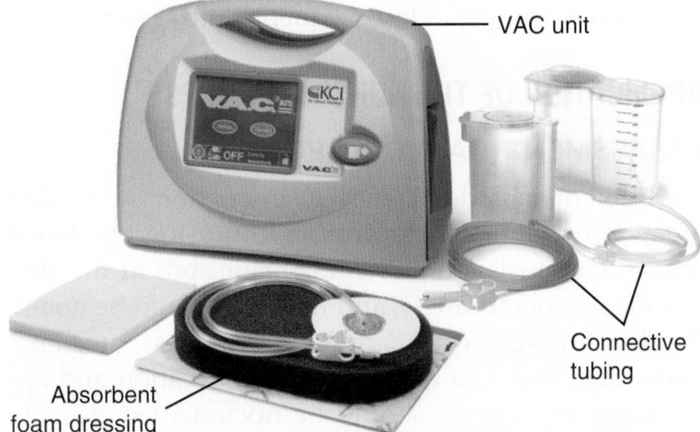

FIGURE 38.13 Wound VAC unit. (Courtesy Kinetic Concepts, Inc., San Antonio, TX.)

NEGATIVE PRESSURE WOUND THERAPY

Wounds that are difficult to heal may respond to negative pressure wound therapy (NPWT). This treatment can increase development of granulation tissue, speed healing rate, and reduce hospitalizations when used to treat open wounds (Huang et al., 2014), while minimizing the need for dressing changes. The therapy, also known as vacuum-assisted closure (VAC), involves applying a suction device to a special wound dressing to institute negative pressure at the wound site, drawing the edges together (Fig. 38.13). Mechanical stretch of cells occurs, which increases cellular proliferation and tissue growth. The negative pressure and suction remove fluid from the wound, allowing increased blood flow, and thereby oxygen and nutrients, to be delivered to the wound (Box 38.3). After a few days of therapy, bacterial counts in the wound bed drop. NPWT keeps the wound moist (Fig. 38.14). The system may be used on a wound before a skin graft is performed to close the wound completely. Dressing changes for the system depend on the type of wound being treated. If the wound is infected, the dressing may be changed every 12 to 24 hours. For a clean wound, the dressing is changed three times a week. Contraindications to the use of a NPWT include bleeding, exposed organs, exposed blood vessels or nerves, and malignant (cancerous) tissue.

Box 38.3 Guidelines for Care of the Negative-Pressure Wound Therapy Dressing

- Observe the dressing area when assessing vital signs.
- Film covering dressing must remain attached to skin in all areas for negative pressure to be maintained.
- Check the setting on the NPWT unit and assess whether it is working properly. Ensure tubing is not pressing against the skin.
- Assess for proper collapse of the dressing, indicating negative pressure is present. A whistling sound may indicate a leak.
- If a leak is present, press down gently around the drape and/or edges of the foam to better seal the drape. Use excess drape to patch over leaks.
- If the dressing needs to be replaced, follow agency protocol and instructions. When changing the dressing, document the wound appearance, wound size, and the presence of erythema or purulent drainage.
- Assess the patient for any complaints or problems in the wound area. If wound has a large amount of exudate, monitor the patient for deficient fluid volume.
- If the NPWT is interrupted for more than 2 hours, remove the old dressing and irrigate the wound prior to resuming therapy.
- Document your findings and that the unit is in place and functioning properly.

NPWT, Negative pressure wound therapy.

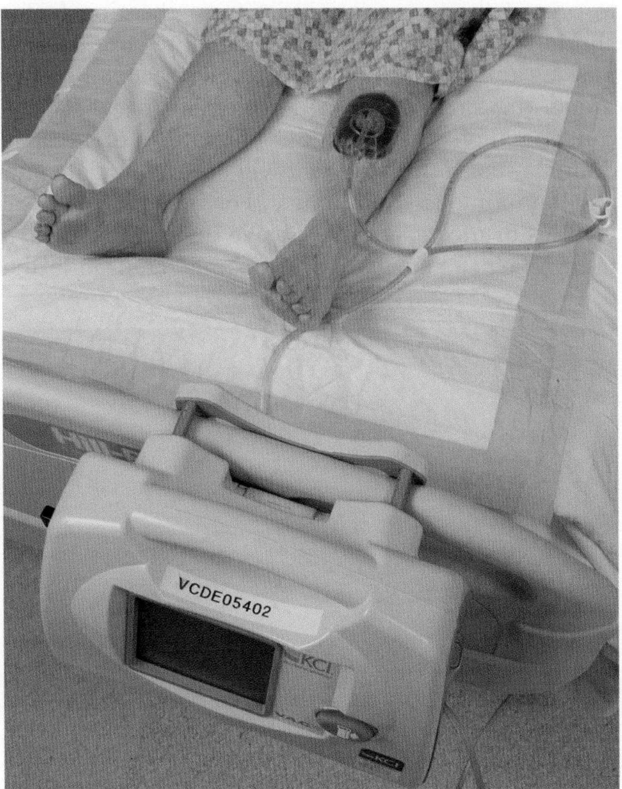

FIGURE 38.14 VAC unit working on a chronic leg wound. (Courtesy Kinetic Concepts, Inc., San Antonio, TX.)

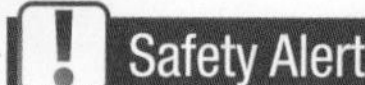

Safety Alert

Serious complications can occur with NPWT, most often related to bleeding and infection; even deaths have occurred, so proper use and patient assessment are crucial.

TREATMENT OF PRESSURE INJURIES OR VASCULAR ULCERS

Causes, staging, and prevention of pressure injuries, along with illustrations, are presented in Chapter 19. Treatment is discussed here along with care for most wounds.

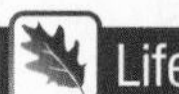

Life Span Considerations

Older Adults

Transparent dressings placed over a reddened area can often prevent skin breakdown in older adults.

Clean ulcers or pressure injuries at each dressing change. Use a syringe and plastic cannula with water, saline, or a nontoxic cleanser to perform pressure irrigation at 4 to 15 psi to prevent damage to new granulation tissue. Use 250 to 500 mL of solution and irrigate using a syringe with a small catheter to reach undermined areas and tunnels (Fig. 38.15). Observe and document the wound characteristics at every dressing change. Cover the wound with a dressing selected according to the wound characteristics. For Stage 1 Pressure Injuries, use protective dressings such as thin film, to protect the pressure injuries from shearing forces and to keep them moist. For Stage 2 Pressure Injuries that are uninfected, use a hydrocolloid, foam, or hydrogel dressing, which will protect against bacterial contamination. For a Stage 3 Pressure Injury that is draining, use a dressing that will absorb exudate and maintain a moist environment. **For infected pressure injuries or ulcers, a nonocclusive dressing is always used.** Chemical enzyme formulas may be used in the wound to help to débride eschar in Stage 4 Pressure Injuries. Sometimes a wet-to-dry dressing may also be applied to help the sloughing of necrotic tissue by mechanical débridement. Occasionally hyperbaric oxygen chamber treatment is used to treat nonhealing wounds. Electrical stimulation may also be used to accelerate wound healing. Growth factors and NPWT have also demonstrated success in healing stage 3 and stage 4 pressure injuries. An unstageable pressure injury needs eschar débridement chemically or mechanically before healing can begin. For a deep tissue pressure injury, aggressive pressure offloading needs to be accomplished. Various techniques are being studied to determine effective methods of pressure reduction, including air fluidized therapy and low frequency ultrasound.

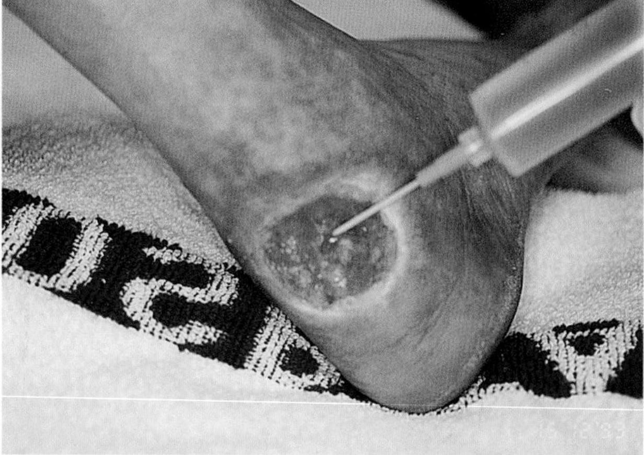

FIGURE 38.15 Wound irrigation using a 35-mL syringe and a 19-gauge plastic intravenous cannula. (From Potter, P. A, & Perry, G. A. [2009]. *Fundamentals of Nursing* [7th ed.]. St. Louis: Mosby.)

APPLICATION OF THE NURSING PROCESS

ASSESSMENT (DATA COLLECTION)

Assessment includes complete inspection of all skin areas. Every abrasion, laceration, contusion, reddened area, ecchymosis (small hemorrhagic spot in the skin or mucous membranes), and incision should be noted. Be alert for signs of inflammation: redness, swelling, pain, heat, and loss of function. The location and appearance of wounds should be documented daily in specific terms because changes can occur rapidly.

During the wound care process, note the number and type of dressings saturated or the diameter of the drainage on the dressing. Assess the wounds by visual inspection, palpation, and smell, noting the wound's appearance and any drainage, swelling, odor, separation, and complaints of pain. Note the color of the wound and surrounding tissue, as well as the **approximation** (degree of closure) of the wound edges. Use the back of a gloved hand to detect increased warmth, tautness of tissue, or edema around the wound. Carefully assess the site for surrounding edema. Gently palpate the periphery of the wound for signs of pain. Assess for drain placement and security, the amount and character of the drainage, and the effectiveness of any suction device.

Assess whether signs or symptoms of local or systemic inflammation or infection are present by reviewing temperature trends, WBC count, and patient report of discomfort. A temperature greater than 101°F (38.3°C), a WBC count greater than 10,000/dL, and a feeling of malaise may indicate wound infection. Assess acute wounds at least once every 8 hours and chronic wounds daily. Measure chronic wounds and pressure injuries every 2 to 4 weeks to determine whether they are healing (Cowan, 2015). It is important to note that in a dark-skinned person, you must rely on localized skin color changes at and around the wound site. The affected skin may be darker or shinier than surrounding skin. Assess the progress of healing by checking decreases in wound size. The size of a nonsurgical wound should be measured and the length, width, and depth recorded as ordered or per facility protocol.

Moderate postoperative pain is normal for 3 to 5 days, but persistent severe pain or sudden onset of new pain may indicate infection or internal hemorrhage.

If the initial dressing is in place, do not touch it until the primary care provider changes it or leaves orders for the nurse to do so. Assess the dressing; its appearance provides some indirect information about the wound underneath it. The dressing may be dry and intact, or it might be soaked with serous or serosanguineous drainage. It is also important to assess the patient's reaction to the wound and readiness to learn to perform wound care. Document your findings after the dressing change.

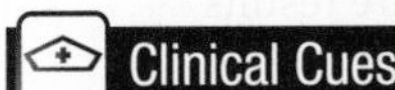

Clinical Cues

Assess for allergy to iodine, medications, cleaning solutions, and tape because many patients are allergic to substances used in wound care.

◆ NURSING DIAGNOSIS

Common nursing diagnoses used for patients with wounds are as follows:

- Impaired skin integrity related to surgical incision (or trauma)
- Risk for infection related to nonintact skin or impaired skin integrity
- Acute pain related to infected wound
- Activity intolerance related to pain and malaise from wound infection
- Disturbed body image related to wound appearance
- Deficient knowledge related to care of wound
- Anxiety related to need to perform wound care

◆ PLANNING

Include time for wound assessment and care in planning the work load. Consideration of whether dressings may become damp from bathing dictates whether wound care is provided before or after a shower or bath. Check orders for directives regarding wound care. **Dressing changes require a medical order, and wound irrigations may be performed only with an order.** Check the medical record for the date of wound occurrence or the surgical procedure to understand how old the wound is. This information is essential to assess the progress of wound healing. Determine what supplies will be necessary for a dressing change or irrigation.

Sample goals and expected outcome statements related to the nursing diagnoses listed above are as follows:

- Incision will be well approximated without disruption.
- Wound will be clean and dry without redness or swelling.
- Pain will resolve when infection is cleared.
- Activity tolerance will improve when infection resolves.
- Patient will verbalize acceptance of wound appearance.
- Patient will learn to properly perform wound care before discharge.
- Practice of wound care before discharge will alleviate anxiety.

A specific time frame for the outcome to be met is individualized to each patient.

◆ IMPLEMENTATION

When implementing wound care, the nurse must use the principles of asepsis presented in Chapters 16 and 17. Careful technique is essential to prevent contamination of the wound and spread of infection, if it is present. Use Standard Precautions for all patient care, particularly during wound care, when one comes into direct contact with body fluids. **Use sterile gloves or sterile forceps whenever you touch an open or fresh surgical wound.** After the wound is closed or sealed, you may use nonsterile disposable gloves. If a dressing becomes wet, it must be changed (Nursing Care Plan 38.1).

Wound Cleansing and Dressing Change

Clean wounds with water, normal saline, or a noncytotoxic wound cleanser. Sometimes antimicrobial solutions are ordered for wound irrigation. Many of these solutions must be kept refrigerated; allow the necessary amount of solution to come to room temperature before performing the irrigation. **Using cold solution lowers the wound temperature, which slows healing.** If an antimicrobial solution is used, dilute it properly. Clean grossly contaminated or infected wounds at each dressing change. Cleaning a healthy wound incorrectly can cause mechanical trauma and delay healing. Use gauze pads rather than cotton balls for cleansing because the cotton fibers can become embedded in the wound and delay healing. For superficial, uninfected wounds, rinse lightly with normal saline rather than using gauze to reduce mechanical trauma. Avoid drying a wound after cleaning because it heals better if it remains moist. Clean surgical wounds from the center outward to avoid pulling microorganisms from the skin into the wound. Change surgical and open wound dressings using sterile technique (Skill 38.1).

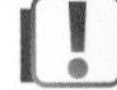

Safety Alert

Solutions That Damage Granulation Tissue

Certain solutions are toxic to growing and normal cells and should not be used to cleanse granulating wounds. Never use Dakin solution (sodium hypochlorite), acetic acid, povidone-iodine, or hydrogen peroxide to clean an uninfected, granulating wound.

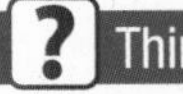

Think Critically

What interventions would you place on the care plan for a patient with a surgical wound? What interventions might be needed for a patient with an open traumatic wound?

Nursing Care Plan 38.1 Care of the Patient with a Vascular Ulcer

SCENARIO Frank Walters, age 72, who smokes one pack of cigarettes a day, has a vascular ulcer on his left lower leg. He had originally bruised the spot when working in the garden. Now he has a stage 4 pressure injury that is not improving. His primary care provider has admitted him for débridement and whirlpool treatments because he lives 175 miles from the hospital.

PROBLEM/NURSING DIAGNOSIS *Open wound*/Impaired skin integrity related to injury and decreased peripheral blood supply.

Supporting Assessment Data *Subjective:* "It's been there for 2 months. It will not heal." ***Objective:*** 5- × 4½-cm open wound on lower lateral aspect of left leg with area of black eschar on upper aspect, yellow tissue, and purulent drainage.

Goals/Expected Outcomes	Nursing Interventions	Selected Rationale	Evaluation
Wound will be without infection within 10 days.	Obtain wound culture as ordered. Administer antimicrobials as ordered.	Culture will determine infecting organism. Antimicrobials will help fight infection.	*Is infection present?* Culture results pending.
	Monitor signs of infection.	Tracking signs of infection will tell whether wound condition is improving.	
	Use whirlpool bath on lower leg daily.	Whirlpool flow will help débride and cleanse wound.	
	Débride mechanically with Travase.	Travase enzymatically breaks down necrotic tissue.	
	Maintain sterile wet-to-damp dressing on wound.	Damp wound environment helps break down eschar.	
	Medicate for pain as needed 30 min before whirlpool treatment and dressing change.	Whirlpool and dressing change on a stage 4 pressure injury may be painful.	
	Measure wound twice a week.	Measurements tell whether wound size is decreasing or increasing.	
	Encourage cessation of smoking to help promote wound healing and prevent further progression of vascular disease.	Smoking contributes to vessel damage that causes vascular disease.	Smoking fewer cigarettes.
	Turn q 2 h.	Turning prevents formation of new pressure injuries.	
Wound will close within 1 month.			*Has wound closed?* Progressing toward expected outcomes Continue plan.

hr, hours; q, every

CRITICAL THINKING QUESTIONS

1. Why is smoking particularly contraindicated for this patient? Explain the pathophysiology of the effect nicotine and smoking have on the body.
2. Why does eschar need to be removed from the wound? Explain the pathophysiology of how eschar interferes with wound healing.

Hydrocolloid Dressings

Hydrocolloid dressings are applied only to uninfected wounds; they keep the wound moist and block entry of microorganisms. A variety of hydrocolloid dressings are available. These are often used on a vascular ulcer or pressure injury to promote healing after the wound is clean (Steps 38.2).

Wound Irrigation, Débridement, and Packing

Irrigation is the flushing out of an area with a liquid. Wound irrigation is performed only with a medical order and requires sterile technique. Using a piston syringe instead of a bulb syringe helps to prevent aspiration of drainage and contamination of the syringe. For deep wounds with small openings, a sterile straight catheter may be attached to the syringe. The wound edges may need to be held open so that the solution can reach the depths of the wound. Skill 38.2 presents the steps in irrigating a wound.

A wound may be packed with gauze to facilitate formation of **granulation tissue** (connective tissue with multiple small vessels) and healing by second intention

Text continues on page 779

Skill 38.1 Sterile Dressing Change

 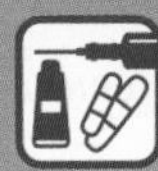 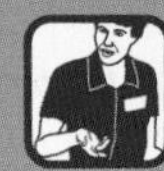  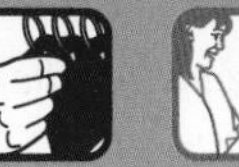 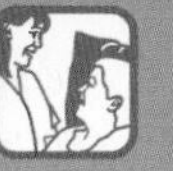 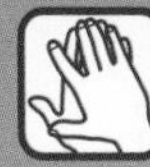 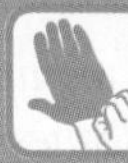

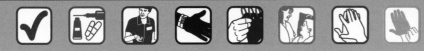

Sterile dressing changes are performed for surgical wounds, open wounds, and pressure injuries or vascular ulcers. The primary care provider orders the frequency of the dressing change and irrigation solutions, if indicated.

SUPPLIES

- Sterile gloves
- Clean gloves
- Tape
- Plastic discard bag
- Scissors
- Dressing supplies
- Gauze sponges
- Telfa dressings
- Abdominal combination dressings
- Sterile normal saline solution
- Antiseptic swabs and solution
- Transparent film dressings
- Cotton-tipped applicators
- Bath blanket

Review and carry out the Standard Steps in Appendix A.

ACTION *(RATIONALE)*

Assessment (Data Collection)

1. Check orders for directions for wound care and dressing change. *(An order is required for wound care and dressing change.)*
2. Determine whether patient is ready for the procedure. *(Saves time if patient is not involved in another activity.)*

Planning

3. Check nurse's notes for the types of supplies needed for the dressing change if in doubt as to what is needed, and visually assess the dressing that is in place. *(Ensures proper supplies will be on hand during the sterile procedure.)*

Implementation

4. Perform hand hygiene. Don clean gloves; loosen the binder or tape; remove the old dressing; pull off the tape toward the wound while stabilizing the skin with the other hand. If tape won't loosen, rub over it with an alcohol swab for several seconds or use adhesive remover. Wet the dressing with normal saline solution if it sticks to the suture line and wait a few minutes before removing it. Assess drainage on the dressings and place them in the plastic discard bag. *(Gloves prevent spread of microorganisms; removing old dressing allows visual assessment of wound and drainage. Pulling tape toward the wound prevents disruption of wound. Alcohol or adhesive remover helps loosen stubborn adhesive.)*

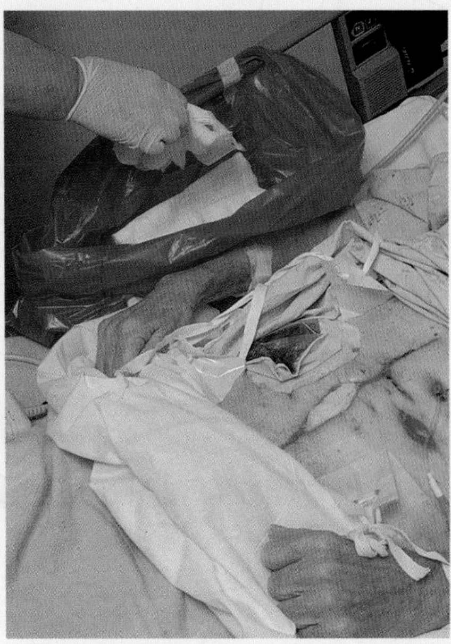

Step **4**

5. Inspect wound, noting degree of healing, presence of purulent exudate, and necrosis; check for odor, drainage, and condition of sutures or drain. Remove gloves and discard them. Perform hand hygiene. *(Provides data for determining progress of wound healing or presence of infection.)*
6. Set up sterile field, placing items in the order in which they will be used. Open the sterile supplies. *(Assists in maintaining a sterile field during the procedure and allows procedure to be done efficiently. Supplies ready for use.)*
7. Don sterile gloves, and clean area around the wound using normal saline or ordered disinfectant. Cleanse by one of the following methods:
   a. Use a separate swab to wipe from top to bottom on each side of incision and continuing outward.
   b. Use a separate swab from the wound edge outward on one side and then on the other side from top to bottom. Do not cleanse directly over the wound unless there is excessive drainage and it is an agency policy. Cleanse drain sites using a circular motion from the drain insertion site, outward.
   c. Use a circular motion from the wound outward in an ever-widening circle. *(Sterile*

Skill 38.1 Sterile Dressing Change—cont'd

technique prevents contamination of the wound. The top of the wound is considered the cleanest area. Cleansing by these methods prevents contaminating the wound. If considerable drainage is present, the wound itself is gently cleansed using a fresh swab for each single stroke.)

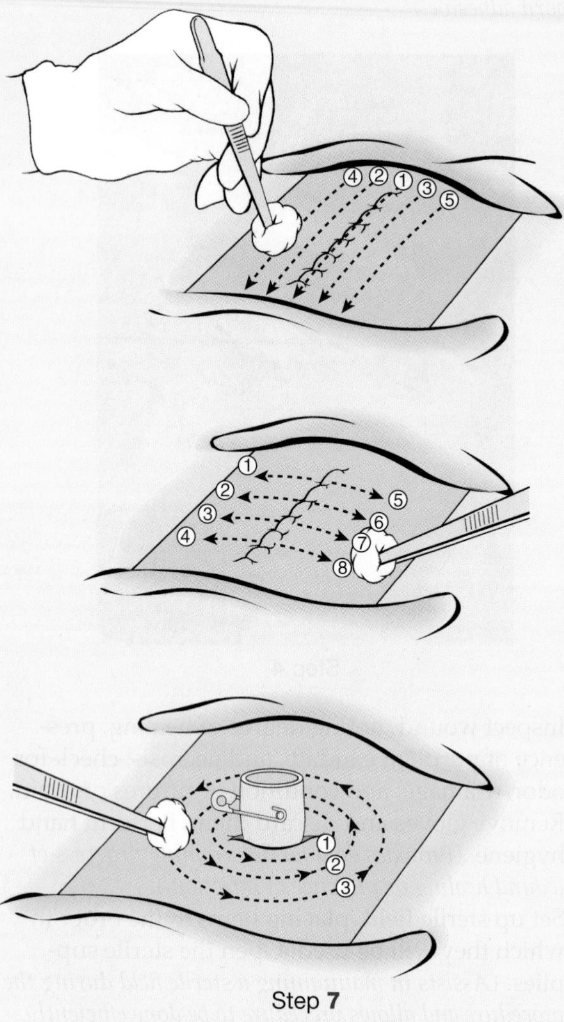

Step 7

8. Apply ointment or medication using applicators if ordered. *(An order is essential for any medication. Using applicators decreases the chance of contamination of the tube or the medication container.)*
9. Apply the dressings by positioning them lightly over the wound area; cover the entire wound, and do not move dressing once it is placed over the wound. Remove and discard gloves. Secure dressing in place. If tape will not stick to the skin, a skin preparation can be used on the skin surface. A binder or Montgomery straps may be used to hold dressings in place. *(Moving the dressing from one area to another may transfer microorganisms; securing the dressing ensures that the wound stays covered.)*

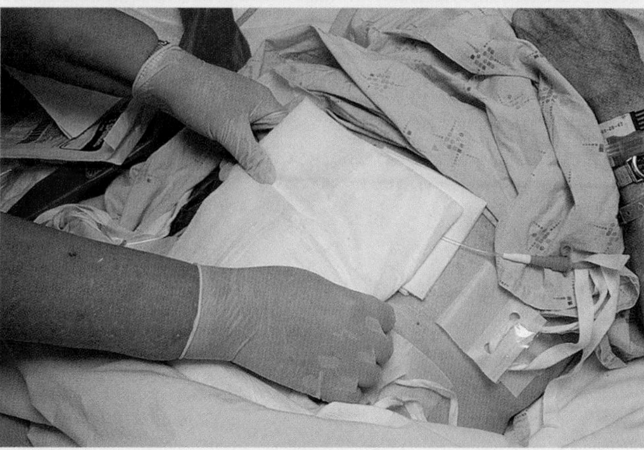

Step 9

10. Contain used dressings in the discard bag and deposit into biohazard trash container. Perform hand hygiene. *(Prevents spread of microorganisms.)*
11. Assist patient in obtaining a comfortable position in bed or, if ambulatory, assist as requested or required. *(Ensures patient's comfort.)*

Evaluation

12. Ask yourself: Are there signs of infection, such as redness and warmth around the wound edges; is thick or colored exudate present? Is the amount of drainage decreasing? Is the wound drain still in place? Had drainage soaked through the dressing? Did the dressing stay intact? *(Answers to these questions provide data regarding wound healing and whether the dressing was sufficient to cover the wound and contain the drainage, or whether the dressing could be discontinued.)*

Documentation

13. Document condition of the wound, including patient's subjective statements and objective observations. Include patient education performed for wound care. *(Provides data regarding would healing and patient education. Documents use of supplies.)*

Documentation Example

Dressing changed with sterile technique using six 4 × 4 gauzes and two combined ABDs. Incision clean, dry, and well approximated. Small amount of serous drainage on dressing. Skin cleansed with alcohol swabs. Reinforced patient education re keeping dressing dry and in place, technique for wound cleansing and dressing change, and signs and symptoms of infection to report immediately. (Nurse's time-stamped electronic signature)

Skill 38.1 Sterile Dressing Change—cont'd

 **Home Care Considerations**

- Wound care instruments can be cleaned with warm, soapy water and boiled for 10 minutes to sterilize. Allow to air dry and store them in a covered container.
- Remind the patient and family to dispose of soiled dressings in impermeable bags to prevent the spread of infection.
- Montgomery straps can be devised by using wide adhesive tape folded back on itself, making holes in the flap ends, and using a shoelace or rubber bands and safety pins to secure the straps together after they are attached to the skin.
- Provide patients with information on where to obtain dressing materials.
- Provide a wound flow sheet to encourage the patient or family to record the wound characteristics when changing dressings. Include columns for date and for a description of wound characteristics.
- For a child, helping the child change a dressing on a stuffed bear or doll helps to decrease anxiety about dressing changes.
- Older adults often have decreased vision and may need more assistance than realized to perform wound care and assess the wound.
- Arthritis in the hands may make it difficult for a person to manage a dressing change independently.

Critical Thinking Questions

1. Why is a wound cleansed from the inside toward the outside? If a wound is infected, would your technique for cleansing change?
2. What would you need to do if tape will not hold the dressing in place on the skin?

ABDs, Abdominal pads.

Steps 38.2 Applying a Hydrocolloid Dressing

Hydrocolloid dressings are used to provide a moist environment for wound healing in uninfected wounds. They occlude air and promote breakdown of necrotic tissue in wounds, thereby providing an alternative to mechanical débridement. These dressings may be left in place for up to 7 days, with 3 to 5 days being the average.

Review and carry out the Standard Steps listed in Appendix A.

ACTION *(RATIONALE)*

1. Clip the hair around wound site and cleanse the wound. *(Dressing will adhere better and be less uncomfortable when removed.)*
2. Choose a large enough dressing to cover a 1¼-inch border of healthy skin around the entire wound. *(For dressing to adhere properly and remain in place while absorbing drainage, a 1¼-inch border is necessary.)*
3. Open the paper from the back of the dressing, and smooth dressing in place from the center outward, peeling back the backing as you progress outward. Do not touch adhesive surface. *(Smoothing the dressing prevents pulling and wrinkling of skin. Adhesive adheres better if not touched.)*
4. Hold your gloved hand over the dressing for a few minutes until all edges have adhered firmly. *(Warmth helps dressing adhere properly.)*
5. If dressing does not firmly adhere, cleanse the skin at the edges of the dressing with a skin prep pad and use hypoallergenic tape around the edges. Do not apply skin prep under the dressing. *(Skin prep makes skin tacky so that tape will adhere well. Tape holds dressing in place. Skin prep over broken skin or wound may damage tissue.)*

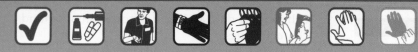

Skill 38.2 Wound Irrigation

 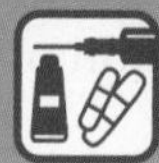 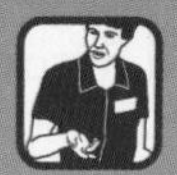 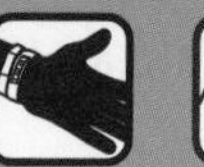 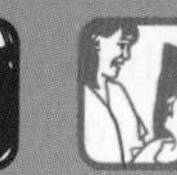 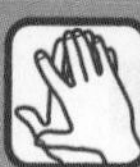 

Wound irrigations are ordered by the primary care provider. They are performed when a wound is infected, has large amounts of drainage, or contains necrotic material.

SUPPLIES

- Sterile gloves
- Protective eyewear
- Mask
- Impermeable gown
- Underpad
- Sterile solution container
- Irrigation set
- Syringe with large bore blunt needle or sterile angiocath
- Normal saline or ordered solution
- Basin to catch solution

Review and carry out the Standard Steps in Appendix A.

ACTION *(RATIONALE)*

Assessment (Data Collection)

1. Check the orders for wound irrigation to determine solution to be used and whether a sterile or clean irrigation is ordered. *(Solution ordered depends on condition of wound and whether infection is present.)*

Planning

2. Determine whether patient is ready for the procedure and whether all dressing and irrigation supplies are on hand. *(Saves time and promotes efficiency.)*

Implementation

3. Perform hand hygiene. Don clean gloves. Using aseptic technique, expose the wound, placing the soiled dressings in the discard bag. Remove gloves and perform hand hygiene. *(Prevents transfer of microorganisms; exposes wound for irrigation.)*
4. Aseptically prepare the irrigation set by pouring the solution into container and checking the action of the syringe plunger. Place an underpad beneath area to be irrigated. Place a basin to catch drainage against the side of the area being irrigated. Have patient hold basin in place if possible. *(Preparing the irrigation set ensures equipment is ready before putting on sterile gloves. An underpad protects linens from moisture. The basin catches most of the irrigation fluid.)*

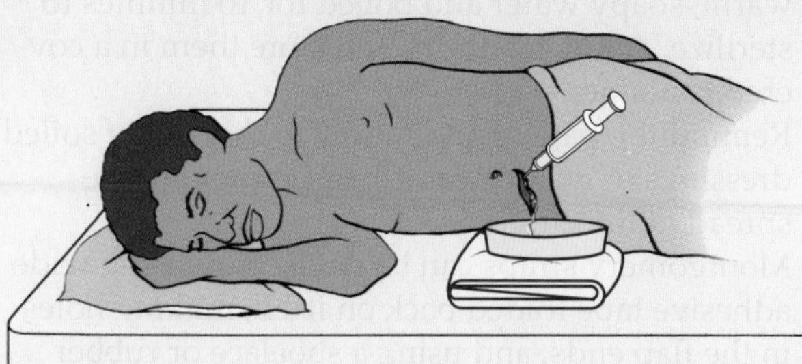

Step 4

5. Don sterile gloves. Draw up solution into the syringe by pulling back on the plunger or squeezing the bulb. Hold tip of the syringe about 1 inch from wound surface, and steadily push on the plunger or squeeze the bulb to eject fluid into the wound. Repeat until all debris is washed from the wound or the amount of solution ordered for irrigation has been used. Irrigate all areas of the wound. *(Keeping the syringe tip 1 inch away from the wound surface prevents contamination of the syringe. Using a 20-gauge needle or angiocath on the syringe causes an effective spray to cleanse the wound. Fluid washes out debris and necrotic tissue.)*

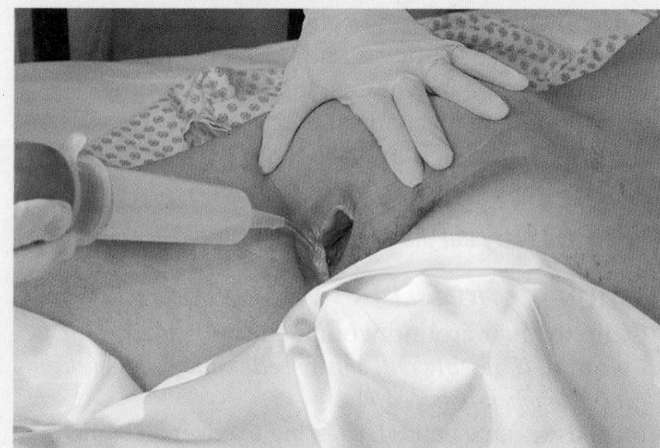

Step 5 (From Leahy, J.M., & Kizilay, P.E. [1998]. *Foundations of Nursing: A Nursing Process Approach.* Philadelphia: Saunders.)

6. Dry skin with gauze sponges so that tape will stick, and apply a sterile dressing. *(Prepares the wound for the dressing; covers the wound.)*
7. Remove gloves and discard them. Perform hand hygiene. *(Prevents transfer of microorganisms.)*

Evaluation

8. Ask yourself: Was sterile technique maintained, if ordered? Was all debris washed from the wound? Were the bed linens kept dry? *(Answers to these questions determine whether the procedure was per-*

Skill 38.2 Wound Irrigation—cont'd

formed correctly or if changes need to be made before irrigating the next time.)

Documentation

9. Document the time of the irrigation and the solution and amount used. *(Notes that ordered procedure was performed. Documents supplies used.)*

Documentation Example

Left buttock wound irrigated with 150 mL normal saline using sterile technique. Wound with pink tissue and serous drainage; no odor noted. Sterile dressing applied. (Nurse's time-stamped electronic signature)

Special Considerations

- When the irrigation is not ordered as a sterile procedure, equipment is kept as clean as possible and reused. This is common in the home environment.
- All irrigations of deep wounds should be performed with sterile technique.
- If the patient cannot hold a basin against the area in which it is needed, use pillows covered with plastic and underpads to position the basin firmly against the skin.

Home Care Considerations

- In the home setting a clean plastic trash bag and a towel can be placed under the area to be irrigated or treated with wet compress dressings to protect the mattress or furniture with each dressing change

Critical Thinking Questions

1. What is a better device for irrigating a wound than a bulb irrigation syringe?
2. If special irrigation solution is ordered and has to be kept refrigerated, why should it be heated? How would you heat it?

or to débride the wound. Usually moistened or medicated non–cotton-filled gauze is used in the form of fluffed (unfolded and loosely placed) 4 × 4s or strips. Either a wet-to-dry or a wet-to-damp technique is used. In the **wet-to-dry** technique the dressings are moistened and packed into the wound and allowed to dry between dressing changes, which are performed every 4 to 6 hours. As the dressings dry, they trap necrotic material and mechanically débride the wound when the dressing is removed. Removal of the dry packing is painful because it may remove some granulation tissue also. This technique is falling out of favor but is still occasionally used. The **wet-to-damp** technique for packing is the preferred treatment for *uninfected* wounds (Skill 38.3). Moistened gauze packing is placed in the wound to absorb exudate but is not allowed to dry before removal and therefore does not damage newly formed tissue.

Clinical Cues

Administer ordered analgesia sufficiently ahead of performing a dressing change on a large or infected wound so that it is effective during the procedure. Wound dressing changes can be painful, especially when débridement and packing are involved.

Débridement of necrotic tissue may be performed by using enzymatic powder, ointment, or granules that are packed into the wound or by cutting away dead tissue (sharp débridement). Enzymes break down the necrotic tissue and wound packing absorbs the debris. Surgical débridement is performed by a surgeon or an advanced practice nurse. The wound heals slowly from the base upward. In many instances the body's own healing processes cause sloughing of the necrotic tissue (autolytic débridement). Petroleum jelly may be used on the skin around the wound to prevent maceration from wet dressings.

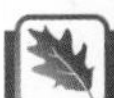

Life Span Considerations

Older Adults

Performing patient education regarding how to perform dressing changes must occur before discharge. Older adults who require dressing changes at home may have difficulty performing this task due to poor vision, loss of joint flexibility, and arthritis. Always assess whether the older adult or a caregiver can be properly taught how to perform a dressing change.

Patient Education for Wound Care

Before the patient is discharged, teach proper technique for cleaning and dressing the wound. Send the patient home with sufficient dressings to last until someone can purchase the needed items. Teach the patient the signs and symptoms of infection, and insist that they be reported immediately, so that intervention can be started quickly to treat the infection. Send written instructions home with the patient to reinforce patient education.

Patient Education

WOUND CARE

Patient education regarding wound care should begin as soon as possible for the hospitalized patient. Home care patients receive ongoing patient education. Include others in the household who will assist with wound care in all instruction. The following points should be covered in the patient education program:

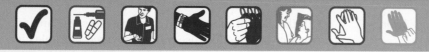

Skill 38.3 Applying a Wet-to-Damp or Wet-to-Dry Dressing

 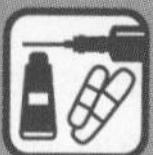 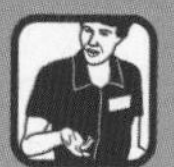 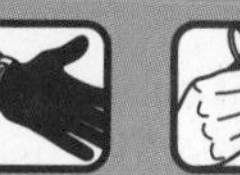 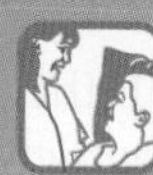 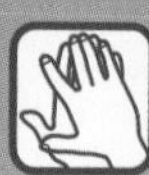 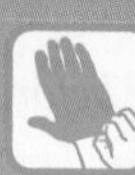

Wet-to-damp dressings are used to keep a wound moist and promote healing; wet-to-dry dressings help to débride wounds and encourage cellular growth from the base of the wound up to the surface. Wet-to-dry dressings have been largely replaced by other methods of débridement because they may harm new cell growth when the dressing is removed.

Supplies

- Gauze sponges
- Sterile basin
- Tape or binder
- Discard bag
- Sterile normal saline
- Sterile gloves
- Clean gloves
- Underpad

Review and carry out the Standard Steps in Appendix A.

ACTION *(RATIONALE)*

Assessment (Data Collection)

1. Check the order, assess the old dressing if one is in place, and determine whether the patient is ready for the procedure. *(Ensures that proper dressing is applied to the right patient.)*

Planning

2. Plan the appropriate time in your work schedule to perform the dressing change. Determine whether all needed supplies are available and on hand at patient's bedside. Wet-to-damp dressings are changed more frequently than wet-to-dry dressings. *(Assists in performing the procedure smoothly and quickly.)*

Implementation

3. Prepare the work space, and open the dressing packages and sterile container for the wetting solution; perform hand hygiene and don clean gloves. *(Readies the dressings and solution for work. Institutes Standard Precautions.)*
4. For wet-to-damp dressing, slowly and carefully remove the gauze. If it is stuck to the wound, add a little normal saline to loosen it. For wet-to-dry dressing, gently and steadily pull the gauze away from the wound because this helps to débride the necrotic tissue. Place used dressings in the discard bag. *(Pulling a stuck dressing loose damages new tissue. A wet-to-dry dressing is not remoistened when removing it.)*
5. Remove dirty gloves, perform hand hygiene, and pour the sterile wetting solution into basin. *(Solution should be poured before putting on sterile gloves.)*
6. Don sterile gloves. *(Prepares hands for sterile procedure.)*
7. Place the needed dressings in the wetting solution or moisten dressing materials by pouring solution on them. *(Dressings should be thoroughly soaked.)*

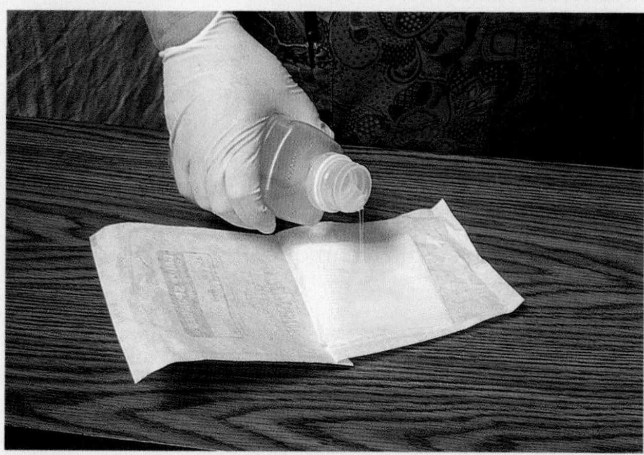

Step 7

8. Wring out dressings one by one and lightly press fluffed gauze into the wound, covering all exposed surfaces. *(Dressings should be moist without dripping. Moisture encourages healthy tissue growth. Gauze pads must be unfolded and lightly packed to be most effective.)*
9. Cover with a second moist dressing for a wet-to-damp dressing and then a dry, sterile 4- × 8-inch combined dressing in a single layer on top of the wet dressings. Additional dry dressings may be added as needed to keep the outside dry. *(To promote wound healing, the entire wet-to-damp dressing must be changed at regular intervals before the inner dressing dries out. The primary care provider may order how frequently this is to be performed; if not, change the entire dressing at least every 2 hours. If moisture reaches the outside of the sterile dressing, it can provide an avenue for pathogens to enter the wound.)*
10. Remove the gloves and discard them; tape the edges of the dressing; perform hand hygiene. *(Secures the dressing. A binder may be used in place of tape.)*

Evaluation

11. Ask yourself: Did the inner dressing stay damp in the wet-to-damp dressing? Did the outer dressing

Skill 38.2 Applying a Wet-to-Damp or Wet-to-Dry Dressing—cont'd

stay dry? Is necrotic tissue being removed from the wound by the wet-to-dry dressing? Is pink granulation tissue appearing in the wound? If the inner dressing for the wet-to-damp dressing is drying, change the dressing more frequently. Add sufficient dressing material to keep the outer dressing dry. *("Yes" answers to these questions determine that the procedure is successful.)*

Documentation

12. Document the times of dressing changes, the procedure, and the appearance of the wound at the completion of the procedure. *(Verifies that orders were carried out and documents the course of wound healing.)*

Documentation Example

Wound packed with fluffed 4 × 4s moistened with normal saline. Sterile technique maintained. Wound 2.2- × 3.4-cm area of black eschar at 3 o'clock position; wound yellow at base. Pink tissue at edges. (Nurse's time-stamped electronic signature)

Special Considerations

- Using a moisture barrier ointment on the skin around the wound protects the skin from **maceration** (softening of tissue from soaking in moisture). Petroleum jelly protects the skin from moisture.
- If a wet-to-dry dressing is ordered, leave out the second moist dressing and cover with only one layer of dry dressing.

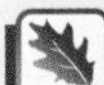

Home Care Considerations

- In the home environment, clean rather than sterile technique may be used.

Life Span Considerations

Older Adults

- Older adults have thinner and more fragile skin that is easily damaged. It is preferable to use a stretch gauze wrap or a binder rather than to repeatedly apply and remove adhesive tape during dressing changes.

Critical Thinking Questions

1. Why would a binder be ideal to use to secure a wet-to-damp dressing?
2. Why must black eschar be removed from a wound for it to heal?

- Factors that assist with wound healing: exercise, nutrition, rest, not smoking
- Where to obtain needed dressing supplies
- Expected appearance of the wound now and as it heals
- Signs and symptoms of infection to report to primary care provider immediately: increased redness, swelling, pain, purulent drainage, persistent increasing fever, increasing malaise
- Importance of keeping the wound and dressing clean and dry
- Limitations on activity related to the wound
- Proper handwashing: before and after doing wound care or touching the wound area
- Disposal of used dressing supplies in a sealable plastic bag, following local guidelines for disposal of biohazardous waste

Instruct the patient in dressing change along with demonstration; seek a return demonstration of dressing change. The following points should be covered:

- Removing dressing
- Assessing the wound
- Cleansing the wound; wound irrigation, shower cleansing if allowed
- Caring for a drain
- Caring for a wound suction device: emptying, activating suction, positioning to prevent pull on drain
- Applying a new dressing
- Disposing of old dressings

When performing patient education about wound care in the home:

- Instruct when it is essential to wear gloves.
- If drainage system is in place, explain its purpose, how to safely use it, and whom to contact if device appears to be malfunctioning.
- Summarize teaching for wound and drain care.
- Provide written instructions in the patient's or caregiver's preferred language.
- Instruct when to call and make an appointment with the primary care provider or surgeon.

Suture and Staple Removal

Although some care providers prefer to remove their own sutures or staples, others write orders for their removal. Suture scissors, forceps, and sterile technique are used to remove sutures (Fig. 38.16). The suture is clipped so that the exposed part will not be pulled through the skin (Steps 38.3). A special staple remover implement is used to remove staples (Fig. 38.17). Inspect the suture after it is pulled out to see that it appears whole. Parts of sutures left under the skin cause inflammation because they are foreign bodies. "Butterfly" closures such as Steri-Strips are often applied to reinforce the incision as sutures are removed (Fig. 38.18). Review with the patient how to care for the wound and stress the importance of allowing the butterfly closures to come off on their own.

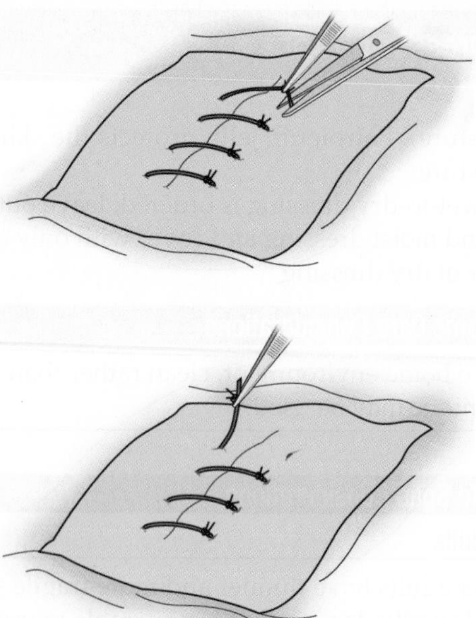

FIGURE 38.16 Clip beneath the knot with scissors to remove the suture.

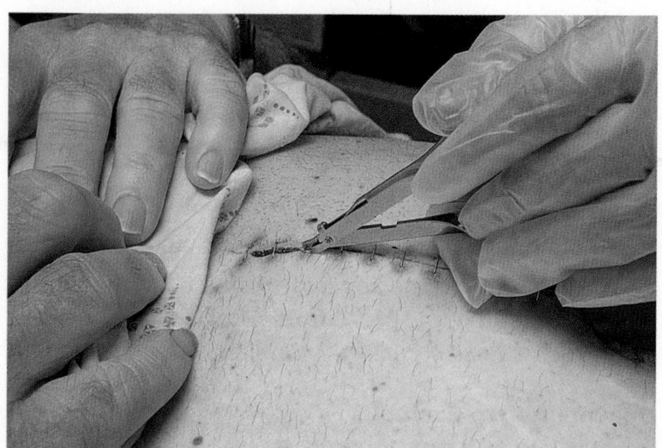

FIGURE 38.17 A special implement is used for staple removal.

Steps 38.3 Removing Sutures or Staples

Sutures or staples are removed when the wound is well sealed and connective tissue has formed. Although the time for suture removal may vary, it usually is performed 7 to 10 days after they have been placed. A medical order is required for removal of sutures or staples.

Review and carry out the Standard Steps in Appendix A.

ACTION *(RATIONALE)*

1. Perform hand hygiene, don clean gloves, and remove the dressing, discarding it in a plastic waste bag. Remove gloves and perform hand hygiene. *(Prevents transfer of microorganisms; exposes the sutures or staples.)*
2. Assess the wound. If crusts or dried blood is on the sutures or staples, apply clean gloves and cleanse wound with sterile gauze dampened with normal saline. *(Lessens the risk of contaminating wound as sutures or staples are removed.)*
3. Open the suture or staple removal set. *(Readies equipment for use.)*

For Sutures

4. Pick up the forceps with the nondominant hand and the suture scissors with the dominant hand. *(This allows good control of instruments.)*
5. Lift the knot of the suture away from the skin with forceps, and slip the curved tip of the scissors under suture beneath the knot. Cut the suture beneath the knot and, using forceps, pull it from the skin in one smooth motion. *(Prevents pulling exposed suture back through skin. The entire suture must be pulled free.)*
6. As long as the skin stays well approximated, remove every other suture. If wound shows no signs of separation, remove remaining sutures. *(Removing every other suture provides a safeguard in case the wound begins to separate.)*

For Staples

4. After opening the equipment, place the lower jaw of the staple remover under the staple. Be certain the tip is all the way under the staple. *(Positions tool to crimp and open the staple.)*
5. Press the handles of the staple remover together all the way to depress the center of the staple. *(The staple must be firmly pressed between the two parts of the staple remover to allow it to be pulled free of the skin.)*
6. When both ends of the staple are visible, lift it up and away from the skin. Drop the staple into the discard bag. *(Removes the staple; prevents transfer of microorganisms and injury by a sharp object.)*

For Sutures and Staples

7. Gently cleanse any dried blood from the suture or staple sites with antiseptic sponge. *(Suture holes are open to the atmosphere and can admit bacteria. Dried blood may contain microorganisms.)*
8. Place Steri-Strips or a dressing over the incisional area as ordered. Often the incision is simply left open to the air. *(Secures the wound.)*
9. Place all used supplies in the discard bag. Remove gloves and discard them. Perform hand hygiene. *(Prevents transfer of microorganisms.)*

Steps 38.4 Irrigating the Eye or Adult Ear

The eye may need irrigating when it has been injured by debris or chemicals. Gently continue irrigation until debris is cleared away or for 10 to 30 minutes after a chemical injury. The ear is irrigated when wax or debris is obstructing the canal and preventing sound from reaching the tympanic membrane.

Review and carry out the Standard Steps listed in Appendix A.

ACTION *(RATIONALE)*

Eye Irrigation

1. For irrigation with a syringe, place patient in a supine position with the head angled in the direction of the affected eye. Position the examination light to illuminate the affected eye. Place an underpad and towel on the bed to protect the linens and clothes. Place an irrigation basin close to the face to catch the irrigation solution. *(Irrigation fluid will run away from the eye and not contaminate the other eye. Good light is needed to visualize the area well.)*
2. Prepare the irrigation set and fluid. *(Fluid should be at room temperature. Sterile normal saline or tap water is used.)*
3. Don gloves, and remove any crusty discharge on the eyelid with a gauze or a cotton ball moistened with sterile normal saline. Discard the used cotton balls in a discard bag. *(Using fresh gauze or a cotton ball for each stroke from the inner canthus to the outer edge maintains aseptic technique.)*
4. Load the irrigation syringe with the prescribed fluid. With the nondominant hand, gently but firmly pull the upper eyelid toward the eyebrow and pull the lower lid down toward the cheek to expose the conjunctival sac. Ask the patient to look downward. *(Assists in maintaining eye in an open position to receive the irrigation fluid.)*
5. Hold the irrigation syringe approximately ½ to 1 inch above the eye, and gently depress the plunger or bulb of the syringe to irrigate the eye, directing the stream from the nasal edge of the eye across to the outer edge. Repeat the irrigation until the desired result occurs or the total amount of solution ordered has been used. Allow patient to close eye between washings if large amount of solution is required. *(Solution removes debris or contaminant from eye. Too much pressure of fluid may damage the cornea. Closing the eye from time to time can help move debris from the upper conjunctival sac to the lower one and help remove the offending item [e.g., eyelash or piece of metal].)*
6. Dry the eyelid with sterile gauze or a cotton ball. Provide a towel to the patient to dry the face. *(Makes the patient comfortable.)*
7. Record the procedure, being certain to include solution used and the amount, appearance of the eye and surrounding tissues, and patient's response to therapy. *(Documents how procedure was performed and how well it was tolerated by patient.)*

Ear Irrigation

1. Place the patient in a sitting position. Drape the shoulder on the side to be irrigated with underpad and towel, and place the light so that the area is well illuminated. *(The syringe is easier to use with the patient sitting. Underpad and towel help keep patient dry.)*
2. Fill the syringe with warm solution (98.6°F [37°C]). Have the patient hold the basin firmly against the neck under the ear. *(Cool water is uncomfortable and causes dizziness and nausea through stimulation of the equilibrium sensors in the semicircular canal. Positioning the basin properly prevents water from running down the neck.)*
3. Straighten the ear canal by grasping the upper portion of the adult pinna and gently pulling upward and backward. *(The canal is straightened so water can penetrate better and debris can be washed out.)*
4. Place the tip of the syringe just into the entrance of the external meatus, and point the tip upward and inward toward the posterior auditory canal; push the plunger or depress the bulb in slowly and carefully. *(The flow of solution is directed forward to wash out debris.)*
5. Inspect the ear canal to see that it is clean. Dry the ear and the neck area. *(Cerumen may still be blocking the canal.)*
6. Repeat until the canal is clean. Be certain solution is still warm. *(Allows visualization of tympanic membrane and allows sound to reach the membrane.)*
7. Document the procedure, including what the drainage looked like and how the patient tolerated the procedure. *(Records how the procedure was performed and the results obtained.)*

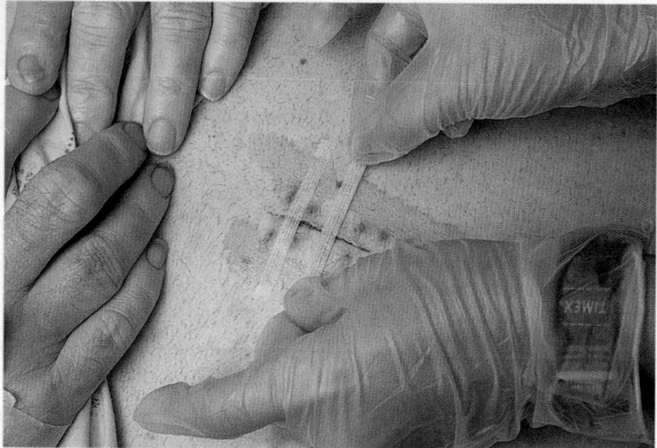

FIGURE 38.18 Apply Steri-Strips to support the incision after suture removal.

 Life Span Considerations

Older Adults

Healing time is slower in older adults with impaired circulation related to atherosclerosis or arteriosclerosis, which can decrease blood flow to the wound area. Sutures may need to be left in a few days longer than in younger or healthier patients.

Eye, Ear, and Vaginal Irrigations

Irrigations must be performed when there is a possibility of debris or caustic substance in or near the eye. Using Standard Precautions, irrigate the affected eye(s) with the prescribed solution, usually sterile saline or tap water. In the emergency department special eyecups and a continuous irrigation system are sometimes used (Steps 38.4).

Ear irrigations are used to remove cerumen or foreign bodies that occlude the ear canal and prevent sound from reaching the tympanic membrane. Ear irrigation is ordered by the primary care provider and should not be performed if there is a possibility that the tympanic membrane is perforated. The irrigation is performed in a fashion similar to the eye irrigation, except the solution is directed toward the roof of the auditory canal while holding the pinna of the older adult up and out with the other hand (see Steps 38.4). The pinna for the child is pulled slightly up and back; for the infant, pull the pinna down and back. Sometimes a Waterpik with a special nozzle is used to irrigate the ear. Only the lowest settings on the irrigation device should be used.

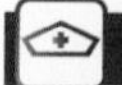 Clinical Cues

Instilling a wax softener, such as carbamide peroxide, per agency protocol before flushing the ear makes flushing quicker and easier on the patient. Allow the patient to rest for 10 to 20 minutes after instilling the drops before flushing the ear.

A vaginal irrigation may be ordered for infection or surgical preparation of the vagina. Frequently, the patient administers the irrigation herself.

Box 38.4 Contraindications for Heat and Cold Applications

HEAT

- Heat should not be applied over an area in which active bleeding is occurring because it will increase the bleeding.
- Heat to the abdomen is contraindicated if there is a chance the patient has appendicitis because it may cause the appendix to rupture.
- If a patient has cardiovascular problems, it is unwise to apply heat to a large part of the body, causing massive vasodilation that may divert blood supply from major organs.

COLD

- Cold is not applied to an injury area if it is already edematous because it will slow circulation and prevent absorption of interstitial fluid.
- When neuropathy is present, cold is not applied because the patient is unable to determine whether tissue becomes too cold.
- If the patient is shivering, cold is not applied. Shivering raises body temperature.

Hot and Cold Applications

Either dry or moist forms of heat and cold can be applied to the body to promote healing. Usually an order is necessary for a treatment because both systemic and local effects occur. The order should include the body site to be treated, the type of treatment, and the frequency and duration of the application. Check your agency's policy for various types of heat and cold treatments.

Assessment of the patient and the area to be treated is essential to identify any contraindications for the treatment (Box 38.4). Assess circulation in and around the area to be treated. Be certain that the patient has intact sensation so that damage will not occur from temperature extremes. When cold is applied to a lower extremity, assess for capillary refill, note skin color, and palpate skin temperature and distal pulses so that a baseline of the area can be documented in the medical record.

Use of heat. Heat is applied to skin surfaces to provide general comfort and to speed the healing process (Table 38.2). Heat is often used for patients with musculoskeletal problems, such as joint strains or low back pain. The amount of blood diverted to the skin through vasodilation reduces the blood circulating through internal organs and tissues. The degree of systemic effect is related to the size of the area to which heat is applied. Systemic circulatory changes may cause faintness, a faster pulse, and some degree of dyspnea. If such changes occur, closely monitor the patient's vital signs. The principles for application are the same for each method used when applying heat (Box 38.5). Heat can be applied locally by means of a hot water bottle, an electric pad, an aquathermia pad, or a disposable heat pack (Fig. 38.19). Moist heat is used in the form of compresses, hot packs, soaks, or a sitz bath (see Chapter 19). Table 38.3

Table 38.2 Therapeutic Effects of Heat and Cold Applications

PHYSIOLOGIC RESPONSE	THERAPEUTIC BENEFIT
	HEAT
Vasodilation	Improves blood flow to injured body part; promotes delivery of nutrients and removal of wastes; lessens venous congestion in injured tissues
Reduced blood viscosity	Improves delivery of leukocytes and antibiotics to wound site
Reduced muscle tension	Promotes muscle relaxation and reduces pain from spasm or stiffness
Increased tissue metabolism	Increases blood flow; provides local warmth
Increased capillary permeability	Promotes movement of waste products and nutrients
	COLD
Vasoconstriction	Reduces blood flow to injured body part, preventing edema formation; reduces inflammation
Local anesthesia	Reduces localized pain
Reduced cellular metabolism	Reduces oxygen needs of tissues
Increased blood viscosity	Promotes blood coagulation at injury site
Decreased muscle tension	Relieves pain

Adapted from Potter, P. A., Perry, A. G., & Stocker, P. A., et al. (2013). *Fundamentals of Nursing* (8th ed., pp. 1211). St. Louis: Elsevier Mosby.

Box 38.5 Principles of Heat Application

- Heat causes dilation of blood vessels and increases the supply of blood to the area.
- Heat stimulates metabolism and the growth of new tissues. Heat is effective in clearing away the debris of infection by bringing antibodies and leukocytes to the site and through **suppuration** (the formation of purulent exudate). Hot packs or compresses applied to infected sites promote earlier healing.
- Extreme temperature changes stimulate pain receptors. Heat application may be painful or soothing.
- Applications of heat to portions of the body activate the autonomic nervous system, which produces systemic responses in the body.
- Vasodilation of superficial vessels of the skin decreases the blood supply elsewhere in the body because the blood volume is constant in a closed system. Vasodilation produces skin redness and warmth.
- Water is more effective than air as a conductor of heat.

provides general ranges of temperature for heat application, but check the agency procedural manual for recommended temperatures.

To protect patients from burns caused by heat applications, measure the temperature of the liquid if possible.

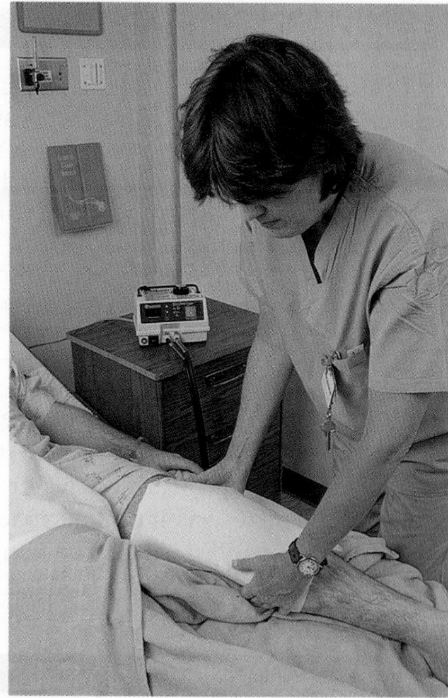

FIGURE 38.19 An aquathermia pad is applied for a heat treatment.

Table 38.3 Temperature Ranges for Heat and Cold Treatments[a]

DESCRIPTION	RANGES
	HEAT TREATMENTS
Warm	93-98°F (33.9-36.7°C)
Hot	98-105°F (36.7-40.6°C)
Very hot	105-110°F (40.6-43.3°C) for at-risk adult or child under age 2 years 105-125°F (40.6-51.7°C) for normal adult, dry heat only
	COLD TREATMENTS
Tepid	80-93°F (26.7-33.9°C)
Cool	65-80°F (18.3-26.7°C)
Cold	55-65°F (12.8-18.3°C)
Very cold	Below 55°F (below 12.8°C)

[a]Discontinue the treatment when numbness occurs.

If no thermometer is available, place the prepared pack against the inner aspect of your own arm. If there is any doubt about whether it is too hot, cool it down. Use a flannel or cloth cover for all hot and cold packs. Observe the condition of the skin frequently for signs of burning or blistering, and be attentive to complaints. Caution the patient and the family not to increase the temperature of heating pads or of water in hot water bottles.

Heat applications. Hot water bottles are filled two-thirds full, the air is expelled, and the plug is attached. A heat lamp is a gooseneck lamp with a 60-watt bulb. A heat lamp provides heat by radiation and is placed 18 to 24 inches (45 to 60 cm) from the area of treatment. Heat applications are left in place for 15 to 30 minutes and may be ordered to be repeated each hour or several times a day.

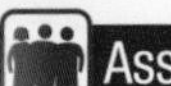 Assignment Considerations

Applying Heat Treatments

In many states, UAPs are allowed to apply heat treatments or warm moist compresses to wounds under the nurse's supervision. When assigning this task, you should remind the UAP of the proper temperature to maintain for the treatment and the specific time the treatment should be applied. The UAP should notify you when the treatment is complete so that you can assess the wound area and the patient's response to the treatment.

An aquathermia pad, or K-pad as it is often called, is constructed with tubes containing water. An electrically controlled unit pumps warmed water through the tubing network. The reservoir of the K-pad is filled to two-thirds full with *distilled* water. The temperature is usually set with a key for 105°F (40.6°C). Cover the pad before application (see Fig. 38.18).

 Safety Alert

PRECAUTIONS WITH HEATING PADS

When the back is treated with a heating pad, do not let the patient lie on the pad. Heat is not dissipated properly if the patient lies on the pad, and burns can occur. Place the patient prone or on the side to apply the pad.

When hot compresses are ordered, heat the solution to the temperature ordered, dip the gauze or cloth in the solution, and wring it out. Use sterile technique, including sterile gloves and supplies, when there is broken skin in the area of treatment. Heat a small amount of solution at a time. You may use petroleum jelly beneath the pack or compress to protect the skin.

In the home, hot compresses can be made with washcloths dipped in hot water and wrung out. After the compress is in place, place a plastic wrap covering on top to help to retain the heat. You may place a towel over the plastic wrap. Gel packs are also available that can be heated in a microwave oven. Carefully follow the instructions to not overheat the device. A freshly boiled egg with the shell removed can be placed inside a sock to apply heat to an eye where inflammation is causing discomfort. The egg can be reheated in hot water. Discard the egg when treatment is finished.

When a soak is ordered, submerge the part to be treated in warm water or solution for 15 to 20 minutes. Use a commercial pack to apply heat to a large area of the body.

Whenever heat is used, you must ensure the patient's safety. Some patients are much more likely to suffer burns: those with sensory impairment; impaired mental status with decreased level of consciousness or confusion; and impaired circulation from peripheral vascular disease, diabetes, or heart failure. When an appliance is no longer in use, return it to central service immediately so that charges to the patient will cease. Document the use of heat or cold devices each shift to ensure insurance payment to the agency.

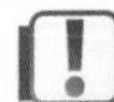 Safety Alert

Safety Factors When Applying Heat

Heat is not usually applied immediately after injury or surgery because it increases bleeding and swelling. Electrical appliances, such as heating pads, must be checked for defects by the agency engineering department. Check the appliance and the cord before use to prevent shock or sparks. Do not use anything with a frayed cord or loose plug. Avoid using safety pins with a heating pad or K-pad. Use an electric pad with moist packs only when the unit is designed to be used with moisture. When a heating pad is in use on a patient, check the temperature setting frequently.

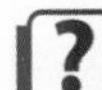 Think Critically

What would you do if you had been giving your patient a heat treatment with a heating lamp and, when you return to discontinue the treatment, you find she has lowered the lamp to within 6 inches of the treatment area and now the skin is very red and she says it is more painful?

Use of cold. Cold is used for two main purposes: (1) to decrease swelling and (2) to decrease pain (see Table 38.2). Cold is often immediately applied to an injury to prevent swelling. When cold is applied to the skin or a part of the body, vasoconstriction causes the skin to become pale and cool. When it interferes with adequate circulation, it can damage body tissues, as in the necrosis caused by frostbite.

Systemic effects of cold are the reverse of those of heat. More blood is sent to the internal organs, and the body acts to conserve heat. The autonomic nervous system is activated, and muscle contractions may produce shivering in an effort to produce heat.

The primary care provider usually indicates the temperature to be used for cold applications (see Table 38.3). Very cold applications are used for 15 to 20 minutes at a time; longer application can damage the skin and underlying tissue.

Cold applications. Cold is applied in the form of compresses, packs, ice bags, ice collars, or hypothermia blankets. Cold compresses consist of gauze or cloth material placed in a basin containing ice chips and a small amount of cold water. The compress is then wrung out and placed on the designated site. The compresses are changed every 15 to 20 minutes.

Cold packs are used for tonsillectomies, perineal wounds, sprains, nosebleeds, fractures of bones, dental extractions, and reduction of postoperative swelling of some parts of the body. Most disposable cold packs are applied directly to the skin, but check the manufacturer's directions. Ice bags or ice collars are reusable. Small ice bags can be made by placing ice chips loosely in a vinyl or nitrile glove and tying it with a knot. This works especially well for applications to the nose or eye. Some gel packs are reusable and are placed in the freezer until frozen. When the gel pack becomes warm, it is either discarded or, if it was placed inside of a sealed plastic bag, in some cases it can be cleansed and returned to the freezer.

A hypothermia blanket is used to lower body heat for patients who are running a persistently high fever. Because this treatment decreases the rate of metabolic processes, it may be used during surgery to reduce blood flow and oxygen requirements and is often used for patients who have severe brain injuries. The cooling blanket is attached to a machine that supplies the blanket with a cooled solution of distilled water and 20% ethyl alcohol. Place the blanket in direct contact with the patient's skin. Continually monitor the patient's temperature when the blanket is in use. Avoid chilling to the point of shivering because this activity causes the body temperature to rise.

Most cold treatments require an order before application. Carefully assess the skin and circulation in the area of application and distal to it, before, during, and after the treatment. Prolonged, very cold applications may cause frostbite. Cold therapy is applied for a maximum of 20 minutes at a time. Precautions taken are the same as those for patients who are at risk with heat applications.

 **Home Care Considerations**

Use of Cold in the Home Setting

In the home, ice bags can be made with crushed ice in tightly closed plastic bags. These should be wrapped in cloth, such as a diaper or dish towel, before application to the skin. A bag of frozen peas or corn also makes an effective cold pack. The vegetables can be refrozen for repeated treatment but should be discarded after the end of treatments. A quick, efficient cold pack can also be made by wetting a washcloth, folding it in quarters, and freezing it inside a zipper-locking plastic bag.

Patient education for hot and cold applications. Assess the caregiver's ability and availability to administer the hot or cold treatment safely. Sterile compresses can be prepared at home in a pressure cooker if one is available. Caution the patient and the family not to heat washcloths or other linens in the microwave oven because fire can occur. This method of heating items in the microwave also provides uneven heat distribution and would increase the danger of burning the patient. Check the cords on home lamps to be used for heat treatments and on heating pads. Instruct the patient to place the heating pad over his body (not under), to never fall asleep when using one, and to never use the high setting to avoid burns.

◆ EVALUATION

Evaluative statements indicating that some previously stated goals and expected outcomes have been met are as follows:

- Wound edges are well approximated.
- Wound is clean and dry without redness or swelling.
- Patient states that pain is gone.
- Patient states that energy has returned and is ambulating in the hall.
- Return demonstration of dressing change was properly performed.

It is important to evaluate the outcome of the heat or cold treatment. Is it producing the desired effect? If not, it should be discontinued or another method tried. When the outcome is such that the initial problem is gone, the primary care provider is notified and the treatment is discontinued.

Get Ready for the NCLEX Examination!

Key Points

- Wounds are open or closed and clean or dirty. Wounds may be partial thickness and heal by epithelialization or full thickness and heal by contraction.
- Surgical wounds heal by first intention because they have little tissue loss at the surface; wounds with tissue loss heal by secondary intention.
- Wound healing is promoted by a diet rich in protein; carbohydrates; lipids; vitamins A, B, and C; and the minerals zinc, iron, and copper, as well as regular exercise. Wound healing is delayed by smoking, medications, and chronic disorders.
- Complications of healing are hemorrhage, infection, dehiscence, and evisceration.
- Negative pressure via NPWT may be used for chronic wounds that are not healing.
- The three basic wound types are red, yellow, and black. Red wounds are clean and ready to heal, yellow wounds contain debris or exudates, and black wounds need débridement.
- Wound drains are placed to provide an exit for blood and fluids that accumulate.
- Dressings protect the wound, prevent microorganisms from entering or escaping, help to support and stabilize tissues, and reduce discomfort. Binders provide support and hold dressings in place.
- Débridement is accomplished surgically or by enzyme or chemical formulas.
- Assessment for signs of infection is important; check for purulent drainage, odor, increased redness, pain, swelling, fever, and leukocytosis. On an extremity, limitation of movement may indicate infection.
- Progress of healing is determined by decrease in size of the wound and improved appearance. Contaminated or infected wounds are cleaned at each dressing change.
- Hydrocolloid dressings are applied only to uninfected wounds; they keep the wound moist and absorb drainage.

- Evaluate the outcome of a heat or cold treatment and wound care; determine whether goals and expected outcomes are being met.

Additional Learning Resources

SG Go to your Study Guide for additional learning activities to help you to master this chapter content.

evolve Go to your Evolve website at http://evolve.elsevier.com/Williams/fundamental for additional online resources.

Review Questions for the NCLEX Examination

*Choose the **best** answer for each question.*

1. Your patient has had abdominal surgery for a ruptured appendix and requires postoperative care and dressing changes. The wound has been left open, and irrigations are ordered. When irrigating a wound, it is *most* important to:
   1. Irrigate slowly to prevent discomfort.
   2. Ensure the solution reaches the depths of the wound.
   3. Prevent wetting of the bed and covers.
   4. Use vigorous irrigation flow from the syringe.
2. If a wound appears infected, you should:
   1. Cleanse it with an antiseptic solution.
   2. Obtain an order for a culture to be performed.
   3. Apply an antibiotic ointment.
   4. Change the dressing every 2 hours.
3. The assessment of the wound indicates healing is occurring when:
   1. The center tissue is white.
   2. Bleeding has stopped.
   3. There is no further drainage from the wound.
   4. Pink granulation tissue is visible.
4. When assessing for wound infection, you know that signs of wound infection may be: *(Select all that apply.)*
   1. A rise in temperature.
   2. Pink granulation tissue.
   3. A WBC count greater than 10,000/dL.
   4. Purulent drainage.
   5. Tenderness around the wound.
5. When caring for a pressure injury, you know that:
   1. Eschar must usually be removed before the wound will heal.
   2. Pink granulation tissue should be cleansed with antiseptic solution.
   3. Keeping the wound dry and covered will aid healing.
   4. Heat treatments hurt new tissue and slow healing.
6. Proper technique for removal of sutures is to:
   1. Clip the suture below the knot.
   2. Assure the patient that suture removal does not hurt.
   3. Refrain from pulling an exposed suture through the wound.
   4. Apply a Steri-Strip before removing the suture.
7. Cold packs applied during the first 24 hours after injury decrease swelling by:
   1. Increasing vasodilation so blood flow will carry away excess fluid.
   2. Causing vasoconstriction and decreasing bleeding from damaged blood vessels.
   3. Decreasing circulating blood volume so that swelling cannot occur.
   4. Dulling pain and thereby reducing cellular enzyme release.
8. Your patient with a leg wound asks about NPWT. You answer her question based on your knowledge that NPWT:
   1. Decreases cellular proliferation.
   2. Is contraindicated in infected wounds.
   3. Can sometimes speed wound healing.
   4. Minimizes mechanical stretch of cells.

Critical Thinking Activities

Read each clinical scenario and discuss the questions with your classmates.

Scenario A

Gregory Hansen requires a sterile dressing change for an abdominal incision.

1. How would you determine what is needed in the way of supplies?
2. How would you set up your sterile field? (Be specific.)
3. Because it is best not to talk while doing a sterile procedure, how would you begin to perform patient education with Mr. Hansen to do the dressing change himself?
4. Describe the factors you would assess to determine whether Mr. Hansen's wound is infected.

Scenario B

Joshua Weintaub just had surgery on his nose for a deviated septum. Ice packs are ordered. What would you use and how would you perform the ice applications?

Scenario C

Heat lamp treatments are ordered for the donor site from which skin graft material was taken on Bruce Herez's leg.

1. What type of lamp is used for this treatment?
2. How would you set up Mr. Herez and the lamp for the treatment?
3. How often would you check on Mr. Herez during the treatment?

chapter 39

Promoting Musculoskeletal Function

http://evolve.elsevier.com/Williams/fundamental

Objectives

Upon completing this chapter, you should be able to do the following:

Theory

1. Discuss the effects of inactivity on respiratory exchange and airway clearance.
2. Describe appropriate care of a cast as it dries.
3. Verbalize the differences among an air fluidized bed, low air loss bed, and continuous lateral rotation bed, listing the reasons for their use.
4. Name at least four pressure relief devices that help prevent skin injury in immobile patients.
5. Describe how to perform a neurovascular assessment on an immobilized extremity.
6. Discuss the use of bandages and slings to immobilize a body part.

Clinical Practice

1. Devise a plan of care for meeting the psychosocial needs of the alert, immobile patient.
2. Correctly care for the patient undergoing skin traction.
3. Use lift sheets and roller or slide devices to move immobilized patients.
4. Teach a patient to properly care for a cast following discharge.
5. Correctly apply an elastic bandage to a stump after an amputation.
6. Transfer a patient using a mechanical lift.
7. Assist a patient with the use of each of the following: walker, crutches, cane, brace, prosthesis, and wheelchair.

Skills & Steps

Skills

Steps

Key Terms

bivalved (BĪ-vălvd, p. 794)
blanch (p. 799)
cast (p. 794)
counter traction force (p. 794)
dorsum (DŎR-sŭm, p. 799)
external fixator (p. 795)
hemiparesis (hĕm-ē-pă-RĒ-sĭs, p. 799)
hemiplegia (hĕm-ē-PLĒ-jă, p. 799)
hydrotherapy (hī-drō-THĔR-ă-pē, p. 806)
hypostatic pneumonia (hī-pō-STĂT-ĭk noo-MŌ-nē-ă, p. 790)
immobilization (ĭ-mō-bĭl-ĭ-ZĀ-shŭn, p. 790)
isometric exercises (ī-sō-MĔT-rĭk, p. 790)
kinetic (p. 796)
moleskin (p. 795)
over-the-bed frame (p. 793)
paraplegics (păr-ă-PLĒ-jĭks, p. 809)
paresthesia (păr-ĕs-THĒ-zē-ă, p. 799)
perfusion (pĕr-FŪ-zhŭn, p. 799)
prosthesis (prŏs-THĒ-sĭs, p. 809)
quadriplegics (kwŏd-rĭ-PLĒ-jĭks, p. 809)
sling (p. 793)
spica casts (SPĪ-kă, p. 794)
splint (p. 792)
traction (p. 790)
trapeze bar (tră-PĒZ, p. 793)

Concepts Covered in This Chapter

- Anxiety
- Functional ability
- Infection
- Mobility
- Nutrition
- Pain
- Patient education

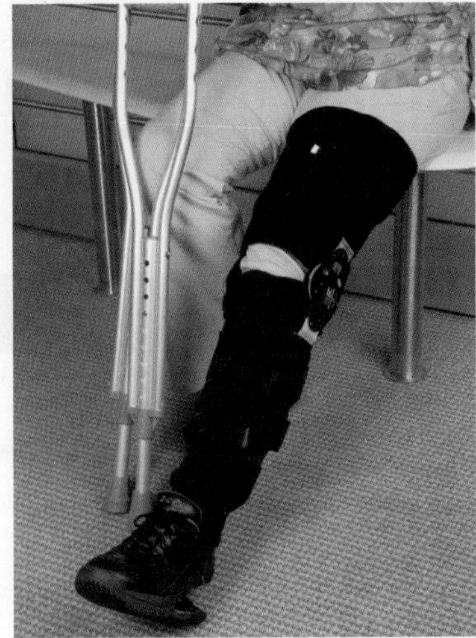

FIGURE 39.1 Patient with a leg brace or splint.

Many conditions, such as strokes, fractures, surgery, and neuromuscular disorders, require bed rest for the patient to heal and recover. These periods of bed rest may result in **immobilization** (prevention or restriction of normal body movement) of the patient. Problems caused by immobilization include pressure injuries, pneumonia, loss of bone mass, and permanent loss of function in the immobilized part. Many supportive or corrective measures necessary for treatment, such as **traction** (exertion of a pulling force), casts, or braces, also restrict mobility and may cause the same types of problems (Fig. 39.1). Good nursing care is critical in preventing complications for immobilized patients.

SYSTEMIC EFFECT OF IMMOBILIZATION

Decrease in muscle strength and coordination, generalized weakness, stiff joints, constipation, and abdominal distention begin within a few days of immobility. Table 39.1 presents the more severe problems that may occur when lack of activity occurs for a longer period of time. Pressure injuries are a frequent consequence of immobility and are presented in Chapter 19.

One of the major concerns when a patient's movement is restricted is the development of respiratory complications. Physical activity causes people to breathe more deeply, expanding their lungs and encouraging clearing of secretions. Without adequate physical activity, these secretions can collect in the lower airways, leading to congestion and ultimately to respiratory illness, particularly **hypostatic pneumonia** (pneumonia caused by stasis of secretions due to inactivity) or hospital-acquired pneumonia.

Range-of-motion (ROM) exercises (Chapter 18), frequent turning, and use of deep breathing exercises can help to prevent pneumonia and increase general oxygenation. Patients experiencing pain may be reluctant to move and breathe deeply; therefore, pain control is essential. However, medications used to control pain may cause sleepiness and further reduce the patient's desire to move about. Opioid analgesics, such as codeine, may depress respirations and further inhibit respiratory clearing (Chapter 31). Measures to promote respiratory function must be included in the plan of care for the immobile patient.

Circulation is also affected by immobilization. Normal movement assists in venous return by compression of the muscles against the venous walls when the muscles are in motion. Healthy, firm muscles provide general support for the venous walls. This is important throughout the body, but especially in the legs, where the force of blood flow is reduced because of the distance from the heart. Various conditions (such as a fracture, trauma, or debilitating illness) and treatments (such as casts, traction, or bed rest) can impair circulation and predispose the patient to pressure injury and permanent loss of function. For these reasons, you must monitor the general circulatory status of the patient and blood flow to the affected areas of the body on a regular basis.

Increasing fluids to at least 3000 mL/day, encouraging adequate nutritional intake, and increasing dietary fiber help prevent gastrointestinal system complications. The fluid increase also helps prevent urinary complications. Stool softeners and laxatives are ordered as needed for constipation.

Life Span Considerations

Older Adult

- Advanced age compromises the respiratory and circulatory systems, which can lead to even greater risk for complications from immobility.
- Inactivity tends to cause anorexia. Interventions for adequate nutritional care should be added to the care plan of the immobile older adult. Frequent small feedings and bedtime nourishments may be needed. Having their favorite foods brought in by family and friends can also be helpful.

Performing active or passive ROM exercises to maintain joint mobility and muscle integrity is the standard of practice for bed rest care. Encouraging active movement of the unaffected extremities throughout the day assists in maintaining muscle tone. When the patient is on extended periods of bed rest, **isometric exercises** (exercises performed against resistance) may be beneficial. Turning the patient every 2 hours, keeping the skin clean and dry, providing smooth and clean linens, and using pressure relief devices help prevent

Table 39.1 **Effects and Problems of Immobility**

BODY PART OR SYSTEM	EFFECT OF IMMOBILITY	PROBLEM OR COMPLICATION
Cardiovascular system	Venous stasis Increased cardiac workload Blood pressure alterations	Thrombus formation Thrombophlebitis Pulmonary embolus Orthostatic hypotension Increased pulse rate
Respiratory system	Stasis of secretions Decreased elastic recoil Decreased vital capacity	Hypostatic pneumonia Bacterial pneumonia Atelectasis Decreased gas exchange
Gastrointestinal tract	Anorexia Metabolic change to catabolism and negative nitrogen balance Decreased peristalsis	Weight loss Protein deficiency Abdominal distention Constipation
Musculoskeletal system	Decreased muscle mass and muscle tension Shortening of muscle Loss of calcium from bone matrix Decrease in bone weight	Fibrosis of connective tissue Atrophy Weakness Joint contracture Osteoporosis Bone pain
Urinary system	Stasis of urine Urinary tract infection Kidney stones	Precipitation of calcium salts Frequency Dysuria
Skin	Decreased circulation from pressure Ischemia and necrosis of tissue	Skin breakdown Pressure injuries
Brain/psychological	Decreased mental activity Decreased sensory input Decreased socialization Decreased independence	Disorientation Confusion Boredom Anxiety Depression Loneliness

pressure injuries. Perform a skin assessment at least every 8 hours and more frequently for the patient at high risk for skin breakdown.

 QSEN Considerations: Teamwork and Collaboration

Teamwork

VALUE THE PERSPECTIVES AND EXPERTISE OF ALL HEALTH TEAM MEMBERS

The systemic effects of immobility can be managed by utilizing multiple members of the health care team. Respiratory therapists, physical therapists, unlicensed assistive personnel, wound, ostomy, and continence nurses (WOCNs), and dietary personnel are all vital members of the patient's health care team.

PSYCHOSOCIAL EFFECTS OF IMMOBILIZATION

Immobilized patients may experience a variety of emotional responses. For example, they may be afraid that they will not be able to return to work and support themselves and those who depend on them. They may fear abandonment by those they love if they cannot function as they did before. Patients who are facing permanent loss, or their significant others, may need professional counseling or support groups. Provide support, use therapeutic techniques of communication that focus on listening, and allow the patient to verbalize concerns. When signs of fear and stress are observed, take time to listen, and refer these patients to social service as appropriate.

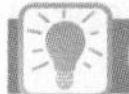 QSEN Considerations: Teamwork and Collaboration

Collaborative Care

APPRECIATE IMPORTANCE OF INTRAPROFESSIONAL AND INTERPROFESSIONAL COLLABORATION

Patients with prolonged immobility or permanent loss may need professional help in dealing with depression. Collaborate with appropriate health care providers to address the psychosocial effects of immobilization and your patient's emotional needs.

Another frequent problem for the alert immobile patient is boredom. Not all patients like television or enjoy reading, and even those who do will become bored with nothing else to do. Chat with patients about things that interest them while providing care. Some patients may want a diversion through the use of a laptop computer or smartphone, or may want to do something creative, such as crocheting or crafts. Encourage family and friends to space visits so the patient avoids long periods of loneliness. Family members can also help by contacting friends and relatives and asking them to send notes and cards on a regular basis. Cards, texts, phone calls, emails, and visits increase the patient's sense of value to others and feelings of self-worth. Positive feelings are known to play an important role in the healing process.

For the immobile patient being cared for at home, it may be helpful to move the bed into the living room or family room to reduce social isolation. This may also save many steps for those providing care, especially if bedrooms are on separate floors. Visits by home health aides and friends or respite caregivers can provide a chance for the caregiver to get out of the house and do errands or spend some time at leisure.

Remember that the nonalert or comatose patient also needs emotional support. Always assume that patients can hear and understand, even when they cannot respond or they respond inappropriately. Talk to the patient in a kind and caring voice. Explain what is being done before and during procedures, and apologize for any unavoidable pain the care may be causing. Talk to the patient about what is going on in the world. If cards or letters arrive, read them to the patient. Patients who have recovered from unconscious states have been known to describe in great detail things that happened while they were unconscious and have expressed thanks to those staff members who continued to treat them as valuable human beings.

Life Span Considerations

Older Adult

Following a stroke, hip fracture, or other condition that causes immobility, older adults may worry about becoming a burden to their families. This feeling may be so strong that they feel that it would be better if they died, and they become depressed. Encouragement and praise from the staff, kindness and patience when they attempt self-care or learn a new task, frequent family visits, and expressions of hope for recovery can help reestablish their sense of self-worth. Consultation with social services may lead to solutions for financial concerns.

TYPES OF IMMOBILIZATION

SPLINTS

A **splint** is a device that protects an injured part of the body by immobilizing or limiting its movement. A splint may be used as a first aid measure before a cast or traction is applied to an injured part, or it may be used instead of a cast. Box 39.1 presents the guidelines for applying a splint. Several types of commercial splints are available: molded splints, immobilizers, inflatable splints, cervical collars, and traction splints (Fig. 39.2). First aid splints are fashioned from materials at hand and require only some rigid material, padding, and something to secure the splint in place. Inflatable splints help control bleeding, as well as immobilize the injured part. The splint should be inflated until fingertips can only indent the device 1½ inches (3.8 cm). Immobilizers are made of cloth and foam with Velcro straps. They are often used on an injured knee to prevent movement while an injury heals or during activity to prevent further injury. Molded splints keep the body part in a functional position to prevent contracture and maintain functional ability. They are used for chronic disorders. Traction splints are applied and hooked to traction ropes, pulleys, and weights to maintain pull on a fracture.

Box 39.1 Applying a First Aid Splint to an Extremity

When a serious injury or fracture occurs in the home or outdoor setting, it is advisable to render first aid by splinting the injured part. To apply a splint to an extremity:

- Handle the injured part gently and do not change its position in any way. This decreases the chance of nerve injury and further bleeding.
- Cover any open wounds with material as clean as can be found to help prevent infection.
- Use a rigid splinting material to immobilize the injured part. Flat boards, broom handles, rolled up newspaper, or similar materials are appropriate. The splint should be long enough to span the joint above and below the injury.
- Pad bony prominences with soft material to prevent pressure wounds.
- Secure the splint with wide bands of material to stabilize the injured limb within the splint.
- Elevate the injured part to decrease edema and swelling.
- Check circulation distal to the injury and loosen the splint ties if tissue becomes pale, cold, or blue.
- Keep the person warm and seek transport to a medical facility.

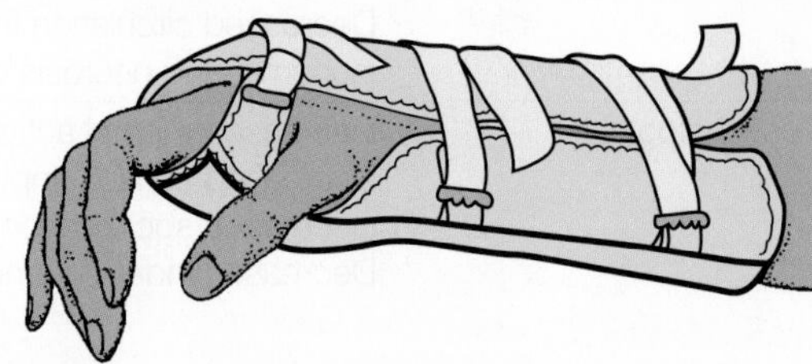

FIGURE 39.2 Wrist and forearm splint. (From deWit, S. C. [2009]. *Medical-surgical nursing: Concepts and practice*. Philadelphia, PA: Saunders.)

TRACTION

Traction is the application of a pulling force, and it is used to maintain parts of the body in extension and alignment. It is used to realign bone ends following fracture and to relieve pain and nerve impairment caused by compression or muscle spasm. There are three types of traction: manual, skin, and skeletal.

The amount of traction is determined by the pull exerted by weights at the end of the traction ropes.

Table 39.2 Principles of Traction with Nursing Interventions

PRINCIPLE	NURSING INTERVENTION
Ropes and weights must be free of friction.	Keep ropes free of entanglement in the linens.
Maintain the correct line of pull.	Keep the patient centered in the bed with the body in good alignment.
Weight and pull of the traction must be continuous and as ordered by the primary care provider.	Remove or add weights only by medical order. Do not interrupt the pull of traction to provide care.
Sufficient counter traction must be maintained.	Keep the patient from sliding down in the bed when in leg or back traction. Keep the patient in sidearm traction in the center of the bed.

The amount of weight must be ordered by the primary care provider and often changes over the course of treatment. Initially the muscles tend to be tight and may go into spasm. A heavier weight is required to overcome the muscular pull and allow the body to resume a normal alignment. As times goes on, the muscles tire and relax; the amount of weight is then reduced. The care provider will leave orders concerning if, and how much, the head of the bed may be raised. The head of the bed should be no higher than 20 degrees (unless ordered) to keep the patient from sliding down in bed and to keep the weights hanging free. A slight Trendelenburg position may be ordered to keep the patient from slipping down in the bed. Tape a sign to the head of the bed indicating any restrictions related to bed positioning. **The weights should swing freely without touching the bed or floor.** The ropes must move freely through the pulleys to prevent injury to the patient and alteration in the effects of the traction. Principles to be followed for traction are listed in Table 39.2.

The patient in traction should have an **over-the-bed frame** (rectangular frame to which traction equipment may be attached) with a **trapeze bar** (overhead bar that patient can grab) attached to the bed (see Fig. 18.9A). The trapeze bar can be grasped by the patient to assist in repositioning. Teach the patient how to tell when body alignment is correct in the bed so that as he becomes more active, he can place himself in correct alignment to maintain the traction.

Manual Traction

In this form of treatment, the hands are used to aid in the realignment of fractured bones. This method should only be used on stable, clean fractures or dislocations. It is typically performed by the physician prior to placing the affected extremity into a splint or cast.

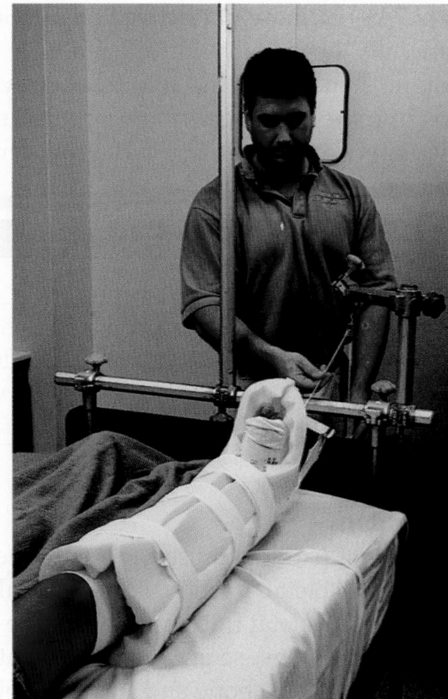

FIGURE 39.3 Buck extension. (From Elkin, M. K., Perry, A. G., & Potter, P. A. [2008]. *Nursing interventions & clinical skills* [4th ed.]. St Louis, MO: Mosby.)

Skin Traction

In patients with hip fractures, recent studies have shown that skin traction has the same effect on pain relief as placing a pillow under the affected extremity. However, skin traction does offer short-term pain relief from muscle spasms due to muscles and tendons pulling the extremity into a shortened position.

QSEN Considerations: Evidence-Based Practice

Decreased Use of Skin Traction

Nurses must differentiate clinical opinion from research and evidence summaries. Recent studies of patients with hip fractures showed that those with skin traction asked for pain medications at the same frequency as those with a pillow propping up the affected extremity

In skin traction a Velcro boot (Buck traction), belt, halter, or **sling** (bandage for supporting a part) is applied snugly to the skin, and the traction is attached to the appliance (Fig. 39.3). Skin traction has the advantage of being noninvasive, and its main purpose is to decrease muscle spasm that accompanies fractures. Damage from skin traction includes blisters, rashes from irritation by adhesives, and skin tears and tissue injuries from the shearing effects of the lateral pull across the skin surface. The amount of weight that can be applied is limited to a maximum of 10 to 15 pounds. Skin traction should not be used if the fracture requires

5 pounds (2.7 kg) or more of tractive weight. Skin traction is generally not used with older adults because of their fragile skin. Check the skin frequently for any indications of injury, and report any problems or skin pain immediately to the primary care provider or traction technician.

 Safety Alert

Safety With Immobilization

Whenever a patient is in an immobilization device, be sure to check for adequacy of circulation in the affected extremity by assessing skin temperature and color, capillary refill when appropriate, and sensation.

Skeletal Traction

Although external fixation is used more frequently for fractures today, skeletal traction is occasionally used for some injuries. Skeletal traction requires the surgical placement of pins, tongs, screws, or wires that are anchored to or through the bone and therefore pierce the skin. Traction is thus applied directly to the bone, which can support more weight than the skin. As much as 30 pounds (14 kg) of tractive force can be used for this type of traction. An orthopedic technician may set up the traction. The LPN/LVN is responsible for maintaining the correct weight and alignment of the traction and for maintaining a balance between traction pull and **counter traction force** (the weight pulling against the weight of the traction). Counter traction is provided by the weight of the patient and the position of the bed. Care of the skin around the openings for the pins, tongs, or wires is performed according to the medical order. Sterile technique is used when performing pin care (Box 39.2). After the sites are healed, they may be left open to the air. Clear fluid drainage is expected initially. Follow the medical order and the policies of the facility, and report immediately any indication of infection at the wound or pin sites. Circulation checks are performed every hour for the first 24 hours and every 4 hours thereafter.

 Think Critically

What interventions would you use to prevent skin breakdown on the back and buttocks of the patient in traction?

CASTS

Patients may be placed directly into a **cast** (a stiff plaster of Paris, fiberglass, or polyester dressing used to immobilize) following a fracture or a variety of orthopedic procedures, or a cast may be applied following a period in traction. The skin is cleansed and inspected and any wounds are treated before a cast is applied. A layer of stockinette is applied first, followed by a thin layer of cotton or synthetic padding and then the cast material. Most casts are made of fiberglass, polyester resin, or thermoplastic material. Plaster of Paris casts are often applied to a lower extremity because they will withstand weight bearing better than the synthetics. Heat may be felt as the casting material is applied, especially with plaster of Paris. Plaster casts can take from a few hours to a couple of days to dry and be fully hardened. Casts made of synthetic material dry rather quickly (7 to 20 minutes) and may be hardened enough to be durable within 30 minutes. **It is critical to protect the cast from uneven pressure during the drying period because the shape or position can be inadvertently changed.**

Box 39.2 Guidelines for Pin Care

Always follow the primary care provider's orders for cleansing or antiseptic solution and use or nonuse of antimicrobial ointment.

- Using sterile swabs, cleanse closest to the pin in a circular motion. Use one swab for each circle. Work your way out in succeeding circles until 1½ inch from the pin.
- Apply antimicrobial ointment with a sterile swab, if ordered.
- Dress with sterile gauze, if ordered.
- Secure ends of wires with cork.
- Monitor for infection, assessing for increased pain, redness, edema, tenderness, or purulent drainage.

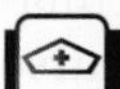 Clinical Cues

When handling the cast during the drying period, use the palm and flat parts of the fingers rather than the fingertips. Dents in the cast can lead to circulatory impairment and pressure injuries, and changes in alignment can alter the position of the healing parts or impede circulation.

Swelling of the tissues is common during the first days after a cast is applied, and if left uncontrolled, this can impair the circulation and cause a pressure injury. A casted extremity should be elevated on pillows. If not padded sufficiently, the edges of the cast may rub or push against bony areas, causing pain and injury. The stockinette may be folded over the outside edge of the cast and taped to protect from chafing, or the cast edge may be "petaled" with waterproof tape. Changing position may relieve the problem, or adding extra padding beneath the edge of the cast may help.

If the cast becomes too tight, it may be **bivalved** (cut in half lengthwise) to relieve the pressure on the tissues. If there is a wound under the cast that needs observation, a window may be cut in the cast over the wound area. When edema has decreased, the cast is secured with outside bandaging or by more casting material. Sometimes after edema subsides, the cast is too loose and must be replaced.

Hip **spica casts** can be particularly challenging for both the patient and caregiver. Hip spica casts encase a portion of the trunk and part or all of both legs (Fig. 39.4). A spreader bar is placed between the legs to maintain the desired angle at the hip and incorporated into the cast. **Do not use the spreader bar as a handle for lifting and turning the patient. It may be dislodged, ruining the cast and causing pain and possible injury to the patient.** Grasp the cast over the leg to assist in turning. Because of their size and thickness, hip spica casts often take longer to dry. Frequent turning is necessary, including prone positioning to ensure complete and uniform drying.

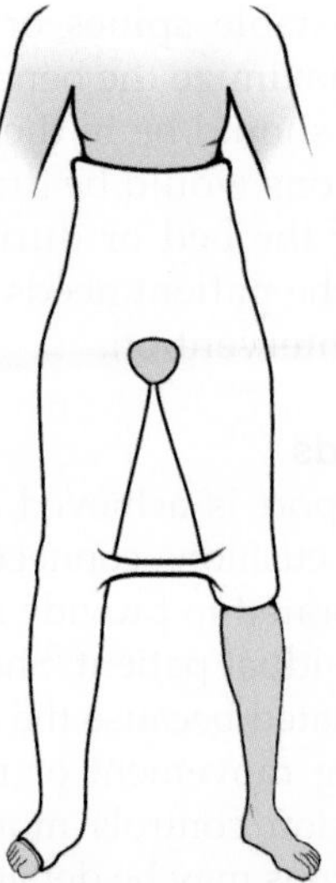

FIGURE 39.4 Hip spica cast. (Courtesy Zimmer, Inc., Warsaw, IN.)

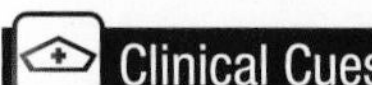 **Clinical Cues**

A hair dryer set on low may be used to assist in drying the plaster of Paris cast. Just be sure to uniformly dry all areas of the cast and lightly touch the cast frequently to make certain that it is not becoming so hot that it will burn the patient's skin.

Toileting can be difficult for the patient with a hip spica cast. Ingenuity is needed to protect the cast from soiling. Using disposable plastic wrap around the perineal opening is one method of protection. Maintaining skin integrity of an incontinent patient in a spica cast is a great challenge for the orthopedic nurse.

Most patients can go home soon after cast placement. If the cast is not yet dry before discharge, instruct the patient and family or caregiver in the proper care of the cast to ensure uniform drying. When elevating a wet cast with pillows, use cloth-covered pillows because plastic-covered ones hamper drying.

Show the patient and family how to check the cast edges for rough spots or crumbling, how to use pillows to elevate the extremity and prevent swelling, and how to pad the rough edges using tape or **moleskin** (thick, durable form of adhesive material). Assess cast condition every 8 hours, checking for cracks, crumbling, or rough edges. A damaged cast may need to be replaced.

Safety Alert

Precautions When the Patient Has a Cast

Caution patients not to place a foreign object under the cast (e.g., wire hanger or stick to scratch an itch). Blowing cool air under the cast with a can of electronic air cleaner may help decrease itching. Discomfort can sometimes be relieved by directing the air of a hair dryer set on "cool" into the cast. Cast Comfort spray is a commercial product that delivers a soothing layer of talc under the cast.

A major concern for patients with casts is bathing. Plaster casts must be kept dry, or they can disintegrate. Even fiberglass casts are a problem if they become thoroughly wet. The outside material tolerates water, but the padding inside tends to stay wet, causing irritation to the skin. Small casts, such as those that immobilize the forearm or lower leg, can often be covered with a large plastic bag taped in place to allow the patient to shower. However, larger casts usually require that the patient take sponge baths until the cast is removed.

When a child is sent home with a cast, it is important to stress the dangers of placing small items inside the cast. These can cause pressure **necrosis** and infection.

Casts are removed using an oscillating saw. The saw is noisy and may frighten the patient. The saw does not cut down to the skin, and the patient needs reassurance about this. After separating the cast material, scissors are used to cut through the stockinette and padding and the cast is removed.

Clinical Cues

Prior to cast removal, inform the patient that the skin underneath will be dry and dirty in appearance, with an unpleasant odor. Washing with warm soapy water, rinsing, and applying cream or lotion removes dead skin cells and helps the skin return to normal. Vitamin E or other recommended ointment rubbed over the healed incisions may also improve appearance.

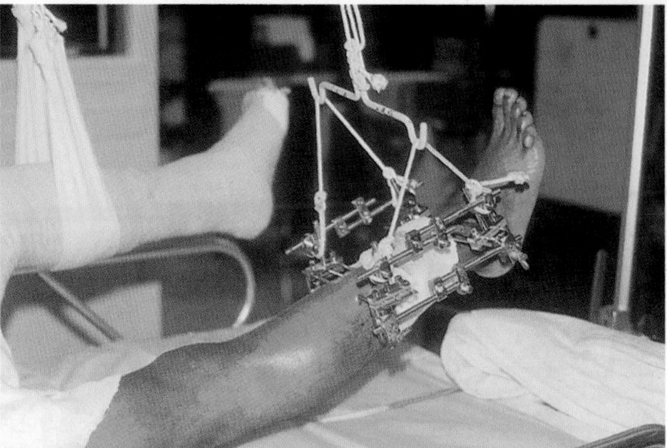

FIGURE 39.5 An external fixator holding fractured bones in place. (From McCance, K. L. [2009]. *Pathophysiology: The biologic basis for disease in adults and children* [6th ed.]. St Louis, MO: Mosby.)

EXTERNAL FIXATORS

An **external fixator** is a metal device, such as a pin, screw, or tong that is inserted into or through one or more bones to stabilize fragments of a fracture while it heals (Fig. 39.5). The metal inserts are attached to a metal frame. This type of immobilization allows the patient to be more active during healing while maintaining immobilization of the fractured area. The pins, screws, or tongs and the frame should be checked for stability every 4 hours. The insertion of the metal device through the skin provides a break in skin integrity that requires regular pin care to prevent infection, which is a common complication of external fixators (see Box 39.2). Pin care is included in Skill 39.2 later in this chapter.

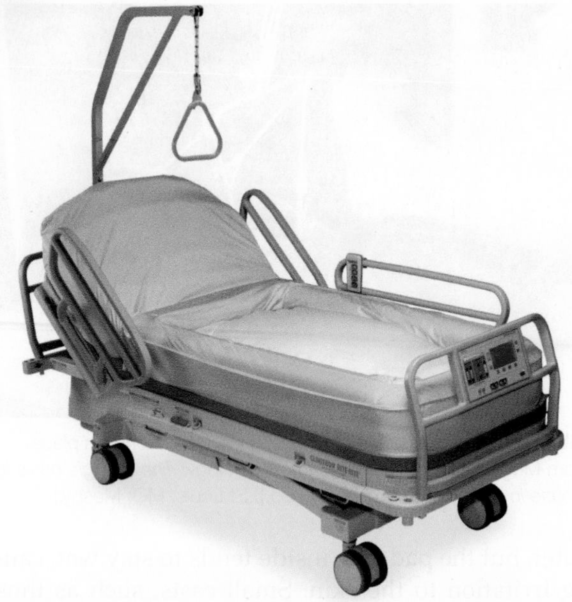

FIGURE 39.6 Clinitron-Elexis air-fluidized therapy unit. (Copyright 2011 Hill-Rom Service, Inc., reprinted with permission. All rights reserved.)

DEVICES USED TO PREVENT PROBLEMS OF IMMOBILITY

SPECIALTY BEDS

On occasion, illness or injury may result in long-term or permanent immobility. The potential complications from permanent immobility can worsen a patient's condition and may require additional interventions. **Kinetic** (moving) and air fluidized beds can be used to help decrease the incidence of these complications. Because their use is very expensive, thorough ongoing documentation of needing this type of bed is essential.

Air Fluidized Beds

Air fluidized beds have tiny silicone beads contained within the bed under a flexible, air permeable filter sheet (Fig. 39.6). Warmed air passes through the small particles, setting them into motion so that they act as a fluid that suspends the patient free from contact with any stationary, hard surface. The flotation or buoyancy of the patient on the air fluidized beads prevents pressure occlusion of blood vessels and shearing of tissues against the mattress during movement, unlike conventional mattresses. The loose filter sheet reduces friction, and the warm air protects the skin from damage by wetness. Air fluidized therapy is effective in the prevention of pressure injury and helps reduce generalized body pain common among bedridden patients. The indications for use include those patients with full-thickness or multiple pressure injuries, fresh grafts, or flap repairs of injuries and immobile patients whose general condition puts them at high risk for skin breakdown. Air fluidized therapy is not recommended for patients with unstable spines or patients who are ambulatory. To maximize the beneficial effects of the therapy, the unit should be in the fluidized mode at all times. Exceptions would be during patient transfer in and out of the bed or during nursing procedures for which the patient needs to be in one stable position for the intervention.

Low Air Loss Beds

Low air loss support is achieved by distributing air through multiple cushions connected in a series. The cushions are calibrated to provide maximum pressure relief for the individual patient. Shear and friction are reduced or eliminated because the cushions give with the patient during movement or rest. A low airflow through the cushion controls moisture on the skin. Segments of cushions may be deflated for patient care. The head of the bed can be raised. This bed is contraindicated for the patient with an unstable spine.

Continuous Lateral Rotation Beds

Lateral-rotation therapy beds, such as the RotoRest bed, are believed to decrease the incidence of lung collapse and hospital-acquired pneumonia, facilitate normal urine flow, and reduce the risk for deep vein thrombosis and pulmonary embolism by encouraging venous flow. This intervention may have a significant positive effect on various body systems of the critically ill patient and improve the overall patient outcome. Skin breakdown is reduced by the pressure reduction foam and gel pack surface. The patient is secured in position on the bed by multiple cushion wedges (Fig. 39.7). The bed turns in an arc up to 80 degrees and can be set to pause on either side for up to 30 minutes. The rotation is stopped and the wedge cushions removed as needed for bathing, procedures, or toileting. There is a built-in scale to allow patient weighing.

The degree and rate of movement are programmed to meet the individual patient's requirements. The constant side-to-side movement prevents the accumulation of respiratory secretions and promotes respiratory clearing. Other lateral rotation beds are combined with low air loss technology to provide relief of tissue pressure.

? Think Critically

What types of problems, if any, do you think you might encounter when caring for a patient in a kinetic or air fluidized bed?

PRESSURE RELIEF DEVICES

There are a variety of accessories that aid in the reduction of skin trauma from pressure for patients in standard hospital beds. These include foam and gel pads, sheepskin pads, and heel and elbow protectors. Pulsating air pads and water mattresses lie on top of the regular mattress, providing additional pressure relief (Figs. 39.8 and 39.9).

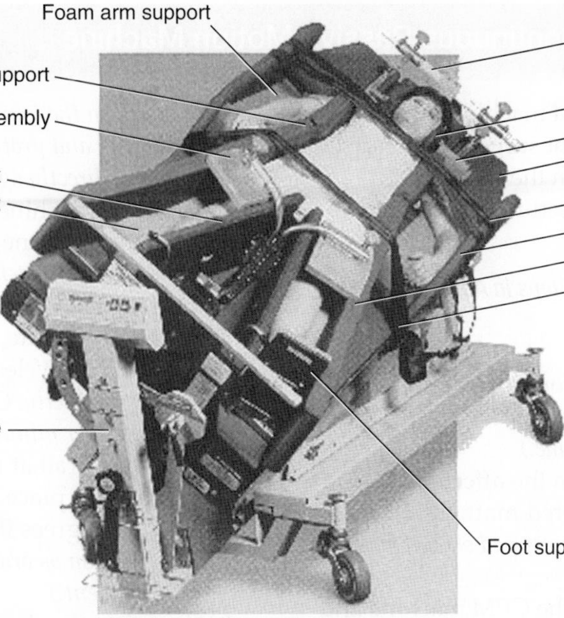

FIGURE 39.7 RotoRest Delta kinetic therapy bed. (RotoRest Delta Advanced Kinetic Therapy System, Courtesy KCI Licensing, Inc.)

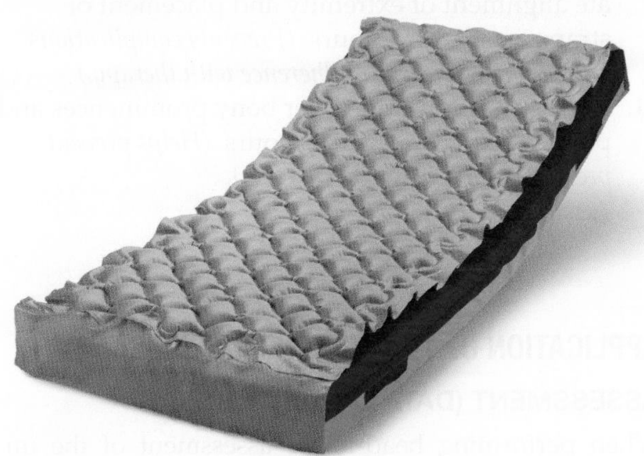

FIGURE 39.8 Alternating air mattress pad. (Courtesy Medline Industries Inc., Mundelein, IL.)

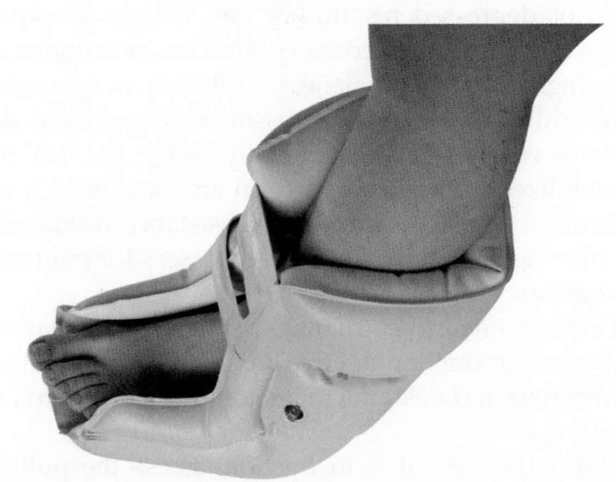

FIGURE 39.9 Heel protector helps to prevent skin breakdown. (Copyright AliMed)

CONTINUOUS PASSIVE MOTION MACHINE

After orthopedic surgery to replace a joint, continuous passive motion (CPM) is often ordered to restore joint function. A purpose of the machine is to exercise the extremity and joint, thus preventing contracture, muscle atrophy, venous stasis, and thrombus formation. The dressing to the extremity must be intact before attaching the patient's extremity to the device. Once in place, the CPM machine extends and flexes the extremity to prescribed angles for a specific period of time. The machine operates continuously as long as it is switched on. Follow Steps 39.1 to initiate therapy. As the degree of joint motion is tolerated, the settings are altered to increase the mobility of the joint (Fig. 39.10).

Clinical Cues

Assess pain level and medicate with ordered analgesia before initiating treatment with this machine. Closely monitor for need of more analgesia throughout exercise. The use of the machine is initially quite painful. **Pain is controlled best when it is treated before it becomes severe.**

THERAPEUTIC EXERCISE

Physical therapy is often ordered for the patient who is immobilized for an extended period of time. The primary care provider indicates what the problems are for the patient, and the therapist performs an evaluation and then designs an exercise program to help the patient and to prevent further musculoskeletal problems from occurring. Full ROM exercises should be

Steps 39.1 Use of a Continuous Passive Motion Machine

The most common use of a CPM machine is for the knee following knee replacement surgery. The nurse is responsible for making certain the machine is attached properly and that the settings are what the surgeon ordered.

Review and carry out the Standard Steps in Appendix A.

ACTION *(RATIONALE)*

1. Check the surgeon's order for flexion and extension limits, speed, and extremity involved. *(Provides data for setting up machine.)*
2. Place machine on the bed on the affected side. Place directly on sheet-covered mattress. *(Provides a stable surface. No extra mattress pad should be under the machine.)*
3. Connect the control box to the CPM machine and set the limits of flexion, extension, and speed control. *(Prepares machine for function.)*
4. Let machine run through one complete cycle then stop the machine at the end of extension. *(Ensures that the CPM is working properly.)*
5. Ensure dressing to wound or incision is intact before attaching extremity to machine. Center the extremity on machine with sheepskin beneath the extremity and adjust the machine to fit the patient. Align patient's joint with the machine joint and strap the extremity in place. *(Prepares machine to work on the joint properly. Avoids pressure on the extremity and protects skin. Intact dressing prevents rubbing directly against wound or incision.)*
6. Start the machine. When it reaches full flexion, stop the machine and check the degree of flexion. *(Ensures that machine is not flexing the joint more than desired, preventing complications.)*
7. Set the cycle rate, start the machine, and observe for two full cycles. *(Ensures that machine is functioning correctly. Cycle rate is usually between 2 and 10 cycles per minute.)*
8. Raise side rail at the foot of the bed to keep CPM machine in place. Keep bed flat with head raised only 20 degrees if necessary. *(Ensures that machine can function as ordered and patient's body will remain in alignment.)*
9. Assess patient's comfort level. *(CPM therapy may initially be painful. Patient should be medicated regularly as ordered for pain. Good pain control allows patient to tolerate increases in speed and flexion.)*
10. Assess the operative site for bleeding and evaluate alignment of extremity and placement of straps every 2 to 4 hours. *(Prevents complications and promotes patient's adherence with therapy.)*
11. Assess skin condition over bony prominences and provide skin care every 2 hours. *(Helps prevent pressure injuries from occurring.)*

CPM, Continuous passive motion.

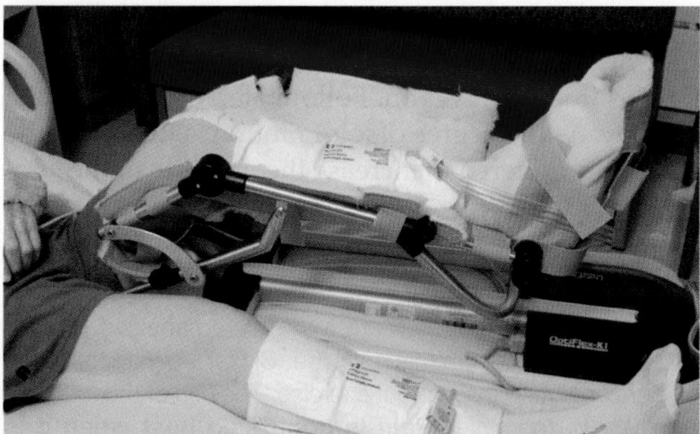

FIGURE 39.10 Continuous passive motion machine for the knee joint. (From DeWit, S. C. [2017]. *Medical-surgical nursing* [3rd ed.]. St. Louis, MO: Mosby.)

performed either actively or passively several times a day (Chapter 18). To prevent joint injury while performing passive ROM exercises, support the limb to be exercised above and below the joint. When the physical therapist is not available, the nurse assists the patient to perform these exercises. A family member or significant other can also be shown how to assist the patient with exercise.

❖ APPLICATION OF THE NURSING PROCESS

◆ ASSESSMENT (DATA COLLECTION)

When performing head-to-toe assessment of the immobilized patient, be alert to indicators of circulatory impairment such as reddened areas, pale or blue skin, coldness, or diminished or absent pulses. Look for signs of respiratory impairment such as shallow breathing, rapid or depressed respiratory rate, cough, abnormal lung sounds, use of accessory muscles, retractions or grunting, generalized paleness, duskiness, or cyanosis.

In addition to regular assessment, you should determine which activities of daily living (ADLs) the immobilized patient can perform and with which assistance is needed. Incorporate assistance needs into the nursing care plan. Continually assess for pain and discomfort.

Perform a neurovascular assessment for any patient with a cast or traction device (Box 39.3). Assess for cultural beliefs and customs that should be considered in planning care.

When the patient is in traction, assess the pulleys and ropes for proper function and free movement. Ensure that the weights are hanging free and the correct

Box 39.3 Neurovascular Assessment

Neurovascular assessment is performed for every patient who has experienced a fracture, whether treated with a cast or traction. It should be performed every hour for the first 24 hours, and after the cast is dry, every 4 to 8 hours. Check agency protocol for specific time schedule.

Skin: Inspect area distal to the injury, noting color. Compare to other extremity. Palpate skin temperature with **dorsum** (back) of the hand; compare with opposite extremity or site.

Movement: Have patient move area distal to the injury, or move it passively. There should be no discomfort.

Sensation: Inquire about feelings of numbness or tingling **(paresthesia)**. Check sensation with a paper clip and compare bilaterally. Sensation should be the same.

Pulses: Palpate pulses distal to the injury. Compare bilaterally if possible.

Capillary refill: Using your thumbnail, press the nail beds distal to the injury to **blanch** (to become pale) and judge time for capillary refill to occur after releasing pressure. Should be within 3 seconds, or within 5 seconds in the older adult.

Pain: Inquire about the degree, location, nature, and frequency of pain, noting any increase in intensity or change in type of pain.

amount of weight is applied. Assess the pin, the wire, or the tong insertion sites for indications of infection.

For the patient in a cast, observe and document any foul or musty odor from the cast. Other indicators of infection are an elevated temperature, purulent drainage, and/or an elevated white blood cell (WBC) count or increased complaints of pain.

All assistive devices and equipment must be checked for structural problems prior to use. Assess the assistive device for correct length or height in relation to the patient's height and posture. Evaluate the patient's ability to use the device correctly and determine if the device provides adequate stability for your patient's safety. Check the foot of the crutch or cane for an intact rubber tip or the walker for properly functioning wheels if they are present (Fig. 39.11).

◆ NURSING DIAGNOSIS

Common nursing diagnoses for patients with immobility are as follows:

- Impaired physical mobility related to **hemiparesis** or **hemiplegia** (one-sided weakness or one-sided paralysis, respectively)
- Impaired physical mobility related to fractured extremity in traction or a cast
- Ineffective peripheral tissue **perfusion** (circulation of blood through tissue) related to decreased circulation in the lower extremities
- Impaired tissue integrity related to skin disruption
- Acute pain related to tissue or bone injury or muscle spasm

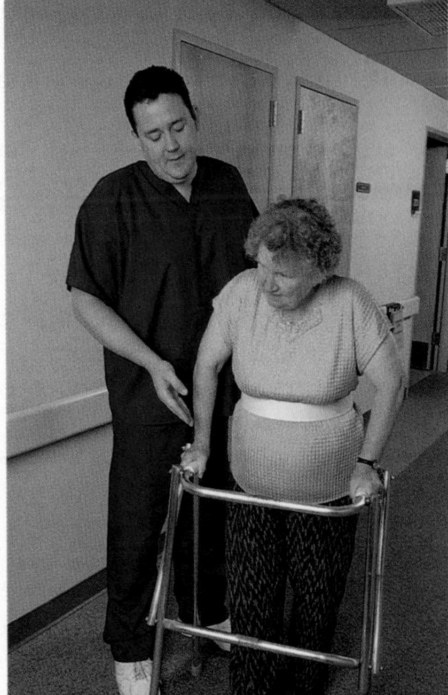

FIGURE 39.11 Assess the gait of the patient learning to use a walker.

- Ineffective airway clearance related to inactivity and bed rest
- Risk for disuse syndrome
- Risk for peripheral neurovascular dysfunction related to fracture and cast application

Nursing diagnoses related to the psychosocial needs of the immobile person are as follows:

- Social isolation related to immobility
- Disturbed body image related to brace or cast
- Deficient diversional activity related to immobility and bed rest
- Situational low self-esteem related to inability to perform usual roles

◆ PLANNING

Planning care for the immobile patient requires careful consideration of the time needed to assist the patient with various aspects of ADLs, the time needed for treatments, and time to be spent providing diversional activity and socialization. Expected outcomes for some of the above nursing diagnoses might be that the patient will:

- Demonstrate the ability to cope with physical mobility limitations as evidenced by resumption of as many self-care activities as possible within 10 days.
- Remain free of pressure-related injuries.
- Have pain controlled with medication and alternative techniques.
- Maintain good respiratory status as evidenced by effective airway clearing and clear breath sounds bilaterally.
- Not experience contracture or muscle atrophy from immobilization.
- Show no evidence of peripheral neurovascular dysfunction from swelling and/or cast application.

- Maintain regular contact with significant others, participating in diversional activities.
- Maintain interest in events occurring in the outside world.
- Evidence self-esteem by positive self-statements and voluntary participation in self-care and attention to grooming.

◆ IMPLEMENTATION

Appropriate interventions related to the identified nursing diagnoses would include regular turning and positioning, use of pressure relief devices, coughing and deep breathing exercises, ROM exercises, assisted ambulation, and visitation or activities addressing the psychosocial needs of the immobile patient. Nursing Care Plan 39.1 presents interventions for a specific patient.

When caring for a patient in a fresh plaster cast, elevate the cast on pillows if possible. This places a soft, yielding surface against the plaster that is less likely to alter the shape of the cast. Elevating the extremity will reduce the likelihood of swelling. Turn the patient hourly so the cast rests on a different area of its surface and will dry evenly. Skill 39.1 presents the points of care for the patient with a cast. For the patient going home with a cast in place, review cast care and assessment of problems with the patient and caregiver.

Patient Education

Fracture and Cast Care

To promote healing of your fracture and care for your cast:

- Keep the casted limb elevated above heart level whenever possible to prevent swelling.
- Call the primary care provider if your fingers or toes become numb, tingle, turn blue, or are cold to the touch.
- Call the primary care provider if you develop a fever, have unusual pain in the casted extremity, or notice a bad odor coming from the cast. These could be signs of infection.
- Regularly perform the exercises your care provider or physical therapist has taught you. These will help you retain your muscle strength while the bone heals.
- If the cast becomes loose or slides, call the primary care provider because it probably needs changing.
- Do not get a plaster cast wet. Check with your care provider about bathing or swimming if you have a synthetic cast.
- Do not insert any object inside the cast to relieve an itch. Doing so may damage the skin and result in an infection.
- Do not bear weight on the cast unless your primary care provider has advised you to do so.

Care of the patient in traction is time consuming because the patient's mobility is severely limited. Skill 39.2 presents the points of care for the patient in traction.

Bandages Used to Support, Apply Pressure, or Immobilize

Elasticized bandages are applied to immobilize a joint, or to apply pressure to reduce swelling. They may also be used to provide support to a wound and hold dressings in place. Elastic bandages are made in rolls of varying widths; the heavy stretch material conforms to the body part and provides support (Box 39.4).

Steps 39.2 show the technique for application of an elastic bandage. The same technique is used for gauze roller bandages. Different bandaging techniques are applied depending on the part to be bandaged.

Circular turn. Circular turns are used to anchor the bandage and to terminate the wrap. This turn is useful for bandaging the proximal aspect of the finger or wrist. Simply hold the free end of the rolled material in one hand and wrap it about the area, bringing it back to the starting point (Fig. 39.12A).

Spiral turn. This turn is used to bandage parts of the body that are uniform in circumference, such as the upper arm or upper leg. The spiral turn partly overlaps the previous turn. The amount of overlap varies from one-half to three-fourths of the width of the bandage (see Fig. 39.12B).

Spiral reverse turn. Spiral reverse turns are used to bandage body parts that are not uniform in circumference, such as the lower leg or forearm. After securing the bandage with circular turns, bring the bandage upward at a 30-degree angle. Place the thumb of the free hand on the upper edge of the bandage to hold it in place while it is reversed on itself. Unroll the bandage approximately 6 inches (15 cm) and turn the hand so that the bandage falls over itself. Continue the bandage around the extremity, overlapping each previous turn by two-thirds the width of the bandage. Make each turn at the same position on the extremity so that the turns of the bandage are all aligned (see Fig. 39.12C). Take care not to apply undue pressure over a major blood vessel.

Figure-of-eight turn. Figure-of-eight turns are used to bandage and stabilize an elbow, knee, or ankle or to immobilize and hold a fractured clavicle in position. Anchor the bandage with two circular turns. Bring the bandage above the joint, around it, and then below it, making a figure-of-eight. Continue bandaging above and below the joint, overlapping the previous turn by one-third to two-thirds the width of the bandage (see Fig. 39.12D). Secure the bandage above the joint with two circular turns and fasten it.

Recurrent turn. This turn is used to cover distal parts of the body, such as the end of a finger, the skull, or the stump left by amputation. Anchor the bandage by two circular turns. Then fold it back on itself and bring

Text continued on page 805

Nursing Care Plan 39.1 Care of the Patient Immobilized by a Stroke

SCENARIO Millie Palmer, age 76, is admitted after suffering an apparent stroke. She has left sided hemiparesis and poor bladder control. She is confused and somewhat groggy. A computed tomography (CT) scan of the brain shows that the problem is from a thrombosis (clot), and she is started on heparin to prevent further thrombi from forming.

***PROBLEM/*NURSING DIAGNOSIS** *Stroke with left sided weakness*/Impaired physical mobility related to weakness of left extremities.

Supporting Assessment Data *Objective:* Weakness of left arm and left leg; stroke.

Goals/Expected Outcomes	Nursing Interventions	Selected Rationale	Evaluation
Patient will maintain muscle tone in all muscles. Patient will maintain joint mobility in all joints.	Passive ROM to left extremities tid.	Passive ROM will help maintain muscle function and joint mobility.	ROM performed.
Patient will maintain muscle tone in all muscles.	Active ROM to other joints bid. Encourage to perform ADLs as possible.	Active ROM will preserve muscle tone and joint function.	*Is muscle tone being maintained?* Some tone to muscle. Actively moving other extremities and joints.
	Assess for muscle spasm each shift.	Muscle spasm may occur with hemiparesis and can be painful.	Progressing toward expected outcomes. Continue plan.

***PROBLEM/*NURSING DIAGNOSIS** *Unable to reposition self*/Risk for impaired skin integrity related to decreased mobility and incontinence.

Supporting Assessment Data
Objective: Left sided weakness, confusion; incontinent of urine.

Goals/Expected Outcomes	Nursing Interventions	Selected Rationale	Evaluation
Skin will remain intact.	Assess skin each shift and when turning, with special attention to pressure points.	Frequent inspection of skin reveals reddened areas before pressure injuries form.	*Is skin intact?* Skin remains intact; area of redness over right ankle; heel protector applied to protect ankle.
	Use cushioning devices under pressure points as needed.	Cushioning reduces pressure over bony prominences.	
	Offer bedpan q 2 h.	Opportunity to void q 2 h helps prevent incontinence.	
	Check absorbent undergarment frequently and change quickly when wet; clean and dry the skin.	Moisture contributes to skin breakdown. Keeping skin clean and dry prevents breakdown.	Meeting expected outcomes. Continue plan.
	Reposition q 2 h.	Repositioning prevents pressure injuries and provides comfort for joints.	

***PROBLEM/*NURSING DIAGNOSIS** *Clot interrupting blood flow in brain*/Risk for ineffective cerebral tissue perfusion related to thrombosis.

Supporting Assessment Data *Objective:* Cerebral thrombus demonstrated on CT scan.

Goals/Expected Outcomes	Nursing Interventions	Selected Rationale	Evaluation
Neurologic deficits will not increase.	Neurologic assessment and vital signs q 2 h.	Assessment will reveal deteriorating condition in a timely fashion.	*Are there neurologic deficits?* Left sided weakness present.

Nursing Care Plan 39.1 Care of the Patient Immobilized by a Stroke—cont'd

Goals/Expected Outcomes	Nursing Interventions	Selected Rationale	Evaluation
	Monitor heparin IV administration.	Heparin IV will help prevent formation of further thrombi.	No change in neurologic status.
	Monitor PTT for therapeutic response to heparin.	PTT levels will demonstrate whether heparin dose is sufficient.	Progressing toward outcomes. Continue plan.

***PROBLEM*/NURSING DIAGNOSIS** *Incontinent of urine*/Functional urinary incontinence related to stroke.

Supporting Assessment Data *Objective:* Left sided weakness, confusion; incontinent of urine.

Goals/Expected Outcomes	Nursing Interventions	Selected Rationale	Evaluation
Patient will regain continence.	Institute bladder training program in 2 days.	Bladder training regimen can reinstitute urinary continence in many stroke patients.	*Is patient continent?* Not completely; some intermittent uncontrolled voiding.
	Offer bedpan q 2 h.	Opportunity to void q 2 h helps prevent incontinence.	Voids in bedpan after meals.
	Obtain order for bedside commode.	With hemiparesis it is easier to transfer to the bedside commode than walk to the bathroom to void.	
	Check absorbent undergarment frequently; change when wet.		Progressing toward outcomes. Continue plan.

CRITICAL THINKING QUESTIONS

1. How might incontinence affect this patient psychologically?
2. If Mrs. Palmer says that she is too tired to do the exercises and all she feels like doing is sleep, how would you respond?

ADLs, Activities of daily living; *PTT,* partial thromboplastin time; *ROM,* range-of-motion; *tid,* three times daily.

Skill 39.1 Cast Care

 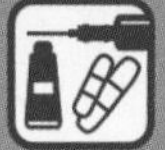 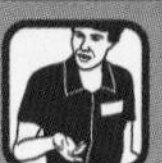   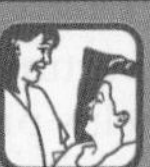 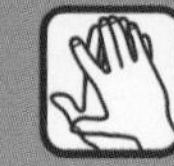 

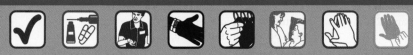

Casts may be applied to almost any area of the body. The larger and thicker the cast, the longer it takes to dry fully. Hip spica and full body casts may take 1 to 2 days to dry completely. Synthetic material casts dry much more quickly than plaster casts.

SUPPLIES

- Tape or moleskin
- Pen for marking drainage
- Lamb's wool for padding

Review and carry out the Standard Steps in Appendix A.

ACTION *(RATIONALE)*

Assessment (Data Collection)

1. Examine cast for any dents. Handle the cast gently with the flats of the fingers and the palms, not the fingertips. *(Dents may cause compression on underlying tissues. Fingertip pressure more easily dents the cast because pressure is on a small area rather than spread over a broader surface.)*
2. Examine cast for any areas where blood may have seeped through. Circle any such areas in ink and write the date and time on the cast. *(Bloodstains seeping through the cast are a common occurrence when surgery has preceded the application of a cast. Marking provides a way to judge further bleeding.)*
3. Assess cast for rough edges and excessive tightness by running a finger along all cast edges and under the edges next to the skin. *(A finger should slip easily under the edge of cast. Checking helps to discover problem areas.)*

Skill 39.1 Cast Care—cont'd

Planning

4. Plan to reassess a new cast every hour for the first 24 hours and every 4 to 8 hours thereafter or per agency policy. *(Swelling may occur in the period after injury or surgery and may cause pressure on nerves and vessels.)*

Implementation

5. Pad any rough edges by petaling with 1½- to 2-inch pieces of tape or moleskin. Place lamb's wool beneath cast to pad under rough spots. *(Rough spots will cause skin chafing, abrasion, and breakdown.)*

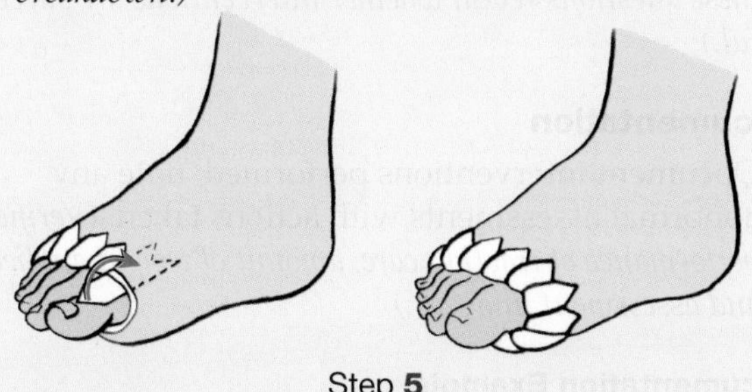

Step **5**

6. Notify the orthopedic technician or primary care provider if any area of cast is too tight. *(Cast may need to be cut to relieve pressure.)*
7. Elevate the casted extremity so that the hand or foot is at or above heart level. *(Aids in reducing or preventing swelling.)*
8. For patients in large casts (e.g., hip spica and body), place the bed in a slight Trendelenburg position for the first day or two to help prevent swelling, unless contraindicated by patient's condition or medical orders. *(Patients in large casts may experience swelling in the legs, thighs, perineum, buttocks, and lower abdomen during the first few days. Placing bed at an approximate 10-degree angle in Trendelenburg position will help prevent this swelling.)*
9. Turn the patient at intervals so that all cast surfaces are exposed to the air to facilitate even drying and prevent skin pressure injuries.
   - When cast is still wet, turn patient hourly.
   - As cast dries, every 2 hours is sufficient unless patient is uncomfortable.
   - Get adequate help when turning patient to prevent injury.
   - Use pillows to prop the patient at different angles as cast dries. *(Air exposure allows moisture to evaporate.)*
10. Instruct patient not to use sharp, pointed, or rigid items to scratch under the cast. *(Skin under the cast often itches. Using such items to scratch can injure skin. If itching is severe, ask for an order for medication to control it.)*
11. Smell the open edges of the cast to assess for infection under the cast. *(Skin injuries may become infected or necrotic and cause a foul or musty odor.)*

Evaluation

12. Evaluate the cast by inspecting for crumbling or cracks. Ask yourself: Is there any discomfort under the cast? Is the cast rubbing the skin anywhere? Are the edges smooth? Is the cast drying evenly? Is swelling in the tissues subsiding? *(Answers to these questions tell whether the interventions are successful in meeting the expected outcomes.)*

Documentation

13. Document assessment findings and interventions. *(Verifies that assessment has been performed and interventions carried out.)*

Documentation Example

Received from recovery room alert and stable. Fresh plaster cast encases right leg from mid-thigh to mid-toes. Toes pink, warm, move well; sensation present; capillary refill less than 2 seconds. Edge of cast easily admits fingertip. Leg elevated on pillows. Rates pain as 3 out of 10. Advised to request pain medication if pain increases. (Nurse's time-stamped electronic signature)

Special Considerations

- Provide full instructions for cast care for the patient discharged home with a cast.
- Instruct to use a hair dryer only on the "cool" setting to help dry the cast or relieve itching.
- Demonstrate how to wrap a cast in plastic for showering, if appropriate.
- Demonstrate how to handle the extremity when repositioning, supporting the joints.

Critical Thinking Questions

1. What would you do if you notice the edge of the cast is crumbling?
2. What would you tell a patient with a long leg cast who keeps slipping a ruler down in the cast to scratch the skin?

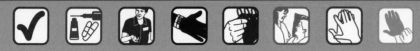

Skill 39.2 Care of the Patient in Traction

 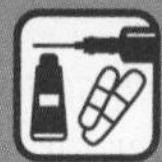 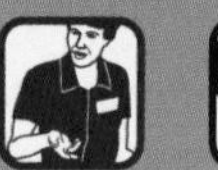 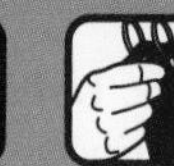 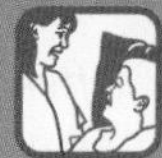 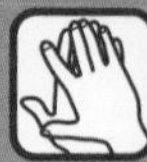 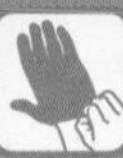

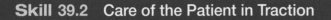

Skin traction is mostly used to decrease muscle spasm after a fracture or back muscle injury. Skin traction may be used on small children with a lower extremity fracture.

SUPPLIES

- Clean gloves (if needed)

Review and carry out the Standard Steps in Appendix A.

ACTION *(RATIONALE)*

Assessment (Data Collection)

1. Check the medical order for desired amount of weight for traction. *(Ensures the correct amount of weight is applied.)*
2. Assess boot, wrap, and traction appliance. Check that ropes and pulleys are working smoothly and weights are hanging free. *(Surface of appliance should be smooth and free of wrinkles or gaps to prevent pressure injury to skin. Appliance should not be rubbing on any skin surface. Traction will not function properly if ropes are hung up in pulleys or weights are resting on floor or bed.)*

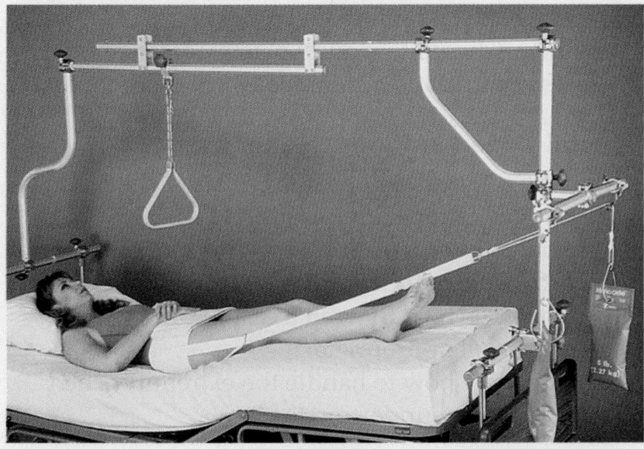

Step 2

3. Assess the skin, distal circulation, and sensation. *(Detects signs of complications.)*

Planning

4. Plan times into work schedule to perform assessments, treatments, and ADLs. *(Care for the immobile patient in traction takes more time.)*

Implementation

5. Realign the patient in the bed as needed to maintain optimal traction pull. *(A direct straight line is needed for traction to be completely effective. Patients need to be pulled up in bed periodically.)*

Evaluation

6. Evaluate for signs of complications. Ask yourself: Is there any sign of irritation where the patient's skin meets the apparatus? Does the patient have a fever? Does the patient complain of pain? Is traction apparatus functioning correctly? *(Answers to these questions reveal whether interventions are successful.)*

Documentation

7. Document interventions performed; note any abnormal assessments with actions taken. *(Verifies performance of traction care, amount of weight applied, and assessment findings.)*

Documentation Example

Slight irritation and erythema on medial aspect of left leg where traction boot meets skin, lateral aspect is clean and without signs or symptoms of infection. Cleansed both aspects of leg with normal saline and dried with 4 × 4 gauze; thin layer of lamb's wool padding inserted between medial aspect of left leg and traction boot. (Nurse's time-stamped electronic signature)

Special Considerations

- It is important to evaluate and medicate the patient in traction for pain, especially in the first few days when muscle spasm occurs.
- Teach family and significant others that they must not tamper with the traction device, ropes, or weights.
- A trapeze bar attached to the over-the-bed frame is very helpful so that the patient may assist in repositioning; it also provides opportunity for exercise of the upper extremities.

Critical Thinking Questions

1. What would you say to a nurse who is helping a patient move up in the bed if she lifts the weights attached to the leg traction?
2. What activities might be good for a patient who is confined to bed in traction to combat boredom?

ADLs, Activities of daily living.

it centrally over the distal end to be covered. Hold it in place with the other hand, and bring the bandage back over the end to the right of the center bandage but overlapping it by two-thirds the width of the bandage. Then bring the bandage back on the left side, overlapping the first turn by two-thirds the width of the bandage. Continue alternating bandaging right and left until the area is well covered.

Box 39.4 Guidelines for Applying an Elastic or Roller Bandage

- Elevate the limb and support it while applying the bandage.
- Face the patient and wrap the bandage from the distal to the proximal area.
- Apply even pressure by exerting equal tension throughout the wrapping of the bandage.
- Overlap turns of the bandage equally.
- Smooth the bandage, removing wrinkles, as you wrap it.
- Secure the end of the bandage with self-adherent portion of the bandage, a safety pin, or tape. (Do not use metal clips, as they may come loose and land in the bed, causing injury to the patient.)
- Check the color and sensation of the part distal and proximal to the bandage when finished and at frequent intervals thereafter.
- Remove the bandage for bathing of the body part; assess the skin for irritation or breaks; rewrap the bandage at least twice a day.

Terminate the bandage with two circular turns and secure the end appropriately (see Fig. 39.12E).

Thumb spica. This is a variation of the figure-of-eight bandage used to support the thumb in neutral position following a sprain or other injury. The technique can also be used to bandage the hip or shoulder. For the thumb, secure the bandage with two circular turns around the wrist. Bring the bandage down to the distal aspect of the thumb and encircle the thumb. If possible, leave the tip of the thumb exposed. Take the bandage back up and around the wrist, and then back down and around the thumb, overlapping the previous turn by two-thirds the width of the bandage. Repeat the above steps, working up the thumb and hand until the thumb is covered (see Fig. 39.12F).

Immobilizing and Supporting With a Sling

A sling may be used to support and immobilize an injured wrist, elbow, or shoulder. The sling holds the extremity in an elevated position to avoid edema of the hand, minimize pain and discomfort, and fatigue. A commercially made arm sling can be placed about the arm and the straps adjusted about the neck. If this type of support is not available, a triangular bandage sling may be used to support the injured upper extremity (Fig. 39.13, Steps 39.3).

Using a Mechanical Lift to Transfer the Immobile Patient

Lifts can be used to move immobile patients from the bed to a stretcher (gurney), a chair, or a wheelchair and back again. Mechanical lifts consist of a sturdy metal

Steps 39.2 Applying of an Elastic Bandage

The type and size of the bandage used will depend on the area to be bandaged and the purpose of the bandage. The primary care provider may order a specific type of bandage.

Review and carry out the Standard Steps in Appendix A.

ACTION *(RATIONALE)*

1. Wash and dry area to be bandaged. *(Helps prevent infection by removing microorganisms.)*
2. Elevate extremity to be bandaged; ask an assistant to help if necessary. *(Elevation encourages venous return and helps prevent swelling. It is easier to wrap the bandage properly if someone else supports extremity.)*
3. Stand in front of patient and unroll the end of the bandage slightly; anchor it in place with the thumb of the nondominant hand on the anterior part of extremity to be bandaged. *(Secures bandage while wrapping is occurring.)*
4. Make two initial circular turns to anchor the bandage in place. *(Securing the bandage end prevents it from becoming loose.)*
5. Use a circular, spiral, spiral reverse, figure-of-eight, recurrent turn, or thumb spica bandaging technique, as appropriate for the area to be bandaged. *(The body part to be bandaged will indicate which style of bandaging is best.)*
6. Apply bandage smoothly and evenly with light to moderate tension. *(Smoothness helps prevent pressure areas; adequate tension is necessary for bandage to stay in place.)*
7. Secure bandage with self-adherent portion of bandage, tape, metal clips, or safety pin. *(Bandage must be secured to remain in place. Place tape on metal clips to minimize risk of coming loose and landing in the bed.)*
8. Assess bandage for fit and circulation distal and proximal to area bandaged. *(A bandage applied too tightly will impede circulation; a loose bandage will fall off.)*

frame with a wide base of support from which a canvas sling is suspended. The lift is on wheels and, when empty, can be easily moved by one person. A hydraulic pump device allows one person to lift the weight of the patient, but it takes two people to use a mechanical lift safely—one to raise and move the lift and one to guide the patient into the chair or onto the bed or stretcher. Such lifts are also used to place patients into a tub or whirlpool bath for bathing or **hydrotherapy** (massage or debridement by moving water).

Never leave a patient requiring the use of a lift unattended while in the lift, in the tub, or in the whirlpool bath. When using a lift, explain to the patient exactly what is being performed. Many patients feel somewhat frightened being lifted off the bed or out of a chair by a mechanical device and may need reassurance. However, the proper use of a mechanical lift allows the nurse to move weak or helpless patients safely while avoiding self-injury (Skill 39.3).

Before placing a patient on the sling, be sure the skin is clean and dry. Protect the sling as needed with a sheet or bath blanket. If soiled, wash the sling with a disinfectant solution before using it again.

Assisting With Aids to Mobilization

Although the use of ambulatory aids is often taught by a physical therapist or kinesiologist, it is important for you to know the proper techniques so that learning can be reinforced. Whenever a patient is using an assistive device for mobility, it is important to keep floors clear of clutter and pathways well lighted. Place the assistive device within easy reach of the patient when not in use. In the home, assess the main pathways the patient will be using and ask for assistance in removing any hazards.

Walkers. A walker is frequently the first mechanical aid used when training an individual to walk following a loss of function or surgical procedure such as a hip or knee replacement. It is particularly helpful for patients who are weak or tend to lose their balance because it offers a broad base of support.

Walkers are rectangular tubular metal frames that are at least waist high and are open on one side. Most walkers have four rubber-capped tips that rest on the floor, although some have wheels on the front. There are handgrips on the side crossbars. Walkers are adjustable in height. The height is correct if the person's elbow is bent at a 15- to 30-degree angle while standing upright and grasping the handgrips. To use a walker, the individual must have the use of both hands and arms and at least one leg. However, generalized weakness may still allow the patient to use a walker effectively.

Crutches. Depending on the person and the need for assistance with ambulation, the use of crutches may follow the use of a walker or be the first aid to ambulation (Fig. 39.14).

Although there are a variety of styles of crutches, three basic types are most commonly seen. These are axillary, Lofstrand, and Canadian crutches. Lofstrand and Canadian crutches are shorter and are designed for patients who will permanently need crutches for mobility. Axillary crutches are commonly used for short-term needs. They are adjustable to a variety of heights and are relatively easy to use. They do present one real danger: **resting the body's weight on the axillary bar puts pressure on vital nerves and can occlude blood vessels in the axilla, causing temporary or permanent damage, including paralysis.** For this reason it is critical that crutches be adjusted to the proper height and the patient be instructed to avoid resting the body's weight on the axillary bar.

Crutches need to adjust both in overall length and from the axillary bar to the handgrip. Measure with the patient standing or supine. If standing, be certain the patient's shoes are on the feet. For standing measurement, position the crutches with tips at a point 4 to 6 inches (10 to 15 cm) to the side and 4 to 6 inches in front of the patient's feet. The pads should be ½ to 2 inches (1.3 to 5 cm) below the axilla. For supine measurement, position the tips 6 inches (15 cm) lateral to the patient's heel. The pad should be three or four fingerbreadths under the axilla. Adjust handgrips for both measurements so that the elbow is flexed 15 or 20 degrees when the palms of the hands are resting on the handgrips. When walking, the patient will need to straighten the elbow and the wrist during weight bearing. This should allow the axilla to pass freely over the axillary bar during forward movement (Box 39.5).

Patient Education

Common Crutch Gaits

GAIT	DESCRIPTION	PATTERN
Four-point gait	Sequence: 1. Advance left crutch. 2. Advance right foot. 3. Advance right crutch. 4. Advance left foot.	Four-point gait 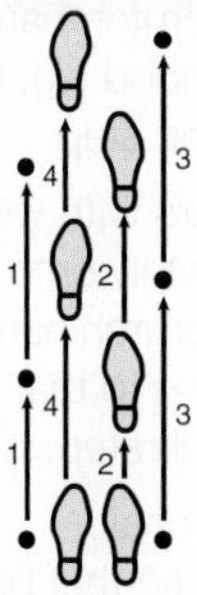
Three-point gait	Sequence: 1. Advance both crutches forward with the affected leg and shift weight to crutches. 2. Advance unaffected leg and shift weight onto it. Advantages: Allows the affected leg to be partially or completely free of weight bearing. Requirements: Full weight bearing on one leg, balance, and upper body strength.	Three-point gait 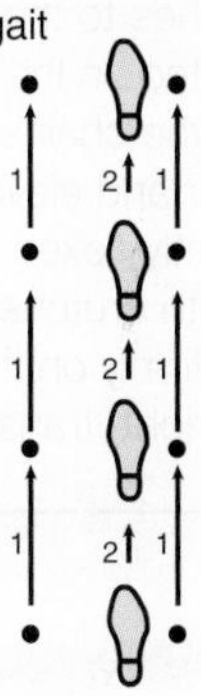
Two-point gait	Sequence: 1. Advance left crutch and right foot. 2. Advance right crutch and left foot. Advantages: Faster version of the four-point gait, more normal walking pattern (arms and legs moving in opposition). Requirements: Partial weight bearing on both legs, balance.	Two-point gait 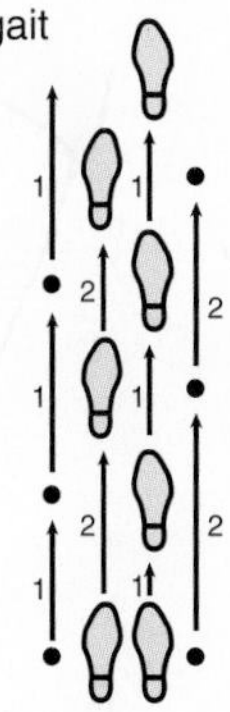
Swing-through gait	Sequence: 1. Move both crutches forward. 2. Move both legs forward, beyond, or even with crutches. Or may keep weight on good foot and move other foot forward and then move good foot forward.	Swing-through gait 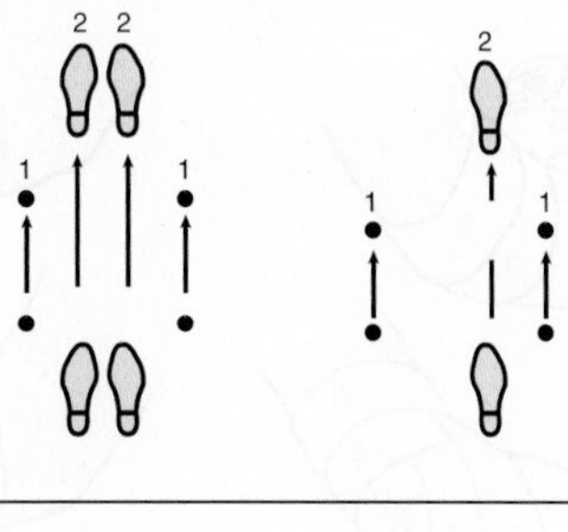

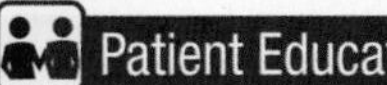 Patient Education

Special Maneuvers on Crutches

MANEUVER	DESCRIPTION
Walking upstairs	1. Stand at foot of stairs with weight on good leg and crutch. 2. Put weight on the crutch handles, and lift the good leg up onto the first step of the stairs. 3. Put weight on the good leg, and lift other leg and the crutches up to that step. 4. Repeat for each stair step.
Walking downstairs	1. Stand at top of stairs with weight on good leg and crutches. 2. Shift weight completely onto the good leg, and put the crutches down on the next step. 3. Put weight on the crutch handles, and transfer injured leg down on the step with the crutches. 4. Bring good leg down to that step. 5. Repeat for each stair step.
Sitting down	1. Crutch walk to the chair. 2. Turn around slowly so that back is to the chair and the backs of the legs touch the seat of the chair. 3. Transfer both crutches to the side with the injured leg, and grasp both hand grips with the one hand. 4. As weight is supported on the crutches and good leg, reach back with free hand and grasp the arm of the chair. 5. Lower slowly onto the chair seat, using the support of both the crutches and the chair. 6. Sit back in the chair and elevate the leg, but not to an angle greater than 90 degrees at the hip. 7. Keep the knee slightly flexed when elevated because too much extension can decrease the circulation. 8. To get up, bring both crutches along the side of the injured leg, and grasp the hand grip firmly. Make sure the crutch tips are firmly on the floor. Place the other hand on the arm of the chair, and push up. 9. After becoming upright, transfer one crutch to the other hand for walking.

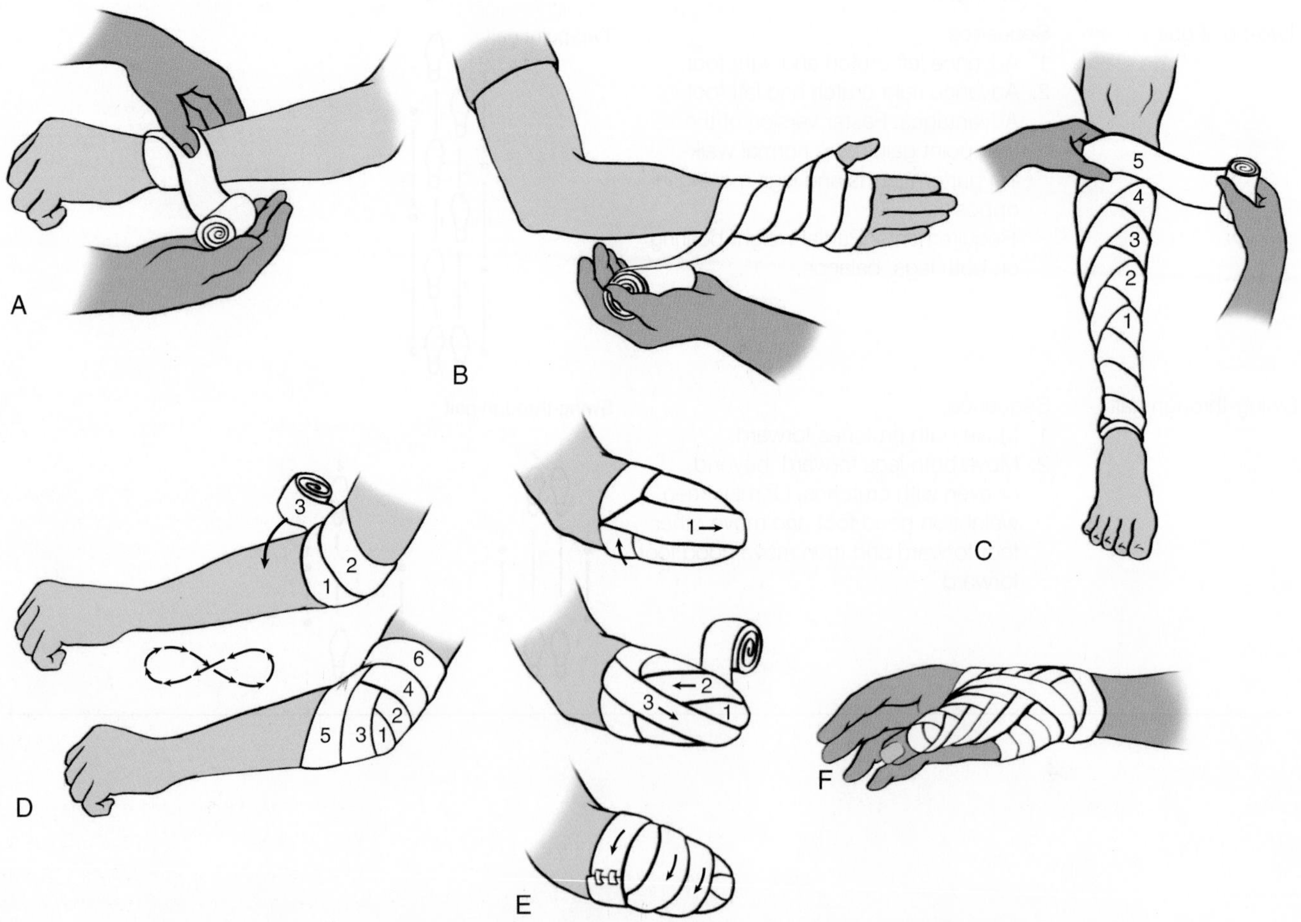

FIGURE 39.12 Applying an Elastic Bandage. (A) Starting a bandage with circular turns. (B) Bandaging with spiral turns. (C) Bandaging with spiral reverse turns. (D) Bandaging a joint with figure-of-eight turns. (E) Recurrent turn bandaging. (F) Thumb spica bandaging.

Canes. The most commonly used canes are the standard (one-point) and the quad (four-point) cane (Fig. 39.15). An advantage of a quad cane is that it will stand up by itself (Box 39.6).

Wheelchairs. Wheelchairs are used for patients who are not able to ambulate either independently or with aids, such as crutches or a walker. Many **paraplegics** (those without use of the legs), **quadriplegics** (those without use of both arms and legs), amputees, and individuals with severe hemiparesis or respiratory problems are dependent on wheelchairs for movement from place to place. Patients who are wheelchair dependent over the long term need chairs that are made specifically to their body measurements. When a patient brings a wheelchair to the hospital, see that it is clearly labeled with the owner's name, and never borrow it for someone else.

When moving someone into or out of a wheelchair, always set the brakes. Be sure the person's feet are correctly placed on the footrests and that clothing or lap robes are tucked safely away from the wheels. Shoes, slippers, or bed socks will protect the feet from direct contact with the footrests. To prevent accidents, keep patients in wheelchairs well away from stairwells, elevators, and doorways if left to sit stationary. **Always lock the brakes when the chair is not in motion.**

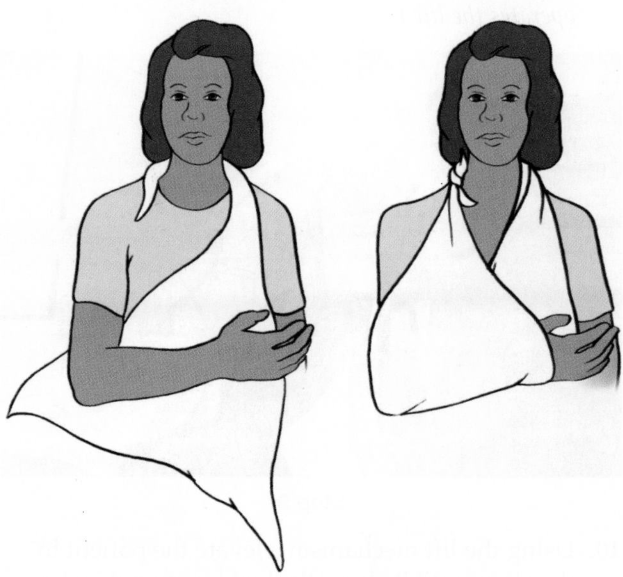

FIGURE 39.13 A triangular sling bandage.

Braces, splints, and prostheses for stabilization. Braces and splints are used to strengthen and support areas of the body affected by weakness or paralysis, such as the legs or back. They may also be used after surgery or trauma to immobilize a part while it heals. Braces and splints are generally made of plastic or metal pieces with padding and straps for attachment. A leg brace may be combined with a shoe. A back brace has metal staves sewn into the fabric; the fabric may be elasticized to provide more support.

A wrist splint is a padded device with an inner metal frame. It is often used to relieve or prevent carpal tunnel syndrome that sometimes occurs with repetitive hand movements and to immobilize a sprained wrist.

A **prosthesis** (artificial substitute for a body part) is used to replace a body part that is missing, either from birth or following amputation. It is specially fashioned to fit the particular patient and assist with lost function. It takes considerable time for a patient to adjust to the use of a prosthesis.

All braces, splints, and prostheses have the potential to irritate and injure the tissues and must be monitored closely. The skin should be carefully evaluated during the initial assessment and then reassessed regularly

Steps 39.3 Applying a Triangular Bandage Sling

When a commercial arm support is not available, use a triangular bandage to form a sling. This will support the upper extremity.

Review and carry out the Standard Steps in Appendix A.

ACTION (*RATIONALE*)

1. Place one end of the triangle over the shoulder on the uninjured side. *(Positions the sling properly.)*
2. Position the point of the triangle toward the elbow. Ask the patient to bend the injured arm horizontally across the body, with the thumb toward the body. Place the bandage under the arm flat against the chest. *(Forms the sling support.)*
3. Bring the other end over the injured arm and shoulder while the patient keeps the elbow bent at right angles across lower chest. The hand should be about 4 inches higher than the elbow. *(Finishes forming the sling support. Elevating the hand prevents the fingers from swelling.)*
4. Tie the two ends at one side of the neck in a square knot. *(Secures the sling; the knot at the side prevents discomfort when the patient lies down and decreases pull on the back of the neck when the arm is in the sling.)*
5. Fold the point of the triangle neatly over the elbow toward the front, and secure with a safety pin. *(Keeps the elbow and sling from slipping back and forth.)*
6. Check the circulation in the fingers, comparing color of the nail beds and temperature of the hand with the other hand. *(Fingers should be pink and warm; cold or bluish fingers indicate impaired circulation.)*

Skill 39.3 Transferring With a Mechanical Lift

 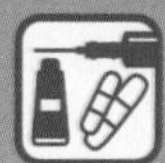 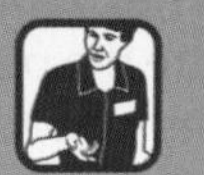 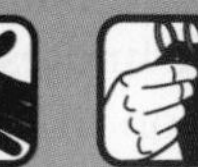 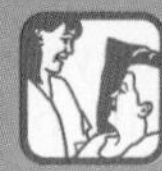 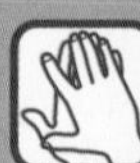 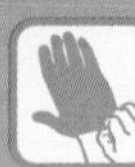

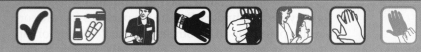

Mechanical lifts allow immobile patients to be moved safely between two points some distance apart. A lift may also be used to elevate helpless patients while the bed is changed under them.

SUPPLIES

- Mechanical lift with sling
- Bath blanket or sheet
- Chair, wheelchair, stretcher, or clean tub (to receive patient)

Review and carry out the Standard Steps in Appendix A.

ACTION *(RATIONALE)*

Assessment (Data Collection)

1. Determine that lift is functioning correctly and that sling is clean. *(Promotes smooth, safe use of the lift.)*
2. Assess patient's readiness to be transferred. Explain to patient exactly what will be performed. *(Patient will experience less anxiety if prepared for the procedure.)*

Planning

3. Obtain the assistance of a second person. *(Two people are needed to safely transfer a patient using a lift.)*

Implementation

4. Position the chair, wheelchair, or stretcher correctly, clearing away any obstructions; set brakes if applicable. *(A clear floor is needed to maneuver the lift. Setting brakes prevents the chair or stretcher from moving while transferring the patient.)*
5. Raise the far side rail, adjust bed to working height, and lock wheels. *(Bed adjustment allows proper use of body mechanics and decreases risk of injury to patient and nurse. Locked wheels prevent bed from moving while transferring.)*
6. Roll the patient onto the side. Instruct patient to hold onto the side rail if possible. Place the sling on the bed positioned from back of the head or the shoulders to mid-thigh; roll patient onto the sling. Assist or have the patient roll to other side so that the sling can be safely unrolled. Assist, or have, the patient lie supine on the sling. *(Supports entire trunk and positions patient in sling for transfer and allows for correct position of sling before attempting to activate the lift.)*
7. Position the lift: Widen the stance of the base of the lift and lock it into place. Position the base under the bed so hooks for the sling are over the patient and in line with the hook openings on the sling. *(Correct positioning prevents lift from tipping during transfer. Allows for easy attachment of hooks to the sling).*
8. Lower the sling hooks in a controlled manner, and attach to the sling. Be certain hooks will not press into patient's skin when sling is elevated. *(Controlling the hooks prevents them from striking the patient. Checking hook location prevents pressure damage to patient's skin).*
9. Ask the patient to fold the arms over the chest; support patient's head. *(Head must be supported if sling is not long enough to do so. One person supports the patient's head and guides the sling as the other operates the lift.)*

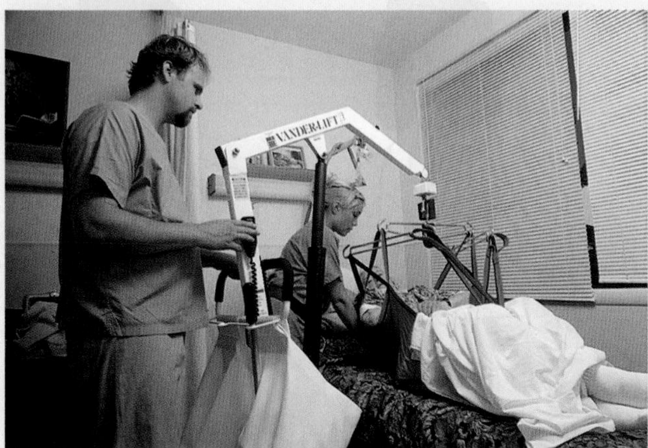

Step 9

10. Using the lift mechanism, elevate the patient in the sling until it clears the bed by several inches. *(Allows unimpeded transfer of the patient to chair or stretcher.)*

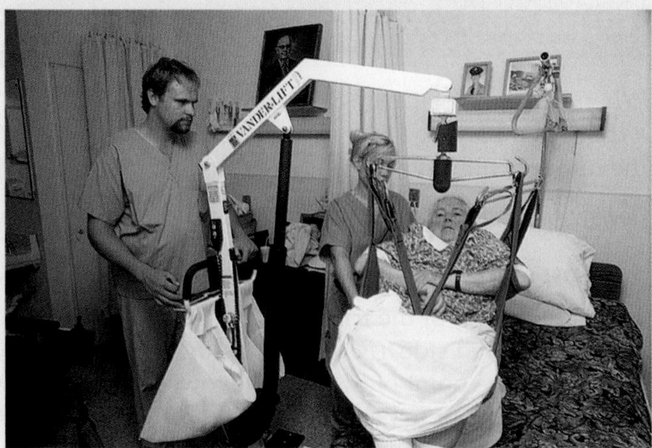

Step 10

11. Roll the lift away from the bed while the second helper safely guides the patient over the chair or stretcher. *(Keeps patient secure and safe. Positions sling for the transfer.)*
12. Use the pressure release valve to lower the patient slowly into the chair or onto the stretcher while

Skill 39.3 Transferring With a Mechanical Lift—cont'd

the helper guides the patient's body. Lower only enough to allow unhooking the sling. *(Safely transfers the patient.)*

13. Unhook the sling, elevate the lift, and roll it away from the patient. *(Prevents hook assembly from striking the patient.)*
14. Position the patient in good alignment. Smooth the sling or remove it. *(Ensures patient is correctly and safely transferred and made comfortable.)*
15. Cover patient with a blanket or sheet; place call light and needed items within reach. Secure patient in the chair with a security vest, or on the stretcher as appropriate. *(Promotes safety and comfort for the patient.)*
16. Monitor at least every 15 minutes for sitting tolerance if the patient is in chair. *(If patient is unable to use a call light, place chair where it is visible to a nurse at all times, such as in the hallway near the nurse's station.)*
17. With the help of an assistant, return the patient to bed using the lift and following the same steps. *(An assistant helps prevent injury to the patient.)*

Evaluation

18. Ask yourself: Was the patient transferred smoothly and without injury? Was the patient excessively frightened? Did the lift work correctly? *(Answers to these questions provide data to evaluate effectiveness of interventions.)*

Documentation

19. Document the procedure, noting the use of an assistant. Include the patient's tolerance of the procedure. *(Notes transfer of patient and tolerance of procedure.)*

Documentation Example

Smooth transfer from bed to wheelchair using mechanical lift and an assistant. Seatbelt in place; chair positioned next to nurse's station. (Nurse's time-stamped electronic signature)

Up in chair X 30 min. Returned patient to bed with assistance and placed into position of comfort, call light within reach. Stated "it felt good to be out of the bed" and rated pain as 2 out of 10. (Nurse's time-stamped electronic signature)

Special Considerations

- Allow patient to see how the lift works before attempting transfer of patient if at all possible.
- In home situation, instruct caregivers thoroughly in use of lift, and provide a demonstration of the equipment.

Critical Thinking Questions

1. How would you handle the situation if your patient, who is to be transferred from the bed to a chair with a lift for the first time, is very frightened of this procedure?
2. Why do you think it is essential that the sling for the lift be attached exactly according to the directions that come with it?

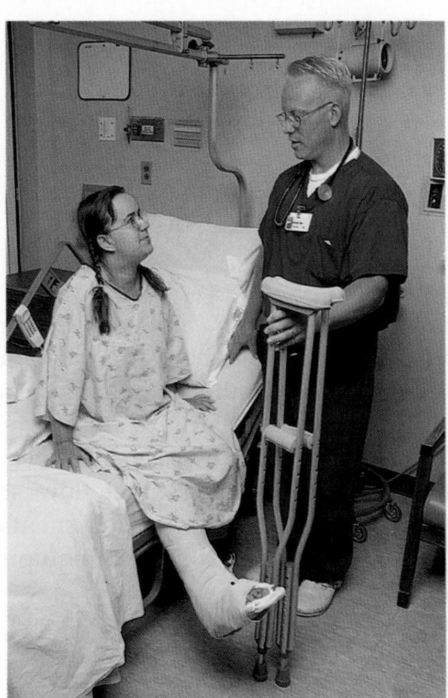

FIGURE 39.14 A patient receiving the beginning of instruction in crutch walking.

throughout the hospital stay or at home. Any problems must both be noted in the medical record and reported promptly to the primary care provider. Handle prosthetic devices carefully as they are made for the specific individual, are expensive, and take many weeks to obtain. Label all the devices with the patient's name and do not allow them out of the room unless in place on the patient.

Rehabilitation

As patients recover from immobilization or from serious illness that restricts usual activity, an exercise prescription may be written to improve muscle tone, joint flexibility, and/or cardiovascular fitness. Parameters for exercise are determined by a target heart rate during activity that is based on age and condition. In a healthy person the target heart rate for aerobic activity is a minimum of 60% of the age-predicted maximum heart rate (subtract the current age from 220 and multiply by the percentage). The ideal training target is 80% of the age-predicted maximum heart rate (American Heart Association, 2015).

Box 39.5 Guidelines to be Considered When Teaching Crutch Walking

- The head is held up, and the eyes look ahead, as in normal walking.
- The crutches are placed slightly ahead of the patient's feet and to the outside of each foot.
- The hands, not the axillae, are used to support the body's weight.
- The back should be kept straight, and the patient should bend at the hips.
- The crutches and affected foot or leg should be moved forward together (at the same time), except when using a swinging gait.
- A smooth, easy rhythm should be achieved in shifting the weight from the crutches to the unaffected (good) leg and then to the crutches again.
- The crutches should be of the proper length and equipped with heavy rubber suction tips to prevent slipping.
- The gait used will depend on the weight-bearing status of the lower extremities and the patient's abilities.

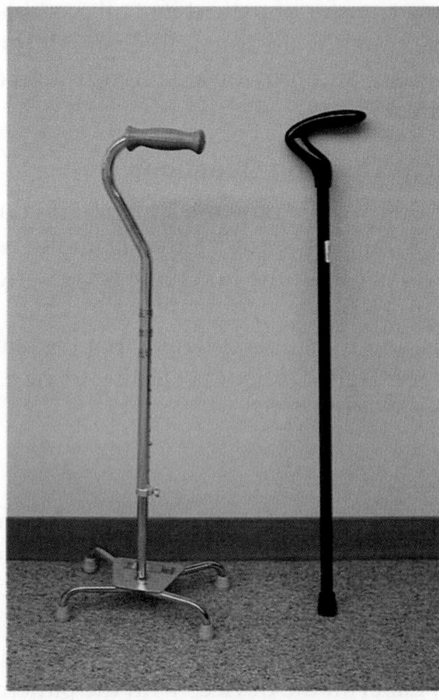

FIGURE 39.15 A regular cane *(right)* provides support, whereas a quad cane *(left)* provides support and stability because of its broad base.

Patients who have had a joint immobilized are often sent to an outpatient physical therapy facility for an individual exercise program to regain maximum strength and mobility of the joint and extremity.

◆ EVALUATION

Evaluation is performed daily by considering whether the specific expected outcomes have been met. Does the skin remain healthy, or are there signs of breakdown? Evaluate the breath sounds, and note any developing cough or signs of dyspnea. Observe the patient's emotional status, including the attitude toward therapy or visitors. Is the patient alert and active in social interactions or withdrawn, hostile, or depressed? If nursing interventions are not achieving the expected outcomes, the care plan needs to be revised. Evaluation statements indicating that some of the expected outcomes stated earlier are being met might be as follows:

- Performing sponge bath, mouth care, and grooming tasks except for left foot.
- Skin is clean, dry, and without redness or abrasion.
- Respirations normal with clear breath sounds bilaterally.
- Demonstrating pleasant interactions with family, friends, and staff.
- Patient is knitting and working on crossword puzzles daily.
- Watching television news show several times a day and discussing events with visitors.
- Asking if a haircut is possible and wants to wear own clothes.
- Checking social media and sending emails and texts to friends, family, and co-workers.

Box 39.6 Guidelines for Using a Cane

Instruction for walking with a cane includes ensuring that:

- The cane has an intact rubber tip.
- The patient uses the cane on the unaffected side unless directed by the therapist or primary care provider to use it on the other side for balance reasons.
- The patient does not lean on or bear full weight on the affected leg.
- The caregiver walks beside the patient on the affected side to provide support in case the patient begins to fall.
- The handgrip is at hip level and the person's elbow is bent at a 15- to 30-degree angle when placing weight on the cane.
- The cane's tip is 6 to 10 inches (15 to 25 cm) to the side and 6 inches (15 cm) in front of the near foot.
- The patient looks straight ahead while walking.

Documentation

Each member of the health care team must maintain a written record of the treatments provided and its effects. Documentation should include any changes in skin integrity, respiratory status, or signs of peripheral circulatory changes. Many assessment aspects can be recorded on an activity/assessment flow sheet. For proper reimbursement, it is vital to document data that indicate a continuing need for use of equipment and ambulation aids.

Get Ready for the NCLEX Examination!

Key Points

- It is essential to include measures to prevent the complications of immobility in the nursing care plan.
- Pay particular attention to respiratory and circulatory function.
- Active or passive exercise is extremely important for the immobilized patient.
- There are special beds and a variety of pressure relief devices available to prevent pressure injuries and other complications of immobility.
- Frequent visitors and inclusion of the patient in family life are important to prevent social isolation.
- The older adult is at higher risk for the complications of immobility and may suffer more psychosocial problems.
- Splints are used for immobilization of an injury or for stabilization of an area with paralysis or weakness.
- Traction is used to treat muscle spasm and fractures. To be effective, the body must be correctly aligned, ropes and pulleys must not be impeded, and weights must hang free.
- Skin traction is applied with a Velcro boot, adhesive strips, slings, or wraps; it is noninvasive, but can be damaging or irritating to the skin.
- External fixators may be used to stabilize a fracture, rather than using a cast, so the patient can be more active during healing.
- Casts are applied to immobilize a particular body part to allow bone healing. They must be handled gently while drying.
- Inspect casts every shift for cracks, crumbling, pressure problems, and signs of infection beneath them. If they become too tight, they may be bivalved.
- The CPM machine is used to exercise the joint after joint replacement surgery.
- Assessment of neurovascular status, of function of an immobilizing device, and of body systems for complications is performed each shift.
- Nursing diagnoses are related to impaired physical mobility, altered tissue perfusion, the risk of complications, and psychosocial problems.
- Elastic bandages are applied to immobilize a joint or to reduce swelling. Perform neurovascular assessment while they are in place.
- To transfer a patient safely with a mechanical lift, two people should perform the procedure. Always follow the facility's policy.
- Never leave a patient alone while suspended in the sling of the lift.
- Aids to mobilization include walkers, crutches, canes, wheelchairs, braces, and prostheses.
- For walkers and canes, the patient's arms should have the elbows placed at a 15- to 30-degree angle when the hands are gripping the device.
- There should be at least two fingerbreadths of space between the top of the crutch and the axilla when the patient's hands are gripping the crutches.
- Crutches, canes, and walkers should have rubber tips on the feet of the device.
- Wheelchairs are placed in locked position when transferring patients in or out of them, and whenever the patient is placed in a stationary position.
- Braces and prostheses must be handled gently and kept with the patient. Tissue under the device should be assessed before application and when the device is removed.
- Evaluation data are collected to determine whether expected outcomes of nursing care plans have been met.
- Documentation is vital for proper reimbursement for equipment and specialty beds.

Additional Learning Resources

SG Go to your Study Guide for additional learning activities to help you master this chapter content.

evolve Go to your Evolve website (http://evolve.elsevier.com/Williams/fundamental/) for the following FREE learning resources:

- Animations
- Answer Guidelines for Think Critically boxes and Critical Thinking Questions and Activities
- Answers and Rationales for Review Questions for the NCLEX Examination
- Concept Map Creator
- Glossary with pronunciations in English and Spanish
- Interactive Review Questions and Exercises for the NCLEX Examination and more!

Review Questions for the NCLEX Examination

*Choose the **best** answer(s) for each question.*

1. You are to perform range-of-motion exercises three times a day with your patient who is immobilized. Range-of-motion exercise promotes circulation by:
   1. Thinning the blood so that it will move freely.
   2. Releasing the one-way valves in the veins and arteries.
   3. Contracting the muscles surrounding a vein, forcing blood to move toward the heart.
   4. Raising the temperature of the tissues, thereby decreasing blood viscosity so it flows more freely.
2. Passive range-of-motion exercises are performed to prevent the problem of:
   1. Formation of a thrombus in the leg.
   2. Sluggish circulation in the extremities.
   3. Skin breakdown over pressure points.
   4. Decreased joint mobility.

3. In addition to good skin care and frequent turning, measures that may help prevent development of pressure injuries in an immobilized patient are: *(Select all that apply.)*
   1. Have family encourage the patient to perform active ROM exercises on unaffected extremities.
   2. Restrict calories to reduce weight gain while immobile.
   3. Encourage adequate nutritional and fluid intake.
   4. Keep the patient's skin clean and dry.
   5. Place the patient on an air fluidized mattress.
4. When assessing the patient with a new cast on the lower arm, if you find that the cast is tight and almost flush to the skin, you would **first**:
   1. Immediately call the orthopedic technician to come and check the cast.
   2. Elevate the extremity on two pillows, making certain it is higher than heart level.
   3. Report the finding to the charge nurse on the unit.
   4. Question the patient as to whether the arm has been kept in an elevated position.
5. A cast that is too tight can directly cause: *(Select all that apply.)*
   1. Pressure on nerves and nerve damage.
   2. Constriction of blood vessels, decreasing circulation.
   3. Blood clot formation.
   4. Numbness and tingling in the extremity.
   5. Faster healing of the fractured bone
6. You notice that the incision on the knee is opening each time the CPM is at its maximum angle. The patient is also complaining of tightness around the sutures. You should:
   1. Pad the portion of the machine that the heel rests on.
   2. Stop the machine and notify the primary care provider.
   3. Reassess the area in 8 hours.
   4. Increase the angle of flexion of the joint to change the pressure on the heel.
7. The LVN is caring for a patient 5 days after falling and breaking his hip. The patient is bedridden and seems bored. The LVN should: *(Select all that apply.)*
   1. Encourage family to visit several different times throughout the day.
   2. Provide long periods of time between visits so patient has time to himself.
   3. Assist patient in finding television programs of interest to him.
   4. Offer newspaper and magazines for reading.
   5. Increase dose of sleep aid so patient can sleep for longer intervals.

Critical Thinking Activities

Read each clinical scenario and discuss the questions with your classmates.

Scenario A

Margaret Thies, age 47, sustained multiple injuries in an automobile accident. She underwent surgery for a lacerated spleen and her right leg has an external fixator due to two fractures. She will be on bed rest for an extended period.

1. For which complications of immobility do you think Margaret is most at risk?
2. For each complication you identified, list the signs and symptoms that might indicate the complication is occurring.
3. What nursing interventions could you use to help prevent each of the complications listed?

Scenario B

Josh Polaski, age 21, has been treated in the outpatient clinic for a fractured ulna. A short-arm fiberglass cast has been applied.

1. Explain to Josh what he can and cannot do while the cast is in place.
2. Teach Josh how to care for the cast and how to assess for complications.
3. How would patient education differ if the patient were sent home with a plaster cast?

Scenario C

Oscar Nunez, age 38, is in traction for a fractured femur suffered in a motorcycle accident. He has been hospitalized for 4 days and is very bored and restless.

1. What assessments would you make to determine whether his restlessness has a physical cause?
2. If his restlessness seems to be psychological in nature, what activities might you suggest to help him occupy the time and his mind?

chapter 40

Common Physical Care Problems of the Older Adult

http://evolve.elsevier.com/Williams/fundamental

Objectives

Upon completing this chapter, you should be able to do the following:

Theory

1. Explain the effect of physical changes on the older adult's lifestyle.
2. Discuss five common age-related physical care problems of the older adult.
3. Identify three ways to promote mobility in older adults.
4. List four ways for the older adult to prevent falls in the home.
5. Review the physical and psychological consequences of chronic incontinence.
6. Discuss how multiple factors affecting older adults may lead to an alteration in nutrition.
7. Explain techniques to facilitate communication and safety for the patient with a sensory deficit.
8. Recognize sexual concerns among the older adult population.
9. Identify five reasons why the older adult is prone to the problem of polypharmacy.

Clinical Practice

1. Perform patient education regarding fall prevention.
2. Formulate a plan to assist an older adult in decreasing or preventing incontinence.
3. Teach an older adult specific ways to enhance nutritional status.
4. Assist a patient in developing a self-medication reminder system.

Key Terms

age-related macular degeneration (AMD) (MĂK-ū-lăr dē-jĕn-ĕr-Ā-shŭn, p. 822)
beta-carotene (BĀ-tă KĂR-ō-tēn, p. 823)
cataracts (KĂT-ă-răkts, p. 822)
dyspareunia (dĭs-pă-RŪ-nē-ă, p. 824)
dysphagia (dĭs-FĀ-zhă, p. 821)
fecal impaction (ĭm-PĂK-shŭn, p. 820)
glaucoma (glăw-KŌ-mă, p. 822)
polypharmacy (pŏl-ē-FĂR-mă-sē, p. 824)
postural hypotension (PŎS-chŭr-ăl hī-pō-TĔN-shŭn, p. 818)
presbycusis (prĕz-bē-KŪ-sŭs, p. 823)
presbyopia (prĕz-bē-Ō-pē-ă, p. 822)
tinnitus (TĪN-ĭ-tŭs, p. 823)
visual accommodation (p. 822)

Concepts Covered in This Chapter

- Development
- Functional ability
- Health promotion
- Mobility
- Nutrition
- Patient education
- Safety
- Sensory perception
- Sexuality

GETTING OLDER

With aging, every body system undergoes some changes that may not necessarily result in disease or illness, but will cause health problems to be more frequent (Table 40.1). Five of the most common physical care problems that plague the older adult population are (1) impaired mobility, (2) alteration in elimination (urinary incontinence, constipation, and fecal impaction), (3) alteration in nutrition, (4) sensory (vision and hearing) deficits, and (5) polypharmacy. Sexuality concerns also are common. Table 40.2 presents the causes of and contributing factors to these problems. Chronic illnesses such as Parkinson disease, arthritis, emphysema, or cardiac disease may compound these problems. Information on these chronic illnesses may be found in a medical-surgical nursing textbook.

IMMOBILITY

Decreased mobility often leads to numerous complications for the older adult. An acute health

Table 40.1 Summary of Common Physiologic Changes of Aging

SYSTEM AFFECTED	COMMON CHANGE WITH AGE
Neurologic and special senses	Fewer and smaller neurons Eye: lens thickens, becomes more yellow and less elastic Ear: decreased ability to hear high-frequency sounds Decreased smell, taste, and touch perception
Cardiovascular	Decreased total body water Increased stiffness of heart muscle and blood vessels Increased incidence of murmurs Slower diastolic filling Moderate increase in systolic blood pressure
Respiratory	Less efficient gas exchange and ability to handle secretions Increased stiffness of chest wall
Gastrointestinal	Taste bud atrophy and loss of teeth Decreased esophageal motility; increased incidence of gastric reflux/gastroesophageal reflux disease (GERD) Increased gastric pH Atrophy of intestinal mucosa and pancreas Decreased liver size and blood flow
Genitourinary	Decreased bladder tone and capacity Increased urine production at night Thinned urethral mucosa after menopause
Integumentary	Decreased elasticity, uneven pigmentation Decreased subcutaneous fat Decreased sebaceous and sweat gland activity Loss of hair follicles; thinning and graying of hair
Musculoskeletal	Average loss in height, typically 3 inches; can be greater with severe osteoporosis Decreased muscle mass; decreased number of muscle fibers
Endocrine	Decreased estrogen production in women (menopause) Decreased testosterone production in men (andropause) Decreased adrenal function (adrenopause) Decreased growth hormone–insulin-like growth factor (somatopause)

From Meiner, S. E. (2011). *Gerontologic nursing* (4th ed.). St. Louis: Elsevier Mosby; Touhy, T., & Jett, K. (2014). *Ebersole & Hess' toward healthy aging: Human needs and nursing responses* (8th ed.). St. Louis: Elsevier. Mosby.

condition requiring bed rest may cause further immobility and, consequently, various other problems associated with immobility (see Chapter 39). Diseases that interfere with adequate circulation and oxygenation contribute to activity intolerance and immobility (Concept Map 40.1). For the person with such a problem, personal hygiene, eating, and socializing may become too difficult because of exhaustion. Poor nutrition may result from immobility or the lack of energy to obtain or prepare food.

NURSING INTERVENTIONS TO PROMOTE MOBILITY

By immediately addressing mobility needs, you can often quickly get the patient back to her former level of activity and avoid potential complications. Educate the older adult about engaging in lifelong activity to maintain optimal mobility. It has been proven that walking 30 minutes a day is beneficial, but doing this even three times a week is better than not walking at all. Strength training with resistance devices, using free weights or weight machines, has been shown to decrease the risk of osteoporosis, muscle wasting, low back pain, and diabetes and to improve the ability to perform activities of daily living (ADLs) needed to maintain functional independence. Strength training also improves balance and walking endurance for older adults even in their 90s. Walking speed, also called gait velocity, is considered to be such an important measurement in the older adult that it has been described by some as the "sixth vital sign" (Peel et al., 2012). Dancing, gardening, home maintenance, and swimming can also promote mobility.

Health Promotion

***HEALTHY PEOPLE 2020* OBJECTIVES FOR PHYSICAL ACTIVITY**

- Reduce the proportion of adults who engage in no leisure-time physical activity.
- Increase the proportion of adults who meet current federal physical activity guidelines for aerobic physical activity and for muscle strengthening activity.

Source: http://www.healthypeople.gov/2020/topics-objectives/topic/physical-activity/objectives

Participating in craft activities and arthritis programs can help preserve fine motor movement. Proper treatment for arthritis and osteoporosis helps prevent immobility problems. Hormone therapy (HT) and adequate dietary or supplemental calcium and vitamin D in combination with weight-bearing exercise are protective against osteoporosis in women. However, HT's potential side effects and risk of breast cancer, heart disease, blood clots, and stroke make its use controversial (Mayo Clinic Staff, 2015). Such

Table 40.2 **Common Physical Care Problems of Older Adults**

PHYSICAL CARE PROBLEM	EFFECT OF AGING ON SYSTEM	OTHER CONTRIBUTING FACTORS AND DISEASES
Impaired mobility	Major loss of calcium, decreased bone density, decreased muscle mass, loss of joint flexibility	Osteoporosis, falls, gout, foot problems, obesity, arthritis, cardiac and respiratory disease, depression, neurologic disorders (e.g., multiple sclerosis)
Urinary incontinence	Altered sphincter control, loss of bladder muscle tone, enlarged prostate, cystocele, rectocele, uterine prolapse, diminished kidney function	Immobility, neurologic disorder (e.g., stroke), urinary tract infection, urinary retention
Constipation	Decreased bowel motility	Immobility, decreased abdominal musculature, insufficient fluid and fiber in diet, hemorrhoids, diverticulosis, depression, nervous system disorders, cognitive impairment, poor dentition, pain medications (e.g., codeine), other medications (e.g., antidepressants and anticholinergics)
Alteration in nutrition	Diseased teeth, poorly fitting dentures, decline in taste buds, decline in sense of smell, dysphagia	Neurologic deficit (e.g., stroke); impaired vision; impaired mobility; anorexia; lack of income, transportation, or facilities; dementia; alcohol abuse; depression; taste alterations (e.g., cancer therapy); multiple medications
Vision deficit	Presbyopia, age-related macular degeneration, glaucoma, cataracts	Inadequate income for eye care, diabetes, arteriosclerosis, long-term steroid use
Hearing deficit	Presbycusis, tinnitus, otosclerosis	Long-term exposure to loud noise, heredity, Ménière disease, labyrinthitis
Polypharmacy	Affects multiple systems	Impaired senses, multiple chronic disorders, impaired cognitive functioning, forgetfulness, multiple providers prescribing, borrowing drugs from others, use of multiple pharmacies, miscommunication or lack of education, use of over-the-counter medications

drugs as alendronate sodium, risedronate sodium, ibandronate sodium, calcitonin-salmon, raloxifene hydrochloride, and denosumab can help to rebuild bone or stop its loss. Anti-inflammatory drugs can also help to maintain mobility. Etanercept, an immunomodulator, may be used for patients with rheumatoid arthritis if they have poor response to other treatment.

The period of bed rest during illness should be as limited as possible. Even transferring a patient from the bed to a chair has beneficial effects. Teach the bed rest patient active range-of-motion (ROM) activities and isometric exercises (applying pressure against resistance). An example of isometric exercise is instructing the patient to push into the bed with her hands and attempt to lift her hips while sitting up in bed. If the patient is too weak to perform these exercises, assist with passive ROM exercises to maintain joint flexibility and help to prevent muscle wasting. If the older adult is noncommunicative, assess for pain using the guidelines in Chapter 31 before implementing ROM exercises.

? Think Critically

ROM exercises may be considered a "chore" for the patient on bed rest. What types of creative exercises or activities can you encourage that would be therapeutic and enjoyable?

With hospital stays so short, begin efforts to restore the patient to her maximum mobility potential as soon as possible. When it is medically indicated, ambulate the patient with assistance. Ensure that appropriate assistance devices, such as sturdy footwear, eyeglasses, walkers, and canes, are brought from home. If the individual is too weak, seek a physical therapy (PT) referral. Such rehabilitative services are essential to promote quality of life for the older adult.

The nursing home setting allows the nurse to monitor and promote mobility over an extended period. All patients should be considered for assisted ambulation unless an underlying condition or illness (e.g., paralysis, severe cardiac disease) prevents it. The older adult who is not ambulated will deteriorate and eventually be unable to walk. Although staff may be reluctant to

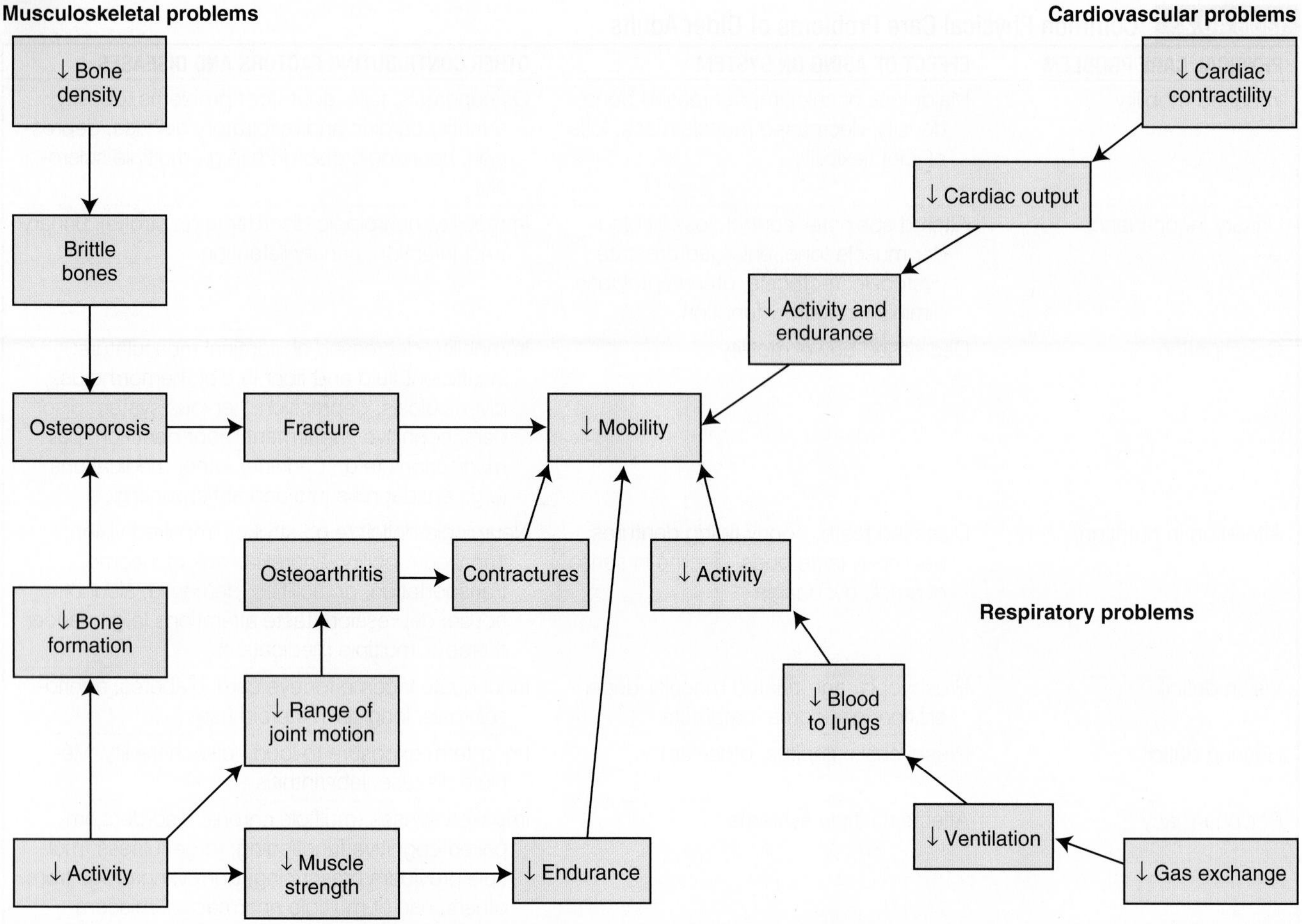

Musculoskeletal problems

↓ Bone density
Brittle bones
Osteoporosis
Fracture
↓ Bone formation
Osteoarthritis
Contractures
↓ Range of joint motion
↓ Activity
↓ Muscle strength
↓ Endurance
↓ Mobility

Cardiovascular problems

↓ Cardiac contractility
↓ Cardiac output
↓ Activity and endurance

Respiratory problems

↓ Activity
↓ Blood to lungs
↓ Ventilation
↓ Gas exchange

CONCEPT MAP 40.1 Relationship of physical changes to decreased mobility.

encourage ambulation of a resident with an unsteady gait, many patients would rather risk a fall than be placed in a wheelchair. You may have to weigh the risk of the older adult falling versus the negative effects of prolonged immobility.

PREVENTING FALLS

Falls are one of the most common safety problems for the older adult. Approximately one-third of those older than 65 years fall each year. For people older than 65, falls are the leading cause of fatal injuries, nonfatal injuries, and hospital trauma admissions. Falls may not always result in serious injury; however, falls can cause hip fractures or traumatic brain injury. Falls often lead to a fear of falling, resulting in physical deconditioning and increased risk of future falls (Centers for Disease Control and Prevention [CDC], 2015). It has been demonstrated that assessing a patient's risk factors for falls and developing targeted nursing interventions based on the assessment are effective strategies for fall prevention (Edelman & Ficorelli, 2012).

Changes in the older adult's posture, balance, gait, and vision contribute to the risk of a fall. Environmental factors, such as clutter in walking areas, inadequate lighting or glare, improper footwear, and unsafe furnishings (such as scatter rugs), predispose the person to falls. Even walkers and canes can increase the risk of falls (Roman de Mettelinge & Cambier, 2015).

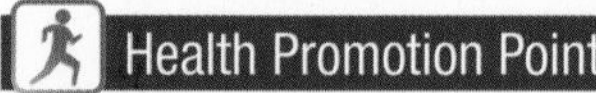

TAI CHI FOR BALANCE

Tai Chi is a form of exercise that has been demonstrated to improve balance. It is also good for improving coordination, stimulating the brain, and decreasing pain in osteoarthritis. Many community recreation centers and colleges offer classes in Tai Chi. Encourage older adults to participate in this activity.

Medications frequently contribute to falls. With each additional medication consumed, the risk of falls is increased. Sedatives, hypnotics, and tranquilizers can decrease alertness and slow reaction time. Diuretics, antihypertensives, and antihistamines increase the risk of **postural (or orthostatic) hypotension** (unusually low blood pressure upon standing), which may cause the patient to become lightheaded and fall.

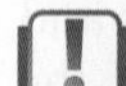

Safety Alert

MEDICATION LISTS

All adults, but especially older adults, should bring in a list of medications and over-the-counter (OTC) preparations they are using when they visit their health care provider. Review the list in light of any new symptom the patient is experiencing. The patient's pharmacist should also have a continually updated copy of this list. This helps prevent adverse events from medication interactions.

Most falls occur in the bedroom or the bathroom. Assess the home environment to see how the patient navigates in these areas during ADLs. Perform patient and family education about risk factors and measures to avoid falls. If the patient is cognitively impaired, implement a toileting schedule to discourage self-toileting and a potential fall. Do not leave patients unattended who unsafely attempt these actions. Hip protectors may prevent falls or reduce the severity of injury if a fall happens (Willy & Osterberg, 2014). Move older adults slowly out of bed to prevent possible orthostatic hypotension. Elastic support stockings may help prevent or lessen such hypotension. Patients should use appropriate footwear. Use a gait belt until independent ambulation is established. Use assistance devices, such as a cane or walker, to provide a wider base of support and increase stability when needed.

Place the call light so it is readily available to the patient who is in bed, in a chair, or in the bathroom. Keep patient beds in the low position with brakes engaged unless a caregiver is at the bedside. Answer lights promptly to avoid unsafe attempts to stand or walk. Maintain clear walking paths, adjust lighting, and wipe up spills from the floor promptly.

Use protective devices only when there is a documented reason and only after the patient or her guardian has given permission and they are ordered by the primary care provider. This includes waist devices, safety belts, and geri chairs. Federal Omnibus Budget Reconciliation Act (OBRA) regulations are specific about when and what types of devices are permissible. Check the guidelines at your place of employment, and follow its policies.

Perform patient and family education about hazards in the home and how to prevent falls in the home. If the older adult is being discharged from the hospital and lives alone, make a referral for a member of the health care team to assess the home for potential safety hazards. Encourage family members and significant others to make regular visits to the older adult's home to check for unsafe conditions.

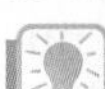

QSEN CONSIDERATIONS: Safety

Fall Prevention

Take the following steps to prevent a fall:

- Use bright, nonglare lighting in each room of the house.
- Keep eyeglasses clean.
- Get up from the bed or chair slowly and stand before walking.
- Avoid tipping the head backward (extending the neck) to obtain something from a shelf, wash a tall window, or hang clothes, since this may cause you to lose your balance.
- Use flat shoes and slippers with nonskid soles. Avoid long, loose-fitting clothing that may cause tripping or get caught on furniture or doorknobs.
- Use a night light in the bedroom and bathroom, or turn on a lamp before getting up at night. Wait for your eyes to adjust to the light before arising.
- If you become dizzy, sit down immediately if possible, or hold on to something solid.
- Avoid using scatter rugs and small bathroom mats that can slide.
- Avoid slick, high polish on floors, and do not walk on wet floor surfaces.
- Use a nonskid mat in the bathtub or shower.
- Install a grab rail in the bath or shower and near the toilet.
- Wipe up spills immediately.
- Watch for pets underfoot.
- Avoid clutter in living spaces.
- Select furniture that provides stability and support such as chairs with arms.
- Check walking aids routinely for worn rubber tips, and replace them as needed.
- Avoid floor coverings with a busy pattern.
- Install handrails on both sides of stairs.

Discourage older adults from climbing a ladder or standing on a chair to reach high places. If a person needs to reach a high area, suggest using a stepstool with a broad base of support. If balance is unsteady, instruct the individual not to reach for objects above head level. Devices to assist with reaching can be purchased to avoid the temptation to reach overhead.

ALTERATION IN ELIMINATION

URINARY INCONTINENCE

Incontinence is one of the most common reasons that older adults are institutionalized. Families who cope with other health problems are often unable to deal with incontinence. Embarrassment, social withdrawal, depression, and low self-esteem are common for the older adult who is incontinent. These factors can be linked to an older adult's ability to self-manage care (Agency for Healthcare Research and Quality [AHRQ], 2012).

Urinary incontinence is *not* a normal consequence of aging. Incontinence can be the result of an acute condition or a chronic problem. Approximately half of noninstitutionalized older women and approximately one-quarter of noninstitutionalized men report urinary incontinence. This number approaches 75% of people who are long-term residents of nursing homes (Centers for Disease Control and Prevention, 2014). Causes and treatment of incontinence are presented in Chapter 29. Temporary incontinence may develop as a result of an acute illness. If the patient is helped to regain continence as soon as the acute episode is over, permanent incontinence can often be avoided. **An underlying cause should always be sought when incontinence occurs.** Bowel incontinence is not as common as urinary incontinence.

Nursing Interventions for Urinary Incontinence

Management of incontinence can be frustrating for both patient and nurse. Incontinence is also costly; annual costs are estimated at $28 billion in the United States (Academy of Women's Health, 2015).

Box 40.1 Behavioral Approaches to Urinary Incontinence

- **Bladder retraining:** *Goal:* Restore normal pattern of voiding by inhibiting or stimulating voiding and by lengthening the time between voidings.
- **Prompted voiding:** *Goal:* Teach the patient to be aware of toileting needs and to request assistance from the caregiver.
- **Habit (timed) voiding:** *Goal:* Take confused or cognitively impaired patients to the toilet at regular intervals.

Treatment is based on the underlying cause and may include such medication as oxybutynin chloride or doxazosin mesylate to relax the smooth muscle of the bladder or prostate. Herbal approaches include the use of saw palmetto and pumpkin seeds, which might reduce prostate swelling; however, in recent studies, saw palmetto demonstrated little or no benefit (Medline Plus, 2015). Treatment may also include surgery or behavioral interventions (Box 40.1). Measures to reduce episodes of incontinence can be found in Chapter 29.

You can help prevent skin breakdown by keeping the patient who is incontinent clean and dry and by using a skin-protecting product. The use of easy-release clothing, protective pads, and condom catheters for men can hinder skin breakdown, avoid the soiling of bed and clothing, and prevent embarrassment for the patient. Encouraging fluids can decrease the urine concentration so it is less irritating, less predisposing to urinary tract infections, and less odoriferous.

Managing urinary incontinence depends not only on effective interventions but also on the health care team's belief that improvement is possible. A continence coordinator can be a valuable resource person in providing information and encouraging staff efforts in achieving patient goals.

CONSTIPATION AND FECAL IMPACTION

Constipation is a common problem among older adults. Many older people believe anything other than a daily bowel movement is abnormal. Before deciding whether constipation is a problem, assess the frequency, the amount, and the consistency of stools and possible contributing factors (see Chapter 30).

Fecal impaction can rapidly develop in the ill older adult who, while on bed rest, is receiving pain medication and not eating a normal diet. It may also develop in the older adult with memory impairment, such as Alzheimer disease, who forgets to heed the urge to defecate. Careful record keeping of bowel movements, especially in those with memory impairment, is important in prevention of fecal impaction. Signs and symptoms may include abdominal cramping or rectal pain, abdominal distention, the passing of small amounts of liquid stool, and loss of appetite. Digital examination of the rectum often reveals a mass. **You must check whether an order is required at your employing institution before performing this procedure.**

QSEN CONSIDERATIONS: Safety

Checking for Fecal Impaction

Perform digital examination with caution, especially in patients with cardiac disease. Digital examination can result in an unusually low heart rate because of vagal stimulation. A low heart rate may lead to cardiac arrhythmia and possibly cardiac arrest.

Nursing Interventions for Constipation and Fecal Impaction

Along with the interventions for constipation (see Chapter 30), patient education should include specific diet remedies such as hot water and lemon juice first thing on arising, prunes, prune juice with carbonated drink, bran cereal or whole grain breads, roughage (such as raw fruits and vegetables), and fluid intake of at least 2500 mL/day. Encourage the patient to adopt an acceptable exercise program, and advise her to heed the urge to defecate quickly to avoid a potential problem. Impacted stool may require manual removal. An oil retention enema should be ordered to soften stool before impaction removal.

Think Critically

Beans are an excellent source of fiber for relieving constipation. Your patient complains that beans give her gas. Can you suggest three alternate high fiber vegetables?

ALTERATION IN NUTRITION

Nutritional needs of older adults are discussed in Chapter 26. Dietary Reference Intake (DRI) tables provide recommendations for older adults (Table 40.3); however, these do not consider requirements for additional nutrients related to decreased absorption, infection, or chronic illness.

It is recommended that older adults reduce their sugar and fat intake and increase the roughage in their diet. Controversy remains as to whether increased nutrients are needed. Some researchers suggest that an increase in whole grain foods, fruits, and vegetables, and additional sources of protein, may help older adults to maintain proper nutrition.

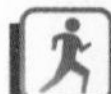

Health Promotion

***HEALTHY PEOPLE 2020* OBJECTIVES FOR NUTRITION**

- Increase the proportion of adults who are at a healthy weight.
- Reduce the proportion of adults who are obese.

Source: http://www.healthypeople.gov/2020/topics-objectives/topic/nutrition-and-weight-status/objectives

Obesity contributes to joint problems and poses a risk for hypertension, heart disease, and stroke. Older adults should adjust their caloric intake to coincide

Table 40.3 **Guidelines for Nutrient Needs of the Older Adult**

NUTRIENT	GENERAL GUIDELINE	RATIONALE/EXPLANATION
Calories	Men: *Not physically active:* 2000 kcal/day *Somewhat active:* 2200-2400 kcal/day *Active:* 2400-2800 kcal/day Women: *Not physically active:* 1600 kcal/day *Somewhat active:* 1800 kcal/day *Active:* 2000-2200 kcal/day	Energy requirements tend to decrease with age. Health problems arise when intake totals are less than 1500 kcal/day.
Protein	0.66 g of protein per kg of weight per day	Adequate protein is needed to maintain a positive nitrogen balance.
Carbohydrate	100 g per day	Impaired glucose tolerance may occur in older adults if too many carbohydrates, especially simple ones such as sugars, are consumed.
Fat	Oil: 5-8 teaspoon/day Solid fats and added sugars: small amounts	Mostly monounsaturated or polyunsaturated fats should be used. Animal fat intake should be limited, and intake of *trans* fatty acids should be virtually eliminated because these tend to contribute to cardiovascular disease.
Calcium	Men age 51-70: 800 mg/day Men age 71 and older: 1000 mg/day Women age 51 and older: 1000 mg/day	Bone demineralization and osteoporosis are common among older adults.
Vitamin D	10 mcg/day	Insufficient vitamin D results in bone demineralization. Sunlight provides vitamin D, but not when sunscreen is used.
Other vitamins and minerals	Nutrients from foods (i.e., 1.5-2.5 cups of fruit and 2-3 cups of vegetables per day) Daily multivitamin-mineral tablet recommended	Vitamins and minerals are needed to maintain optimal nutritional status and health. Older adults typically do not consume sufficient fruits and vegetables per day; therefore, a multivitamin-mineral tablet is recommended.
Water	Men: 3.7 L/day Women: 2.7 L/day	Older adults are susceptible to dehydration. When fluid loss is excessive, water and electrolytes must be replaced.

From: US Department of Agriculture. (2015). Dietary reference intakes: Recommended intakes for individuals. <https://fnic.nal.usda.gov/dietary-guidance/dietary-reference-intakes/dri-tables-and-application-reports>; National Institute on Aging. (2015). Healthy eating after age 50. <http://www.nia.nih.gov/health/publication/healthy-eating-after-50>.

with their activity to maintain a weight that is appropriate for their height and body build.

NURSING INTERVENTIONS FOR NUTRITIONAL SUPPORT

Make meals more enjoyable for the patient in a long-term care setting by serving the food in an attractive manner and by making the environment as pleasant as possible. Assess for social problems, such as annoying or disruptive people at the table, and appropriately address the issue. A nutritionist can assist in determining the nutritional needs of the institutionalized person. A liquid dietary supplement may be necessary to help the older adult meet dietary needs. Tube feedings or parenteral feedings may have to be used if attempts at oral feedings are unsuccessful. Patients with **dysphagia** (difficulty swallowing) are at high risk for developing a nutritional deficit. A management plan developed from a formal swallowing evaluation may be in place (see Chapter 27, Assisted Feeding). To avoid aspiration, position patients with dysphagia upright or in a high Fowler position and feed very small amounts. You may thicken liquids if recommended by the swallowing evaluation.

QSEN CONSIDERATIONS: Safety

Dysphagia

Assess patients with dysphagia for adequate hydration. Research has shown that thickened liquids may lead to inadequate fluid intake (Ackley & Ladwig, 2014).

Instruct the dysphagia patient to tuck her chin when swallowing. Keep the patient in an upright position for 45 to 60 minutes after eating. Provide a stress-free environment because stress can make dysphagia more pronounced.

Think Critically

Your 75-year-old hemiplegic patient with dysphagia is depressed and anxious over her recent stroke. She motions for you to take away her food. What can you do to maintain her nutritional intake?

SENSORY DEFICITS

VISION DEFICITS

Age-related eye changes can be debilitating if they are not recognized and corrected, and they may result in a severe limitation of the patient's overall independence. **Visual accommodation** (the ability to focus on near and far objects) decreases with age as a result of weakening of the muscles that control the lens. Beginning in their 40s, most people need bifocals or reading glasses to correct **presbyopia** (age-related decreased ability to focus on near objects) and to compensate for loss in accommodation.

The lens of the eye may yellow with age, causing a decline in color perception in older adults. Because the iris has decreased ability to respond to light changes, the older adult may experience difficulty adjusting from light to dark.

As the blood supply to the retina decreases, depth perception, peripheral vision, and night vision decrease. Any loss of peripheral vision should be further evaluated to rule out glaucoma. **Glaucoma,** a common disorder of the aging eye, is the accumulation of fluids inside the eye that exert pressure on the optic nerve, eventually causing blindness. It is often asymptomatic and a frequent cause of preventable blindness.

Older adults frequently develop **cataracts,** a clouding of the lens. Cataracts occur to some extent in almost all older adults, especially those with diabetes. Perhaps the most debilitating eye disorder is **age-related macular degeneration (AMD),** in which the older adult gradually loses acute, central, and color vision. There is no cure for AMD, although some recently developed therapies can delay progression and possibly restore some vision. One sign of AMD is the presence of drusen, which are yellow deposits beneath the retina. Small drusen are common with aging, but larger ones could indicate AMD (see Table 40.4).

Table 40.4 Age-Related Macular Degeneration (AMD)

Risk Factors	Smoking Race: more common in Caucasians Genetics
Signs	Drusen: medium to large Pigment changes beneath retina
Symptoms (vision loss)	Early/intermediate stages: no Late stage: yes
Stages	Early: medium-size drusen Intermediate: large drusen; pigment changes Late: vision loss—two types • Geographic atrophy ("dry" AMD): breakdown of macular cells and supporting cells • Neovascularization ("wet" AMD): new blood vessels grow beneath retina, leaking fluid and blood, leading to edema and damage to macula
Treatment	Early stages: comprehensive, annual dilated eye examination Intermediate/late stages: Age-Related Eye Disease Studies (AREDS and AREDS2) identified specific nutrient combinations that may help slow progression of the disease: • 500 mg of vitamin C • 400 international units of vitamin E • 80 mg zinc as zinc oxide (25 mg in AREDS2) • 2 mg copper as cupric oxide • 15 mg beta-carotene, OR 10 mg lutein and 2 mg zeaxanthin Advanced neovascular: • Drug injections into the eye • Photodynamic therapy using lasers • Laser surgery

Source: National Eye Institute (2015).

Nursing Interventions for the Visually Impaired

Measures to enhance vision include the use of medications, surgery, and prosthetic devices. There are many degrees of vision loss, and interventions are geared to promote the individual's maximum independence.

You must orient the patient with vision loss to any new environment to avoid potential confusion and anxiety and reduce the risk of accidents. It is imperative to use bright lights and bed rails and remove hazards in the room. Inform all health team members about the patient's vision deficit. All people should identify themselves on entering the patient's room and state when they are leaving to be certain the patient knows of their departure.

Do not rearrange the room or the patient's personal belongings without permission or explanation. Speak before handing an object to her. To promote independence in eating, describe the positions of food on the plate in relation to clock position (e.g., 3 o'clock, 6 o'clock).

When walking with the patient with a visual impairment, offer your arm for guidance. Pause and explain any environmental changes, such as steps, to decrease fear of new surroundings.

For the patient with low vision, devices such as a closed-circuit TV system and the low vision enhancement system (LVES), are available to magnify and illuminate reading material. Telescopic lenses, TV screen magnifiers, large print books, talking books, large-number watches, clocks, and telephones are examples of aids that can be beneficial. Bright, glare-free light is necessary for older adults to move about safely. Night lights may also be helpful. During the day, natural light may be preferable.

Regarding patient and family education, all interventions to assist the patient with independence must be explained to family member who live with the older adult at home. Additional patient education or referrals (e.g., to a blind rehabilitation center) may be necessary for someone who is completely blind. A common concern is the visually impaired older adult who continues driving. This creates a psychosocial issue that involves not only the older adult and the family but society as well. In coping with this concern, many states and provinces now require special testing before reissuing licenses to those over a certain age (ranging from 70 to 80 years of age). Individuals may be given limited licenses that restrict driving to specific distances and areas. Encourage older people who continue to drive to avoid night driving and to wear prescribed hearing aids or glasses to help enhance sensory awareness. Advise older adults to not drive under the influence of alcohol or drugs and to avoid driving in bad weather to avoid an accident.

Encourage the wearing of sunglasses when outside and supplementation with vitamin and mineral antioxidants which may help protect against AMD. Encourage a diet rich in antioxidant foods, such as **beta-carotene,** vitamin E, vitamin C, and selenium (synergistic with vitamin E), as beneficial food choices.

HEARING DEFICIT

The inability to hear high-frequency sounds usually becomes noticeable by late middle age. **Presbycusis** is the inability to hear high-pitched sounds and the inability to hear spoken words. This problem is often intensified with the presence of background noise. **Tinnitus,** or ringing in the ears, may cause further loss of hearing.

Presbycusis is commonly exacerbated by cerumen (earwax) accumulation. **Removal of a wax impaction can make a significant difference in the older adult's hearing ability.** It is of utmost importance to frequently assess whether cerumen is contributing to the hearing loss. Wax can often be softened using mineral oil or baby oil (or a commercial product) and removed at home. Occasionally someone may need to go to an otolaryngologist where suction and miniature instruments may be used to remove the cerumen.

Hearing loss can lead to ongoing frustration and embarrassment for the individual. The person with a hearing deficit may complain of others mumbling and have a reduced tolerance for loud noises. She may pretend to hear when she really does not understand what has been said. This becomes an important concern when attempting to communicate about health-related issues. Hearing should be checked periodically.

Nursing Interventions for the Hearing Impaired

If the patient has a hearing aid, the nurse should know how to operate it. The hearing aid should be free of earwax and fit properly in the ear canal to function correctly. Chapter 19 describes hearing aid care. Periodic irrigation of the auditory canal to remove impacted cerumen is a high priority.

Communication with a person with hearing loss can be difficult for both patient and nurse. Face the patient so she knows you are present, and speak clearly and distinctly in low tones, rephrasing sentences as needed (Fig. 40.1). Facial expressions and gestures can be helpful in communicating messages.

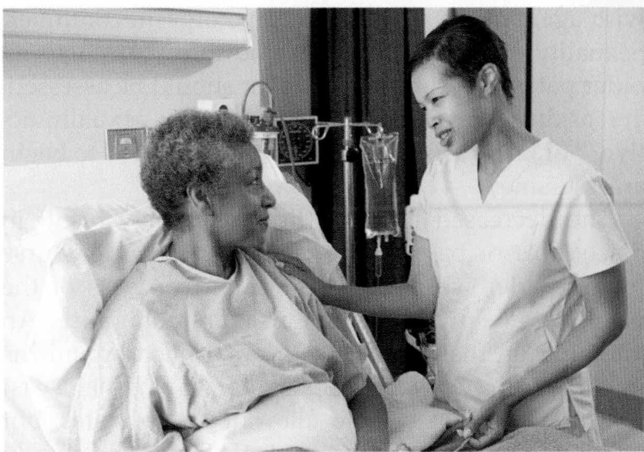

FIGURE 40.1 Communication with the older adult with a vision or hearing deficit. Position yourself in front of the patient where your lips can be seen to communicate. (Photo copyright istock.com)

Conduct your conversations in a well lit area with minimal outside distractions. Do not stand or sit in front of bright lights or windows. Speak toward the patient's "good ear" if possible. If the patient wears glasses, she should have them on to aid in seeing facial expressions and reading lips. Keep environmental noise to a minimum to avoid confusion and improve the clarity of conversation. Use a pad and pencil if messages are still unclear. Under the Americans with Disability Act, facilities must provide reasonable communication accommodations including a qualified sign language interpreter when caring for a patient who is deaf (Cunha, 2013).

Clinical Cues

When working with a patient with a known hearing deficit, seek feedback regarding instructions given. Do not assume that the patient heard correctly even if a hearing aid is worn.

Family members may become frustrated with an older adult who will not get a hearing aid or who will not wear the hearing aid to communicate. As a result, the individual may gradually stop participating in conversation and become isolated. Work with patients and families to enhance communication techniques. Some patients may benefit from a cochlear implant.

? Think Critically

What types of safety measures could you teach the hearing-impaired older adult who lives alone?

SEXUALITY

Despite the general view of the younger generation, the need for sexual expression does not disappear with age. People continue sexual activity into old age. Changing health status, age-related physical changes, and loss of a sex partner do have an effect on the sexual practices of older adults. Sexual response time slows with age, but the ability to achieve orgasm continues. Sexuality may be difficult for you to discuss with an older patient, but it is an area that should be assessed. Try asking questions such as "Are you sexually active?" or "Are you happy with your sex life?" to begin an assessment.

The decreased levels of hormones may result in discomfort or pain (**dyspareunia**) during intercourse for the older woman. Thinning and dryness of the vaginal walls predispose the woman to vaginitis. An alteration in the numbers of normal microorganisms in the vagina may predispose her to vaginal yeast infection. HT can help to alleviate these issues, but because of potential side effects, HT must be closely monitored. Topical vaginal moisteners can be helpful. There has been US Food and Drug Administration (FDA) approval of a medication to enhance sexual drive in women (flibanserin), but it has been approved only for premenopausal women, alcohol is contraindicated when taking the drug, and it has potentially dangerous side effects of hypotension and loss of consciousness.

The older man may experience a slower sexual arousal. Erection is often less firm than when younger. It takes longer for the man to reach an orgasm, and less seminal fluid is released. Diabetes may contribute to impotence. Many resources are available to help the man to achieve erection. Sildenafil citrate, vardenafil, and tadalafil have been successful in promoting a satisfying sex life for older men. Vacuum pumps, penile implants, and penile injections are other aids to achieve an erection. An elastic ring can help a man to maintain an erection once it is achieved. New medications and therapies are being studied, including medications via nasal spray and gene therapy.

Chronic illness or disability may affect one partner's ability to participate in sexual activity. The nurse should explore other ways to help a couple express their sexuality and achieve sexual satisfaction.

A concern is the rise of human immunodeficiency virus (HIV) infection and other sexually transmitted infections (STIs) in the older population. Older adults may not practice safe sex because pregnancy is no longer an issue. It is imperative to perform patient education about the dangers of unprotected sex and the possibility of the transmission of HIV and other STIs. Older women may be at greater risk of HIV infection because of vaginal thinning and dryness leading to tearing of the vaginal area. It is not uncommon for some older adults to strike up a romance within an assisted living facility or a long-term care facility. Chlamydia infections have increased 31% and syphilis 52% in recent years among people age 65 and older (Emanuel, 2014). People with HIV are living longer; almost one-fourth of people with HIV are older than age 50. People may mistake signs of acquired immune deficiency syndrome (AIDS) for normal aging or diseases, such as Alzheimer disease, and care providers may neglect asking the older adult about risky behaviors.

POLYPHARMACY

The greater the number of medications consumed by an individual, the greater the risk of undesirable reactions, drug interactions, and toxicity. **Polypharmacy** is the use of multiple medications, often inappropriately and excessively, at the same time. This often occurs when the patient sees multiple care providers and each is unaware of what the other is prescribing. Patients may use a local pharmacy *and* a mail-order pharmacy, so the pharmacist is unaware of all the drugs the patient is consuming. Individuals older than 65 are the largest users of prescription and OTC drugs and therefore are more likely to experience a polypharmacy situation (Fig. 40.2).

> **Safety Alert**
>
> Nearly half of all emergency department visits by older adults are related to the following medication groups: antiplatelet agents (e.g., aspirin, clopidogrel), anticoagulant medications (e.g., warfarin), and antidiabetic agents (e.g., insulin). These medications are important, but the older adult must be monitored carefully (AHRQ, 2015).

In the older person, drug interactions and toxicity can result in behavioral or cognitive changes that may be mistaken for dementia. Unfortunately, when older people experience adverse drug effects, these problems are often overlooked, inappropriately blamed on the aging process, or treated with yet another medication.

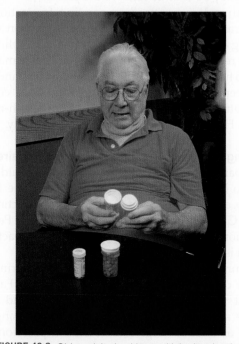

FIGURE 40.2 Older adult checking multiple drug bottles.

Clinical Cues

Whenever an older adult patient develops confusion or a new symptom, it is wise to first check to see if a new medication or supplement has been taken. A patient may build up a toxic level of a drug after being on it for a few days or weeks and show symptoms of adverse effects.

Many factors related to aging alter the rate at which drugs are metabolized and excreted. Absorption, storage, and serum-binding factors all affect the way a drug is used within the body. Decreased body water, increased ratio of fat to muscle, and a low serum albumin all predispose the older patient to drug toxicity and extended duration of drug action (Table 40.5). Alterations in enzyme function, cardiac output, and circulatory function can reduce blood flow to the liver. These changes decrease the liver's effectiveness and speed in metabolizing drugs. Because most drugs are metabolized in the liver, the risk for toxicity increases. The risk for toxicity can significantly increase if the older adult is malnourished, because medications are metabolized more slowly when the diet is inadequate.

Aging kidneys are significantly less effective in excreting drugs, resulting in elevated drug levels and symptoms of toxicity. Some medications, such as digoxin, cause retention of other drugs in the presence of diminished renal function. The use of substances such as alcohol and nicotine can also cause changes in drug elimination in older adults.

NURSING INTERVENTIONS FOR POLYPHARMACY

A thorough medication history is the initial step in preventing polypharmacy. A comprehensive assessment can help maintain a therapeutic medication regimen, identify educational needs, eliminate unnecessary medications, and reduce the risk of adverse drug reactions (Nursing Care Plan 40.1). Specifically, ask questions to obtain information about the patient's current prescriptions, OTC drugs, and any vitamins and herbal preparations being taken. Instruct the patient to bring a bag with all the drugs she takes at home. Assessment data should also include the patient's current administration schedule, knowledge about her medications, medication-related problems, nonadherence problems, frequency of care provider visits, sensory deficits, mental and physical disabilities, ability to purchase and obtain medication, and use of alcohol and caffeine. Ideally, a pharmacist, primary care provider, or nurse practitioner should address these questions. However, the nurse should be prepared to initially assess the patient's drug history and continue to gather information so that a therapeutic medication regimen may be maintained.

In a long-term care facility you must continually assess the number of medications, side effects, and the necessity for each being administered to avoid a potentially dangerous situation.

Assignment Considerations

Medication Administration

If your facility uses nursing assistants who are certified in medication administration, recognize that it remains your responsibility to monitor the patient for correct response and side effects to the medications administered.

Think Critically

Your patient mentions to you that she has been using several pharmacies to get the best price for the six prescriptions and four OTC drugs she takes each day. What types of questions might you ask her in your assessment?

Attempt to reduce the complexity of the medication regimen by improving self-medication practices. Develop a drug reminder system and a schedule that is compatible with the individual's lifestyle to help to decrease confusion and increase adherence. Refer the patient to a home health nurse for monitoring of adherence at home. One frequently used medication reminder system is the daily or weekly pill container, available at pharmacies. Other reminder tactics include the use of check-off systems, calendars, color- or symbol-coded medication bottles, an alarm clock, or a voicemail system. The use of queuing medications with daily events, such as brushing teeth, can also help to promote adherence.

Table 40.5 Age-Related Changes Affecting Drug Therapy in Older Adults

CHANGE	IMPACT	NURSING MEASURES
Drier mucous membrane of oral cavity	Tablets and capsules may stick to roof or sides of mouth and not be swallowed; can dissolve in and irritate mouth.	Offer fluids before drug administration to moisten mouth and ample fluids during and following administration. Inspect mouth or advise patient to inspect mouth for any tablet or capsule that may not have been swallowed. Unless contraindicated, break large tablets to facilitate swallowing.
Decreased circulation to lower bowel and vagina; lower body temperature	Suppositories require longer time to melt and risk being expelled undissolved.	Explore possibility of using alternative route. Allow longer time for suppository to melt. Check or advise patient to check that suppository has melted before getting out of bed to resume activities.

Continued

Table 40.5 Age-Related Changes Affecting Drug Therapy in Older Adults—cont'd

CHANGE	IMPACT	NURSING MEASURES
Decreased tissue elasticity	Patient has poor seal of tissues and oozing after injection; poor absorption.	Use ventrogluteal or vastus lateralis sites for intramuscular injections and rotate sites. Shorter needle may be needed if the patient has decreased muscle mass. Use Z-track injection technique for injections to facilitate sealing. Cleanse any medication that has oozed onto skin.
Decreased pain sensation	Infection or other problem at injection site may not be detected.	Check injection sites regularly.
Decreased cardiac efficiency	Patient has greater risk of circulatory overload during intravenous administration of medications.	Monitor intravenous drip closely. Observe for signs of circulatory overload (e.g., rise in blood pressure, rapid respirations, coughing, shortness of breath).
Less gastric acid	Absorption is slower for drugs that require low gastric pH.	Administer antacids 1-2 hours apart from other medications.
Increase in adipose tissue compared to lean body mass; decreased cardiac output	Drugs stored in adipose tissue (lipid-soluble drugs) have increased tissue concentrations and decreased plasma concentrations and accumulate and remain in body for longer duration; plasma levels of drugs can increase while less is deposited in reservoirs (particularly true of water-soluble drugs).	Ensure dosages are age adjusted. Become familiar with adverse effects of drugs administered and observe for these effects.
Reduced serum albumin levels	Administering several protein-bound drugs together can cause drugs to compete for same protein molecules; some drugs may not effectively bind and may be less effective.	Advise prescribing provider of other protein-bound drugs patient is taking when new protein-bound drug is prescribed; highly protein-bound drugs include phenytoin, warfarin, naproxen, ibuprofen, furosemide, and digitoxin. Ensure serum albumin level is evaluated along with blood level of drug (if serum albumin level is low, patient has greater risk for becoming toxic despite normal or low blood levels of drug).
Reduced number of functioning nephrons; decreased glomerular filtration rate; reduced blood flow	Biologic half-life is extended; drugs take longer to be filtered from body; increased risk of adverse reactions.	Ensure age-adjusted dosages are prescribed for drugs excreted through renal system.

From Touhy, T. & Jett, K. (2014). *Ebersole & Hess' toward healthy aging: Human needs and nursing responses* (8th ed.). St. Louis: Elsevier. Mosby; Edmunds, M. W., & Mayhew, M. S. (2014). *Pharmacology for the primary care provider* (4th ed.). St. Louis: Mosby.

Nursing Care Plan 40.1 Care of the Patient at Risk for Polypharmacy

SCENARIO Alice Woo, age 75, who has a history of emphysema, will be discharged on bumetanide, digoxin, and theophylline after treatment for symptoms related to her failure to correctly follow her prescribed medication protocol. When the nurse was reviewing medications during hospitalization, Mrs. Woo consistently confused the medications and exhibited difficulty remembering when to appropriately take each medication.

PROBLEM AND NURSING DIAGNOSIS *Confused about medications*/Ineffective health management.

Supporting Assessment Data ***Subjective:*** "Sometimes I just can't remember which ones to take in the morning and which ones to take at night." ***Objective:*** Patient cannot correctly identify three pills by name or use. Hospitalized for symptoms related to improper medication use.

Nursing Care Plan 40.1 Care of the Patient at Risk for Polypharmacy—cont'd

Goals/Expected Outcomes	Nursing Interventions	Selected Rationale	Evaluation
Patient will communicate an understanding of need to follow treatment regimen before discharge.	Determine readiness and ability to learn. Reinforce relationship between not following treatment and present hospitalization.	People who are not ready to learn do not learn nearly as well as those who are ready.	*Does patient verbalize an understanding of her treatment regimen?* States she understands the reason for her present hospitalization. Meeting outcome.
Patient will correctly identify all three medications 100% of the time before discharge.	Assess patient's ability to read a medication label. If patient cannot see or read labels, use symbol code system on mock medicine bottles marked with large "B," "D," and "T" (referring to medication names) for easy identification. Review identification method with patient three times a day before discharge. Have significant other or pharmacy label patient's medications with letter symbols.	Patient must be able to read medication labels to correctly identify the medication.	Despite visual impairment, patient is now able to easily recognize the coded letters on medication bottles and correctly identify each medication. Meeting outcome.
Patient will state the correct dose, frequency, and major side effects of each medication.	Teach patient correct dosage, number of pills to take at each dose, and any potential side effects. Reinforce verbal information using large "flash cards." Ask patient to read each card.	To take medication correctly, patient must know this information.	*Can patient state the correct dosage, frequency, and major side effects of each medication?* Patient correctly recites dosage of each medication, number of pills to take at each dose of each medication, and general side effects of each medication. Meeting outcome.
Patient will demonstrate ability to monitor effects of medication by return demonstration of taking pulse correctly and using weight record sheet.	Teach patient to count radial pulse for 1 full minute, noting regularity, and have patient do return demonstration. Teach patient to record daily weight using a sample calendar form.	Accurately counting the radial pulse allows patient to know when not to take the digoxin or when to report an abnormality to the primary care provider. Tracking daily weight is essential to determine whether condition is worsening.	*Is patient monitoring pulse and weight accurately?* Monitoring pulse and weight correctly. Meeting outcome.
Patient will state intent to call primary care provider if pulse is irregular or below 60; if weight changes by more than 5 lb; if ankle edema develops; or if she experiences gastrointestinal symptoms, neurologic changes, or visual problems.	Instruct patient to promptly call primary care provider if side effects occur or general condition changes. Reinforce instructions; provide clearly printed card with primary care provider's telephone number.	Knowing specific signs and symptoms that indicate a change in condition or side effect will reinforce need to call primary care provider.	*Is patient able to verbalize what to report to the primary care provider?* Able to verbalize when to call primary care provider. Meeting outcome.
Patient will state intent to avoid foods and habits that will affect theophylline level, and increase foods that will help prevent potassium loss from bumetanide.	Instruct patient to increase fluids and to limit caffeine products, smoking, and charbroiled foods.	Increasing fluids helps prevent dehydration. Limiting listed items helps maintain a steady theophylline level.	*Can patient identify which foods to avoid and which to increase in diet?* Patient correctly names several foods to avoid, potassium-rich foods, and states understanding of the need to limit caffeine, smoking, and charbroiled foods. Meeting outcome.

Continued

Nursing Care Plan 40.1 Care of the Patient at Risk for Polypharmacy—cont'd

Goals/Expected Outcomes	Nursing Interventions	Selected Rationale	Evaluation
Patient will identify various types of caffeine products and potassium-rich sources.	Encourage patient to decrease consumption of caffeine and increase consumption of potassium-rich foods.	Intake of potassium-rich foods helps prevent hypokalemia.	Patient correctly names several foods to avoid and identifies potassium-rich foods to increase. Meeting outcome.
Patient will state intent to avoid taking antacid products within 1 h of taking digoxin.	Give patient list of foods to avoid or increase to promote drug effectiveness. Instruct patient to avoid concurrent use of antacids with digoxin to avoid ineffective absorption.	A printed list will aid memory and make it easier for patient to adhere to.	*Does patient refrain from taking antacid products inappropriately?* Yes; waits for an hour after taking digoxin to take her antacid.
Patient will demonstrate ability to self-administer prescribed medications.	Give written directions for all medications, doses, and times on a note card in large bold letters.	A reference card helps if patient cannot remember the prescribed dosage.	*Is patient able to administer her medications on schedule?* Able to administer medications correctly from 7-day medication planner. Meeting outcome.
	Referring to written instructions, teach method of monitoring self-administration of medication using a pill box system.	Monitoring the patient's self-administration of medications is essential to adherence.	
	Allow patient to learn at own rate in a distraction-free environment.	Rushing someone to learn causes anxiety and decreases learning. Learning occurs best in a distraction-free environment, especially for an older adult.	

CRITICAL THINKING QUESTIONS

1. How would you determine Mrs. Woo's readiness to learn?
2. What questions would it be necessary to ask Mrs. Woo to reduce the risk for polypharmacy?

Get Ready for the NCLEX Examination!

Key Points

- Common health problems that affect mobility include respiratory and cardiovascular diseases, osteoporosis, gout, foot conditions, obesity, neurologic disorders, and psychosocial and emotional disorders.
- Immediately addressing mobility needs can allow the patient to quickly resume her former activity level and prevent undesirable consequences.
- Changes in the older adult's posture, balance, gait, and vision coupled with chronic conditions and the use of multiple medications greatly increase the risk of a fall.
- Enhance home safety by performing patient and family education about environmental factors that contribute to falls.
- Incontinence is not a normal consequence of aging, but a condition that is secondary to pathologic, physiologic, and functional contributing factors; it is one of the most common reasons for institutionalization.
- True constipation can be identified only after assessing the frequency, the amount, and the consistency of stools, along with possible contributing factors.
- Patient education for prevention of constipation includes specific diet remedies and a physical exercise plan.
- Physical, social, and psychological factors affect the nutritional status of older adults.
- The older adult with a sensory deficit may quickly become confused in a new environment, become subject to safety problems and self-care deficits, and experience difficulty socializing.
- Many people continue sexual activity as they age. STIs are increasing in the older adult population.
- Individuals over 65 years of age are most likely to experience a polypharmacy situation and are at risk for drug toxicity.

Additional Learning Resources

SG Go to your Study Guide for additional learning activities to help you master this chapter content.

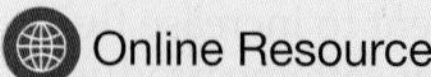
Go to your Evolve website at http://evolve.elsevier.com/Williams/fundamental for additional online resources.

Online Resources

- Academy of Nutrition and Dietetics, www.eatright.org
- Alzheimer's Association, www.alz.org
- American Macular Degeneration Foundation, www.macular.org
- Health Canada, Division of Aging and Seniors, www.hc-sc.gc.ca/hl-vs/seniors-aines/index-eng.php
- International Foundation for Functional Gastrointestinal Disorders, www.aboutincontinence.org

Review Questions for the NCLEX Examination

*Choose the **best** answer for each question.*

1. Regarding sexuality and the older adult: *(Select all that apply.)*
   1. Rates of HIV infection are decreasing but other STIs are increasing in the older population.
   2. Older women are more vulnerable than older men to acquiring a new HIV infection.
   3. Health care providers are less likely to ask the older patients about their sex practices.
   4. People living with HIV/AIDS typically do not live into their older adult years.
   5. Older adults are at low risk for STIs because condom use is a well developed habit.
2. Your neighbor asks your advice on nutrition for her aging parents. You consider your response based on your knowledge that:
   1. Older adults require more protein for wound healing.
   2. Decreasing fluids can reduce one's risk of urinary incontinence.
   3. Increased amounts of high fiber foods can lead to constipation.
   4. In general, older adults require fewer calories.
3. Which statement is true regarding sensory deficits in the older adult? *(Select all that apply.)*
   1. Cleaning excess cerumen can improve hearing.
   2. Age-related macular degeneration can always be prevented.
   3. Blindness is the leading cause of institutionalization.
   4. High-frequency hearing loss occurs to some degree in all older adults.
   5. Most older adults experience difficulty focusing on near objects.
4. The older adult with a sensory impairment as a result of the aging process may:
   1. Experience an abrupt awareness of the sensory loss.
   2. Be subject to safety problems.
   3. Increase socialization patterns.
   4. Easily adapt to new environments.
5. Measures to try to prevent age-related macular degeneration include:
   1. Sunglasses and a diet of antioxidant foods.
   2. Sunglasses and a diet low in calcium oxidate.
   3. Artificial tears and a low roughage diet.
   4. Eye exercises and a diet high in vitamin A.
6. Drug toxicity occurs more easily in older adults because of: *(Select all that apply.)*
   1. Decreased kidney function.
   2. Slower liver metabolism.
   3. Others overdosing them.
   4. Diet interaction with drugs.
   5. Age-related changes in brain chemistry.
7. Drug use assessment to identify concerns related to polypharmacy should include:
   1. Names of the pharmacies used.
   2. Types of insurance coverage.
   3. Usual diet consumed.
   4. Type of drug reminder system used.

Critical Thinking Activity

Read the clinical scenario and discuss the questions with your classmates.

Your patient is a 79-year-old widowed woman being discharged from the rehabilitation unit to her home after recovery from a fractured hip secondary to a fall. She states, "I'm having trouble swallowing these big 'horse pills' for my osteoporosis."

1. What nutritional counseling could you do for this individual?
2. What safety concerns would you have for this individual?
3. What community services could be helpful to this individual during her recovery?

chapter

41 Common Psychosocial Care Problems of the Older Adult

http://evolve.elsevier.com/Williams/fundamental

Objectives

Upon completing this chapter, you should be able to do the following:

Theory

1. Discuss general principles of care for older adults with altered cognitive functioning.
2. Assist with assessment of cognitive changes in the older adult.
3. Differentiate characteristics of delirium, dementia, and depression.
4. Identify options for keeping the cognitively impaired older adult safe.
5. Implement strategies to decrease agitation, wandering, sundowning, and eating problems in patients.
6. Discuss the interrelationship among alcoholism, depression, and suicide in the older adult.
7. Identify the four main categories of elder abuse.
8. List five crimes commonly perpetrated on older adults.
9. Discuss two future psychosocial issues for older adults.

Clinical Practice

1. Formulate a plan of care for the cognitively impaired older adult.
2. Demonstrate the ability to interact therapeutically with patients with depression and suicidal tendencies.
3. Teach crime prevention suggestions to a group of older adults.

Key Terms

age-associated memory impairment (p. 830)
Alzheimer disease (AD) (ĂWLZ-hī-mĕr, p. 834)
behavior modification (p. 836)
benign senescent forgetfulness (bē-NĪN sĕ-NĔS-ĕnt, p. 830)
creative behavioral therapies (p. 833)
delirium (dĕ-LĬR-ē-ŭm, p. 831)
dementia (dē-MĔN-shē-ă, p. 832)
depression (dē-PRĔSH-ŭn, p. 837)
electroconvulsive therapy (ECT) (ē-LĔK-trō-kŏn-VŬL-sĭv, p. 838)
nocturnal delirium (nŏk-TŬR-năl, p. 831)
paranoia (păr-ă-NŎY-ă, p. 836)
selective serotonin reuptake inhibitors (SSRIs) (p. 838)
serotonin/norepinephrine reuptake inhibitors (SNRIs) (p. 838)

Concepts Covered in This Chapter

- Anxiety
- Caregiving
- Coping
- Family dynamics
- Functional ability
- Health promotion
- Patient education
- Safety

The psychosocial status of the older adult is influenced by several factors, including functional ability and external forces. Cognitive impairments, such as dementia, and physical care problems, such as altered mobility, are two examples of functional limitations. External forces may include economic and environmental factors, such as income, housing, technology, geographic area, community resources, and crime. Individual life circumstances, such as the lack of a support system or loneliness and depression leading to alcohol abuse, can also influence the older adult's overall well-being. These factors, individually or in combination, all affect the way older adults perceive the health care system and ultimately respond to illness.

CHANGES IN COGNITIVE FUNCTIONING IN OLDER ADULTS

Many misconceptions exist about the mental functioning of older adults, given the negative attitudes of our American society toward growing old. People often assume that mental confusion and forgetfulness are typical of aging. However, few cognitive changes are attributable to age-related factors alone.

The terms **benign senescent forgetfulness** and **age-associated memory impairment** are often used to describe age-related changes in mental processes. These changes include a modest decline in short-term memory and a slight and gradual decline in cognitive skills, such as word fluency, logical analysis, selective attention (maintaining attention in the presence of numerous stimuli), naming of objects, and complex visuospatial skills (such as drawing or building furniture) (Ellison et al., 2015). **Older adults are just as capable of learning new things as younger people, but their speed of processing information is slower.**

Examples of mental changes that are not due to the normal aging process include confusion, disorientation, inappropriate behavior, depression, and the inability to concentrate or follow directions. Major declines in cognitive functioning typically result from dementia and metabolic disorders; stress, such as that associated with relocation; alcohol abuse or undesirable medication effects; and vision or hearing impairments. Dispiritedness and depression result from becoming withdrawn and detached from social interaction.

Think Critically

Can you think of a time you heard someone attribute confusion in an older adult to "getting old"?

ASSESSMENT OF COGNITIVE CHANGES IN OLDER ADULTS

The older adult with significant changes in mental functioning should be given a comprehensive mental status examination using a tool such as the Short Portable Mental Status Questionnaire (SPMSQ), Mini-Cog, or the Mini-Mental State Examination (MMSE). A detailed and accurate medical history and physical examination should be performed before making a judgment about the cause of altered mental functioning.

As a nurse, you need to understand that disorientation and other mental symptoms can have a physiologic basis. Carefully observe older and confused patients and question them and significant others about events preceding admission. Be patient and allow enough time for the older adult to respond to questions. Compensate for sensory limitations during all interactions. Assess for factors that may contribute to an altered mental state, such as medication effects, a new environment, disease processes such as infection, fluid and electrolyte imbalance, or psychosocial stressors. Promptly report all information to assist in the appropriate diagnosis and treatment.

Clinical Cues

An older adult who is experiencing a situation that makes him anxious may demonstrate temporary decreased cognitive function. Ask the patient, "Is anything causing you to worry at this time?"

COMMON COGNITIVE DISORDERS IN OLDER ADULTS

CONFUSION

Patients with confusion have difficulty remembering, learning, following directions, and communicating their needs. Mental confusion can significantly influence a patient's dignity, independence, personality, and support system and may complicate diagnosis and treatment of an illness. It can be caused by delirium, dementia, or numerous other often reversible conditions (Box 41.1).

Think Critically

Can you imagine how frustrating it would be to have difficulty remembering your own address? Do you ever experience difficulty remembering something?

DELIRIUM

Delirium is an acute confusional state that can occur suddenly or over a long period as a result of an underlying biologic cause or psychological stressor. Causes include stroke, tumors, infection, fluid and electrolyte imbalance, acute inflammatory disorders, alcohol, drug reactions, toxins, sensory deprivation or overload, hospitalization or surgery, and depression. If left untreated, delirium can lead to coma or death. Delirium should be assessed using a validated tool, such as the Confusion Assessment Method (CAM), 3D-CAM (3-dimensional CAM that can be performed in 3 minutes), or CAM-S (CAM-Severity that ranks delirium according to severity) because undetected delirium will go untreated. **Nocturnal delirium,** also known as sundown syndrome or sundowning, is the appearance or increase of symptoms of confusion or agitation in the

Box 41.1 Conditions Associated with Confusion

- Atypical presentation of illness (e.g., urinary tract infection, pneumonia)
- Vascular insufficiency
- Trauma
- Tumors
- Central nervous system infections
- Hypotension
- Systemic disorders
- Pulmonary or cardiovascular diseases
- Metabolic disorders
- Electrolyte imbalance
- Anemia
- Altered renal function
- Drug toxicity
- Endocrine disorders
- Nutritional deficiencies
- Stress
- Pain
- Anesthesia
- Altered body temperature
- Dehydration
- Anxiety
- Depression or grief
- Fatigue
- Sensory deprivation or overload
- New environment
- Toxic substances

late afternoon or early evening hours and usually continuing into the night (Box 41.2). Little is known about this disorder, which poses a management problem for caregiving, although it is sometimes associated with faster cognitive decline in the patient with Alzheimer disease (AD) (Ferrazzoli et al., 2013). Impaired mental status, dehydration, fatigue, low lighting or increased shadows, and disruption in the internal body clock may contribute to sundowning.

DEMENTIA

Dementia is generally a permanent condition characterized by several cognitive deficits. It is characterized by a slow, insidious onset that affects memory, intellectual functioning, and the ability to problem-solve. Primarily seen in patients with AD, it also occurs with brain tumors or with serious medical or surgical disorders. Symptoms of dementia may mask depression. The reverse is also true: the depressed person may be seen with symptoms similar to dementia, such as confusion and disorientation. Furthermore, depression can serve as a risk factor for dementia, and it can also contribute to development of dementia (Aziz & Steffens, 2013). Careful assessment is therefore essential to determine the cause of the patient's symptoms. Table 41.1 differentiates delirium, dementia, and depression.

Box 41.2 Signs and Symptoms of Sundown Syndrome

These behaviors, which occur later in the day, may indicate sundown syndrome in the person with dementia:

- Restlessness
- Increased anxiety
- Increased agitation
- Increased confusion
- Uncooperativeness
- Argumentativeness

The cognitive losses associated with dementia, delirium, and depression are similar; however, patients with each condition experience cognitive changes at different rates, and each responds differently to interventions.

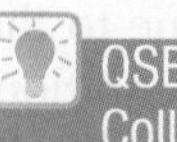

QSEN CONSIDERATIONS: Teamwork and Collaboration

Hypoxemia

Interventions to compensate for cognitive losses must be individualized, with ongoing commitment from both the health care team and the family.

General principles of care for older adults with altered cognitive functioning are summarized in Box 41.3.

Specific Interventions for Confusion and Disorientation

Psychosocial Measures. A behavioral approach is essential to enhance the quality of life for an older adult with confusion or disorientation. Two basic types of behavioral management are psychosocial interventions and medication. The plan of care should also include considerations for the patient's family.

The primary goal of psychosocial interventions is to produce a feeling of well-being in the confused and disoriented older adult. Although therapy is usually implemented by a social worker or the activity department, you can support therapy during patient care and evaluate changes in the patient's behavior to revise the plan of care as needed.

A variety of therapies can help patients who are experiencing confusion and disorientation to regain their sense of who they are and what is happening in the environment around them. Once a therapy is initiated, it should be used consistently by everyone in contact with the patient, including the family, to

Table 41.1 Differentiation of Delirium, Dementia, and Depression

	DELIRIUM	DEMENTIA	DEPRESSION
Onset	Sudden	Gradual	Gradual or rapid
Orientation	Disoriented, clouding of consciousness, fluctuating level of awareness	Disoriented	Oriented or disoriented
Affect, mood	Varies	Labile, inappropriate	Despair, worry
Behavior	Agitation; inability to perform ADLs; changes in sleep-wake cycle; can experience delusions or paranoia	Agitation or apathy; inability to perform ADLs	Apathy, agitation, self-neglect, appetite change
Speech	May be incoherent and inappropriate or coherent and appropriate	Sparse, repetitive; may initially lie to cover deficits; later does not conceal	Coherent; may not want to talk
Memory	Impaired for recent events; memory disturbed	Impaired for recent events, intact remote memory	Impaired; decreased ability to concentrate; sometimes called "pseudodementia"
Prognosis	Good; resolves with treatment	Poor; no return to predemented state	Resolves with treatment of cause or treatment of depression

ADL, activities of daily living.

avoid further confusion. Table 41.2 presents several types of psychosocial approaches, their purpose, and related activities.

Other psychosocial interventions include **creative behavioral therapies,** such as art, music, and humor that can allow for self-expression and alleviate anxiety and depression. The goal of creative therapies is to slow the rate of deterioration and prevent institutionalization as long as possible. Having pets available can also meet many needs, such as companionship and the need for touch. Pets may help a person deal with the loneliness caused by the many losses experienced in old age, such as decreased income, death of a spouse, and loss of independence (Fig. 41.1).

Box 41.3 Principles of Nursing Care for the Cognitively Impaired Older Adult

- Monitor and maintain physical well-being.
- Recognize the underlying meaning of actions and behaviors.
- Adjust the environment accordingly.
- Use concise, direct interactions.
- Maintain and enhance self-esteem and socialization.
- Implement strategies to enhance orientation.
- Maintain adequate nutrition.

Table 41.2 Psychosocial Approaches for Confusion and Disorientation

PURPOSE	ACTIVITIES
Reality Orientation	
Orient patient to person, place, and time.	Consistent 24 h/day interaction with staff and family Continual reminders of day, year, time Consistent mealtimes, activities of daily living, treatment Memory aids, such as television, radio, newspaper, clock, calendar
Validation Therapy	
Decrease stress, promote self-esteem and communication, reduce chemical and physical restraints, and delay institutionalization.	Group support to encourage respect for the feelings of the individual from his perspective Activities such as singing favorite songs, reminiscing, sharing a memento or family photo
Reminiscence	
Reexamine past to promote socialization and mental stimulation; wrap up unresolved issues.	Individual or group sharing of information about past life and experiences
Remotivation Therapy	
Stimulate senses and provide new motivation in life through factual information rather than feelings.	Introduction of pictures, plants, animals, fish, or sounds to encourage interaction
Resocialization	
Encourage socialization patterns within a group.	Assigned socialization roles in a group, such as serving each other refreshments

 **Think Critically**

How could you use reminiscence to help an older adult adapt to relocating to a nursing home?

Pharmacotherapy. Before administering medications to deal with problem behaviors, first implement all other types of nursing interventions and document their effectiveness. It is important to use drugs for valid psychological problems, and not just for annoying behaviors.

Adaptation is necessary when using psychotropic drugs with older adults. Many psychotropic drugs require an extended time to have a therapeutic effect. Toxicity and undesirable side effects, such as constipation and orthostatic hypotension, may occur. Because of chronic health problems in an individual, some medications may be contraindicated or require careful administration. Thus, patient and family education about medications is essential.

Major tranquilizers, also known as antipsychotics, such as chlorpromazine or haloperidol, are sometimes prescribed to manage the anxiety, agitation, hostility, and paranoia associated with dementia. The US Food and Drug Administration (FDA) ordered that a boxed ("black box") warning be placed on all antipsychotics indicating they are not approved to treat dementia symptoms (Alzheimer's Association, 2015), and they increase the risk of death in the older adult (Blue Cross/Blue Shield of Texas, 2012). The "black box" warning is the strongest advisory the FDA makes, indicating a serious or life-threatening risk to the consumer. Legislators and hospital officials are scrutinizing the

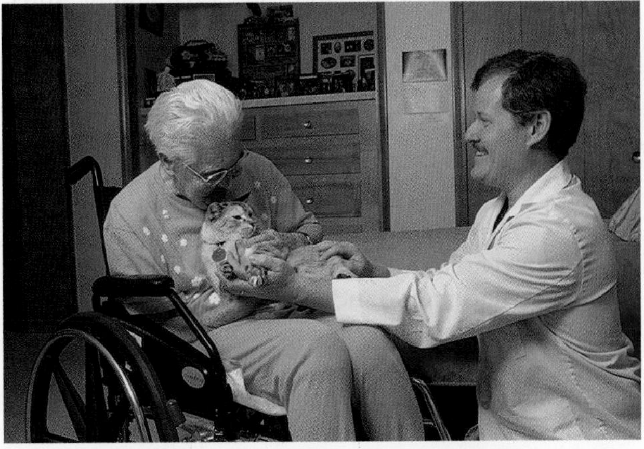

FIGURE 41.1 Pet therapy for the lonely older adult.

use of antipsychotics in nursing home residents. If an antipsychotic is prescribed, patients need to be closely monitored. **Minor tranquilizers** may also be used to treat symptoms of agitation and anxiety, although many medications in this category appear on the Screening Tool of Older Person's Prescriptions (STOPP) criteria list. **Antidepressants**, such as citalopram or duloxetine, may be used if depression coexists with dementia. These drugs may improve appetite and sleep habits, enhance socialization, and increase energy levels. Assess carefully for side effects, such as arrhythmias and orthostatic hypotension. Hypnotics, antianxiety drugs, and anticonvulsants may also be helpful.

? Think Critically

What interventions could you try before medicating a patient for anxiety or agitation?

Family Support. It is important to provide emotional and social support to the patient with dementia and to significant others. As caregivers, the entire family often experiences changes in lifestyle, privacy, socialization, and family dynamics. The caregiver may experience physical and mental exhaustion from providing round-the-clock care.

Adjusting to the reality that dementia is a chronic, irreversible condition that may result in a lingering death can be difficult. This places families in a situation of dealing with grief over a long time. Acceptance of a relative with dementia depends on personal coping strategies, support, and past experiences. Integrate the care of the family into the nursing care plans to enhance adjustment. Family members need ongoing support by the entire health care team. They may need an explanation regarding the disease or condition to help them better cope with the future.

Financial problems and multiple role responsibilities add to the burden of caregiving by the spouse or the adult children. Caregivers can experience loneliness, depression, and social isolation. An assessment of the caregiver's health and functional ability, nutrition, and exercise patterns can allow development of strategies to help families to cope more effectively with caregiving. Encourage caregivers to take time out and attend to their own well-being.

Nurses can encourage families to consider adult day services or respite care if the older adult resides at home. These types of care can provide for much-needed psychological and physical rest for the caregivers. Provide guidance in locating resources to explore. Referrals may include health care professionals, community mental health centers, area agencies on aging, or support groups for specific diseases, such as AD.

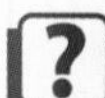 **Clinical Cues**

Most large communities have respite care for those with dementia where the family caregivers can take the patient while they have a short break. For qualified veterans, the Department of Veterans Affairs facilities can provide respite care for up to 30 days each year. Often these are special units attached to a hospital or long-term care facility.

Social implications for the resident in long-term care whose abilities continue to deteriorate relate to maintaining interactions with others for as long as possible. It is important to realize that the family will continue to require support from the health care team.

? Think Critically

What type of personal stress management strategies could you suggest to a caregiver of an Alzheimer patient?

ALZHEIMER DISEASE

Alzheimer disease (AD) is the most common form of dementia (estimates range from 50% to 80% of dementia patients) in older adults and is the fifth leading cause of death in this population. With the graying of America, this disorder may pose a significant public health concern in future years.

The loss of neurons in the frontal and temporal lobes accounts for the AD patient's inability to process and integrate new information and retrieve memory. Although many diagnostic tools are available to rule out some cognitive diseases, few can diagnose AD. Positron emission tomography (PET) has shown reduced lobe activity early in the disease. The diagnostic criteria for AD have been revised and now include three stages: preclinical AD, mild cognitive impairment, and dementia (Box 41.4). These stages are expected to be further refined, identifying specific biologic changes (biomarkers) for the disease.

Box 41.4 Stages of Alzheimer Disease

PRECLINICAL ALZHEIMER DISEASE

- Measurable biologic changes (in the brain's β-amyloid plaque); specific biomarkers (such as the APOE gene) may include brain imaging studies and protein in spinal fluid
- No obvious symptoms of memory loss or confusion
- Occurs years to perhaps decades before the next stage

MILD COGNITIVE IMPAIRMENT CAUSED BY ALZHEIMER DISEASE

- Mild changes in memory, reasoning, and visual perception
- Noticeable to person affected, friends, and family
- Capable of carrying out everyday activities

DEMENTIA CAUSED BY ALZHEIMER DISEASE

- Memory impairment
- Behavioral symptoms
- Impaired ability to function in daily life

APOE, Apolipoprotein E.

Treatment and Nursing Interventions for Alzheimer Disease

Treatment is primarily symptomatic. Three cholinesterase inhibitor drugs—donepezil, galantamine, and rivastigmine—produce modest benefits early in the disease by improving memory, alertness, and social engagement. These drugs work by increasing acetylcholine in the cerebral cortex. Memantine is another type of medication, thought to protect nerve cells from excess stimulation from the neurotransmitter glutamate and delay progression of symptoms; it was the first treatment option for moderate to severe AD. Several new drugs and therapies are being studied for AD, including the antioxidant found in chocolate and red wine, resveratrol (Storrs, 2015). Researchers in Sweden are placing nerve growth factor implants into the brain in a study attempting to stop the breakdown of cholinergic neurons.

Estrogen was once considered to protect the brain from cognitive decline, but study results have been inconsistent and controversial. Other medications found to enhance cognitive functioning, improve behavioral problems, or delay the effects of the disease include vitamin E, folic acid, and possibly nonsteroidal anti-inflammatory drugs (NSAIDs) and the cholesterol-lowering statin drugs. General nursing interventions for AD patients depend on the severity of illness. Early in the disease process, nursing care for a confused patient (previously discussed) is necessary. Later in the disease process, nursing care is primarily supportive. One novel idea in England is the "REM Room," in which nurses re-create simulated environments from an older adult's past to decrease anxiety in dementia patients. The simulated environments include painted backdrops and props; for example, there is a "pub" REM room with nonalcoholic drinks, and a "potting shed" REM room with artificial plants and potting supplies. Nurses report decreased anxiety in the patients. See www.rempods.co.uk/ for an example. Box 41.5 lists some nursing diagnoses appropriate for the cognitively impaired older patient.

Box 41.5 Selected NANDA-I Nursing Diagnoses for the Cognitively Impaired Older Adult

- Acute confusion
- Anxiety
- Fatigue
- Functional urinary incontinence
- Imbalanced nutrition: less than body requirements
- Impaired memory
- Impaired social interaction
- Impaired verbal communication
- Risk for injury
- Self-care deficit
- Sleep deprivation

NANDA-I, NANDA International, Inc.

SAFETY FOR THE COGNITIVELY IMPAIRED

When an older adult is cognitively impaired, home safety becomes an issue. When the impairment is mild, the patient may be able to safely remain in his own home. Otherwise, there must be adjustments to the living situation. When a person with dementia goes to live with relatives, they should attach alerting systems to outside doors to prevent the person from wandering out alone.

 **QSEN CONSIDERATIONS: Safety**

Identification of Personal Items

Identification should be sewn into clothes and placed in a wallet or purse. An identification bracelet that is not easily removed is helpful if the person wanders.

Measures need to be taken to alert the household if the person leaves the bedroom area at night so that the stove is not used without supervision. Sometimes residential placement is needed. Options include an assisted-living facility, a board-and-care facility, or a long-term care facility.

If the person still owns a car, driving is another safety issue and many states have limitations on older adult driving. No one wants to give up independence. Families have great difficulty getting an older adult to stop driving. One way to help is to suggest that a family member take the person wherever he wants to go for 1 month so that it becomes apparent that giving up the car does not mean staying at home. Another option is to research what alternative transportation is available and have a family member accompany the person the first few times that transportation is used. If that works well, then it can be pointed out that the person does not need to drive anymore to maintain his present lifestyle and independence. Another method is to see whether the person will consent to having an outside evaluation by a driver's education firm to determine safe driving capability. Of course, the person should drive only if confusion about direction is not an issue. Helpful information is available in the American Medical Association guide, *Physician's Guide to Assessing and Counseling Older Drivers*. Driver rehabilitation specialists can be hired to help sharpen driving skills (see online resources at end of the chapter for web addresses).

BEHAVIORS ASSOCIATED WITH COGNITIVE DISORDERS

Agitation, Hostility, and Paranoia

Violent behavior in older adults may be the result of a lifelong psychological pattern, an organic condition, or an adverse reaction to medication. Aggressive behavior may also occur as a self-protective response to confusion, fear, pain, or sensory loss. Frequently it is associated with delirium, dementia, stroke, metabolic disorders, or hypoxia. In patients with dementia,

behavior is a form of communication. Nonverbal behavior, such as agitation or restlessness, may be an expression of unmet needs, such as thirst or pain. It is the nurse's responsibility to facilitate communication and determine if there are such unmet needs.

Agitation can be prevented and managed by watching carefully for signs, such as increasing irritability or sudden, explosive outbursts. Notice if patients are talking loudly, pacing more or faster, or making threats. Before an actual outburst occurs, try to engage the patient in conversation, using therapeutic communication skills (see Chapter 8). If seeing reflections in a mirror causes agitation, cover or remove the mirrors.

Matching the tone of the patient's voice may be calming. It may be advisable to step back 4 to 6 feet while conversing. With a patient who is disoriented or has a sensory deficit, you may want to approach more closely to maintain eye contact and touch. This must be done cautiously for everyone's protection. Move other patients or visitors out of the way as necessary.

Behavior modification is an intervention used to change agitated behavior by giving positive feedback for desired behaviors and negative feedback for undesired behaviors. Use distraction for the older adult not responding to behavior modification.

If a patient becomes violent, you must remember to protect the patient from his own behavior. You must call for help and, as a team member, decide what intervention will be most effective.

Points to consider for intervention are the patient's right to the least restrictive treatment and the federal and state regulations regarding the use of chemical (medication) and physical protective devices. Before giving medications, it is necessary to try behavioral approaches and document their effectiveness. When all else fails and the patient poses a threat to his well-being or to others, protective devices may be necessary.

Paranoia can also be caused by delirium, dementia, or psychological conditions, such as schizophrenia. Patients with paranoia may misinterpret their environment and believe others are untrustworthy and out to get them. These patients may sound convincing and logical in their suspicious behaviors.

For the patient with paranoia, developing trust is the most important approach. Being consistent and reliable is perhaps the best way to develop trust in the relationship with the paranoid patient. Do not make promises you cannot keep. If you say you will do something, follow up with it. Never put any medication in a drink or food without the patient's knowledge to maintain trust.

? Think Critically

Why would it be especially important for you to offer explanations to a hearing impaired patient experiencing paranoia or thinking that others are talking about him?

Wandering

Wandering may be a problem for the patient affected with a cognitive disorder. Wanderers tend to be individuals who were active before the onset of disease. For some, wandering may be goal directed, such as looking for the bathroom. Others may wander to combat boredom or restlessness. Nursing interventions include ensuring the environment is safe for wandering, informing and educating others about this problem, ensuring the patient has an identification bracelet, frequently checking the patient, observing for behaviors that trigger the wandering, diverting his attention, and maintaining a regular activity program. Many units are designed for wandering patients and even include gated outside areas in which to enjoy nature.

? Think Critically

What type of diversional activities could you use for a wandering patient who is trying to go home?

Sundown Syndrome

To alleviate the confusion and fears associated with sundowning, it is important for you to help the patient feel safe in his environment. Using a night light, placing the call light within reach, reducing stimulation in the environment, and moving the patient closer to the nurses' station can help to minimize nocturnal confusion (Box 41.6). Protective devices should be used as a

Box 41.6 Proven Strategies and Interventions to Minimize Sundowning

- Limit outings and activities to the morning hours.
- For the person with AD, keep times of sensory stimulation short. Prevent sensory overload (e.g., television, noisy children, activity of others in the vicinity), but keep the home well lit in the evening.
- Avoid nicotine, caffeinated drinks or foods, concentrated sugars, and large meals in the afternoon and evening.
- Prevent excessive napping during the day, but keep the person well rested.
- Advise caregivers to be mindful of their own stress and fatigue at the end of the day, because the person with AD can pick up on this and become agitated or confused.
- Provide soothing music as dusk approaches and through the evening.
- Provide stimulating activities during the day along with exercise, but prevent exhaustion. Maintain a consistent schedule.
- Make certain physical needs are met and that the person is not hungry, thirsty, wet, soiled, hot, or cold.
- Obtain treatment for arthritis, shortness of breath, urinary tract infection, cold or flu symptoms, or other discomforts.
- Provide a private "time-out" place for the person subject to sundowning.
- Keep surroundings as simple and familiar as possible with an uncluttered appearance. Remove mirrors and pictures if they cause the person distress. Avoid changing things in the environment once simplified.

last resort safety measure because they may add to the patient's anxiety.

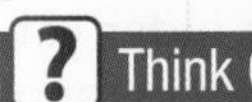

Think Critically

What would it feel like to awaken at night and think that the shadow cast on the wall is someone leaning over you with a knife?

Eating Problems

Adequate nutrition often becomes a problem for the patient with dementia. Common feeding challenges include loss of appetite, refusing to open the mouth, holding food in the mouth (keeping it between the upper teeth and cheek), refusing to swallow food, and choking when swallowing.

Patient Education

Strategies to Improve Nutritional Status of the Cognitively Impaired Older Adult

- Provide mealtime companionship in a stress-free environment.
- Provide proper oral hygiene and properly fitting dentures.
- Inspect the mouth for gum or dental problems.
- Identify the "hungry time" of day.
- Serve meals in same place and at the same time.
- Provide frequent small meals and nutritious snacks.
- Serve favorite foods if possible.
- Limit food choices, and serve them in an attractive manner.
- Serve one food at a time to decrease confusion.
- Use liquid thickeners to prevent aspiration.
- Remind the patient to open mouth, chew, and swallow.
- Avoid hurrying the patient to eat.

DEPRESSION, ALCOHOLISM, AND SUICIDE

Depression (feelings of sadness, despair, or discouragement) in the older adult is often overlooked and untreated. It is the most common functional mental illness in older adults but is often mistaken for delirium or dementia. Almost half of older adults in hospital and long-term care settings have depression (Aziz & Steffens, 2013).

Depression is often difficult to recognize because symptoms may be attributed to the aging process. Instead of complaining of a depressed mood, older adults may complain of anorexia, sleep disturbances, lack of energy, and loss of interest and enjoyment in life. Depression in older adults occurs to a great degree as a result of situational factors such as multiple losses. It is helpful to assess the older adult's mood periodically (Box 41.7). Undiagnosed and untreated depression is a major contributor to alcoholism and suicide in older adults.

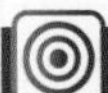

Focused Assessment

Assessment of Depression in Older Adults

Signs and symptoms to look for include:

PHYSICAL ASSESSMENT

- Fatigue
- Headaches
- "Not feeling good"
- Memory impairment
- Vague aches and pains

PSYCHOSOCIAL ASSESSMENT

- Social withdrawal
- Loss of motivation and energy
- Envy or criticism of others
- Increasing demands on others
- Feelings of worthlessness and helplessness
- Appetite changes
- Sleep pattern changes
- Indecisiveness
- Obsessive worrying
- Poor outlook on life

Alcohol abuse, suicide, and depression are interrelated in that they each have similar risk factors associated with multiple losses. Loss of status and power, income, spouse, friends, health, and mobility contribute to feelings of despair and hopelessness. The older adult's outlook on life is distorted, preventing him from exploring acceptable solutions to his problems. Older adults with suicidal thoughts are more likely to act on them when compared with younger people with similar thoughts (Aziz & Steffens, 2013).

Alcohol misuse is a serious concern in the older adult because it can interfere with the management of chronic diseases and heighten the risk of adverse drug reactions because of diminishing liver and kidney function. Alcoholism is often overlooked because so many older adult problem drinkers are retired and hidden at home. Clues to alcoholism include

Box 41.7 Questionnaire to Determine Presence of Depression

MOOD SCALE (SHORT FORM)

Choose the best answer for how you have felt over the past week:

1. Are you basically satisfied with your life? YES/NO
2. Have you dropped many of your activities and interests? YES/NO
3. Do you feel that your life is empty? YES/NO
4. Do you often get bored? YES/NO
5. Are you in good spirits most of the time? YES/NO
6. Are you afraid that something bad is going to happen to you? YES/NO
7. Do you feel happy most of the time? YES/NO
8. Do you often feel helpless? YES/NO
9. Do you prefer to stay at home, rather than going out and doing new things? YES/NO
10. Do you feel you have more problems with memory than most? YES/NO
11. Do you think it is wonderful to be alive now? YES/NO
12. Do you feel pretty worthless the way you are now? YES/NO
13. Do you feel full of energy? YES/NO
14. Do you feel that your situation is hopeless? YES/NO
15. Do you think that most people are better off than you are? YES/NO

depression, insomnia, mental confusion, frequent falls, self-neglect, and uncontrollable hypertension or diabetes, along with gastritis and anemia.

INTERVENTIONS FOR DEPRESSION, ALCOHOLISM, AND SUICIDE PREVENTION

Patients who are depressed are usually treated with psychotherapy and antidepressants. Hospitalization may be necessary if the patient is at risk of suicide.

Complementary & Alternative Therapies

OMEGA-3 FATTY ACIDS

Many studies have demonstrated the potential benefit of omega-3 fatty acids in alleviating depression without dangerous side effects. Omega-3 fatty acids also aid cognition. Cod liver oil is rich in omega-3 fatty acids. Eating fish such as salmon, sardines, mackerel, and tuna can increase omega-3 intake. For those who do not like fish, supplement capsules of omega-3 fatty acids are available (Mazza et al., 2015).

The five main categories of medications used to treat depression are the three newer categories of antidepressants (usually "first line therapy"): the **selective serotonin reuptake inhibitors (SSRIs)**, the **serotonin/norepinephrine reuptake inhibitors (SNRIs)**, and the atypical antidepressants; and the older categories: the tricyclic antidepressants and the monoamine oxidase inhibitors (MAOIs). Table 41.3 lists examples and important considerations for these medications.

Electroconvulsive therapy (ECT) is a treatment option for those patients who have severe forms of depression and have not responded to several regimens of medication. ECT consists of electric shock to the brain delivered via electrodes attached to the patient's temples, intentionally triggering a brief seizure that seems to alter brain chemistry and improve symptoms. How this mechanism works is not fully understood, although it is speculated that it alters neurotransmitters or stress hormone regulation (University of Michigan, 2015). The patient usually receives two or three treatments per week for several weeks.

The primary nursing responsibility for a depressed patient is to protect him from self-injury, especially *after* the patient has initiated antidepressant therapy.

Table 41.3 Antidepressants Used with Older Adults

	SELECTIVE SEROTONIN REUPTAKE INHIBITORS (SSRIS)	SEROTONIN/ NOREPINEPHRINE REUPTAKE INHIBITORS (SNRIS)	TRICYCLIC ANTIDEPRESSANTS	MONOAMINE OXIDASE (MAO) INHIBITORS (MAOIS)	ATYPICAL ANTIDEPRESSANTS
Examples	Sertraline Paroxetine Fluoxetine	Duloxetine Venlafaxine Desvenlafaxine	Amitriptyline Doxepin	Phenelzine Selegiline	Bupropion Trazodone Amoxapine
Mode of Action	Block reuptake of serotonin	Block reuptake of serotonin and norepinephrine	Block reuptake of serotonin and norepinephrine	Affect monoamine neurotransmitter system	Affect a variety of receptors
Side effects; older adult considerations	Nausea, agitation/ insomnia, sexual dysfunction; start with low dose, may increase fall risk	Nausea, anorexia, dizziness, diaphoresis; hyponatremia in older adults, may increase fall risk	Sedation, orthostatic hypotension, anticholinergic symptoms (dry mouth, blurred vision, constipation); long half life	CNS stimulation, orthostatic hypotension	Vary by drug; some cause GI symptoms and anticholinergic symptoms
Contraindications, precautions, alerts	Contraindicated if taking MAOIs: risk for **serotonin syndrome** (potentially fatal)	Risk for **serotonin syndrome** if taken with MAOIs; may increase **stroke** risk	**Overdose can be life-threatening**. Not typically the first choice category for older adults	Must maintain tyramine-free diet to avoid **hypertensive crisis**	Varies by drug: cautious use with cardiac disorders (trazodone), caution in patients with seizures (amoxapine)
Other	Taper therapy; do not discontinue abruptly	Taper therapy; do not discontinue abruptly	Interacts with numerous medications	Rarely prescribed	**Suicide risk** can increase with all antidepressant medications

CNS, central nervous system; From: Bankhead (2012), Burchum & Rosenthal (2016), and Thorlund et al. (2015).

Before that time, he may not have the energy to commit suicide.

It may be difficult to communicate with a depressed patient because of his negative thoughts and behaviors. Genuine concern for the patient is essential. You need to help him to set realistic, achievable goals. Start with small goals, such as grooming, and slowly work toward larger goals. Remember that goal setting and problem solving take concentration and energy that may not be available to the person who is still somewhat depressed. Providing a quiet environment conducive to sleep can help to restore energy for individuals who complain of sleep deprivation.

Caregivers need to be alert to signs of potential suicide, such as meticulous planning of personal affairs, giving away of treasured possessions, sudden euphoria, or statements of death wishes. Assisting the patient in improving self-esteem and taking part in meaningful activities may resolve the intent of suicide. You must build a trusting relationship with the suicidal patient to let him know you care. Spend time with your patient and actively listen to demonstrate your concern.

If the patient makes references to suicide, ask him directly if he is planning to end his life. Referral to a mental health care provider or immediate crisis intervention is important for evaluation and treatment of suicidal behavior. However, as with any individual who believes suicide is the only answer, the older adult may eventually carry out this act. In such cases, caregivers and family need support and possible counseling to resolve their grief.

? Think Critically

What response would you have for the older adult who tells you he wishes he could go to sleep for the last time?

During the admission patient interview, assess the use of alcohol by depressed older adults. Making a diagnosis of alcohol dependency is not necessarily difficult, but unless the patient admits he has a problem, long-term recovery is unlikely. Initial treatment for the older adult may consist of detoxification and stabilization in the hospital with reduced doses of benzodiazepines or shorter-acting benzodiazepines and vitamin supplements, along with intravenous (IV) hydration. Once the patient is stable, therapy may consist of group, behavioral, or individual therapy to help with depression, loneliness, and loss and to help build a social network.

Patient and family education must include information about the effects of alcohol on medications and on chronic health conditions. Referral to a 12-step program, such as Alcoholics Anonymous (AA) for the patient and Al-Anon for family members, can also be a beneficial part of treatment.

CRIMES AGAINST OLDER ADULTS

ELDER ABUSE

Abuse is defined as the intentional infliction of physical or emotional discomfort or the deprivation of basic necessities for comfort or survival. It is estimated that only 1 in 14 cases of elder abuse is reported.

Elder abuse is most often inflicted by a spouse or adult children in the home, and it is often undetected. It is often related to caregiving stress, unresolved family conflicts, unhealthy family dynamics, or families with a history of abuse. All forms of abuse are destructive and at the very least reduce the victim's self-esteem. Box 41.8 identifies the five different categories of abuse.

? Think Critically

Can you remember an incident when you suspected abuse of a friend or an acquaintance?

The nurse's responsibilities include identifying those at risk and reporting suspected abuse. During assessment of potential abuse, avoid a condescending tone of voice or judgmental expression. Establish a confidential, trusting relationship. Demonstrate willingness to also listen to the caregiver's perspective. Assess the caregiver's early memories of relationships with the older adult to learn of possible long-term conflicts.

Focused Assessment

ASSESSMENT OF SUSPECTED SIGNS AND SYMPTOMS OF ABUSE IN OLDER ADULTS

When working with the older adult, be observant for:

- Unkempt, inappropriate dress and hygiene
- Malnourishment, dehydration
- Bruises or fractures of undetermined cause; cigarette burns
- Conflicting explanations of an older adult's condition
- Unusual fear exhibited by the older adult
- Confusion not attributable to other causes
- Abnormal behavior in the caregiver
- Hostility displayed by the caregiver in response to questions

Box 41.8 Categories of Elder Abuse

- **Physical:** Infliction of physical pain and injury via assault and battery. Using physical restraints or confining people against their will is also classified as physical abuse. It may also include the inappropriate use of drugs.
- **Sexual:** Infliction of nonconsensual sexual contact of any kind.
- **Psychological:** Verbal harassment, including intimidation, defamation, and isolation. It may also include threats of abandonment or physical violence. Psychological abuse laws vary from state to state.
- **Material:** Theft of older adult's money, misuse of funds, or theft or misuse of possessions.
- **Neglect:** Failure to meet the needs of the older adult, including leaving the person alone; withholding medication, food, or other necessities; and not assisting with activities of daily living or providing inadequate care.

You have a legal obligation to report elder abuse and are accorded protection from civil liability in most states that mandate reporting of suspected abuse, as long as you made the report based on reasonable suspicion and in good faith (Brent, 2013). Report suspected abuse immediately to the appropriate agency for investigation. **The standard for reporting is usually a reasonable belief that an individual has been or is likely to be abused, neglected, or exploited.** Be aware that advocacy for the abused may be difficult because you may receive threats from those who resent your involvement. A common frustrating situation is the competent older adult with full legal rights who refuses help or desires to remain in an environment that is unsafe or unacceptable. In this case the health care team must provide counseling about potential dangers but then honor the person's decision. If a person is legally incompetent, steps must be taken for appropriate guardianship. Testifying in court about an abusive situation can be stressful for everyone involved.

Individual and/or group psychotherapy is often used to treat both victims and abusers. The victim should be removed from the home before entering treatment to avoid retaliation. Intensive psychotherapy may be necessary for the abuser with psychopathology. Support groups are also available for both victims and abusers. Long-term follow-up is essential to prevent further abuse.

SCAMS AND WHITE COLLAR CRIME

Crime is of particular concern to older adults because of their sense of vulnerability. Older adults do not suffer any greater physical injury or financial loss than younger people; however, the effects of crime, such as fear, isolation, loneliness, and feelings of powerlessness, may be more detrimental. Older adults may even fall prey to Internet scams, such as receiving email from someone posing as a relative emailing from a foreign country who has "lost their wallet and passport." Some of the crimes against older adults are listed in Box 41.9.

Box 41.9 Crimes or Scams Against Older Adults

- Personal or household theft
- Vehicular theft
- Purse snatching, pickpocketing
- Investment theft
- Mailbox theft
- Rape
- Assault
- Fraudulent schemes through white collar crime
- Donations, fundraisers
- Investments
- Toll-free numbers
- Prize offers
- Funeral planning
- Home improvements
- Telemarketing
- Timesharing
- Auto repair
- Medical quackery

Nurses can help to reduce fear of crime and assist older adults in exploring security-conscious behaviors to decrease vulnerability to victimization.

Patient Education

CRIME REDUCTION SUGGESTIONS FOR OLDER ADULTS

Teach patients and people in the community:

- Attend a crime prevention program.
- Identify police or security personnel available in high-risk areas.
- Institute an informal surveillance or buddy system among neighbors.
- Keep doors locked with deadbolt locks.
- Do not attach identification to key rings.
- If keys are lost, have locks changed.
- Lock windows; draw blinds or curtains at night.
- Keep all hidden entries such as garage or basement doors locked.
- Use a peephole. Confirm service person's identity by calling the service agency first before opening the door.
- Install a video doorbell that allows you to see who is at your door before answering it.
- Do not let strangers at your door or on the telephone know that you are alone.
- Beware of telephone tricks; do not give information to strangers. Hang up on and report nuisance callers.
- Consider a pet to provide protection.
- Travel in groups.
- Carry a whistle or wear one around your neck.
- Carry few valuables on yourself; hide key and other valuables in inside pockets.
- Protect assets; keep money in the bank; use direct deposit of Social Security and pension funds.

Think Critically

Can you think of a situation in which an older adult you know was subtly scammed by a business?

Nurses also need to learn about referral programs in crime protection, prevention, and victim assistance. Federal programs through the US Department of Housing and Urban Development offer crime prevention and victim counseling. State offices of aging and organizations such as AARP (formerly the American Association of Retired Persons) and the National Crime Prevention Council have also proved beneficial in enhancing awareness of crime prevention.

FUTURE ISSUES OF CONCERN TO OLDER ADULTS

It is not easy to predict the future, but the most appropriate word for the older population may be *increasing*, in both number and age. Older adults will be the fastest growing segment of the population and will have the greatest effect on the delivery of health care. Older adults of tomorrow will be better educated, more involved in community and political activities, more Internet savvy, and more knowledgeable consumers of health care.

What will be the priorities in the future? How much funding will go toward research of life-threatening diseases of older adults versus solving environmental problems that affect all populations? With the nation's long list of priorities, what decisions will be made?

? Think Critically

What health care issues do you think **you** might face when you become older?

PLANNING FOR THE FUTURE

Expanding present services and developing new delivery systems will be challenges for the future. Safe housing and efficient mass transportation to stores and recreational facilities will continue to be needed, along with one-stop shopping senior centers. This concept can allow for care coordination of multiple services, such as home-delivered meals and chore services, at a nominal cost, which can make a difference as to whether a person can remain at home or must be institutionalized.

Planning for the future will need to include lifelong learning opportunities that assist the older adult with maintaining wellness, preparing for retirement and leisure time, financial planning, and coping with advances in technology. Other considerations are job training and retraining for "early retirees" who wish to remain employed. Health issues to be addressed include the rapidly rising rate of acquired immune deficiency syndrome (AIDS) and sexually transmitted infections (STIs) in the older adult population and the health problems specific to the growing proportion of older women.

As we have discussed throughout this book, *Healthy People 2020* is a federal campaign designed to encourage people to adopt healthy lifestyles to maintain or improve their health. Emphasis is on health promotion, protection, and prevention. The overall goal for older adults is to "improve the health, function, and quality of life of older adults."

Will the programs and services discussed become realities? The answer lies partially with older adults of today. Individuals over 65 comprise a powerful political group with real voting power that can effectively make change happen. Combined with the advocacy of nursing power to access necessary resources, the new goals of *Healthy People 2020* can realistically be achieved.

Get Ready for the NCLEX Examination!

Key Points

- Mental confusion and forgetfulness are not age-related processes.
- A comprehensive mental status examination, medical history, and physical examination are necessary before making a judgment about the cause of altered cognitive functioning.
- Confusion can be caused by delirium, dementia, or numerous other, often reversible, conditions.
- Cognitive changes associated with dementia, delirium, and depression are similar and must be differentiated through careful assessment.
- Behavioral management of the confused patient includes psychosocial approaches first and then medication, if psychosocial approaches are ineffective.
- A significant consideration in managing dementia is providing emotional and social support to both the patient and significant others.
- AD is the most common form of dementia and the fifth leading cause of death in older adults.
- Common behaviors associated with cognitive disorders include agitation, hostility, paranoia, wandering, and sundown syndrome.
- Depression is the most common functional mental illness in older adults. It is often undertreated because symptoms may be attributed to aging.
- Alcohol abuse, suicide, and depression are interrelated and have similar risk factors.
- The exact number of abused older adults is difficult to determine due to underreporting.
- Protection from civil liability is accorded to nurses who report abuse in good faith.
- Crimes and scams against older adults include white-collar fraudulent schemes by professional people.
- Planning for the future for older adults should include lifelong learning opportunities that address maintaining wellness; retirement, leisure, and financial planning; job training or retraining; and coping with advances in technology.

Additional Learning Resources

SG Go to your Study Guide for additional learning activities to help you master this chapter content.

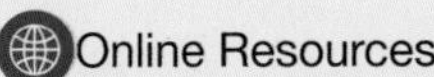

evolve Go to your Evolve website at http://evolve.elsevier.com/Williams/fundamental for additional online resources.

Online Resources

- *Alzheimer's Association,* www.alz.org
- American Medical Association (2010). *The Physicians Guide to Assessing and Counseling Older Drivers,* http://geriatricscareonline.org/ProductAbstract/physicians-guide-to-assessing-and-counseling-older-drivers/B013
- *Association for Driver Rehabilitation Specialists,* http://www.driver-ed.org/
- National Institute on Aging (2013). Caring for a person with Alzheimer disease. https://www.nia.nih.gov/sites/default/files/caring_for_a_person_with_alzheimers_disease_2.pdf
- *National Crime Prevention Council,* www.ncpc.org

Review Questions for the NCLEX Examination

*Choose the **best** answer for each question.*

1. When it comes to learning, older adults are:
   1. As capable as younger people, but slower to learn.
   2. Less able to learn than younger people.
   3. Able to learn as well as younger people.
   4. About one-third less efficient at learning than a younger person.
2. Confusion is often a reversible condition in patients with:
   1. Dementia.
   2. Depression.
   3. Delirium.
   4. Alzheimer disease.
3. Measures to keep the cognitively impaired older adult safe in a home environment include: *(Select all that apply.)*
   1. Placing alarms on the outside doors.
   2. Removing knobs from the stove burners and oven at night.
   3. Having the person carry a cell phone at all times.
   4. Placing an identification bracelet on the person.
   5. Getting the person a guide dog.
4. Which symptoms is the nurse most likely to observe in a depressed, older adult? *(Select all that apply.)*
   1. Anger
   2. Poor memory
   3. Insomnia
   4. Loss of motivation
   5. Pacing
5. Medications that work by increasing acetylcholine in the cerebral cortex may produce:
   1. A calming effect and less hostility.
   2. Greater ability to organize and carry out tasks.
   3. Greater ability to concentrate and learn new things.
   4. Improved memory, alertness, and social engagement.
6. You recently admitted a patient with Alzheimer disease to your long-term care nursing unit. This patient appears restless and agitated. What should you do first?
   1. Obtain an order for restraints.
   2. Medicate the patient with haloperidol.
   3. Assist the patient in attending his scheduled music group therapy.
   4. Obtain an order for duloxetine.
7. When you suspect an older adult is considering suicide, the most appropriate intervention is to:
   1. Discuss suspicions with a significant other.
   2. Ask the patient directly about such plans.
   3. Constantly watch the patient.
   4. Refer the patient for mental health counseling.
8. The usual standard for reporting elder abuse is one:
   1. Of 100% certainty.
   2. Of reasonable belief that abuse has occurred or may occur.
   3. That is beyond a shadow of a doubt.
   4. With testimony of one or more eyewitnesses.
9. Long-term recovery from alcohol abuse is most likely to occur when:
   1. The family is supportive and kind.
   2. The patient uses disulfiram.
   3. The patient undergoes detoxification with benzodiazepines.
   4. The patient admits to having a problem.
10. Strategies to help prevent crime include: *(Select all that apply.)*
    1. Changing door locks after losing keys.
    2. Using direct deposit for pension funds.
    3. Using an informal buddy system in the neighborhood.
    4. Checking a service person's identification after letting him in.
    5. Avoiding clicking on an e-mail link from an unexpected or unknown sender.

Critical Thinking Activity

Read the clinical scenario and discuss the questions with your classmates.

Your 75-year-old male patient who is being discharged to his daughter's home has just been diagnosed with mild cognitive impairment. He has a history of alcohol abuse but has "not had a drink in a couple of years." Donepezil has been prescribed in hopes of slowing disease progression.

1. What pharmacologic concerns might you have for this individual?
2. What type of education could you do with his family?
3. To what type of community services could you refer the patient's daughter for help in managing this disorder?

appendix A

Standard Steps for All Nursing Procedures

AT THE BEGINNING OF THE PROCEDURE

STEP A: PERFORM THE TASK ACCORDING TO PROTOCOL

Mentally review the steps of the task beforehand. If you are uncertain how to do a task, ask your team leader, resource nurse, instructor, or charge nurse. If you are uncertain, ask your instructor.

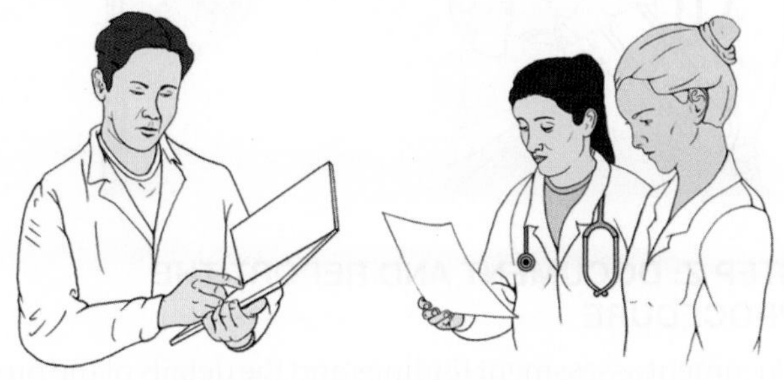

STEP B: CHECK THE ORDER, COLLECT THE EQUIPMENT AND SUPPLIES, AND PERFORM HAND HYGIENE

Verify that the procedure is to be done for the patient. Check the agency's policies and procedures manual for the accepted method of performing the procedure. Process equipment and supply charges. Take all equipment and supplies to the patient's room. Perform hand hygiene.

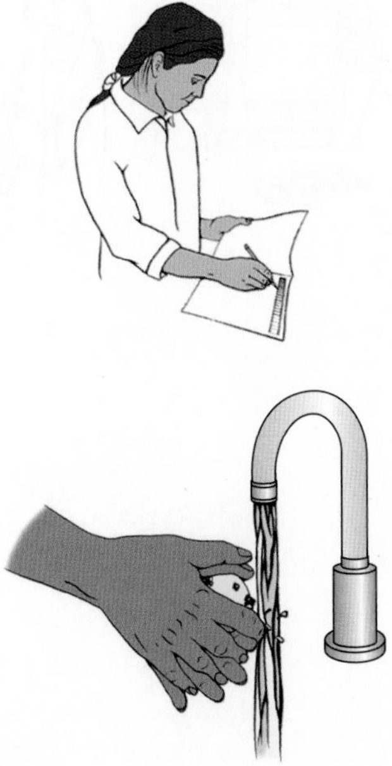

STEP C: IDENTIFY AND PREPARE THE PATIENT; INTRODUCE YOURSELF

Greet the patient, introduce yourself, and check the patient's identification band. Use two identifiers during the identification process. Explain what you are going to do in terms the patient can understand. Elicit questions and answer questions clearly. Provide necessary patient education related to the procedure to be performed.

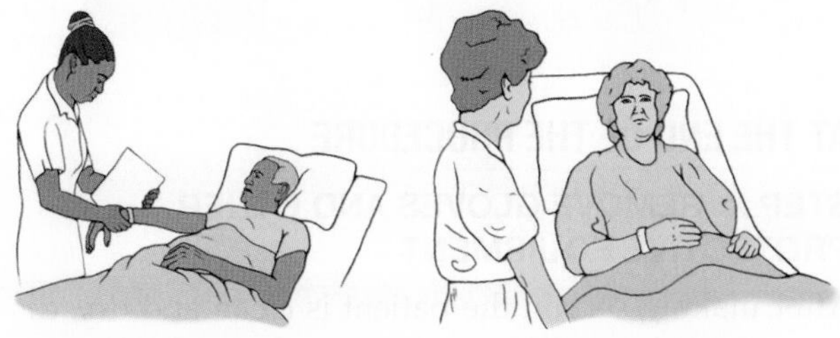

STEP D: PROVIDE PRIVACY AND INSTITUTE SAFETY PRECAUTIONS; ARRANGE THE SUPPLIES AND EQUIPMENT

Close the door or curtains and drape the patient before beginning the procedure or discussing information the person might want kept confidential. Check equipment for breaks or wear and for safety. Set up the equipment and supplies in an orderly, methodical fashion. Raise the bed to an appropriate working height. Raise the side rail before turning the patient and be certain that the wheels are locked. Perform hand hygiene to prevent contaminating the patient with organisms from the computer, the nurses' station, and the supply room.

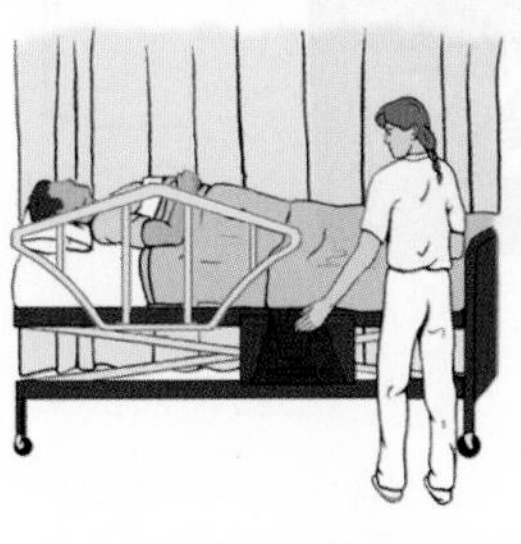

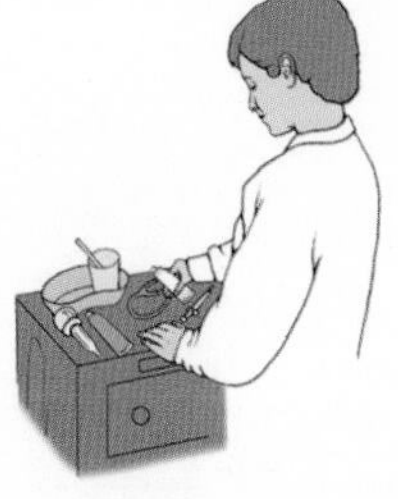

DURING THE PROCEDURE

STEP E: USE STANDARD PRECAUTIONS AND ASEPTIC TECHNIQUE AS APPROPRIATE

Protect yourself from blood and body fluids by wearing gloves. If there is a danger of splashing blood or body fluids, wear protective glasses or goggles and an impermeable cover gown or apron. Be very careful with sharp instruments and needles to prevent nicking your skin. (See Appendix D: Standard Precautions.)

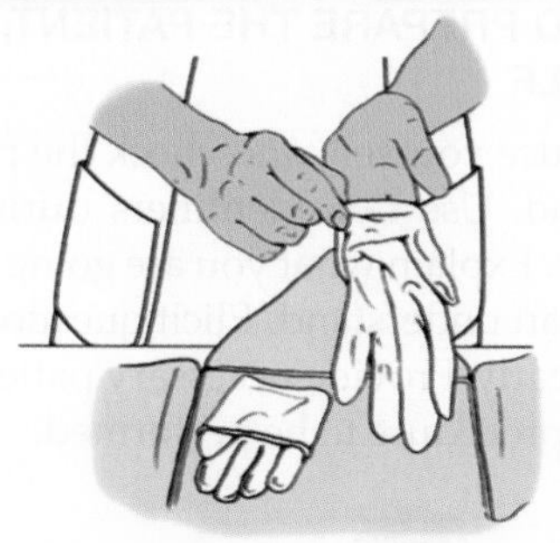

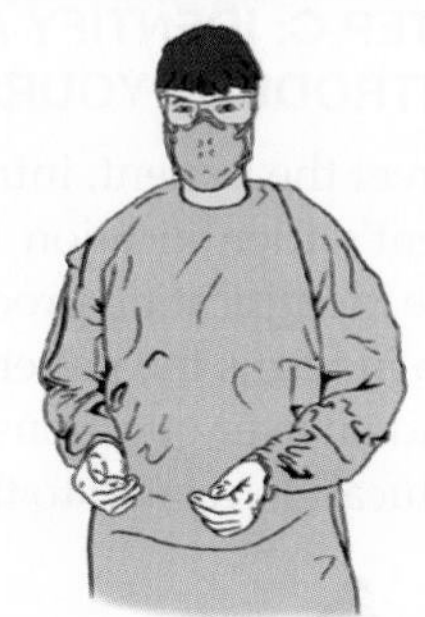

AT THE END OF THE PROCEDURE

STEP X: REMOVE GLOVES AND OTHER PROTECTIVE EQUIPMENT

After making certain the patient is clean and dry, dispose of used supplies, remove goggles and other protective equipment, and discard or store appropriately. To remove gloves without contaminating yourself, begin by pulling one glove off without touching your skin; hold the removed glove in the palm of the remaining gloved hand and then reach to the inside of the other glove and roll it down the hand. Dispose of the gloves in the trash. Perform hand hygiene immediately.

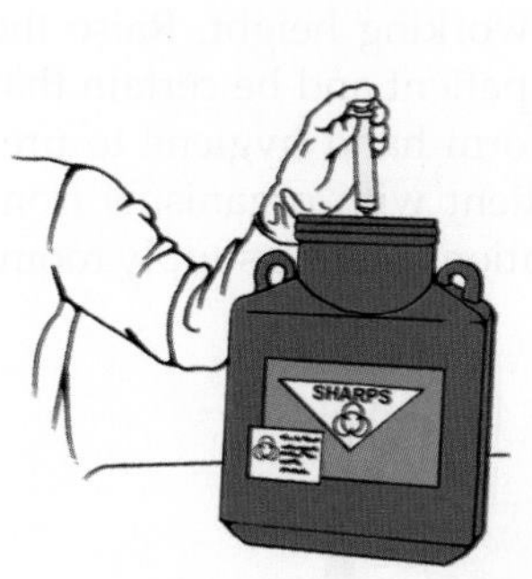

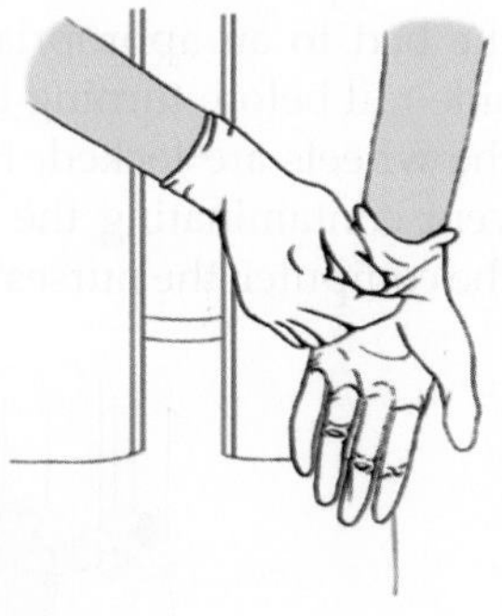

STEP Y: RESTORE THE UNIT. COLLECT THE USED EQUIPMENT; DISPOSE OF, CLEAN, OR STORE ITEMS IN THE PROPER PLACES

Make the person comfortable, tidy the bed and unit, place the call light and personal items within reach, and provide for safety by lowering the bed. Remove used equipment. Soiled linens are placed in a soiled linen hamper. Reusable items are cleaned and returned to the storage or processing area (central supply). Discontinue use of the equipment on the computer so no further charges will be made. Remove unsightly, odorous, or potentially infectious trash from the room. Inquire if anything else is needed. Perform hand hygiene before leaving the room.

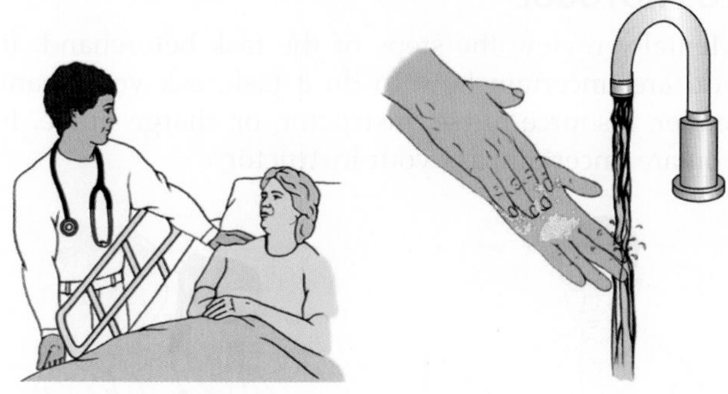

STEP Z: DOCUMENT AND REPORT THE PROCEDURE

Document assessment findings and the details of the procedure performed, or care given, in the medical record. Include any problems encountered and the patient's response to the care or treatment. The recording should be accurate, specific, concise, and appropriate and should include the specific time the procedure was performed and how it was done. Report abnormalities encountered to the charge nurse or the primary care provider.

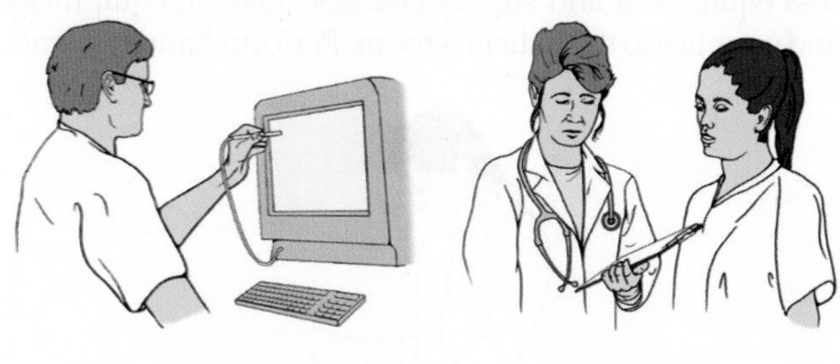

appendix B

NFLPN Nursing Practice Standards for the Licensed Practical/Vocational Nurse

"*Nursing Practice Standards*" is one of the ways that NFLPN meets the objective of its bylaws to address principles and ethics and also to meet another Article II objective, "To interpret the standards of practical (vocational) nursing."

In recent years, LPNs and LVNs have practiced in a changing environment. As LPNs and LVNs practice in expanding roles in the health care system, "*Nursing Practice Standards*" is essential reading for LPNs, LVNs, PN, and VN students and their educators, and all who practice with LPNs and LVNs.

NURSING PRACTICE STANDARDS FOR THE LICENSED PRACTICAL/VOCATIONAL NURSE

PREFACE

The Standards were developed and adopted by NFLPN to provide a basic model whereby the quality of health service and nursing service and nursing care given by LP/VNs may be measured and evaluated.

These nursing practice standards are applicable in any practice setting. The degree to which individual standards are applied will vary according to the individual needs of the patient, the type of health care agency or services, and the community resources.

The scope of licensed practical nursing has extended into specialized nursing services. Therefore specialized fields of nursing are included in this document.

THE CODE FOR LICENSED PRACTICAL/VOCATIONAL NURSES

The code, adopted by NFLPN in 1961 and revised in 1979, provides a motivation for establishing, maintaining, and elevating professional standards. Each LP/VN, upon entering the profession, inherits the responsibility to adhere to the standards of ethical practice and conduct as set forth in this code.

1. Know the scope of maximum utilization of the LP/VN as specified by the nursing practice act and function within this scope.
2. Safeguard the confidential information acquired from any source about the patient.
3. Provide health care to all patients regardless of race, creed, cultural background, disease, or lifestyle.
4. Uphold the highest standards in personal appearance, language, dress, and demeanor.
5. Stay informed about issues affecting the practice of nursing and delivery of health care and, when appropriate, participate in government and policy decisions.
6. Accept the responsibility for safe nursing by keeping oneself mentally and physically fit and educationally prepared to practice.
7. Accept responsibility for membership in NFLPN and participate in its efforts to maintain the established standards of nursing practice and employment policies that lead to quality patient care.

INTRODUCTORY STATEMENT

Definition

Practical/vocational nursing means the performance for compensation of authorized acts of nursing that use specialized knowledge and skills and that meet the health needs of people in a variety of settings under the direction of qualified health professionals.

Scope

Licensed practical/vocational nurses represent the established entry into the nursing profession and include specialized fields of nursing practice.

Opportunities exist for practicing in a milieu where different professions unite their particular skills in a team effort: to preserve or improve an individual patient's functioning and to protect health and safety of patients.

Opportunities also exist for career advancement within the profession through academic education and for lateral expansion of knowledge and expertise through both academic/continuing education and certification.

STANDARDS

Education

The Licensed Practical/Vocational Nurse

1. Shall complete a formal education program in practical nursing approved by the appropriate nursing authority in a state.
2. Shall successfully pass the National Council Licensure Examination for Practical Nurses.
3. Shall participate in initial orientation within the employing institution.

Legal/Ethical Status

The Licensed Practical/Vocational Nurse

1. Shall hold a current license to practice nursing as an LP/VN in accordance with the law of the state wherein employed.
2. Shall know the scope of nursing practice authorized by the Nursing Practice Act in the state wherein employed.
3. Shall have a personal commitment to fulfill the legal responsibilities inherent in good nursing practice.
4. Shall take responsible actions in situations wherein there is unprofessional conduct by a peer or other health care provider.
5. Shall recognize and have a commitment to meet the ethical and moral obligations of the practice of nursing.
6. Shall not accept or perform professional responsibilities that the individual knows he or she is not competent to perform.

Practice

The Licensed Practical/Vocational Nurse

1. Shall accept assigned responsibilities as an accountable member of the health care team.
2. Shall function within the limits of educational preparation and experience as related to the assigned duties.
3. Shall function with other members of the health care team in promoting and maintaining health, preventing disease and disability, caring for and rehabilitating individuals who are experiencing an altered health state, and contributing to the ultimate quality of life until death.
4. Shall know and use the nursing process in planning, implementing, and evaluating health services and nursing care for the individual patient or group.
   a. Planning: The planning of nursing includes the following:
      1) Assessment/data collection of health status of the individual patient, the family, and community groups.
      2) Reporting information gained from assessment/data collection.
      3) The identification of health goals.
   b. Implementation: The plan for nursing care is put into practice to achieve the stated goals and includes the following:
      1) Observing, recording, and reporting significant changes that require intervention or different goals.
      2) Applying nursing knowledge and skills to promote and maintain health, to prevent disease and disability, and to optimize functional capabilities of an individual patient.
      3) Assisting the patient and family with activities of daily living and encouraging self-care as appropriate.
      4) Carrying out therapeutic regimens and protocols prescribed by personnel pursuant to authorized state law.
   c. Evaluations: The plan for nursing care and its implementations are evaluated to measure the progress toward the stated goals and will include appropriate person[s] and/or groups to determine the following:
      1) The relevancy of current goals in relation to the progress of the individual patient.
      2) The involvement of the recipients of care in the evaluation process.
      3) The quality of the nursing action in the implementation of the plan.
      4) A reordering of priorities or new goal setting in the care plan.
5. Shall participate in peer review and other evaluation processes.
6. Shall participate in the development of policies concerning the health and nursing needs of society and in the roles and functions of the LP/VN.

Continuing Education

The Licensed Practical/Vocational Nurse

1. Shall be responsible for maintaining the highest possible level of professional competence at all times.
2. Shall periodically reassess career goals and select continuing education activities that will help achieve these goals.
3. Shall take advantage of continuing education and certification opportunities that will lead to personal growth and professional development.
4. Shall seek and participate in continuing education activities that are approved for credit by appropriate organizations, such as the NFLPN.

Specialized Nursing Practice

The Licensed Practical/Vocational Nurse

1. Shall have had at least 1 year's experience in nursing at the staff level.
2. Shall present personal qualifications that are indicative of potential abilities for practice in the chosen specialized nursing area.
3. Shall present evidence of completion of a program or course that is approved by an appropriate agency to provide the knowledge and skills necessary for effective nursing services in the specialized field.
4. Shall meet all of the standards of practice as set forth in this document.

NFLPN, National Federation of Licensed Practical Nurses; LPN, licensed practical nurse; LVN, licensed vocational nurse; PN, practical nurse; VN, vocational nurse

appendix C

American Nurses Association Code of Ethics for Nurses

- The nurse practices with compassion and respect for the inherent dignity, worth, and unique attributes of every person.
- The nurse's primary commitment is to the patient, whether an individual, family, group, community, or population.
- The nurse promotes, advocates for, and protects the rights, health, and safety of the patient.
- The nurse has authority, accountability, and responsibility for nursing practice; makes decisions; and takes action consistent with the obligation to promote health and to provide optimal care.
- The nurse owes the same duties to self as to others, including the responsibility to promote health and safety, preserve wholeness of character and integrity, maintain competence, and continue personal and professional growth.
- The nurse, through individual and collective effort, establishes, maintains, and improves the ethical environment of the work setting and conditions of employment that are conducive to safe, quality health care.
- The nurse, in all roles and settings, advances the profession through research and scholarly inquiry, professional standards development, and the generation of both nursing and health policy.
- The nurse collaborates with other health professionals and the public to protect human rights, promote health diplomacy, and reduce health disparities.
- The profession of nursing, collectively through its professional organizations, must articulate nursing values, maintain the integrity of the profession, and integrate principles of social justice into nursing and health policy.

Adapted from: <http://nursingworld.org/DocumentVault/Ethics-1/Code-of-Ethics-for-Nurses.html>

appendix

D Standard Precautions

RECOMMENDATIONS

IV STANDARD PRECAUTIONS

Assume that every person is potentially infected or colonized with an organism that could be transmitted in the health care setting and apply the following infection control practices during the delivery of health care.

IV.A Hand Hygiene

IV.A.1: During the delivery of health care, avoid unnecessary touching of surfaces in close proximity to the patient to prevent both contamination of clean hands from environmental surfaces and transmission of pathogens from contaminated hands to surfaces.

IV.A.2: When hands are visibly dirty, contaminated with proteinaceous material, or visibly soiled with blood or body fluids, wash hands with either a non-antimicrobial soap and water or an antimicrobial soap and water.

IV.A.3: If hands are not visibly soiled, or after removing visible material with non-antimicrobial soap and water, decontaminate hands in the clinical situations described in IV.A.3.a–f. The preferred method of hand decontamination is with an alcohol-based hand rub. Alternatively, hands may be washed with an antimicrobial soap and water. Frequent use of alcohol-based hand rub immediately following handwashing with non-antimicrobial soap may increase the frequency of dermatitis. Perform hand hygiene:

- *IV.A.3.a:* Before having direct contact with patients.
- *IV.A.3.b:* After contact with blood, body fluids or excretions, mucous membranes, nonintact skin, or wound dressings.
- *IV.A.3.c:* After contact with a patient's intact skin (e.g., when taking a pulse or blood pressure or lifting a patient).
- *IV.A.3.d:* If hands will be moving from a contaminated body site to a clean body site during patient care.
- *IV.A.3.e:* After contact with inanimate objects (including medical equipment) in the immediate vicinity of the patient.
- *IV.A.3.f:* After removing gloves.

IV.A.4: Wash hands with non-antimicrobial or antimicrobial soap and water if contact with spores (e.g., *Clostridium difficile* or *Bacillus anthracis*) is likely to have occurred. The physical action of washing and rinsing hands under such circumstances is recommended because alcohols, chlorhexidine, iodophors, and other antiseptic agents have poor activity against spores.

IV.A.5: Do not wear artificial fingernails or extenders if duties include direct contact with patients at high risk for infection and associated adverse outcomes (e.g., those in intensive care units [ICUs] or operating rooms).

- *IV.A.5.a:* Develop an organizational policy on the wearing of non-natural nails by health care personnel who have direct contact with patients outside of the groups specified above.

IV.B Personal Protective Equipment

IV.B.1: Observe the following principles of use:

- *IV.B.1.a:* Wear Personal Protective Equipment (PPE), as described in IV.B.2–4, when the nature of the anticipated patient interaction indicates that contact with blood or body fluids may occur.
- *IV.B.1.b:* Prevent contamination of clothing and skin during the process of removing PPE.
- *IV.B.1.c:* Before leaving the patient's room or cubicle, remove and discard PPE.

IV.B.2: Gloves

- *IV.B.2.a:* Wear gloves when it can be reasonably anticipated that contact with blood or other potentially infectious materials, mucous membranes, nonintact skin, or potentially contaminated intact skin (e.g., of a patient incontinent of stool or urine) could occur.
- *IV.B.2.b:* Wear gloves with fit and durability appropriate to the task.
  - *IV.B.2.b.i:* Wear disposable medical examination gloves for providing direct patient care.
  - *IV.B.2.b.ii:* Wear disposable medical examination gloves or reusable utility gloves for cleaning the environment or medical equipment.
- *IV.B.2.c:* Remove gloves after contact with a patient and/or the surrounding environment (including medical equipment) using proper technique to prevent hand contamination. Do not wear the same pair of gloves for the care of more than one patient. Do not wash gloves for the purpose of reuse since this practice has been associated with transmission of pathogens.

IV.B.2.d: Change gloves during patient care if the hands will move from a contaminated body site (e.g., perineal area) to a clean body site (e.g., face).

IV.B.3: Gowns

IV.B.3.a: Wear a gown, that is appropriate to the task, to protect skin and prevent soiling or contamination of clothing during procedures and patient-care activities when contact with blood, body fluids, secretions, or excretions is anticipated.

IV.B.3.a.i: Wear a gown for direct patient contact if the patient has uncontained secretions or excretions.

IV.B.3.a.ii: Remove gown and perform hand hygiene before leaving the patient's environment.

IV.B.3.b: Do not reuse gowns, even for repeated contacts with the same patient.

IV.B.3.c: Routine donning of gowns upon entrance into a high-risk unit (e.g., ICU, neonatal intensive care unit [NICU], hematopoietic stem cell transplantation [HSCT] unit) is not indicated.

IV.B.4: Mouth, nose, eye protection

IV.B.4.a: Use PPE to protect the mucous membranes of the eyes, nose, and mouth during procedures and patient-care activities that are likely to generate splashes or sprays of blood, body fluids, secretions, and excretions. Select masks, goggles, face shields, and combinations of each according to the need anticipated by the task performed.

IV.B.5: During aerosol-generating procedures (e.g., bronchoscopy, suctioning of the respiratory tract [if not using in-line suction catheters], endotracheal intubation) in patients who are not suspected of being infected with an agent for which respiratory protection is otherwise recommended (e.g., *Mycobacterium tuberculosis*, SARS, or hemorrhagic fever viruses), wear one of the following: a face shield that fully covers the front and sides of the face, a mask with attached shield, or a mask and goggles (in addition to gloves and gown).

IV.C Respiratory Hygiene/Cough Etiquette

IV.C.1: Educate health care personnel on the importance of source control measures to contain respiratory secretions to prevent droplet and fomite transmission of respiratory pathogens, especially during seasonal outbreaks of viral respiratory tract infections (e.g., influenza, RSV, adenovirus, parainfluenza virus) in communities.

IV.C.2: Implement the following measures to contain respiratory secretions in patients and accompanying individuals who have signs and symptoms of a respiratory infection, beginning at the point of initial encounter in a health care setting (e.g., triage, reception and waiting areas in emergency departments, outpatient clinics and physician offices).

IV.C.2.a: Post signs at entrances and in strategic places (e.g., elevators, cafeterias) within ambulatory and inpatient settings with instructions to patients and other persons with symptoms of a respiratory infection to cover their mouths/noses when coughing or sneezing, use and dispose of tissues, and perform hand hygiene after hands have been in contact with respiratory secretions.

IV.C.2.b: Provide tissues and no-touch receptacles (e.g., foot pedal–operated lid or open, plastic-lined wastebasket) for disposal of tissues.

IV.C.2.c: Provide resources and instructions for performing hand hygiene in or near waiting areas in ambulatory and inpatient settings; provide conveniently located dispensers of alcohol-based hand rubs and, where sinks are available, supplies for handwashing.

IV.C.2.d: During periods of increased prevalence of respiratory infections in the community (e.g., as indicated by increased school absenteeism, increased number of patients seeking care for a respiratory infection), offer masks to coughing patients and other symptomatic persons (e.g., persons who accompany ill patients) upon entry into the facility or medical office and encourage them to maintain special separation, ideally a distance of at least 3 feet, from others in common waiting areas.

IV.C.2.d.i: Some facilities may find it logistically easier to institute this recommendation year-round as a standard of practice.

IV.D Patient Placement

IV.D.1: Include the potential for transmission of infectious agents in patient placement decisions. Place patients who pose a risk for transmission to others (e.g., uncontained secretions, excretions or wound drainage; infants with suspected viral respiratory or gastrointestinal infections) in a single-patient room when available.

IV.D.2: Determine patient placement based on the following principles:

- Route(s) of transmission of the known or suspected infectious agent
- Risk factors for transmission in the infected patient
- Risk factors for adverse outcomes resulting from an HAI in other patients in the area or room being considered for patient placement
- Availability of single-patient rooms
- Patient options for room sharing (e.g., cohorting patients with the same infection)

IV.E Patient-Care Equipment and Instruments/Devices

IV.E.1: Establish policies and procedures for containing, transporting, and handling patient-care equipment and instruments/devices that may be contaminated with blood or body fluids.

IV.E.2: Remove organic material from critical and semi-critical instruments/devices, using recommended cleaning agents before high-level disinfection and sterilization to enable effective disinfection and sterilization processes.

IV.E.3: Wear PPE (e.g., gloves, gown) according to the level of anticipated contamination, when handling patient-care equipment and instruments/devices that are visibly soiled or may have been in contact with blood or body fluids.

IV.F Care of the Environment

IV.F.1: Establish policies and procedures for routine and targeted cleaning of environmental surfaces as indicated by the level of patient contact and degree of soiling.

IV.F.2: Clean and disinfect surfaces that are likely to be contaminated with pathogens, including those that are in close proximity to the patient (e.g., bed rails, over bed tables) and frequently touched surfaces in the patient care environment (e.g., doorknobs, surfaces in and surrounding toilets in patients' rooms) on a more frequent schedule compared to that for other surfaces (e.g., horizontal surfaces in waiting rooms).

IV.F.3: Use EPA-registered disinfectants that have microbicidal (i.e., killing) activity against the pathogens most likely to contaminate the patient-care environment. Use in accordance with manufacturer's instructions.

IV.F.3.a: Review the efficacy of in-use disinfectants when evidence of continuing transmission of an infectious agent (e.g., rotavirus, *C. difficile*, norovirus) may indicate resistance to the in-use product and change to a more effective disinfectant as indicated.

IV.F.4: In facilities that provide health care to pediatric patients or have waiting areas with child play toys (e.g., obstetric/gynecology offices and clinics), establish policies and procedures for cleaning and disinfecting toys at regular intervals. Use the following principles in developing this policy and procedures:

- Select play toys that can be easily cleaned and disinfected.
- Do not permit use of stuffed furry toys if they will be shared.
- Clean and disinfect large stationary toys (e.g., climbing equipment) at least weekly and whenever visibly soiled.
- If toys are likely to be mouthed, rinse with water after disinfection; alternatively wash in a dishwasher.
- When a toy requires cleaning and disinfection, do so immediately or store in a designated labeled container separate from toys that are clean and ready for use.

IV.F.5: Include multiuse electronic equipment in policies and procedures for preventing contamination and for cleaning and disinfection, especially those items that are used by patients, those used during delivery of patient care, and mobile devices that are moved in and out of patient rooms frequently (e.g., daily).

IV.F.5.a: No recommendation for use of removable protective covers or washable keyboards. Unresolved issue.

IV.G Textiles and Laundry

IV.G.1: Handle used textiles and fabrics with minimum agitation to avoid contamination of air, surfaces, and persons.

IV.G.2: If laundry chutes are used, ensure that they are properly designed, maintained, and used in a manner to minimize dispersion of aerosols from contaminated laundry.

IV.H Safe Injection Practices

The following recommendations apply to the use of needles, cannulas that replace needles, and where applicable, intravenous delivery systems:

IV.H.1: Use aseptic technique to avoid contamination of sterile injection equipment.

IV.H.2: Do not administer medications from a syringe to multiple patients, even if the needle or cannula on the syringe is changed. Needles, cannulas, and syringes are sterile, single-use items; they should not be reused for another patient or to access a medication or solution that might be used for a subsequent patient.

IV.H.3: Use fluid infusion and administration sets (i.e., intravenous bags, tubing, and connectors) for one patient only, and dispose appropriately after use. Consider a syringe or needle/cannula contaminated once it has been used to enter or connect to a patient's intravenous infusion bag or administration set.

IV.H.4: Use single-dose vials for parenteral medications whenever possible.

IV.H.5: Do not administer medications from single-dose vials or ampules to multiple patients or combine leftover contents for later use.

IV.H.6: If multidose vials must be used, both the needle or cannula and syringe used to access the multidose vial must be sterile.

IV.H.7: Do not keep multidose vials in the immediate patient treatment area and store in accordance with the manufacturer's recommendations; discard if sterility is compromised or questionable.

IV.H.8: Do not use bags or bottles of intravenous solution as a common source of supply for multiple patients.

IV.I Infection Control Practices for Special Lumbar Puncture Procedures

Wear a surgical mask when placing a catheter or injecting material into the spinal canal or subdural space (i.e., during myelograms, lumbar puncture, and spinal or epidural anesthesia).

IV.J Worker Safety

Adhere to federal and state requirements for protection of health care personnel from exposure to bloodborne pathogens.

EPA, environmental protection agency; HAI, health care-associated infection; RSV, respiratory syncytial virus; SARS, severe acute respiratory syndrome

appendix E

Most Common Laboratory Test Values

Complete Blood Count

TEST	CONVENTIONAL UNITS	SI UNITS
Erythrocytes (Red Blood Cells [RBCs])		
Males	4.7-6.1 million/mm^3	4.7-6.2 × 10^{12}/L
Females	4.2-5.4 million/mm^3	4.2-5.4 × 10^{12}/L
Children (varies with age)	4.5-5.1 million/mm^3	4.5-5.1 × 10^{12}/L
	4,500-11,000/mm^3	4.5-11.0 × 10^9/L
Red Cell Indices		
Mean corpuscular hemoglobin (MCH)	27-31 pg	27-31 pg
Mean corpuscular volume (MCV)	80-95 fL	80-95 fL
Mean corpuscular hemoglobin concentration (MCHC)	32-36 g/dL	320-360 g/L
Hemoglobin		
Males	14.0-18.0 g/dL	8.7-11.2 mmol/L
Females	12.0-16.0 g/dL	7.4-9.9 mmol/L
Newborns	16.5-19.5 g/dL	10.2-12.1 mmol/L
Children (varies with age)	11.2-16.5 g/dL	7.0-10.2 mmol/L
Hematocrit		
Males	42-52 mL/dL	0.42-0.52
Females	37-47 mL/dL	0.37-0.47
Newborns	49-54 mL/dL	0.49-0.54
Children (varies with age)	35-49 mL/dL	0.35-0.49
Leukocytes (white blood cells [WBCs])	5,000-10,000/mm^3	5.0-10.0 × 10^6/L
Leukocyte Differential Counts		
Band neutrophils	3-5%	150-400 × 10^6/L
Segmented neutrophils	54-62%	3,000-5,800 × 10^6/L
Lymphocytes	28-33%	1,500-3,000 × 10^6/L
Monocytes	3-7%	300-500 × 10^6/L
Eosinophils	1-3%	50-250 × 10^6/L
Basophils	0-1%	15-50 × 10^6/L
Platelets	150,000-400,000/mm^3	150-400 × 10^9/L

fL, Femtoliter

Urinalysis

TEST	CONVENTIONAL UNITS	TEST	CONVENTIONAL UNITS
Appearance	Clear	Ketones	Negative
Color	Yellow amber	Bilirubin (urobilinogen)	Negative
Odor	Aromatic	Glucose	Negative
pH	4.6-8.0	WBCs	0-4 per low-power field
Specific gravity	1.003-1.030	RBCs	0-2 per high-power field
Protein	0-0.8 mg/dL	Casts	None
Nitrites	Negative	Crystals	None

RBCs, Red blood cells; *WBCs,* white blood cells.

Blood Chemistry Panel (SMA, Astra-7, Chem-7, Basic Metabolic Panel, Electrolytes)

TEST	CONVENTIONAL UNITS	SI UNITS
Albumin	3.5-5.0 g/dL	35-50 g/L
Alkaline phosphatase (ALP)	30-120 units/L	30-120 units/L
Aspartate aminotransferase (AST)	0-35 units/L	0-35 units/L
Bilirubin, conjugate	0.1-0.4 mg/dL	1.7-6.8 mcg mol/L
Bilirubin, total	0.3-1.1 mg/dL	5.1-19.0 mcg mol/L
Blood urea nitrogen (BUN)	11-23 mg/dL	8.0-16.4 nmol/L
Calcium	8.4-10.6 mg/dL	2.10-2.65 mmol/L
Carbon dioxide	4-31 mEq/L	24-31 mmol/L
Chloride	96-106 mEq/L	96-106 mmol/L
Creatinine	0.6-1.2 mg/dL	50-110 mcg mol/L
Glucose	70-100 mg/dL	3.9-5.55 nmol/L
Potassium	3.5-5.0 mEq/L	3.5-5.0 mmol/L
Protein	6.0-8.0 g/dL	60-80 g/L
Sodium	135-145 mEq/L	135-145 mmol/L
Triglycerides	40-150 mg/dL	0.4-1.5 g/L
Uric Acid		
Males	2.5-8.0 mg/dL	150-480 mcg mol/L
Females	2.2-7.0 mg/dL	130-420 mcg mol/L

SMA, sequential multiple analysis.

Lipid Panel

TEST	CONVENTIONAL UNITS	SI UNITS
Cholesterol, total	<200 mg/dL	<5.20 mmol/L
Low-density lipoprotein (LDL)	<130 mg/dL	<3.4 mmol/L
High-density lipoprotein (HDL)	>45 mg/dL (men)	>1.16 mmol/L (men)
	>55 mg/dL (women)	>1.42 mmol/L (women)

Thyroid Tests

TEST	CONVENTIONAL UNITS	SI UNITS
Thyrotropin (TSH)	0.3-5.0 mcg IU/mL	0.3-5.0 mIU/L
Thyroxin (T_4)	4.0-12.0 mcg/dL	51-154 nmol/L
Thyroxine, free (FT_4)	0.8-2.8 ng/dL	10-36 pmol/L

Miscellaneous Commonly Performed Tests

TEST	CONVENTIONAL UNITS	SI UNITS
Digoxin level	0.8-2.0 ng/mL	0.8-2.0 ng/mL
Prothrombin time (PT)	12.0-14 s; INR 1.5-2 times control value	85-100%; INR 20-30%
Activated partial thromboplastin time (APPT)	20-25 s	20-35 s

INR, International normalized ratio; *pg*, pictograms.
Data from Pagana, K., & Pagana, T. (2014). *Mosby's manual of diagnostic and laboratory tests* (5th ed.). St. Louis, MO: Mosby.
Additional data from: *Mayo Clinic Staff. Cholesterol test*. (2016). http://www.mayoclinic.org/tests-procedures/cholesterol-test/details/results/rsc-20169555.

appendix F

NANDA-I Approved Nursing Diagnoses, 2015-2017*

Activity intolerance: Insufficient physiological or psychological energy to endure or complete required or desired daily activities.

Acute pain: An unpleasant sensory and emotional experience associated with actual or potential tissue damage, or described in terms of such damage (International Association for the Study of Pain); sudden or slow onset of any intensity from mild to severe with an anticipated or predictable end.

Anxiety: Vague, uneasy feeling of discomfort or dread accompanied by an autonomic response (the source is often nonspecific or unknown to the individual); a feeling of apprehension caused by anticipation of danger. It is an alerting sign that warns of impending danger and enables the individual to take measures to deal with threat.

Bathing self-care deficit: Impaired ability to perform or complete bathing activities for self.

Bowel incontinence: Change in normal bowel habits characterized by involuntary passage of stool.

Chronic low self-esteem: Longstanding negative self-evaluating/feelings about self or self-capabilities.

Chronic pain: Unpleasant sensory and emotional experience associated with actual or potential tissue damage, or described in terms of such damage (International Association for the Study of Pain); sudden or slow onset of any intensity from mild to severe, constant or recurring without an anticipated or predictable end and a duration of greater than three (>3) months.

Constipation: Decrease in normal frequency of defecation accompanied by difficult or incomplete passage of stool and/or passage of excessively hard, dry stool.

Decisional conflict: Uncertainty about course of action to be taken when choice among competing actions involves risk, loss, or challenge to values and beliefs.

Decreased cardiac output: Inadequate blood pumped by the heart to meet the metabolic demands of the body.

Deficient diversional activity: Decreased stimulation from (or interest or engagement in) recreational or leisure activities.

Deficient fluid volume: Decreased intravascular, interstitial, and/or intracellular fluid. This refers to dehydration, water loss alone without change in sodium level.

Deficient knowledge: Absence or deficiency of cognitive information related to a specific topic.

Diarrhea: Passage of loose, unformed stools.

Disturbed body image: Confusion in mental picture of one's physical self.

Dressing self-care deficit: Impaired ability to perform or complete dressing activities for self.

Excess fluid volume: Increased isotonic fluid retention.

Fatigue: An overwhelming, sustained sense of exhaustion and decreased capacity for physical and mental work at the usual level.

Fear: Response to perceived threat that is consciously recognized as a danger.

Feeding self-care deficit: Impaired ability to perform or complete self-feeding activities.

Functional urinary incontinence: Inability of a usually continent person to reach the toilet in time to avoid unintentional loss of urine.

Grieving: A normal complex process that includes emotional, physical, spiritual, social, and intellectual responses and behaviors by which individuals, families, and communities incorporate an actual, anticipated, or perceived loss into their daily lives.

Hyperthermia: Core body temperature above the normal diurnal range due to failure of thermoregulation.

Hypothermia: Core body temperature below normal diurnal range due to failure of thermoregulation.

Imbalanced nutrition: less than body requirements: Intake of nutrients insufficient to meet metabolic needs.

Impaired gas exchange: Excess or deficit in oxygenation and/or carbon dioxide elimination at the alveolar-capillary membrane.

Impaired physical mobility: Limitation in independent, purposeful physical movement of the body or of one or more extremities.

Impaired skin integrity: Altered epidermis and/or dermis.

Impaired social interaction: Insufficient or excessive quantity or ineffective quality of social exchange.

Impaired spontaneous ventilation: Decreased energy reserves resulting in an inability to maintain independent breathing that is adequate to support life.

*NANDA International, Inc. terms and definitions used in this text. For the complete list, please refer to Herdman TH (Ed.) Nursing Diagnoses – Definitions and Classifications 2015-2017. Copyright © 2014, 1994-2014 NANDA International.

Impaired swallowing: Abnormal functioning of the swallowing mechanism associated with deficits in oral, pharyngeal, or esophageal structure or function.

Impaired urinary elimination: Dysfunction in urine elimination.

Impaired verbal communication: Decreased, delayed, or absent ability to receive, process, transmit, and/or use a system of symbols.

Impaired walking: Limitation of independent movement within the environment on foot.

Ineffective airway clearance: Inability to clear secretions or obstructions from the respiratory tract to maintain a clear airway.

Ineffective breathing pattern: Inspiration and/or expiration that does not provide adequate ventilation.

Ineffective coping: Inability to form a valid appraisal of the stressors, inadequate choices of practiced responses, and/or inability to use available resources.

Ineffective health management: Pattern of regulating and integrating into daily living a therapeutic regimen for the treatment of illness and its sequelae that is unsatisfactory for meeting specific health goals.

Ineffective peripheral tissue perfusion: Decrease in blood circulation to the periphery that may compromise health.

Ineffective role performance: A pattern of behavior and self-expression that does not match the environmental context, norms, and expectations.

Ineffective thermoregulation: Temperature fluctuation between hypothermia and hyperthermia.

Noncompliance: Behavior of person and/or caregiver that fails to coincide with a health-promoting or therapeutic plan agreed on by the person (and/or family and/or community) and health care professional. In the presence of an agreed-on, health-promoting, or therapeutic plan, person's or caregiver's behavior is fully or partly non-adherent and may lead to clinically ineffective or partially effective outcomes.

Overflow urinary incontinence: Involuntary loss of urine associated with overdistention of the bladder.

Readiness for enhanced comfort: A pattern of ease, relief, and transcendence in physical, psychospiritual, environmental, and/or social dimensions, which can be strengthened.

Readiness for enhanced nutrition: A pattern of nutrient intake, which can be strengthened.

Readiness for enhanced sleep: A pattern of natural, periodic suspension of relative consciousness to provide rest and sustain a desired lifestyle, which can be strengthened.

Reflex urinary incontinence: Involuntary loss of urine at somewhat predictable intervals when a specific bladder volume is reached.

Risk for aspiration: Vulnerable to entry of gastrointestinal secretions, oropharyngeal secretions, solids, or fluids to the tracheobronchial passages, which may compromise health.

Risk for deficient fluid volume: Vulnerable to experiencing decreased intravascular, interstitial, and/or intracellular fluid volumes, which may compromise health.

Risk for disuse syndrome: Vulnerable to deterioration of body systems as the result of prescribed or unavoidable musculoskeletal inactivity, which may compromise health.

Risk for dry eye: Vulnerable to eye discomfort or damage to the cornea and conjunctiva due to reduced quantity or quality of tears to moisten the eye, which may compromise health.

Risk for falls: Vulnerable to increased susceptibility to falling, which may cause physical harm and compromise health.

Risk for imbalanced fluid volume: Vulnerable to a decrease, increase, or rapid shift from one to the other of intravascular, interstitial, and/or intracellular fluid, which may compromise health. This refers to body fluid loss, gain, or both.

Risk for impaired skin integrity: Vulnerable to alteration in epidermis and/or dermis, which may compromise health.

Risk for ineffective cerebral tissue perfusion: Vulnerable to a decrease in cerebral tissue circulation, which may compromise health.

Risk for infection: Vulnerable to invasion and multiplication of pathogenic organisms which may compromise health.

Risk for injury: Vulnerable to physical damage due to environmental conditions interacting with the individual's adaptive and defensive resources, which may compromise health.

Risk for peripheral neurovascular dysfunction: Vulnerable to disruption in the circulation, sensation, and motion of an extremity, which may compromise health.

Risk for unstable blood glucose level: Vulnerable to variation in blood glucose/sugar levels from the normal range, which may compromise health.

Risk-prone health behavior: Impaired ability to modify lifestyle/behaviors in a manner that improves health status.

Situational low self-esteem: Development of a negative perception of self-worth in response to a current situation.

Sleep deprivation: Prolonged periods of time without sleep (sustained natural, periodic suspension of relative consciousness).

Social isolation: Aloneness experienced by the individual and perceived as imposed by others and as a negative or threatening state.

Spiritual distress: A state of suffering related to the impaired ability to experience meaning in life through connections with self, others, world, or a superior being.

Stress urinary incontinence: Sudden leakage of urine with activities that increase intra-abdominal pressure.

Toileting self-care deficit: Impaired ability to perform or complete self-toileting activities.

Urge urinary incontinence: Involuntary passage of urine occurring soon after a strong sense of urgency to void.

Urinary retention: Incomplete emptying of the bladder.

Reader References

CHAPTER 1

Academy of Medical-Surgical Nurses. (2014). *Evidence-Based Practice*. www.amsn.org/practiceresources/evidence-based-practice.

Benner, P., & Wrubel, J. (1989). *The Primacy of Caring: stress and Coping in Health and Illness*. Upper Saddle River, NJ: Prentice-Hall.

Centers for Medicare & Medicaid Services. (2015). *Closing the Coverage Gap: medicare Prescription Drugs Are Becoming More Affordable*. www.medicare.gov/Pubs/pdf/11493.pdf.

Cliff, B. (2012). The evolution of patient-centered care. *Journal of Healthcare Management*, *57*(2), 86–88.

Epstein, B., & Turner, M. (2015). The nursing code of ethics: its value, its history. *OJIN: the Online Journal of Issues in Nursing*, *20*(2), Manuscript 4.

Hawkins, J. E., & Shell, E. (2012). *Magnet® hospitals are attracted to the BSN but what's in it for nurses?* www.nursingcenter.com/lnc/journalarticle?Article_ID=1307122#sthash.jITptiu9.dpuf.

Henderson, V. A. (1955). Definition of nursing. In B. Harmer (Ed.), *Textbook of the Principles and Practice of Nursing*. New York, NY: MacMillan Pub. Co.

Johnson, D. E. (1968). *One conceptual model of nursing. Unpublished Lecture*. Nashville, TN: Vanderbilt University.

Koloroutis, M., Manthey, M., Felgen, J., et al. (2004). *Relationship-Based Care: a Model for Transforming Practice*. Minneapolis, MN: Creative Health Care Inc.

National League for Nursing. (2014). *A Vision for Recognition of the Role of Licensed Practical/Vocational Nurses in Advancing the Nation's Health*. www.nln.org/docs/default-source/about/nln-vision-series-%28position-statements%29/nlnvision_7.pdf?sfvrsn=4.

Neuman, B., & Young, R. J. (1972). A model for teaching total person approach to patient problems. *Nursing Research, May/June*, *21*(3), 264–269.

Orem, D. E. (1971). *Nursing: concepts of Practice*. New York, NY: McGraw-Hill.

Parse, R. R. (1987). *Nursing Science: major Paradigms, Theories, and Critiques*. Philadelphia, PA: Saunders.

Patient Centered Primary Care Collaborative. (2014). *Defining the Medical Home*. www.pcpcc.org/about/medical-home.

Petiprin, A. (2016). *Nursing Theories and Models*. www.nursing-theory.org/theories-and-models/.

QSEN.org. (2015). *Pre-Licensure KSAs*. http://qsen.org/competencies/pre-licensure-ksas/.

Quealy, K., & Sanger-Katz, M. (2014). *Obama's Health Law: who Was Helped Most*. www.nytimes.com/interactive-/2014/10/29/upshot/obamacare-who-was-helped-most.html?_r=0&abt=0002&abg=1.

Rogers, M. E. (1970). *An Introduction to the Theoretical Basis of Nursing*. Philadelphia, PA: F.A. Davis.

Roy, C. (1976). *Introduction to Nursing: an Adaptation Model*. Upper Saddle River, NJ: Prentice-Hall.

Stevens, K. R. (2013). The impact of evidence-based practice in nursing and the next big ideas. *OJIN: online Journal of Issues in Nursing*, *18*(2), 4.

UCLA Department of Nursing. (2015). *Relationship Based Care (RBC)*. http://nursing.uclahealth.org/body.cfm?id=67.

University of Iowa College of Nursing. (2015a). *Evidence Based Practice Guidelines*. www.nursing.uiowa.edu/excellence/evidence-based-practice-guidelines.

University of Iowa College of Nursing. (2015b). *HCGNE: best Practices for Healthcare Professionals*. www.nursing.uiowa.edu/hartford/best-practices-for-healthcare-professionals.

Watson, J. (1979). *Nursing: the Philosophy and Science of Caring*. New York, NY: Little, Brown and Co.

CHAPTER 2

Cannon, W. B. (1967). *The Wisdom of the Body. Revised and enlarged edition*. New York, NY: Norton.

Dickens, C., & Piano, M. R. (2013). Health literacy and nursing: an update. *American Journal of Nursing*, *113*(6), 52–57.

Dunn, H. L. (1973). *High Level Wellness*. Arlington, VA: Beatty.

Maslow, A. H. (1970). *Motivation and Personality*. Upper Saddle River, NJ: Prentice Hall.

Richards, E. A. (2016). The evolution of physical activity promotion. *American Journal of Nursing*, *115*(8), 50–54.

Selye, H. (1974). *Stress Without Distress*. Philadelphia, PA: Lippincott.

US Department of Health and Human Services. (2010). *Healthy People 2020: a Society in Which All People Live Long Healthy Lives*. http://healthypeople.gov/2020/about/DOHAbout.aspx.

CHAPTER 3

American Hospital Association. (2003). *The patient care partnership: understanding expectations, rights and responsibilities*. http://www.aha.org/advocacy-issues/communicatingpts/pt-care-partnership.shtml.

Brent, N. J. (2013). *Who can give informed consent and what is the nurse's role in obtaining consent for treatment?* www.cphins.com/blog/post/who-can-give-informed-consent-and-what-is-the-nurses-role-in-obtaining-consent-for-treatment.

Children's Bureau. (2012). *Abandoned infants assistance*. www.acf.hhs.gov/programs/cb/resource/abandoned-infants-assist.

Child Welfare Information Gateway. (2015). *Definitions of child abuse and neglect in federal law*. https://www.childwelfare.gov/topics/can/defining/federal/.

National Council of State Boards of Nursing [NCSBN]. (August 7, 2011). *White Paper: a Nurses Guide to the Use of Social Media*. www.ncsbn.org/11_NCSBN_Nurses_Guide_Social_Media.pdf.

Patients Rights Council. (February 6, 2012). *Assisted Suicide Laws in the United States*. www.patientsrightscouncil.org/site/assisted-suicide-state-laws/.

QSEN Institute. (2014). *Interactive Teaching Strategy Using I-SBAR-R to Improve Communication and Quality and Safety in Patient Care*. Roe v. Wade. (1972) http://qsen.org/an-interactive-teaching-strategy-using-i-sbar-r-to-improve-communication-and-quality-and-safety-in-patient-care-7/. www.law.cornell.edu/supremecourt/text/410/113.

Saccomano, S. J., & Zipp, G. P. (2014). Integrating delegation into the undergraduate curriculum. *Creative Nursing*, *20*(2), 106–115.

US Department of Health and Human Services. (1996). *Health Information Privacy*.

US Department of Labor. (1970). *Occupational Safety & Health Administration*.https://www.osha.gov/pls/oshaweb/owadisp.show_document?p_table=OSHACT&p_id=2743.

CHAPTER 5

Moorhead, S., Johnson, M., Maas, M., et al. (2013). *Nursing Outcomes Classification* (5th ed.). St. Louis, MO: Elsevier.

NANDA International (NANDA-I). (2015). *Nursing Diagnoses: definitions and Classification*. www.nanda.org/nanda-international-nursing-diagnoses-definitions-and-classification.html.

Wilkinson, J. M. (2014). *Pearson Nursing Diagnosis Handbook with NIC Interventions and NOC Outcomes*. London, UK: Pearson.

CHAPTER 6

Centers for Medicare and Medicaid Services. (2012). *CMS's RAI Version 3.0 Manual*. www.cms.gov/Medicare/Quality-Initiatives-Patient-Assessment-Instruments/NursingHomeQualityInits/Downloads/MDS-30-RAI-Manual-v1-09-Replacement-Manual-Pages.pdf.

CHAPTER 7

American Medical Informatics Association. (2015). *Nursing Informatics*. www.amia.org/programs/working-groups/nursing-informatics.

Centers for Medicare and Medicaid Services. (2015). *eHealth Programs Interactive Timeline*. http://cms.gov/apps/interactive-timeline/.

HealthIT.gov. (2014). *What is an electronic medical record (EMR)?* www.healthit.gov/providers-professionals/electronic-medical-records-emr.

International Health Terminology Standards Development Organisation. (2015). *SNOMED CT: the global language of healthcare*. www.ihtsdo.org/snomed-ct.

Shepard, S. (2015). *Frequently asked questions: medical records issues*. www.thedoctors.com/KnowledgeCenter/PatientSafety/articles/CON_ID_001699.

CHAPTER 8

Gesundheit, B., Zlotnick, E., Wygoda, M., et al. (2015). Truth telling to patients: a discussion of Jewish sources. *Harefuah*, *154*(3), 209.

Giroux, J. (2013). Making the communication connection. *Urologic Nursing*, *33*(6), 265.

Holt, D., Cassidy, B., Yue, X., et al. (2014). Neural correlates of personal space intrusion. *Journal of Neuroscience*, *34*(12), 4123–4134.

Mayo Clinic Staff. (2013). *Stress relief from laughter? It's no joke*. www.mayoclinic.org/healthy lifestyle/stress-management/in-depth/stress-relief/art-20044456.

Medline Plus. (2014). *Health information in multiple languages*. www.nlm.nih.gov/medlineplus/languages/languages.html.

My Jewish Learning.org. (2015). *Ask the expert: jews in the hospital: what should nurses know?* www.myjewishlearning.com/article/ask-the-expert-jews-in-the-hospital/.

National Aphasia Association. (2015). *Communication tips*. www.aphasia.org/aphasia resources/communication-tips/.

Quality & Safety Education for Nurses (QSEN). (2014a). *Definitions and pre-licensure KSAs for patient-centered care*. http://qsen.org/competencies/pre-licensure-ksas/.

Quality & Safety Education for Nurses (QSEN). (2014b). *Video Presentations: the Lewis Blackman Story and Chasing Zero: winning the War on Healthcare Harm*. http://qsen.org/faculty-resources/videos/.

The Joint Commission. (2016). Update: texting orders. *Joint Commission Perspectives*, *36*(5), 15.

CHAPTER 9

Health Canada. (2014). *About Health Canada*. www.hc-sc.gc.ca/ahc-asc/activit/about-apropos/index-eng.php.

CHAPTER 10

Healthcare Consulting. (2012). *Patient safety tip of the week*. January 10, 2012 verbal orders http://www.patientsafetysolutions.com/docs/January_10_2012_Verbal_Orders.htm.

CHAPTER 11

Ackley, B. J., & Ladwig, G. B. (2014). *Nursing Diagnosis Handbook: an Evidence-Based Guide to Planning Care* (10th ed.). St. Louis, MO: Mosby.

Bureau of Labor Statistics. (2016). *Employment Characteristics of Families Summary*. www.bls.gov/news.release/famee.nr0.htm.

Centers for Disease Control and Prevention (CDC). (2013). Trends in the prevalence of marijuana, cocaine, and other illegal drug use. *National YRBS 1991–2013*. www.cdc.gov/healthyyouth/data/yrbs/pdf/trends/us_drug_trend_yrbs.pdf.

Centers for Disease Control and Prevention (CDC). (2014). *Current Contraceptive Status Among Women Aged 15–44: united States, 2011–2013*. www.cdc.gov/nchs/data/databriefs/db173.htm.

Centers for Disease Control and Prevention (CDC). (2015a). *About teen pregnancy: teen pregnancy in the United States*. www.cdc.gov/teenpregnancy/about/index.htm.

Centers for Disease Control and Prevention (CDC). (2015b). *Sexual risk behavior: HIV, STD, & teen pregnancy prevention*. www.cdc.gov/healthyyouth/sexualbehaviors/.

Centers for Disease Control and Prevention, National Center for Health Statistics. (2016). *Teen births*. http://www.cdc.gov/nchs/fastats/teen-births.htm.

Guttmacher Institute. (2015). *FACT SHEET: american teens' sexual and reproductive health*. www.guttmacher.org/pubs/FB-ATSRH.html.

Kaufman, S. B. (2013). *American education and the IQ trap*. http://articles.latimes.com/2013/jul/20/opinion/la-oe-0721-kaufman-gifted-psychology-iq-20130721.

Newport, F. (2015). *Americans greatly overestimate percent gay, lesbian in U.S.* www.gallup.com/poll/183383/americans-greatly-overestimate-percent-gay-lesbian.aspx.

Patchin, J. (2015). *The summary of our research (2004–2015). The Cyberbullying Research Center*. http://cyberbullying.us/summary-of-our-research/.

Potera, C. (2015). U.S. teens are smoking less, but the increase in e-cigarettes is dragging down the gains. *American Journal of Nursing*, *115*(8), 17.

Reports. Sexual orientation and health among U.S. adults: national health interview survey. (2013). Number 77. *Centers for Disease Control and Prevention (CDC)*. www.cdc.gov/nchs/data/nhsr/nhsr077.pdf.

Shaffer, D. R., & Kipp, K. (2010). *Developmental Psychology: childhood and Adolescence*. Belmont, CA: Wadsworth, Cengage Learning.

Ward, B. W., Dahlhamer, J. M., Galinsky, A. M., et al. (2015). *National Health Statistic*.

Wisnieski, D. M., & Matzo, M. (2013). Promoting healthy sexual behavior in adolescents. *American Journal of Nursing*, *113*(6), 67–70.

CHAPTER 12

American Cancer Society. (2015a). *American Cancer Society Releases New Breast Cancer Guideline*. www.cancer.org/cancer/news/news/american-cancer-society-releases-new-breast-cancer-guidelines.

American Cancer Society. (2015b). *American Cancer Society Guidelines for the Early Detection of Cancer*. www.cancer.org/healthy/findcancerearly/cancerscreeningguidelines/american-cancer-society-guidelines-for-the-early-detection-of-cancer.

Centers for Disease Control and Prevention. (2015a). *Leading causes of death*. www.cdc.gov/nchs/fastats/leading-causes-of-death.htm.

Centers for Disease Control and Prevention. (2015b). *Leading causes of death in males United States*. www.cdc.gov/men/lcod/index.htm.

Centers for Disease Control and Prevention/National Center for Health Statistics. (2015). *National Vital Statistics System National marriage and divorce rate trends*. www.cdc.gov/nchs/nvss/marriage_divorce_tables.htm.

Health Professional/National Vital Statistic Report. (2015). *Births: final data for 2013*. www.cdc.gov/nchs/data/nvsr/nvsr64/nvsr64_01.pdf.

Henderson, T. (2014). *More Americans living alone, census says*. www.washingtonpost.com/politics/more-americans-living-alone-census-says/2014/09/28/67e1d02e-473a-11e4-b72e-d60a9229cc10_story.html.

Houghton, K. (2013). *Why (most) successful women are childless*. www.huffingtonpost.com/kristen-houghton/childless_b_2630389.html.

Institute for Women's Policy Research. (2015). *The status of women in the states: 2015—employment and earnings*. www.iwpr.org/publications/pubs/the-status-of-women-in-the-states-2015-2014-employment-and-earnings#sthash.QVKjz4GE.dpuf.

National Institutes of Health. (2013). *Calcium*. https://ods.od.nih.gov/factsheets/Calcium.

Schaie, K. W. (1996). *Intellectual Development in Adulthood: the Seattle Longitudinal Study*. Cambridge, UK: Cambridge University Press [classic reference].

United States Census Bureau. (2014). *Median age at first marriage, by sex: 1890 to present*. https://www.census.gov/hhes/families/files/graphics/MS-2.pdf.

United States Census Bureau. (2015). *Millennials outnumber baby boomers and are far more diverse, census bureau reports*. www.census.gov/newsroom/press-releases/2015/cb15-113.html.

CHAPTER 13

Administration on Aging. (2014). *A Profile of Older Americans: 2014*. Washington, DC: U.S. Department of Health and Human Services. http://www.aoa.acl.gov/Aging_Statistics/Profile/2014/docs/2014-Profile.pdf.

Alzheimer's Association. (2015). *Types of dementia*. www.alz.org/dementia/types-of-dementia.asp.

Aziz, R., & Steffens, D. C. (2013). What are the causes of late life depression? *Psychiatric Clinics of North America*, *36*(4), 497–516.

Central Intelligence Agency. (2014). *The World Factbook*. www.cia.gov/library/publications/the-world-factbook/fields/2102.html.

Federal Interagency Forum on Aging Related Statistics. (2012). *Older Americans 2012: key Indicators of Well-being*. www.agingstats.gov/agingstatsdotnet/Main_Site/Data/2012_Documents/Docs/EntireChartbook.pdf.

Hoover, R. M., & Polson, M. (2014). Detecting elder abuse and neglect: assessment and intervention. *American Family Physician—March 15, 2014*, *89*(6), 453–460.

Jacobs, J. M., Cohen, A., Ein-Mor, E., et al. (2014). Gender differences in survival in old age. *Rejuvenation Research*, *17*(6), 499–506.

Livingston, G. (2013). *At grandmother's house we stay: one-in-ten children are living with a grandparent. Pew Research Center*. www.pewsocialtrends.org/2013/09/04/at-grandmothers-house-we-stay/.

National Institute on Aging. (2015). *Exercise and physical activity: your everyday guide from the National Institute on Aging*. www.nia.nih.gov/health/publication/exercise-physical-activity/sample-exercises-strength.

Pellicano, M., Buffa, S., Goldeck, E., et al. (2014). Evidence for less marked potential signs of T-cell immunosenescence in centenarian offspring than in the general age-matched population. *Journals of Gerontology. A Biological Sciences and Medical Sciences*, *69*(5), 495–504.

Pew Research Center. (2014). *Number of older Americans in the workforce is on the rise*. www.pewresearch.org/fact-tank/2014/01/07/number-of-older-americans-in-the-workforce-is-on-the-rise/.

US Census Bureau. (2015). *FFF: older Americans Month: may 2015*. http://www.census.gov/newsroom/facts-for-features/2015/cb15-ff09.html.

US Census Bureau. (2012). *Statistical abstract of the United States: 2012*. Retrieved from www.census.gov/compendia/statab/2012/tables/12s0104.pdf.

CHAPTER 15

American Nurses Association (ANA). (2013). *Position Statements: euthanasia, Assisted Suicide and Aid in Dying*. Washington, DC: Author.

Belvins, M. A. (2008). A personal journey through the grief and healing process with Virginia Satir, Dr. E. Kűbler-Ross, and J. William Worden. *The Satir Journal*, *2*(2), 89–105.

Centers for Disease Control and Prevention (CDC). (2015). *Life expectancy*. www.cdc.gov/nchs/fastats/life-expectancy.htm.

Coyle, N. (2014). Palliative care, hospice care, and bioethics. *Journal of Hospice & Palliative Nursing*, *16*(1), 6–14.

Hospice and Palliative Nurses Association (HPNA). (2015). *Certified Hospice and Palliative Licensed Nurse (CHPLN®)*. http://hpcc.advancingexpertcare.org/competence/lpvn-chpln/.

Kübler-Ross, E. (1969). *On Death and Dying*. New York, NY: Scribner Classics.

Lakasing, E., Kulkarni, S., Sparkes, C., et al. (2014). A practice-based survey of patients dying in hospital: can we do more to support end-of-life care at home? *British Journal of Community Nursing*, *19*(3), 130–133.

Maciejewski, P. K., Zhang, B., Block, S. D., et al. (2007). An empirical examination of the stage theory of grief. *JAMA: the Journal of the American Medical Association*, *297*(7), 716.

Mayer, D. M., & Winters, C. A. (2016). Palliative care in critical access hospitals. *Critical Care Nurse*, *36*(1), 72–78.

National Hospice and Palliative Care Organization (NHPCO). (2015). *History of hospice care*. www.nhpco.org/history-hospice-care.

Perrin, K. O., & MacLeod, C. E. (2013). *Understanding the Essentials of Critical Care*. Upper Saddle River, NJ: Prentice Hall.

Statistics Canada. (2012). *Life expectancy at birth, by sex, by province*. www.statcan.gc.ca/tables-tableaux/sum-som/l01/cst01/health26-eng.htm.

United Network for Organ Sharing (UNOS). (2015). *About us*. http://transplantpro.org/about/about-us/.

Wagner, K. D., & Hardien-Pierce, M. G. (2014). *High Acuity Nursing*. Upper Saddle River, NJ: Prentice Hall.

Williams, P. A. (2016). *Basic Geriatric Nursing*. St. Louis, MO: Elsevier.

World Health Organization. (2015a). *WHO definition of palliative care*. www.who.int/cancer/palliative/definition/en/.

World Health Organization. (2015b). *Treatment guideline on pain*. www.who.int/medicines/areas/quality_safety/guide_on_pain/en/.

CHAPTER 16

Centers for Disease Control and Prevention (CDC). (2002). *Guideline for hand hygiene in the health-care settings*. www.cdc.gov/mmwr/PDF/rr/rr5116.pdf.

Centers for Disease Control and Prevention (CDC). (2015). *Carbapenem-resistant enterobacteriaceae (CRE) infection: patient FAQs*. www.cdc.gov/hai/organisms/cre/cre-patientFAQ.html.

World Health Organization. (2009). *WHO guidelines on hand hygiene in health care*. http://apps.who.int/iris/bitstream/10665/44102/1/9789241597906_eng.pdf.

CHAPTER 17

Centers for Disease Control and Prevention (CDC). (2015). *Healthcare-associated infections (HAIs)*. www.cdc.gov/HAI/surveillance/.

Institute for Healthcare Improvement (IHI). (2012). *How-to guide: prevent ventilator-associated pneumonia*. www.ihi.org/resources/pages/tools/howtoguidepreventvap.aspx.

Institute for Healthcare Improvement (IHI). (2015). *Ventilator bundle checklist*. www.ihi.org/resources/Pages/Tools/VentilatorBundleChecklist.aspx.

Munro, N., & Ruggiero, M. (2014). Ventilator-associated pneumonia bundle: reconstruction for best care. *AACN Advanced Critical Care, 25*(2), 163–175.

Shang, J., Larson, E., Liu, J., et al. (2015). Infection in home health care: results from National Outcome and Assessment Information Set data. *American Journal of Infection Control, 43*(5), 454–459.

Shen, N. J., Pan, S. C., Sheng, W. H., et al. (2015). Comparative antimicrobial efficacy of alcohol-based hand rub and conventional surgical scrub in a medical center. *Journal of Microbiology, Immunology and Infection, 48*(3), 322–328.

CHAPTER 18

Gattinoni, L., Taccone, P., Carlesso, E., et al. (2013). Prone position in acute respiratory distress syndrome: rationale, indications, and limits. *American Journal of Respiratory and Critical Care Medicine, 188*(11), 1286–1293.

Liebenthal, J. A., Wu, S., Rose, S., et al. (2015). Association of prone position with sudden unexpected death in epilepsy. *Neurology, 84*(7), 703–709.

CHAPTER 19

Clark, T. C. (2012). Zero HAPUs: reaching for the moon. *Nursing Management, 43*(3), 11–12.

Heavey, E. (2014). Oral health in primary care. *Nursing, 44*(3), 59–62.

National Pressure Ulcer Advisory Panel, European Pressure Ulcer Advisory Panel and Pan Pacific Pressure Injury Alliance. (2014). *Prevention and Treatment of Pressure Ulcers: quick Reference Guide*. In E. Haesler (Ed.). Osborne Park, Western Australia: Cambridge Media.

National Pressure Ulcer Advisory Panel. (2016). National Pressure Ulcer Advisory Panel (NPUAP) announces a change in terminology from pressure ulcer to pressure injury and updates the stages of pressure injury. http://www.npuap.org/national-pressure-ulcer-advisory-panel-npuap-announces-a-change-in-terminology-from-pressure-ulcer-to-pressure-injury-and-updates-the-stages-of-pressure-injury/.

Powers, J., & Fortney, S. (2014). Bed baths: much more than a basic nursing task. *Nursing, 44*(10), 67–68.

Waters, T. M., Daniels, M. J., Bazzoli, G. J., et al. (2015). Effect of Medicare's nonpayment for hospital-acquired conditions. *Journal of the American Medical Association Internal Medicine, 175*(3), 347–354.

CHAPTER 20

Centers for Disease Control and Prevention (CDC) Smoking & Tobacco Use. (2015a). *Secondhand smoke(SHS) facts*. www.cdc.gov/tobacco/data_statistics/fact_sheets/secondhand_smoke/general_facts/.

Centers for Disease Control and Prevention (CDC) Ebola (Ebola Virus Disease). (2015b). *Ebola 101 for Healthcare Professionals*. www.cdc.gov/vhf/ebola/healthcare-us/index.html.

Daniels, K. (2014). Fighting bed alarm fatigue in orthopedic units. *Nursing, 44*(9), 66–67.

Landro, L. (2013). *Hospitals work on patients' most-frequent complaint: noise*. www.wsj.com/articles/SB10001424127887324634304578537350035525538.

Sendelback, S., & Funk, M. (2013). Alarm fatigue: a patient safety concern. *American Association of Critical-Care Nurses, 24*(4), 378–386.

U. S. Army Medical Research Institute of Infectious Diseases. (2012). *Quick Bio-agents Guide* (1st ed.). www.usamriid.army.mil/education/docs/Quick_Bio-Agents_Giude.pdf.

US Food and Drug Administration. (2014). *CMS/CDRH letter regarding physical restraint definition*. www.fda.gov/MedicalDevices/ProductsandMedicalProcedures/GeneralHospitalDevicesandSupplies/HospitalBeds/ucm123678.htm.

World Health Organization. (2015). *Lassa fever*. www.who.int/mediacentre/factsheets/fs179/en.

CHAPTER 21

A blood pressure study is stopped early because of important results. *American Journal of Nursing, 115*(12), (2015), 19.

KeithRN. (2016). *Does my patient have orthostatic changes?* http://www.keithrn.com/2016/02/orthostatic-hypotension/.

National Heart, Lung, and Blood Institute. (2012). *Who is at risk for high blood pressure?* www.nhlbi.nih.gov/health/health-topics/topics/hbp/atrisk.

The Joint Commission. (2014). *Clarification of the pain management standard*. www.jointcommission.org/assets/1/18/Clarification_of_the_Pain_Management__Standard.pdf.

Williams, P. (2016). *Basic Geriatric Nursing*. St. Louis, MO: Elsevier.

Wold, G. H. (2012). *Basic Geriatric Nursing*. St. Louis, MO: Elsevier.

CHAPTER 24

Carlisle, H. (2015). Promoting the use of capnography in acute care settings: an evidence-based practice project. *Journal of Perianesthesia Nursing, 30*(3), 201–208.

The Joint Commission. (2016). *Hospital National Patient Safety Goals*. www.jointcommission.org/assets/1/6/2016_NPSG_HAP.pdf.

CHAPTER 25

Fulop, T. (2014). *Hypomagnesemia*. http://emedicine.medscape.com/article/2038394-overview#a5.

Gunnerson, K. J. (2015). *Lactic acidosis*. http://emedicine.medscape.com/article/167027-overview#a4.

Lederer, E. (2014). *Hypokalemia*. http://emedicine.medscape.com/article/242008-overview#a1.

Lewis, J. L. (2013). *Hypomagnesemia*. www.merckmanuals.com/professional/endocrine-and-metabolic-disorders/electrolyte-disorders/hypomagnesemia.

Soifer, J. T., & Kim, H. T. (2014). Approach to metabolic alkalosis. *Emergency Medicine Clinics of North America, 32*(2), 453–463.

Thomas, E. Y., & Johns Hopkins Hospital. (2015). Fluids and electrolytes. In *The Harriett Lane Handbook*. Philadelphia, PA: Saunders.

Zipursky, J., MacDonald, E. M., Hollands, S., et al. (2014). Proton pump inhibitors and hospitalization with hypomagnesemia: a population-based case-control study. *PLoS Medicine, 11*(9), e1001736.

CHAPTER 26

Budd, G. M. (2015). The obesity epidemic, part 2: nursing assessment and intervention. *American Journal of Nursing, 115*(2), 38–45.

Cullum-Dugan, D. (2014). Top questions vegetarians ask RDs: here's how to answer them with ingenuity and expertise. *Today's Diet, 16*(10), 28.

DiNicolantonio, J. J., Lucan, S. C., & O'Keefe, J. H. (2016). The evidence for saturate fat and for sugar related to coronary heart disease. *Prog Cardiovasc Dis, 58*(5), 464–472.

Donaldson, A. A. (2013). Bone health in adolescents. *Contemporary Pediatrics*. http://contemporarypediatrics.modernmedicine.com/contemporary-pediatrics/news/modernmedicine/welcome-modernmedicine/bone-health-adolescents?page=full.

HealthyPeople.gov. (2015). http://www.healthypeople.gov/2020/topics-objectives/topic/nutrition-and-weight.

Kirkey, S. (2015). *Juice becomes the latest food target as Health Canada appears poised to cut fruit drinks from nutritional guide.* http://news.nationalpost.com/news/canada/health-canada-appears-poised-to-cut-fruit-juice-from-nutrition-guide.

Mauldin, K., & O'Leary-Kelley, C. (2015). New guidelines for assessment of malnutrition in adults: obese critically ill patients. *Critical Care Nurse, 24*(4), 24–30.

Riddle, M. S., Murray, J. A., Cash, B. D., et al. (2013). Pathogen-specific risk of celiac disease following bacterial causes of foodborne illness: a retrospective cohort study. *Digestive Diseases and Sciences, 58*(11), 3242–3245.

Roeder, A. (2013). *Skip the juice, go for whole fruit.* http://news.harvard.edu/gazette/story/2013/08/reduce-type-2-diabetes-risk/.

Simon, S. (2015). *World Health Organization says processed meat causes cancer.* www.cancer.org/cancer/news/news/world-health-organization-says-processed-meat-causes-cancer.

US Department of Agriculture. (2015). *Individual dietary assessment.* https://fnic.nal.usda.gov/dietary-guidance/individual-dietary-assessment.

Zolot, J. (2015). Plant-based diet reduces weight and cholesterol levels in obese children [abstract]. *American Journal of Nursing, 115*(11), 62–63.

CHAPTER 27

Abbott Laboratories. (2015). *Best practices for managing tube feeding: a nurses pocket manual.* http://static.abbottnutrition.com/cms-prod/abbottnutrition.com/img/M4619.005%20Tube%20Feeding%20manual.pdf.

American College of Obstetricians and Gynecologists. (2013, reaffirmed 2015). Committee Opinion No. 548: weight gain during pregnancy. *Obstetrics and Gynecology*, 121, 210–212.

American Diabetes Association. (2014). *Age, race, gender & family history.* www.diabetes.org/are-you-at-risk/lower-your-risk/nonmodifiables.html.

American Diabetes Association. (2015). *Fats.* www.diabetes.org/food-and-fitness/food/what-can-i-eat/making-healthy-food-choices/fats-and-diabetes.html.

American Psychiatric Association. (2013). *Diagnostic and Statistical Manual of Mental Disorders* (5th ed.). Washington, DC: American Psychiatric Association.

American Society for Metabolic and Bariatric Surgery. (2013). *Metabolic and bariatric surgery.* http://asmbs.org/resources/metabolic-and-bariatric-surgery.

Boeykens, K., Steeman, E., & Duysburgh, I. (2014). Reliability of pH measurement and the auscultatory method to confirm the position of a nasogastric tube. *International Journal of Nursing Studies, 51*(11), 1427–1433. http://dx.doi.org/10.1016/j.ijnurstu.2014.03.004.

Carvalho, L. S. F., & Sposito, A. C. (2015). Vitamin D for the prevention of cardiovascular disease: are we ready for that? *Atherosclerosis, 241*, 729–740.

DiNicolantonio, J. J., Lucan, S. C., & O'Keefe, J. H. (2016). The evidence for saturate fat and for sugar related to coronary heart disease. *Prog Cardiovasc Dis, 58*(5), 464–472.

Fawzi, W. W., Msamanga, G. I., Spiegelman, D., et al. (2004). A randomized trial of multivitamin supplements and HIV disease progression and mortality. *The New England Journal of Medicine, 351*, 23–32.

Institute of Medicine. (2009). *Weight Gain During Pregnancy: reexamining the Guidelines.* www.iom.edu/~/media/Files/Report%20Files/2009/Weight-Gain-During-Pregnancy-Reexamining-the-Guidelines/Report%20Brief%20-%20Weight%20Gain%20During%20Pregnancy.pdf.

Macht, M., Wimbish, T., Bodine, C., et al. (2013). ICU-acquired swallowing disorders. *Critical Care Medicine, 41*(10), 2396–2405.

Mayo Clinic Staff. (2013). *DASH diet: healthy eating to lower your blood pressure.* www.mayoclinic.org/healthy-lifestyle/nutrition-and-healthy-eating/in-depth/dash-diet/art-20048456.

National Health Service (NHS). (2013). *How to get vitamin D from sunlight.* www.nhs.uk/Livewell/Summerhealth/Pages/vitamin-D-sunlight.aspx.

National Institutes of Health. (2013). *Calcium: dietary supplement fact sheet.* https://ods.od.nih.gov/factsheets/Calcium-HealthProfessional/.

The Centers for Disease Control and Prevention. (2015). *Adult obesity facts.* www.cdc.gov/obesity/data/adult.html.

van der Maarel-Wierink, C. D., van der Putten, C. J., De Visschere, L. M., et al. (2015). Risk of aspiration in care home residents and associated factors. *Journal of Gerontological Nursing, 41*(2), 26–31.

Zgambo, M., He, G., & Wang, H. (2012). Effects of nutritional supplementation on children with HIV/AIDS in China. *Journal of Central South University, 37*(3), 305–310.

CHAPTER 28

Ackley, B. J., & Ladwig, G. B. (2014). *Nursing Diagnosis Handbook: an Evidence-Based Guide to Planning Care* (10th ed.). Maryland Heights, MO: Elsevier Mosby.

American Heart Association. (2015). *Highlights of the 2015 AHA Guidelines Update for CPR and ECC.* www.heart.org/idc/groups/heart-public@wcm/@ecc/documents/downloadable/ucm_317350.pdf. http://ccguidelines.heart.org/wp-content/uploads/2015/10/2015-AHA-Guidelines-Highlights-English.pdf.

Nance-Floyd, B. (2011). Tracheostomy care: an evidence-based guide to suctioning and dressing changes. *American Nurse Today, 6*(7), 14–16.

CHAPTER 29

Bardsley, A. (2015). Safe and effective catherisation for patients in the community. *British Journal of Community Nursing, 20*(4), 166.

Buswell, J. (2013). Practice question: dignity and continence care. *Nursing Older People, 25*(3), 12.

Chenoweth, C. E., Gould, C. V., & Saint, S. (2014). Diagnosis, management, and prevention of catheter-associated urinary tract infections. *Infectious Disease Clinics of North America, 28*(1), 105–119.

Cheung, R. Y., Shek, K. L., Chung, T. K., et al. (2015). Pelvic floor muscle biometry and pelvic organ mobility in East Asian and Caucasian nulliparae. *Ultrasound in Obstetrics and Gynecology, 45*(5), 599–604.

Derpapas, A., Ahmed, S., Vijaya, G., et al. (2012). Racial differences in female urethral morphology and levator hiatal dimensions: an ultrasound study. *Neurourology and Urodynamics, 31*(4), 502–507.

Foxman, B. (2014). Urinary tract infection syndromes. *Infectious Disease Clinics of North America, 28*(1), 1–13.

Geerlings, S. E., Beerepoot, M. A. J., & Prins, J. M. (2014). Prevention of recurrent urinary tract infections in women. *Infectious Disease Clinics of North America, 28*(1), 135–147.

Gokula, M., & Gaspar, P. M. (2014). Implementation of the FIRM (Foley Insertion, Removal, and Maintenance) protocol in skilled nursing facilities. *Translation: the University of Toledo Journal of Medical Sciences* Vol. 1, Article 6.

Hall, B., & Woodward, S. (2015). Pelvic floor muscle training for urinary incontinence postpartum. *British Journal of Nursing, 24*(11), 576–579.

Halm, M. A., & O'Connor, N. (2014). Do system-based interventions affect catheter-associated urinary tract infection? *American Journal of Critical Care: an Official Publication, American Association of Critical-Care Nurses, 23*(6), 505–509.

Huber, K., Sood, G., & Maygers, J. (2015). Get those Foleys out: successful reduction of catheter utilization through use of a nurse driven Foley discontinuation protocol. *AJIC: American Journal of Infection Control*, *43*(6), S52–S52.

Islam, M. S., Luby, S. P., Sultana, R., et al. (2014). Family caregivers in public tertiary care hospitals in Bangladesh: risks and opportunities for infection control. *AJIC: American Journal of Infection Control*, *42*(3), 305–310.

Kennedy, E. H., Greene, M. T., & Saint, S. (2013). Estimating hospital costs of catheter associated urinary tract infection. *Journal of Hospital Medicine*, *8*(9), 519–522.

McCarron, K. (2011). Renal labs: putting it all together. *Nursing Made Incredibly Easy*, *9*(5), 15–17.

Mody, L., & Juthani-Mehta, M. (2014). Urinary tract infections in older women: a clinical review. *Journal of the American Medical Association*, *311*(8), 844–854.

National Kidney and Urologic Diseases Information Clearinghouse. (2012). *Urinary incontinence in women*. www.niddk.nih.gov/health-information/health-topics/urologic-disease/urinary-incontinence-women/Pages/ez.aspx#difference.

Newman, D. K., & Willson, M. M. (2011). Review of intermittent catheterization and current best practices. *Urologic Nursing*, *31*(1), 12–48.

Shaw, C., & Logan, K. (2013). Psychological coping with intermittent self-catheterisation (ISC) in people with spinal injury: a qualitative study. *International Journal of Nursing Studies*, *50*(10), 1341–1350.

The Joint Commission. (2011). *Catheter-associated urinary tract infections. R3 Report1 Requirement, Rationale, Reference 2*. www.jointcommission.org/assets/1/18/R3_Report_Issue_2_9_22_11_final.pdf.

CHAPTER 30

American Cancer Society. (2013). *Colon cancer prevention and early detection: what you need to know*. www.cancer.org/cancer/news/features/coloncancer-prevention-and-early-detection-what-you-need-to-know.

Bowles, T., & Readding, L. (2013). Caring for people with arthritis and a stoma. *British Journal of Nursing (Mark Allen Publishing)*, *22*(16), S14–S17.

Burch, J. (2014a). Looking after the stoma and the surrounding peristomal skin. *Nursing & Residential Care*, *16*(4), 190–195.

Burch, J. (2014b). Management of peristomal skin complications. *British Journal of Healthcare Management*, *20*(6), 264–269.

Burch, J. (2014c). Stoma appliances and accessories: getting it right for the patient. *British Journal of Nursing*, *23*, S4–S10.

Centers for Disease Control and Prevention. (2013). *Global diarrhea burden: diarrhea: common illness, global killer*. www.cdc.gov/healthywater/global/diarrhea-burden.html.

Cronin, E. (2013). Dietary advice for patients with a stoma. *Gastrointestinal Nursing*, *11*(3), 14–24.

Gardiner, A., & Hilton, A. (2016). Managing constipation in adults with co-morbidities. *Independent Nurse*. http://www.independentnurse.co.uk/clinical-article/managing-constipation-in-adults-with-co-morbidities/141940/.

Gillibrand, W. (2012). Faecal incontinence in the elderly: issues and interventions in the home. *British Journal of Community Nursing*, *17*(8), 364–368.

Hall, M. (2014). For optimal health, increase fiber-rich foods. *Environmental Nutrition*, *37*(7), 7.

Hande, K. (2014). Are you screening your patients for colorectal cancer? *Journal for Nurse Practitioners*, *10*(9), 757–758.

Harvard Health Letter. (Eds.). (2014). Caffeine IQ: how much is too much? *Harvard Health Letter*, *39*(7), 5.

Hempel, S., Newberry, S. J., Maher, A. R., et al. (2012). Probiotics for the prevention and treatment of antibiotic-associated diarrhea: a systematic review and meta-analysis. *Journal of the American Medical Association*, *307*(18), 1959–1969.

International Foundation for Functional Gastrointestinal Disorders (IFFGD). (2014). *Managing Diarrhea*. www.iffgd.org/site/gi-disorders/functional-gi-disorders/diarrhea/management/. Adapted from: thompson, W. G. IFFGD Publication #201.

Iqbal, F., Zaman, S., & Bowley, D. M. (2013). Editorial: the Journal of Wound, Ostomy and Continence Nursing at 40: living on a global stage. *Journal of Wound, Ostomy and Continence Nursing*, *40*(6), 563–564.

Kamm, K. B., Feikin, D. R., Bigogo, G. M., et al. (2014). Associations between presence of handwashing stations and soap in the home and diarrhea and respiratory illness, in children less than five years old in rural western Kenya. *Tropical Medicine & International Health*, *19*(4), 398–406.

Lewis, S. L., Dirksen, S. R., & Heitkemper, M. M. (2014). *Medical-Surgical Nursing: assessment and Management of Clinical Problems*. St. Louis, MO: Mosby.

Prichard, D., & Bharucha, A. (2015). Management of opiod-induced constipation for people in palliative care. *International Journal of Palliative Nursing*, *21*(6), 272–280.

Prynn, P. (2011). Managing adult constipation. *Practice Nurse*, *41*(17), 23–28.

Rao, S. S. C. (2015). *Constipation in the older adult*. www.uptodate.com/contents/constipation-in-the-older-adult.

Scemons, D. (2014). Managing fecal incontinence in adults. *Nursing Made Incredibly Easy!* *12*(2), 18–24.

Shanahan, D. J. (2012). Bedrails and vulnerable older adults: how should nurses make 'safe and sound' decisions surrounding their use? *International Journal of Older People Nursing*, *7*(4), 272–281.

CHAPTER 31

Cong, X., McGrath, J. N., et al. (2013). Pain assessment and mesaurement in neonates: an updated review. *Advances in Neonatal Care*, *13*(6), 379–395.

Dolan, R., Huh, J., et al. (2016). A prospective analysis of sleep deprivation and disturbance in surgical patients. *Annals of Medicine and Surgery*, *6*, 1–5.

Healthy People 2020. (2015). Sleep Health: objectives. http://www.healthypeople.gov/2020/topics-objectives/topic/sleep-health.

Kumar, K. H., & Elavarasi, P. (2016). Definition of pain and classification of pain disorders. *Journal of Advanced Clinical and Research Insights*, *3*(3), 87–90.

Malec, M., & Shega, J. W. (2015). Pain management in the elderly. *Medical Clinics of North America*, *99*(2), 337–350.

Moayedi, M., & Davis, K. (2013). Theories of pain: from specificity to gate control. *Journal of Neurophysiology*, *109*(1), 5–12.

National Institutes of Health, Medline Plus. (2012). *Fentanyl nasal spray*. https://www.nlm.nih.gov/medlineplus/druginfo/meds/a612015.html.

Rahu, M. A., Grap, M. J., et al. (2015). Validity and sensitivity of 6 pain scales in critically ill, intubated adults. *American Journal of Critical Care*, *24*(6), 514–523.

The Joint Commission. (2014). Clarification of the pain management standard. *Joint Commission Perspectives*, *34*(11), 11.

Wang, C. F., Sun, Y. L., et al. (2014). Music therapy improves sleep quality in acute and chronic sleep disorders: a meta-analysis of 10 randomized studies. *International Journal of Nursing Studies*, *51*(1), 51–62.

CHAPTER 32

Lynch, M. L., Sawynok, J., Hiew, C., et al. (2012). A randomized controlled trial of qigong for fibromyalgia. *Arthritis Research and Therapy*. www.biomedcentral.com/content/pdf/ar3931.pdf.

Sawynok, J., & Lynch, M. (2014). Qigong and fibromyalgia: randomized controlled trials and beyond. *Evid Based Complement Alternative Medicine*, *2014*, 379715.

UHN Multi-Organ Transplant Program. (2015). *Using herbal and other natural health products before and after transplant*. www.uhn.ca/PatientsFamilies/Health_Information/Health_Topics/Documents/Using_Herbal_Natural_Health_Products_Transplant.pdf.

Wagner, J. (2015). Incorporating acupressure into nursing practice. *American Journal of Nursing, 115*(12), 40–45.

CHAPTER 33

Agency for Healthcare Research and Quality. (2013a). *Computerized provider order entry cuts medication error likelihood in half*. www.ahrq.gov/news/newsletters/e-newsletter/370.html.

Agency for Healthcare Research and Quality. (2013b). *Multiple interventions offer pathways to improved medication adherence*. www.ahrq.gov/news/newsletters/research-activities/13aug/0813RA5.html.

Agency for Healthcare Research and Quality. (2015). *Medication reconciliation*. https://psnet.ahrq.gov/primers/primer/1/medication-reconciliation.

Cleveland Clinic. (2015). *Minimizing interruptions during medication administration*. http://consultqd.clevelandclinic.org/2015/05/minimizing-interruptions-during-medication-administration/.

Institute for Healthcare Improvement. (2015). *Kaiser Permanente MedRite Program*. www.ihi.org/resources/pages/tools/kpmedriteprogram.aspx.

Kreitz, C., Schnuerch, R., Furley, P. A., et al. (2015a). Does semantic preactivation reduce inattentional blindness? *Attention, Perception & Psychophysics, 77*(3), 759–767.

Kreitz, C., Schnuerch, R., Gibbons, H., et al. (2015b). Some see it, some don't: exploring the relation between inattentional blindness and personality factors. *PLoS One, 10*(5), e0128158.

Leung, A. A., Denham, C. R., Gandhi, T. K., et al. (2015). A safe practice standard for barcode technology. *Journal of Patient Safety, 11*(2), 89–99.

Mayo Clinic Staff. (2015). *Lactose intolerance*. www.mayoclinic.org/diseases-conditions/lactose-intolerance/basics/risk-factors/con-20027906.

National Institute for Health and Care Excellence. (2015). *Medicines optimisation: the safe and effective use of medicines to enable the best possible outcomes*. www.nice.org.uk/guidance/NG5/chapter/1-recommendations.

Rochon, P. A. (2015). *Drug prescribing for older adults*. www.uptodate.com/contents/drug-prescribing-for-older-adults.

The Joint Commission. (2015a). *Facts about the official "Do Not Use" list of abbreviations*. www.jointcommission.org/facts_about_do_not_use_list/.

The Joint Commission. (2015b). *National patient safety goals effective January 1, 2015: hospital accreditation program*. www.jointcommission.org/assets/1/6/2015_NPSG_HAP.pdf.

US Food and Drug Administration. (2012). *A guide to safety terms at FDA*. www.fda.gov/downloads/ForConsumers/ConsumerUpdates/UCM107976.pdf.

US Food and Drug Administration. (2013). *Strategies to reduce medication errors: working to improve medication safety*. www.fda.gov/Drugs/ResourcesForYou/Consumers/ucm143553.htm.

US Food and Drug Administration. (2014). *Preventable adverse drug reactions: a focus on drug interactions*. www.fda.gov/Drugs/DevelopmentApprovalProcess/DevelopmentResources/DrugInteractionsLabeling/ucm110632.htm.

Williams, T., King, M. W., Thompson, J. A., et al. (2014). Implementing evidence-based medication safety interventions on a progressive care unit. *The American Journal of Nursing, 114*(11), 53–61.

CHAPTER 34

Agency for Healthcare Research and Quality. (2014). *Root cause analysis*. https://psnet.ahrq.gov/primers/primer/10/root-cause-analysis.

American Association of Critical-Care Nurses. (2011). *Prevention of aspiration. AACN practice alert. 2011*. www.aacn.org/wd/practice/docs/practicealerts/prevention-aspiration-practice-alert.pdf?menu=aboutus. www.aacn.org/wd/practice/content/practicealerts/aspiration-practice-alert.pcms?menu=practice.

Cleveland Clinic. (2015). *Medical devices: inhalers*. https://my.clevelandclinic.org/health/medicaldevices/hic_How_to_Use_a_Metered_Dose_Inhaler.

Cohen, H. (2013). Prevent adverse drug events from topical medications. *Nursing, 43*(7), 68–69.

Grissinger, M. (2013). Oral syringes: making better use of a crucial and economical risk reduction strategy. *Pharmacy and Therapeutics, 38*(1), 5–6.

Habib, W. A., Alanizi, A. S., Abdelhamid, M. M., et al. (2014). Accuracy of tablet splitting: comparison study between hand splitting and tablet cutter. *Saudi Pharmaceutical Journal, 22*(5), 454–459. www.sciencedirect.com/science/article/pii/S1319016413001254.

Institute for Safe Medication Practices. (2011). Building patient safety skills: common pitfalls when conducting a root cause analysis. *Nurse Advise-ERR, 9*(3), 1–4.

Lahue, B. J., Pyenson, B., Iwasaki, K., et al. (2012). National burden of preventable adverse drug events associated with inpatient injectable medications: healthcare and medical professional liability costs. *American Health and Drug Benefits, 5*(7), 1–10.

Leapfrog. (2014). *leapfrog hospital survey results*, 2014. www.LeapfrogGroup.org/HospitalSurveyReport. www.leapfroggroup.org/media/file/2014LeapfrogReport_CPOE_FINAL.pdf.

Potera, C. (2015). Misuse of autoinjectors and inhalers. *The American Journal of Nursing, 115*(3), 17.

Rambhade, S., Chakarborty, A., Shrivastava, A., et al. (2012). A survey on polypharmacy and use of inappropriate medications. *Toxicology International, 19*(1), 68–73.

Rassool, G. H. (2015). Cultural competence in nursing Muslim patients. *Nursing Times, 111*(14), 12–15.

Siu, H. K. (2015). Effective inpatient medication reconciliation: the 10 commandments. *HospitalPractice, 43*(2), 65–69. www.tandfonline.com/doi/pdf/10.1080/21548331.2015.1023159.

Smeulers, M., Verweij, L., Maaskant, J. M., et al. (2015). Quality indicators for safe medication preparation and administration: a systematic review. *PLoS One, 10*(4), e0122695. http://dx.doi.org/10.1371/journal.pone.0122695. www.ncbi.nlm.nih.gov/pubmed/25884623.

CHAPTER 35

Boyle, T. (2014). *Experts warn against use of multi-dose vials in wake of hepatitis C outbreak at colonoscopy clinics*. www.thestar.com/life/health_wellness/2014/09/30/experts_warn_against_use_of_multidose_vials_in_wake_of_hepatitis_c_outbreak_at_colonoscopy_clinics.html.

Centers for Disease Control and Prevention. (2015). *Vaccines and immunizations*. www.cdc.gov/vaccines/pubs/pinkbook/vac-admin.html#route.

deWit, S., & Kumagai, C. (2012). *Medical-Surgical Nursing: concepts & Practice* (2nd ed.). Philadelphia, PA: Saunders.

Hanan, Z. I., & Durgin, J. M. (2015). *Pharmacy Practice for Technicians* (5th ed., p. 347). Clinton Park, NY: Cengage Learning.

Holland, K. (2014). *Insulin pens*. www.healthline.com/health/type-2-diabetes/insulin-pens#Overview1.

Hopkins, U., & Arias, C. Y. (2013). Large volume IM injections: a review of best practices. *Oncology Nurse Advisor, 4(1)*, 32. www.oncologynurseadvisor.com/chemotherapy/large-volume-im-injections-a-review-of-best-practices/article/281208/.

Immunize.org. (2015). *Administering vaccines: dose, route, site, and needle size*. www.immunize.org/catg.d/p3085.pdf.

Institute for Safe Medication Practices. (2014). *ISMP list of high-alert medications in acute care settings*. https://www.ismp.org/tools/institutionalhighAlert.asp.

Lee, S. (2012). *Why insulin injection site rotation is important*. www.diabetesmonitor.com/supplies/insulin/insulin-site-rotation.htm.

McNew, R. (2013). *Emergency Department Compliance Manual*, 2013 edition. New York, NY: Wolters Kluwer Law & Business.

Morris, S. Y. (2014). *Insulin injection sites: where and how to inject*. www.healthline.com/health/diabetes/insulin-injection.

Perry, A. G., Potter, P. A., & Ostendorf, W. (2016). *Nursing Interventions & Clinical Skills* (6th ed.). St. Louis, MO: Elsevier Mosby.

Sisson, H. (2015). Aspirating during the intramuscular injection procedure: a systematic literature review. *Journal of Clinical Nursing, 24*, 2368–2375.

World Health Organization. (2010). *WHO Best Practices for Injections and Related Procedures Toolkit*. http://apps.who.int/iris/bitstream/10665/44298/1/9789241599252_eng.pdf.

CHAPTER 36

Beck, C. E., Choong, K., Puligandla, P. S., et al. (2013). Avoiding hypotonic solutions in paediatrics: keeping our patients safe. *Paediatrics and Child Health, 18*(2), 94–95.

Bentley, J., Heard, K., Collins, G., et al. (2015). Mixing medications: how to ensure patient safety. *The Pharmaceutical Journal, 294* (7859). http://dx.doi.org/10.1211/PJ.2015.20068289. www.pharmaceutical-journal.com/learning/learning-article/mixing-medicines-how-to-ensure-patient-safety/20068289.article.

Centers for Disease Control and Prevention. (2016). *Central Line-associated Bloodstream Infection (CLABSI)*. https://www.cdc.gov/HAI/bsi/bsi.html.

Centers for Disease Control and Prevention. (2011). *Guidelines for the prevention of intravascular catheter-related infections, 2011*. www.cdc.gov/hicpac/pdf/guidelines/bsi-guidelines-2011.pdf.

Chiu, P., Lee, Y., et al. (2015). Establish a perioperative check forum for peripheral intravenous access to prevent the occurrence of phlebitis. *Kaohsiung Journal of Medical Sciences, 31*(4), 215–221.

Goulette, C. (2011). Blasting BSI. *Advance for Nurses, 13*(6), 26.

Hadaway, L. (2015). *Peripheral catheter assessment: components and frequency*. http://www.hadawayassociates.com/1/post/2015/02/peripheral-catheter-assessment-components-and-frequency.html.

Harnage, S. (2012). Seven years of zero central-line-associated bloodstream infections. *British Journal of Nursing*, 21(21), S6-S12.

Institute for Healthcare Improvement. (2011). *Implement the Central Line Bundle*. www.ihi.org/IHI/topics/criticalcare/intensivecare/changes/implementthe central linebundle.htm.

Institute for Safe Medical Practices. (2015). *ISMP Safe Practice Guidelines for Adult IV push Medications: a Compilation of Safe Practices From the ISMP Adult IV Push Medication Safety Summit*. www.ismp.org/Tools/guidelines/ivsummitpush/ivpushmedguidelines.pdf.

IV House. (2016). *Ergonomic armboard reduces injuries, increases efficiency*. http://www.pedagogyeducation.com/Main-Campus/Student-Union/Campus-Blog/July-2016/Ergonomic-Armboard-Reduces-Injuries,-Increases-Eff.aspx.

Kamangar, N. (2015). *Bacterial Pneumonia Treatment & Management*. http://emedicine.medscape.com/article/300157-treatment.

Kirkey, S. (2015). *Hooking up to an IV Drip Is the Latest Health Fad, But Critics Say There Is Little Proof it Works*. http://news.nationalpost.com/news/canada/0801-na-vitamin-drip.

Kornbau, C., Lee, K. C., et al. (2015). Central line complications. *International Journal of Critical Illness Science, 5*(3), 170–178.

Kreidieh, F. Y., Moukadem, H. A., et al. (2016). Overview, prevention and management of chemotherapy extravasation. *World Journal Clinical Oncology, 7*(1), 87–97.

O'Grady, N. P., Alexander, M., Burns, L. A., et al. (2011). *Guidelines for the prevention of intravascular catheter-related infections*. www.cdc.gov/hicpac/BSI/01-BSI-guidelines-2011.html.

Pharmacy & Therapeutics Committee, Marquette General Hospital. (2014). Safe use of promethazine injection. *P&T Committee Newsletter, 4*(3), 1–4.

Rangel-Castilla, L. (2014). *Closed Head Trauma Treatment & Management*. http://emedicine.medscape.com/article/251834-treatment.

Reynolds, P. M., MacLaren, R., Mueller, S. W., et al. (2014). Management of extravasation injuries: a focused evaluation of noncytotoxic medications. *Pharmacotherapy, 34*(6), 617–632.

Stupnytskyi, C., Smolarek, S., Reeves, C., et al. (2014). Changing blood transfusion policy and practice. *The American Journal of Nursing, 114*(12), 50–59.

Talati, E. (2012). *Pushing the Boundaries: revisiting Transfusion of Blood Products in the Children of Jehovah's Witnesses*. http://blogs.law.harvard.edu/billofhealth/2012/09/11/pushing-the-boundaries-revisiting-transfusion-of-blood-products-in-the-children-of-jehovahs-witnesses/.

The Joint Commission. (2013). *Preventing central line-associated bloodstream infections: useful tools, an international perspective*. http://www.jointcommission.org/CLABSIToolkit.

US Food and Drug Administration (FDA). (2015). *Infusion pump risk reduction strategies for facility administrators and managers*. www.fda.gov/MedicalDevices/ProductsandMedicalProcedures/GeneralHospitalDevicesandSupplies/InfusionPumps/ucm205410.htm.

CHAPTER 37

Glickman-Simon, R., & Tessier, J. (2014). Guided imagery for postoperative pain, energy healing for quality of life, probiotics for acute diarrhea in children, acupuncture for postoperative nausea and vomiting, and animal-assisted therapy for mental disorders. *Explore: the Journal of Science and Healing, 10*(5), 326–329.

Johnstone, R. E. (2013). NPO: never precisely originated, not prudently ordered. *Anesthesiology News, 39*(10). www.anesthesiologynews.com/ViewArticle.aspx?d=Commentary&d_id=449&i=October+2013&i_id=1002&a_id=24177.

Phillips, N., Chettle, C. C., & Barzoloski-O'Connor, B. (2015). Reducing the risk of surgical site infections with the surgical care improvement project (SCIP). *Nurse.com West, 28*(5), 78–83.

Steelman, V. M., & Graling, P. R. (2013). Top 10 patient safety issues: what more can we do? *Association of periOperative Registered Nurses Journal, 97*(6), 679–701.

CHAPTER 38

Cowan, L. (2015). *Wound Series Part 2: approaches to Treating Chronic Wounds*. https://ceufast.com/course/wound-series-part-2-approaches-to-treating-chronic-wounds.

Grady, H. (2014). *Wound Care 101*. Palm Springs, CA: Presented at California Association of Physician Assistants Conference.

Kirman, C. N. (2015). *Pressure ulcers and wound care treatment & management: treatment*. http://emedicine.medscape.com/article/190115-treatment.

National Pressure Ulcer Advisory Panel. (2015). *NPUAP pressure ulcer stages/categories*. www.npuap.org/resources/educational-and-clinical-resources/npuap-pressure-ulcer-stagescategories/.

CHAPTER 39

American Heart Association. (2015). *Target heart rates*. www.heart.org/HEARTORG/GettingHealthy/PhysicalActivity/FitnessBasics/Target-Heart-Rates_UCM_434341_Article.jsp.

CHAPTER 40

Academy of Women's Health. (2015). *Overactive bladder and urinary incontinence*. http://academyofwomenshealth.org/overactive-bladder-and-urinary-incontinence/.

Ackley, B. J., & Ladwig, G. B. (2014). *Nursing Diagnosis Handbook: an Evidence-Based Guide to Planning Care* (10th ed.). Maryland Heights, MO: Elsevier Mosby.

Agency for Healthcare Research and Quality (AHRQ). (2012). Depression, hearing impairment, and health literacy influence older adults' abilities to self-manage their care. *Agency for Healthcare Research and Quality, 378*, 16.

Agency for Healthcare Research and Quality (AHRQ). (2015). *Medication errors*. https://psnet.ahrq.gov/primers/primer/23/medication-errors.

Centers for Disease Control and Prevention. National Center for Health Statistics. (2014). *Prevalence of incontinence among older Americans*. www.cdc.gov/nchs/data/series/sr_03/sr03_036.pdf.

Centers for Disease Control and Prevention (CDC). (2015). *Older adult falls: get the facts*. www.cdc.gov/homeandrecreationalsafety/falls/adultfalls.html.

Cunha, S. (2013). Bridging communication gaps with the deaf. *Nursing, 43*(11), 24–29.

Edelman, M., & Ficorelli, C. T. (2012). Keeping older adults safe at home. *Nursing, 42*(1), 65–66.

Emanuel, E. J. (2014). *Sex and the single senior*. www.nytimes.com/2014/01/19/opinion/sunday/emanuel-sex-and-the-single-senior.html?_r=0.

Mayo Clinic Staff. (2015). *Hormone therapy: is it right for you?* www.mayoclinic.org/diseases/conditions/menopause/in-depth/hormone-therapy/art-20046372.

Medline Plus, (2015). *Saw palmetto*. https://www.nlm.nih.gov/medlineplus/druginfo/natural/971.html.

National Eye Institute. (2015). *Facts about age-related macular degeneration*. https://nei.nih.gov/health/maculardegen/armd_facts.

Peel, N. M., Kuys, S. S., & Klein, K. (2012). Gait speed as a measure in geriatric assessment in clinical settings: a systematic review. *Journals of Gerontology A Biological Sciences and Medical Sciences, 68*(1), 39–46. http://dx.doi.org/10.1093/gerona/gls174.

Roman de Mettelinge, T., & Cambier, D. (2015). Understanding the relationship between walking aids and falls in older adults: a prospective cohort study. *Journal of Geriatric Physical Therapy, 38*(3), 127–132.

Willy, B., & Osterberg, C. M. (2014). Strategies for reducing falls in long-term care. *Annals of Long-Term Care, 22*(1). www.annalsoflongtermcare.com/article/strategies-for-reducing-falls-long-term-care.

CHAPTER 41

Alzheimer's Association. (2015). *Treatments for behavior*. www.alz.org/alzheimers_disease_treatments_for_behavior.asp.

Aziz, R., & Steffens, D. C. (2013). What are the causes of late-life depression? *Psychiatric Clinics of North America, 36*, 497–516.

Bankhead, C. (2012). *SSRIs linked to risk of stroke*. www.medpagetoday.com/Cardiology/Strokes/35387.

Blue Cross/Blue Shield of Texas. (2012). *Medicare Part D update: utilization of antipsychotics in the elderly population*. www.bcbstx.com/provider/news/2012_11_14.html.

Brent, N. J. (2013). *Nurses and mandatory reporting laws*. www.cphins.com/blog/post/nurses-and-mandatory-reporting-laws.

Burchum, J. R., & Rosenthal, L. D. (2016). *Lenhe's Pharmacology for Nursing Care*. St. Louis, MO: Elsevier Saunders.

Ellison, D., White, D., & Farrar, F. C. (2015). Aging population. *Nursing Clinics of North America, 50*(2015), 185–213.

Ferrazzoli, D., Sica, F., & Sancesario, G. (2013). Sundowning syndrome: a possible marker of frailty in Alzheimer's disease? *CNS and Neurological Disorders Drug Targets, 12*(4), 525–528.

Mazza, M., Marano, G., Traversi, G., Di Nicola, M., Catalano, V., & Janiri, L. (2015). The complex interplay of depression, inflammation and omega-3: state of the art and progresses in research. *Clin Ter, 166*(3), e242–e247.

Storrs, C. (2015). *For Alzheimer's patients, reservatrol brings new hope*. www.cnn.com/2015/09/11/health/resveratrol-hope-for-alzheimers-patients/.

Thorlund, K., Druyts, E., Wu, P., et al. (2015). Comparative efficacy and safety of selective serotonin reuptake inhibitors and serotonin-norepinephrine reuptake inhibitors in older adults. *Journal of the American Geriatrics Society, 63*(5), 1002–1009.

University of Michigan Department of Psychiatry. (2015). *Electroconvulsive therapy program: how does ECT work?* www.psych.med.umich.edu/ect/how-does-ect-work.asp.

Glossary

A

abduction Moving a limb away from the midline of the body.
abortion Ending a pregnancy before the fetus is viable.
abscess Localized infection consisting of an accumulation of purulent material made up of debris from phagocytosis when microorganisms have been present.
absorption The uptake of substances into or across tissues (e.g., skin, intestine, and kidney).
acceptance Admission of reality, as in the reality of death; the final stage in the process of dealing with dying and death.
accountability Taking responsibility for one's actions.
accountable Responsible.
achievement stage Life stage dealing with learning and successfully using your abilities.
acidosis Excess of acid or depletion of alkaline substances in the blood and body tissues.
active listening Listening with great concentration and focused energy.
active transport Force that can move molecules into cells regardless of their electrical charge or the concentrations already in the cell.
acupressure Technique that involves applying pressure to various points in the body to relieve pain or other symptoms.
acupuncture Technique that involves the insertion of extremely fine, sterile needles into various points of the body to relieve pain or other symptoms, restoring balance.
acute Sharp, severe; having rapid onset, severe symptoms, and short course.
acute illness Illness that develops suddenly and resolves in a short time.
acute radiation sickness (ARS) Illness that results when most or all of the body is exposed to a high dose of radiation, usually over a short period of time.
adaptation Adjustment in structure or habits.
adduction Moving a limb toward the midline of the body.
adhesion Fibrous band that holds parts together that are normally separated.
adipose Fatty; composed of fat cells.
ADLs Activities of daily living: bathing, dressing, grooming, cleansing teeth, shaving, toileting, etc.
advance directive Consent constructed before the need for it arises; it spells out a patient's wishes regarding surgery and diagnostic and therapeutic treatments.
adventitious Acquired; arising sporadically.
adventitious sounds Abnormal lung sounds elicited upon auscultation of the lungs during assessment.
adverse drug reaction (ADR) (or adverse drug event [ADE]) Unintended effect on the body resulting from therapeutic drug use, drug abuse, or interaction of drugs.
adverse effects Very undesirable side effects with more serious consequences.
advocate Standing up for your patient's rights; acting in the patient's behalf; being a representative of your patient.
aerobic Needing oxygen to live and grow.
afebrile Without a fever.
affective domain Learning domain in which the material is presented in a way that appeals to the learner's beliefs, feelings, and values.
age-associated memory impairment Age-related changes in mental processes, such as a decline in short-term memory and cognitive skills.
ageism Prejudice against aging and older adults.
age-related macular degeneration (AMD) Disorder associated with age in which there is a gradual loss of acute, central, and color vision.
aging Continual process of biologic, cognitive, and psychosocial change.
agnostic Person who doubts the existence of God because it cannot be proved or disproved.
agonists Drugs that produce a response.
AHRQ Agency for Healthcare Research and Quality, which develops standards of practice based on research.
Airborne Infection Isolation Precautions Same as Standard Precautions plus the following: place the patient in a private room with negative air pressure or in a room with a patient with the same infectious organism; wear a respirator when in the room with the patient; keep susceptible persons out of the patient's room; and limit the patient's movement outside the room.
alarm fatigue The phenomenon of nurses becoming desensitized to patient care alarms and missing or delaying their response to the alarm.
alignment Arrangement in a straight line; bringing a line into order.
alkalosis Excess of alkaline or decrease of acid substances in the blood and body fluids.
allergen Substance (antigen drug, foreign protein, or toxin) that produces an anaphylactic (allergic) reaction.
alternative therapies Therapies that are not mainstream or commonly used in medicine in a particular country.
Alzheimer disease Progressive, degenerative disease of the brain of unknown origin, resulting in the person's inability to process and integrate new information and retrieve memory.
ambulate Walk.
amino acid Organic compound; protein is composed of 20 amino acids.
ampule Small, sterile, all-glass or plastic container used for medication.
anaerobic Able to live and grow only when oxygen is absent.
analgesic Drug that relieves pain without causing loss of consciousness.
anaphylactic shock Serious and profound state of shock brought about by hypersensitivity to an allergen.
anaphylaxis Severe allergic reaction (hypersensitivity).
andropause The emotional and physical changes that happen to many men with age; male menopause.
anemia Low red blood cell count.
anesthesia The loss of sensory perception.
angiography Method of injecting a dye into an artery and then obtaining an x-ray of blood vessels, tumors, and lesions.
anorexia nervosa Disorder in which the focus is on remaining thin, causing restriction of food intake to the point of danger.

anoxia Condition of being without oxygen.
antagonists Drugs that block a response.
antibiotic Agent that is capable of killing or inhibiting the growth of microorganisms.
antibody Immunoglobulin molecule that has a specific amino acid sequence that gives it the ability to adhere to and interact only with the antigen that induced its synthesis.
anticipatory grieving Grieving that occurs before the loss actually happens.
antimicrobial Substance capable of killing or suppressing the multiplication and growth of microorganisms.
antipyretic Relieving or reducing fever.
antiseptic Chemical compound used on skin or tissue to eliminate microorganisms.
anuria Absence of urine.
anus Opening of the rectum at the skin.
apex The lowest superficial part of the heart, usually located at the fifth intercostal space.
aphasia Difficulty expressing or understanding language.
apical pulse Pulse found over the apex of the heart; created as the left ventricle rotates against the chest wall during systole (part of the cardiac cycle).
apnea Absence of breathing.
apothecary system System used for measuring and weighing drugs and solutions.
appliance Device or apparatus used for therapy or to improve function, including a pouch (bag) that attaches to the skin over an ostomy stoma to collect fecal matter or urine.
apprenticeship Situation where a worker learns a trade or profession by working with a master of the trade or profession; learning by doing.
approximate To close together, as in wound healing.
approximation Degree of closure of a wound.
aromatherapy The use of selected fragrances in lotions and inhalants in an effort to affect mood and promote health.
arrhythmia Any variation from the normal rhythm of a heartbeat; also called *dysrhythmia*.
arteriography Radiography of an artery or arterial system after injection of a contrast medium into the bloodstream.
ascites Abnormal accumulation of serous fluid within the peritoneal cavity.
asepsis Destruction and/or containment of infectious agents after they leave the body of a patient with an infectious disease.
aseptic Free of microorganisms.
aseptically Without introducing infectious material.
aspiration Withdrawal of fluid or cells.
assault The threat to harm another, or even to threaten to touch another without that person's permission.
assessment (data collection) Data-gathering activities for the purpose of collecting a complete, relevant database from which a nursing diagnosis can be made.
assignment The asking of ancillary, unlicensed personnel to perform certain duties or tasks.
assimilation The process by which members of a culture change their lifeways to become totally integrated into another culture.
assisted suicide Making available to patients the means to end their lives with knowledge that suicide is their intent.
asymptomatic Without symptoms.
atelectasis Collapsed or airless part of the lung; collapse of alveoli.
atheist Person who does not believe in the existence of God.
atherosclerosis The accumulation of fatty deposits on the walls of blood vessels.
atrophy Decrease in size or a wasting away of a cell, tissue, organ, or part.
auditory learning Learning through what is heard.
auscultation Listening for sounds produced within the body, usually with a stethoscope.
auscultatory gap Period where no sound is heard.
authority Power or right delegated or given.
autocratic Leadership style of tight control and unlimited power.
autologous From one's own body.
autonomic Not subject to voluntary control.
autonomy Ability to function independently.
autopsy Examination of the body organs and tissues to determine the cause of death.
autotransfusion Reinfusion of a patient's own blood.
axillary Pertaining to the armpit.

B

baby boomers People born between 1946 and 1964.
bacteria Single-celled microorganisms lacking a nucleus, which can reproduce as quickly as every few minutes, depending on conditions.
baptism Religious sacrament marked by the symbolic use of water resulting in admission of the recipient into the community of Christians.
baptized When someone has been the recipient of a baptism.
bargaining Attempt to make an arrangement whereby one gives something in order to gain something in return; the third stage in Kübler-Ross stages of the grieving process.
basal metabolic rate (BMR) The rate at which heat is produced when the body is at rest.
battery Actual physical contact that has been carried out against a person's will.
behavior modification In psychology, a form of treatment used to change behavior by giving positive feedback for desired behavior and negative feedback for undesirable behavior.
behavioral objective Statement of desired change in behavior or addition to current behaviors and attitudes.
being present Focusing on the moment.
belief Conviction or opinion that one considers to be true.
benign senescence Normal physical changes of aging.
benign senescent forgetfulness Term used to describe age-related changes in mental processes, including a slight decline in short-term memory and cognitive skills.
bereavement The state of having suffered a loss by death.
beta-carotene Fat-soluble hydrocarbon found in dark green leafy vegetables and deep orange vegetables and fruits; converts to vitamin A in humans.
bevel Slanted part of a needle tip.
bile Orange or yellow digestive fluid produced by the liver.
binder Support bandage that wraps around the breasts or abdomen and is secured with ties, Velcro, or elastic.
binge eating Episodes of continuous eating, often followed by purging.
bioavailability The degree to which a drug or other substance becomes available to the target tissue after administration.
biofeedback Specialized relaxation technique using a machine that measures the degree of muscular tension with skin electrodes.
biohazard Biologic agent or condition that can be harmful to a person's health.
biologic theories Theories based on cellular function and body physiology.
biopsy Surgical excision of a small amount of tissue.
bioterrorism The release of pathogenic microorganisms into a community to achieve political and/or military goals.
Biot respirations Respirations that are shallow for two or three breaths with a period of variable apnea.
bivalve Cut in half lengthwise.
"black box" warning Warning on a prescription medication to alert the patient and health care provider about important safety concerns, such as serious side effects or life-threatening risks.
blanch To turn skin white, or on darker skin, to become pale.

bleb Bump, or visible elevation of the epidermis.
body language Nonverbal communication.
body mass index (BMI) Ratio that uses height and weight to estimate fat values at which the risk for disease increases.
bolus Concentrated dose given in a short period of time.
bonding Sense of attachment between two people.
bone Dense and hard type of connective tissue.
boomerang children Those who return to the parental home for a period of time.
bore Internal diameter of a needle.
bowel training program Program of timing bowel movements and then scheduling toileting to promote a regular evacuation time.
brachial pulse Pulse found over the brachial artery that can be felt in the upper arm.
bradycardia Pulse that is less than 60 beats per minute.
bradypnea Slow and shallow breathing.
brain death The permanent stopping of integrated functioning of the person as a whole; cessation of brain functioning.
bronchoscopy Inspection of the interior of the tracheobronchial tree through a bronchoscope.
bronchovesicular sounds Those lung sounds heard over the central chest or back.
bruit Abnormal sound heard on auscultation of an artery, a "swishing" sound.
buccal Pertaining to or directed toward the cheek.
buffer Substance that by its presence in solution increases the amount of acid or alkali necessary to produce a unit change in pH.
bulimia nervosa Eating disorder characterized by episodic binge eating, followed by behaviors designed to prevent weight gain, including purging, fasting, laxatives use, and excessive exercise.
burette Tubelike chamber that holds 150 mL of fluid.
bursa Small fluid-filled sac that provides a cushion at friction points in freely movable joints.

C

cachexia Profound and marked state of constitutional disorder; general ill health and malnutrition.
cannula Tube for insertion into a duct or cavity.
capitated cost Set fee is paid for every patient enrolled in the health network each year.
carbohydrate Chemical substance containing only carbon, oxygen, and hydrogen; category of food.
carcinogen Any cancer-producing substance.
cardiac catheterization Introduction of a catheter into the heart chambers for diagnostic purposes.
cardiac output The pulse rate multiplied by the stroke volume.
career Work that requires specific training; one's occupation or profession.
caries Dental cavities.
carotenoids Antioxidants that protect cells and tissues from damage by free radicals; shown to increase immunity, improve vision, and have a role in cancer prevention.
carotid pulse Pulse found over the carotid artery on the front side of the neck.
carrier Individual who harbors the specific organism of disease without manifesting symptoms and is capable of transmitting the infection.
cartilage Fibrous connective tissue that acts as a cushion.
case management system charting Documentation that tracks variances from the clinical pathway.
cast Rigid dressing, molded to the body while pliable, that hardens as it dries to give firm support.
catabolism Metabolic process of breaking down complex substances into simple compounds.
cataract Opacity (not letting light through) of the lens of the eye, which impairs vision.
cathartics Agents that cause bowel evacuation.
catheter embolus Piece of catheter that travels through a vessel and lodges, obstructing blood flow.
catheterization Insertion of a tube into a body channel or cavity.
cellulitis Acute, spreading inflammation of the deep subcutaneous tissues and sometimes muscle, which may be associated with abscess formation.
centenarians People over age 100.
cephalocaudal Proceeding from head to tail.
cerumen Waxy substance secreted by the ceruminous glands; earwax.
chart *n.* Medical record; *v.* to document in the medical record.
charting Documentation of the nursing process, treatment, and associated care.
charting by exception Documentation that focuses on deviations from predefined norms, using preset protocols and standards of care.
Cheyne-Stokes respirations Respirations that gradually become more shallow and are followed by periods of apnea (no breathing), with repetition of the pattern.
chi'i Universal life force or energy.
chills Sensations of cold and shaking of the body.
chiropractic Science based on the theory that health and disease are related to the function of the nervous system; chiropractic manipulation involves adjustment and manipulation of the joints and adjacent tissues, particularly the spinal column.
cholesterol Component of fat found only in animal products.
chronic Persisting for a long time.
chronic illness Illness that develops slowly over a long period and lasts throughout life.
chyme Liquefied food and digestive juices.
clinical practice guidelines Systematically developed statements to assist practitioner and patient decisions about appropriate health care in specific clinical circumstances.
circadian rhythm Biologic rhythmic pattern that is regularly repeated every 24 hours.
circumcision Surgical removal of all or part of the penile foreskin.
circumduction Circular movement of a limb or of an eye.
clinical judgment The outcome of clinical reasoning; the conclusion, decision, or opinion reached by the care provider.
clinical pathway/care map Collaborative type of plan of care referred to as an interdisciplinary care plan that provides a step-by-step approach to care of the patient.
clinical reasoning Critical thinking in the clinical setting.
closure To say goodbye to those people and things that are important.
cognitive The mental process of knowing, remembering, and relating; connected thinking.
cognitive domain Learning domain in which the learner takes in and processes information by listening to or reading the material.
collaborate To work or cooperate with another.
collaboration Working together in a joint intellectual effort.
collagen Fibrous structural protein of all connective tissue.
colon The part of the large intestine extending from the cecum to the rectum.
colonization Development of a bacterial infection; microorganisms take up residence and grow.
colonoscopy The inspection of the entire large intestine for polyps, areas of inflammation, and malignant lesions.
colostomy Artificial opening (stoma) created in the large intestine and brought to the surface of the abdomen for evacuating the bowels.
colostrum The first breast fluid.
colposcopy Gynecologic examination that uses the colposcope to examine the walls of the vagina and the cervix.
comfort care Identifying symptoms that cause the patient distress and adequately treating those symptoms.

commode chair Chair with a container inserted to catch urine or feces.
communication The exchange of information and ideas by speech, writing, gesture, expression, body posture, intonation, and general appearance.
communion Christian sacrament in which the bread of the Eucharist is distributed and consumed.
competence Possession of required skills or knowledge.
competent Legally fit (mentally and emotionally).
complementary protein Protein from plant sources.
complementary therapies Therapies that are used along with medical therapies to promote health.
complete blood count (CBC) Includes type and number of red blood cells, white blood cells, platelets, and hemoglobin.
complete protein One that contains all nine essential amino acids.
compliance Implementation by the patient of the therapeutic plan that has been established.
compress Pad of gauze or similar dressing, for application of pressure or medication to a restricted area, or for local applications of heat or cold.
computed tomography scan (CT scan) Through use of a computer, cathode ray tubes emit radiation at different depths to show density of tissues and organs, indicating abnormalities; also called computed axial tomography (CAT) scan.
computer-assisted charting Documentation in which data are input via the computer.
computerized provider order entry (CPOE) The entering of provider orders into the medical record via computer.
concept Idea, thought, or notion derived from experiences and information acquired from one's external environment; an element used in the development of a theory.
conception Union of ovum and sperm.
condom catheter Condom with a tube attached to the distal end that is attached to a drainage bag.
confidence Belief in oneself and one's abilities.
confidential Kept private.
confidentiality The principle of keeping private all information about a patient.
conflict resolution Resolving a conflict.
congenital Condition present before or at birth.
congruent In agreement.
conization Coring or removal of the mucous lining of the cervical canal and its glands by means of cutting with a high-frequency current; may be performed when a Pap smear indicates abnormal cells.
conscious Having awareness of oneself and one's acts and surroundings.
consent Permission given by the patient or his or her legal representative.
constipation Decreased frequency of bowel movement or passage of hard, dry feces.
constructive criticism Helpful comments to assist the person to improve some plan, action, or interaction.
Contact Precautions Standard Precautions plus the following: never touch with bare hands anything wet that comes from a body surface or cavity; use gloves, impermeable gowns, masks, and protective eyewear when necessary.
contaminate To make unclean.
continuous positive airway pressure (CPAP) Gas (oxygen) delivered at positive pressure to keep alveoli open that would normally close upon expiration.
continuous quality improvement Process of continually evaluating nursing care to identify specific areas that need changes for improvement.
contracture Adaptive shortening of skeletal muscle tissue rendering the muscle highly resistant to stretching; prevents normal joint movement.
contraindications Reasons not to administer (a drug).
convalescence The process of recovering after an illness and regaining health.
convalescent Recovering, getting well.
co-pay The amount an insurance carrier requires the patient to pay for care.
coping Adjusting to or adapting to challenges.
core Circular piece cut out by the sharp edges of a needle; the center.
core temperature Temperature deep within the body.
coroner Person with legal authority to determine cause of death.
countertraction force The weight pulling against the weight of the traction.
crackles Abnormal, nonmusical sound heard on auscultation of the lungs during inspiration; also called rales.
creative behavioral therapy Psychosocial intervention that includes art, music, and humor, and that can allow for self-expression and alleviate anxiety and depression.
Credé maneuver Massage from top of bladder to bottom by starting above the pubic bone and rocking the palm of the hand steadily downward.
crisis Abrupt decline in fever.
critical pathway/care map Step-by-step approach to the total care of the patient.
critical thinking Directed, purposeful, mental activity by which ideas are created and evaluated, plans are constructed, and desired outcomes decided. It can occur inside and outside of the clinical setting.
cross-contamination Transmission of infectious microorganisms from one person or object to another.
cues Pieces of data or information that influence decisions.
cultural awareness Knowledge of a people's history and ancestry and an appreciation for their artistic expressions, foods, and celebrations.
cultural competence Knowing yourself, examining your own values, attitudes, beliefs, and prejudices.
cultural sensitivity Refraining from using offensive language, respecting accepted patterns of communication, and refraining from speaking in ways that are disrespectful of a person's cultural beliefs.
culture (1) The propagation of living organisms or tissue in special media conducive to their growth; (2) values, beliefs, and practices shared by most individuals within a group of people.
culture shock Confusion and anxiety confronting a person who is suddenly exposed to a foreign culture.
curandero, curandera Hispanic-American folk healer.
curative surgery Surgery that alleviates or cures a problem.
custom Practice that is followed by a particular group or region.
cyanosis Bluish discoloration or skin color changes, particularly around the mouth and in the nail beds, due to lack of oxygen.
cystitis Inflammation of the bladder.
cystoscopy The visual inspection of the interior of the bladder for the collection of biopsy specimens, collection of urine separately from each ureter, and treatment of various conditions.
cytology The study of the structure, function, and pathology of cells.

D

dangling The patient position of sitting on the side of the bed with the legs and feet hanging over the side.
data Pieces of information on a specific topic.
database Collection of facts and figures for analysis from which conclusions may be drawn.
death, dying The cessation of all physical and chemical processes that invariably occurs in all living organisms; a stage of life.
debridement Removal of foreign or unhealthy tissue from a wound.

debris Dead tissue or foreign matter.
decision making Choosing the best actions to meet a desired goal.
deductible The amount an insurance carrier requires the patient to pay for care before beginning to pay expenses.
defamation Remarks made by one person about another person that are untrue, and the remarks damage that person's reputation.
defecate Expel feces.
defense mechanisms Strategies used to protect us from increasing anxiety.
defervescence Abatement of fever.
defining characteristics Signs and symptoms that must be present for a particular nursing diagnosis to be appropriate.
degrade Break down.
dehiscence Separation of the layers of the surgical wound; spontaneous opening of an incision.
dehydration Removal of water from a tissue.
delegate Authorize another person to do something; entrust to another.
delegation The assignment of duties to another person.
delirium Acute confusional state that can occur suddenly or over a long period as a result of an underlying biologic cause or psychological stressor.
dementia Neurologic condition characterized by the following cognitive defects: impaired memory, disturbed intellectual function, and inability to problem solve.
democratic Leadership style practicing social equality or majority rule.
demographics Statistics about populations.
denial Defense mechanism in which the existence of intolerable conditions is unconsciously rejected; first stage in the acceptance of death.
dependent nursing action Action requiring a provider's order.
depression Mental state characterized by feelings of sadness, despair, and discouragement, ranging from mild to major symptoms.
dermis The inner, fibrous layer of skin beneath the epidermis.
diabetes mellitus Disturbance of the metabolism of carbohydrates and the use of glucose by the body.
diagnosis-related groups (DRGs) Use of a system by which a hospital receives a set amount of money for a patient who is hospitalized with a certain diagnosis.
dialects Regional variations of a language with different pronunciation, grammar, or word meanings.
diaphoresis Excessive sweat production; perspiration.
diarrhea Frequent loose stool.
diastole The phase or part of the cardiac cycle when the ventricles relax and fill with blood.
diastolic pressure The lower pressure exerted on the artery when the heart is at rest between contractions.
Dietary Reference Intakes (DRIs) Guidelines for estimating nutrient intake for planning and evaluating diets of healthy people.
diffusion The process by which substances move back and forth across a membrane until they are evenly distributed throughout the available space.
digestion The process of converting food into chemical substances that can be absorbed into the blood and used by the body tissue.
diluent Specified fluid used to dissolve a solute.
diplopia The perception of two images of a single object.
direct contact Contact of the caregiver's hands with a microorganism or with equipment and supplies that have been soiled by body secretions.
discharge planner Registered nurse or social worker who implements and organizes the plan for patient discharge.
discrimination To make a decision or treat persons based on a class or group to which they belong, such as race, religion, or sex.
disease Pathologic process with a definite set of signs and symptoms; disease causes illness.
disinfectant Agent that destroys infection-producing organisms.
distention The state of being stretched out or inflated.
distraction Technique of purposeful focusing of attention away from undesirable sensations and/or pain.
diuresis Increased excretion of urine.
do-not-resuscitate (DNR) order Order written by a physician or other authorized provider when the patient has indicated a desire to be allowed to die if breathing ceases or the heart stops.
document/documentation To record/the recording of pertinent data on the clinical record.
dorsalis pedis pulse Pulse found over the dorsalis pedis artery, which is located just lateral to and parallel with the extensor tendon of the big toe in the foot.
dorsiflexion Backward flexion or bending, as of the hand or foot.
dorsum Back.
douche Stream of water or air directed against a part of the body or into a cavity.
Droplet Precautions Same as Standard Precautions plus the following: place the patient in a private room with negative air pressure or in a room with a patient with the same infectious organism; wear a mask when in the patient's room; and transport the patient outside the room only when necessary, with the patient wearing mask if possible.
drug interaction Process occurring when one drug modifies the action of another drug.
dual-energy x-ray absorptiometry (DXA) Imaging technique used to quantify density.
durable power of attorney for health care Legal document that appoints a person chosen by the patient to carry out his or her wishes as expressed in an advance directive.
dysfunctional Not natural or normally functioning.
dyspareunia Abnormal pain during sexual intercourse.
dysphagia Difficulty swallowing.
dyspnea Difficult and labored breathing.
dysrhythmia Abnormal cardiac rhythm.
dysuria Painful urination.

E

ecchymosis Flat, hemorrhagic, blue or purplish patch on the skin or mucous membrane; bruising.
edema Fluid in interstitial spaces.
effluent Discharged fecal matter.
egalitarian Family/household with shared equality between men and women.
ego The problem solver and reality tester portion of the mind that develops with the person's interaction with the environment and the demands of the id. A component of the mind as postulated by Freud.
ego integrity Positive aspect of last psychosocial stage of life in which one reflects on one's achievements and feels self-satisfaction.
egocentric One who perceives everything from his or her own viewpoint and in his or her own way.
elder abuse Any type of abuse of older adults.
elective Voluntary.
electroconvulsive therapy (ECT) Treatment that consists of electric shock to the brain, for severe depression that fails to respond to medication or psychotherapy.
electroencephalogram (EEG) Tracing of the brain waves.
electrolyte Mineral or a salt that is dissolved in body fluid.
electronic health record (EHR) Health record entered into a computer's software program that is updated via the computer.
electronic medication administration record (eMAR) Electronic medical record of drug orders and administration, in which nurses record the times at which doses of medication are given.

embolus Clot that travels and lodges in a vessel.
embryonic Early formation stage of fetal development.
emergency admission Admission for which there is no prior planning.
empathy The ability to understand by seeing the situation from another's perspective.
empty nest syndrome Psychological syndrome occurring when children have left home, causing a sense of loss and sadness.
enculturation Learning the concepts, values, and behavioral standards of a culture.
endorphins Naturally occurring opiate-like peptides that modify the perception of pain.
endoscope Instrument used to view inside a body cavity.
endoscopic retrograde cholangiopancreatography (ERCP) Examination of the biliary system done through a flexible endoscope following instillation of contrast medium into the ampulla of Vater of the pancreas.
endotoxin Heat-stable toxin associated with the outer membranes of certain gram-negative bacteria that is released when the cells are disrupted.
endotracheal Within the trachea.
enteral Within the small intestine.
environment The total of all elements and conditions that surround us and influence our development.
epidemiology Study of the distribution and determinants of health-related states and events in populations, and the application of this study to the control of health problems.
epidermis The outer, thicker layer of skin.
epidural Outside or above the dura mater.
epidural analgesia Analgesia injected into the epidural space outside the dura mater to relieve pain.
erythema Redness of the skin caused by congestion of the capillaries in the lower layers of the skin that occurs with any skin injury, infection, or inflammation.
eschar Slough produced by a thermal burn, corrosive material, or gangrene.
esophagogastroduodenoscopy (EGD) Endoscopic examination of the esophagus, stomach, and duodenum.
essential amino acid Amino acid that must be consumed through food sources.
ethical code Actions and beliefs approved of by a particular group of people.
ethical principles Rules of right and wrong from a moral view.
ethics Actions and beliefs approved of by a particular group of people.
ethics committee Committee that looks at ethical issues of patient care and makes decisions as to whether unethical conduct has occurred, or whether a procedure or treatment would be ethical.
ethnic Referring to a group within a race usually differentiated by geographic, religious, social, or language differences.
ethnicity One's distinct culture based on shared ancestry, social experience, regional and/or national history.
ethnocentrism The tendency of human beings to feel that their way of thinking, believing, and doing things is the only way or the only right way.
etiologic factors The causes of a problem.
etiology Study of the cause of disease; origin.
eupnea Normal, relaxed breathing pattern.
euthanasia Easy or painless death; *active euthanasia*, or mercy killing, is the deliberate ending of the life of a person who is incurably and terminally ill; *passive euthanasia* is the withholding of heroic measures and allowing the person to die.
evaluation Judgment of the effectiveness of the intervention or plan.
evidence-based nursing Nursing practice based on validated research.
evisceration Extrusion of the viscera through a surgical incision; protrusion of an internal organ through the incision.
exacerbation Increase in severity of a disease or any of its symptoms.
excoriation Abrasion of the skin.
executive substage Stage of cognitive development of middle adults in which they delegate appropriately, juggle roles, and manage complex situations.
expected outcome Specific statement of the goal the patient is expected to achieve as a result of nursing intervention.
expectorate Cough up and spit out.
expiration Movement of air out of the lungs.
expire To breathe out or exhale; to die.
extension posture Arms are stiffly extended, adducted, and hyperpronated with hyperextension of the legs and plantar flexion of the feet; indicates disruption of the motor fibers in the midbrain and brainstem; formerly called decerebrate posture.
external fixator Metal device inserted into or through one or more bones to stabilize fragments of a fracture while it heals.
extracellular Outside of the cell.
extravasation Infiltration of a drug from an intravenous line.
exudate Fluid in or on tissue surfaces that has escaped from blood vessels in response to inflammation, and that contains protein and cellular debris.

F

faith Belief that cannot be proven, or for which no material evidence exists.
false imprisonment Preventing a person from leaving a facility or restricting his or her movements within the facility.
fat Essential nutrient made up of fatty acids and glycerol that supplies a concentrated form of energy.
febrile Stage of fever in which the body temperature rises to the new set point established by the hypothalamus and remains there until there is resolution of the cause of the fever.
fecal impaction Collection of hardened feces in the rectum or colon.
fecal incontinence Involuntary passage of feces.
feces Intestinal waste material.
feedback Return of information and how it was interpreted.
feeding pump Pump used in continuous feedings that pumps the liquid formula, drop by drop, into the feeding tube.
femoral pulse Pulse found over the femoral artery in the groin.
fetal Late stage of prenatal development.
fever Elevated temperature.
fiber That portion of carbohydrate that cannot be broken down by intestinal enzymes and juices.
fibrin Insoluble protein essential to clotting.
fibrosis Formation of fibrous tissue.
filtration The movement of water and suspended substances outward through a semipermeable membrane.
first intention Type of wound healing (closure) for wounds with little tissue loss, such as a surgical incision.
fissure Narrow slit.
fistula Abnormal, tubelike passage within body tissue, usually between two internal organs or leading from an internal organ to the body surface.
flatus Intestinal gas released from the anus.
flexion posture Internal rotation and adduction of the arms with flexion of the elbows, wrist, and fingers, resulting from neurologic injury and interruption of voluntary motor tracts; extension of the legs may also be seen; formerly called decorticate posture.
fluoroscopy Examination by means of a fluoroscope using x-rays displayed on a fluorescent screen.
focus charting Documentation that centers on the patient from a positive perspective; this form of documentation has three components: data, action, and response.
fornix/fornices Archlike structure(s).
Fowler position Position arranged by elevating the head of the bed 60 to 90 degrees.

fructose Fruit sugar.
fungi Tiny, primitive organisms of the plant kingdom that contain no chlorophyll and reproduce by means of spores; present in soil, air, and water.

G

gait Style of walking.
gait belt Sturdy belt made of tightly webbed canvas material that is used to ambulate and/or transfer the weak or unsteady patient.
gastrocolic reflex Increase in intestinal and colonic peristaltic activity following the arrival of food into the empty stomach.
gastroscopy The visual inspection of the upper digestive tract and the stomach to obtain specimens of gastric contents, and perform a biopsy on the stomach tissues.
gastrostomy tube Feeding tube placed directly into the stomach through the abdominal wall.
gate control theory View of pain transmission as being controlled by a gate mechanism in the central nervous system.
gauge Scale of measurement.
gender The sex of an individual, male or female.
gender roles Behaviors and attitudes that a culture expects and approves for males or females.
generalization The formation of a general principle or idea.
generativity Stage of life in which the person guides the lives of the next generation.
generic name Drug name not protected by trademark.
genes Segments of DNA that carry the blueprints of development.
germinal Initial stage of prenatal development.
gerontologist Specialist in the study of older adults.
gingiva The part of the oral mucosa covering the tooth-bearing border of the jaw; the gum.
glaucoma The accumulation of fluid inside the eye, which exerts pressure on the optic nerve, eventually causing blindness.
glomerulus Small tuft or cluster of capillaries; it is the integral part of the nephron (the basic unit of the kidney), the function of which is to bring blood to the nephron.
glucometer Small device used to measure glucose content of capillary blood.
glucose The metabolized form of sugar in the body.
gluteal Pertaining to the buttocks.
glycemic index Ranking of foods based on the response of postprandial blood glucose as compared with a reference food, usually white bread or glucose.
glycosuria Glucose in the urine.
goal Broad statement describing what is to be accomplished over a specified period.
gram-negative Bacteria that lose the stain in the Gram method of staining.
gram-positive Bacteria that retain the stain in the Gram method of staining.
granulation tissue Connective tissue with multiple small blood vessels.
grief The total emotional response of pain and distress that a person experiences as a reaction to loss.
grieving process Process that occurs over a period of time as a person adapts to and moves through the pain of loss.
guaiac Reagent to test for blood in the stool.
guided imagery Guidance to use the imagination.
gurgles Wet sounds heard when auscultating the lungs; formerly called rhonchi; gurgle sounds also occur in the bowel.

H

half-life The time required for the plasma level of a drug to fall to half of a certain measured level.
halitosis Bad breath.
health The state of functioning well physically and mentally and expressing the full range of one's potentialities.
health care agent Person designated by the patient to make health care decisions when the patient is incapacitated (not able to make those decisions).
health care–associated infections (HAIs) Infection that occurs within a health care facility or because of a treatment or procedure.
health care proxy Person chosen by the patient to carry out the patient's wishes as expressed in an advance directive.
health literacy The ability to obtain, process, and understand information related to health and illness.
health maintenance organization (HMO) Type of group practice that enrolls patients for a set fee per month and provides a limited network of doctors, hospitals, and other health care providers from which to choose.
heart failure Pump failure of the right or left ventricle associated with abnormal retention of fluid.
helminths Parasitic worms or flukes that belong to the animal kingdom.
hematemesis The vomiting of blood.
hematology Study of blood and its components.
hematoma Localized collection of clotted blood underneath the skin.
hematuria Blood in the urine.
hemiparesis Muscular weakness or partial paralysis affecting one side of the body.
hemiplegia One-sided paralysis.
hemolysis Rupture of erythrocytes with release of hemoglobin into the plasma.
hemoptysis Coughing up and spitting out of blood as a result of bleeding from the respiratory tract.
hemorrhoids Enlarged veins inside or just outside the rectum.
hemostasis Arrest of the escape of blood by natural (clot formation or vessel spasm) or artificial (compression) means, or the interruption of blood flow to a part.
hemothorax Collection of blood in the pleural cavity.
herbals Substances composed of herbs for health promotion.
hernia The abnormal protrusion of part of an organ or tissue through the structures normally containing it.
hierarchy The arrangement of objects, elements, or values in a graduated series.
HIPAA Health Insurance Portability and Accountability Act.
hirsutism Abnormal hairiness, especially in women.
histology Division of anatomy dealing with the structure, composition, and function of tissues.
HMO Health maintenance organization.
holistic Approach to health care that considers the biologic, psychological, sociologic, and spiritual aspects and needs of the person.
homeostasis Tendency of biologic systems to maintain stability in their internal environment while continually adjusting to changes necessary for survival.
hope Inner positive life force, a feeling that what is desired is possible.
hospice Program that provides a continuum of home and inpatient care for terminally ill patients and their families.
host Animal or plant that harbors and provides sustenance for another organism (a parasite).
human immunodeficiency virus (HIV) The causative agent for acquired immunodeficiency syndrome (AIDS).
humidifier Device that supplies moisture to a gas.
humidity The amount of moisture in the air.
hydrostatic pressure Pressure exerted by fluid.
hydrotherapy Massage or debridement by moving water.
hygiene The practice of cleanliness that is conducive to the preservation of health.
hypercalcemia Above-normal level of calcium in the blood.
hypercapnia Excess carbon dioxide in the blood.
hyperchloremia Abnormally high chloride in the blood.
hyperemia Excess of blood in a part.

hyperextension Extension of a limb or a part beyond the normal joint limit.
hyperglycemia Excess of glucose (sugar) in the blood.
hyperkalemia Excessive amount of potassium in the blood.
hypermagnesemia Excess magnesium in the blood.
hypernatremia Excess of sodium in the blood or a loss of body water.
hyperosmolality Increased concentration of solutes within the fluid.
hyperphosphatemia Excess phosphate in the blood.
hypertension Blood pressure elevated above the normal range.
hyperthermia Above-normal body temperature; *malignant hyperthermia*: a syndrome affecting patients undergoing general anesthesia, marked by a rapid rise in body temperature, signs of increased muscle metabolism, and rigidity.
hypertonic Of greater concentration; having a greater tonicity than blood.
hyperventilation Pattern of breathing in which there is an increase in the rate and depth of breaths and carbon dioxide is "blown off," causing the blood level of carbon dioxide to fall.
hypervolemia Abnormal increase in the volume of circulating blood.
hypnosis Therapeutic suggestion, involving inducing a trance-like state using focusing and relaxation techniques and giving the patient suggestions that may be helpful after the return to an alert state of consciousness.
hypocalcemia Below-normal level of calcium in the blood.
hypochloremia Abnormally low chloride in the blood.
hypoglycemia Abnormally low level of glucose (sugar) in the blood.
hypokalemia Abnormally low potassium in the blood.
hypomagnesemia Abnormally low magnesium in the blood.
hyponatremia Abnormally low sodium in the blood.
hypophosphatemia Decreased phosphate in the blood.
hypostatic pneumonia Pneumonia caused by stasis of lung secretions due to inactivity, which provides a medium for bacterial growth.
hypotension Abnormally low blood pressure.
hypothalamus The portion of the diencephalon lying beneath the thalamus at the base of the cerebrum, and forming the floor and part of the lateral wall of the third ventricle of the brain.
hypothermia Subnormal body temperature.
hypotonic Of lesser concentration; containing less solute than extravascular fluid.
hypoventilation Reduction in the amount of air entering the pulmonary alveoli, which causes an increase in the arterial carbon dioxide level.
hypovolemia Decreased volume of circulating blood.
hypoxemia Decreased amount of oxygen in the bloodstream.
hypoxia State of insufficient oxygen in the blood.

I

iatrogenic Referring to any adverse condition in a patient resulting from medical or surgical treatment.
id The body's basic primitive urges as postulated by Freud.
ideology Belief or value system.
idiopathic Of unknown origin.
ileostomy Opening surgically created at the ileum to divert intestinal contents after lower portions of the bowel have been surgically removed.
ileum The distal (farthest) portion of the small intestine, extending from the jejunum to the cecum.
illness Disease of body or mind.
illness period The third stage of infection, where localized and systemic signs and symptoms appear.
imagery Set of mental pictures or images.
immobilization Rendering a part incapable of moving.
immune response Reaction of the body to substances interpreted as non-self.
immunity Security against a particular disease; nonsusceptibility to the invasive or pathogenic effects of foreign microorganisms or to the toxic effect of antigenic substances.
immunocompromised Having poorly functioning immune systems.
impervious Not affording a passage.
implement To put into action.
implementation Performing an intervention and assessing the response.
incident report Documentation of an incident or occurrence that is out of the ordinary, including the facts, who was involved, and who discovered it.
incomplete protein One that does not contain all essential amino acids.
incongruent Verbal and nonverbal messages that do not agree.
incontinence (fecal) Lack of voluntary control over the anal sphincter.
incontinence (urinary) Inability to prevent passing urine.
incubation period The time from invasion of the body by the microorganisms to the onset of symptoms.
independent nursing action Action that does not require a medical order, but does require critical thinking.
individualized aging Describes how older adults should be viewed as individuals, not as a stereotypical member of the group.
induration Area of the skin that feels hard.
infection Invasion and multiplication of microorganisms (e.g., bacteria and viruses) in body tissues, causing cellular injury.
infection prevention and control The use of medical and surgical asepsis and Standard Precautions to prevent or control the spread of microorganisms.
inferences Conclusions made based on observed data.
infiltrated When solution is deposited in tissue outside the vein.
inflammation Localized protective response brought about by injury or destruction of tissues, which serves to destroy or wall off the injurious agent.
infusion Slow introduction of fluid into a vein.
infusion pump Electronic pump that regulates the flow of an intravenous infusion.
inhaler Apparatus for administering vaporized or volatilized agents by inhalation, or for protecting the lungs from harmful substances in the air.
initiative Willingness to try.
injection The act of forcing a liquid into a part or organ of the body.
input Information put in.
insomnia Difficulty in getting to sleep or staying asleep at night.
inspection Visual examination for detection of abnormal signs or qualities.
inspiration Movement of air into the lungs.
instillation Administration of a liquid drop by drop.
Institute for Safe Medication Practices (ISMP) Institute formed to find ways to prevent medication errors.
insulin pump Programmable pump that delivers insulin directly into the body.
integrated delivery network Set of providers and services organized to deliver coordinated care to promote wellness, care for illness, and promote rehabilitation.
integrative medicine The delivery of complementary and alternative care along with conventional medicine, providing a holistic approach.
integument The skin covering the body.
integumentary System containing the skin (the largest organ of the body), hair, nails, and sweat and sebaceous glands.
intelligence Combination of verbal ability, reasoning, memory, imagination, and judgment.

interdependent action Action that comes from collaborative care planning.
interferon Biologic response modifier that affects cellular growth.
interpersonal relationships Association or connection between two people.
interstitial Placed or lying between.
interstitial fluids Body fluids that are located in the tissue spaces around the cells.
interventions Nursing actions taken to improve, maintain, or restore health or prevent illness.
interview Conversation in which facts are obtained.
intimacy Close, meaningful relationship.
intracellular Within the cell.
intracellular fluid Body fluid that is within the cell walls.
intractable pain Pain that is resistant to treatment.
intradermal (ID) Into the dermis.
intramuscular (IM) Into the muscle.
intrathecal Pertaining to or within the spinal canal.
intrauterine Within the uterus.
intravascular Within a vessel or vessels.
intravenous (IV) Within a vein or veins.
intravenous pyelography (IVP) Injection of a dye into a vein to show urine flow through the renal pelvis, ureters, and bladder on x-ray.
interventions Nursing actions aimed at accomplishing a goal or expected outcome.
invasion of privacy Violation of the confidential and privileged nature of a professional relationship.
invasive procedures Procedures that require entry into the body.
irrigation Washing by a stream of water or other fluid.
ISBAR-R Technique for communication between members of the health care team; the acronym stands for **I**ntroduction, **S**ituation, **B**ackground, **A**ssessment, **R**ecommendation, and **R**eadback.
ischemia Deficiency of blood in a part, usually due to functional constriction or actual obstruction of a blood vessel.
isolation The separation of infected individuals from those uninfected for the period of communicability of a particular disease; quarantine.
isometric Maintaining the same measurements; of equal dimensions.
isometric exercises Exercises performed against resistance.
isotonic Of equal solute concentration; solutions that have the same concentration, or osmolality, as blood and are used to expand the fluid volume of the body.

J

jaundice Yellowness of the skin, sclera, mucous membranes, and excretions resulting from hyperbilirubinemia and deposition of bile pigments; also called icterus.
jejunostomy or duodenal tube Feeding tube placed directly into the intestines through the abdominal wall.
jejunum That portion of the small intestine that extends from the duodenum to the ileum.
joint The union of two or more bones in the body.
jugular venous distention (JVD) Visible thickening of the jugular veins when the patient is positioned sitting in bed at a 15- to 35-degree angle; assessed as a sign of heart failure or overhydration.

K

keloid Permanent raised, enlarged scar.
ketonuria Acetone bodies in the urine.
kinesiology The study of the movement of body parts, also known as body mechanics.
kinesthetic learning Learning by performing a task or handling items.
kinetic Moving.
Korotkoff sounds Sounds that relate to the effect of arterial wall vibrations during auscultation of blood pressure.
kosher Properly prepared in accordance with Jewish dietary laws.
KUB x-ray X-ray of the kidneys, ureters, and bladder.
Kussmaul respirations Respirations having an increased rate and depth with panting and long, grunting exhalations.
kwashiorkor Condition occurring in infants and young children soon after weaning from breast milk, due to severe protein deficiency.
kyphosis Increased curve in the thoracic spine.

L

laceration Torn, ragged, or mangled wound.
lactation The secretion of milk.
lacto-ovo-vegetarian Diet consisting of dairy products, eggs, and plant foods.
lactose Sugar derived from milk.
lactovegetarian Diet consisting of dairy products and plant foods.
laissez-faire Leadership style that is based on noninterference with what others desire.
laser Acronym for *l*ight *a*mplification by the *s*timulated *e*mission of *r*adiation.
last rites Religious rite performed by a clergyman for the individual just prior to death.
lateral position Positioned on the side.
law Rule of conduct established by government.
lesion Damaged tissue.
lethargy Abnormal drowsiness or stupor.
leukocyte White blood cell.
leukocytosis Increase in the number of leukocytes in the blood, due to infection or other causes.
leukoplakia White patch on a mucous membrane that will not rub off.
liability Responsibility.
liable Responsible.
libel Written defamation.
libido The sex drive.
life span The number of years of a person's life.
ligaments Strong, fibrous connective tissues that support and strengthen the bones of joints.
lipids Group of substances comprising fatty, greasy, oily, and waxy compounds that are insoluble in water and soluble in nonpolar solvents, such as hexane, ether, and chloroform.
living will Document detailing the measures desired for treatment or to prolong life if the person becomes incapacitated; also called advance directives.
logrolling Technique used to turn a patient in bed as a single unit while maintaining straight body alignment at all times.
longevity Length of life.
lordosis Exaggerated lumbar curve.
loss To no longer have or possess an object, person, or situation.
lumbar puncture Insertion of a hollow needle into the subarachnoid space between the third and fourth lumbar vertebrae to withdraw samples of cerebrospinal fluid for analysis and to measure the pressure; also called spinal puncture and spinal tap.
lumen Opening or interior diameter of a needle; channel within a tube.
lymphocyte Any of the mononuclear, nonphagocytic leukocytes, found in the blood, lymph, and lymphoid tissues, that comprise the body's immunologically competent cells and their precursors.
lysis Breakdown, disintegration; also reduction or abatement.

M

maceration The softening of tissue that increases the chance of trauma or infection.
macrobiotic Type of diet consisting mostly of whole grains and beans.
macrodrops 10 gtt/mL of fluid.
macrophage Any of the mononuclear phagocytes found in tissues.
macular degeneration Disorder resulting in a loss of acute, central, and color vision.
magnetic resonance imaging (MRI) Noninvasive diagnostic method based on use of magnetic fields to visualizing soft tissue without the use of contrast media or ionizing radiation.
maladaptation Lack of adjustment.
malaise Discomfort, uneasiness, or indisposition, often indicative of infection.
malnutrition Poor nourishment resulting from improper diet or from some deficit in nutrition that prevents the body from using its food properly.
malpractice When a professional causes harm by failing to meet the standard of care; failure to do what a reasonable and prudent person in a similar situation would do.
managed care plan Health care plan in which all medical care is managed by the insuring group.
marasmus Form of protein-calorie malnutrition occurring chiefly in the first year of life, characterized by growth retardation and wasting of subcutaneous fat and muscle.
massage Stimulation of the skin and underlying tissues with varying degrees of hand pressure to decrease pain, produce relaxation, and/or improve circulation.
mastication The act of chewing.
matriarchal Female dominated family/household.
maturity State of being fully developed physically or emotionally.
meconium Dark green mucilaginous material in the intestine of the full-term fetus; it constitutes the first stools passed by the newborn infant.
mediate To resolve or settle differences by working with all the conflicting parties.
Medicaid State medical care coverage for individuals and families with reduced or poverty-level income.
medical asepsis The practice of reducing the number of organisms present or reducing the risk for transmission of organisms.
medical record Paper or electronic record that contains all orders, tests, treatments, and care that occurred during the time a person was under the care of a health care provider.
medical social worker (MSW) Individual who provides counseling and information regarding long-term planning, financial assistance, or available community services.
Medicare Health care provided through the Social Security Administration primarily for the retired older adult.
medication administration record (MAR) Patient record of drug orders and administration, in which nurses record the times at which doses of medication are given.
medication reconciliation Procedure used to compare medications ordered currently with those the patient normally takes at home or during the previous medical facility admission.
meditation Focusing on an image or thought.
melanin The main determinant of skin color.
melena Blood that has changed into a dark, tarry substance as it moves through the stomach or small intestine.
meniscus The curved, upper surface of a liquid being poured for dosage administration.
menopause Cessation of menstruation.
mentor Wise and trusted teacher or coach.
meridian Lines or passageways.
metabolism Cellular chemical reactions in the body.
metered-dose inhaler (MDI) Device that delivers a measured dose of an inhalant medication.
microdrops 60 gtt/mL of fluid.
microorganism Organism only visible with a microscope.
micturition Urination.
mindful Being highly aware and alert to another's feelings; considerate.
mineral Inorganic substance contained in animals and plants.
minister One who is authorized to perform religious functions in a Christian church.
mobility The ability to move in one's environment with ease and without restriction.
moleskin Soft material, often with an adhesive backing, used especially on the feet to protect against chafing.
morals Rules or standards regarding what is right or wrong.
Moro reflex Startle response of the newborn.
murmur Periodic sound of short duration of cardiac or vascular origin.
myocardial infarction (MI) Loss of blood supply to the heart muscle.
MyPlate The US Department of Agriculture (USDA) schematic and description of recommended foods and exercise for a healthy diet and lifestyle.

N

NANDA-I NANDA International, which identifies, develops, and classifies nursing diagnoses; founded in 1973.
narcolepsy Recurrent, uncontrollable brief episodes of sleep during hours of wakefulness.
narcotic Drug that produces insensibility or stupor; legal definition refers to habit-forming drugs such as opiates and any of many synthetic drugs such as meperidine.
nasogastric (NG) tube Type of tube that is placed through the nose into the stomach.
nebulizer Device that dispenses liquid in a fine spray, used in inhalation therapy.
necrosis Local death of tissue from disease or injury.
necrotic Of or pertaining to necrosis.
negligence Departure from the standard of care which, under similar circumstances, would have ordinarily been exercised by a similarly trained and experienced professional.
neonate Newborn.
nephron The structural and functional unit of the kidney, each nephron is capable of forming urine by itself.
neurotransmitter Substance (e.g., norepinephrine) that is released from the axon terminal of a presynaptic neuron on excitation, and that travels across the synaptic cleft to excite or inhibit the target cell.
nocturia Voiding during the night.
nocturnal delirium The appearance of or increase of symptoms of confusion or agitation associated with the late afternoon or early evening hours, usually continuing into the night; also known as sundowning or sundown syndrome.
nonadherence When a patient does not or is unable to adhere to the medical and treatment plan.
noncompliance When patients do not take the drugs that are prescribed for them on the schedule indicated by the prescription or do not adhere to a prescribed treatment regimen.
nonjudgmental Refraining from judgment; an attitude of openness.
nondisclosure agreement Legal agreement between two parties (e.g., a nursing student and a hospital) in which the parties promise to protect the confidentiality of information.
nonessential amino acid Amino acid that can be manufactured by the liver.
non-rapid eye movement (NREM) sleep The state of sleep when the body receives the most rest.
nonsteroidal anti-inflammatory drugs (NSAIDs) Drugs with anti-inflammatory properties that do not contain steroids.
nonverbal Without words.

nosocomial Infection acquired during hospitalization.
NPO No food or fluids by mouth.
nurse licensure compact Agreements that allow mutual recognition of a nursing license between the different states that are members of the compact. A nurse who is licensed in one compact state is allowed to practice nursing in another compact state without obtaining another nursing license.
nurse practice act State law defining the scope of nursing practice and the regulation of the profession by a state board for nursing.
nursing audit Examination of a series of patient records to determine if nursing care for those patients met particular standards.
nursing diagnosis Statement that indicates the patient's actual health status or the risk of a problem developing, the causative or related factors, and specific defining characteristics.
nursing implications Points that the nurse needs to remember about a drug or needs to teach patients.
nursing process Goal-directed series of activities whereby the practice of nursing accomplishes its goal of alleviating, minimizing, or preventing real or potential health problems.
nursing theory Statement about relationships among concepts or facts, based on existing information.
nutrient Biochemical substance used by the body that must be supplied in adequate amounts from foods consumed.
nutrition The sum of processes involved in taking in nutrients and absorbing and using them.
nystagmus Involuntary, rapid, rhythmic movement of the eyeball.

O

obesity Excessive accumulation of body fat.
obituary Notice of death, often published in newspapers.
objective data Information obtained through the senses or measured by instruments.
observe To see or notice; to watch attentively.
obturator Curved guide that is inserted into the trachea to facilitate placement of a tube.
occult Hidden or concealed.
Occupational Safety and Health (OSH) Act Law passed in 1970 to improve the work environment in areas that affect the worker's health or safety.
Occupational Safety and Health Administration (OSHA) The main federal agency responsible for the enforcement of safety and health legislation.
olfaction Smelling.
oliguria Diminished amount of urine formation.
omega-3 fatty acid Fatty acid with a double bond at the third carbon; appear to have protective functions against formation of blood clots and coronary heart disease.
one-time (single) order Order written for a drug to be given just one time.
ophthalmic Having to do with the eyes.
ophthalmoscope Lighted instrument used for viewing the interior of the eye.
ordinal position Birth order.
orientation Awareness of one's environment with reference to place, time, and people.
orthopnea The ability to breathe easily only in the upright position.
orthostatic hypotension Fall in blood pressure associated with dizziness, syncope (fainting), and blurred vision, which occurs upon standing; also called postural hypotension.
osmolality The concentration of a solution in terms of osmoles of solute per kilogram of solvent.
osmoreceptors Specialized neurons in the thalamus that are stimulated by increased extracellular fluid osmolality to release antidiuretic hormone (ADH) from the posterior pituitary.
osmosis The movement of pure solvent (liquid) across a membrane.
ostomy Diversion of intestinal contents from their normal path, resulting in an artificial opening into the intestine.
otic Having to do with the ear.
otoscope Lighted instrument used to visualize the tympanic membrane and interior of the ear canal.
ototoxic Having a damaging effect on the eighth cranial nerve (vestibulocochlear) or on the organs of hearing and balance.
outcome-based quality improvement (OBQI) Type of nursing audit that compares actual patient outcomes with desired outcomes so that measures to improve care can be devised.
outcomes Results of actions.
overhydration Excess fluid volume.
over-the-bed frame Rectangular frame to which traction equipment may be attached.
over-the-counter (OTC) Drugs that may be purchased without a prescription.
oximeter Device that measures oxygen in the blood.
oximetry Measurement of oxygen.

P

pain Feeling of distress or suffering, caused by the stimulation of nerve endings.
palliation The act of treating symptoms to relieve pain and provide comfort.
palliative Relieving symptoms when a disease cannot be cured.
palliative surgery Surgery to relieve pain or complications.
pallor Paleness of the skin.
palpate Feel.
palpation Touching with the hands and fingers.
panel Group of tests.
Papanicolaou (Pap) smear Microscopic laboratory examination used to determine the presence of malignant cells using body secretions (from the respiratory, genitourinary, or digestive tract).
paracentesis Needle puncture of the abdomen to remove ascites fluid, perform a lavage, or initiate peritoneal dialysis.
paralytic ileus Obstruction of the intestines from inhibition of bowel motility.
paranoia Behavior characterized by delusions of persecution and/or delusions of grandeur.
paraplegic Person who is paralyzed in the legs and lower part of the body.
parenteral Introduction of a substance into the body by some means other than the gastrointestinal tract.
paresthesia Feeling of numbness or tingling.
pastor Christian minister.
patent Freely open (e.g., a patent drain).
pathogen Any disease-producing organism.
pathologic fracture Fracture due to weakening of the bone structure brought on by pathologic process, such as cancer and other diseases.
patient advocate One who speaks for, and protects the rights of, the patient.
patient-centered care Recognizing the patient as the source of control and full partner in providing compassionate and coordinated care based on respect for the patient's values, needs, and preferences.
patient-controlled analgesia (PCA) Analgesia doses controlled by the patient.
patriarchal Male-dominated family/household.
peak action The blood level at which a drug delivers its greatest action.
peak and trough The highest and lowest blood level of a drug.
peers Others of similar age and background.
peripheral parenteral nutrition (PPN) Nutrition delivery using a peripheral vein.

perception Being aware of something through the senses of seeing, hearing, feeling, tasting, and smelling.
percussion Light, quick tapping on the body surface to produce sounds.
percutaneous endoscopic gastrostomy (PEG) tube Feeding tube placed directly into the stomach.
perfusion The act of pouring over or through, especially the passage of a fluid through the vessels of a specific organ; circulation of blood through tissue.
perioperative Period from the time of the decision to have surgery through recovery from the procedure.
periostomal Area around a stoma.
peripheral Situated away from a center or central structure.
peristalsis The action caused by muscle fibers in a tubular organ that propels contents through the organ in waves.
personal protective equipment (PPE) Items such as gloves, gowns, masks, protective eyewear, and hair covering used to protect the health care team member from infectious organisms.
petechiae Pinpoint, round, purplish-red spots that are not raised; caused by intradermal or submucous hemorrhage; a significant sign for various diseases.
phagocytes Cells capable of ingesting particulate matter (e.g., macrophages).
phagocytosis The engulfing of microorganisms and foreign particles by phagocytes.
pharmacodynamics The study of a drug's effect on cellular physiology and biochemistry and the mechanism of action.
pharmacokinetics The study of how drugs enter the body, are metabolized, reach their site of action, and are excreted.
phimosis Constriction of the foreskin orifice causing an inability to push the foreskin back over the end of the penis.
phlebitis Inflammation of a vein.
photophobia Abnormal visual intolerance of light.
phytotherapy Treatment by use of plants.
PIE charting Method of documentation in which "P" means problem identification, "I" means interventions, and "E" means evaluation.
pigmentation The deposition of coloring matter in the skin.
pivot Turn or change direction with your feet while remaining in a fixed place.
placebo Medicinal preparation having no specific pharmacologic activity against the patient's illness or complaint, given solely for the psychophysiologic effects of the treatment; a dummy treatment.
planning Determining specific desired outcomes for each nursing diagnosis.
plantar flexion Reflex bending of the toes and foot.
platelet aggregation Clumping of platelets during wound healing.
pleural friction rub Grating or scratchy sound heard on auscultation of the lungs; caused when irritated pleural membranes rub over each other.
pneumonia Inflammation and consolidation of the lung with exudate.
pneumothorax Accumulation of air or gas in the pleural space, which may occur spontaneously, or as a result of trauma or a pathologic process, or be introduced deliberately.
PO By mouth; orally.
poison Substance that, when ingested, inhaled, absorbed, applied, injected, or developed within the body, may cause functional or structural disturbances.
polypharmacy The use of multiple medications, often inappropriately and excessively, at the same time.
polyps Growths protruding from a mucous membrane.
polyuria Production of an excessive amount of urine.
popliteal pulse Pulse found over the popliteal artery at the posterior surface of the knee.
posterior tibial pulse Pulse found over the posterior tibial artery between the malleolus and the Achilles tendon in the ankle.
postmortem After death.
postoperative After surgery.
postural drainage Removal of lung secretions by changes in the patient's position.
postural hypotension Fall in blood pressure associated with dizziness, syncope (fainting), and blurred vision that occurs upon standing; also called orthostatic hypotension.
practice act Defines activities in which nurses may engage, states the legal requirements and titles for nursing licensure, and establishes the education needed for licensure.
preferred provider organization (PPO) Organization that offers discounted insurance fees in return for a large pool of potential patients who choose a doctor from the list of those associated with the PPO.
prejudice Positive or negative attitude or opinion that is unsupported by evidence.
preoperative Before surgery.
prepuberty Beginning sexual development.
presbycusis Inability to hear high pitched sounds and some spoken words; occurs in old age.
presbyopia Age-related decreased ability to focus the eye on nearby objects.
prescription Written direction for the preparation and administration of a remedy.
pressure injury Localized damage to the skin and/or underlying soft tissue usually over a bony prominence or related to a medical or other device.
priest In many Christian churches, a member of the clergy who may administer the sacraments; in any number of religions, any person having the authority to perform and administer religious rites.
primary illness Illness that develops without being caused by another health problem.
primary intention Type of wound healing (closure) for wounds with little tissue loss, such as a surgical incision.
prions Proteinaceous particles believed to be responsible for transmissible neurodegenerative diseases.
prioritize To put in order of importance.
priority Right of first consideration established on the basis of emergency or need.
privilege Permission to do what is usually not permitted in other circumstances.
PRN Order written to give a medication when the patient requires it.
problem-oriented medical record (POMR) charting Documentation that focuses on patient status, emphasizes the problem-solving approach to patient care, and provides a method for communicating what, when, and how things are to be done to meet the patient's needs.
proctoscopic examination Examination of the rectum with a lighted instrument.
proctosigmoidoscopy Examination of the rectum and sigmoid colon with a sigmoidoscope.
prodromal period Early or very beginning stage of an illness.
productive cough Cough that produces sputum or mucus.
prolapse The falling down or sinking of a part.
pronation Applied to the hand, the act of turning the palm posteriorly, performed by medial rotation of the forearm; applied to the foot, a combination of eversion and abduction movements.
prone position When the patient is lying face down.
prosthesis Artificial body part.
protective device Mechanical device that prevents a person from getting out of a room, bed, or chair (no longer called a restraint); or drugs such as sedatives or tranquilizers used to sedate the patient so that he or she is unable to move about (no longer called chemical restraint).
protein One of a class of complex nitrogenous compounds that occur naturally in plants and animals and yield amino acids when hydrolyzed.

proteinuria Excess of serum proteins in the urine.
protocols Standard procedures.
protozoa One-celled microscopic organisms belonging to the animal kingdom.
proximal Nearest; closer to a point of reference.
prudent Sensible and careful.
psychomotor domain Learning domain in which the learner processes the information by doing.
psychosocial Pertaining to both psychological and social aspects.
psychosocial theories Theories related to socialization and life satisfaction.
ptosis Drooping of the upper eyelid from paralysis of the third nerve or from sympathetic innervation.
ptyalin Form of amylase in the saliva of human beings and some animals that catalyzes the hydrolysis of starch into maltose and dextrin.
puberty Sexual maturation.
pulse deficit Deficit between the apical and radial pulse.
pulse pressure The difference between the systolic and the diastolic pressure.
purulent Containing thick typically white-yellow or yellow exudate, caused by infection.
pyrexia Fever; when a body temperature rises above 100.2°F (38.0°C).
pyrogen Substance that causes fever.
pyuria Purulent exudate in the urine.

Q

qi In traditional Chinese medicine, the vital energy of the human body.
qi gong Type of exercise and stimulation therapy emphasizing breathing, coordination, and relaxation.
Quality and Safety Education for Nurses (QSEN) project National project started in 2005 designed to better prepare nurses to have the knowledge, skills, and attitudes they need to improve the quality and safety of the health care systems in which they work.
quality improvement Evaluating nursing care to identify specific areas that need changes for improvement.
quadrant Quarter.
quadriceps muscles The large muscles of the thigh.
quadriplegics Individuals who are paralyzed in all four limbs.

R

rabbi Chief religious official of a synagogue (Jewish religious temple).
race Biologic way of categorizing people based on physical characteristics, such as skin color and texture, facial characteristics, and body proportions.
racism Form of prejudice that takes place when individuals, groups, and/or institutions exercise power against groups that are judged to be inferior.
radial pulse Pulse found over the radial artery in the wrist at the base of the thumb.
radiation Energy transmitted by waves through space or through some medium.
radiography The making of film records of internal structures of the body by exposure of film sensitized to x-rays.
radioimmunoassay (RIA) Use of radionuclides, following principles of immunology, to measure materials present in blood in minute amounts.
radionuclides Radioactive substances that disintegrate with the emission of electromagnetic radiation.
radiopharmaceutical Radioactive pharmaceutical substance used for diagnostic or therapeutic purposes.
rapid eye movement (REM) sleep The period of sleep during which the brain waves are fast and of low voltage, and autonomic activities (heart rate and respiration) are irregular; type of sleep associated with dreaming.
rapport Relationship of mutual trust or affinity.
reactive hyperemia Process in which the blood rushes to where there is a decrease in circulation.
reasoning The use of reason to form conclusions, inferences, or judgments; evidence or arguments used in thinking.
reciprocity Recognition of one state's nursing license in another state.
recommended daily allowances (RDAs) Recommended amounts of various nutrients for diet planning.
rectum Distal portion of the large intestine where feces are stored.
reflex Autonomic (automatic) response mediated by the nervous system and not requiring conscious movement.
Reiki Therapy in which a practitioner acts as a conduit for healing energy that is directed into the patient's energy field or body.
relaxation Technique for release of tension, which is helpful in reducing pain and in allowing the patient to obtain greater relief from pain medications.
release Legal document that records the patient's permission to perform a treatment or surgery, or to give information to insurance companies or other health care providers; or a legal form to excuse one party from liability.
religion Formalized system of belief and worship.
religious Showing belief in God or a higher power.
reminiscence Reviewing one's life.
remission Abatement of the symptoms of a disease; also, the period during which such an abatement occurs.
residual urine Urine left in the bladder after urination.
residue Remains after digestion or evaporation.
respiration The exchange of oxygen and carbon dioxide in the lungs and tissues, which is initiated by the act of breathing.
respite care Nursing care allowing the caregiver time away from caregiving responsibilities.
responsibility The state of being responsible or accountable.
responsibility stage Stage of middle adulthood concerned with real-life problems and with being in charge of self and others.
retraction Inward movement of respiratory muscles upon inspiration.
return demonstration Review or patient demonstration of what has previously been learned or demonstrated.
rhonchi Continuous dry, rattling sounds heard on auscultation of the lungs; caused by partial obstruction. Newer term: gurgles.
Rickettsia Genus of small, rod-shaped to round microorganisms found in tissue cells of lice, fleas, ticks, and mites and transmitted to humans by their bites.
rigor mortis The stiffness that occurs in dead bodies as chemical changes take place.
Rinne test Test to compare bone and air conduction of sound, performed with a tuning fork.
risk management Putting into action policies or procedures that reduce inherent or possible risks.
ritual Ceremonial act.
root cause analysis Structured method used to analyze serious adverse events in patient care.
routine admission Admission that is scheduled in advance.

S

sandwich generation Persons having dependent children at home and dependent older adults needing care.
sanguineous Bloody.
saturated fats Fatty acids that come from animal food sources, coconut oil, and palm oil.
SBAR Situation, Background, Assessment, and Recommendation format for accurate communication between health care professionals.
scar Mark remaining after the healing of a wound.

scientific method Step-by-step process used by scientists to solve problems.
scoliosis Pronounced lateral curvature of the spine.
"scrub the hub" Slogan to emphasize the importance of using a sterile alcohol pad and applying friction for 15 seconds to cleanse the skin when accessing a central line injection port or intravenous (IV) connection, and to exceed the standard of care by scrubbing the hub when accessing a peripheral IV line.
sebaceous Gland that secretes an oily substance called sebum.
sebum Oily substance secreted by the sebaceous glands.
secondary illness Illness that results from or is caused by a primary illness.
second intention Type of wound healing for wounds with tissue loss, as in pressure injuries; the wound remains open and fills with scar tissue.
selective serotonin reuptake inhibitors (SSRIs) Medications, such as fluoxetine, sertraline, paroxetine, and venlafaxine, used to treat depression.
self-actualization Reaching one's full potential.
self-concept The way one views oneself.
self-esteem Pride in yourself.
semi-Fowler position Position arranged by elevating the head of the bed 30 to 60 degrees and raising the knees up to 15 degrees.
sensorimotor The first cognitive stage.
sensory deficit Lack or deficiency in one of the senses.
sensory deprivation Condition in which a person receives less than normal sensory input.
sensory overload Condition in which a person receives an excessive or intolerable amount of sensory stimuli.
sentinel event Event of major gravity and importance according to The Joint Commission.
sequential multiple assay (SMA) Chemical analyzer that performs assay tests for a variety of chemical substances on a single blood or serum sample one after another.
serosanguineous Composed of serum and blood.
serotonin/norepinephrine reuptake inhibitors (SNRIs) Medications, used for depression, that block reuptake of both serotonin and norepinephrine.
sexual harassment Unwelcome sexual advances, requests for sexual favors, and other verbal or physical conduct of a sexual nature.
sexual orientation Sexual preference.
sexuality The constitution of an individual in relation to sexual attitudes or activity.
shaman Member of certain tribal societies who acts as a medium between the visible world and an invisible spirit world and who practices for purposes of healing, divination, and control over natural events.
shearing force Applied force that causes a downward and forward pressure on the tissues beneath the skin.
shift report Report on the details of a patient's condition and treatment.
shock Condition of circulatory failure.
shroud Dress or garment for the dead; winding sheet.
sibling Brother or sister.
side effects Results of unintended actions.
side-lying (lateral) position When the patient is resting on his or her side.
sigmoidoscopy Examination of the sigmoid colon using a lighted instrument.
sign Any objective evidence of disease or dysfunction.
Sims position Side-lying position in which the weight is distributed over the anterior ilium, humerus, and clavicle.
sinus Canal or passageway leading to an abscess.
skeletal muscles Striated muscles that are made of bundles of muscle fibers surrounded by a connective tissue sheath.
slander Oral (spoken) defamation.
sleep apnea Condition in which a person will stop breathing for brief periods during sleep.
sleep disorder Chronic disorder involving sleep.
sling Bandage for supporting a part.
sloughing When a layer of dead tissue separates from living tissue; to shed dead tissue.
smears Specimens for microscopic and cytologic study.
smegma The cheesy secretion of sebaceous glands, especially secretions found under the penile foreskin.
social competence Comfort in public, ability to get along with others.
socialization The process by which society integrates the individual, and the individual learns to behave in socially acceptable ways.
solute Solid material that has been dissolved in a solution.
sore Lesion of the skin or mucous membranes.
source-oriented (narrative) charting Documentation that is organized by the "source" or author of the documentation.
spansule Medication in the form of tiny time-release pellets within a capsule.
speculum Short, funnel-like tube for examining canals, such as the nasal canal and the vaginal canal.
sphincter Circular muscle that closes an orifice.
sphygmomanometer Device used to indirectly measure blood pressure.
spica cast Figure-of-eight cast.
spiritual distress Feelings of guilt and unworthiness, abandonment, anger, despair, or hopelessness; need to seek forgiveness; conflict between one's religious or spiritual beliefs and medical treatment.
spirituality Intangible element of religion that concerns the spirit or soul.
splint Device that protects an injured body part by immobilizing it.
spores Oval bodies formed within bacteria as a resting stage during the life cycle of the cell; characterized by resistance to environmental changes (humidity or temperature).
sputum Mucous secretions of the lungs ejected through the mouth.
stagnation Inactivity; self-absorption.
Standard Precautions Precautions that protect both the nurse and the patient from infection and are to be used for every patient contact.
standards of care (practice) Rules as defined in nursing procedure books, institutional manuals of procedures or protocols, and nursing journals that outline current skills or techniques.
standing order Order that is carried out until it is canceled by the provider or until the prescribed number of doses have been given.
stasis Stoppage of flow.
stat Immediately.
stat order Order for a single dose of a medication to be given immediately.
statute Legal term for a law.
steatorrhea Stools with an abnormally high fat content.
stereotype Set opinion or belief about a group of people that is applied to an individual.
sterile Without pathologic organisms.
sterilization The process of rendering an article free of microorganisms and their pathogenic products.
stertor Snoring sound produced when patients are unable to cough up secretions from the trachea or bronchi.
stethoscope Device that augments sound.
stoma Opening.
stool Waste eliminated from the colon.
stress The sum of biologic reactions that take place in response to any adverse stimulus.
stressor Adverse stimulus.
stricture Narrowed lumen.

stridor Shrill, harsh sound on inspiration; caused by obstruction of the upper air passages, as occurs in croup or laryngitis.
stroke volume The volume of blood pushed into the aorta per heartbeat.
subculture Smaller group within the culture whose members have similar views and goals in addition to or in place of those of the main culture.
subcutaneous Beneath the skin layers.
subjective Perceived only by the person; not perceptible to the senses of another.
subjective data Data obtained orally.
sublingual Under the tongue.
sucrose Table sugar.
superego Further development of the ego that represents the moral component as postulated by Freud.
supination The act of turning the palm of the hand forward or upward.
supine position Resting on the back.
suppuration The formation of purulent matter.
suprapubic Above the pubic bone.
surgical asepsis The practice of preparing and handling materials in a way that prevents the patient's exposure to living microorganisms.
suture Material used in closing a surgical or traumatic wound with stitches.
symmetry Equality in size, form, and arrangement of parts on opposite sides of a plane; a mirror image.
symptom Any indication of disease perceived by the patient; subjective information.
syncope Fainting.
synergistic effect Combined interaction of drugs.
systole The phase or part of the cardiac cycle when blood is pumped from the ventricles and fills the pulmonary and systemic arteries.
systolic pressure The maximum pressure exerted on the artery during left ventricular contraction.

T

tachycardia Heart rate greater than 100 beats per minute.
tachypnea Increased or rapid breathing.
tactile Pertaining to touch.
technique The method of a procedure.
temporal pulse Pulse found over the temporal artery just in front of the ear.
tenacious Adhesive, sticky.
tendons Cords of fibrous connective tissue that connect a muscle to a bone to allow for joint movement.
terminal illness Illness for which no cure is available; it ends in death, usually within a short period of time.
tertiary intention Type of wound healing; delayed or secondary closure, such as a draining abdominal wound.
tetany Continuous tonic spasm of a muscle; characterized by severe muscle cramps, carpopedal spasms, laryngeal spasms, and stridor.
thanatology The medicolegal study of the dying process and death.
theory Belief, policy, or principle proposed or followed as a basis of action; an idea formed by reasoning from facts.
therapeutic Having medicinal or healing properties.
therapeutic communication Communication that promotes understanding between the sender and the receiver.
therapeutic range Range or level of a drug in the blood that will produce a desired effect without causing toxic effects.
thermoregulation The regulation of heat, such as the body heat of a warm-blooded animal.
third intention Type of wound healing; delayed or secondary closure, such as a draining abdominal wound.
thoracentesis Insertion of a needle through the chest wall to the pleural space to drain fluid or air or to instill medication.
thrombophlebitis Blood clot causing inflammation of a vessel.
thrombosis Formation of a thrombus (blood clot).
time-fixed Tasks that must be done at a set time.
time-flexible Tasks that can be done any time.
time-out Quiet time alone without toys.
tinnitus Noise in the ears such as ringing, buzzing, or roaring.
topical Pertaining to a particular surface area of skin or mucous membrane.
tort Violation of civil law.
total parenteral nutrition (TPN) The technique of providing needed nutrients intravenously.
toxic effects Harmful effects.
toxicity Degree of virulence of a poison.
toxin A poison; a poisonous protein produced by certain bacteria.
tracheostomy Opening into the trachea.
traction The act of drawing or exerting a pulling force, as along the axis of a structure.
trade name Manufacturer's name for a drug or device, protected by trademark.
transcellular Secretions and excretions that move through cell membranes and eventually leave the body.
transcultural nursing Multicultural nursing care that recognizes cultural diversity and is sensitive to the needs of the patient and family.
transcutaneous electrical nerve stimulation (TENS) Form of pain treatment that uses a small electrical stimulator attached to electrodes, which serves to block pain.
transdermal Through the skin.
transducer Wand that emits sound waves.
transfer belt Sturdy belt made of tightly webbed canvas material that is used to ambulate and/or transfer the weak or unsteady patient.
transfusion The introduction of whole blood or a blood component directly into the bloodstream.
transition to practice Program for newly licensed nurses involving a 6-month preceptorship and ongoing support during the first year of professional practice.
Transmission-Based Precautions Precautions that are based on interrupting the mode of transmission by identifying the specific secretions, body fluids, tissues, or excretions that might be infective.
trapeze bar Overhead bar on a bed, which the patient can grab.
treadmill stress test Test that measures heart rate and blood pressure response to clinically controlled active exercise on a treadmill with a moving belt (a machine on which one walks while staying in one place).
tremors Involuntary fine movement of the body or limbs.
trimester Period of 3 months.
trochanter roll Roll of material used to support the upper legs and hips to prevent external rotation of the legs.
tuberculin syringe Syringe with graduated measurements to 1 mL.
tuning fork Forked metal instrument used to test hearing and the sense of vibration.
turgor Normal tension of a cell; swelling, distention; elastic condition of skin.
tympanic membrane Eardrum.

U

ultrasonography Technique in which deep structures of the body are visualized by recording the reflections (echoes) of ultrasonic waves directed into the tissues.
unconscious Insensible; incapable of responding to sensory stimuli and of having subjective experiences.
unit dose Drugs packaged in single (individual) doses.
unlicensed assistive personnel Unlicensed personnel who, after some training, perform tasks usually performed by nurses.

unsaturated fats Fatty acids that come from vegetables, nuts, or seeds.
urinary incontinence Involuntary emission of urine from the body.
urinary retention Urine retained in the bladder after voiding.
urination Expelling urine.
urinometer Instrument that measures the specific gravity (thinness or thickness) of urine.
urostomy Artificial opening on the abdomen through which urine drains.
urticaria Reaction characterized by reddened, slightly elevated patches known as wheals.

V

vagal response Activation of the vagal nerve.
Valsalva maneuver Closure of glottis and tightening of abdominal muscles after intra-abdominal pressure increases when one holds one's breath; may result in voluntary defecation.
values Measure of worth or efficiency; an ideal, custom, or institution of a society toward which the members of the group have an affective regard (emotional connection).
varicosities Swollen, distended, and knotted veins, usually in the subcutaneous tissues of the leg.
vascular access devices Devices such as needles, cannulas, or catheters that allow direct access to the circulatory system.
vasoconstriction Decrease in the caliber of blood vessels.
vasodilation Dilation of a blood vessel.
vector Carrier that transports an infective agent from one host to another, such as animals, insects, and rodents.
vegan Vegetarian diet in which all animal food sources are excluded.
vegetarian One whose diet is lacto-ovo-vegetarian, lactovegetarian, or vegan.
venesection Phlebotomy.
venipuncture Puncture of the vein with a needle.
ventilation (1) The process or act of supplying a house or room continuously with fresh air; (2) exchange of air between the lungs and atmosphere.
verbal In words; expressed orally.
vernix caseosa Cheesy, waxy substance that protects the skin in fetal life.
vertigo Sensation of rotation or whirling movement; dizziness.
vesicant Chemical irritant that causes tissue destruction.
vesicular sounds Soft, rustling sounds heard in the periphery of the lung fields.
viable Capable of living; able to survive outside the womb.
vial Small bottle.
virulence Degree to which a microorganism can cause infection in the host or invade the host.
viruses Extremely small particles of nucleic acids, either DNA or RNA, with a coat of protein, and in some cases a membranous envelope, that can trigger an immune reaction or damage cells in other ways.
viscous Sticky or gummy; having a high degree of viscosity or resistance to flow; thick.
visual accommodation The ability to focus on both near and far objects.
visual learning Learning through what is seen.
vital signs The signs of life, namely pulse, respiration, and temperature.
vitamin Essential nutrient that must be taken in through food sources or supplements.
vocational Related to trade, profession, or occupation.
void Excrete urine.

W

walking rounds When nurses perform shift report by off-going and oncoming nurses walking together, room to room.
Weber test Test of bone conduction of sound performed with a tuning fork placed in the center of the forehead or the skull.
wellness Dynamic and active movement toward fulfillment of one's potential.
wheeze High pitched whistling sound of air forced past a partial obstruction, as found in asthma or emphysema.
whistle-blowing Reporting illegal or unethical actions.
wisdom Having good judgment based on accumulated knowledge.
worldview The perspective a culture takes of the world that is shared by cultural group members, and that influences health and illness beliefs.
wound Bodily injury caused by physical means with disruption of the skin or other structure.

Y

yang Force that is positive, light, warm, or masculine.
yin Force that is negative, dark, cold, or feminine.
yoga Hindu discipline aimed at training the consciousness for a state of perfect spiritual insight and tranquility; a system of exercises practiced as part of the discipline to promote control of the mind and body.

Z

Z-track technique Injection technique causing a needle track, or pathway, in the shape of a "Z."
zygote Fertilized egg.

Index

Page numbers followed by *b*, *t*, and *f* indicate boxes, tables, and figures, respectively.

C

U